GRABB AND SMITH'S PLASTIC SURGERY

SIXTH EDITION

Editor-in-Chief

Charles H. Thorne, MD

Associate Professor of Plastic Surgery
NYU Medical Center
New York, New York

Editors

Robert W. Beasley, MD

Professor of Surgery, New York University, New York, New York
Director of New York University Hand Surgery Services, Institute of Reconstructive
Plastic Surgery and Bellevue Hospital Center, New York, New York
Hand Surgery Consultant, Veteran's Administration, New York, New York
Consulting Surgeon, Hackensack University Hospital, Hackensack, New Jersey
and Impartial Advisor to Chairman, New York State Workers' Compensation Board

Sherrell J. Aston, MD

Professor of Surgery (Plastic)
New York University School of Medicine
Chairman, Department of Plastic Surgery
Manhattan Eye Ear and Throat Hospital
New York, New York

Scott P. Bartlett, MD

Professor of Surgery, University of Pennsylvania
Mary Downs Endowed Chair in Pediatric Craniofacial Treatment and Research,
Children's Hospital of Philadelphia
Philadelphia, Pennsylvania

Geoffrey C. Gurtner, MD, FACS

Associate Professor of Surgery, Department of Surgery, Division of Plastic Surgery
Stanford University School of Medicine
Stanford, California

Scott L. Spear, MD, FACS

Professor and Chief
Division of Plastic Surgery
Georgetown University Medical Center
Washington, DC

Wolters Kluwer | Lippincott Williams & Wilkins
Health
Philadelphia · Baltimore · New York · London
Buenos Aires · Hong Kong · Sydney · Tokyo

Acquisitions Editor: Brian Brown
Developmental Editor: Cotton Coslett and Keith Donnellan, Dovetail Content Solutions
Managing Editor: Julia Seto
Project Manager: Alicia Jackson
Senior Manufacturing Manager: Benjamin Rivera
Associate Director of Marketing: Adam Glazer
Design Coordinator and Cover Designer: Terry Mallon
Production Service: Techbooks
Printer: Edwards Brothers

Library of Congress Cataloging-in-Publication Data

Grabb and Smith's plastic surgery.—6th ed. / editor-in-chief, Charles H. Thorne ... [et al.].
        p. ; cm.
    Includes bibliographical references and index.
    ISBN 978-0-7817-4698-4
    ISBN 0-7817-4698-1
    1. Surgery, Plastic. I. Thorne, Charles, 1952- II. Grabb, William C. III. Title: Plastic surgery.
    [DNLM: 1. Surgery, Plastic. 2. Reconstructive Surgical Procedures. WO 600 G7265 2007]
    RD118.G688 2007
    617.9′5—dc22   2006033593

To purchase additional copies of this book, call our customer service department at (800) 638-3030 or fax orders to (301) 223-2320. International customers should call (301) 223-2300.

Visit Lippincott Williams & Wilkins on the Internet: at LWW.com. Lippincott Williams & Wilkins customer service representatives are available from 8:30 am to 6 pm, EST.

10 9 8 7 6 5 4 3 2 1

TO MY WIFE OF 25 YEARS, ALISA, AND
TO GOOD TEACHERS EVERYWHERE. IN MY CASE:
ALISA, WELLS, MODE, KEED, NATE, GITCH,
JOHN SIEBERT, PETE NEWELL, LES OTTINGER,
AND MANY MORE

Charles H. Thorne, MD

Valerie J. Ablaza, MD, FACS
Assistant Professor
Department of Surgery
Columbia University
College of Physicians and Surgeons
New York, New York

Al Aly, MD, FACS
Attending
Department of Plastic Surgery
Iowa City Plastic Surgery
Coralville, Iowa

P.G. Arnold, MD
Professor of Plastic Surgery
Department of Surgery, Division of Plastic Surgery
Mayo Clinic
Rochester, Minnesota

Christopher E. Attinger, MD
Professor
Department of Plastic Surgery
Georgetown University
Medical Director
The Limb Center
Georgetown University Hospital
Washington, District of Columbia

Alberto Aviles, MD
Resident in Plastic Surgery
Department of Plastic Surgery
Medical College of Wisconsin
Milwaukee, Wisconsin

Stephen B. Baker, MD, DDS, FACS
Associate Professor
Associate Program Director
Department of Plastic Surgery
Georgetown University Hospital
Washington, District of Columbia
Co-Director, Craniofacial Clinic
Inova Fairfax Hospital for Children
Falls Church, Virginia

Scott P. Bartlett, MD
Professor of Surgery
University of Pennsylvania
Mary Downs Endowed Chair in Pediatric
Craniofacial Treatment and Research
Children's Hospital of Philadelphia
Philadelphia, Pennsylvania

Steven J. Bates, MD
Chief Resident
Division of Plastic Surgery
Stanford University Medical Center
Stanford, California

Bruce S. Bauer, MD, FACS, FAAP
Professor of Surgery
Department of Surgery
Division of Plastic Surgery
The Feinberg School of Medicine Northwestern University
Chief
Division of Plastic Surgery
Children's Memorial Hospital
Chicago, Illinois

John D. Bauer, MD
Assistant Professor, Division of Plastic Surgery
Department of Surgery
UTMB at Galveston
Galveston, Texas

Robert W. Beasley, MD
Professor of Surgery, New York University
Director of New York University Hand Surgery Services,
    Institute of Reconstructive Plastic Surgery and Bellevue
    Hospital Center
Hand Surgery Consultant, Veteran's Administration
Impartial Advisor to Chairman, New York State Workers'
    Compensation Board, New York, New York
Consulting Surgeon, Hackensack University Hospital,
    Hackensack, New Jersey

Michael S. Beckenstein, MD, FACS
Birmingham, Alabama

Sean Boutros, MD
Attending Surgeon
Houston Plastic and Craniofacial Surgery
Hermann Hospital and Children's Memorial Hermann
    Hospital
Houston, Texas

James P. Bradley, MD
Associate Professor, Sarnat Craniofacial Chair
Division of Plastic Surgery
UCLA David Geffen School of Medicine
Chief Pediatric Plastic Surgery
Division of Plastic Surgery
Mattel Children's Hospital
Los Angeles, California

Lawrence E. Brecht, DDS
Clinical Assistant Professor of Surgery
Department of Surgery
New York University School of Medicine
Co-Director of Craniofacial Prosthetics
Institute of Reconstructive Plastic Surgery
New York University Medical Center
Clinical Associate Professor of Prosthodontics
Director of Maxillofacial Prosthetics
Advanced Education Program in Prosthodontics
New York University College of Dentistry
New York, New York

Arnold S. Breitbart, MD, FACS
Assistant Professor of Clinical Surgery
Adjunct Assistant Professor of Surgery
Columbia University College of Physicians and Surgeons
Weill Cornell University Medical College
New York, New York

Duc T. Bui, MD
Department of Surgery
Stony Brook University Medical Center
Stony Brook, New York

Charles E. Butler, MD
Associate Professor
The University of Texas
M.D. Anderson Cancer Center,
Department of Plastic Surgery, Houston, Texas

Peter E. M. Butler, MB, BSc (Hons)
Consultant Plastic Surgeon
Royal Free Hospital
University College London
London, England

Grant W. Carlson, MD
Professor
Department of Surgery
Emory University
Chief of Surgical Services
Crawford W. Long Hospital
Atlanta, Georgia

Benjamin Chang, MD, FACS
Associate Professor of Clinical Surgery
Division of Plastic Surgery
University of Pennsylvania School of Medicine
Attending Surgeon
Division of Plastic Surgery
Hospital of the University of Pennsylvania
Philadelphia, Pennsylvania

James Chang, MD
Associate Professor
Division of Plastic Surgery
Stanford University Medical Center
Attending Surgeon
Lucile Packard Children's Hospital at Stanford
Stanford University Medical Center
Palo Alto, California

Raymond R. Chang, MD
Assistant Professor of Surgery
Department of Surgery, Division of Plastic Surgery
George Washington University
Attending
Department of Surgery, Division of Plastic Surgery
George Washington University Hospital
Washington, District of Columbia

James J. Chao, MD, FACS
Associate Professor of Plastic Surgery
Department of Surgery
University of California,
    San Diego School of Medicine
San Diego, California

Mihye Choi, MD
Assistant Professor
Department of Surgery
New York University
New York, New York

Mark A. Codner, MD
Clinical Assistant Professor
Department of Plastic and Reconstructive
    Surgery
Emory University
Atlanta, Georgia

Sydney R. Coleman, MD
Assistant Clinical Professor
Department of Plastic Surgery
New York University School of Medicine
New York, New York

Peter G. Cordeiro, MD
Professor of Surgery
Department of Surgery
Weill Medical College of Cornell University
Chief, Plastic & Reconstructive Surgery Service
Department of Surgery
Memorial Sloan-Kettering Cancer Center
New York, New York

Alfred Culliford IV, MD
Division of Plastic, Reconstructive and Hand Surgery
Staten Island University Hospital
Staten Island, New York

Court Cutting, MD
Professor of Surgery-Plastic Surgery
Director, Cleft Lip and Palate Program
Institute of Reconstructive Plastic Surgery
NYU Medical Center
New York, New York

Genevieve de Bese, MD
General Manager and Director of Research
American Hand Prostheses
New York, New York

Mark DeLacure, MD
Associate Professor of Otolaryngology and Surgery
    (Plastic Surgery)
New York University Medical Center
New York, New York

Joseph J. Disa, MD, FACS
Associate Attending Surgeon
Plastic and Reconstructive
    Surgery Service
Memorial Sloan-Kettering Cancer Center
New York, New York

Matthias B. Donelan, MD
Associate Clinical Professor of Surgery
Harvard Medical School
Chief of Plastic Surgery
Shriners Burns Hospital
Boston, Massachusetts

Ivica Ducic, MD, PhD
Associate Professor
Chief–Peripheral Nerve Surgery
Department of Plastic Surgery
Georgetown University Hospital
Washington, District of Columbia

Gregory A. Dumanian, MD, FACS
Associate Professor of Surgery
Department of Surgery, Division of Plastic Surgery
Feinberg School of Medicine, Northwestern University
Associate Professor of Surgery
Department of Surgery, Division of Plastic Surgery
Northwestern Memorial Hospital
Chicago, Illinois

Charles J. Eaton, MD
Hand Surgeon
Department of Surgery
Jupiter Medical Center
Jupiter, Florida

Charles R. Effron, MD
Rochelle Park, New Jersey

L. Franklyn Elliott II, MD
Atlanta Plastic Surgery, P.C.
Atlanta, Georgia

Gregory R. D. Evans, MD, FACS
Professor of Surgery and Biomedical Engineering
Chief Aesthetic Plastic Surgery
University of California Irvine
Professor of Surgery and Biomedical Engineering
Chief Aesthetic Plastic Surgery
UCI Medical Center
Orange, California

Maryam Feili-Hariri, PhD
Assistant Professor
Surgery and Immunology
University of Pittsburgh
Pittsburgh, Pennsylvania

Derek T. Ford, MD, FRCSC
Private Practice
Toronto, Ontario, Canada

M. Felix Freshwater, MD
Miami, Florida

David W. Friedman, MD
Assistant Professor
Department of Surgery-Plastic
New York University
Fellowship Director
Hand Surgery
New York University Medical Center
New York, New York

Jeffrey D. Friedman, MD
Assistant Professor
Department of Plastic Surgery
Baylor College of Medicine
The Methodist Hospital
Houston, Texas

Robert D. Galiano, MD
Institute of Reconstructive Plastic Surgery
New York University
New York, New York

Roy G. Geronemus, MD, PC
Laser and Skin Surgery Center of New York
Clinical Professor
Department of Dermatology
New York Medical Center
New York, New York

Giulio Gherardini, MD, PhD
Rome, Italy

Mary K. Gingrass, MD, FACS
Assistant Clinical Professor
Department of Plastic Surgery
Vanderbilt University School of Medicine
Chief of Plastic Surgery
Department of Plastic Surgery
Baptist Hospital
Nashville, Tennessee

Cornelia N. Golimbu, MD
Professor of Radiology
Department of Radiology
New York University Medical Center
New York, New York

Arun K. Gosain, MD
Professor
Department of Surgery
Case Western Reserve University
University Hospital (Lakeside)
Chief
Section of Craniofacial and Pediatric Plastic Surgery
Rainbow Babies and Childrens Hospital
Cleveland, Ohio

Barry Grayson, DDS
Associate Professor of Surgery (Orthodontics)
Institute of Reconstructive Plastic Surgery
New York University School of Medicine
Tisch Hospital
New York, New York

Arin K. Greene, MD, MMSc
Craniofacial Fellow
Department of Plastic Surgery
Children's Hospital Boston, Harvard Medical School
Boston, Massachusettes

Geoffrey C. Gurtner, MD, FACS
Associate Professor of Surgery
Department of Surgery, Division of Plastic Surgery
Stanford University School of Medicine
Stanford, California

J. Joris Hage, MD, PhD
Chief
Department of Plastic and Reconstructive Surgery
Netherlands Cancer Institute-Antoni van Leeuwenhoek
    Hospital
Amsterdam, The Netherlands

Elizabeth J. Hall-Findlay, MD, FRCSC
Plastic Surgeon
Mineral Springs Hospital
Banff Alberta, Canada

Dennis C. Hammond, MD
Center for Breast & Body Contouring
Grand Rapids, Michigan

Michael Hausman, MD
Assistant Professor
Department of Orthopaedics
Chief, Hand Service Mount Sinai Hospital
New York, New York

Robert J. Havlik, MD
Professor
Department of Surgery-Section of Plastic Surgery
Indiana University School of Medicine
Chief Section of Plastic Surgery
Riley Hospital for Children
Indianapolis, Indiana

Alexes Hazen, MD
Attending, Plastic Surgery
Department of Plastic Surgery
NYU Medical Center
Chief Plastic Surgery
Manhattan Veterans Administration Hospital
New York, New York

David A. Hidalgo, MD
New York, New York

Larry Hollier, Jr., MD
Associate Professor/Residency Program Director
Department of Plastic Surgery
Baylor College of Medicine
Texas Children's Hospital
Ben Taub General Hospital
Houston, Texas

Richard A. Hopper, MD, MS
Associate Professor
Department of Surgery
University of Washington
Surgical Director
The Craniofacial Center
Seattle Children's Hospital
Seattle, Washington

Christopher J. Hussussian, MD
Plastic Surgery Associates
Waukesha, Wisconsin

Alamgir Isani, MD
Clinical Assistant Professor
Plastic Surgery
New York University Medical Center
New York, New York

Jeffrey E. Janis, MD
Assistant Professor
Chief of Plastic Surgery
Parkland Health
Hospital System Co-Director
Plastic Surgery Residency Program
University of Texas Southwestern Medical Center
Dallas, Texas

John N. Jensen, MD
Department of Plastic Surgery
Medical College of Wisconsin
Milwaukee, Wisconsin

Neil F. Jones, MD, FRCS
Professor
Division of Plastic & Reconstructive Surgery
Department of Orthopedic Surgery
University of California Los Angeles
Chief of Hand Surgery
UCLA Hand Center
UCLA Medical Center
Los Angeles, California

Michael A. C. Kane, MD, BS
Attending Surgeon
Department of Plastic Surgery
Manhattan Eye, Ear & Throat Hospital
New York, New York

Nolan S. Karp, MD
Associate Professor of Plastic Surgery
NYU School of Medicine
New York, New York

Armen K. Kasabian, MD
Assistant Professor of Plastic Surgery
Department of Plastic Surgery
New York University Medical Center
Chief, Section of Microsurgery
Institute of Reconstructive Plastic Surgery
New York, New York

Henry Kawamoto, Jr., MD, DDS
Clinical Professor
Department of Surgery, Division
   of Plastic Surgery
UCLA
Los Angeles, California

Patrick Kelley, MD
Medical Director
Craniofacial Center
Children's Hospital of Austin
Austin, Texas

Amy Kells, MD, PhD
Microsurgery Fellow
Department of Plastic Surgery
University of Mississippi
Jackson, Mississippi

Karen H. Kim, MD
Director of Research
Laser and Skin Surgery Center of New York
New York, New York

Arnold William Klein, MD
Professor of Medicine and Dermatology
Department of Medicine and Dermatology
David Geffen School of Medicine at UCLA
Beverly Hills, California

Matthew B. Klein, MD
Assistant Professor
Department of Plastic Surgery
University of Washington
Associate Director
University of Washington Burn Center
Harborview Medical Center
Seattle, Washington

David M. Knize, MD
Associate Clinical Professor of Plastic Surgery
Department of Surgery
University of Colorado Health Sciences Center
Denver, Colorado
Former Chief of Plastic Surgery
Department of Surgery
Swedish Medical Center
Englewood, Colorado

James Knoetgen, III, MD
Consultant in Plastic Surgery
Department of Surgery, Division of Plastic Surgery
Mayo Clinic
Rochester, Minnesota

Howard N. Langstein, MD
Department of Plastic Surgery
The University of Texas
M. D. Anduson Cancer Center
Houston, Texas

W. P. Andrew Lee, MD
Professor of Surgery
University of Pittsburgh
Chief
Division of Plastic Surgery
University of Pittsburgh Medical Center
Pittsburgh, Pennsylvania

Salvatore C. Lettieri, MD
Instructor
Department of Plastic Surgery
Mayo Graduate School
Rochester, Minnesota
Chief
Department of Plastic Surgery
Maricopa Medical Center
Phoenix, Arizona

Jamie Levine, MD
Assistant Professor
Division of Plastic Surgery
New York University
Chief Plastic and Microsurgery
Department of Surgery
Bellevue Hospital
New York, New York

J. William Littler, MD
Professor Emeritus of Clinical Surgery
Columbia University Department of Surgery; and Retired
    Senior Attending Physician, Chief of Plastic and
    Reconstructive Surgery
St. Luke's-Roosevelt Hospital Center
New York, New York

Otway Louie, MD
House Staff
Institute of Reconstructive and Plastic Surgery
NYU Medical Center
New York, New York

David W. Low, MD
Associate Professor of Surgery
Division of Plastic Surgery
University of Pennsylvania School of Medicine
Philadelphia, Pennsylvania

Susan E. Mackinnon, MD
Shoenberg Professor and Chief
Division of Plastic and Reconstructive Surgery
Washington University in St. Louis
Barnes-Jewish Hospital
St. Louis, Missouri

John S. Mancoll, MD
Fort Wayne, Indiana

Ralph T. Manktelow, MD, FRCS(c)
Professor of Surgery
University of Toronto
Staff Surgeon
Department of Surgery
Toronto General Hospital
Toronto, Ontario, Canada

Stephen J. Mathes, MD
Institute of Reconstructive Plastic Surgery
New York University Medical Center
New York, New York

Joseph G. McCarthy, MD
Lawrence D. Bell Professor of Plastic Surgery
Institute of Reconstructive Plastic Surgery
NYU School of Medicine
Director
Institute of Reconstructive Plastic Surgery
NYU Medical Center
New York, New York

Babak J. Mehrara, MD
Assistant Professor
Department of Surgery
Columbia University New York Hospital-Cornell
    MedicalCenter
Assistant Attending
Memorial Sloan-Kettering Cancer Center
New York, New York

Frederick J. Menick, MD
Associate Clinical Professor
Division of Plastic Surgery
University of Arizona
Staff Surgeon
Division of Plastic Surgery
St. Joseph's Hospital
Tucson, Arizona

Timothy A. Miller, MD
Professor and Chief Plastic Surgery
University of California School of Medicine
David Geffen School of Medicine at UCLA
Department of Surgery
UCLA Medical Center
Los Angeles, California

Blake A. Morrison, MD
Private Practice
North Texas Hand Surgery
Dallas, Texas

Hannan Mullett, MD, FRCS (TR & ORTM)
Consultant Orthopaedic Surgeon
Department of Orthopaedic Surgery
Beaumont Hospital
Dublin, Ireland

John B. Mulliken, MD
Professor of Surgery
Harvard Medical School
Director Craniofacial Centre
Department of Plastic Surgery
Children's Hospital
Boston, Massachusetts

Thomas A. Mustoe, MD
Professor
Department of Surgery, Division of Plastic Surgery
Feinberg School of Medicine, Northwestern University
Chief
Department of Plastic Surgery
Northwestern Memorial Hospital
Chicago, Illinois

Terence M. Myckatyn, MD, FRCSC
Assistant Professor
Department of Plastic and Reconstructive Surgery
Washington University School of Medicine
St. Louis, Missouri

Randall Nacamuli, MD
Resident
Division of Plastic and Reconstructive Surgery
Oregon Health Sciences University
Portland, Oregon

James D. Namnoum, MD
Atlanta Plastic Surgery, P.C.
Atlanta, Georgia

Peter C. Neligan, MB, FRCSC, FACS
Wharton Chair in Reconstructive Plastic Surgery
Professor and Chair, Division of Plastic Surgery
University of Toronto
Toronto, Canada

Martin I. Newman, MD
Active Staff
Department of Plastic & Reconstructive Surgery
Cleveland Clinic Florida
Weston, Florida

John A. Perrotti, MD
Clinical Assistant Professor
Department of Surgery
New York Medical College
Valhalla, New York
Attending Surgeon
Department of Plastic Surgery
Manhattan Eye, Ear and Throat Surgery
New York, New York

John A. Persing, MD
Professor and Chief Plastic Surgery, Professor of
    Neurosurgery
Yale University School of Medicine
Chief
Plastic Surgery
Yale-New Haven Hospital
New Haven, Connecticut

Linda G. Phillips, MD
Truman G. Blocker Distinguished Professor and Chief
Division of Plastic Surgery
UTMB Galveston
Galveston, Texas

Michael L. Reed, MD
Associate Clinical Professor
Department of Dermatology
New York University School of Medicine
Attending Physician
Department of Dermatology
New York University Medical Center
New York, New York

Rod J. Rohrich, MD, FACS
Professor and Chairman
Department of Plastic Surgery
The University of Texas Southwestern Medical Center
Chief of Plastic Surgery
Department of Plastic Surgery
University Hospital – Zale Lipshy
Dallas, Texas

Harvey M. Rosen, MD, DMD
Clinical Associate Professor
Department of Surgery
University of Pennsylvania
Chief
Division of Plastic Surgery
Pennsylvania Hospital
Philadelphia, Pennsylvania

George H. Rudkin, MD, FACS
Clinical Associate Professor
Department of Plastic Surgery
UCLA Medical Center
Chief, Plastic Surgery
Department of Plastic Surgery
VA West Los Angeles
Los Angeles, California

Pierre B. Saadeh, MD
Assistant Professor
Attending Physician
Department of Surgery, Plastic Surgery
New York University School of Medicine
New York, New York

Hrayr K. Shahinian, MD, FACS
Director
Skull Base Institute
Cedars-Sinai Medical Office Towers
Los Angeles, California

Sheel Sharma, MD
Faculty
Department of Plastic and Reconstructive Surgery
Hackensock, New Jersey

Joseph H. Shin, MD
Associate Professor of Surgery
Director Yale Craniofacial Center
Department of Plastic Surgery
Yale University School of Medicine
Attending Physician
Yale New Haven Hospital
New Haven, Connecticut

Sumner A. Slavin, MD
Division of Plastic Surgery
Beth Israel Deaconess Medical Center
Harvard Medical School
Brookline, Massachusetts

Hooman Soltanian, MD, FACS
Attending
Specialties of Plastic Surgery
Hartford, Connecticut

Scott L. Spear, MD
Chairman
Department of Plastic Surgery
Georgetown University
Professor and Chairman
Department of Plastic Surgery
Georgetown University Hospital
Washington, District of Columbia

Henry M. Spinelli, MD
Clinical Professor of Surgery
Department of Surgery
Weill Medical College of Cornell University
Attending Surgeon
Department of Plastic Surgery
New York Presbyterian Hospital – Weill Cornell
New York, New York

G. Ian Taylor, AO
Professor
Department of Anatomy and Cell Biology
University of Melbourne
Senior Consultant
Department of Reconstructive Plastic Surgery
Royal Melbourne Hospital
Parkville, Victoria, Canada

Alisa C. Thorne, MD
Professor of Clinical Anesthesiology
Weil Cornell School of Medicine
Director of Ambulatory Anesthesia
Memorial Sloan Kettering Cancer Center
New York, New York

Charles H. Thorne, MD
Associate Professor
Department of Plastic Surgery
NYU School of Medicine
New York, New York

John T. Tymchak, MD, FACS
Clinical Assistant Professor
Department of Surgery
SUNY Health Science Center at Brooklyn
Director, Division of Plastic Surgery and Hand Surgery
   Services
Department of Surgery, Division of Plastic Surgery
The Brookdale University Hospital and Medical Center
Brooklyn, New York

Lok Huei Yap, MD
Department of Plastic Surgery
The University of Texas
M.D. Anderson Cancer Center
Houston, Texas

Michael J. Yaremchuk, MD
Clinical Professor
Department of Surgery
Harvard Medical School
Chief of Craniofacial Surgery
Department of Plastic Surgery
Massachusetts General Hospital
Boston, Massachusetts

Paul Zidel, MD, MS, FACS
Clinical Faculty
Department of Surgery
Nova Southeastern University
Fort Lauderdale, Florida
Attending
Department of Surgery
University Hospital
Tamarac, Florida

Ronald M. Zuker, MD, FRCSC, FACS
Professor of Surgery
Department of Surgery
University of Toronto
Staff Surgeon
Division of Plastic Surgery
The Hospital for Sick Children
Toronto, Ontario, Canada

Although I can vouch that the editors are humble, our task was not: to produce a comprehensive text covering all of plastic surgery in a single volume. Grabb and Smith's *Plastic Surgery* is now the *only* single-volume text that attempts such a feat. In fact, the book was based on the belief that with proper editing, our single volume could contain all the essential information of any multiple-volume text.

The second challenge was to make the book sufficiently new to justify calling it a "new" edition. Of the 93 chapters, over two thirds (64) are completely new, with new authors. The remaining 29 chapters were re-written, in many cases completely. The number of topics covered increased in all areas except Hand, with the largest expansion in the Breast and Cosmetic sections. We grouped ten chapters within a newly titled section, Congenital Anomalies and Pediatric Plastic Surgery. Every chapter is shorter than its counterpart in the previous edition, and references were limited to 15. Our authors are experts in their fields, and their skills in surgery are equaled by their writing skills. I am grateful that they accepted my editing,

some of which was quite deep in my attempts to keep chapters pithy.

The downside of a single volume that is comprehensive enough for examination preparation is its weight! As our senior co-editor Dr. Beasley warned, "It should be light enough to take to bed with you." In this regard, we may have failed, but we feel comfortable blaming the scope of the field rather than the competence of the editors.

The book is intended for medical professionals and trainees at all levels: Practicing plastic surgeons, surgeons in related fields such as Ophthalmology, Otolaryngology, Oral Surgery, Orthopedics and General Surgery, surgery residents in all subspecialties, medical students, physicians assistants, nurses, and nurse practitioners.

My thanks to the co-editors, authors, Lippincott Williams and & Wilkins, and Dovetail Content Solutions for their contributions to this worthy endeavor.

Charles H. Thorne, MD

CONTENTS

PART IV ■ HEAD AND NECK

PART V ■ AESTHETIC SURGERY

PART VI ■ BREAST

GRABB AND SMITH'S
PLASTIC SURGERY

SIXTH EDITION

PART I ■ PRINCIPLES, TECHNIQUES, AND BASIC SCIENCE

CHAPTER 1 ■ TECHNIQUES AND PRINCIPLES IN PLASTIC SURGERY

CHARLES H. THORNE

Plastic surgery is a unique specialty that defies definition, has no organ system of its own, is based on principles rather than specific procedures, and, because of cosmetic surgery, is the darling of the media.

What is plastic surgery? No complete definition exists. Joe McCarthy defines it as the "problem-solving specialty." My wife, an anesthesiologist, calls plastic surgeons the "finishers" because they come in when "the other surgeons have done all they can do and the operation has to be finished." An even more grandiose definition is the following from a plastic surgery resident: "Plastic surgery is surgery of the skin and its contents." There is no way to define this specialty that has acquired "turf" through a combination of tradition and innovation. What is the common denominator between craniofacial surgery and hand surgery? Between pressure sore surgery and cosmetic surgery?

Unlike other surgical specialties, plastic surgery is not organized around a specific organ system. Plastic surgery has only traditional areas of expertise and principles on which to rely for its existence and future. Because plastic surgery has loose boundaries and no specific anatomic region, it faces competition from regionally oriented specialties. Traditional areas of expertise can be lost as other specialties acquire the skills to perform the procedures developed by plastic surgeons. Consequently, plastic surgery has both freedom and vulnerability. It is this vulnerability that makes plastic surgery dependent on both the maintenance of superiority in the traditional areas of expertise and on continued innovation and acquisition of new techniques, new procedures, new problems to solve—that is, new turf.

Plastic surgery is based more on principles than on the details of specific procedures. This allows the plastic surgeon to solve unusual problems, to operate from the top of the head to the tip of the toe, to apply known procedures to other body parts, and to be innovative.

No specialty receives the attention from the lay press that plastic surgery receives. At the same time, no specialty is less-well understood. Although the public equates plastic surgery with cosmetic surgery, the roots of plastic surgery lie in its reconstructive heritage. Cosmetic surgery, an important component of plastic surgery, is but one piece of the plastic surgical puzzle.

Plastic surgery consists of reconstructive surgery and cosmetic surgery but the boundary between the two, like the boundary of plastic surgery itself, is difficult to draw. The more one studies the specialty, the more the distinction between cosmetic surgery and reconstructive surgery disappears. Even if one asks, as an insurance company does, about the functional importance of a particular procedure, the answer often hinges on the realization that the **function of the face is to look like a face** (i.e., function = appearance). A cleft lip is repaired so the child will **look,** and therefore hopefully **function,** like other children. A common procedure such as a breast reduction is enormously complex when one considers the issues of appearance, self-image, sexuality, and womanhood, and defies categorization as simply cosmetic or necessarily reconstructive.

This chapter outlines basic plastic surgery principles and techniques that deal with the skin. Cross-references to specific chapters providing additional information are provided. Subsequent chapters in the first section will discuss other concepts and tools that allow plastic surgeons to tackle more complex problems. Almost all wounds and all procedures involve the skin, even if it is only an incision, and therefore the cutaneous techniques described in this text are applicable to virtually every procedure performed by every specialty in surgery.

OBTAINING A FINE-LINE SCAR

"Will there be a scar?" Even the most intelligent patients ask this preposterous question. **When a full-thickness injury occurs to the skin or an incision is made, there is always a scar.** The question should be, "Will I have a relatively inconspicuous fine-line scar?"

The final appearance of a scar is dependent on many factors, including the following: (a) Differences between individual patients that we do not yet understand and cannot predict; (b) the type of skin and location on the body; (c) the tension on the closure; (d) the direction of the wound; (e) other local and systemic conditions; and, lastly, (f) surgical technique.

The same incision or wound in two different patients will produce scars that differ in quality and aesthetics. Oily or pigmented skin produces, as a general rule, more unsightly scars (Chapter 2 discusses hypertrophic scars and keloids). Thin, wrinkled, pale, dry, "WASPy" skin of patients of English or Scotch-Irish descent usually results in more inconspicuous scars. Rules are made to be broken, however, and an occasional patient will develop a scar that is not characteristic of his or her skin type.

Certain anatomic areas routinely produce unfavorable scars that remain hypertrophic or wide. The shoulder and sternal area are such examples. Conversely, eyelid incisions almost always heal with a fine-line scar.

Skin loses elasticity with age. Stretched-out skin, combined with changes in the subcutaneous tissue, produces wrinkling, which makes scars less obvious and less prone to widening in older individuals. Children, on the other hand, may heal faster but do not heal "better," in that their scars tend to be red and wide when compared to scars of their grandparents. In addition, as body parts containing scars grow, the scars become proportionately larger. Beware the scar on the scalp of a small child!

Just as the recoil of healthy, elastic skin in children may lead to widening of a scar, tension on a closure bodes poorly for the eventual appearance of the scar. The scar associated with a simple elliptical **excision** of a mole on the back will likely result

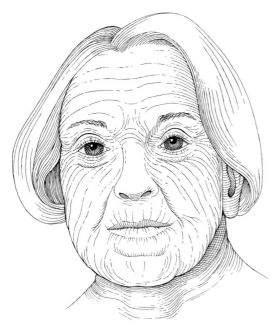

FIGURE 1.1. Relaxed skin tension lines. (Reproduced with permission from Ruberg R. L. In: Smith DJ, ed. *Plastic Surgery, A Core Curriculum.* St. Louis: Mosby, 1994.)

in a much less appealing scar than an **incisional** wound. The body knows when it is missing tissue.

The direction of a laceration or excision also determines the eventual appearance of the scar. The lines of tension in the skin were first noted by Dupuytren. Langer also described the normal tension lines, which became known as "Langer lines." Borges referred to skin lines as "relaxed skin tension lines" (Fig. 1.1).

Elective incisions or the excision of lesions are planned when possible so that the final scars will be parallel to the relaxed skin tension lines. Maximal contraction occurs when a scar crosses the lines of minimal tension at a right angle. Wrinkle lines are generally the same as the relaxed skin tension lines and lie perpendicular to the long axis of the underlying muscles.

Other issues, which are not related to the scar itself but to perception, determine if a scar is noticeable. Incisions and scars can be "hidden" by placing them at the junction of aesthetic units (e.g., at the junction of the lip and cheek, along the nasolabial fold), where the eye expects a change in contour (Chapter 38). In contrast, an incision in the midcheek or midchin or tip of the nose will always be more conspicuous.

The shape of the wound also affects ultimate appearance. The "trapdoor" scar results from a curvilinear incision or laceration that, after healing and contracture, appears as a depressed groove with bulging skin on the inside of the curve. Attempts at "defatting" the bulging area are never as satisfactory as either the patient or surgeon would like.

Local conditions, such as crush injury of the skin adjacent to the wound, also affect the scar. So, too, will systemic conditions such as vascular disease or congenital conditions affecting elastin and/or wound healing. Nutritional status can affect wound healing, but usually only in the extreme of malnutrition or vitamin deficiency. Nutritional status is probably overemphasized as a factor in scar formation.

Technique is also overemphasized (by self-serving plastic surgeons?) as a factor in determining whether a scar will be inconspicuous, but it is certainly of some importance. Minimizing damage to the skin edges with atraumatic technique, debridement of necrotic or foreign material, and a tension-free closure are the first steps in obtaining a fine-line scar. Ultimately,

however, scar formation is unpredictable even with meticulous technique.

Two technical factors are of definite importance in increasing the likelihood of a "good" scar. First is the placement of sutures that will **not leave permanent suture marks** or the **prompt removal** of skin sutures so disfiguring "railroad tracks" do not occur. In other words, removing the sutures may be more important than placing them! Plastic surgeons have been known to mock other specialists for using heavy-gauge suture for skin closure, but the choice of sutures is irrelevant if the sutures are removed soon enough. Sutures on the face can usually be removed in 3 to 5 days and on the body in 7 days or less. Except for wounds over joints, sutures should rarely be left in for more than 1 week. A subcutaneous layer of closure and Steri-Strips are usually sufficient to prevent dehiscence.

The second important technical factor that affects the appearance of scars is wound-edge eversion. In wounds where the skin is brought precisely together, there is a tendency for the scar to widen. In wounds where the edges are everted, or even hypereverted in an exaggerated fashion, this tendency is reduced, possibly by reducing the tension on the closure. In other words, the ideal wound closure may not be perfectly flat, but rather bulging with an obvious ridge, to allow for eventual spreading of that wound. Wound-edge eversion **ALWAYS** goes away. The surgeon need not ever worry that a hypereverted wound will remain that way; it will always flatten over time.

CLOSURE OF SKIN WOUNDS

While the most common method of closing a wound is with sutures, there is nothing necessarily magic or superior about sutures. Staples, skin tapes, or wound adhesives are also useful in certain situations. Regardless of the method used, precise approximation of the skin edges without tension is essential to ensure primary healing with minimal scarring.

Wounds that are deeper than skin are closed in layers. The key is to eliminate dead space, to provide a strong enough closure to prevent dehiscence while wound healing is occurring, and to precisely approximate the skin edges without tension. Not all layers necessarily require separate closure. A closure over the calf, however, is subject to motion, dependence, and stretching with walking, requiring a stronger closure than the scalp, which does not move, is less dependent, and not subject to tension in daily activities.

Except for dermal sutures, which are placed with the knot buried to prevent it from emerging from the skin during the healing process, sutures should be placed with the knot superficial to the loop of the suture (not buried), so that the tissue layers can be everted (Fig. 1.2A).

Buried dermal sutures provide strength so the external sutures can be removed early, but do not prevent the scar from spreading over time. There is no technique that reliably prevents a wound that has an inclination to widen from doing so.

Suturing Techniques

Techniques for suturing are illustrated in Figure 1.2 and are listed below.

Simple Interrupted Suture

The simple interrupted suture is the gold standard and the most commonly employed suture. The needle is introduced into the skin at an angle that allows it to pass into the deep dermis at a point further removed from the entry of the needle. This allows the width of suture at its base in the dermis to be wider

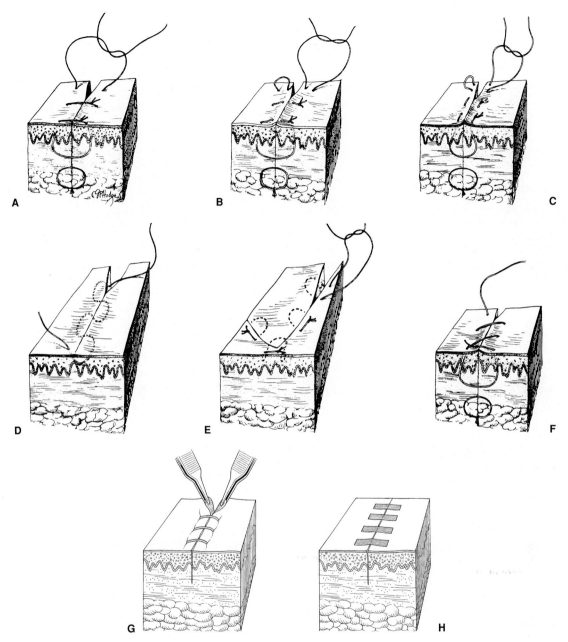

FIGURE 1.2. Types of skin closure. **A:** Simple interrupted. **B:** Vertical mattress. **C:** Horizontal mattress. **D:** Subcuticular continuous. **E:** Half-buried horizontal mattress. **F:** Continuous over-and-over. **G:** Staples. **H:** Skin tapes (skin adhesive performs a similar function).

than the epidermal entrance and exit points, giving the suture a triangular appearance when viewed in cross section and everting the skin edges. Care must be taken to ensure that the suture is placed at the same depth on each side of the incision or wound, otherwise the edges will overlap. Sutures are usually placed approximately 5 to 7 mm apart and 1 to 2 mm from the skin edge, although the location and size of the needle and caliber of the suture material make this somewhat variable.

Vertical Mattress Suture

Vertical mattress sutures may be used when eversion of the skin edges is desired and cannot be accomplished with simple sutures alone. **Vertical mattress sutures tend to leave the most obvious and unsightly cross-hatching if not removed early.**

Horizontal Mattress Suture

Horizontal mattress sutures also provide approximation of the skin edges with eversion. They are particularly advantageous in thick glabrous skin (feet and hand). **In the author's opinion, horizontal mattress sutures are superior to their vertical counterparts.**

Subcuticular Suture

Subcuticular (or intradermal) sutures can be interrupted or placed in a running fashion. In a running subcutaneous closure, the needle is passed horizontally through the superficial dermis parallel to the skin surface to provide close approximation of the skin edges. Care is taken to ensure that the sutures are placed at the same level. Such a technique obviates the need for external skin sutures and circumvents the possibility of suture marks in the skin. Absorbable or nonabsorbable suture can be used, with the latter to be removed at 1 to 2 weeks after suturing.

Half-Buried Horizontal Mattress Suture

Half-buried horizontal mattress sutures are used when it is desirable to have the knots on one side of the suture line with no suture marks on the other side. For example, when insetting the areola in breast reduction, this method leaves the suture marks on the dark, pebbly areola instead of on the breast skin.

Continuous Over-and-Over Suture

Continuous over-and-over sutures, otherwise known as *running simple sutures* can be placed rapidly but depend on the wound edges being more-or-less approximated beforehand. **A continuous suture is not nearly as precise as interrupted sutures.** Continuous sutures can also be placed in a locking fashion to provide hemostasis by compression of wound edges. They are especially useful in scalp closures.

Skin Staples

Skin staples are particularly useful as a time saver for long incisions or to position a skin closure or flap temporarily before suturing. Grasping the wound edges with forceps to evert the tissue is helpful when placing the staples to prevent inverted skin edges. Staples must be removed early to prevent skin marks and are ideal for the hair-bearing scalp.

Skin Tapes

Skin tapes can effectively approximate the wound edges, although buried sutures are often required in addition to skin tape to approximate deeper layers, relieve tension, and prevent inversion of the wound edges. Skin tapes can also be used after skin sutures are removed to provide added strength to the closure.

Skin Adhesives

Skin adhesives have been developed, and may have a role in wound closure, especially in areas where there is no tension on the closure, or where strength of closure has been provided by a layer of buried dermal sutures. Adhesives, by themselves, however, do not evert the wound edges. Eversion must be provided by deeper sutures.

Methods of Excision

Lesions of the skin can be excised with *elliptical, wedge, circular, or serial excision.*

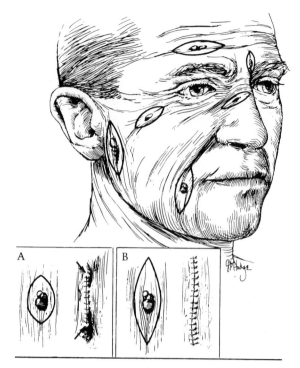

FIGURE 1.3. Elliptical excision. **A:** If the ellipse is too short, dog-ears (*arrows*) form at the ends of the closed wound. **B:** Correct method with length of ellipse at least three times the width.

Elliptical Excision

Simple elliptical excision is the most commonly used technique (Fig. 1.3). Elliptical excision of inadequate length may yield "dog-ears," which consist of excess skin and subcutaneous fat at the end of a closure. There are several ways to correct a dog-ear, some of which are shown in **Figure 1.4.** Dog-ears are the bane of plastic surgical existence and one must be facile with their elimination. **Dog-ears do not disappear on their own.**

Wedge Excision

Lesions located at or adjacent to free margins can be excised by wedge excision. In some elderly patients, one third of the lower lip and one fourth of the upper lip can be excised with primary closure (Fig. 1.5)

Circular Excision

When preservation of skin is desired (such as the tip of the nose) or the length of the scar must be kept to a minimum (children), circular excision might be desirable. Figure 1.6 shows some closure techniques. Figure 1.6 is included because these techniques

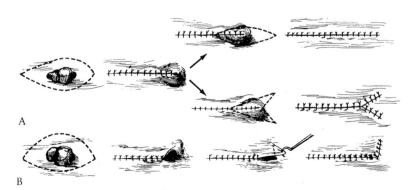

FIGURE 1.4. Three methods of removing a dog-ear caused by making the elliptical excision too short. **A:** Dog-ear excised, making the incision longer, or converted to a "Y". **B:** One method of removing a dog-ear caused by designing an elliptical excision with one side longer than the other. Conversion to an "L" effectively lengthens the shorter side.

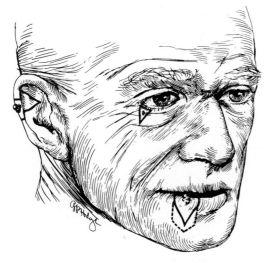

FIGURE 1.5. Wedge excisions of the ear, lower eyelid and lip.

may be of value, as well as for historical purposes. Circular defects can also be closed with a purse-string suture that causes significant bunching of the skin. This is allowed to mature for many months and may result in a shorter scar on, for example, the face of a child.

Serial Excision

Serial excision is the excision of a lesion in more than one stage. Serial excision and tissue expansion (Chapter 10) are frequently employed for large lesions such as congenital nevi. The inherent viscoelastic properties of skin are used, allowing the skin to "stretch" over time. These techniques enable wound closure to be accomplished with a shorter scar than if the original lesion was elliptically excised in a single stage.

SKIN GRAFTING

Skin grafts are a standard option for closing defects that cannot be closed primarily. A skin graft consists of epidermis and some or all of the dermis. By definition, a graft is something that is removed from the body, is completely devascularized, and is replaced in another location. Grafts of any kind require vascularization from the bed into which they are placed for survival. Any tissue which is not completely removed prior to placement is not a graft.

Skin Graft Types

Skin grafts are classified as either split-thickness or full-thickness, depending on the amount of dermis included. Split-thickness skin grafts contain varying amounts of dermis, whereas a full-thickness skin graft contains the entire dermis (Fig. 1.7).

All skin grafts contract immediately after removal from the donor site and again after revascularization in their final location. **Primary contraction** is the immediate recoil of freshly harvested grafts as a result of the elastin in the dermis. The more dermis the graft has, the more primary the contraction that will be experienced. **Secondary contracture**, the real nemesis, involves contraction of a healed graft and is probably a result of myofibroblast activity. A full-thickness skin graft contracts more on initial harvest (primary contraction) but less on healing (secondary contracture) than a split-thickness skin

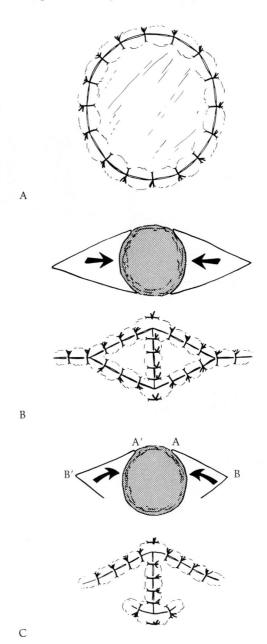

FIGURE 1.6. Closure of wounds following circular excision. **A:** Skin graft. **B:** Sliding triangular subcutaneous pedicle flaps can be advanced to close the circular defect; the triangular defect is closed in a V-Y fashion. **C:** Transposition flaps based on a skin pedicle and rotated toward each other can also be used. Circular defects can also be closed by other local flaps (Figs. 1.10–1.15) or by pursestring suture.

graft. The thinner the split-thickness skin graft, the greater the secondary contracture. Granulating wounds left to heal secondarily, without any skin grafting, demonstrate the greatest degree of contracture and are most prone to hypertrophic scarring.

The number of epithelial appendages transferred with a skin graft depends on the thickness of the dermis present. The ability of grafted skin to sweat depends on the number of glands transferred and the sympathetic reinnervation of these glands from the recipient site. Skin grafts are reinnervated by ingrowth of nerve fibers from the recipient bed and from the periphery. Full-thickness skin grafts have the greatest sensory return because of a greater availability of neurilemmal sheaths. Hair follicles are also transferred with a full-thickness

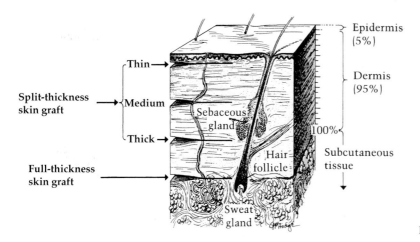

FIGURE 1.7. Skin graft thickness.

skin graft. In general, full-thickness skin grafts demonstrate the hair growth of the donor site whereas split-thickness skin grafts, especially thin split-thickness skin grafts, are generally hairless.

Requirements for Survival of a Skin Graft

The success of skin grafting, or "take," depends on the ability of the graft to receive nutrients and, subsequently, vascular ingrowth from the recipient bed. Skin graft revascularization or "take" occurs in three phases. The first phase involves a process of serum imbibition and lasts for 24 to 48 hours. Initially, a fibrin layer forms when the graft is placed on the recipient bed, binding the graft to the bed. Absorption of nutrients into the graft occurs by capillary action from the recipient bed. The second phase is an inosculatory phase in which recipient and donor end capillaries are aligned. In the third phase, the graft is revascularized through these "kissing" capillaries. Because the full-thickness skin graft is thicker, survival of the graft is more precarious, demanding a well-vascularized bed.

To optimize take of a skin graft, the recipient site must be prepared. Skin grafts require a vascular bed and will seldom take in exposed bone, cartilage, or tendon devoid of their periosteum, perichondrium, or paratenon. There are exceptions, however, as skin grafts are frequently successful inside the orbit or on the temporal bone, despite removal of the periosteum. Close contact between the skin graft and its recipient bed is essential. Hematomas and seromas under the skin graft will compromise its survival, and immobilization of the graft is essential.

Skin Graft Adherence

For the skin graft to take, it must adhere to the bed. There are two phases of graft adherence. The first begins with placement of the graft on the recipient bed, to which the graft adheres because of fibrin deposition. This lasts approximately 72 hours. The second phase involves ingrowth of fibrous tissue and vessels into the graft.

Meshed versus Sheet Skin Grafts

Multiple mechanical incisions result in a meshed skin graft, allowing immediate expansion of the graft. A meshed skin graft covers a larger area per square centimeter of graft harvest and allows drainage through the numerous holes. Meshed

skin grafts result in a "pebbled" appearance that, at times, is aesthetically unacceptable. In contrast, a sheet skin graft has the advantage of a continuous, uninterrupted surface, often leading to a superior aesthetic result, but has the disadvantages of not allowing serum and blood to drain through it and the need for a larger skin graft.

Skin Graft Donor Sites

The donor site epidermis regenerates from the immigration of epidermal cells originating in the hair follicle shafts and adnexal structures left in the dermis. In contrast, the dermis never regenerates. Because split-thickness skin grafts remove only a portion of the dermis, the original donor site may be used again for a subsequent split-thickness skin graft harvest. Thus, the number of split-thickness skin grafts harvested from a donor site is directly dependent on the donor dermis thickness. Full-thickness skin graft donor sites must be closed primarily because there are no remaining epithelial structures to provide re-epithelialization.

Skin grafts can be taken from anywhere on the body, although the color, texture, thickness of the dermis, vascularity, and donor site morbidity of body locations vary considerably. Skin grafts taken from above the clavicles provide a superior color match for defects of the face. The upper eyelid skin can also be used, as it provides a small amount of very thin skin. Full-thickness skin graft harvest sites are closed primarily and are therefore of smaller size. The scalp, abdominal wall, buttocks, and thigh are common donor sites for split-thickness skin grafts. Surgeons should avoid the mistake of harvesting split-thickness skin grafts from the most accessible locations such as the anterior thigh. Although donor sites heal by re-epithelialization, there is always visible evidence that an area was used as a donor site. This can vary from keloids to simple hyper- or hypopigmentation. Less-conspicuous donor sites are the buttocks or scalp. Split-thickness skin grafts harvested from the scalp will have hair in them initially but no hair follicles and therefore will ultimately be hairless. The hair in the scalp donor site will return after re-epithelialization because the hair follicles were left undisturbed.

Postoperative Care of Skin Grafts and Donor Sites

Causes of graft failure include collection of blood or serum beneath the graft (raising the graft from the bed and preventing revascularization), movement of the graft on the bed

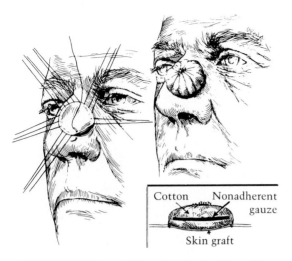

FIGURE 1.8. Tie-over bolster dressing for skin grafts.

Biologic Dressings

Skin grafts can also be used as temporary coverage of wounds as biologic dressings. This protects the recipient bed from desiccation and further trauma until definitive closure can occur. In large burns where there is insufficient skin to be harvested for coverage, skin substitutes can be used (Chapter 18). Biologic skin substitutes include human allografts (cadaver skin), amnion, or xenografts (such as pig skin). Allografts become vascularized (or "take") but are rejected at approximately 10 days unless the recipient is immunosuppressed (e.g., has a large burn), in which case rejection takes longer. Conversely, xenografts are rejected before becoming vascularized. Synthetic skin substitutes such as silicone polymers and composite membranes can also be applied, and new skin substitutes are constantly being developed. Human epidermis can be cultured in vitro to yield sheets of cultured epithelium that will provide coverage for large wounds. The coverage is fragile as a result of the lack of a supporting dermis.

interrupting revascularization (immobilization techniques include the use of bolster dressings as shown in Fig. 1.8), and infection. The risk of infection can be minimized by careful preparation of the recipient site and early inspection of grafts applied to contaminated beds. Wounds that contain more than 10^5 organisms per gram of tissue will not support a skin graft. In addition, an infection at the graft donor site can convert a partial-thickness dermal loss into a full-thickness skin loss.

The donor site of a split-thickness skin graft heals by re-epithelialization. A thin split-thickness harvest site (less than 10/1,000 of an inch) generally heals within 7 days. The donor site can be cared for in a number of ways. The site must be protected from mechanical trauma and desiccation. Xeroform, OpSite, or Adaptic can be used. **Because moist, occluded wounds (donor sites) heal faster than dry wounds, the older method of placing Xeroform and drying it with a hairdryer is not optimal.** An occlusive dressing, such as semipermeable polyurethane dressing (e.g., OpSite), will also significantly decrease pain at the site.

SKIN FLAPS

Unlike a skin graft, a skin flap has its own blood supply. Flaps are usually required for covering recipient beds that have poor vascularity; covering vital structures; reconstructing the full thickness of the eyelids, lips, ears, nose, and cheeks; and padding body prominences. Flaps are also preferable when it may be necessary to operate through the wound at a later date to repair underlying structures. In addition, muscle flaps may provide a functional motor unit or a means of controlling infection in the recipient area. Muscle flaps and microvascular free flaps are discussed in Chapters 5 and 8.

In an experimental study, Mathes et al. compared musculocutaneous flaps with "random" skin flaps to determine the bacterial clearance and oxygen tension of each (Fig. 1.9). Placement of 10^7 *Staphylococcus aureus* underneath random skin flaps in dogs resulted in 100% necrosis of the skin flaps within 48 hours; the musculocutaneous flaps, however, demonstrated long-term survival. The quantity of viable bacteria placed in wound cylinders under these flaps demonstrated an immediate reduction when placed deep to musculocutaneous flap. Oxygen

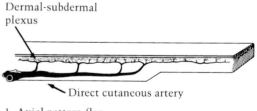

1. Axial pattern flap

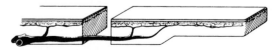

2. Island axial pattern flap

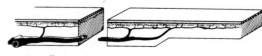

3. Free flap

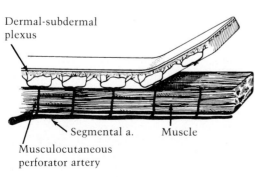

A. RANDOM PATTERN SKIN FLAP

B. AXIAL PATTERN SKIN FLAPS

FIGURE 1.9. "Old-fashioned" classification of skin flaps. **A:** Random pattern. **B:** Axial pattern.

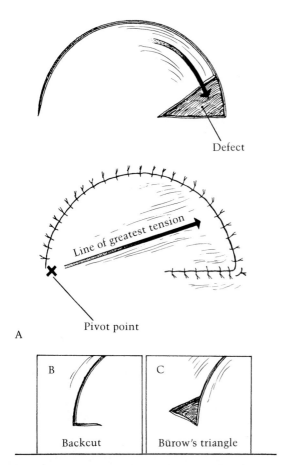

FIGURE 1.10. Rotation flap. The edge of the flap is four to five times the length of the base of the defect triangle. A back-cut or a Burow triangle can be used if the flap is under excessive tension. **A:** Pivot point and line of greatest tension. **B:** Backcut. **C:** Bürow's triangle.

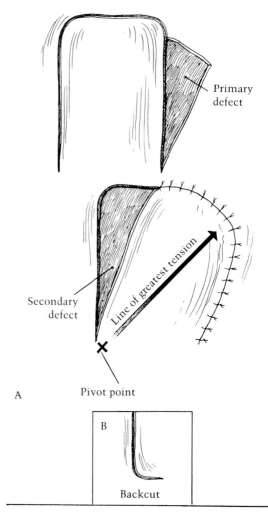

FIGURE 1.11. Transposition flap. The secondary defect is often closed by a skin graft. A back-cut can be used if the flap is under excessive tension.

tension was measured at the distal end of the random flap and compared to that underneath the muscle of the distal portion of musculocutaneous flap as well as in its subcutaneous area. It was found that the oxygen tension in the distal random flap was significantly less than in distal muscular and cutaneous portions of the musculocutaneous flap. This study has been used to justify transfer of muscle flaps in infected wounds. It may be that well-vascularized skin flaps would be equally efficacious as muscle flaps.

Finally, a flap may be chosen because the aesthetic result will be superior. For example, a nasal defect from a skin cancer could be closed with a skin graft, leaving a visible patch. A local skin flap may require incisions in the adjacent nasal tissue, but may be aesthetically preferable in the long-term. There is no better tissue to replace nasal tissue than nasal tissue. **Replace like with like.**

A skin flap consists of skin and subcutaneous tissue that are transferred from one part of the body to another with a vascular pedicle or attachment to the body being maintained for nourishment. Proper planning of a flap is essential to the success of the operation. All possible sites and orientations for the flap must be considered so that the most suitable option is selected.

Planning the flap in reverse is an important principle. A pattern of the defect is transferred onto a piece of cloth toweling. The steps in the operative procedure are carried out in reverse order, using this pattern until the donor site is reached. The flap is designed slightly longer than needed, as some length will be lost in the rotation process and slight redundancy may avoid

kinking of the flap blood supply. The process is repeated, being certain each time the base is held in a fixed position and not allowed to shift with the flap. **Measure twice, cut once.** It is easier to trim a flap that is slightly long than to add to one that is too small.

Planning a transposition or rotation flap requires attention to ensure that the line of greatest tension from the pivot point to the most distal part of the flap is of sufficient length (Figs. 1.10, 1.11 and 1.12).

Local skin flaps are of two types: flaps that rotate about a pivot point (rotation, transposition, and interpolation flaps) (Figs. 1.10 and 1.11) and advancement flaps (single-pedicle advancement, V-Y advancement, Y-V advancement, and bipedicle advancement flaps) (Figs. 1.17 and 1.18).

Flaps Rotating About a Pivot Point

Rotation, transposition, and interpolation flaps have in common a pivot point and an arc through which the flap is rotated. The radius of this arc is the line of greatest tension of the flap. The realization that these flaps can be rotated only about the pivot point is important in preoperative planning.

The rotation flap is a semicircular flap of skin and subcutaneous tissue that rotates about a pivot point into the defect to be closed (Fig. 1.10). The donor site can be closed by a skin graft or by direct suture of the wound.

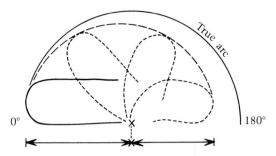

FIGURE 1.12. Importance of the pivot point. A skin flap rotated about a pivot point becomes shorter in effective length the farther it is rotated. Planning with a cloth pattern is helpful when designing such a flap.

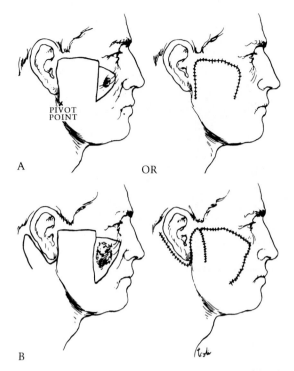

FIGURE 1.13. Transposition flap that can be used to close defects on the anterior cheek. **A:** Small defects can be closed by a single transposition cheek flap that follows the skin lines. **B:** Large defects can be closed by a double transposition flap that uses a flap of postauricular skin to close the secondary defect left by the cheek flap.

A flap that is too tight along its radius can be released by making a short back-cut from the pivot point along the base of the flap. Because this back-cut decreases the blood supply to the flap, its use requires some degree of caution. With some flaps it is possible to back-cut only the tissue responsible for the tension, without reducing the blood supply to the flap. Examples of this selective cutting are found in the galea aponeurotica of the scalp and in areas over the trunk where the fascia within the thick subcutaneous layer can be divided. The necessity for a back-cut may be an indication of poor planning. A triangle of skin (Burow triangle) can be removed from the area adjacent to the pivot point of the flap to aid its advancement and rotation (Fig. 1.10c). This method is of only modest benefit in decreasing tension along the radius of the flap.

The transposition flap is a rectangle or square of skin and subcutaneous tissue that also is rotated about a pivot point into an immediately adjacent defect (Fig. 1.11). This necessitates that the end of the flap adjacent to the defect be designated to extend beyond it (Figs. 1.12 and 1.13). As the flap is rotated, with the line of greatest tension as the radius of the rotation arc, the advancing tip of the flap will be sufficiently long. The flap donor site is closed by skin grafting, direct suture of the wound, or a secondary flap from the most lax skin at right angles to the primary flap. An example of this latter technique is the ingenious bilobed flap (Fig. 1.14). The key to a successful bilobed flap is an area of loose skin to permit direct closure of the secondary flap defect. Pinching the skin between the examiner's fingers helps find the loosest skin, for example, in the glabellar area and lateral to the eyelids.

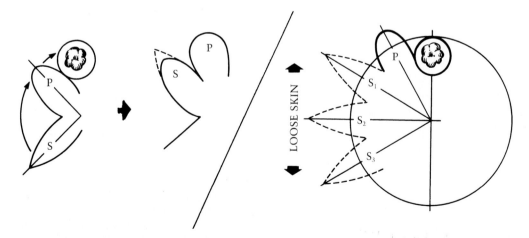

FIGURE 1.14. Bilobed flap. After the lesion is excised, the primary flap (*P*) is transposed into the initial defect. The secondary flap (*S*) is then transposed into the defect left after the primary flap has been moved. The primary flap is slightly narrower than the defect caused by excision of the initial lesion, and the secondary flap is half the diameter of the primary flap. For the bilobed flap to be successful, the secondary flap must come from an area of loose skin so that the defect remaining after moving the secondary flap can be closed by approximation of the wound edges. Three possible choices for the secondary flap (*S1*, *S2, S3*) are depicted. The surgeon chooses the location of the secondary flap based on the skin laxity and the location of the eventual scar.

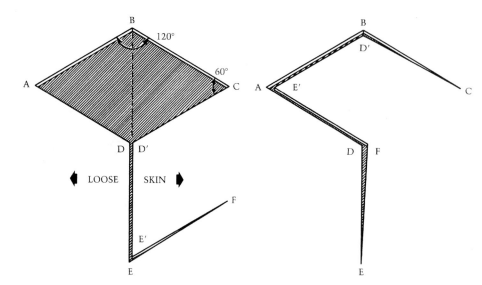

FIGURE 1.15. Planning a rhomboid (Limberg) flap. The rhomboid defect must have 60- and 120-degree angles. The flap is planned in an area of loose skin so that direct closure of the wound edges is possible. The short diagonal *BD* (which is the same length as each side) is extended by its own length to point *E*. The line *EF* is drawn parallel to *CD* and is of the same length. After the flap margins have been incised, the flap is transposed into the rhomboid defect.

The Limberg flap is a type of transposition flap. This flap, like the bilobed flap and the Z-plasty (discussed below), depends on the looseness of adjacent skin, which can be located by pinching various areas of skin between thumb and forefinger. Fortunately, most patients who require local skin flaps are in the older age group and therefore have loose skin. A Limberg flap is designed for rhomboid defects with angles of 60 and 120 degrees, **but most wounds can be made rhomboid, or imagined as rhomboid, so the principle is applicable to most facial wounds.** The flap is designed with sides that are the same length as the short axis of the rhomboid defect (Figs. 1.15 and 1.16).

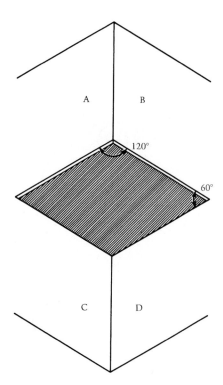

FIGURE 1.16. Four Limberg flaps are available for any rhomboid defect with 60- and 120-degree angles. The choice is made based on the location of the eventual scar, skin laxity, and blood supply of the flap.

Advancement Flaps

All advancement flaps are moved directly forward into a defect without any rotation or lateral movement. Modifications are the single-pedicle advancement, the V-Y advancement, and the bipedicle advancement flaps. Advancement flaps are also used in the movement of expanded skin (Chapter 10).

The single-pedicle advancement flap is a rectangular or square flap of skin and subcutaneous tissue that is stretched forward. Advancement is accomplished by taking advantage of the elasticity of the skin (Fig. 1.17A) and by excising Burow triangles lateral to the flap (Fig. 1.17B). These triangular excisions help to equalize the length between the sides of the flap and adjacent wound margins.

The V-Y advancement technique has numerous applications. It is not an advancement in the same sense as the forward movement of a skin flap just described. Rather, a V-shaped incision is made in the skin, after which the skin on each side of the V is advanced and the incision is closed as a Y (Fig. 1.18). This V-Y technique can be used to lengthen such structures as the nasal columella, eliminate minor notches of the lip, and, in certain instances, close the donor site of a skin flap.

Z-PLASTY

Geometric Principle of the Z-Plasty

The Z-plasty is an ingenious principle that has numerous applications in plastic surgery (Chapter 18). Z-plasties can be applied to revise and redirect existing scars or to provide additional length in the setting of scar contracture. The principle involves the transposition of two triangular flaps (Fig. 1.19). The limbs of the Z must be equal in length to the central limb, but can extend at varying angles (from 30 to 90 degrees) depending on the desired gain in length. The classic Z-plasty has an angle of 60 degrees (Table 1.1) and provides a 75% theoretical gain in length of the central limb by recruiting lateral tissue.

Gain in length is in the direction of the central limb of the Z and depends on the angle used and the length of the central limb. Although the theoretical gain can be determined

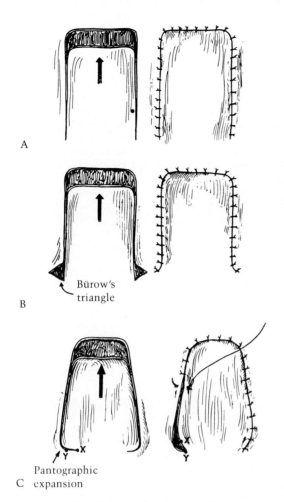

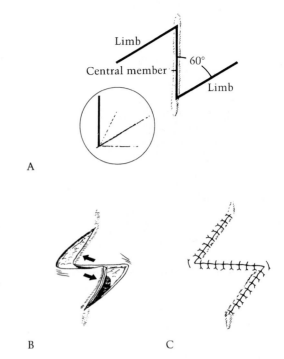

FIGURE 1.19. Classic 60-degree-angle Z-plasty. Inset shows the method of finding the 60-degree angle by first drawing a 90-degree angle, then dividing it in thirds by sighting. The limbs of the Z must be equal in length to the central member. **A:** Design. **B:** Transposition of flaps. **C:** Final result. Note central limb has changed direction by 90 degrees.

FIGURE 1.17. Single-pedicle advancement flaps. **A:** Advancement by taking advantage of the skin elasticity. **B:** Advancement by excising Burow triangles of skin laterally to equalize the length of the flap and the adjacent wound edge. **C:** Pantographic expansion. This method is frequently used after the skin expansion but is risky as the back cuts decrease the blood supply.

mathematically, the actual gain is based on the mechanical properties of the skin and is always less.

Planning and Uses of the Z-Plasty

The resulting central limb, after flap transposition, will be perpendicular to the original central limb. In scar revision, the final central limb should lie in the direction of the skin lines and should be selected first. The Z-plasty is then designed.

The Z-plasty principle can be used to increase the length of skin in a desired direction. For example, it is useful for release of scar contractures, especially in cases in which the scar crosses a flexion crease. Any number of Z-plasties can be designed in series, especially in cosmetically sensitive areas (such

as the face) to break up the appearance of a straight line or to release a contracture. Large Z-plasties, however, do not look good on the face and it is better to use many tiny Z-plasties. Congenital skin webs can also be corrected with Z-plasties. U-shaped or "trapdoor" scars may be improved by breaking up the contracting line. Circumferential scars are amenable to lengthening using Z-plasties, especially in constricting bands of the extremities. These deformities are best released one-half at a time because of concern over interruption of blood supply to the extremity.

Borges described the W-plasty as another method of revising a scar. It is useful occasionally, but lacks the applicability and universality that Z-plasty has. This technique simply involves excising the scar in multiple small triangles that are so situated that they interdigitate (Fig. 1.20). Although the W-plasty changes the direction of the linear scar, it would only be by chance that one of the limbs of the W would lie in the same direction as the skin lines. Because a W-plasty does not lengthen a contracted scar line, it is best to use the Z-plasty for this purpose.

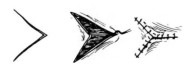

FIGURE 1.18. V-Y advancement. It is the skin on each side of the V that is actually advanced.

TABLE 1.1

Z-PLASTY, ANGLES, AND THEORETICAL GAIN

Angles of Z-plasty (degrees)	Theoretical gain in length (%)
30–30	25
45–45	50
60–60	75
75–75	100
90–90	120

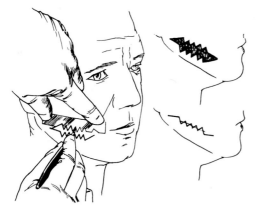

FIGURE 1.20. The W-plasty can also be used to break up a long scar that does not lie in the direction of the skin lines.

Both the Z-plasty and the W-plasty have the additional attribute of breaking up a linear scar into an accordion-like scar that has some degree of elasticity to it. This change permits the skin to be more mobile in its contribution to facial expressions. To their detriment, both techniques more than double the length of the scar. If the W-plasty is employed, the triangles

must be made very small to avoid worsening the appearance of the scar.

RECONSTRUCTIVE LADDER

The techniques described above are applicable to cutaneous defects. Plastic surgeons often are consulted regarding closing more complex defects. When analyzing a wound, whether cutaneous or more complex, the options for closure are evaluated beginning with the simplest and progressing up the "reconstructive ladder" to the more complex (Fig. 1.21). This progression from primary closure, to skin graft, to local flap, to regional flap, to microvascular free flap provides a framework that can be applied to any reconstructive situation. Application of the simplest option that meets the reconstructive requirements ensures a "lifeboat" should the procedure fail. In many situations, however, a higher "rung" on the ladder is intentionally chosen. For example, a local flap may be selected over a skin graft for a defect on the nose because it may provide a superior result, or a free flap may be chosen for a breast reconstruction when an attached, pedicled flap would suffice because the blood supply of the former is superior.

CONCLUSION

The application of fundamental principles in the practice of plastic surgery allows the surgeon to approach even the most complex problem in an organized, systematic fashion. This chapter presents fundamental principles that can be applied to any wound closure situation.

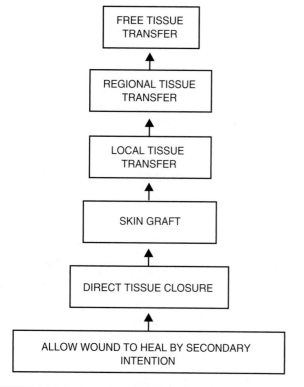

FIGURE 1.21. Reconstructive ladder demonstrating the fundamental principle in planning closure of a defect from simple to more complex.

Suggested Readings

Birch J, Branemark PI. The vascularization of a free full thickness skin graft: a vital microscopic study. *Scand Plast J Surg.* 1969;3:1.

Borges AF. *Elective Incisions and Scar Revision.* Boston: Little, Brown; 1973.

Capla J, Ceradini D, Tepper O, et al. Skin graft vascularization involves precisely regulated regression and replacement of endothelial cells through both angiogenesis and vasculogenesis. *Plast Reconstr Surg.* 2005. In press.

Converse JM, Rapaport FT. The vascularization of skin autografts and homografts: an experimental study in man. *Ann Surg.* 1956;143:306.

Edgerton MT. *The Art of Surgical Technique.* Baltimore: Williams & Wilkins; 1988.

Edgerton MT, Hansen FC. Matching facial color with split thickness skin grafts from adjacent areas. *Plast Reconstr Surg.* 1960;25:455.

Furnas DW, Fischer GW. The Z-plasty: biomechanics and mathematics. *Br J Plast Surg.* 1971;24:144.

Krizek TJ, Robson MC. Evolution of quantitative bacteriology in wound management. *Am J Surg.* 1975;130:579.

Mathes S, Alpert B, Chang N. Use of the muscle flap in chronic osteomyelitis: experimental and clinical correlation. *Plast Reconstr Surg.* 1982;69:815.

Robson MC, Krizek TJ, Heaggars JP. Biology of surgical infections. In: Ravitch MM, ed. *Current Problems in Surgery.* Chicago: 1973.

Rudolph R. Inhibition of myofibroblasts by sham skin grafts. *Plast Reconstr Surg.* 1979;63:473.

Tanner JC, Vandeput J, Olley JF. The mesh skin graft. *Plast Reconstr Surg.* 1964;34:287.

Vogt PM, Andree C, et al. Dry, moist and wet skin wound repair. *Ann Plast Surg.* 1995;34:493.

CHAPTER 2 ■ WOUND HEALING: NORMAL AND ABNORMAL

GEOFFREY C. GURTNER

THE RESPONSE TO INJURY

What is wound healing? Definitions include the repair or re-constitution of a defect in an organ or tissue, commonly the skin. However, it is clear that the process of wounding activates systemic processes that alter physiology far beyond the confines of the defect itself. Inflammatory cascades are initiated that impact nearly every organ system and have potentially dire consequences for survival, as illustrated by multisystem organ failure. Furthermore, recent research implicating the participation of stem and progenitor cells in the wound-healing process requires a broader perspective than one that focuses solely on the defect itself (1,2). Wound healing is best understood as an organism's global response to injury, regardless of whether the location is in skin, liver, or heart. Seen from this perspective, it is not an exaggeration to regard the response to injury as one of the most complex physiologic processes that occurs in life.

The complexity of the process is easily demonstrated in cutaneous wound healing. During the progression from a traumatic injury to a stable scar, the intrinsic and extrinsic clotting systems are activated, acute and chronic inflammatory responses occur, neovascularization proceeds through angiogenesis and vasculogenesis, cells proliferate, divide, and undergo apoptosis, and extracellular matrix is deposited and remodeled. These (as well as other events) occur simultaneously, and also interact and influence each other at the level of gene transcription and protein translation in a dynamic and continuous fashion. On top of this, normally sterile tissues are encountering and interacting with bacteria and other elements of the external environment in a way that never occurs except following injury. It is not surprising that wound healing and the response to injury remain poorly understood by scientists and clinicians, except at a purely descriptive or empiric level. **The number of commercially available products of unproven efficacy (see Chapter 3) is a testament to the lack of mechanistic understanding regarding this most common surgical problem.**

Most textbook chapters on wound healing are an encyclopedic catalogue of the phenomenology of wound healing. They list the multitude of cytokines and growth factors that are observed during wound healing, usually based on experimental data, or in in vitro systems that are prone to artifact. With the increasing sensitivity of new technologies such as quantitative polymerase chain reaction (Q-PCR), the list of cytokines, growth factors, chemokines, and the like that appear during wound healing continues to grow.

How will we ever make sense of this mountain of data so that we can intervene and predict or alter the outcome of wound healing/response to injury? In this chapter, a theoretical framework is proposed for classifying wound healing. The broad biologic transitions that occur during cutaneous wound healing (i.e., inflammatory phase, proliferative phase, remodeling phase) are described. An abbreviated list of major "factors" is provided but not discussed in detail as it remains unclear which of these factors are of primary or incidental importance in either functional or abnormal wound healing. Finally, there is a discussion of abnormal human healing within the proposed theoretical context. For a more detailed list of the myriad events occurring in wound healing, the reader is referred to a number of excellent recent reviews (3,4). However given the inherent lag in book publication and the rapid pace of the field, the reader should refer to Medline (www.ncbi.nlm.nih.gov/entrez/query.fcgi) and search for the latest reviews in the field of wound healing to obtain the most up-to-the-minute information.

SCAR FORMATION VERSUS TISSUE REGENERATION

Wound healing is a broad and complex topic that covers a variety of responses to injury in a variety of different organ systems. However, some common features exist. Generally, wound healing represents the response of an organism to a physical disruption of a tissue/organ to re-establish homeostasis of that tissue/organ and to stabilize the entire organism's physiology. There are essentially two processes by which this re-establishment of homeostasis occurs. The first is the substitution of a different cellular matrix as a patch to immediately re-establish both a physical and physiologic continuity to the injured organ. This is the process of *scar formation*. The second process is a recapitulation of the developmental processes that initially created the injured organ. By reactivating developmental pathways the architecture of the original organ is recreated. This is the process of *regeneration* (5).

The dynamic balance between scarring and tissue regeneration is different in different tissues and organs (Fig. 2.1). For example, neural injury is characterized by little regeneration and much scarring, whereas hepatic and bone injury usually heals primarily through regeneration. It is important to note, however, that the liver can respond to injury with scarring as it does in response to repetitive insults with alcohol during hepatic cirrhosis. Moreover, the same injury in phylogenetically related species can result in very different responses. Thus, limb amputation in newts results in limb regeneration, whereas in humans, only scarring can occur.

It is important to realize that the balance between scar and regeneration are likely subject to evolutionary pressures and may, in fact, be functional. Thus, a cutaneous injury in our prehistoric predecessors disrupted their homeostasis with respect to thermoregulation, blood loss, and, most importantly, prevention of invasive infection. In an era before antibiotics and sterility, invasive infection was clearly a threat to life. As such, a very rapid and dramatic recruitment of inflammatory

15

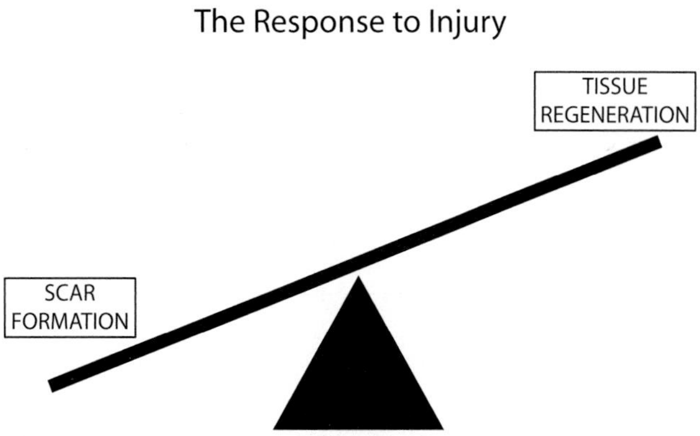

The Response to Injury

FIGURE 2.1. The different ways organisms and organ systems respond to injuries. Scar formation refers to the patching of a defect with a different or modified tissue (i.e., scar). Tissue regeneration refers to the complete recreation of the original tissue architecture. Most processes involve both, but usually one predominates and may be the source of undesirable side effects. For cutaneous wounds, scar formation usually predominates (except in the unique situation of fetal wound healing) and is the source of many of the problems plastic surgeons address.

cells and a proliferative/contractile burst of activity to close the wound as quickly as possible was adaptive. The more leisurely pace of tissue regeneration was a luxury that could not be afforded. In the modern world, however, these adaptive responses often lead to the disfigurement and functional disability characteristic of burn scars. What was once functional has become unwanted, in part because of our ability to close wounds with sutures, circumventing the need for a vigorous contractile response following wound formation.

In the same way that scar formation is not always bad, tissue regeneration is not always good. Peripheral nerve neuromas are dysfunctional and some attempts at regeneration of organ systems results in disabling conditions that threaten the entire organism. In these cases, scar formation is preferable. Indeed, the ablative measures used to treat these neuromas are attempts to *prevent* further regeneration.

When analyzing an undesirable or dysfunctional response to injury in a tissue or organ system, it is useful to consider (a) what is the undesirable portion of the response to injury and (b) whether substitution of a new tissue (scar) or recreation of the pre-existing tissue (regeneration) is responsible for this undesirable effect. It is important to consider the possible adaptive role that the dysfunctional process might have. In the case of a neuroma, the case can be made that the occasional return of protective or functional sensibility following a partial nerve injury is more adaptive and has a survival advantage over the occurrence of complete anesthesia in a peripheral nerve territory. Similarly, with respect to fetal wound healing, in the sterile intrauterine environment, the predominance of regenerative pathways may be adaptive, whereas for the adult organism existing in a microbe-filled environment, it may not be.

Such an analysis suggests strategies to correct the undesirable end result in a given tissue or organ. If the problem is overexuberant scar formation, then it is likely that measures to decrease scarring would be helpful. However, as this balance is a dynamic one, efforts at accelerating regeneration might also be effective. Perhaps even better still would be the simultaneous decrease in scar formation and increase in tissue regeneration.

It is clear that the response to injury in different tissues involves different proportions of scar formation and tissue regeneration. By understanding the differences using the approach described above, we begin to understand why different organs and tissues respond to injuries in very different ways. Just as a

corneal ulcer, a myocardial infarction, and a stage IV pressure sore have different functional implications for the organism, the dynamic balance of scarring and regeneration will be different in the attempt to re-establish homeostasis. The failure of either scar formation or regeneration may lead to similar appearing clinical problems that have a completely different underlying etiology. Hopefully, this type of analysis will lead to a more organized approach to the classification and treatment of injuries in a variety of different organ systems. Most importantly, it may suggest strategies for intervention to optimize the response to injury and prevent the undesirable sequelae of wound healing.

SEMANTICS OF WOUND HEALING

The nomenclature of both scientific and clinical wound healing research is imprecise and confusing. For example, what is the difference between a chronic wound and a nonhealing wound? For purposes of this chapter, several terms are defined. The vast majority of surgical wounds are incisional wounds that are reapproximated by sutures or adhesives and in the absence of complications will heal *primarily* or by *primary intention*. Generally such wounds heal with a scar and do not require special wound care or the involvement of a specialist in wound healing. This is in contrast to wounds that are not reapproximated (for any reason) and the subsequent defect is "filled in" with granulation tissue and then re-epithelialized. This is referred to as healing by *secondary intention* and generally results in a delay in the appearance of a healed or "closed" wound. Often these wounds require special dressings and treatments (discussed in detail in Chapter 3) and have a higher likelihood of progressing to a chronic wound. The discussion of normal wound healing that follows discusses healing by secondary intention, although the same phases occur in all wounds.

An *acute wound* is a wound that has occurred within the past 3 to 4 weeks. If the wound persists beyond 4 to 6 weeks it is considered a *chronic wound*, a term that also includes wounds that have been present for months or years. *Nonhealing wound* or *delayed healing wounds* are terms used interchangeably to describe chronic wounds. In addition, chronic wounds are often referred to as a "granulating." This refers to the appearance in the wound cavity of granulation tissue (see discussion of proliferative in Table 3.3) and is a sign that suggests that the wound is progressing, albeit slowly.

PHASES OF NORMAL WOUND HEALING

The normal mammalian response to a break in cutaneous defect integrity occurs in three overlapping, but biologically distinct, phases (Fig. 2.2). Following the initial injury, there is an initial *inflammatory phase* the purpose of which is to remove devitalized tissue and prevent invasive infection. Next, there is a *proliferative phase* during which the balance between scar formation and tissue regenerations occurs. Usually, scar formation predominates, although in fetal wound healing an impressive amount of regeneration is possible. Finally, the longest and least understood phase of wound healing occurs, the *remodeling phase*, the purpose of which is to maximize the strength and structural integrity of the wound.

Inflammatory Phase

The inflammatory phase (Fig. 2.3) of wound healing begins immediately following tissue injury. The functional priorities

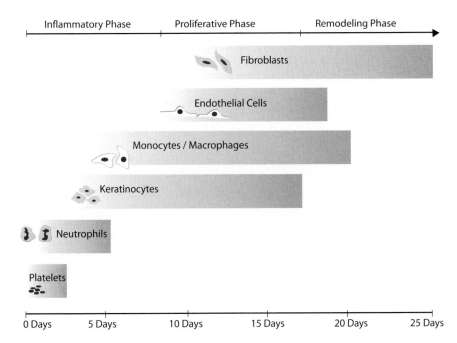

FIGURE 2.2. The three phases of wound healing (inflammatory, proliferative, remodeling), the timing of these phases in adult cutaneous wound healing, and the characteristic cells that are seen in the healing wound at these time points.

during this phase are attainment of hemostasis, removal of dead and devitalized tissues, and prevention of colonization and invasive infection by microbial pathogens, principally bacteria.

Initially, components of the injured tissue, including fibrillar collagen and tissue factor, act to activate the extrinsic clotting cascade and prevent ongoing hemorrhage. Disrupted blood vessels allow blood elements into the wound, and platelets clump and form an aggregate to plug the disrupted vessels. During this process, platelets degranulate, releasing growth factors such as platelet-derived growth factor (PDGF) and transforming growth factor-β (TGF-β). The end result of the intrinsic and extrinsic coagulation cascades is the conversion of fibrinogen to fibrin and subsequent polymerization into a gel. This provisional fibrin matrix provides the scaffolding for cell migration required during the later phases of wound healing. Removal of the provisional fibrin matrix will impair wound healing.

Almost immediately, inflammatory cells are recruited to the wound site. During the initial stages of wound healing, inflammatory cells are attracted by activation of the complement cascade (C5a), TGF-β released by degranulating platelets, and products of bacterial degradation such as lipopolysaccharide (LPS). For the first 2 days following wounding, there is neutrophilic infiltrate into the fibrin matrix filling the wound cavity. The primary role of these cells is to remove dead tissue by phagocytosis and to prevent infection by oxygen-dependent and -independent killing mechanisms. They also release a variety of proteases to degrade remaining extracellular matrix to prepare the wound for healing. It is important to realize that although neutrophils play a role in decreasing infection during cutaneous wound healing, their absence does not prevent the overall progress of wound healing (6). However, their prolonged persistence in the wound has been proposed to be a primary factor in the conversion of acute wounds into nonhealing chronic wounds.

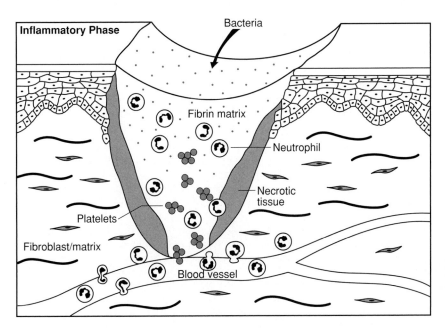

FIGURE 2.3. The inflammatory phase of wound healing begins immediately following tissue injury and serves to obtain hemostasis, remove devitalized tissues, and prevent invasive infection by microbial pathogens.

TABLE 2.1

GROWTH FACTORS, CYTOKINES, AND OTHER BIOLOGICALLY ACTIVE MOLECULES IN WOUND HEALING

Name	Abbreviation	Source	Description
Vascular endothelial growth factor	VEGF	Endothelial cells	Promotes angiogenesis
Fibroblast growth factor 2	FGF-2	Macrophages, mast cells, endothelial cells, T lymphocytes	Promotes angiogenesis. Stimulates endothelial cell migration and growth Promotes epithelialization via keratinocyte and fibroblast migration and proliferation
Platelet-derived growth factor	PDGF	Platelets, macrophages, endothelial cells	Enhances proteoglycan and collagen synthesis Recruits macrophages and fibroblasts
Keratinocyte growth factor	KGF	Fibroblasts	Controls keratinocyte growth and maturation Induces epithelial secretion of other growth factors
Epidermal growth factor	EGF	Platelets, macrophages	Stimulates collagenase secretion by fibroblasts to remodel matrix
Transforming growth factor-β	TGF-β	Platelets, macrophages, T and B cells, hepatocytes, thymocytes, placenta	Promotes angiogenesis Establishes chemoattractant gradients, induces adhesion molecule expression, and promotes proinflammatory molecules that stimulate leukocyte and fibroblast migration Induces extracellular matrix synthesis by inhibiting protease activity and up-regulating collagen and proteoglycan synthesis
Tumor necrosis factor-α	TNF-α	Macrophages, T and B cells, natural killer (NK) cells	Induces collagen synthesis in wounds Regulates polymorphonuclear (PMN) leukocyte margination and cytotoxicity
Granulocyte colony-stimulating factor	G-CSF	Stromal cells, fibroblasts, endothelial cells, lymphocytes	Stimulates granulocyte proliferation, survival, maturation, and activation Induces granulopoiesis
Granulocyte-macrophage colony-stimulating factor	GM-CSF	Macrophages, stromal cells, fibroblasts, endothelial cells, lymphocytes	Stimulates granulocyte and macrophage proliferation, survival, maturation, and activation Induces granulopoiesis
Interferon-α	IFN-α	Macrophages, B and T cells, fibroblasts, epithelial cells	Activates macrophages; inhibits fibroblast proliferation
Interleukin-1	IL-1	Macrophages, keratinocytes, endothelial cells, lymphocytes, fibroblasts, osteoblasts	Proinflammatory peptide Induces chemotaxis of PMN leukocytes, fibroblasts, and keratinocytes Activates PMN leukocytes
Interleukin-4	IL-4	T cells, basophils, mast cells, bone marrow stromal cells	Activates fibroblast proliferation Induces collagen and proteoglycan synthesis
Interleukin-8	IL-8	Monocytes, neutrophils, fibroblasts, endothelial cells, keratinocytes, T cells	Activates PMN leukocytes and macrophages to begin chemotaxis Induces margination and maturation of keratinocytes
Endothelial nitric oxide synthase	eNOS	Endothelial cells, neurons	Synthesizes nitric oxide in endothelial cells with multiple downstream effects
Inducible nitric oxide synthase	iNOS	Neutrophils, endothelial cells	Synthesizes nitric oxide by macrophages and basal keratinocytes; multiple downstream effects

Monocyte/macrophages follow neutrophils into the wound and appear 48 to 72 hours after injury. They are recruited to healing wounds primarily by expression of monocyte chemoattractant protein 1 (MCP-1). Monocyte/macrophages are key regulatory cells for this and later stages of wound repair. Tissue macrophages originate from the circulation, where they are known as monocytes, and alter their phenotype following egress into the tissue. By the third day after wounding they are the predominant cell type in the healing wound. Macrophages phagocytose debris and bacteria, but are especially critical for the orchestrated production of the growth factors necessary for production of the extracellular matrix by fibroblasts and the production of new blood vessels in the healing wound. Table 2.1 provides only a partial listing of chemokines,

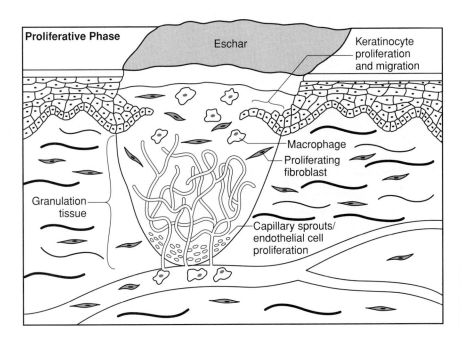

FIGURE 2.4. The proliferative phase of wound healing occurs from days 4 to 21 after wounding. During this phase, granulation tissue fills the wound and keratinocytes migrate to restore epithelial continuity.

cytokines, and growth factors present in the healing wound, as the list grows daily (7). The exact function for each of these factors is incompletely understood, and the literature is filled with contradictory data. **However, it is clear that, unlike the neutrophil, the absence of monocyte/macrophages has severe consequences for healing wounds (8).**

The lymphocyte is the last cell to enter the wound and enters between 5 and 7 days after wounding. Its role in wound healing is not well defined, although it has been suggested that populations of stimulatory CD4 and inhibitory CD8 cells may usher in and out the subsequent proliferative phase of wound healing (9). Similarly, the mast cell appears during the later part of the inflammatory phase, but, again, its function remains unclear. Recently, it has become an area of intense research inquiry because of a correlation between mast cells and some forms of aberrant scarring.

Given the consistent and precise appearance of different subsets of inflammatory cells into the wound, it is likely that soluble factors released in a stereotypic pattern underlie this phenomenon. The source of these factors, the upstream regulators for their production and the downstream consequences of their activity, is a complex topic and the subject of intense ongoing research. Again, Table 2.1 provides a partial list of growth factors thought to be important during wound healing. All are targets for the development of therapeutics to augment or block their action and either accelerate wound healing or decrease scar formation (10). However the biologic relevance of any one factor in isolation remains unclear.

Proliferative Phase

The proliferative phase of wound healing is generally accepted as occurring from days 4 to 21 following injury. However, the phases of wound healing overlap. Certain facets of the proliferative phase, such as re-epithelialization, probably begin almost immediately following injury. Keratinocytes adjacent to the wound alter their phenotype in the hours following injury. Regression of the desmosomal connections between keratinocytes and to the underlying basement membrane frees the cells and allows them to migrate laterally. Concurrent with this is the formation of actin filaments in the cytoplasm of keratinocytes, which provides them with the locomotion to actively migrate

into the wound. Keratinocytes then move via interactions with extracellular matrix proteins (such as fibronectin, vitronectin, and type I collagen) via specific integrin mediators as they proceed between the desiccated eschar and the provisional fibrin matrix beneath (Fig. 2.4).

The provisional fibrin matrix is gradually replaced by a new platform for migration: granulation tissue. Granulation tissue is composed of three cell types that play critical and independent roles in granulation tissue formation: fibroblasts, macrophages, and endothelial cells. These cells form extracellular matrix and new blood vessels, which histologically are the ingredients for granulation tissue. Granulation tissue begins to appear in human wounds by about day 4 postinjury. Fibroblasts are the workhorses during this time and produce the extracellular matrix that fills the healing scar and provides a platform for keratinocyte migration. Eventually this matrix will be the most visible component of cutaneous scars. Macrophages continue to produce growth factors such as PDGF and TGF-β_1 that induce fibroblasts to proliferate, migrate, and deposit extracellular matrix, as well as stimulating endothelial cells to form new vessels. Over time the provisional matrix of fibrin is replaced with type III collagen, which will, in turn, be replaced by type I collagen during the remodeling phase.

Endothelial cells are a critical component of granulation tissue and form new blood vessels through angiogenesis and the newly described process of vasculogenesis, which involves the recruitment and assembly of bone marrow derived progenitor cells. Proangiogenic factors that are released by macrophages include vascular endothelial growth factor (VEGF), fibroblast growth factor (FGF)-2, angiopoiten-1, and thrombospondin, among others. The upstream activator of gene transcription of these growth factors may be hypoxia via HIF-1a protein stabilization. The relative importance of these different vascular growth factors and the precise timing of their arrival and disappearance is an area of active investigation. However, it is clear that the formation of new blood vessels and subsequent granulation tissue survival is important for wound healing during the proliferative phase of wound healing. Blocking this process with angiogenesis inhibitors impairs excisional wound healing and can be rescued with growth factors such as VEGF.

One interesting element of the proliferative phase of wound healing is that at a certain point all of these processes need to be turned off and the formation of granulation tissue/extracellular

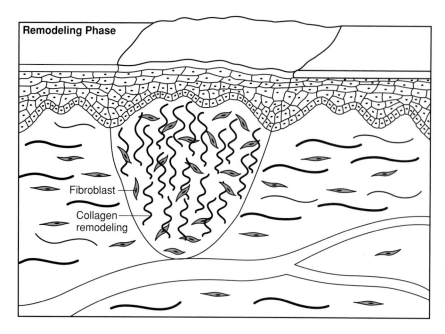

Remodeling Phase

Fibroblast

Collagen remodeling

FIGURE 2.5. The remodeling phase of wound healing is the longest phase and lasts from 21 days to 1 year. Remodeling, although poorly understood, is characterized by the processes of wound.

matrix halted. It is clear that this is a regulated event because once collagen matrix has filled in the wound cavity, fibroblasts rapidly disappear and newly formed blood regress, resulting in a relatively acellular scar under normal conditions. So how do these processes turn off? It seems likely that these events are programmed and occur through the process of gradual self-destruction called apoptosis. The signals that activate this program are unknown but must involve environmental factors as well as molecular signals. Because dysregulation of this process is believed to underlie the pathophysiology of fibrotic disorders such as hypertrophic scarring, understanding the signals for halting the proliferative phase is of obvious importance for developing new therapeutics for these disabling conditions.

Remodeling Phase

The remodeling phase is the longest part of wound healing and in humans is believed to last from 21 days up to 1 year. Once the wound has been "filled in" with granulation tissue and after keratinocyte migration has re-epithelialized it, the process of wound remodeling occurs. Again, these processes overlap, and the remodeling phase likely begins with the programmed regression of blood vessels and granulation tissue described above.

Despite the long duration of the remodeling phase and the obvious relevance to ultimate appearance, it is by far the least-understood phase of wound healing.

In humans, remodeling is characterized by both the processes of wound contraction and collagen remodeling (Fig. 2.5). The process of wound contraction is produced by wound myofibroblasts, which are fibroblasts with intracellular actin microfilaments capable of force generation and matrix contraction. It remains unclear whether the myofibroblast is a separate cell from the fibroblast or whether all fibroblasts retain the capacity to "trans-differentiate" to myofibroblasts under the right environmental conditions. Myofibroblasts contact the wound through specific integrin interactions with the collagen matrix.

Collagen remodeling is also characteristic of this phase. Type III collagen is initially laid down by fibroblasts during the proliferative phase, but over the next few months this will be replaced by type I collagen. This slow degradation of type III collagen is mediated through matrix metalloproteinases se-

creted by macrophages, fibroblasts, and endothelial cells. The breaking strength of the healing wound improves slowly during this process, reflecting the turnover in collagen subtypes and increased collagen crosslinking. At 3 weeks, the beginning of the remodeling phase, wounds only have approximately 20% of the strength of unwounded skin, and will eventually only possess 70% of the breaking strength of unwounded skin.

ABNORMAL RESPONSE TO INJURY AND ABNORMAL WOUND HEALING

Just as it is overly simplistic to consider all the different responses to injury seen in different tissues as simply "wound healing," it is naïve to try to classify all the manifestations of abnormalities in this process as simply "abnormal wound healing." To more accurately classify all the different types of abnormal wound healing, it is useful to consider the balance between attempts to replace tissue defects with new, substitute tissues (scar formation) against the recreation of the original tissue in situ (regeneration) as illustrated in Figure 2.1. It is also helpful to determine where within the normal phases of wound healing the problem occurs. The goal is to understand each abnormal process in terms of the dynamic balance and to propose therapeutic strategies to restore homeostasis.

The process is not merely a semantic exercise but has potential therapeutic implications. Although a corneal ulcer, a peripheral neuroma, and stage IV pressure sores are all examples of abnormal healing, the treatment, as guided by an understanding of the mechanism underlying the abnormality, will vary. For the corneal ulcer, which represents a defect in epithelial regeneration, growth factor therapy to augment the potential for regeneration make senses. It makes less sense for a defect such as a peripheral neuroma. For the neuroma, treatments aimed at preventing nerve regeneration make more sense. In the following paragraphs, the various types of abnormal wound healing are classified using the dynamic balance between scar formation and regeneration. Such an analysis will elucidate and clarify new therapeutic opportunities targeting one component or the other, as illustrated in Figure 2.1.

Inadequate Regeneration Underlying an Abnormal Response to Injury

The classic example of inadequate regeneration is found in central nervous system injuries. The response to injury in these cases is usually characterized by virtually no restoration or recovery of functional neural tissue. The absence of neural regeneration is compensated by a normal physiologic process of replacement with scar tissue, but in most cases this process does not appear excessive or overexuberant. Although attempts to decrease scar formation have been attempted, it is currently thought that these will be ineffective unless neural regeneration can also be achieved. Consequently, current efforts are focused on strategies to increase regeneration of central nervous system (CNS) components. Current modalities under investigation include the use of implanted neural stem/progenitor cells and the use of developmental morphogens to recapitulate the processes of neural development. Techniques to decrease neural scar formation might also be useful to provide a window of opportunity for regeneration to occur, but they are unlikely to be successful in and of themselves. Other examples of inadequate regeneration include bone nonunions and corneal ulcers.

Inadequate Scar Formation Underlying an Abnormal Response to Injury

Many examples of impaired wound healing seen by plastic surgeons belong in this category. In most cases, these diseases result from a failure to replace a tissue defect with a substitute patch of scar (i.e., inadequate scar formation). In these conditions, stable scar tissue is sufficient to restore cutaneous integrity and eliminate the pathology. Regeneration of the skin, although perhaps ideal, is not required for an adequate functional outcome. Examples of these types of conditions include diabetic foot ulcers, sacral pressure sores, and venous stasis ulcers. In all these cases, restoration of cutaneous integrity is sufficient; thus, efforts must be made to understand and correct the defects in scar formation that are occurring in these disease states.

Once the defect in scar formation is understood, therapy can be rationally designed. At times, it is useful to subdivide the scar formation defects further and examine whether the primary defect occurs in the inflammatory, proliferative, or remodeling phases of wound healing. For instance, in humans and experimental models, diabetic ulcers occur because of defects in the inflammatory and proliferative phases of wound healing. Accordingly, therapeutics are targeted toward these phases (10). In contrast, wounds occurring because of vitamin C depletion (i.e., scurvy) are a result of abnormal collagen crosslinking that occurs during the remodeling phase of wound healing. Treatment is best directed to this later phase. Although in both cases therapeutic efforts are focused on correcting defects in scar formation (as opposed to augmenting tissue regeneration), the targets will be different.

Excessive Regeneration Underlying an Abnormal Response to Injury

These situations are relatively rare. In these cases, pathways of tissue regeneration lead to the recreation of the absent tissue but there are functional problems reintegrating the tissue into the systemic physiology. They often occur in peripheral nerve tissue, such as peripheral nerve regeneration leading to neuroma. Other examples include the hyperkeratosis that occurs in cutaneous psoriasis or adenomatous polyp formation in the colon. It is plausible that conditions we consider "precancerous" are the result of overexuberant attempts at tissue regeneration, leading to disordered and uncontrolled growth. In these situations, scar formation would be preferable to regeneration because of possible loss of growth control and transformation to overt cancer.

In these disease states, therapeutic measures are targeted toward decreasing cellular proliferation and blocking or impeding the aberrant regenerative pathways. Irritant strategies to maximize scar formation may also play a role, as when alcohol is injected into a neuroma. The goal is to limit the ability of the tissue to activate pathways leading to regeneration. It is sobering to realize that although much current effort is focused on maximizing tissue regeneration, there are circumstances where this already occurs and has proven to be dysfunctional. It also illustrates the need for care and strict control of the technology of tissue generation using stem and progenitor cells.

Excessive Scar Formation Underlying an Abnormal Response to Injury

When these conditions affect the skin, they are commonly treated by plastic surgeons, but they can occur elsewhere, as in pulmonary fibrosis or cirrhosis. "Excessive" cutaneous scar formation remains a poorly understood and ubiquitous disease for which there are few treatment options. Abnormal scarring is classified as either hypertrophic scarring or keloid formation. Both are manifestations of overexuberant scarring, although the upstream etiology is probably different. Keloids are less common, and have a genetic component that limits them to <6% of the population, primarily the black and Asian populations. **Histologically, keloids are differentiated by the overgrowth of dense fibrous tissue beyond the borders of the original wound with large, thick collagen fibers composed of numerous fibrils closely packed together.** However, keloids are less likely to produce dysfunctional contractures than hypertrophic scars, which can potentially affect all humans.

The etiology and pathophysiology of both hypertrophic scarring and keloid formation remain unknown. Many theories have been proposed to account for hypertrophic scar and keloid formation, including mechanical strain, inflammation, bacterial colonization, and foreign-body reaction. Unfortunately, investigation of the mechanisms underlying these diseases is hindered by the absence of an animal model that reproduces the characteristics of human hypertrophic scars. As recently as 2004, it was stated in a major review of burns and trauma that "Hypertrophic scarring remains a terrible clinical problem ... understanding the pathophysiology and developing effective treatment strategies have been hindered by the absence of an animal model" (11). Decreasing the process of scar formation are the prime goals of therapy for both disease states. Modalities employed include steroid injections, pressure therapy with silicone sheeting, and external beam irradiation. However, with current treatment modalities, recurrence rates approach 75%. Theoretically, attempts to augment regeneration are potentially appealing and underlie the interest in fetal wound healing research (12). However, it seems likely that efforts to decrease scar formation will also be essential components to the solution for these unsolved problems.

CONCLUSION

This chapter proposes a theoretical framework with which to understand and classify the normal responses to injury that occur in different tissues and different species. These responses can be conceptualized as favoring replacement of injured tissue with a patch, otherwise known as scar formation, or recapitulating developmental processes to duplicate the original architecture, otherwise referred to as regeneration. The dynamic balance between these two processes may underlie the myriad abnormal responses to injury that occur in human disease states. It is hoped that such a framework will suggest new therapeutic strategies to correct imbalances, by either augmenting or suppressing one component or the other. This may provide a basis for accelerated progress in the care of patients with abnormal or dysfunctional responses to injury that result in human disease.

ACKNOWLEDGMENTS

I would like to thank NYU medical students Sharam Aarabi and Matthew Grieves, who assisted with the preparation of the graphics in this chapter. In addition, I would like to thank Kristen Wienandt Marzejon for the artwork in Figures 2.1, 2.2, and 2.3.

References

1. Van Bekkum DW. Phylogenetic aspects of tissue regeneration: role of stem cells: a concise overview. *Blood Cells Mol Dis.* 2004;32:11–16.
2. Galiano RD, Tepper OM, Pelo CR, et al. Topical vascular endothelial growth factor accelerates diabetic wound healing through increased angiogenesis and by mobilizing and recruiting bone marrow-derived cells. *Am J Pathol.* 2004;164(6):1935–1947.
3. Singer AJ, Clark RAF. Mechanisms of disease: cutaneous wound healing. *N Engl J Med.* 1999;341(10):738–746.
4. Grose R, Werner S. Wound healing studies in transgenic and knockout mice. *Mol Biotechnol.* 2004;20:1–19.
5. Woolley K, Martin P. Conserved mechanisms of repair: from damaged single cells to wounds in multicellular tissues. *Bioessays.* 2000;22(10):911–919.
6. Simpson DM, Ross R. The neutrophilic leukocyte in wound repair: a study with antineutrophil serum. *J Clin Invest.* 1972;51:2009–2023.
7. Werner S, Grose R. Regulation of wound healing by growth factors and cytokines. *Physiol Rev.* 2003;83:835–870.
8. Leibovich SJ, Ross R. The role of the macrophage in wound repair: a study with hydrocortisone and antimacrophage serum. *Am J Pathol.* 1992;78:71–100.
9. Park JE, Barbul A. Understanding the role of immune regulation in wound healing. *Am J Surg.* 2004;187:11S–16S.
10. Goldman R. Growth factors and chronic wound healing: past, present, and future. *Adv Skin Wound Care.* 2004;17:24–25.
11. Sheridan RL, Tompkins RG. What's new in burns and metabolism. *J Am Coll Surg.* 2004;198(2):836–837.
12. Dang C, Ting K, Soo C, et al. Fetal wound hearing current perspectives. *Clin Plast Surg.* 2003;30(1):13–23.

CHAPTER 3 ■ WOUND CARE

ROBERT D. GALIANO AND THOMAS A. MUSTOE

A wound is a microcosm of the patient. Most wounds will heal with minimal intervention in a healthy individual. Conversely, the incidence of nonhealing wounds is higher in patients with systemic diseases, particularly those who are hospitalized. In general, the plastic surgeon is consulted to evaluate three types of wounds: (a) the acute wound where the final appearance may be the principal concern, (b) the wound in a patient whose medical status and/or mode of injury predisposes her to wound-healing difficulties and the threat of a problem wound, or (c) the established chronic wound refractory to past interventions. A solid foundation in the basics of wound care is imperative to treat the broad spectrum of wounds encountered by plastic surgeons and to make sense of the advances in wound treatments that have been made or are on the horizon.

The strides made in understanding the biochemical and cellular aspects of tissue repair have been married to advances in biomaterial design and clinical know-how. The importance of proper wound care in maximizing rates of limb salvage has led to the creation of wound care centers and specialists. In addition, factors such as convenience to the patient and practitioner have evolved as valid variables that should be addressed when choosing a wound-care modality. This is a natural outcome of the evolution and sophistication present in this dynamic and expanding field. Some recent advances in this field are described in this chapter and summarized in Table 3.1.

FUNDAMENTALS

All wounds, whether acute or chronic, should be evaluated initially by a physician to determine the mechanism and to outline an approach to treatment. Tetanus prophylaxis is administered. A history and physical are performed, with an emphasis placed on determining the cause of the wound and identifying any comorbid conditions that might influence healing. The term *wound* encompasses a broad range of lesions without consideration of etiology, and the list of possible causes is vast. Table 3.2 lists the systemic and local factors that can interfere with healing.

The history, physical, and critical evaluation of the possible etiologies of the wound will direct subsequent diagnostic tests. Some useful clinical laboratory tests to assist in the care of the problem wound patient include albumin, prealbumin, and transferrin levels (to determine nutritional status), C-reactive protein and the erythrocyte sedimentation rate (markers of inflammation), glucose and hemoglobin A_{1C} (to determine glucose control in diabetic patients), and a complete blood count (to determine if white blood cell numbers are elevated or if anemia is present). In addition, some useful laboratory tools include transcutaneous oxygen pressure ($tcPO_2$) measurements, toe pressures, neurofilament testing, and ankle–brachial indices (ABI), to name a few. These may direct the need for procedures such as surgical revascularization or nerve decompressions. Wound documentation is also extremely useful to monitor the progression of healing in an objective manner.

The basics of care for most wounds can be summarized as follows:

- Optimize systemic parameters
- Debride nonviable tissue
- Reduce the wound bioburden
- Optimize blood flow
  - Warmth
  - Hydration
  - Surgical revascularization
- Reduce edema
  - Elevation
  - Compression
- Use dressings appropriately, and selectively use biologic dressings, with attention to cost-effectiveness of overall treatment. Aims include:
  - Moist wound healing
  - Exudate removal
  - Avoid trauma to wound or pain to patient with dressing changes
- Use pharmacologic therapy when necessary
- Close wounds surgically with grafts or flaps as indicated

To attain these goals, it is useful to emphasize the common causative factors that are shared by chronic wounds, as opposed to isolating the differences between diverse types of wounds. With this framework in mind, it is remarkable that the majority of problem wounds share the following causative factors: age, ischemia (often exacerbated by repeated episodes of ischemia–reperfusion injury), and bacterial infection. Addressing these three factors will allow the surgeon to effectively manage most problem wounds.

Age and Wound Healing

Most chronic wounds occur in the aged population (older than age 60 years). Although most wounds heal without incident in aged patients, there is a slight, but consistent, decline in wound healing rates in the elderly. The effect of aging declares itself when a variable such as ischemia or infection is superimposed on an injury. Laboratory studies reveal a decline in molecular processes important for tissue repair in aged fibroblasts and endothelial cells. These include accelerated senescence, diminished production of growth factors, decreased ability to survive hypoxic and toxic stresses, and decreased production of collagen and other matrix molecules. Interestingly, cells in diabetic subjects and in irradiated beds share many of these molecular characteristics, and it is useful to consider cells in patients with these conditions as being prematurely aged or senescent.

Because age cannot be reversed, wounds in these patients are best approached by aggressively optimizing systemic parameters, and by directed supplementation when appropriate. Consequently, avoidance of ischemia and infection is particularly

TABLE 3.1

ADVANCES IN WOUND CARE

Old paradigm	New paradigm
Acute wounds versus chronic wounds	Appreciation that not all problem wounds are chronic. Some acute wounds deserve to be treated as intensively as chronic wounds from the onset, if systemic or local factors are expected to impact on healing.
Problem wounds are segregated by underlying disease process	A unifying hypothesis that most problem wounds share the burdens of age, episode of ischemia with reperfusion, and infection.
Wet to dry dressings	Moist wound healing.
Reliance on H_2O_2, Dakin solution (bleach), Povidine-iodine solutions	Products with cadexomer iodine and silver, strategically developed to decrease the bioburden in the wound, are key elements in the wound-care arsenal.
Surgical debridement	Autolytic debridement, enzymatic debridement, and pressurized water tools as adjuncts to "sharp" debridement.
Underappreciation of pain relief	Importance of pain relief for healing and compliance with therapy.
Unna boot as "one-size-fits all" therapy for venous stasis ulcers	Multilayered, sustained, graduated compression therapy products, customized to fit each patient, to better assist in edema control and wound healing.
Air mattresses	Pressure reducing and pressure-relieving products.
Gauze as the universal surgical dressing	Dressings are now tailored to wounds to manage various levels of exudate and bacterial burdens.
Dressings or surgery as sole options for wound care	Negative-pressure wound therapy has introduced a new option for wound care, allowing both temporizing of wounds and definitive treatment.
Lack of pharmacologic agents to accelerate healing of problem wounds	Growth factors as biotech-derived products indicated in the therapeutic treatment of problem wounds.
Limited options for treatment of scars	Scar modulation and prevention of hypertrophic scars with compression garments, compression dressings, and silicone sheets.
Skin grafts	Bioengineered skin products available to stimulate the wound-healing process in hard-to-heal or stalled wounds. Some are available as dermal replacements, others are available as combined epidermal–dermal replacements. They will on occasion permit coverage of exposed bone or tendons.

critical in aged patients, and growth factors may be helpful in select patients.

Hypoxia and Wound Healing

An understanding of the role of hypoxia in wound repair is important, as tissue hypoxia is a characteristic of most chronic wounds. Surgical and nonsurgical interventions can be undertaken to maximize oxygen delivery to tissues. It is known that the diffusion of oxygen and nutrients from capillaries to cells is limited to a distance of 60 to 70 μm in a person breathing room air. The damage to small vessels that occurs in a wound ensures that a wound is hypoxic relative to the surrounding tissues, with oxygen tensions averaging 25 mm Hg in the wound and 40 mm Hg in normal tissues. This hypoxia can be chronic in the settings of periwound fibrosis, which is commonly found in problem wounds. The benefits of ensuring adequate oxygen delivery to a wound are not restricted to established wounds. Adequate oxygenation is also essential to *prevent* complications from occurring. A major emphasis of proper wound care is predicated, intentionally or otherwise, on assuring adequate

delivery of oxygen to the wound. Thus maneuvers such as elevation (reduction of edema), offloading (reduction of pressure-induced ischemia and cyclical reperfusion injury), debridement (removal of dead spaces, foreign bodies, and barriers to oxygenation), pain control (reduction of the constriction of sympathetically innervated cutaneous resistance vessels), warmth (improving perfusion to the skin by directly stimulating the *active* vasodilatation of the cutaneous arteriovenous anastomoses), cessation of smoking, and hydration all act to increase oxygen delivery at the cellular level within the injured tissue.

Ischemia–Reperfusion Injury and Wound Healing

Most problem wounds are characterized by episodes of chronic episodic ischemia followed by reperfusion. The detrimental effects of the release of free radicals has been documented in other organ systems, such as the heart, but has not been as well appreciated in the pathogenesis of problem wounds. Reperfusion

TABLE 3.2

CONDITIONS THAT CONTRIBUTE TO IMPAIRMENTS IN WOUND HEALING

Age
Ischemia
Reperfusion injury
Infection or bacterial burden
Malnutrition
    Global
    Nutrient-specific
Foreign bodies
Diabetes
Steroids
Uremia
Jaundice
Cancer
Genetic causes (e.g., Ehlers-Danlos, Werner syndromes)
Irradiation
Chemotherapy
Tobacco use
Alcohol use
Edema
Pressure

damage is particularly prevalent in lower-extremity wounds, where walking and standing can lead to localized ischemia in pressure-bearing areas in diabetic feet, or can increase edema in patients with venous stasis. The relief of pressure from resting or foot elevation can lead to the resumption of flow and the onset of reperfusion injury. This cycle can occur multiple times each day, and over the span of several days can result in extensive cellular damage and an inflammatory milieu from which wounds cannot recover. Similar cycles of ischemia–reperfusion may also occur in patients with pressure sores, as they shift about in bed.

Modalities such as total contact casting and compression therapy with elevation of the affected extremity minimize these repetitive traumatic events and ameliorate one potent cause of wound damage.

Bacteria and Wound Healing

All wounds are contaminated; however, the presence of excessive numbers of bacteria will interfere with wound healing. A quantitative culture of 10^5 bacteria per gram of tissue is usually diagnostic of an infection. However, this tool is rarely used because few microbiology laboratories perform this test reliably. Furthermore, the value of 10^5 is relative and not universally applicable. Certain bacterial species such as β-hemolytic streptococci can establish an infection at lower densities. The presence of diabetes or ischemia will lower the threshold needed to establish a true infection to an unknown extent. Likewise, the presence of a foreign body will lower the counts needed to establish a true infection by a factor of 10^3.

An important mechanism by which tissue hypoxia predisposes wounds to infection is by impairing the "oxidative burst" essential to micro-organismal killing by leukocytes. This enormously elevated production of oxygen-derived radicals is a self-regulated process that is important in clearing the wound of bacteria. Interestingly, this process of radical production, which is normally limited to the early stages of wound repair, can be aberrantly prolonged in the setting of constant infection or inflammation as persistent bacterial colonization sets

up a cycle of continuous free radical release (Fig. 3.1). This can result in bystander damage to the body's normal cells, and in many cases characterizes the microenvironment of the indolent wound.

Bacteria exert their adverse effects on healing in several ways. They set up an environment of free radicals, of secreted toxins, and of proteases. These enzymes degrade growth factors, prevent the ordered assembly of matrix constituents, and result in the manufacture of the proteinaceous debris that will constitute the pseudoeschar. As importantly, they place a strain on the wound that the host may not be able to overcome. *Bioburden* represents the metabolic demands placed on the healing wound by bacteria, and is in part the sum of the by-products produced by bacteria, the competitive exhaustion of nutrients and oxygen by bacteria, and the toxic proteases and reactive oxygen species generated by the inflammatory cells of the host defense. The level of the wound bioburden is stratified. Wounds may be *contaminated* (bacteria present without proliferation), *colonized* (bacteria present and multiplying without an overt host reaction), *critically colonized* (the point where host resistance is beginning to be overcome by the bacteria), or *infected* (expanding bacterial numbers with a host reaction). These definitions permit a prognosis for the wound to be made and proper therapy to be undertaken. Wound cleansers are useful in decreasing bacterial counts in colonized and contaminated wounds. Surface irrigation with saline and these cleansers may be all that is needed for contaminated wounds, whereas surgical debridement is essential for infected wounds.

Antibiotics are unnecessary for most wounds. However, there are settings where they are helpful. For example, many venous stasis ulcers develop a cellulitis that is difficult to control without antibiotic therapy. Critical colonization of a wound or infection is often heralded by stasis in the progression of a wound that was previously healing. In fact, if the rate of healing decreases in any wound, it should be considered infected until proven otherwise. Increased pain is another indication of infection. Another sign of infection is the appearance straw-colored "oozing" from the skin; this is actually likely evidence of an underlying *Staphylococcus* cellulitis or lymphangitis. Any patient with significant lymphedema and an open wound should be considered for antibiotic therapy. Antibiotics should also be used in contaminated wounds (oral flora, animal bites), as well as in patients with mechanical implants. However, it must be recognized that systemic antibiotics are only delivered to perfused tissues; consequently, topical antibiotics and/or removal of bioburden by cleansing play a critical role.

ADJUNCTS TO WOUND TREATMENT

Debridement

Debridement prepares the wound for healing by reducing the bioburden. Without an adequate debridement, a wound is persistently exposed to cytotoxic stressors and competes with bacteria for scarce resources such as oxygen and nutrients. As mentioned previously, this step is crucial, as most problematic wounds afflict aged patients and occur in the setting of ischemia. Although nonsurgeons and wound-product manufacturers have rediscovered the importance of debridement in the care of both acute and chronic wounds, many surgeons underappreciate the importance of adequate debridement. That many surgeons still allow wounds to heal under a "biologic dressing" or eschar suggests an underappreciation of the deleterious side effects that occur during the process of eschar formation.

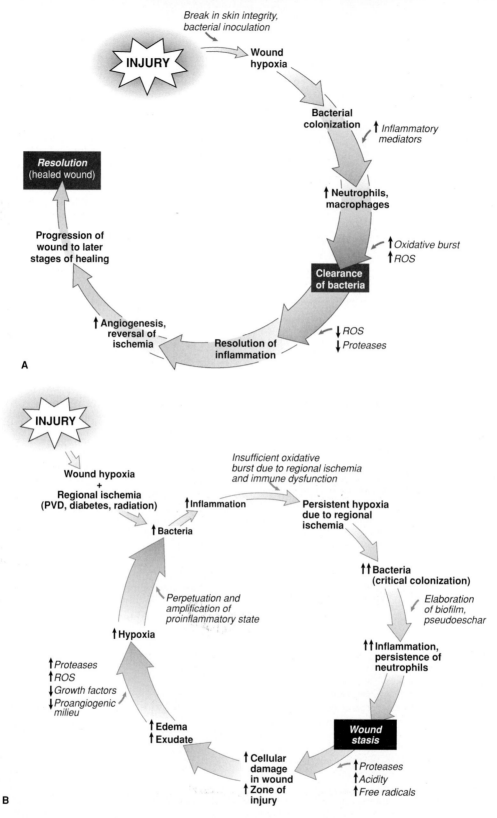

FIGURE 3.1. The normal inflammatory cascade of wound healing (**A**) in a healthy patient. In the limb or body area with normal perfusion there is an early neutrophil-derived burst of reactive oxygen species *(ROS)* that help clear bacteria. Because the bacterial numbers subsequently decline, this oxidative burst is self-limited, minimizing bystander cellular damage. The wound exits the inflammatory phase of healing, permitting angiogenesis with resolution of wound hypoxia, and the wound progresses to the latter stages of healing. In the setting of regional ischemia (**B**), bacteria are not efficiently cleared, partly because of an ineffective oxidative burst (which requires oxygen). Bacteria multiply until a level of critical colonization is reached. In the absence of an adequate debridement and therapy, bacteria continue to accumulate in a biofilm, resulting in an amplified and/or prolonged inflammatory response with wound stasis. The persistent inflammatory response and cellular damage will eventually result in the vicious cycle depicted. PVD, peripheral vascular disease.

An eschar begins as a *pseudoeschar* or *slough*, which is essentially a provisional matrix formed from exudated serum components at the wound–air interface. If allowed to dry, the gelatinous composition of the pseudoeschar will harden to form the true eschar, or scab. While most practitioners recognize the importance of debridement of grossly nonviable or foreign material, the role that a pseudoeschar may play in prolonging the inflammatory stage of wound healing, and hence setting the wound up for persistent bacterial colonization, is not fully appreciated. The proteinaceous components of the pseudoeschar are a meal for bacteria; hence pseudoeschar should be debrided when it accumulates. This layer can be quite tenacious because proteins are "sticky" and the biofilm generated by bacteria (comprised of complex carbohydrates) is also sticky and not degraded by most proteases. An effective way to do this as the wound heals is through the proper use of dressings and debriding agents, as detailed below.

Debridement is typically considered to be surgical, but it may also be enzymatic, mechanical, or autolytic (occurring through the action of leukocytes). Enzymatic and proautolytic agents prevent the crosslinking of exudated components and impede the bacteria-sequestering pseudoeschar and biofilms from forming. Some dressings (notably hydrocolloid dressings) have the advantageous ability to rehydrate partially dehydrated and hardened scab tissue, which are then phagocytosed by wound leukocytes. A particularly useful mechanical debrider is the pressurized water jet (VersaJet, Smith & Nephew, Largo, FL), which has the ability to penetrate into microcrevasses in the wound bed to flush out entrapped particulate matter as well as bacteria. A Waterpik (Waterpik Technologies, Fort Collins, CO), or even a handheld shower spray, is a low-tech device that patients can use at home. Similarly, a syringe with a 20-gauge needle will generate the 15 psi necessary to lower bacteria counts in tissue.

Another means of achieving wound debridement is through the use of maggot therapy, which can be remarkably efficacious in removing devitalized material while sparing viable, well-perfused tissue. Some centers use this form of biologic debridement extensively.

Negative-Pressure Wound Therapy

Negative-pressure wound therapy (NPWT), or vacuum-assisted wound closure, has been a tremendous advance for the wound-care practitioner. It consists of the use of a porous sponge within the wound, covered by an airtight occlusive dressing, to which a vacuum is applied. This modality has many uses, but should perhaps best be thought of as an adjunct to assist in surgical closure of a problem wound. It can certainly be used to completely heal a wound, but this use is expensive, time-consuming, and not always effective. A more practical use is to expeditiously prepare a wound bed for surgical closure by tertiary intent.

NPWT works through a combination of mechanisms. One important action is relief of edema. The process of inflammation from healing and from immunologic-mediated mechanisms releases a series of chemical mediators that dilate blood vessels and open up junctions between endothelial cells, enabling the efflux of fluid into the perivascular space. Furthermore, injured vessels and lymphatics have a tendency to continue to leak blood and fluid. NPWT removes this pericellular transudate and wound exudate, thereby improving interstitial diffusion of oxygen to cells.

NPWT also removes deleterious enzymes from the wound. Many chronic wounds are characterized by the presence of collagenases and matrix metalloproteinases (MMPs) and other proteases related to inflammatory cells, as well as bacterially derived proteases, which serve to degrade nascent matrix proteins and growth factors. By removing the wound fluid and bacteria that inhibit wound healing, NPWT modifies the wound microenvironment toward one more conducive to healing. In addition, the cyclic compression and relaxation of the wound tissue likely stimulates mechanotransductive pathways that result in increased growth factor release, matrix production, and cellular proliferation.

NPWT needs to be carefully and properly used. The sponge should not be placed on normal skin, or in areas sensitive to pressure and ischemia. The suction port should be tunneled away from the wound and connected by an umbilicus of foam in wounds that have marginally adequate perfusion. The pressure is extremely important. Whereas most wounds will heal optimally with a pressure of 125 mm Hg, other wounds may only tolerate a setting of 75 mm Hg before capillary flow is occluded.

Clinical situations amenable to NPWT include lymphatic leaks, venous stasis ulcers, diabetic wounds, and wounds with fistulae. NPWT has also greatly assisted the plastic surgeon in managing sternal wounds, orthopedic wounds, and abdominal wounds. By reliably encouraging the growth of granulation tissue, NPWT permits these wounds to be managed in a nonemergent fashion and allows for medical stabilization and optimization of these patients. In some instances, it has enabled avoidance of free flaps, thereby assuring a place in the reconstructive ladder of the plastic surgeon. Other advances, such as the instillation of antimicrobials into the sponge and the development of NPWT for home use have continued to broaden the usefulness of this modality even further. NPWT can also be used to assist the neovascularization of skin grafts and tissue engineered skin substitutes.

There are several contraindications to the use of NPWT, including the presence of a malignancy, use on wounds characterized by ischemia, and inadequately debrided or badly infected wounds. There are reports of extension of the zone of necrosis when used on ischemic wounds; for this reason, these patients should be revascularized prior to application of NPWT.

Hyperbaric Oxygen

The use of hyperbaric oxygen (HBO) (typically, 100% O_2 saturation at 2 to 3 ATA) raises the dissolved oxygen saturation in plasma from 0.3% to nearly 7%. This rise in oxygen increases the interstitial diffusion distance of oxygen four- to fivefold. The initial enthusiasm for HBO led to indiscriminate and unscientific use of HBO for unjustified indications. This led to a significant controversy with a predictable backlash on the part of referring physicians, surgeons, and third-party payers. However, it is now clear that an appreciation of the wound microenvironment, with a focus on the microcirculation, can direct the proper use of this oftentimes valuable modality. The broadening use of transcutaneous oximetry has permitted evaluation of patients that will likely benefit from HBO. Broadly speaking, if the periwound area/extremity demonstrates a rise in $tcPO_2$ when the patient inspires supplemental oxygen, the patient is likely to benefit from HBO. This diagnostic maneuver eliminates the two groups of patients that will not benefit from HBO: those with a normal environmental perfusion, and those with ischemic limbs who need a bypass to restore blood flow to a limb. Occasionally, HBO may be used as a means of limb salvage in a patient with an ischemic wound who is not a candidate for a surgical or endovascular procedure. It must be recognized that there are still a paucity of prospective randomized studies that support its use and the duration and frequency of treatment remains empiric. More recently, there has been some interest in regional oxygen therapy to the wound itself, with even less supporting evidence.

Growth Factors

The first growth factor approved by the FDA in the United States is platelet-derived growth factor (PDGF), marketed under the name becaplermin (Regranex). It is approved for the treatment of diabetic foot ulcers. It has been widely used "off-label" for the treatment of a variety of other wound types, such as irradiated wounds and in aged patients. It appears to be effective only in the context of a well-prepared wound bed, which is logical, as an infected bed filled with proteases will rapidly degrade this peptide growth factor. Other growth factors, including vascular endothelial growth factor (VEGF), are currently in clinical trials.

Enzymes

The rationale for using enzymatic debriding agents is that they will selectively digest necrotic, devitalized tissue and prevent slough and eschar from accumulating. These agents include such products as papain with urea, and are general proteases useful for breaking up developing proto-eschars and accumulated biofilms characteristic of many open wounds. Their use is sometimes associated with pain, which may limit their use. Another enzyme widely used is collagenase. These products are not substitutes for mechanical debridement; however, when properly used, they are less traumatic to healthy tissue than surgical debridement.

Dressings

The types of dressings can be broadly divided into films, composites, hydrogels, hydrocolloids, alginates, foam, and other absorptive dressings, including NPWT. Within these categories of dressings, there are few, if any, prospective, randomized clinical trials that definitively prove the superiority of one type of wound dressing over the other, emphasizing the need for further research in this area. There is a dizzying array of choices currently available, and to add to the confusion many indications for the use of dressings are promoted by industry. The choice of one over another is best made by considering wound characteristics and treatment goals (Table 3.3). The goal in clean wounds that are to be closed primarily or are granulating well is to provide a moist healing environment to facilitate cell migration and prevent desiccation of the wound. Consequently, films can be used for incisions, and hydrogels or hydrocolloids can be used for open wounds. The amount and type of exudate that is present in the wound will direct the dressing used in wounds that have some degree of bacterial colonization. In general, hydrogels, films, and composite dressings are best for wounds with light amounts of exudates; hydrocolloids are used for wounds with moderate quantities; and alginates, foams, and NPWT are best used for wounds with heavier volumes of exudate. NPWT is also useful for wounds with heavy amounts of lymph as a consequence of a leak, as well as for fistulae. Wounds with large volumes of necrotic material should not be treated with a dressing until a surgical debridement has been performed.

Gauze

Gauze dressings suffer the burden of being the traditional first choice for the generic care of wounds. The realization that the practice of moist to dry dressings for wound care is actually traumatic and proinflammatory has led to a decline in the use of these dressings in the arena of wound care. In addition, the costs associated with these dressings, particularly in personnel expenses, are high compared with modern dressings that need to be changed less frequently. These are often painful to remove, and are nonselective debriders that cause significant bystander damage to healthy tissue. Furthermore, many of them leave behind fine microfibers that can act as irritants and as foci of a source of infection. However, the material expense of these dressings is very low, and they may be purchased in any drugstore. They are excellent as surgical bandages and can be used in small, noncomplicated wounds or as secondary dressings. They may also be purchased impregnated with petrolatum, iodinated compounds, or other materials useful for keeping the wound bed moist. It should be noted that most dressings have been approved by the FDA as "substantially equivalent" to gauze in their efficacy. There is no definitive evidence that other dressings will heal a wound faster than moist gauze, although they have other advantages, which are discussed below.

Semiocclusive Dressings

These are sheets that are impermeable to fluids but permit the passage of small gas molecules. They are typically used in combination with gauze or other dressings, and act to maintain the moisture content of clean wounds. Semiocclusive dressings are commonly used to cover and protect freshly closed incisions and skin graft donor sites, and likely enhance epithelialization when used this way. They should not be used in wounds known to be significantly contaminated, and should be cautiously used in patients with fragile skin prone to tearing.

Hydrogel Dressings

Hydrogel dressings are particularly useful in maintaining a moist wound bed and rehydrating wounds to facilitate healing as well as autolytic debridement. Thus, they are useful in wounds with small amounts of eschar or that are predisposed to dessication. Their usefulness is achieved by their intrinsic moisture content and hydrophilic nature. They are usually composed of complex polysaccharides (e.g., starch). Unlike alginates and hydrocolloids, they are not dependent on wound secretions to maintain a moist wound microenvironment. Yet, like these other dressings, they can absorb moderate amounts of fluid from the wound. An additional benefit is that they can be used in infected wounds. They are nonadhesive, and therefore cause minimal pain with dressing changes. Because they do not adhere well to the wound or skin, they usually require a secondary dressing.

Hydrocolloids

Typically, these are pastes, powders, or sheets that are placed within the wound and covered with a dressing (in the case of pastes or powders) to form an occlusive barrier that gels as it absorbs mild amounts of exudates. Hydrocolloids consist of gel-forming agents (typically gelatin, carboxymethylcellulose, or pectin) that are impermeable to gases and liquids. They may be left on the wound for 3 to 5 days; during this time, they provide a moist environment that promotes cell migration and wound debridement by autolysis. However, because of their occlusive nature, hydrocolloids are not to be used in the presence of wounds that are heavily colonized with bacteria, particularly anaerobic strains. These are not highly absorbent, and hence should not be used for highly exudative wounds.

Foam Dressings

Foam dressings are made of nonadhering polyurethane, which is hydrophobic, and an occlusive cover. The polyurethane is highly absorptive and acts as a wick for wound fluids, making foam dressings useful in highly exudative wounds. However, because of their high wicking ability, they are not to be used on nonexudating or minimally exudating wounds.

TABLE 3.3

TYPES OF DRESSINGS, THEIR CHARACTERISTICS AND APPLICATIONS

Dressing material	Absorption level	Adhesive quality	Conformability (Surface vs. cavity)	Hydration/ debridement ability	Odor control ability	Clinical application
Films	None	Fully adhesive surface	Conformable to surface anatomy	Will hydrate slowly	None	Superficial, lightly exuding wounds, as a secondary dressing
Hydrogel sheets	Low	Nonadhesive or adhesive borders	Conformable to surface anatomy	Will hydrate moderately	None	Superficial, light to moderately exuding wounds, painful wounds
Amorphous gels	Low to moderate	Non-adhesive	Conformable to cavities	Will hydrate quickly	None	Superficial to deep, light to moderately exuding wounds
Hydrocolloids	Low to moderate	Fully adhesive surface, may be aggressive	Conformable to surface anatomy	Will hydrate moderately to quickly depending on water content	May exacerbate odor (without ill effect)	Superficial, light to moderately exuding wounds
Foams	High	Nonadhesive, fully adhesive surface, adhesive borders	Some versions conformable to cavities	Not hydrating	Slight because of absorption; some versions contain charcoal for active control	Superficial to deep, moderately to heavily exuding wounds
Alginates	High	Nonadhesive	Conformable to cavities	Not hydrating	Anecdotal evidence for minor effect; charcoal version exists	Superficial to deep, moderately to highly exuding wounds
Collagen	Moderate to high	Nonadhesive	Conformable to cavities	Not hydrating	None	Superficial to deep, light to moderately exuding wounds
Contact layers	None	Nonadhesive	Conformable to surface anatomy	Slightly hydrating, depending on cover dressings	None	Superficial wounds of any exudates level

From Ovington LG. Wound dressings: their evolution and use. In: Falanga V, ed. *Cutaneous Wound Healing*. London, UK: Martin Dunitz; 2001:221–232, with permission.

Alginates

Alginates (derived from brown seaweed) are particularly useful in wounds characterized by significant amounts of exudate. Their use permits the desired removal of exudated fluids from the wound environment and yet frees the practitioner from the burden of daily or multiple dressing changes per day. These products are not to be used in nonexudative wounds, as they can dry out the wound bed. They come in several forms, including a rope/ribbon form that is useful for packing wounds with deep pockets. These dressings can absorb approximately 20 times their dry weight in fluid. They should be covered with a semiocclusive dressing. If the practitioner desires to use these alginate dressings on dry wounds, they should be hydrated with sterile saline prior to being placed on the wound to maintain wound moisture and permit epithelialization and autolysis. A particularly useful alginate dressing is manufactured impregnated with silver.

Antimicrobials

Antimicrobial dressings are a generic term for a dressing that contains an antimicrobial agent. The most beneficial agent appears to be silver. Silver is ionized in the moist environment of the wound, and it is the silver ion that has biologic activity. This agent has a broad spectrum of microbicidal activity with low toxicity to human cells. It is further advantageous in that its tri-pronged mechanism of activity (cell membrane permeabilizer, inhibitor of cellular respiration, and nucleic acid denaturer) means that it is active against a broad range of micro-organisms in addition to bacteria, and also maintains activity against vancomycin-resistant *Enterococcus* (VRE) and methicillin-resistant *Staphylococcus aureus* (MRSA). These dressings fill a true need; although it is axiomatic that surgical debridement is the best way to decrease the bioburden of a wound, wounds are rapidly colonized following a seemingly sterile debridement. Furthermore, for certain types of ulcers characterized by an impaired blood supply (ischemic, irradiated wounds) these dressings can be useful as a wound treatment and as a temporizing measure while the patient is optimized for definitive surgical therapy. Cadexomer iodine is another antimicrobial agent and is a slow-release form of iodine formulated to achieve consistently bactericidal levels within the wound bed without the wound cell-damaging effects seen with the use of Povidine-iodine products. Other antimicrobials include silver sulfadiazine, mupirocin, and topical antibiotics, including neomycin, gentamicin, metronidazole, and bacitracin ointments and creams.

Skin Substitutes or Human Tissue Equivalents

These are among the first tissue-engineered products applied to clinical use. Besides providing wound coverage, some of these products contain living cells that are cellular factories, secreting a broad panoply of growth factors and other bioactive molecules that assist in healing. A downside is their expense. They need to be applied to meticulously clean wounds with adequate vascularity and the site needs to be immobilized to prevent shearing and graft loss. Representative products include cultured autologous keratinocyte sheets (Epicel, Genzyme Corporation, Cambridge, MA); dermal constructs such as Biobrane (Mylan Laboratories, Canonsburg, PA), Oasis (Cook Biotech, West Lafayette, IN), AlloDerm (LifeCell Corp, Branchburg, NJ), Integra (Integra Life Sciences Corp, Plainsboro, NJ), TransCyte (Smith & Nephew, Largo FL), and Dermagraft (Smith & Nephew, Largo FL); and bilayered tissue engineered constructs consisting of keratinocytes and fibroblasts such as OrCel (Ortec International, New York, NY) and Apligraf (Organogenesis, Canton, MA). The indications for their use are highly patient and center specific. We are impressed with Integra, as it is especially useful for sites prone to contracture (neck, axillae) and to replenish contour in burn wounds and donor sites. In addition, it can enable coverage of tendons, bone, and surgical hardware, and in select situations can obviate the need for more complex wound closures, such as flaps.

Scar Therapy

The use of silicone sheets improves the appearance of scars. This is likely a result of the increased moisture and slightly increased warmth provided by the continuous application of the silicone sheet, as this increases slightly the rate of collagenolysis. Other useful tools include steroids and pressure garments. Calcium channel blockers are used, but they are unproven, as are topical formulations of salicylic acid, an anti-inflammatory, although the theoretical basis underlying the use of this agent appears sound.

Clinical Wound Care of Uncomplicated Wounds

The rate of healing following elective operations with clean incisions is a direct reflection of the kinetics of collagen deposition and remodeling within the wound. Classic experiments in humans and in preclinical models demonstrated that approximately 30% to 50% of the final strength of a wound is achieved in 42 days. It is for this reason that elective surgery patients are told to refrain from strenuous activity or heavy lifting for at least 6 weeks. This curve, representing the expected course of healing, is shifted to the right in patients with underlying comorbidities, including renal failure, ischemia, and steroid use (Fig. 3.2). Therefore, in patients with wound-healing abnormalities, postoperative instructions should be adjusted to reflect the anticipated delay in healing. Note that in healthy patients, no pharmacologic agent has been demonstrated to shift the curve to the left; that is, healing rates are for most purposes maximized in healthy people, particularly in incisions closed primarily. However, it still may be possible to modify the *quality* of the healing, and research on scar modulation and manipulation is currently an area of significant future promise.

Clinical Wound Care of Problem Wounds

Timing

In an ideal world, problem wounds would be seen by a wound care specialist as soon as possible. Unfortunately, in practice it is difficult to identify the incipient problem wound. Furthermore, not all problem wounds are actually *chronic* wounds. The development of biomarkers for wounds that will not heal is of tremendous importance, and is an area of promising research. This has practical importance, as many third-party reimbursement agents will not cover specialized care of wounds unless they have been present for a defined period of time. The standard definition of a chronic wound is one that has been present for 3 months but such a definition is seized upon by insurance carriers to deny specialized care to impaired wounds. Unfortunately, this condemns the patient to months of unnecessary waiting, morbidity, and time away from work, and may even worsen outcomes in cases of threatened limb loss. It is, therefore, perhaps time to redirect the conceptualization of a problem wound to de-emphasize chronicity and re-emphasize its fall off the trajectory of expected healing. The majority of problem wounds seem to share the traits of advanced age, infection, and ischemia with reperfusion injury, as described above. Some unique traits are detailed below.

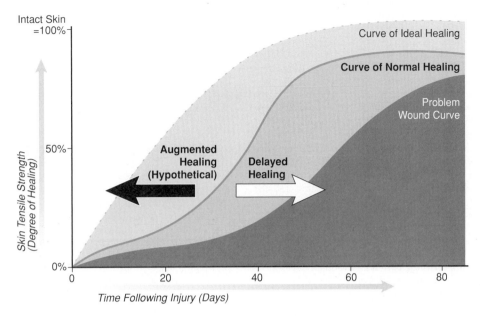

FIGURE 3.2. The healing trajectories of a normal wound, a problem wound, and a hypothetical ideal wound are depicted. Most normal wounds heal with a slight lag phase, an exponential phase of active gain in tensile strength with active matrix deposition, and a protracted resolution phase. This wound heals with a scar that does not achieve the strength of normal unwounded skin. The curve on the right represents a "typical" problem wound curve. The exact shape of the curve varies among different patients, and vagaries are to be expected in the duration of the lag phases, the slope of the active-healing phase, and likely in the ultimate percent of tensile strength achieved. Ideally, all wounds would heal according to the kinetics of the hypothetical curve on the left, where there is a minimal lag phase and an expeditious gain of tensile strength and regeneration of normal skin with ultimate tensile strength similar to that of unwounded skin.

Wound Care in Patients with Irradiated Skin or Steroids. Patients who are on steroids should receive vitamin A (25,000 IU daily by mouth or 200,000 IU topically t.i.d.), as experimental models of steroid-impaired healing have shown this vitamin to be useful. Wounds in patients receiving steroids are prone to infection, and show decreased rates of angiogenesis, collagen deposition, and cellular proliferation. It is important to remember that steroids may impair healing even long after their use is discontinued. Maintenance of a clean wound with minimal bacterial colonization should be the main goal of care for these wounds.

Irradiated wounds present a challenging problem. The progressive endarteritis obliterans and microvascular damage, along with fibrotic interstitial changes, results in a wound marked by ischemia, hampered by cellular senescence, and prone to infection. These wounds need to be gingerly debrided, as further surgical injury often results simply in a larger nonhealing wound. The use of antimicrobial dressings, capable of maintaining moist wound healing while promoting autolysis, is ideal for these wounds, as is the use of growth factors and even hyperbaric oxygen therapy. These wounds will often need a microvascular free flap to attain stable wound coverage.

Wound Care in Patients with Pressure Sores. Patients with pressure sores are often debilitated. This is not necessarily a contraindication to surgery, as clinical experience shows that most cachectic, chronically malnourished patients are capable of successful healing. However, patients who have recently shown an *acute* episode of weight loss or malnourishment are more likely to have problems with wound repair; these patients are the subset that should be aggressively nourished and receive vitamin supplementation. Consideration should be given to the administration of growth hormone or anabolic steroids, such as oxandrolone, as this steroid counteracts the catabolic state

of these patients. The pressure sore needs to be debrided as thoroughly as possible. Given the debilitated state of these patients, debridements are often performed "at the bedside" in a less-than-thorough manner. A formal debridement should ideally be done, with multiple return visits to the operating room as needed. A frustrating aspect of the care of these patients is the high rate of ulcer recurrence.

Spasm should be controlled, either medically or, in extreme cases, surgically. Dressings are used strategically. Because the priority in stage 1 and stage 2 ulcers is to maintain a moist, clean environment, film dressings are appropriate. More absorptive dressings (hydrocolloids, alginates, or foams) are used for stages 2 through 4 ulcers, depending on the level of wound drainage, and should be covered with a film dressing to prevent desiccation and to exclude soilage.

A tremendous advance has been the evolution of support surface therapies. These are pressure-reducing (reduction of pressure at the ulcer site to a level less than that exerted by a regular surface) and pressure-relieving devices (relief of pressure to a level less than the capillary closing pressure). These devices include air-fluidized beds, air mattresses, air flotation and water flotation devices, and low air-loss beds. The variables they control, in addition to pressure, include moisture retention, shear forces, and temperature. A drawback is their expense, which can be formidable.

Wound Care in Patients with Diabetes. The foundation of care in the patient with diabetes is recognition that most of the ulcers seen are actually pressure sores that have occurred in a setting of neuropathy. The neuropathic ulcer is a multietiologic lesion, with components of pressure necrosis, functional microangiopathy, and true neuropathic derangements. We prefer the term "functional microangiopathy" because although diabetics do not have anatomic abnormalities in their arterioles and capillaries (hence the fallacy of *diabetic small-vessel* *disease*), they nevertheless do have a dysfunctional microvasculature, with impairments in vasodilatation and compensatory angiogenesis in response to ischemia. The treatment of the diabetic foot is tailored to address these varied components. Selective debridement, control of glucose levels, pressure offloading (either through noncontact orthotics or surgically in the case of Charcot feet, or with the use of an Achilles tendon lengthening procedure), revascularization when there is a significant arterial lesion, use of growth factors such as becaplermin (Regranex), and, in certain instances, tibial nerve decompression, are all modalities that should be considered to maximize healing rates. Given the varied treatments and derangements found in the so-called diabetic foot, these patients are best served by care in a dedicated multidisciplinary wound/limb salvage clinic.

Wound Care in Patients with Venous Stasis Ulcers. Compression therapy is essential for venous stasis ulcers. This is as true for patients who have undergone vascular surgery as for those who have not. More sophisticated and individualized compression garments for these patients have been developed. A caveat to the use of compression therapy is that this modality is contraindicated in patients with an ABI <0.7 and should be used under close medical supervision in extremities with an ABI between 0.7 and 0.9.

Rigid compression products include Unna boot-paste dressings and low-stretch bandages. Elastic compression dressings are more applicable for nonambulatory patients, as they have a higher resting pressure than rigid products. Types of compression products include stockings, elastic wraps, and multilayer wraps. Use of combination dressings incorporating an elastic component and an absorptive minimally stretching component have achieved widespread acceptance as superior to the traditional Unna boot, which does not achieve optimal pressure by itself, although it can be quite useful when combined with an elastic compression dressing.

These garments are individualized to the patient. Although ideally the pressures exerted should be between 30 and 40 mm Hg, there are situations when more or less pressure can be used. The rationale for this level of pressure is experimental evidence showing that venous stasis ulceration is greatly increased when the ambulatory venous pressure rises above 30 mm Hg. Care should be taken not to exceed the pressure recommended for the clinical indication, as ulceration may result. A key to the use of compression therapy is the commitment on the part of the patient that she may need multiple changes and resizing to accommodate the changes in limb girth as treatment progresses. Compression therapy should be continued for several weeks following successful closure of the wound to permit remodeling and strengthening of the neomatrix.

Compression therapy is often supplemented by the use of dressings. The choice of dressing is again dictated by the amount of drainage present. Because many compression products are worn for days at a time, the dressing chosen must be capable of absorbing the high levels of exudate and transudate produced by these types of wounds. When the edema is controlled, closure is often expedited by the use of tissue-engineered skin substitutes.

The indication for vascular surgical intervention remains superficial venous insufficiency with insufficiency of the perforating system. All patients with venous stasis ulcers resistant to compression therapy merit vascular studies to determine suitability for these interventions. The use of subfascial endoscopic perforator surgery is under intensive study in association with more traditional vascular approaches such as vein stripping.

FUTURE MODALITIES

It may be possible in the future to augment healing in elderly, diabetic, or irradiated patients with the use of autologous stem cells. Even more exciting is the potential manipulation of the healing response to direct the wound "program" less toward rapid healing with an amorphous scar, and more toward the recapitulation of developmental programs that will result in true regeneration. The directed and precisely manipulated growth of appendages such as sebaceous glands and follicles, and the precise modulation of melanocytes, could potentially result in imperceptible scars.

CONCLUSION

Intensive research into the pathophysiology of chronic wounds and exciting advances in stem cells and regenerative medicine will undoubtedly be translated into novel, exciting treatment approaches for wound care. However, much of the use of wound care products has been market and industry driven. Neutral, unbiased evaluations of these products, ideally with prospective, randomized studies, are urgently needed. The concept of wound care centers has been aggressively marketed, and if properly directed, can be a benefit to patient care. However, the potential for conflicts of interest exists, in that many are company organized and are biased in their treatment options. The ideal wound care center is multidisciplinary with the participation of interested surgeons. A movement by organized nursing societies into autonomous patient management is being aggressively played out in the arena of wound care. The overall benefit for patients with problem wounds, particularly those wounds that require a surgical intervention, remains to be determined.

Suggested Readings

Falanga V, ed. *Cutaneous Wound Healing*. London: Martin Dunitz; 2001.

Hess CT, ed. *Clinical Guide: Wound Care*. Philadelphia: Lippincott Williams & Wilkins; 2005.

Hunt TK, Hopf HW. Wound healing and wound infection. What surgeons and anesthesiologists can do. *Surg Clin North Am*. 1997;77:587.

Mustoe T. Understanding chronic wounds: a unifying hypothesis on their pathogenesis and implications for therapy. *Am J Surg*. 2004;187:65S.

Robson MC, Steed DL, Franz MG. Wound healing: biologic features and approaches to maximize healing trajectories. *Curr Probl Surg*. 2001;38:72.

CHAPTER 4 ■ THE BLOOD SUPPLY OF THE SKIN

G. IAN TAYLOR

Knowledge of the cutaneous arteries and veins is fundamental to the design of skin flaps and incisions. Although detailed studies of these vessels were performed by such anatomists as Manchot in 1889 (1), Spalteholz in 1893 (2), and Salmon in 1936 (3), they were published in either German, Italian, or French. The English-speaking world paid little attention to the anatomy of the cutaneous vessels so that surgeons designed skin flaps randomly on whatever vessels happened to be in the area (random flaps), citing the necessity for rigid length-to-breadth ratios. It was not until the last four decades that interest reawakened to the intricacies of the vascular pathways to and from the skin. It is ironic that the description of muscle flaps and fascial flaps distracted surgeons from the organ they were trying to keep alive—the skin!

There has been a bewildering explosion of terms and attempts to classify the cutaneous circulation, often based on flap design rather than vascular anatomy. It is worth stating, however, that many of the "new" flaps—whether island, fascial, neurocutaneous, direct, indirect, axial, random, super, septal, arterial, musculocutaneous, perforator, or otherwise—are essentially the same flaps, just viewed through different eyes. Converse stated that "the anatomical vascular basis of the flap provides the most accurate approach for classification." Time has supported the veracity of this statement.

OVERVIEW

The skin is the largest organ of the body. Temperature regulation to maintain homeostasis is one of its major roles. This important function is provided by a rich network of cutaneous arteries and veins, especially in the dermal and subdermal plexus, which supply the sweat glands and allow for heat exchange by convection, conduction, and radiation. Although the cutaneous circulation is rich and vast, the metabolic demands of the skin elements are low so that only a small fraction of the potential cutaneous circulation is necessary for skin viability, a fact that is pertinent to the design and survival of various skin flaps.

The *cutaneous arteries* arise *directly* from the underlying source arteries, or *indirectly* from branches of those source arteries to the deep tissues, especially the muscles (Fig. 4.1). From here the cutaneous arteries follow the connective tissue framework of the deep tissues, either between or within the muscles, and course for a variable distance beneath the outer layer of the enveloping "body suit" of deep fascia. They then pierce that structure, usually at fixed skin sites, as cutaneous perforators. After emerging from the deep fascia, the arteries course on its superficial surface for a variable distance, supplying branches to the fascia and the undersurface of the fat. They then worm their way between the lobules of the subcutaneous fat, ultimately reaching the subdermal plexus, where they again travel for variable distances to supply the overlying skin. During their subcutaneous course the cutaneous arteries (and veins) often travel with the cutaneous nerves, either as long channels or as a chain-linked system of vessels.

The density, size, and direction of the cutaneous perforators varies from region to region of the body, being modified by growth, differentiation, and the functional demands of the part, factors that provide the basis for the various anatomic concepts that follow. In general, the vessels of the head, neck, torso, and proximal limbs are larger and more widely spaced than their counterparts in the forearms, legs, hands, and feet (Fig. 4.1A). Although the size and length of the cutaneous perforators may vary, they all interconnect to form a three-dimensional "body carpet" that has a particularly well-developed horizontal strata of vessels in the dermis, in the subdermis, on the undersurface of the subcutaneous fat, and on the outer surface of the deep fascia.

The connection between adjacent cutaneous arteries is by either true anastomoses, without change in caliber, or by reduced-caliber choke anastomotic vessels (Fig. 4.2). The latter are plentiful in the integument (skin and subcutaneous tissues) and may be important in regulating the blood flow to the intact skin. These choke vessels play an important role in skin-flap survival, where, like resistors in an electrical circuit, they provide an initial resistance to blood flow between the base and the tip of the flap. **When a skin flap is delayed by the strategic division of cutaneous perforators along its length, these choke vessels dilate to the dimensions of true anastomoses (see later), thus enhancing the circulation to the distal flap.** Although some dilation of the choke vessels occurs because of the relaxation of sympathetic tone, the major effect is seen between 48 and 72 hours after surgery (4,5). This is due to an active process resulting in hypertrophy and hyperplasia of the elements of the vessel wall and an increase in diameter of its lumen.

The **cutaneous veins** also form a three-dimensional plexus of interconnecting channels with dominant strata in the subdermis (Figs. 4.3 to 4.5). Although many of these veins have valves that direct the blood in a particular direction, they are often connected by avalvular veins. These avalvular (oscillating) vessels allow bidirectional flow between adjacent venous territories whose valves may be oriented in opposite directions, thus providing for the equilibration of flow and pressure. Indeed, there are many veins whose valves direct flow initially in a distal direction, away from the heart, before joining veins whose flow is proximal. The superficial inferior epigastric veins that drain the lower abdominal integument toward the groin are good examples. In some regions, valved channels direct flow radially away from a plexus of avalvular veins as, for example, in the venous drainage from the vertex of the scalp or the nipple–areolar summit of the breast. In other areas valved channels direct flow toward a central focus, seen in the groin or in the stellate limbs of the cutaneous perforating veins (Fig. 4.3).

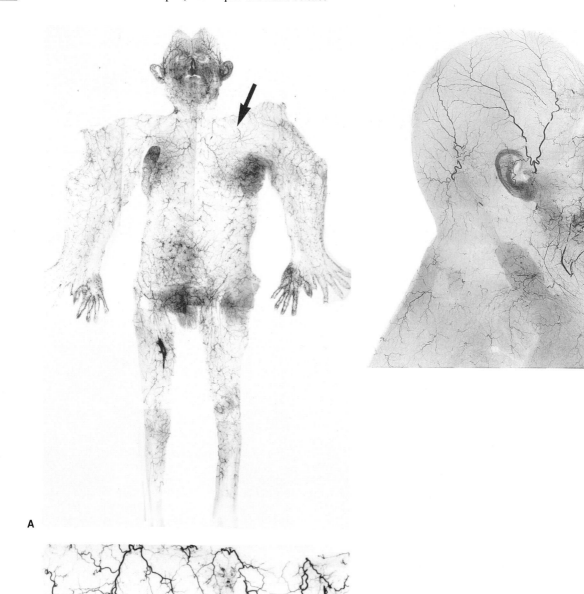

FIGURE 4.1. Cutaneous arteries. **A:** Montage of the cutaneous arteries of the body. The skin has been incised along the ulnar border in the upper extremities and the integument has been removed, with the deep fascia on the left side and without it on the right. **B:** A closer view of the vessels of the head and the neck from the side. Note (a) the direction, size, and density of the perforators, which are large on the torso and head and get progressively smaller and more numerous toward the periphery of the limbs, and (b) the reduced-caliber (choke) anastomotic arteries that link the perforators into a continuous network. **C:** Enlargement of the area depicted by the arrow in (A). (Reproduced with permission from Taylor GI, Palmer JH. The vascular territories (angiosomes) of the body: experimental study and clinical applications. *Br J Plast Surg.* 1987;40:113.)

In general the cutaneous veins accompany the arteries. However, the venous drainage of the skin is established in the embryo in two stages that overlap, but which are separated in time by approximately 1 week of development (Fig. 4.4). The primary system of veins develops first in the human embryo at about 5 weeks in the subectodermal region and is represented in the adult by large-caliber veins such as the cephalic, saphenous, and external jugular veins. These veins often course at some distance from the cutaneous arteries. Often they are accompanied by cutaneous nerves, and they travel for long distances before piercing the deep fascia (Fig. 4.4).

The secondary system of veins develops approximately 1 week later in the embryo. This network consists of central axial source veins that accompany the axial source arteries and receive perforating veins from the subectodermal region, which accompany the developing cutaneous arteries (Fig. 4.4). In the adult, they are represented by the venae comitantes of the cutaneous perforating arteries with which they travel in close proximity. Thus from the dermal and subdermal venous plexus, the veins collect into either a horizontal "freeway" of large-caliber veins, where they are often related to the cutaneous nerves and a longitudinal system of chain-linked arteries, or,

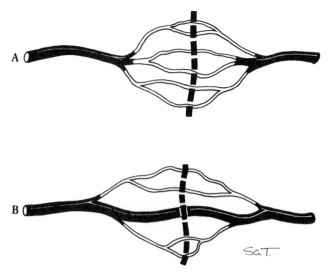

FIGURE 4.2. Choke vessels. **A:** Schematic of choke anastomoses (**A**) and true anastomoses (**B**) between adjacent arteries. (Reproduced with permission from Taylor GI, Minabe T. The angiosomes of the mammals and other vertebrates. *Plast Reconstr Surg.* 1992;89:181.)

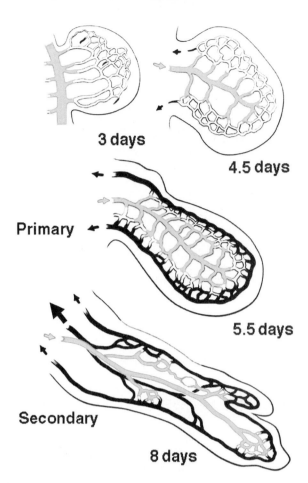

FIGURE 4.4. Diagram of developing arteries and veins in the forelimb of a quail embryo. Approximately 1 day in the quail equates to 1 week in the human embryo. Note the primary venous system, which develops first (independent of the arteries); it drains the ectoderm (later the dermis) and the deep tissues along the surface of the embryo. The secondary venous system develops centrally (along with the arteries), connects with the primary system, and drains areas of the ectoderm (dermis) radially and then axially along the limb.

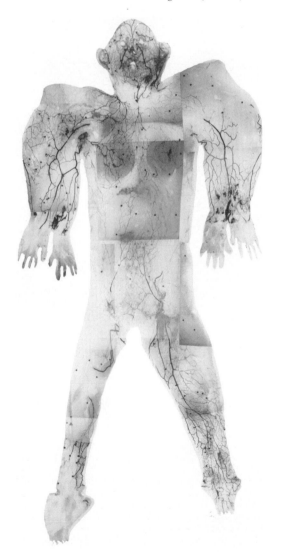

FIGURE 4.3. The venous network of the integument of a female subject. (Reproduced with permission from Taylor GI, Caddy CM, Watterson PA, et al. The venous territories (venosomes) of the human body: experimental study and clinical implications. *Plast Reconstr Surg.* 1990;86:185.)

alternatively, they collect in centripetal or stellate fashion into a common channel that passes vertically down in company with the cutaneous arteries to pierce the deep fascia (Fig. 4.5). These perforating veins remain in company with the direct and indirect cutaneous arteries, ultimately draining into the vena comitantes of the source arteries in the deep tissue. Thus, the skin is fed and drained by a continuous network of arteries and of veins formed by vessels whose size, shape, density, and direction vary from region to region in the body. The following observations provide for a better understanding of this variation in vessel anatomy.

ANATOMIC CONCEPTS

The Angiosome Concept

A review of the works of Manchot (1) and Salmon (3) combined with our own total-body studies of the blood supply to the skin and the underlying deep tissues, enabled us to segregate the body anatomically into three-dimensional vascular territories that I named "angiosomes" (6). These three-dimensional anatomic territories are supplied by a source (segmental or distributing) artery and its accompanying vein(s) that span

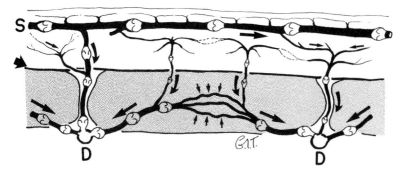

FIGURE 4.5. Composite diagram of the integument and underlying muscle *(shaded)* illustrating the superficial *(S)* and deep *(D)* venous systems with their interconnections. A large vena communicans *(C)* connects these systems; the alternative pathways of four venae comitantes of the perforating arteries are shown. Note the bidirectional system of veins within the muscle *(small arrows)* and the diverging direction of flow of the muscular veins as determined by the orientation of their valves. (Reproduced with permission from Taylor GI, Caddy CM, Watterson PA, et al. The venous territories (venosomes) of the human body: experimental study and clinical implications. *Plast Reconstr Surg.* 1990;86:185.)

between the skin and the bone (Figs. 4.6 to 4.8). Each angiosome can be subdivided into matching arteriosomes (arterial territories) and venosomes (venous territories). Initially I described 40 angiosomes, but this was an intentional oversimplification as many of these territories can and have been subdivided further into smaller composite units.

These composite blocks of skin, bone, muscle, and other soft tissue fit together like the pieces of an intricate jigsaw puzzle. In some angiosomes there is a large, overlying cutaneous "crust" and a relatively small deep-tissue region; in others, the reverse pattern exists. In some regions the territory does not reach the skin and is confined to the deep tissues, as seen, for example, in more recent studies of the head and neck. Each angiosome is linked to its neighbor, in each tissue, by a fringe of either true (simple) anastomotic arteries without change in caliber or by reduced-caliber choke (retiform) anastomotic vessels. On the venous side avalvular (bidirectional or oscillating) veins often match the anastomotic arteries and define the boundaries of the angiosome, especially in the deep tissues.

Clinical Applications

The angiosome concept has many implications. For example:

1. Each angiosome defines the safe anatomic boundary of tissue in each layer that can be transferred separately or combined together on the underlying source artery and vein as a composite flap. Furthermore, the anatomic territory of each tissue in the adjacent angiosome can usually be captured with safety when combined in the flap design.
2. Because the junctional zone between adjacent angiosomes occurs usually within the muscles of the deep tissues rather than between them, these muscles provide a vital anastomotic detour if a main source artery or vein is obstructed.
3. Similarly, because most muscles span across two or more angiosomes and are supplied from each territory, one is able to capture the skin island from one angiosome via the muscles supply in the adjacent territory.

This anatomic fact provides the basis for the design of many musculocutaneous flaps.

Vessels Follow the Connective Tissue Framework of the Body

The fact that vessels follow the connective tissue framework is fundamental to the design of all flaps, but especially to the "fasciocutaneous" and "septocutaneous" flaps.

Developmentally the vascular system appears in the mesoderm of the embryo as a continuous network of vessels. The specialized tissues develop within the interstices of that vascular network. As growth and differentiation progress, vessels

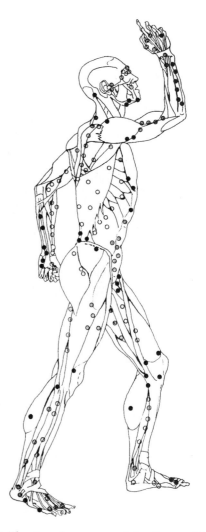

FIGURE 4.6. The sites of emergence of the direct and indirect cutaneous arterial perforators of 0.5 mm or greater averaged from all studies. Note their concentration near the dorsal and ventral midlines, around the base of the skull, and over the intermuscular septa. Direct perforators are more common in the limbs, whereas indirect perforators predominate in the torso. The vessels were color coded to match their underlying source arteries and to correlate with the angiosomes of the body. Compare with Figure 4.10. (Reproduced with permission from Taylor GI, Palmer JH. The vascular territories (angiosomes) of the body: experimental study and clinical applications. *Br J Plast Surg.* 1987;40:113.)

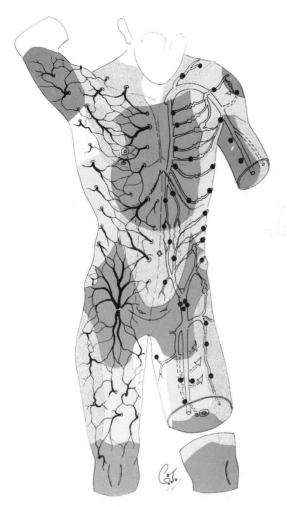

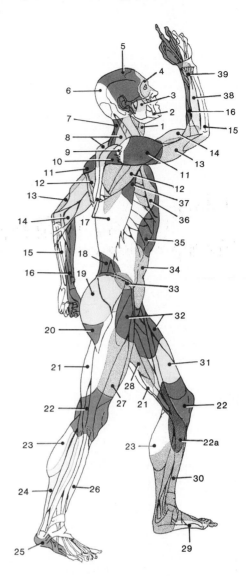

FIGURE 4.7. Schematic of the cutaneous perforators *(left)* and their interconnections. The underlying source arteries, their interconnections, and the sites of origin of the cutaneous vessels are shown on the *right*. Only the major perforators are illustrated. The vascular territories of the source arteries then have been defined in the integument *(left)* and in the deep tissues *(right)* by lines drawn around their perimeter, across the choke connecting arteries and arterioles. Note how the territories correspond in each layer. When taken together they constitute the angiosomes. (Reproduced with permission from Taylor GI, Palmer JH. The vascular territories (angiosomes) of the body: experimental study and clinical applications. *Br J Plast Surg.* 1987;40:113.)

FIGURE 4.8. The three-dimensional vascular territories—angiosomes—encompassing all tissues between skin and bone from *(1)* thyroid, *(2)* facial, *(3)* buccal (internal maxillary), *(4)* ophthalmic, *(5)* superficial temporal, *(6)* occipital, *(7)* deep cervical, *(8)* transverse cervical, *(9)* acromiothoracic, *(10)* suprascapular, *(11)* posterior circumflex humeral, *(12)* circumflex scapular, *(13)* profunda brachii, *(14)* brachial, *(15)* ulnar, *(16)* radial, *(17)* posterior intercostals, *(18)* lumbar, *(19)* superior gluteal, *(20)* inferior gluteal, *(21)* profunda femoris, *(22)* popliteal, *(22a)* descending geniculate (saphenous), *(23)* sural, *(24)* peroneal, *(25)* lateral plantar, *(26)* anterior tibial, *(27)* lateral femoral circumflex, *(28)* adductor (profunda), *(29)* medial plantar, *(30)* posterior tibial, *(31)* superficial femoral, *(32)* common femoral, *(33)* deep circumflex iliac, *(34)* deep inferior epigastric, *(35)* internal thoracic, *(36)* lateral thoracic, *(37)* thoracodorsal, *(38)* posterior interosseous, *(39)* anterior interosseous, and *(40)* internal pudendal source territories. (Reproduced with permission from Taylor GI, Palmer JH. The vascular territories (angiosomes) of the body: experimental study and clinical applications. *Br J Plast Surg.* 1987;40:113.)

become encased within the various tissues and are continuous with vessels coursing between the tissues by way of vascular pedicles at various sites. These sites, in turn, are determined by the mobility or fixity of those tissues. The connective tissue can be regarded as what is "left over" after the specialized tissues have developed. Like a honeycomb, the connective tissues house and support the specialized tissues, and in so doing, support the vascular system of the body with which they have developed an intimate relationship. It is important to differentiate between the superficial and the deep fascia, as these terms are often confused (Fig. 4.9).

The superficial fascia is a loose connective tissue honeycomb that connects the dermis to the outer layer of the deep fascia. It houses the subcutaneous fat, the breast, and remnants of the panniculus carnosus where it still exists (for example the muscles of facial expression in the head, the platysma in the neck, the palmaris brevis in the hand, and the dartos muscle in the scrotum). In the lower abdomen, it is separated into two layers by the fascia of Scarpa.

The deep fascia is also a honeycomb of connective tissue that is usually more rigid than its superficial counterpart. It has a tough outer layer that surrounds and sometimes provides origin to the muscles as a sheath on the torso and a stocking in the limbs. Often referred to as *the* deep fascia, this is only the outer layer. Radiating intermuscular septa of the deep fascia, dense in some areas and looser in other areas, anchor the outer layer to the skeleton where the deep fascia becomes

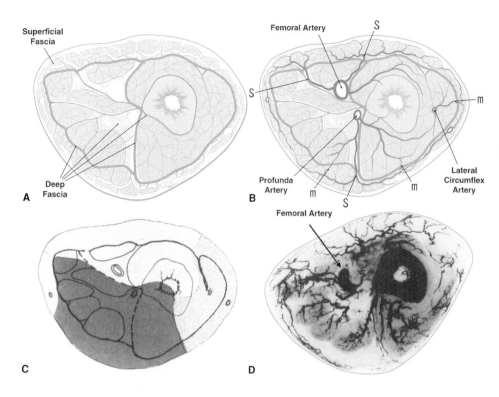

FIGURE 4.9. Cross-sectional studies to illustrate the origin and the course of the cutaneous perforators from their source arteries in the deep tissues. **A to D:** Schematic diagrams and radiographic study at mid-thigh level. **A:** The connective tissue network of the superficial and deep fascia. **B:** The same as (A) but the vessels have been added that follow this connective tissue framework. **C:** The angiosomes supplied by each of the source vessels are shown. **D:** The lead oxide cadaver injection study that corresponds with (B). Note the large direct cutaneous perforators that follow the intermuscular septa *(s)* and the large and small indirect musculocutaneous perforators *(m)*. (Reproduced with permission from Taylor GI, Palmer JH. The vascular territories (angiosomes) of the body: experimental study and clinical applications. *Br J Plast Surg.* 1987;40:113.)

continuous with the periosteum. From these septa and from the periosteum the deep fascia is continued into the muscles as intramuscular septa.

In the adult, the major arteries are closely related to the bones of the axial skeleton. Their branches follow the intermuscular connective tissues, where they divide to supply the muscles, bones, tendons, nerves, and deep fat deposits, in each instance following the connective tissue framework of that structure down to the cellular level.

The cutaneous perforators exhibit the same pattern. They usually arise from the source artery or from one of its muscle branches, either before or after entering the muscle, and follow the intermuscular or intramuscular connective tissues of the deep fascia as direct or indirect cutaneous vessels, respectively, to pierce the outer layer of the deep fascia (Fig. 4.9). Some cutaneous vessels, however, are derived from branches to other deep structures, such as the nerves, the periosteum of bones, the joints, and some glands. After emerging from the deep fascia, the cutaneous vessels follow the connective tissue framework of the superficial fascia to reach another connective tissue structure, the dermis of the skin.

In some regions the connective tissue is loose areolar, in which case the vessels travel within the connective tissue to allow the arteries to pulsate and the veins to dilate. In other regions, the connective tissue forms dense fibrous sheets, such as the outer layer of the deep fascia, some intermuscular septa, and the periosteum of bone. In these cases, the vessels course beside or on the dense fasciae, not within them.

Clinical Applications

This vessel relationship to the different types of connective tissue achieves special significance when the surgeon raises a cutaneous flap that includes the outer layer of the deep fascia (termed *fasciocutaneous flap*) or when the design is extended to include the intermuscular septa (the septocutaneous flaps).

In the former case, the deep fascia should be included in the design of the fasciocutaneous flap in those sites where the

skin is relatively fixed to the deep fascia, for example, in the limbs or the scalp (Fig. 4.10B). In these instances the dominant cutaneous vessels course on, or lie adjacent to, the deep fascia. Although they can be dissected free in some cases, it is safer and more expedient to include the deep fascia with the flap. However, where the skin and subcutaneous tissues are mobile over the deep fascia, for example, in the iliac fossae or the breast, it is unnecessary to include this fascial layer as the major cutaneous vessels have already left its surface (Fig. 4.10A).

The term *septocutaneous* is sometimes misleading, especially when used to describe a surgically created entity rather than a true anatomic structure. This may occur, for example, when the cutaneous perforators of a radial or an ulnar flap are dissected within an envelope of loose areolar tissue between the flexor tendons. Furthermore the septocutaneous flap may provide traps for the unwary surgeon. In some cases the cutaneous artery and its accompanying vein leave the underlying source vessels and course toward the surface in a surgically favorable position adjacent to a true white fibrous intermuscular septum. This is typical of the blood supply to the skin of the lateral arm flap, where cutaneous perforators arise from descending branches of the profunda brachii vessels and follow the lateral intermuscular septum toward the skin. This pattern of supply usually exists where the muscles glide on either side of the intermuscular septum. However, if the muscles attach to either side of the intermuscular septum, then the course of the cutaneous perforator may be quite variable.

This variability of anatomy is evident, for example, in the lateral aspect of the upper calf, as during an osteocutaneous fibula harvest. If a compound skin-and-bone flap is placed over the lateral intermuscular septum, based on the cutaneous perforators of the peroneal vessels, these skin vessels may course directly to the surface, traveling in a favorable position, adjacent to the septum. Alternatively, they may arise indirectly from branches to the soleus muscle as terminal twigs of muscle branches that have arisen from the peroneal vessels at considerable distance from the lateral intermuscular septum.

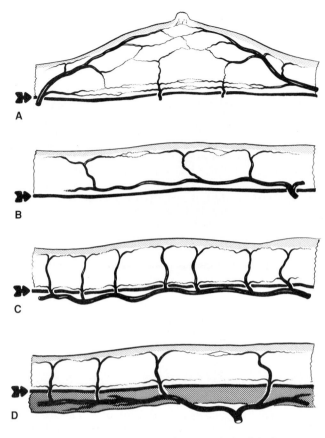

FIGURE 4.10. Schemata of the perforator pattern of the breast (**A**), thigh (**B**), sole of the foot (**C**), and buttock (**D**), including the underlying gluteus maximus muscle. The schemata illustrate the dominant horizontal axis of vessels, which provides the primary supply to the skin in each case and the relationship to the deep fascia *(arrow)*. In **A**, the vessels predominate in the subdermal plexus. Note from left to right the internal thoracic perforator and lateral thoracic artery converging on the nipple *(arrow)* in the radiograph of the loose skin region of the torso. In **B**, the vessels are coursing on the surface of the deep fascia in this relatively fixed skin area. In **C**, the source artery itself is the dominant horizontal vessel supplying the skin, coursing beneath the deep fascia in this rigidly fixed skin region. In **D**, the horizontal vessel is again the source artery (inferior gluteal), but this time its branches have to pierce muscle indirectly to reach this fixed skin region. (Reproduced with permission from Taylor GI, Palmer JH. The vascular territories (angiosomes) of the body: experimental study and clinical applications. *Br J Plast Surg.* 1987;40:113.)

In these instances, a painful and laborious intramuscular dissection of the cutaneous supply awaits the unfortunate surgeon. These two pathways provide the basis for classifying the various "perforator flaps."

Vessels Radiate from Fixed to Mobile Areas

Vessels cross tissue planes at or near their fixed margins and radiate to mobile areas. This concept is well illustrated in the blood supply to the skin because vessels emerge from the deep fascia where the skin is fixed or tethered. From here they travel for variable distances, depending on the mobility of the skin. The more mobile the integument is, the longer the vessels. These fixed-skin sites are seen in a well-muscled individual at skin crease lines, over intermuscular septa, or near the fixed attachments of muscles to bone (Fig. 4.6).

Clinical Applications

It follows that long, robust flaps should be based where the skin is fixed, with their axes oriented along the lines of maximal skin mobility. The further the distance between fixed points, the longer the safe dimensions of the flap. There are many instances in which this applies in practice. For example, long flaps can be based at the groin, the paraumbilical region of the abdomen, or the parasternal region of the chest (Figs. 4.1 and 4.6). Additional precision to flap design can be obtained by the use of the Doppler ultrasonic probe to locate these perforators as they emerge from the deep fascia (7). **In this way a viable flap can be designed by basing it on a significant perforator that is located with the probe, by finding the next dominant perforator along the desired flap axis, and then simply joining these two points, as I have found experimentally that one adjacent vascular territory can be captured with safety (4,5,8,9).**

Vessels Hitchhike with Nerves

Recent work confirms that the intimate relationship between nerves and blood vessels that is known to exist in the deep tissues and in some areas of the integument is, in fact, present in all regions of the skin and subcutaneous tissues of the body (10). The cutaneous nerves are accompanied by a longitudinal system of arteries and veins that are often the dominant blood supply to the region. The veins, in company with the nerves, are frequently large "primary" venous freeways, such as the cephalic, basilic, long saphenous, and short saphenous systems. The arteries are either long vessels—for example, the supraorbital, lateral intercostal, or saphenous arteries—or they exist as a chain-linked system of cutaneous perforators, often joined in series by true anastomoses without change in caliber.

Clinical Applications

This neurovascular relationship presents another basis for designing long flaps with the added potential for providing sensation at the repair site. Many of the current "axial" or "fasciocutaneous" flaps are in fact neurovascular flaps. The original long and short saphenous flaps in the calf described by Ponten are cases in point.

Vessel Size and Orientation Are a Product of Tissue Growth and Differentiation

More than 200 years ago, John Hunter suggested that at some stage of fetal development, and certainly at birth, an individual has a fixed number of arteries in the body, the size, length, and direction of which are modified by subsequent growth and differentiation of the parts. This helps to explain why long vessels radiate from the skull base toward its vertex as the brain and skull expand, why long vessels course on the torso as the lungs expand and the fetus extends from the flexed position, and why long vessels converge on the nipple from the periphery as the breast develops in the female (Fig. 4.11).

Clinical Application

This information provides the basis for the logical planning of the various breast-reduction operations. Each technique revolves around the design of a flap of skin and subcutaneous tissue (including breast) that is based on one or more vessels as they pierce the deep fascia around the perimeter of the pectoralis major muscle. Tissue expansion is another example. Here existing vessels in the skin and subcutaneous tissues, like the vessels in the abdominal wall during pregnancy, hypertrophy and elongate as the fluid is introduced into the expander.

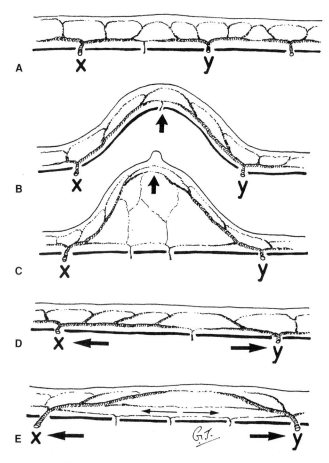

FIGURE 4.11. Schematic to illustrate John Hunter's hypothesis of a fixed number of cutaneous arteries in the fetus and how growth and differentiation of the tissues could modify the definitive size and relationship of the arteries *X* and *Y* in different regions of the body after they pierce the deep fascia. **A:** The "resting state." **B:** The vessels are stretched by expansion of structures beneath the deep fascia, for example, the skull and brain. **C:** The vessels are stretched and compressed toward the dermis by the developing breast above the deep fascia. **D:** The vessels are stretched apart by the developing long bones but still retain a dominant relationship to the deep fascia. **E:** Growth again stretches the vessels apart, but this time a gliding plane develops between the deep fascia and the subcutaneous fat in this loose skin area, for example, the iliac fossa. (Reproduced with permission from Taylor GI, Palmer JH. The vascular territories (angiosomes) of the body: experimental study and clinical applications. *Br J Plast Surg.* 1987;40:113.)

Therefore, if possible, the expander should be placed beneath mobile skin and between fixed skin sites to take maximal advantage of the inherent vascular anatomy of the region.

Vessels Obey "The Law of Equilibrium"

This concept was described by Debreuil-Chambardel and is referred to constantly by Michel Salmon (3) in his description of the cutaneous arteries. Basically, this concept states that "the anatomical territories of adjacent arteries bear an inverse relationship to each other yet combine to supply the same region." If one vessel is small, its partner is large to compensate, and vice versa. This is well illustrated in the variability in size between each of the parasternal perforators of the internal mammary artery and between the internal mammary perforators and the cutaneous perforator of the adjacent angiosome: the acromio-

thoracic (Fig. 4.1). It is likely that the same relationship occurs between the cutaneous veins.

Clinical Applications

The deltopectoral flap of Bakamjian is an excellent example. It is based medially over the second to fourth intercostal spaces so as to embrace the variable sizes of the internal thoracic (internal mammary) perforators. Designed below and parallel to the clavicle, it is usually dissected medially from its tip at the shoulder. If small perforators are noted over the deltoid muscle, and in particular from the deltopectoral groove, the dissection is continued to the flap base on the assumption that the internal thoracic perforators will be large. If, however, a large cutaneous perforator is seen emerging from the deltopectoral groove, then this pedicle is usually ligated and further dissection of the flap is delayed for 1 week because of the possibility that the adjacent internal thoracic perforators will be small. This delay procedure is employed because of the risk of flap necrosis, especially if the flap tip spans beyond the point of the shoulder.

Vessels Have a Relatively Constant Destination but May Have a Variable Origin

This is typical of the vessels that emanate from the groin to supply the skin of the lower abdomen and upper thigh. The superficial inferior epigastric artery (SIEA) and the superficial circumflex iliac artery (SCIA), for example, may arise either separately from the common femoral artery, as a combined trunk from that vessel or from one of its branches (11). Whichever is the case, their destination is constant to supply the integument of the lower abdomen and the hip (Fig. 4.1).

Clinical Application

Although this variability in vessel origin may not be important when designing a pedicled flap at the groin, it certainly becomes so if the flap is to be isolated on its feeding vessels for microvascular transfer.

The Vessels Form a Continuous Unbroken Network

This fact has been referred to already but is highlighted because it is fundamental to the understanding of the various flap designs where, for example, the same area of skin and subcutaneous tissue can be raised as either a "cutaneous," "fasciocutaneous," "septocutaneous," "musculocutaneous," or "perforator flap." In each case, regardless of the flap design, the vessels that enter the flap at its base connect into the same vascular network. What may vary between flap designs, however, are the size and site of entry of the cutaneous perforators, thus influencing flap survival.

Clinical Applications

There are numerous instances whereby the surgeon knowingly or unwittingly takes advantage of this anatomic fact. For example, the skin and subcutaneous fat over the pectoralis major muscle can be designed (a) as a musculocutaneous flap on small perforators emerging from the underlying muscle, (b) as a fasciocutaneous flap based either medially on the large internal thoracic (internal mammary) perforators or laterally on the dominant perforator(s) of the acromiothoracic axis, or (c) as a neurovascular fasciocutaneous flap when based superiorly on the supraclavicular neurovascular pedicles that flow down over the clavicle from the neck.

Other important considerations are the anastomotic vascular "keystones," which are usually formed by reduced-caliber choke arteries that link adjacent primary cutaneous perforators to form the arterial network. When a flap is elevated, these choke vessels, which initially impede flow from one arterial territory to the next along the flap, enlarge to the caliber of the cutaneous arteries they connect. However, this process of vessel enlargement is an active event and takes time. It involves multiplication and elongation of the cells in each layer of the vessel wall with its maximal effect occurring between 48 and 72 hours after the operation.

Clinically, it has been noted that one adjacent anatomic vascular territory can be captured with safety on the cutaneous artery at the flap base and that necrosis usually occurs at the level of the next choke anastomosis in the arterial network or the one beyond. Surgically, flap survival can be extended by the strategic division of vascular pedicles at various time intervals along the length of the proposed flap—the "flap-delay" procedure.

CLASSIFICATION OF THE CUTANEOUS BLOOD SUPPLY

I have left the contentious subject of classification of the cutaneous blood supply until the end, as I believe it is more important to understand the pure and the applied (functional) anatomy of the cutaneous arteries than to be concerned about which classification is the best. It is essential, however, to differentiate between classifications based correctly on the anatomy and physiology of the cutaneous supply rather than antiquated terms that focus on flap design, such as axial, random, cutaneous, fasciocutaneous, septocutaneous, and musculocutaneous, each of which describes the method by which the flap is planned and dissected.

One of the oldest, simplest, and best classifications was offered by Spalteholz (2) in 1893. He subdivided the cutaneous vessels into two groups, depending on whether they were the main (dominant) supply to the area or whether they had a relatively minor (supplementary) role. Recently, this classification was modified, stimulated by the resurgence of interest on the anatomically based "perforator flaps."

Direct Cutaneous Vessels

These vessels contribute to the primary (dominant) cutaneous supply to the area and are particularly well developed in the limbs. They arise from the underlying source artery or from one of its muscle branches before they enter the muscle. They pass between the muscles and other deep structures in the intermuscular septa and rapidly reach and perforate the outer layer of the deep fascia, where their main destination is the skin. They are usually large and spaced well apart in the torso, head, neck, arms, and thighs, especially where the skin is mobile. They are smaller and more numerous in the forearms and legs except where they accompany cutaneous nerves. In the palm of the hands and the soles of the feet they are evident as a dense network of small vessels (Figs. 4.1 and 4.9).

In each case these direct cutaneous vessels follow the connective tissue framework of the deep tissue to the skin. They pass between the muscles and tendons, sometimes closely related to true intermuscular septa, as "septocutaneous vessels." If the source artery is close to the surface, for example the radial, ulnar, or common femoral arteries, their course to the outer layer of the deep fascia may be short. Conversely if the source artery is deeply situated, their length is longer, for example, the direct cutaneous perforators of the profunda brachii, lateral femoral circumflex, and peroneal arteries.

When the cutaneous perforators are traced to the underlying source vessels to provide "septocutaneous" perforator flaps, the septum may be well formed, as seen in the lateral arm and thigh, or consist of loose areolar tissue, as occurs in the forearm over the radial or ulnar vessels.

Indirect Cutaneous Vessels

These vessels arise from the source arteries and penetrate the deep tissues, usually muscle, vertically or obliquely before piercing the outer layer of the deep fascia (Fig. 4.11). They can be quite large, contribute to the primary (dominant) blood supply to the skin, and are particularly well developed on the torso (e.g., the internal thoracic, intercostal, and deep inferior epigastric musculocutaneous perforators). Alternatively, they may emerge as small, "spent" terminal branches to provide the secondary (supplementary) supply to the skin. These are small vessels, often quite numerous, which emerge as terminal twigs of vessels whose predominant supply is to the various deep tissues, especially the muscles.

Whatever their origin and size, these indirect cutaneous perforators provide the basis for the musculocutaneous perforator flaps, which require a more tedious dissection with the potential to preserve muscle function. Large or small they enter, and become continuous with, the same vascular network that is formed by the direct cutaneous arteries. Often the smaller indirect cutaneous vessels are the main blood supply to some musculocutaneous flaps, especially where the skin island is sited over muscle to which it is loosely attached, for example, the gracilis and the gastrocnemius musculocutaneous flaps.

CONCLUSION

Knowledge of the basic anatomy of the cutaneous vessels coupled with an appreciation of the factors that influence its structure in different regions of the body provides for the logical planning of flaps and incisions. In the sage words of Michel Salmon: "*Entre l'anatomie et la physiologie, il y a place pour une anatomie de fonction, pour une anatomie physologique*" ("Between anatomy and physiology there is room for a functional anatomy, for a physiologic anatomy").

References

1. Manchot C. *The Cutaneous Arteries of the Human Body*. New York: Springer-Verlag, 1983.
2. Spalteholz W. Die vertheilung der blutgefasse in der haut. *Arch Anat.* 1893.
3. Salmon M. Arteries of the skin. In: Taylor GI, Tempest M, eds. London: Churchill-Livingstone; 1988.
4. Dhar SC, Taylor, GI. The delay phenomenon: the story unfolds. *Plast Reconstr Surg.* 1999;104(7):2079–2091.
5. Morris SF, Taylor GI. The time sequence of the delay phenomenon: when is a surgical delay effective? An experimental study. *Plast Reconstr Surg.* 1995; 95(1):526.
6. Taylor GI, Palmer JH. The vascular territories (angiosomes) of the body: experimental study and clinical applications. *Br Plast Surg.* 1987;40:113.
7. Taylor GI, McCarten G, Doyle M. The use of the Doppler probe for planning flaps: anatomical study and clinical applications. *Br J Plast Surg.* 1990;43:1.
8. Callegari PR, Taylor GI, Caddy CM, et al. An anatomical review of the delay phenomenon: 1. Experimental studies. *Plast Reconstr Surg.* 1992;89:397.
9. Taylor GI, Corlett RJ, Caddy CM, et al. An anatomical review of the delay phenomenon: II. Clinical applications. *Plast Reconstr Surg.* 1992;89:408.
10. Taylor GI, Gianoutsos MP, Morris SF. The neurovascular territories of the skin and muscles: anatomic study and clinical implications. *Plast Reconstr Surg.* 1994;94:1.
11. Taylor GI, Daniel RK. The anatomy of several free flap donor sites. *Plast Reconstr Surg.* 1975;56:243.
12. Esser JFS. *Artery Flaps*. Antwerp: De Vos-van Kleef; 1929.

CHAPTER 5 ■ MUSCLE FLAPS AND THEIR BLOOD SUPPLY

STEPHEN J. MATHES AND JAMIE LEVINE

FLAPS

A *flap* is a unit of tissue that may be transferred from a donor to a recipient site while maintaining its blood supply. Numerous types of flaps and classification schemes exist. Flaps can be characterized by their component parts (e.g., cutaneous, musculocutaneous, osseocutaneous), their special relationship to the defect (local, regional, or distant), the nature of the blood supply (random versus axial), or by the movement placed on the flap (e.g., advancement, pivot, transposition) to fill an associated defect. This chapter focuses on axial-pattern muscle flaps; that is, flaps with a known blood vessel oriented longitudinally within the flap.

HISTORY

Skin and subcutaneous tissue was initially elevated as "random" pattern flaps either from a site adjacent to the wound or from a distant site. Because of poor and inconsistent circulation, these flaps often went on to partial or complete flap necrosis. Subsequently, vascular pedicles were identified in select cutaneous locations (e.g., dorsalis pedis, groin flap). Because these flaps could be elevated with a defined vascular pedicle, it became possible to use a flap with greater dimensions than was possible with the random pattern flap. These early axial flaps were a significant improvement with regard to size and reliability, but were limited to specific topographic locations. Nevertheless, these flaps had a significant impact on reconstructive surgery.

The identification of muscle flaps as a source of tissue offered tremendous flexibility and more options anatomically for wound coverage and defect reconstruction (1). Muscles are available in almost all topographic areas. As the vascular anatomy to these muscles were elaborated, it became possible to detach the muscle origin, insertion, or both, and to transfer the muscle to a new site as a flap while maintaining vascular perfusion. The choice of which muscle is best to use to cover a given defect takes into account multiple factors, including the size and location of the defect, damage to regional tissues, and the presence of exposed vital structures. The potential to use muscle for defect coverage has changed the way physicians can manage complex wounds of any variety.

The increasing interest in muscle circulation resulted in recognition of the contribution of muscle flap circulation to the overlying skin, which advanced our ability to close complex, composite defects with improved function, cosmesis, and variability within the donor options. Each superficial muscle provides vascular connections via musculocutaneous perforating vessels to the overlying skin. Identification of vascular connections to the skin made it possible to include a segment of skin with the muscle flap (2). Prior to identification of the muscle

skin territory, which allows its design as a musculocutaneous flap, the muscle flap was inset into the wound and exposed portions were skin grafted for coverage. With a composite of muscle and its overlying skin, defect closure can be accomplished with muscle, subcutaneous tissue, and skin. As understanding of cutaneous blood supply increased, fasciocutaneous flaps were also described. Finally, Ian Taylor was able, through ink injection analysis, to put the various concepts of skin circulation together in its most coherent form, thereby defining the concept of the angiosome (Chapter 4). These studies have helped to define the vascular territories of the more than 300 cutaneous perforators found in the average body (3), thereby providing a reliable guide to composite flap design based on cutaneous vascular anatomy.

BLOOD SUPPLY

Random Flaps

All flaps require an intact blood supply at the time of transfer to ensure viability and successful healing. Random cutaneous flaps are based on random, nondominant contributions from the dermal and subdermal plexus. The combined contributions of experimental studies and clinical experience resulted in the observation that the ratio of flap length to width is critical for flap survival. These restrictions limit their ability to reliably cover large defects. When used appropriately and their limitations respected, random flaps are reliable first choices for coverage of smaller defects throughout the body.

Axial Flaps

In contrast to random-pattern flaps, axial-pattern flaps are based on a reliable, anatomically defined vascular territory that is oriented longitudinally within the flap and that extends beyond the base of the flap. Since the description of the first axial flap (the deltopectoral flap) nearly 40 years ago, the knowledge of the body's various cutaneous angiosomes and subsequent exploitation of axially based flaps has grown exponentially (4). The advances in anatomic science increased the reliability of axial flaps and eventually fostered the development of microsurgical free flap transfer. Because of their significantly greater reliability, axial flaps are preferred for coverage of moderate to large defects.

The reliability and volume of tissue that can be placed into a defect is markedly greater than any random-pattern circulation-based flap. Because of the axially oriented circulation, delay procedures are often unnecessary when mobilizing large tissue volumes in a single procedure based on this direct circulation. Axial flaps have had a significant impact on reconstructive surgery and have revolutionized the management of large composite tissue defects. Their only limitation, when pedicled, is the limited topographic arc of rotation. These limitations have been essentially overcome by microvascular free tissue transfer techniques, where the only limitations are based on the availability of recipient-site blood vessels.

Delay Phenomenon

To extend the somewhat restricted size of random flaps, surgeons rely on the *delay phenomenon*. This vascular delay is most commonly achieved by interrupting a portion of the normal blood supply to the flap without transferring the flap from its native position. **The associated sublethal ischemia results in (a) opening of "choke" vessels that are normally closed, allowing blood flow into the ischemic region of the flap, (b) reorientation of the vessels within the flap to a more longitudinal pattern, and (c) sprouting of new vessels within the flap through angiogenesis and, perhaps, via vasculogenesis.**

Vessels within the flap also respond to the stress of delay by increasing in caliber. Most surgeons find it prudent to delay a flap for at least 10 days to 3 weeks prior to final transfer, thereby permitting a maturation of the process of neovascularization.

Incorporating a planned delay can significantly improve the chances of complete survival of a large, random-pattern, cutaneous flap in patients with an impaired microcirculation, such as smokers and diabetics. Furthermore, a delay should always be considered a safety net if a flap demonstrates signs of ischemia or venous congestion after elevation. The reconstruction in such cases is best performed in a staged manner, following a period of delay.

Vascular delay can also be used to maximize survival of extended axial-type flaps. A significant delay and maximization of the tissue in a pedicled axial flap will occur by either preincising the skin and subcutaneous tissue in a musculocutaneous or fasciocutaneous flap, or by dividing the nondominant or codominant vascular pedicles. An example is the delay of a pedicled transverse rectus abdominis musculocutaneous (TRAM) flap. As the inferior epigastric vessels are the pri-

mary vascular supply to the TRAM, division of this pedicle and flap based on the superior pedicle often leads to areas of congestion or ischemia in the skin beyond zone one. By ligating the deep inferior epigastric vessels with or without incising the skin paddle 1 to 2 weeks prior to breast reconstruction surgery, a much larger and more reliable skin paddle can be transferred.

PATTERNS OF MUSCLE CIRCULATION

The most universally accepted system of muscle flap blood supply was developed by Mathes and Nahai. Every muscle, in part or as a whole, has potential for use as a muscle flap. Muscle circulation is based on specific pedicles that enter the muscle between its origin and insertion and consist of an artery and single or paired venae comitantes (5). The position, number, and size of the vascular pedicles influence both the likelihood of flap survival and the flap design. The relative importance of each vascular pedicle to muscle circulation has been determined in cadavers by colored latex and barium injections, allowing evaluation of each vascular pedicle with regard to its length, diameter, location, and regional source. Subsequent use of the muscles as flaps has confirmed the relative importance of each pedicle to muscle survival and the potential for various flap modifications. If a pedicle to a muscle is critical to muscle survival based on its size and distribution to the internal vascular architecture of the muscle, it is specified as a dominant (where multiple pedicles are present) or major (where more than one pedicle is dominant) pedicle. Nondominant pedicles are labeled as minor pedicle(s). When a series of segmental smaller vessels are identified that may support muscle flap survival despite ligation of dominant or major pedicles, these minor pedicles are considered secondary pedicles. Variations in major and dominant pedicle anatomy are uncommon, although the location and number of minor pedicles is quite variable.

Five patterns of circulation to muscle have been identified and are the basis of the classification system using patterns of vascular anatomy (Fig. 5.1): types I, II, III, IV, and V.

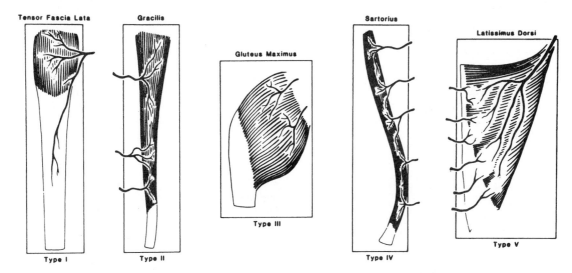

FIGURE 5.1. Patterns of vascular anatomy: type I, one vascular pedicle; type II, dominant pedicle(s) and minor pedicle(s); type III, two dominant pedicles; type IV, segmental vascular pedicle; type V, one dominant pedicle and secondary segmental pedicle. (From Mathes SJ, Nahai F. Classification of the vascular anatomy of muscles: experimental and clinical correlation. *Plast Reconstr Surg.* 1981;67:177, with permission.)

Type I: Single Vascular Pedicle

A single vascular pedicle enters the muscle. The muscle may be safely elevated on this pedicle. Muscles identified with this pattern of circulation include the abductor digiti minimi (hand); abductor pollicis brevis; anconeus; first dorsal interosseous; gastrocnemius; genioglossus; hyoglossus; longitudinalis linguae; styloglossus; tensor fascia lata (TFL); transversus and verticalis linguae; and vastus lateralis.

Type II: Dominant Vascular Pedicle(s) and Minor Vascular Pedicle(s)

Use of a type II flap generally requires division of part or all of the minor pedicles with preservation of the dominant pedicle. The muscle survives when elevated based on the dominant vascular pedicle. Muscles with a type II vascular pattern include the following: the abductor digiti minimi (foot); abductor hallucis; brachioradialis; coracobrachialis; flexor carpi ulnaris; flexor digitorum brevis; gracilis; hamstring (biceps femoris); peroneus brevis; peroneus longus; platysma; rectus femoris; soleus; sternocleidomastoid; trapezius; triceps; and vastus medialis.

Type III: Dominant Pedicles

Type III muscles contain two large vascular pedicles, each of which can support the entire muscle. Muscles with a type III vascular pattern include the following: gluteus maximus; intercostal; orbicularis oris; pectoralis minor; rectus abdominis; serratus; and temporalis.

Type IV: Segmental Vascular Pedicles

This group of muscles contains a series of segmental pedicles—generally of equal size—that enter the muscle along its course. Each segmental pedicle provides circulation to a portion (segment) of the muscle. Generally, division of two or more pedicles is feasible for transposition of a portion of the muscle as a flap. However the muscle generally will not survive if an excessive number of the segmental pedicles are divided during flap elevation. Muscles with a type IV vascular pattern include the following: the extensor digitorum longus; extensor hallucis longus; external oblique; flexor digitorum longus; flexor hallucis longus; sartorius; and tibialis anterior.

Type V: Dominant Vascular Pedicle and Secondary Segmental Vascular Pedicles

In this pattern of circulation, the muscle receives a large vascular pedicle that will reliably provide circulation to the muscle when it is elevated solely based on this particular vascular pedicle. However, the muscle has secondary vascular pedicles, which generally enter the muscle at its opposite end from the site of entry of the dominant vascular pedicle. These secondary pedicles will also support the muscle if the dominant vascular pedicle is divided. Thus, the muscle may be used as a flap based on two separate sources of circulation. Muscles with a type V pattern include the following: internal oblique; latissimus dorsi; and pectoralis major.

ARC OF ROTATION

Each muscle and myocutaneous flap has a limited arc of rotation when based as a pedicle flap. These limitations are based from the point of the pedicle circulation to the most distant region of muscle or skin that is being elevated. A muscle that can be based on a dominant vascular pedicle can reach adjacent areas that fall within the radius created by the pedicle and the most distal portion of muscle that is supplied by that circulation. Generally, the muscle is released from either its origin or its insertion. The muscle is then elevated to the point of rotation, generally located adjacent to the major or dominant pedicle. To avoid injury and kinking in pedicle flap elevation, the pedicle is not skeletonized. These limitations should be incorporated into the surgical plan so that defect coverage is maximized. With progressive mobilization of the pedicle, the arc of rotation of the flap is increased. Release of the bony attachments overlying the point of entry of the vascular pedicle allows muscle elevation as an island flap based only on its vascular pedicle, with subsequent increase in its arc of rotation (Fig. 5.2).

A specific knowledge of anatomic landmarks, including muscle insertion and origin and where the vascular pedicle enters the muscle, enables better planning of adjacent defect coverage. A template can be made of the defect and then the arc of rotation of candidate regional muscles can be plotted. Based on these approximations appropriate coverage can be chosen for a defect. Certain defects can require two or more regional flaps, but a strong knowledge of the muscular anatomy enables the surgeon to reliably plan coverage based on these principles. Muscle flap elevation based on the dominant pedicle is designated as the standard flap. A muscle flap that is elevated on its secondary pedicles, which requires division of its dominant pedicle, is classified as a reverse flap. An example of this is using a pectoralis muscle flap, which is normally elevated on its dominant axial pedicle— the thoracoacromial vessels— but is now raised as a turnover flap based on the secondary vessels coming from the internal mammary circulation, to cover a midline sternal defect.

In a rotation advancement flap such as a gluteal flap for sacral wound coverage, the arc of rotation is based more on the pivot point of the cutaneous incision and any associated back-cut instead of the vascular pedicle alone. Clearly, these flaps are limited by distance, as a large cutaneous component remains attached.

SKIN TERRITORY

Musculocutaneous flaps are composite axial flaps that consist of muscle and overlying subcutaneous tissue and skin. In most cases, the muscle at the base of the flaps is supplied by a single dominant vessel, which gives off one or more perforating vessels to supply the overlying subcutaneous tissue and skin. Two examples of musculocutaneous flaps are the TRAM flap and the latissimus dorsi flap. Topographically, nearly any muscle in the direct subcutaneous location provides perforators to the skin either directly through or adjacent to the muscle. This subcutaneous tissue and overlying skin can be incorporated into a multilayered type of reconstruction. The skin territory of each superficial muscle is defined anatomically as that segment of skin extending between the origin and insertion of the muscle and located between its edges along the course of the muscle, and can even be extended beyond this territory. The pedicled musculocutaneous flap may be designed with the skin left intact (skin rotation flap) at the flap base; alternatively, a skin island (skin island flap) may be designed over the flap. Generally, the more narrow muscles, such as the gracilis, have a greater limitation in skin territory because of the decreased number of perforating vessels to the overlying skin and the increased importance of septocutaneous vessels to the skin territory in proximity to the muscle.

These musculocutaneous flaps can be reliably raised as free flaps. Similarly, these skin islands can be raised without muscle

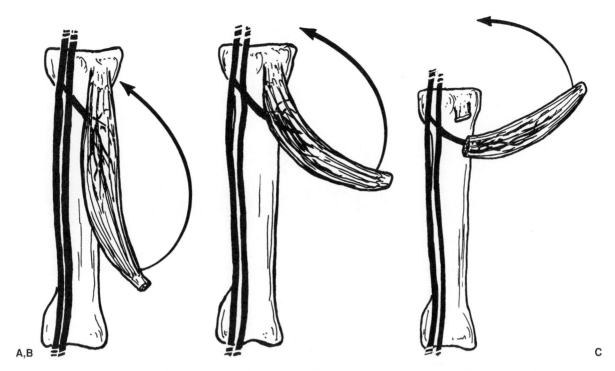

A,B

C

FIGURE 5.2. Arc of rotation. **A:** Arc of rotation with flap elevation to point of entrance of vascular pedicle to flap. **B:** Extended arc of rotation based on flap elevation with dissection of pedicle to regional source. **C:** Extended arc of rotation based on flap elevation with pedicle dissection and release of proximal fascia and/or muscle origin or insertion. (From Mathes SJ, Nahai F. *Reconstructive Surgery Principles, Anatomy and Technique*, vol. 1. New York: Churchill Livingstone; 1997:115, with permission.)

as perforator flaps. These techniques are discussed later in this chapter (see Perforator Flap subsection).

FLAP MODIFICATIONS

The goals of reconstructive surgery include safety as well as restoration of form and function. The donor site must also be considered when planning a reconstruction. Repair of a defect in one region by creating an equally problematic defect in the donor site is not a satisfactory trade-off. Anatomic knowledge of the vascular territory of the donor muscle based on either dominant or segmental supply help to define which portion of the muscle can successfully be transferred or survive regional mobilization. Limitations of fascial harvest and muscle dissection can offer a functional benefit to certain donor regions and should be taken into account when designing the reconstruction. A classic example of this is muscle and fascial harvest in TRAM flaps and the associated risks of abdominal wall laxity and weakness. Although the standard design of the muscle flap often represents the most appropriate method to reach these goals, alterations in flap design might avoid problems at the donor site. Muscle-sparing and perforator approaches help to decrease the abdominal wall morbidity associated with this type of flap harvest, and minimize the need for alloplastic (mesh) reconstruction of the donor site.

Segmental Flap

As noted above, use of part of a muscle has potential advantages, including functional preservation, decreased bulk at the recipient site, and potential use of the remaining muscle as a secondary flap. Type III muscles, especially the gluteus maximus,

are ideally suited for segmental design because these muscles have a dual blood supply. Thus, it is possible to split the muscle, leaving half of it attached to its origin, insertion, and motor nerve. The other half of the muscle can then be elevated as a transposition flap. This type of muscle flap modification may be used for both type I and type II muscles because the muscle is divided based on branches of the dominant vascular pedicle.

Type IV muscle, in particular, requires elevation as a segmental flap, because the entire flap generally does not survive based on a single segmental vascular pedicle. Only a portion of the muscle can be divided and used as a transposition flap. Use of the superior part of the sartorius muscle for groin vessel coverage is an example of segmental muscle flap design. The sartorius is elevated by ligating one to two (as many as needed) perforators and rotating the proximal muscle medially to cover the femoral vessels. Additional ligation of distal perforators may compromise the blood supply to the proximal flap, which is required for the vessel coverage.

Distally Based Flaps

Design of a flap on minor pedicles located opposite to the base of the standard flap is classified as a distally based flap. Generally, the entire muscle will not survive division of the dominant pedicle and, therefore, only a small part of the muscle is elevated on a specific, identified, minor pedicle. Surgical delay of the dominant pedicle by ligation prior to flap elevation helps in successful elevation of a distally based flap, including the proximal muscle (see Blood Supply section of this chapter). **The main problem for these distally based flaps can be venous drainage, especially in the lower extremity.** Elevation of the extremity to allow for postural drainage and surgical delay, as mentioned above, helps the distally based flap to adapt the venous circulation to its new circuitous pathway.

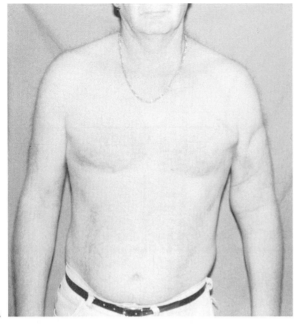

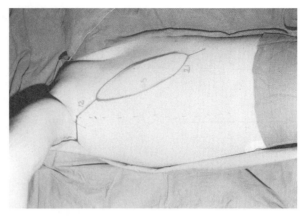

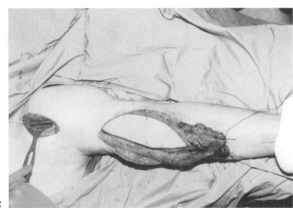

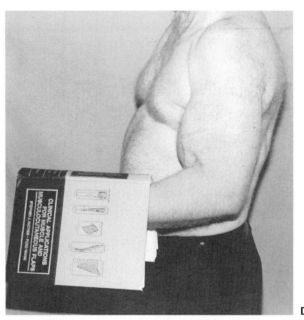

FIGURE 5.3. Functional muscle modification. **A:** The patient suffered traumatic avulsion of the biceps muscle, the overlying skin, and the soft tissue. **B:** Posterior view demonstrates the skin island designed over the latissimus dorsi muscle in preparation for functional muscle transfer. **C:** Transposition of the latissimus dorsi musculocutaneous flap into position for coverage of an upper extremity defect and to reestablish muscle origin in the proximal ulna. **D:** The patient demonstrates active flexion of the elbow based on the functional muscle transfer.

Neurotized-Functional Muscle Flap

A muscle flap may be used to provide motor function at the site of reconstruction (6). Flap design requires preservation of both the dominant vascular pedicle and the motor nerve (examples include the latissimus and the gracilis). **To maintain effective muscle function, the muscle must be inset so that its resting length and tension is the same as it was in the donor site.** A muscle may be designed to provide both coverage of a defect and to restore function at the defect site. An example of this is use of the latissimus dorsi muscle in the upper extremity. In the upper arm-biceps region, it may be used as a pedicled flap leaving its motor unit (thoracodorsal nerve) intact or anastomosing to the musculocutaneous nerve. In the forearm region, it can be used as a free flap (Fig. 5.3).

Sensory Flap

Sensory reinnervation of cutaneous islands after transfer is unpredictable. A musculocutaneous flap may be designed to in-clude a sensory nerve to the cutaneous portion of the flap. If the sensory nerve does not enter the skin territory of the flap adjacent to the dominant or major vascular pedicle, the nerve may require division during pedicled or free flap elevation. If divided, a neurorrhaphy may be performed to another sensory nerve at the recipient site. Examples of this exist with breast reconstruction. The eleventh intercostal nerve, which is involved in sensation to the rectus myocutaneous flap, and the cutaneous branches of the seventh thoracic nerve, which provides sensation to the cutaneous component of the latissimus flap, can be anastomosed to the lateral cutaneous branch of the fourth intercostal nerve, which provides the major contribution to sensation of the breast. Clinical and research studies have shown more consistent sensory return to the recipient site when a sensory neurorrhaphy is performed (7). The difficulty with this approach is that sensory return is not a functional requirement in all territories of the body. Even in areas such as the plantar aspect of the foot, where sensation is important for protection and proprioception, function can be preserved without sensory reconstruction. Also, sensory nerves supplying a given cutaneous territory may not be clearly visible or consistent on dissection. The indications for sensory reconstruction in these flaps must be individualized and should be planned to help guide the flap dissection and the patient's expectations. Division of sensory nerves must be performed appropriately to avoid neuroma formation. Regional dysesthesia is a potential consequence with injury to, or harvest of, sensory nerves supplying a cutaneous area.

Vascularized Bone

Vascular connections between muscle and bone are generally observed at the muscle–bone interface. If these vascular connections are preserved, it is possible to elevate a segment of vascularized bone with the flap. A segment of the sixth rib with the pectoralis major muscle and a segment of the iliac bone with the internal oblique muscle (deep circumflex iliac artery flap) are examples of muscle flaps that may include bone. When considering a free fibula flap harvest, the flexor hallucis longus is vascularly supplied by the peroneal vessels and interconnected through this vasculature with the fibula bone (Fig. 5.4). Although the muscle dissection can be limited during the flap harvest, it is often incorporated to supply extra internal or cutaneous coverage, bulk, and vascular supply.

Tissue Expansion

Although rarely used because of surgical staging difficulties and risk of complications, insertion of a tissue expander beneath a musculocutaneous flap allows for both an increase in skin island dimensions and assists in donor-site closure. In flap cover-

age surgery, tissue expansion is more commonly used in preparation of fasciocutaneous advancement flaps. Tissue expansion can be used to increase the useable skin island in a latissimus musculocutaneous flap and allow for primary closure of the defect. When used for breast reconstruction, the tissue expander increases the dimensions of both the remaining skin envelope and the associated overlying pectoralis major muscle.

Free Flaps

Free flaps are the natural extension of axially based muscle and musculocutaneous flaps and have further advanced our ability to provide reconstructive options. Pedicled flaps are limited regionally by their arc of rotation, whereas microvascular free tissue transfer broadens the flap's usefulness to all areas of the body. Free tissue transfer should, like all reconstructive techniques, be performed in a well-planned fashion and should not be performed in lieu of appropriate regional options. The reasons for using muscles as free flaps are essentially fourfold. First, in cases where limited regional options for muscle rotation exist, such as in distal third tibial and foot defects. Second, the volume of the defect is larger than local tissues can reconstruct. Microvascular transplantation is frequently used in the head and neck region where there is a lack of suitable regional muscles to satisfy the reconstructive need for combined facial, oral, and nasal cavity defects. Third, when functional deficits from using the regional muscle supply may limit the outcome, nonessential muscle can be used from a distant location and maintain the functional outcome. Fourth, for infectious or prosthetic coverage even when local, fasciocutaneous coverage can be performed. In cases where flap re-elevation is

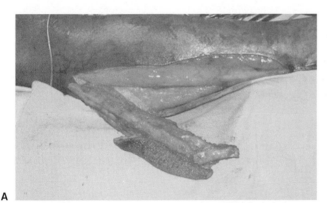

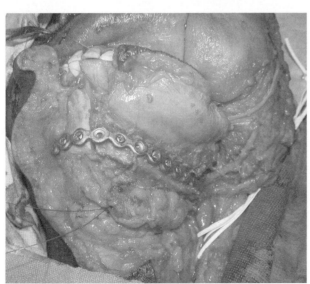

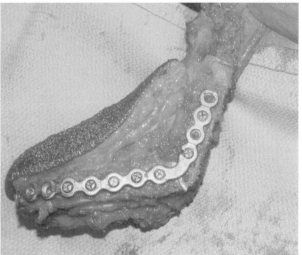

FIGURE 5.4. **A:** Fibula harvest for mandible reconstruction including a portion of the flexor hallucis longus muscle, which is supplied by the peroneal vasculature. **B:** Fibula osteotomized and plated while remaining attached to its pedicle in situ. **C:** Fibula transferred and revascularized. Bone inset has been performed and soft-tissue inset is next. Included is a skin island (osteomyocutaneous) for intraoral reconstruction.

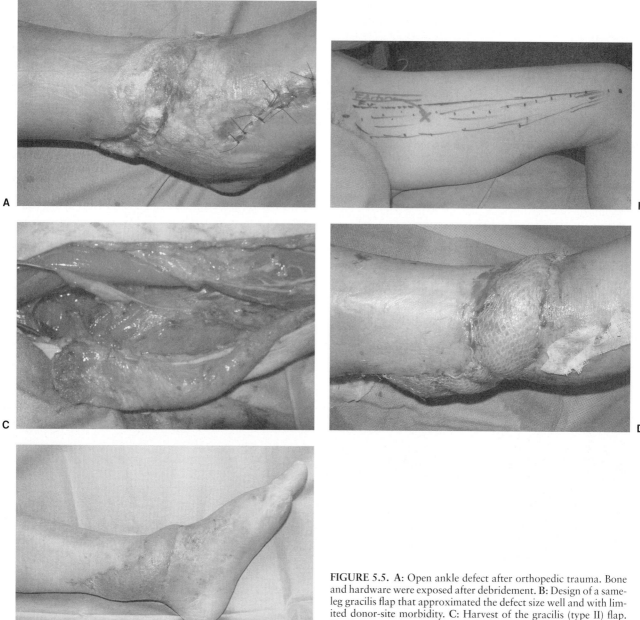

FIGURE 5.5. A: Open ankle defect after orthopedic trauma. Bone and hardware were exposed after debridement. **B:** Design of a same-leg gracilis flap that approximated the defect size well and with limited donor-site morbidity. **C:** Harvest of the gracilis (type II) flap. **D:** Intraoperative coverage of this small defect with well-vascularized muscle. **E:** Several-month postoperative picture showing excellent healing and recontouring.

known or likely, it is used to provide excess coverage so that reliable coverage on re-exploration can be assured.

Flap design is essentially the same for both regional transposition and microvascular transplantation of muscle and musculocutaneous flaps. The reconstructive needs are analyzed and treated in a composite fashion. Like tissues are chosen to reconstruct the defect for both functional and aesthetic purposes. The consistent long vascular pedicle to most types I, II, and V muscles allows rapid elevation of the muscle with its vascular pedicle to be used for microvascular transplantation (Fig. 5.5).

Perforator Flaps

A muscle's axial blood vessel provides perforators that first branch and supply the muscle and then proceed superficially to supply the overlying skin and subcutaneous tissue. These vessels can be meticulously dissected free from the surrounding muscle to produce a direct cutaneous perforator flap (Fig. 5.6). These perforator flaps are cutaneous flaps that are based on the vessels known to traverse various muscle flaps, such as the deep inferior epigastric, thoracodorsal, and superior gluteal vessels. These flaps also demonstrate that unnamed cutaneous/perforating vessels arise from larger, named vessels and travel through muscles or muscle septums to supply a large cutaneous territory. The reliability of these flaps is clearly more robust than previously thought. The problem of anatomic variability to these cutaneous perforators is greater when not following known muscle territories. Perforator flaps, although technically challenging, may decrease some of the functional morbidity associated with the harvest of muscles and overlying muscle fascia in myocutaneous flap harvest. These flaps are widely used for breast reconstruction but can be used throughout the body (8).

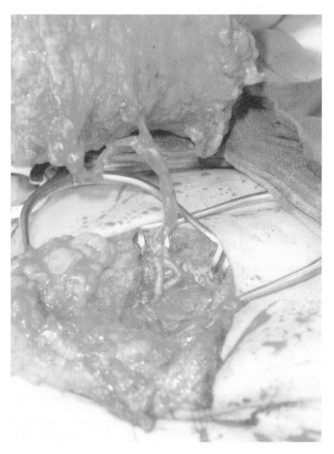

FIGURE 5.6. Perforator TRAM (transverse rectus abdominis musculocutaneous) flap anastomosed to the internal mammary vessels.

Prefabricated Flaps

Prefabrication represents the future of flap-based reconstruction and is in vivo tissue engineering. The goal of this type of reconstruction is to provide all missing components of a given defect by positioning support lining and coverage tissues in preplanned positions and allowing them to vascularize prior to transfer (9). Descriptions of prefabrication have been mostly focused to the head and neck region, but can be translated to all parts of the body. The complexity of the head and neck region with multiple-layered tissues results in defects that can involve mucosal loss from the oral, nasal, and pharyngeal cavities, structural loss of the bony or cartilaginous skeleton, and skin loss. For larger defects there is no one flap that facilitates the reconstruction for all of these missing layers. Precise, planned flap prefabrication can permit these defects to be reconstructed. Currently, the use of thinned flaps with the placement of autologous or bioengineered structural elements such as bone and cartilage by pregrafting and the creation of new vascular bundles in desired donor sites is well reported in the literature. The scientific and clinical advancement of in vivo and ex vivo tissue engineering is the next frontier for reconstructive surgery.

COMPLEX WOUNDS

Muscle and musculocutaneous flaps appear to be ideal for treating difficult soft-tissue, bony, and prosthetic infections. Although treatment to decrease the bacterial inoculum below 10^6 per gram of tissue is necessary, subsequent coverage with well-vascularized muscle appears to further decrease the bac-

terial load, protect against recurrence of infection, and maintain wound closure. Planned treatment of complex wounds with staged debridements to viable, minimally infected tissue, followed by coverage with well-vascularized tissue and appropriate therapy with antibiotics, has revolutionized wound management and is the standard of care in most situations. Experimental studies comparing bacterial resistance in musculocutaneous to cutaneous and fasciocutaneous flaps demonstrate superior resistance to bacterial invasion and subsequent flap necrosis in the muscle and musculocutaneous flaps (10). As muscle flaps appear to provide protection from progressing bacterial injury to the soft tissues and to improve tissue vascularity, muscle flaps have enabled management of complex wounds that traditionally did not respond well to local wound care.

Osteomyelitis

Following debridement of the infected bone associated with chronic osteomyelitis, a muscle flap is transposed as a regional flap or transplanted by microvascular technique into the defect. The flap fills the area of bone debridement with well-vascularized tissue and provides stable wound coverage. As noted above (see Complex Wounds section), short-term culture-specific antibiotic therapy is used simultaneously. This approach has resulted in successful management of chronic infection in the site of bone or cartilage injury (11) (Fig. 5.7). Debridements can be performed in a staged fashion depending on the amount of infection and stability of the patient. Coverage with the muscle flap should be planned immediately after the final debridement. Sternal wounds are a common and problematic example of osteomyelitis. Treatment as noted above with serial debridements, antibiotics, and coverage, usually with a muscle flap such as the pectoralis and/or the rectus, is necessary for ultimate wound closure, chest wall stabilization, and patient survival.

Vascular Insufficiency

Nonhealing wounds associated with vascular insufficiency frequently require extremity amputation. Revascularization of the leg may salvage the extremity, but wound management will still necessitate flap coverage. Although revascularization provides macroscopic blood flow to an extremity, the area of a specific wound may still not have enough microvascular tissue perfusion or may be too large a defect to heal on its own. Muscle flap placement provides transplanted microcirculation and tissue bulk that enables these wounds to functionally heal and, ultimately, provides for limb salvage. Either simultaneous or delayed muscle flap transplantation will allow preservation of a functional extremity despite wound complexity (Fig. 5.8).

Chronic Radiation Wound

Wounds associated with radiation injury do not respond to local wound care and can be some of the most difficult wounds to treat (Chapter 3). Tissue that has undergone high-dose ionizing radiation therapy has limited resistance to injury and ability to regenerate. The effects of this type of radiation are longstanding. Radiated tissue can remain intact for decades, but any form of tissue stress or injury can form a chronic wound with critical structures ultimately being exposed. Treatment of these wounds usually requires wide debridement of necrotic skin, affected soft tissue, and sclerotic or infected bone, and results in a complex wound usually associated with exposure of vital structures. If adjacent muscle units have vascular pedicles

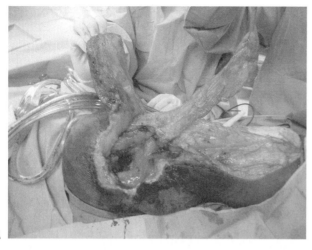

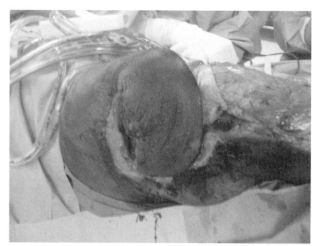

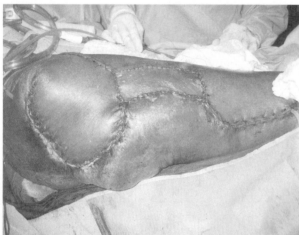

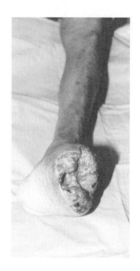

FIGURE 5.7. A: Large, chronic, trochanteric wound with osteomyelitis requiring debridement, proximal femoral head resection, and flap closure using both TFL (tensor fascia lata) and vastus lateralis rotation flap elevation and coverage. **B:** Deep coverage using the vastus lateralis muscle to fill the trochanteric cavity and superficial coverage with a myocutaneous TFL flap. **C:** Coverage completed with flaps and skin graft at the cutaneous donor site.

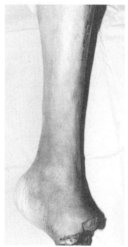

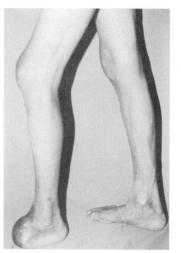

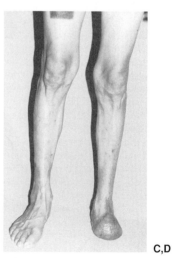

FIGURE 5.8. Muscle transplantation for complex wound associated with extremity revascularization. **A:** Diabetic patient with a renal transplant who has severe peripheral vascular disease. **B:** Nonhealing transmetatarsal amputation site. **C:** Lateral view. Postoperative view 6 months after microvascular transfer of the serratus muscle to the amputation site with end-to-side anastomoses to posterior tibial vessels. **D:** Anterior view. Despite severe vascular insufficiency, the amputation site has healed and the patient remains ambulatory.

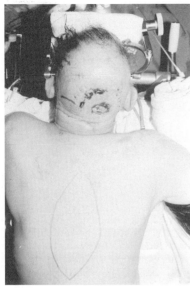
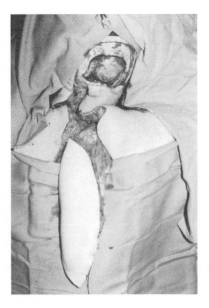
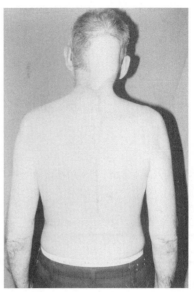

A,B   C

FIGURE 5.9. Muscle transposition for management of chronic osteoradionecrosis. **A:** Design of left trapezius musculocutaneous flap. **B:** Elevated trapezius musculocutaneous flap. (Note: Proximal fibers between the occiput and acromial clavicular joint are maintained in the normal position, providing function preservation.) **C:** One-year postoperative view demonstrates stable coverage at site of musculocutaneous flap inset.

located distant to the radiation port, regional muscle flaps are frequently useful and required for vascularized coverage (12). In areas with poor local muscle availability, such as the head and neck region, particularly in the skull, microvascular transplantation of a muscle flap is generally required for coverage (Fig. 5.9).

Exposed or Infected Prosthesis

When wound coverage overlying the site of a vascular or orthopedic prosthesis fails, early wound debridement, muscle flap coverage, and culture-specific antibiotic therapy frequently allow salvage of the prosthesis while providing stable defect coverage. Once infection is established in the prosthesis, however, it is usually necessary to remove the prosthesis. More common areas of exposure for vascular grafts are in the groin and lower extremity. Groin coverage is usually accomplished reliably with a sartorius muscle flap, but larger flaps can also be mobilized if needed. Orthopedic hardware is more commonly exposed in the midline from spine surgery or over a joint with limited coverage, such as the knee. Spine hardware can usually be well covered with myocutaneous advancement flaps, whereas joint coverage usually requires rotation flaps, such as the gastrocnemius muscle. Lastly, hardware exposure can occur in combination with trauma such as in lower-extremity injuries or after radiation injury leading to exposure of underlying bony or vascular prostheses. In any of these cases, reconstruction with either a local or free muscle flap is almost always indicated.

CONCLUSION

Muscle and musculocutaneous flaps are available in all body regions. With the selection of muscles with a suitable vascular pedicle, the muscle may be safely elevated to provide coverage and simultaneously restore form and function. Thorough knowledge of the muscular anatomy, vascular circulation, and the arc of rotation is required in order to select the optimal mus-

cle unit for specific defects throughout the body. When regional muscle flaps are unavailable or undesirable, the surgeon may elect to transfer distant muscle or musculocutaneous flaps microsurgically. Muscle and musculocutaneous flaps also provide a method to treat complex wounds—such as osteomyelitis and radiation necrosis—that in the past were recalcitrant to wound care. Use of muscle and musculocutaneous flaps broadens the options for defect closure in every area of the body. Nearly any defect can be closed with a careful analysis and a planned approach for reconstruction. Flap reconstruction continues to become more refined with the use of perforator flaps and flap prefabrication.

References

1. Mathes SJ, Nahai F. *Clinical Applications for Muscle and Musculocutaneous Flaps.* St. Louis: CV Mosby, 1982.
2. McCraw JB, Dibbell DG, Carraway JH. Clinical definition of independent myocutaneous vascular territories. *Plast Reconstr Surg.* 1977;60:341.
3. Taylor GI, Palmer JH. The vascular territories (angiosomes) of the body: experimental study and clinical applications. *Br J Plast Surg.* 1987;40(2):113–141.
4. Bakamjian VY, Long M, Rigg B. Experience with the medially based deltopectoral flap in reconstructive surgery of the head and neck. *Br J Plast Surg.* 1971;24(2):174–183.
5. Mathes SJ, Nahai F. Classification of the vascular anatomy of muscles: experimental and clinical correlation. *Plast Reconstr Surg.* 1981;67:177.
6. Terzis JK, Sweet RC, Dykes RW, et al. Recovery of function in free muscle transplants using microneurovascular anastomoses. *J Hand Surg.* 1978;3:37.
7. Yap LH, Whiten SC, Forster A, et al. Sensory recovery in the sensate free transverse rectus abdominis myocutaneous flap. *Plast Reconstr Surg.* 2005; 115(5):1280–1288.
8. Geddes CR, Morris SF, Neligan PC. Perforator flaps: evolution, classification, and applications [review]. *Ann Plast Surg.* 2003;50(1):90–99.
9. Garfein ES, Orgill DP, Pribaz JJ. Clinical applications of tissue engineered constructs. *Clin Plast Surg.* 2003;30(4):485–498.
10. Gosain A, Chang N, Mathes S, et al. A study of the relationship between blood flow and bacterial inoculation in musculocutaneous and fasciocutaneous flaps. *Plast Reconstr Surg.* 1990;86(6):1152–1162, discussion 1163.
11. Mathes SJ, Alpert BS, Chang N. Use of the muscle flap in chronic osteomyelitis: experimental and clinical correlation. *Plast Reconstr Surg.* 1982;69:185.
12. Mathes SJ, Alexander J. Radiation injury [review]. *Surg Oncol Clin N Am.* 1996;5(4):809–824.

CHAPTER 6 ■ TRANSPLANT BIOLOGY AND APPLICATIONS TO PLASTIC SURGERY

W.P. ANDREW LEE, MARYAM FEILI-HARIRI, AND PETER E.M. BUTLER

Allogeneic transplantation is a clinical reality. Although there is potentially no limit to the possibilities for allogeneic reconstructive transplantation, nonautologous tissue is susceptible to immunologically mediated rejection and possible graft loss. At present, the only way to attain long-term allograft survival is the use of prolonged, systemic immunosuppression.

HISTORY

The history of plastic surgery is heavily interwoven with that of transplantation and abounds with myth and legend. The modern era in transplantation started with Tagliacozzi of Bologna, who, in 1597, described a forearm flap to reconstruct the nose. British colonial expansion into India led to the rediscovery of the ancient plastic surgical methods as described in the *Sushruta Samheta*, with the result that forehead flaps were reintroduced into the West by Carpue in the early 19th century. Success with full-thickness skin autografts was reported by Baronio in Milan, who described a series of famous autologous skin grafting experiments in sheep. It was not until 1869 that the problem of graft loss was overcome, when Reverdin made the grafts thinner. In parallel work, Bert demonstrated that for a graft to survive it required ingrowth of new host vessels from the recipient bed. The development of a consistent method for harvesting split-thickness skin grafts was reported by Thiersch in 1886. The question of survival of allogeneic and xenogeneic skin grafts in human recipients was answered by Schone in 1912 and Lexer in 1914, who demonstrated that these grafts did not survive more than 3 weeks after transplantation. Further evidence was provided by Padgett in 1932, when he reported rejection of all skin allografts within 35 days in 40 patients. However, he also demonstrated that skin grafts exchanged between identical twins survived indefinitely.

World War II accelerated progress in transplantation. Gibson, a plastic surgeon at the Glasgow Royal Infirmary, described the "second-set rejection" of skin allografts when treating pilots with burn injuries. (**Today, second-set rejection is defined as the accelerated rejection of allogeneic tissue because of the presence of humoral antibodies from prior exposure to the same allogeneic source.**) Medawar joined Gibson to investigate this phenomenon and, in combination with Billingham and Brent, laid the foundation of modern immunology. In 1955, Murray et al. reported the first successful kidney transplant between identical twins. Subsequent development of tissue typing and more sophisticated methods of immunosuppression transformed organ allograft transplantation into a routine clinical occurrence. Today kidney, liver, heart, and lung allografts achieve prolonged survival with lifelong immunosuppression. Between the years 2000 and 2006, approximately 18 hand transplants and a laryngeal transplant have been successfully carried out. **A partial face transplant was performed successfully in France in 2005.** Others have transplanted knee joints, nerves, tongue, scalp, and ears, and even the flexor tendon apparatus of the hand. The principal ethical dilemma is that reconstructive transplantation requires a level of immunosuppression roughly equivalent to organ transplants, but is performed in healthy patients who have a normal life expectancy. The exposure to lifelong immunosuppression may shorten their life expectancy. Immunologic research has focused on the induction of tolerance to allogeneic and xenogeneic tissues, which would remove the need for long-term immunosuppression. Such an advance would significantly reduce the risk inherent in allogeneic reconstructive transplantation and initiate the next revolution in plastic and reconstructive surgery.

NOMENCLATURE

A *graft* is tissue separated from its donor bed that relies on ingrowth of new vessels from the recipient tissues. A *vascularized graft* (or *flap*) remains attached to its blood supply or becomes revascularized via microvascular anastomoses to recipient vessels. An *autograft* refers to tissue transplanted from one location to another within the same individual. An *isograft* is transplanted between genetically identical individuals, such as transplants between syngeneic mice or human monozygotic twins. An *allograft* (*homograft* in older terminology) is tissue transplanted between unrelated individuals of the same species. A *xenograft* (*heterograft* in older terminology) is transplanted between different species. Transplantation can also be described according to the site into which the tissue is transferred. An *orthotopic* transplant is transferred into an anatomically similar site, whereas a *heterotopic* transplant is transferred into a site different from its origin.

TRANSPLANT IMMUNOLOGY

Transplantation Antigens

Immune responses against tissue grafts are a barrier to successful transplantation; consequently, learning how to suppress these responses is a major goal of transplant immunologists. The antigens of the grafts are proteins that are the principal determinant of acceptance or rejection of tissue grafts exchanged between individuals. These antigens are encoded in the major histocompatibility complex (MHC). T lymphocytes recognize antigens bound to the MHC on the surface of antigen-presenting cells (APCs). There are two types of MHC molecules: class I antigens, which are expressed on all nucleated cells, and class II antigens, which are only expressed on APCs such as B lymphocytes, monocytes, macrophages, dendritic cells (DCs), endothelial cells, and activated human and rat T cells. Every individual is likely to express some MHC proteins that appear foreign to another individual's immune system, except in the case of identical twins. Thus the MHC polymorphism causes rejection of transplants. The MHC antigens in humans are called the human leukocyte antigens (HLAs). The genes coding for these antigens are located on the short arm of chromosome 6. Each individual has two MHC regions, one of paternal and one of maternal origin. Each MHC has an inherited group of HLA genes or haplotypes. HLA class I genes are known as HLA-A, -B, and -C, and HLA class II genes are known as HLA-DP, -DQ, and -DR.

Allogeneic Transplantation

Rejection of transplanted tissue occurs through cellular and humoral immune responses. These responses are generated when the host APC and T lymphocytes respond to the genetic differences in the MHC molecules expressed by the donor cells. After transplantation of the tissue or organs, the host's immune system will mount a response directed against the donor cells in the graft, a process called *transplant rejection*. T cells have fundamental roles in graft rejection, and their responses are rapid and lead to inflammation and tissue destruction. There are two pathways by which the host T cells recognize alloantigens. Following transplantation, at the site of tissue injury, donor APCs migrate toward host lymphoid tissues and directly activate T cells. Once T cells are activated they become effector T cells and migrate to the graft and mediate graft rejection. **This is called the direct pathway of allorecognition and causes acute allograft rejection.** The direct allorecognition can be demonstrated in a mixed leukocyte reaction (MLR) in vitro. In contrast to the direct pathway, host APCs play a significant role in the indirect pathway of allorecognition where they present processed donor antigens to host T cells. Although both pathways of allorecognition are important in mediating graft rejection, the indirect pathway is thought to be of greater significance in the pathogenesis of chronic graft rejection.

DCs are the most efficient APCs and have the capacity to take up and present antigens to T cells in vivo. Because DCs reside in most tissues and have the capacity to endocytose foreign antigens, they serve as the major APCs. DCs rapidly respond to inflammatory stimuli, microbial products, or alloantigens following transplantation, and express high levels of MHC class II and costimulatory molecules essential for T-cell activation.

Successful allogeneic transplantation, without alteration of the immune system, is only possible in transplantation between identical twins. Tissue typing is beneficial in human visceral organ transplantation. Because transplantation between related individuals is not feasible in limb or composite tissue transplantation, long-term immunologic modification is necessary to achieve allograft survival.

Xenogeneic Transplantation

Although the shortage of suitable donor organs is a major problem in transplantation, xenogeneic transplantation offers a possible solution. It is feared that xenografts risk the introduction of pathogenic retroviruses into the human population. Additionally, experimental studies show that hyperacute rejection is a major problem with these grafts and occurs within the first few minutes to hours after transplantation. The presence of "natural" antibodies (i.e., preformed antibodies to xenogeneic tissues in the recipient before exposure to the xenoantigens) is widespread. These antibodies are produced against microorganisms to which nearly everyone has been exposed and which cross-react with cells of other species. Hyperacute rejec-

tion is caused by antibodies against a carbohydrate antigen (α-1,3-galactosyltransferase enzyme), generally termed anti-GAL antibodies. This antigen is present on pig and most mammal cells, whereas it is absent on cells from humans and the highest nonhuman primates (i.e., baboon). **This precludes xenogeneic transplantation of tissues into humans from most species except the highest nonhuman primates.**

Immunosuppression

Progress in experimental transplantation of limb tissues (skin, muscle, bone cartilage, nerve cartilage, nerve, whole limb) mirrors the development of immunosuppressive regimens for visceral organ transplantation. Some of the methods for immune suppression include total-body, thymic, and graft irradiation. Total-body irradiation has been used experimentally in rodents for bone marrow transplantation but produces unacceptable side effects in humans at equivalent doses. Thymic irradiation is directed at lymphoid elements without damage to other tissues, especially the long bones. Attempts to use graft irradiation to reduce antigenicity via γ or ultraviolet (UV) irradiation resulted in the destruction of the radiosensitive and potent antigenic Langerhans cells in skin. It has also been shown experimentally to prolong survival of skeletal tissue allografts. Consequently, graft irradiation can serve as a useful adjunct in combination with other immunosuppressive therapy.

Several pharmacologic drugs are used to control graft rejection. It is important to note that these drugs lack selectivity, cause generalized immunosuppression, and render transplant patients highly susceptible to infections and certain types of malignancies. There are three main groups of immunosuppressive drugs:

- Steroids with anti-inflammatory actions, namely prednisone, inhibit activation of nuclear factor κ B (NF-κB) transcription factor, thus inhibiting cellular activation and cytokine production. Prednisolone was one of the first pharmacologic agents used in allogeneic organ transplantation. Steroids are still used today in combination with other immunosuppressive agents.
- Cytotoxic drugs, namely, cyclophosphamide, methotrexate, and azathioprine, interfere with DNA replication and kill proliferating lymphocytes that are activated by alloantigens.
- Fungal or bacterial products, namely, cyclosporine, tacrolimus (FK506), and sirolimus. Cyclosporine and FK506 inhibit the signaling pathways of T-cell activation by interfering with calcineurin activation and interleukin (IL)-2 gene transcription. Cyclosporine is a metabolic extract from the fungus *Tolypocladium inflatum gamus*, which was described in 1976. Its discovery revolutionized the field of visceral organ transplantation by significantly increasing survival of kidney, heart, and liver allografts. Cyclosporine has been shown to prolong limb allograft survival in various experimental animal models. FK506 is a macrolide lactone antibiotic isolated from the soil fungus. Sirolimus is the newest drug that inhibits multiple biochemical pathways critical for cellular proliferation, with the main target being T cells.

These immunosuppressive agents are reported to allow successful allogeneic transplantation in clinical organ and experimental limb transplants. Although FK506 may have fewer adverse effects, prolonged administration remains too toxic to justify its use in limb tissue transplantation.

Although T cells are the most widely recognized targets for pharmacologic agents, these drugs also have influence on DC phenotype and function. These agents induce a degree of immune tolerance by inhibiting DC maturation and their capacity to stimulate T cells.

Another approach for the generation of an immune-suppressed host environment is depletion of T cells. Polyclonal antithymoglobulin (ATG) and antilymphocyte sera (ALS) have been used in several studies for depletion of recipient T cells and prevention of graft rejection. Furthermore, studies using monoclonal antibodies against T-cell receptors (TCRs), Campath-1H (anti-CD52), a monoclonal antibody to deplete lymphocytes, or anti-CD3 immunotoxin, an anti-CD3 monoclonal antibody conjugated to a mutant form of the diphtheria toxin protein, have yielded beneficial results for prolongation of graft survival. **Immunosuppressive agents may serve as useful adjuncts in limb-tissue transplantation, but the clinical feasibility ultimately hinges on development of immunologic tolerance in the allograft recipient.**

Immunologic Tolerance

Tolerance refers to the state of immunologic acceptance or unresponsiveness of the recipient to the donor allograft or xenograft. Induction of tolerance allows transplantation without the need for prolonged immunosuppression. Acceptance or tolerance of one's own tissues first develops in utero, along with an immunologic ability to recognize foreign tissue. The ability of the immune system to distinguish between self and foreign antigens is controlled by two mechanisms called *central* and *peripheral tolerance*. The thymus plays a major role in the maintenance of tolerance to self and also the induction of tolerance to alloantigens. The mechanism of T-cell tolerance in the thymus is called central tolerance and results from deletion of self or alloreactive T cells upon interaction with bone marrow-derived APCs in the thymus. Because deletion causes the elimination of donor-reactive T cells, it is the most robust mechanism for tolerance induction. Deletion of T cells can be induced by direct injection of donor antigens into the thymus. Following intrathymic injection, donor antigens are presented by APCs to thymocytes, which allows for activation of alloreactive T cells in the thymus and their deletion. Intrathymic injection has been successful in rodents but as yet has been of limited efficacy in larger animals. The most widely used studies for the induction of tolerance is the use of mixed hematopoietic bone marrow transplantations. The combination of total-body irradiation to remove some of the recipient's bone marrow cells is generally followed by donor bone marrow cells, depleted of donor T cells before transplantation, to induce a state of mixed "chimerism." The term *chimera* is derived from the Greek mythologic figure comprised of the parts of different animals. Chimeric animals develop an immune system that is tolerant of both donor and recipient antigens.

Immunologic tolerance is also controlled in the periphery. The mechanisms of peripheral tolerance include T-cell anergy (nonresponsiveness), induction of T-regulatory/suppressor cells, and T-cell deletion. The induction of T-cell anergy has been demonstrated by prevention of T-cell activation. This can be achieved by blockade of T cells and costimulatory molecule interactions. In this approach, monoclonal antibodies against costimulatory molecules on either APCs or T cells are used for the inhibition of T-cell activation. The induction of T-regulatory/suppressor cells is another mechanism to induce T-cell tolerance to donor antigens. The T regulatory cells play a key role in the maintenance of tolerance to both self and foreign antigens. Studies in recent years have demonstrated the potential role for DCs to promote and maintain peripheral tolerance to transplantation antigens. The induction of immunologic tolerance holds promise for the transplantation of limb or composite tissues by reducing or possibly eliminating systemic immunosuppression.

CURRENT TRANSPLANTATION IN PLASTIC SURGERY

Skin

Skin Autograft

The mechanism of autologous skin graft "take" is covered in Chapter 1. The full-thickness skin graft was the first skin graft described. It provides a superior cosmetic result with limited graft contraction but has the disadvantage of less reliable graft "take." The amount of full-thickness skin graft available is also limited if primary closure of donor site is to be achieved. In cases where large areas are to be covered with a full-thickness graft, as in resurfacing a face after burns, the donor area can be increased by preoperative tissue expansion or the donor area can be covered with a split-thickness skin graft. Autologous split-thickness skin grafting as first described by Thiersch is the most commonly practiced form of tissue transplantation in plastic surgery today. The graft can be taken at different thicknesses, depending on the level at which it is harvested through the dermis. It has the advantages of large available donor areas and better graft "take," but is prone to increased graft contraction and hypertrophic scarring, especially in children. Expansion of the split-thickness skin graft by meshing with expansion ratios from 1:1.5 to 1:9 can be useful, and sometimes essential, in extensive burns (see Chapter 18). This method improves graft bed drainage but leads to poorer scar appearance.

Skin Allograft

Skin allografts were the first "organ" transplants and research regarding these allografts provided the foundation of modern transplant immunology. **Skin, however, is strongly antigenic and is subject to rejection even in the presence of surviving visceral organ allografts in the same experimental animal.** This phenomenon is attributed to the "skin-specific antibody," an antigen that is theorized either to be present only in skin, or to exist in all tissues but is presented only by skin following transplantation. The use of skin allografts has been found to be beneficial in large burns with or without concurrent skin autografts. **The immunocompromised state of patients after a major burn delays rejection of allografts, sometimes for several weeks.** Techniques such as using widely meshed autologous split-thickness skin grafts with a meshed allograft overlay improve healing in comparison to autologous graft alone. The availability of skin allografts has increased with the formation of regional tissue banks. Allogeneic skin can be frozen and stored in a manner that maintains its viability for a protracted period of time. There are two factors that prevent its widespread use at present: (a) Harvesting and banking services are not uniformly available, yet demand exceeds supply; and (b) there is a small risk of disease transmission. Cultured allogeneic keratinocytes have also been used as a temporary covering and do survive with immunosuppressive drugs. Such grafts can be grown in culture preemptively for burn treatment but are susceptible to rejection in addition to the problems associated with cultured autografts.

Skin Xenograft

Porcine xenograft has been used as a temporary dressing and, in a technique similar to human allograft, with seeding of autologous grafts beneath it in large burns. The application of xenogeneic dermis has also been found valuable in preparing a wound for subsequent grafting by stimulation of granulation tissue formation. The acellular artificial skin described by Burke uses a bovine collagen "dermis" that is repopulated by recipient fibroblasts. Xenogeneic tissue has limited uses in skin grafting at present, and its cellular components are susceptible to hyperacute rejection, especially in porcine-derived products.

Bone

Bone has two components: (a) inorganic material (largely calcium salts) and (b) a collagen matrix. Two-thirds of bone by weight is represented by inorganic components. Structurally, all bone consists of an outer compact or cortical bone and an inner spongy or cancellous bone. The structural unit of dense cortical bone is the osteon, in which an osteocyte is centrally located and surrounded by concentric layers of bone or lamellae with a system of haversian canals housing nutrient vessels. Resorption of bone is accomplished by osteoclasts, which are multinucleated giant cells. Osteoclasts form new haversian systems by forming a resorptive wedge or "cutting" cone into which osteoblasts and vascular elements migrate and form new bone. Normal bone undergoes a constant cycle of formation and resorption termed the *remodeling cycle*. Cancellous bone is found between the internal lamellae of flat bones and in the metaphysis of long bones. The structure of cancellous bone is more open and consists of trabeculae and spicules. The osteocytes reside on the surfaces of trabeculae and are also found in lacunae in regions of functional stress. The axes of trabeculae are oriented perpendicularly to the stress of external forces such as weight bearing and muscle contracture.

Bone Autograft

A series of histologic events follows transplantation of a bone graft. The classical healing cascade occurs with infiltration of inflammatory cells followed by ingrowth of new vessels and replacement of necrotic tissues. These events vary, depending on the status of graft vascularity (vascularized versus nonvascularized), the characteristics of the graft (cortical versus cancellous), and the condition of the recipient bed. Nonvascularized grafts undergo necrosis, as only the osteocytes on the surface reestablish blood supply and survive. The remainder of the graft is infiltrated by blood vessels from the recipient site and is repopulated by recipient mesenchymal stem cells. Vascular ingrowth in cortical bone grafts occurs through pre-existing haversian canals. There is an initial expansion in osteoclast resorptive activity that increases the porosity and decreases the strength of the graft. Revascularization of cortical grafts may take many months. By comparison, cancellous grafts are more rapidly revascularized within 2 to 3 days by virtue of their open structure. **The process by which vascular tissue invades the graft and brings osteoblasts that deposit new bone has been termed *creeping substitution*.** The strength of cortical and cancellous grafts varies according to the time period. Cancellous grafts are structurally weaker than cortical bone at the outset, but there is early bone formation in cancellous grafts, so the strength of the bone remains relatively constant whereas the necrotic elements are resorbed and remodeled. Cortical bone grafts show incomplete resorption of necrotic bone, and the final mixture of living and dead bone does not approach the strength of a cancellous graft.

Other factors may also influence bone graft survival. Stress is important in bone remodeling by maintaining graft volume and strength. Despite early reports to the contrary, it is currently believed that there is no difference over the long-term between endochondral and membranous bone grafts. The presence of periosteum also affects graft survival. A greater number of osteocytes are present in grafts with preserved periosteum.

Blood supply of bone comes from a dual source of periosteal covering and endosteal or medullary blood vessels that enter the cavity as nutrient vessels. This vascular basis permits transfer of vascularized bone grafts on a vascular pedicled or microvascular manner. Vascularized bone grafts obviate the reparative phase of nonvascularized grafts and do not depend on recipient bed vascularity. The vascularized bone graft is particularly suitable after extensive trauma, chronic scarring, or prior irradiation. Biomechanically, vascularized bone grafts are also superior to nonvascularized grafts (see Chapter 41).

Reconstruction of large bony defects is limited by available autologous donor sites. Although allogeneic bone grafts have been used, another alternative being investigated experimentally is autologous osteocytes expanded in culture and grown in the recipient on polymer scaffolds. No clinical studies have been conducted.

Bone Allograft

Reconstruction of large bony defects in the axial and peripheral skeleton with nonvascularized allogeneic bone has been widely practiced. This has been made possible by well-organized tissue banks and improved methods of bone sterilization and preservation. Very few of the donor cells, if any, in the nonvascularized bone allograft survive. These donor cells express antigens similar to other allogeneic tissues and are susceptible to rejection. The remaining bone acts as a scaffold for ingrowth of recipient mesenchymal stem cells (osteocyte precursors), which repopulates the donor by "creeping substitution." Because of slow union, long-term fixation is required of bone allograft, which is prone to stress fracture and loosening of fixation hardware. In studies of retrieved human allografts, however, union was seen at the graft–host interface.

Vascularized bone allograft is susceptible to immunologic rejection. The humoral and cellular response generated were found to be similar in intensity and timing as those generated by other vascularized allogeneic limb tissues, such as skin and muscle. Although individual bone cells express antigens, the predominant antigenic stimulus in a bone allograft is thought to be derived from the marrow. **Removal of bone marrow by irradiation or replacement with recipient marrow has been shown experimentally to prolong allograft survival.** Like any other allogeneic tissue, this rejection process can be ameliorated with immunosuppression, and long-term survival of orthotopic vascularized skeletal allograft has been achieved in animal models. However, the adverse effects of prolonged immunosuppression required for survival of a vascularized bone allograft preclude its clinical application currently.

Cartilage

Cartilage is composed of chondrocytes within lacunae dispersed throughout a water-laden matrix. The matrix is composed predominantly of proteoglycans and type II collagen. Water is important, as cartilage has no intrinsic blood supply and relies on diffusion of nutrients and oxygen through the matrix. The combination of water and proteoglycans imparts the characteristic of viscoelasticity, depending on the relative concentrations of both elements. The variable water content in the matrix causes a balanced tension within it and helps maintain its three-dimensional shape. The viscoelastic property of the matrix confers "memory" such that cartilage returns to its original shape after deformation. Surgical manipulation or scoring disrupts this equilibrium. In contrast to osteocytes, chondrocytes have little reparative ability and heal by forming fibrous scar tissue. Histologically, there are three types of cartilage: hyaline, elastic, and fibrocartilage.

Cartilage Autograft

The use of cartilage autografts is widespread and includes nasal, auricular, and craniofacial skeleton and joint reconstruction. As for bone grafts, potential autologous cartilage donor sites are limited, and therapeutic options include the use of allogeneic or xenogeneic cartilage. Recent developments in tissue-engineering techniques have enabled the expansion of chondrocytes in culture. These cells were seeded experimentally onto biodegradable polymers to form new autologous cartilage. **Unlike bone allografts, cartilage grafts do not resorb and, unless infected, maintain their exact stage indefinitely.** An interesting adjunct involves the use of an injectable polymer, which ultimately would allow delivery of autologous cartilage percutaneously or arthroscopically.

Cartilage Allograft

Chondrocytes express HLA antigens on their surface and are thus immunogenic in isolation. Cartilage, however, is immunologically privileged as a consequence of the shielding of chondrocytes by its matrix, which is only weakly antigenic. Surgical scoring or dicing of cartilage allograft with resultant exposure of allogeneic cells hastens cartilage resorption.

Cartilage allografts have been used successfully for similar applications as autologous cartilage. Allogeneic cartilage can be either preserved or fresh. Preserved cartilage has the advantage of a more abundant supply and decreased risk of infection in comparison to fresh cartilage. Although immunologically privileged, cartilage allografts are still susceptible to loss of volume through resorption. It is a matter of debate whether this is caused by immunologic rejection or lack of viable cells following preservation. It has also been noted that small allografts are less prone to volume loss than larger grafts.

Cartilage Xenograft

Some authors advocate the use of bovine-derived cartilage xenografts. However, both chondrocytes and matrix are subject to xenogeneic mechanisms of rejection with a generally poorer outcome in comparison to autologous or allogeneic cartilage grafts. Attempts to modify these xenogeneic responses by altering the graft's immunologic stereotactic structure has been reported as being beneficial.

Nerve

Nerve Autograft

The best clinical outcome following nerve transection is achieved with primary repair. More extensive injuries or a delay in repair may result in a nerve gap following debridement of damaged nerves, and a nerve graft may be necessary to achieve neurorrhaphy without tension. The nerve graft undergoes the same degenerative process as in the distal nerve after division (see Chapter 8). The myelin sheath remains, with Schwann cells that act as a biologic conduit for the regenerating axons. Vascularized nerve grafts are theoretically advantageous, particularly in scarred beds. Other "conduits" used as nerve grafts include autologous vein, silicone tubes seeded with Schwann cells, and freeze-fractured autologous muscle.

Nerve Allograft

Autologous nerve grafts with acceptable donor-site morbidity are limited, and extensive nerve reconstruction might require other sources, such as nerve allografts. Immunologic rejection of nerve allograft can be ameliorated experimentally with immunosuppressive drugs, and in rodents, axons were found to traverse the allogeneic nerve graft. A similar result has also been demonstrated in primates. Immunosuppression was necessary during axonal regeneration, but in some studies could be terminated afterwards with satisfactory nerve functions. In the only clinical experience, Mackinnon reported return of motor and sensory functions in the upper or lower limbs of six of seven patients following nerve allograft reconstruction.

Limb

The ability to use allogeneic limb tissues would revolutionize the field of reconstructive surgery. Transplantation of vascularized limb tissue allograft is technically achievable because of well-developed microvascular techniques. Allograft survival has been achieved experimentally with various immunosuppressive regimens. Normal wound healing and bony growth occur following experimental transplantation. Return of neuromuscular function has been observed in limb allografts of animals treated with immunosuppression, including those of nonhuman primates. The tissue components of a limb allograft (such as skin, subcutaneous tissue, muscle, bone, and blood vessel) were found to possess differing immunogenic mechanisms and encounter rejections that vary in timing and intensity. Techniques that selectively decreased the antigenicity of its component parts were found to prolong overall allograft survival.

The first hand transplant, which was performed in Lyon, France, demonstrated that limb transplantation was possible with modern immunosuppressive drugs. When the transplanted hand was amputated as a consequence of patient noncompliance with the immunosuppressive regime, it further demonstrated that patient selection criteria must be objective and robust. Between 1998 and 2003, 18 patients received hand transplants, including six bilateral transplants. Preliminary results demonstrate return of protective sensation and hand motor function from extrinsic (host) muscles. However, fine sensibility, such as two-point discrimination and intrinsic muscle function, were observed in only a small minority of transplanted hands by an independent observer. Hand-transplant recipients have generally experienced an enhanced body image and greater independence in daily activities, particularly in bilateral recipients. However, as mentioned earlier, reconstructive transplantation is very different from other forms of transplantation. It is performed in healthy patients who have a normal life expectancy. The allograft they receive may increase the *quality* of their life, but because of immunosuppressive complications, the *quantity* of life may be affected. So far these procedures have required a level of immunosuppression equivalent to organ transplants. This exposes the patient to the same risks as other allograft recipients face, including organ toxicity, opportunistic infection, and malignancy.

In the case of hand transplantation, many surgeons consider unilateral hand transplants difficult to justify, whereas some believe the indication exists for bilateral amputees. The justification is functional benefit, as it has been reported that the transplanted hands perform better than a prosthesis and comparable to the function of a replanted hand. However, chronic rejection may be a long-term obstacle to limb transplantation. In solid organs, chronic rejection from progressive fibrosis as high as 50% has been reported over a 10-year period after transplantation. In the limb, chronic rejection would result in loss of function. Furthermore, episodes of rejection occurring throughout the life of the transplant might lead to scarring in muscle and nerve, thus worsening function in the limb. When this occurs in other composite tissue transplants, such as the face, the risk-to-benefit assessment becomes even more difficult. Nevertheless, it is difficult to make judgments about the risk-to-benefit balance of composite tissue transplants for reconstructive purposes because the improvement in quality of life cannot be measured objectively.

Face

The consideration for transplantation of face, or any face or nonorgan body part, is similar to that for the hand transplant. Although the partial face transplant in France in 2005 demonstrated its technical feasibility, the debate on reconstructive transplantation is increasingly focused on the risk-to-benefit balance. It has also become more evident that there are many patients who cannot be reconstructed adequately with autogenous tissues yet who stand to benefit from composite-tissue transplants. Many questions remain unanswered regarding face transplant, such as the optimal tissue layers (skin, subcutaneous fat, muscle) for transplantation and the degree of resultant facial expression.

FUTURE TRANSPLANTATION

The risks of chronic immunosuppression along with the prospect of chronic rejection make allogeneic reconstruction a high-risk undertaking. However, development of specific and less-toxic immunosuppressive agents or effective tolerance induction regimens may alter the risk-to-benefit ratio to realize widespread transplantation of composite-tissue allografts. Genetic matching between donor and recipient has been shown to be of benefit in swine limb transplantation. Site-specific immunosuppression, whereby the immunosuppressant is delivered to the site of action with a reduced systemic administration is being investigated. Development of monoclonal antibodies that block a specific step in the rejection cascade provides a potential additional adjunct.

The focus of research in transplantation is on the development of immunologic tolerance. Clinical tolerance has been achieved to renal allografts. Tolerogenic regimens have reduced the need for immunosuppression in other organ transplants. In a swine model, chimeras possessing both donor and recipient cells have been created via donor marrow infusion that accepted limb allografts without long-term immunosuppression in the prenatal and adult animals. If successful, this could be the prerequisite for the widespread clinical use of transplantation in reconstructive surgery.

Suggested Readings

Colson Y, Zadach K, Nalesnik M, et al. Mixed allogeneic chimerism in the rat: donor-specific transplantation tolerance without chronic rejection for primarily vascularized cardiac allografts. *Transplantation*. 1995;60:971.

Cupps TR, Fauci AS. Corticosteroid-mediated immunoregulation in man. *Immunol Rev*. 1982;65:133.

Dunn DL. Problems related to immunosuppression. Infection and malignancy occurring after organ transplantation. *Crit Care Clin*. 1990;6:955.

Hettiaratchy S, Melendy E, Randolph MA, et al. Tolerance to composite tissue allograft across a major histocompatibility barrier in miniature swine. *Transplantation*. 2004;77:514.

Lee WPA, Mathes DW. Hand transplantation: pertinent data and future outlook. *J Hand Surg*. 1999;24A:906.

Lee WPA, Nguyen VT. Perspective on hand transplantation. *Clin Plast Surg*. 2005;32:463.

Lee WPA, R JP, Bourget JL, et al. Tolerance to limb tissue allografts between swine matched for major histocompatibility complex antigens. *Plast Reconstr Surg*. 2001;107:1482.

Lee WPA, Yaremchuk MJ, Pan Y-C, et al. Relative antigenicity of components of a vascularized limb allograft. *Plast Reconstr Surg*. 1991;87:401.

Mackinnon SE, Doolabh VB, Novak CB, et al. Clinical outcome following nerve allograft transplantation. *Plast Reconstr Surg*. 2001;107:1419.

Morel PA, Feili-Hariri M, Coates PT, et al. Dendritic cells, T-cell tolerance, and therapy of adverse immune reactions. *Clin Exp Immunol*. 2003;133(1):1.

Petit F, Paraskevas A, M AB, et al. Face transplantation: where do we stand? *Plast Reconstr Surg*. 2004;113:1429.

Silvers WK, Bartlett ST, Chen HD, et al. Major histocompatibilitty complex restriction and transplantation immunity. A possible solution to the allograft problem. *Transplantation*. 1984;37(1):28.

CHAPTER 7 ■ IMPLANT MATERIALS

ARNOLD S. BREITBART AND VALERIE J. ABLAZA

The history of implant materials can be traced to 3000 B.C., when the Incas of Peru used gold and silver to repair trephination defects. Petronius offered an early description of the use of alloplastic materials in 1565 when he described closure of a cranial defect with a gold plate. Over the next 300 years, the use of implants was sporadic and often complicated by infection. The use of synthetic materials as bioimplants did not become widespread until after the 1940s, when advances in biomaterial science led to the development of numerous materials suitable for implantation.

Alloplastic implantation is indicated for the stabilization of fractures and for the reconstruction or augmentation of soft tissue defects or bony deformities. **The ideal implant material produces no foreign-body inflammatory response, does not support the growth of microorganisms, and should be sterilizable, nontoxic, nonallergenic, noncarcinogenic, and biologically compatible.** Other criteria for the ideal implant material include resistance to strain and deformation, ease of removal, ease of shaping into the desired form, and, in certain circumstances, radiolucency.

The selection of a particular implant depends on the specific requirement for its use. Certain implants are more appropriate for soft-tissue augmentation, whereas others are used for bone contouring or reconstruction. The possibility of encapsulation or tissue ingrowth is also relevant to the choice of an implant. For example, the strength of integrated polypropylene mesh and the rigid incorporation of a bone substitute are often desirable, whereas the encapsulation of a silicone Hunter rod allows for free gliding of a subsequent tendon graft.

The use of autologous tissue, particularly vascularized autologous tissue, may be more appropriate in many circumstances, especially when conditions for implantation are not optimal. These include a history of radiotherapy, marginal blood supply of the surrounding tissue, or tenuous soft-tissue coverage over the implant. In these circumstances, the risk of implant-related complications, including infection and implant extrusion, are significant, and the use of an alloplastic implant should be avoided. Implants are less likely to tolerate overlying wound-healing problems than autologous tissue, and in such circumstances may require removal of the implant when a reconstruction with autologous tissue might have been salvaged. In addition, because the complications of alloplastic materials may develop long-term, one must not make early assumptions about the safety of these implants.

Implants, however, can be used as alternatives to autogenous tissue in selected cases, and as such, have the advantages of avoiding operative time for graft harvesting, the absence of donor site morbidity, and an unlimited supply. Unlike autologous tissue, implants can be fabricated in such a manner that they undergo no resorption, and therefore may be preferable to autologous grafts in certain cases. In particular, implants have been used as bone graft substitutes with much success in orbital floor reconstruction, cranioplasty, and maxillofacial reconstruction.

The basic classification of implant materials most commonly used includes metals, calcium ceramics, polymers, and biologic materials (Table 7.1).

METALS

Metals are primarily used in plating systems for craniomaxillofacial internal fixation and hand surgery, and as Kirschner wires (K-wires), cranial plates, hemoclips, rods, and artificial joints. Stainless steel, cobalt-chromium, and titanium are the principal metals currently available for biologic implantation. Characteristics of a desirable metal implant include biocompatibility, strength, resistance to corrosion, and imaging transparency.

Stainless steel is an alloy composed of iron, chromium, nickel, molybdenum, manganese, and silicone; it was first used in biomedical implants in the 1920s. Although all of the metals are biocompatible, stainless steel miniplates for rigid fixation in craniofacial surgery were found to undergo corrosion with the potential for implant failure after several years. With regards to magnetic resonance imaging (MRI), stainless steel may have the potential to cause artifacts or movement.

The development of Vitallium (Howmedica, Rutherford, NJ) helped to overcome the problem of corrosion. Vitallium is composed primarily of cobalt and chromium, with molybdenum, nickel, manganese, and silicone added to increase strength. The superior corrosion resistance of Vitallium is partially a result of the surface formation of a protective oxide film. Although Vitallium alloys have the greatest tensile strength of the metals in terms of fracture and resistance to fatigue, they are difficult to bend or shape. Compared to stainless steel, Vitallium has no magnetic properties and causes less artifact on computerized tomography (CT) or MRI scans than does stainless steel.

Titanium is the most recently developed alloy and has generally replaced the use of stainless steel and Vitallium in craniofacial plating systems. It is available as pure titanium, as well as a stronger alloy of titanium in combination with aluminum and vanadium. In the unalloyed form, titanium is more malleable than stainless steel or Vitallium, which facilitates easy and precise molding to fit the contours of the facial skeleton. Despite its malleability, titanium's tensile strength is similar to that of Vitallium. The protective oxide layer that forms on the surface of titanium makes it the least corrosive metal for implantation. **It also induces significantly less scatter on CT and MRI scans than either stainless steel or Vitallium, thereby allowing for postoperative imaging with minimal bone distortion.**

Gold has also been used as an implant material, but with limited applications. Although gold is resistant to corrosion, its lack of strength and high cost has generally made it a suboptimal choice as an implant. It is, however, used as an upper eyelid weight in cases of facial nerve dysfunction.

TABLE 7.1

IMPLANT MATERIALS

Metals
  Stainless steel
  Vitallium (cobalt-chromium)
  Titanium
  Gold
Calcium ceramics
  Hydroxyapatite
  Tricalcium phosphate
  Hydroxyapatite cement
  Bioactive glass
Polymers
  Silicone
  Polymethylmethacrylate
  Hard tissue replacement (HTR) polymer
  Polyesters (Dacron, Mersilene)
  Biodegradable polyesters (polyglycolic acid,
    poly-L-lactic acid)
  Polyamides (Supramid, Nylamid)
  Polyethylene (Medpor)
  Polypropylene (Prolene, Marlex)
  Cyanoacrylates
  Polytetrafluoroethylene (Teflon, Gore-Text)
Biologic materials
  Collagen
  AlloDerm
Discontinued materials
  Polyurethane
  Proplast

Metals are also used as osseointegrated implants to attach dental and facial prostheses. Most of the available implants are composed of titanium. Because bone grows into the implant and bonds to its surface, the implant becomes rigidly fixed (osseointegrated) and is resistant to infection. The development of osseointegrated implants was pioneered in Sweden by Branemark. They have been used as bone anchors to which epitheses are secured, most commonly for dental, auricular, ocular, and nasal restoration.

CALCIUM CERAMICS

Calcium phosphate ceramics are extensively used as bone graft substitutes. They are biocompatible, can be fabricated into different shapes, and, depending on the porosity, are osteoconductive, providing a scaffold for bone ingrowth. The primary calcium phosphate ceramics in clinical use are hydroxyapatite, tricalcium phosphate, and calcium phosphate bone cements.

Hydroxyapatite $[Ca_{10}(PO_4)_6(OH)_2]$ is converted as a replica from naturally occurring calcium carbonate coral by a hydrothermal exchange process. Its porous structure has parallel channels and interconnecting fenestrations and has a macroscopic architecture resembling that of human cancellous bone (1). It is commercially available in both block form and as granules (Interpore, Cross International, Irvine, CA) and does not resorb.

Tricalcium phosphate $[Ca_3(PO_4)_2]$ is prepared synthetically, and its pore structure is more random than that of hydroxyapatite. Unlike hydroxyapatite, tricalcium phosphate is resorbable, with resorption rates ranging from 30% to 85% by 6 months, depending on the porosity and implantation con-

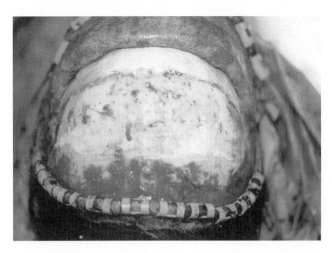

FIGURE 7.1. Secondary reconstruction of post-traumatic frontal bone deformity with onlay hydroxyapatite cement.

ditions. Tricalcium phosphate is also available in block form and in granules, and has been used clinically in the repair of traumatic defects of long bones.

Hydroxyapatite has been widely used as a bone graft substitute, most successfully as an interpositional graft. It has also been used in its block form as an onlay graft, but with somewhat less success. Hydroxyapatite granules, when mixed with blood and microfibrillar collagen to form a paste, have been used for craniofacial skeletal augmentation.

The principal disadvantages of calcium phosphate ceramics are that they are brittle, have low tensile and compressive strength, and may be difficult to fix into position. However, because they are osteoconductive, they are incorporated into surrounding tissue by both bone and fibrous tissue ingrowth, and become vascularized.

Calcium phosphate bone cements are among the most recently developed bone graft substitutes (2). These materials can be used in the repair of cranial defects and in the restoration or augmentation of bony contours of the craniofacial skeleton for non–stress-bearing applications (Fig. 7.1). The commercially available materials (Norian CRS Bone Cement, BoneSource, and Mimix) are supplied as variations of calcium phosphate powders, which are mixed intraoperatively with a solution to form a puttylike substance. These substances can then be used to fill cranial defects or as onlay materials for craniofacial augmentation or restoration. It generally hardens within 5 to 10 minutes to become a structurally stable osteoconductive implant. Norian CRS Bone Cement (Synthes, Paoli, PA) is comprised of a powder of monocalcium phosphate monohydrate, α-tricalcium phosphate, and calcium carbonate, which is mixed intraoperatively with sodium phosphate solution. It hardens within 10 minutes and forms dahllite, the primary mineral component of bone. BoneSource (Stryker-Leibinger, Kalamazoo, MI) is similarly prepared by mixing calcium phosphate salts and sodium phosphate solution, and converts to hydroxyapatite. Mimix (W. Lorenz Surgical, Jacksonville, FL) is a mixture of tetracalcium phosphate and tricalcium phosphate, which is mixed with citric acid to form a hydroxyapatite material. The calcium phosphate-based bone cements undergo a limited degree of resorption and replacement with bone at the periphery. These bone cements are also used in conjunction with resorbable miniplates (see Biodegradable Polyesters below) in order to provide additional structural stability in the reconstruction of larger cranial defects.

Calcium phosphate ceramics have been combined with bone growth factors in an attempt to increase the amount of bone ingrowth within the implant. This improves both the incorporation and fixation of the implant. Tricalcium phosphate combined with osteogenin, one of the bone morphogenetic proteins, has potential as a bone graft substitute because it is replaced by new bone ingrowth as the tricalcium phosphate resorbs. Experimentally, tricalcium phosphate-osteogenin composite maintains its volume over time, while being replaced by new bone (3).

Bioactive glass is a related material; it forms a surface layer of apatite in vivo, which promotes the formation and attachment of bone. Nova Bone (Porex Surgical, Fairburn, GA) is a synthetic bioactive glass consisting of 45% sodium oxide, 45% silica dioxide, 5% calcium, and 5% phosphate. This material is osteoconductive and promotes bone formation at the bioactive glass–bone interface. It has been used for periodontal and alveolar ridge repair, orbital floor reconstruction, and, when mixed with autogenous bone particles, for cranial vault reconstruction (4).

POLYMERS

Polymers are the most extensively used alloplastic materials and have applications in both bone and soft-tissue reconstruction and augmentation. The structure of polymers consists of long chains of repeating basic units that can reach high molecular weights.

Commonly used polymer biomaterials include silicone, polymethylmethacrylate, polyesters, nylon, polyethylene, polypropylene, cyanoacrylates, and polytetrafluoroethylene.

Silicone

Silicone, or dimethylsiloxane, consists of a monomer backbone of interlinked silicone and oxygen molecules, with methyl and, occasionally, vinyl or phenyl side groups, in a varying number of repeating units. This material is very stable, highly biocompatible, nontoxic, and insoluble in body fluids. Although silicone is considered biologically inert, it does elicit a mild foreign-body reaction, which is followed by encapsulation, but without tissue ingrowth.

The viscosity of silicone is determined by the extent of polymerization. Short polymer chains result in liquid silicone with less viscosity, lengthening of the chains results in gel-type substances, and cross-linking of the polymer chains results in high-viscosity silicone rubber.

Liquid silicone was developed in 1963 and used for augmentation of the breast and face prior to the development of a purer grade of injectable silicone, which was available for investigational purposes. This new formulation was in the process of being considered as an investigational new drug by Dow-Corning in 1976, when the accumulation of reported adverse effects, including inflammation, induration, discoloration, ulceration, migration, and silicone granuloma formation led Dow-Corning to withdraw its application. **Liquid silicone is not Food and Drug Administration (FDA) approved and its use should be condemned.**

The polymerization of dimethylsiloxane into longer chains results in silicone gel. This form of the polymer has been used primarily for filling breast implants, and has also been used in buttock implants and in the correction of contour deficiencies. The use of silicone gel, however, has been surrounded by the controversy related to concerns about migration, toxicity, and an unproven association with human adjuvant disease, leading to restriction of the use of silicone gel implants by the FDA in 1992. As they await FDA approval for unrestricted use, silicone gel breast implants are currently available in the United States only as part of a protocol for use in breast reconstruction, or

in cases where implant-related complications necessitate implant replacement. Although the initial clinical experience and early data related to the newer generation of silicone gel breast implants are quite favorable, additional longer-term data are currently being accumulated. Cohesive gel implants, made with a higher-viscosity silicone gel have also been developed, and, although available in Europe and elsewhere, are not yet FDA approved for use in the United States.

The cross-linking of polymerized chains of dimethylsiloxane results in a silicone rubber elastomer. This high-viscosity silicone is used for fabricating tissue expanders, the outer shell of both saline-filled and silicone gel-filled breast implants, and as an onlay material for the augmentation of the bony skeleton and soft tissues. Solid silicone implants are commonly used for chin and malar augmentation, and have been used in nasal, chest, and calf augmentation, as well as in joint replacement and tendon reconstruction.

The use of silicone elastomer implants has been associated with capsule formation and contracture, particularly with breast implants, which may lead to implant distortion and hardness. Texturing of the implant surface was thought to minimize this potential for capsular contracture, but it is still not clear if it offers any advantage. Silicone synovitis is a recognized complication of silicone implant arthroplasty, which usually requires removal of the implant.

Polymethylmethacrylate

Polymethylmethacrylate (PMMA) is a high-molecular-weight polymer used as a replacement for bone. It is biocompatible, biologically inert, and rigid. When liquid methylmethacrylate monomer is added to powdered granules of methylmethacrylate polymer, a moldable dough forms as the monomer polymerizes and binds together pre-existing polymer particles, which hardens in about 10 minutes. **Because the polymerization process results in an exothermic reaction that can generate high temperatures, saline irrigation should be used to cool the surrounding tissues during the curing process.** PMMA can be custom-made preoperatively or prepared intraoperatively.

PMMA is a widely used alloplastic material for cranial bone reconstruction (5). It can be used alone or in combination with wire or mesh reinforcement (Fig. 7.2). The immobility and relatively low stresses intrinsic to the calvarium are responsible for the low morbidity of PMMA cranioplasty.

Most of the potential complications are related to the exothermic reaction produced during the curing process, which may result in local tissue damage, including bone necrosis and soft-tissue injury. Local and systemic allergic reactions have on occasion been observed and are attributed to the toxic effects of the unbound monomer.

Hard tissue replacement (HTR) polymer (W. Lorenz Surgical, Jacksonville, FL) is a nonresorbable composite of PMMA beads fused with polyhydroxyethylmethacrylate, which is then coated with calcium hydroxide. HTR polymer is biocompatible and demonstrates remarkable compressive strength in spite of its extensive porosity. Although it has not been widely used, applications for HTR include chin and malar augmentation, as well as correction of the temporal "hourglass" deformity following postsurgical temporalis atrophy. It has also been used as a prefabricated computer-generated implant based on three-dimensional CT scan images for cranial defect reconstruction (6).

Polyesters (Dacron, Mersilene)

Dacron (polyethylene terephthalate) is a biocompatible, flexible, nonabsorbable polymer that is used as a suture material,

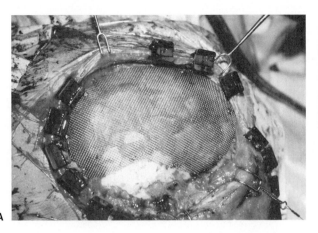
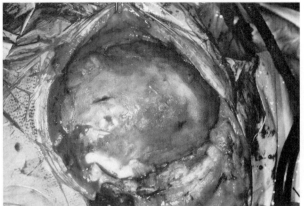

A   B

FIGURE 7.2. Reconstruction of cranial defect with titanium mesh-reinforced polymethylmethacrylate. A: Placement of titanium mesh. B: Polymethylmethacrylate applied to mesh.

as a prosthetic material for arterial replacement, and as a mesh (Mersilene mesh, Ethicon, Inc., Somerville, NJ). It is a suitable implant for applications requiring both tensile strength and stability, and has been used for abdominal and chest wall reconstruction, as well as for chin and nasal augmentation.

Biodegradable Polyesters (Polyglycolic Acid, Poly-L-Lactic Acid)

In contrast to the aromatic polyester Dacron, the biodegradable polyesters are aliphatic compounds that are more susceptible to hydrolysis. Polyglycolic acid (PGA) and poly-L-lactic acid (PLLA) are two of these polymers that are degraded in the body at physiologic pH over the course of several months. These resorbable polymers are available as mesh sheets for body wall reconstruction, and as rods for the internal fixation of fractures and osteotomies.

Biodegradable polyesters have been widely used in the fabrication of resorbable miniplates and screws for the fixation of bones of the craniofacial skeleton, and as orbital floor implants (7). They are especially indicated for use in pediatric craniofacial fixation, because the potential for intracranial migration (as sometimes seen with permanent metallic plates, screws, and wires) is avoided (Fig. 7.3). These biodegradable polymers have also been used as components of resorbable craniofacial distraction devices. LactoSorb (W. Lorenz Surgical, Jacksonville, FL) plates and screws are composed of a copolymer of 82% L-lactic acid and 18% glycolic acid. They retain most of their strength for 6 to 8 weeks and absorb within 12 months. Similar resorbable fixation devices fabricated from a copolymer of 70:30 poly (L-lactide-co-D, L-lactide) are also commercially available (Macropore Biosurgery, San Diego, CA).

Endotine Forehead fixation device and Endotine Midface ST 4.5 (Coapt Systems, Inc., Palo Alto, CA) consist of 82% PLLA and 18% PGA and are easy to use, bioabsorbable implants designed to create sutureless soft-tissue fixation during brow lift and midface suspension surgery. The absorbable tines of both these devices allow for multiple points of contact to grasp and elevate soft tissue, holding it in position until the soft tissues adhere to the underlying bone.

PGA has also been applied in the fabrication of resorbable matrices in the tissue engineering of both cartilage and bone, and as tubes for guided nerve regeneration. PGA implants seeded with chondrocytes or genetically modified mesenchymal stem cells have been used as scaffolds in the tissue engineering of articular cartilage (8). PGA matrices seeded with cultured periosteal cells have been used in the tissue-engineered bone repair of calvarial defects (9).

Polyamide (Supramid, Nylamid)

The polyamide compound nylon is available as a woven mesh implant (SupraFOIL, Sepramesh, S. Jackson, Inc., Alexandria, VA). It consists of long chains of amide units that are twisted and then woven. Nylamid is biocompatible, can be easily shaped and sutured, possesses stability as a result of fibrous tissue ingrowth, and has been used successfully as an implant for the repair of orbital floor defects. Polyamide compounds do, however, undergo resorption over time, limiting their applications in facial reconstruction and augmentation.

Polyethylene, Polypropylene (Medpor, Prolene, Marlex)

Polyethylene is an inert material with a high degree of biocompatibility. There are several types of polyethylene compounds available with different biochemical properties, based on the density of the material. Chemical resistance, tensile strength, and hardness increase with increasing density from the low-density polyethylene, to the ultrahigh-molecular-weight polyethylene.

Medpor (Porex) is a high-density porous polyethylene implant that is used in facial reconstruction. It is nonantigenic, nonallergenic, nonresorbable, highly stable, easy to fixate, and is available in a wide variety of preformed shapes (Fig. 7.4). It is produced through a sintering process that produces a contiguous porous polyethylene framework. This porosity allows for vascular and soft tissue ingrowth with incorporation of the implant.

Medpor is most commonly used in the restoration or augmentation of bony contour in the craniofacial skeleton for both reconstructive and aesthetic applications (Fig. 7.5). Medpor has been used as malar, chin, nasal, orbital rim, orbital floor, and cranial implants, as well as an auricular framework in postburn ear reconstruction (10).

Complications of Medpor are unusual, but include exposure and infection. Although the ingrowth of fibrous tissue offers the advantage of positional stabilization, it also creates difficulty should the implant need to be removed.

The substitution of one methyl group for a hydrogen atom in each polyethylene unit results in a loosely woven, high-density polypropylene polymer with biologic properties similar

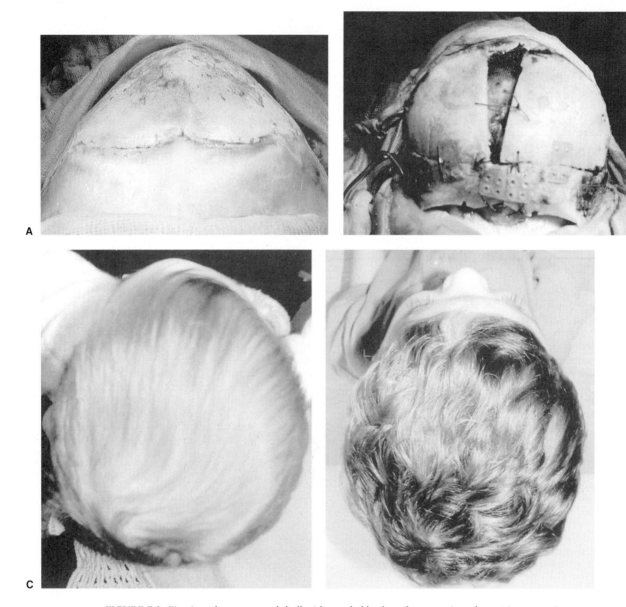

FIGURE 7.3. Fixation of reconstructed skull with resorbable plates for correction of metopic synostosis. A: Trigonocephalic appearance of metopic synostosis. B: Fixation of advanced fronto-orbital segment with resorbable plates and screws. C: Appearance of patient before (*left*) and 1 year after (*right*) surgical treatment of metopic synostosis using resorbable fixation.

to polyethylene. Polypropylene is one of the most inert biomaterials used in surgery, and is available as a woven mesh (i.e., Marlex, Prolene). It is easy to suture, has good tensile strength, and demonstrates early fibrous tissue ingrowth that serves to fix and incorporate the mesh. Polypropylene mesh is commonly used to repair abdominal fascial defects. It is also used in the reconstruction of chest wall defects, either alone or sandwiched around a polymethylmethacrylate core (Fig. 7.6).

Cyanoacrylates

The cyanoacrylates are quick-setting, biodegradable, polymeric tissue adhesives that have become useful tissue-bonding agents. They form a strong, durable bond with most human tissue, particularly those tissues containing a large amount of protein, such as skin and tendon. In addition to their role in

bonding tissues, these polymers are also used as hemostatic and embolic agents.

The cyanoacrylate tissue adhesives polymerize by an exothermic reaction in the presence of water and hydroxyl groups on the wound surface, and thus are effective on moist surfaces. The first of the cyanoacrylate compounds to be synthesized was methyl-2-cyanoacrylate, which was followed by the development of other adhesives, including ethyl-2-cyanoacrylate (Krazy Glue), isobutyl cyanoacrylate (Bucrylate), and butyl-2-cyanoacrylate (Histoacryl). Experimental and clinical applications of cyanoacrylates in plastic surgery include sutureless skin closure for incisions and lacerations, fixation of bone and cartilage grafts, fixation of craniofacial fractures, tendon repair, and tarsorrhaphy.

The FDA approval of Dermabond (2-octyl cyanoacrylate, Ethicon, Inc., Somerville, NJ) as a topical skin adhesive in 1998 has contributed to the increased use of the polymeric tissue adhesives. The liquid polymerizes within minutes after

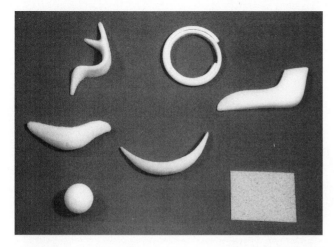

FIGURE 7.4. A variety of Medpor implants, including (clockwise from top left) auricular framework, auricular helix, mandibular angle/body, orbital floor, chin, enucleation, and malar implants.

application to the skin, setting as a thin film that covers the wound edges and peels away in 7 to 10 days. In vitro studies show Dermabond to be an effective barrier against the penetration of bacteria. Indermil tissue adhesive (n-Butyl-2-cyanoacrylate, U.S. Surgical, Norwalk, CT) received FDA approval in January 2004, with the additional claim that it acts as a barrier to microbial penetration as long as the adhesive film is intact.

Polytetrafluoroethylene (Teflon, Gore-Tex)

The basic unit of the polytetrafluoroethylene (PTFE) polymer consists of an ethylene monomer backbone with four covalently bound fluorine molecules. This material is inert and highly biocompatible.

Teflon is synthesized from the polymerization of tetrafluoroethylene gas under high temperature and pressure. It is a

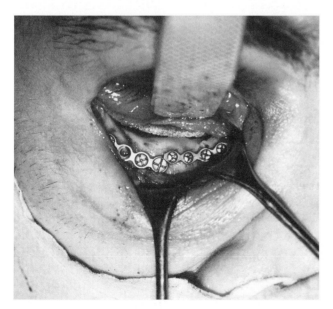

FIGURE 7.5. Medpor implant used to reconstruct orbital floor. Orbital rim fracture has been repaired with titanium plates.

chemically inert polymer with favorable handling characteristics. The main application for Teflon has been in the reconstruction of orbital floor defects.

Gore-Tex (W.L. Gore, Flagstaff, AZ) is an expanded synthetic polymer composed of solid PTFE nodes with interconnecting thin PTFE fibrils that form a grid pattern. It is a pliable, durable, inert, biocompatible material that demonstrates some tissue ingrowth, little inflammatory reaction, and almost no encapsulation. It is available as sheets that are easily contoured or stacked to a desired thickness, as well as solid blocks (SAM Facial Implant, W.L. Gore, Flagstaff, AZ) that can be carved to customized shapes (11). Applications of Gore-Tex in plastic surgery include abdominal fascial reconstruction (Fig. 7.7); chest wall reconstruction; soft-tissue filler for lip, nasal, chin, and malar augmentation; and as treatment for nasolabial and glabellar creases. Composite sheets of polypropylene mesh and expanded PTFE are also available for abdominal wall reconstruction. In this application, the PTFE side is placed on the side in closest proximity to the bowel so as to avoid the adherence of the polypropylene mesh to the underlying bowel.

BIOLOGIC MATERIALS (COLLAGEN, ALLODERM)

Collagen is a large, rod-shaped protein composed of three polypeptide chains arranged in a triple-helix configuration. It is the most common protein in the body and is a widely used biologic implant material (see Chapter 45).

AlloDerm (LifeCell Corp., Branchburg, NJ) is an acellular, structurally and biochemically intact human dermal graft that is used for cosmetic and reconstructive soft-tissue augmentation. Donated human skin is denuded of epithelium, freeze-dried, and decellularized through a special process that preserves the bioactive components without damaging the extracellular dermal matrix and basement membrane architecture. The resulting graft serves as a framework to support cellular repopulation, revascularization at the surgical site, and soft-tissue regeneration by the recipient's own cells (12). Animal studies demonstrate that AlloDerm is nontoxic with no elicitation of an inflammatory response. It has a shelf-life of up to 2 years under standard refrigeration and is rehydrated immediately before use with normal saline or lactated Ringer solution.

The most common uses for AlloDerm include fascial defect repair, wound coverage, lip enhancement, dorsal nasal augmentation, correction of depressed scars and liposuction defects, and nipple augmentation. Depending on the degree of soft-tissue replacement needed, AlloDerm can be used as a single layer or stacked in multiple layers. The graft can be pulled through subdermal tunnels created through small incisions. Cymetra (LifeCell Corp., Branchburg, NJ) is a particulate form of AlloDerm delivered by injection and is most commonly used (as is collagen and hyaluronic acid) for lip augmentation and the filling of prominent nasolabial folds.

DISCONTINUED IMPLANT MATERIALS

The polyurethanes and Proplast are implant materials that are no longer available for clinical use but deserve mention for historical reasons. The polyurethanes are a group of polymers consisting of a diisocyanate and an alcohol. An intense foreign-body giant cell reaction, followed by tissue adhesion, was responsible for the connective tissue ingrowth that resulted in the low capsular contracture rates seen with polyurethane-covered breast implants. Concerns regarding the effect of

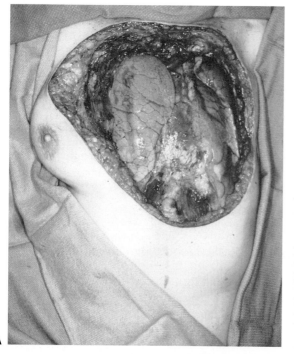

A

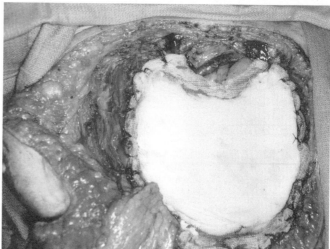

B

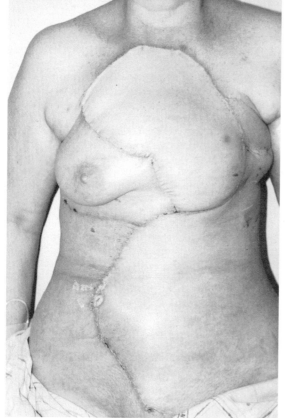

C

FIGURE 7.6. A: Exposure of heart and lungs following resection of sternum and ribs for recurrent chest wall sarcoma. **B:** Reconstruction of chest wall with Marlex-polymethylmethacrylate sandwich. **C:** Coverage with free rectus myocutaneous flap.

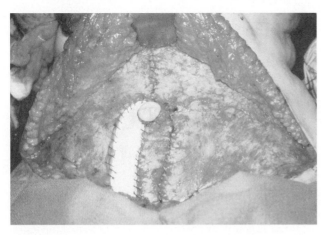

FIGURE 7.7. Abdominal fascial reconstruction with Gore-Tex sheet following harvest of transverse rectus abdominis myocutaneous flap.

toluene-diamine, the breakdown product of polyurethane, resulted in the FDA request for a voluntary delay of production and sales of polyurethane-covered breast implants in 1991, and production was subsequently discontinued.

Proplast I (Vitek, Houston, TX) was introduced as a highly porous, black Teflon and carbon composite with a spongy consistency. Proplast II, a more rigid, white Teflon and alumina compound, was developed as an alternative to Proplast I. Although Proplast was previously regarded favorably, with a wide variety of applications including the correction of bony deformities of the face, skull, and rib cage, the subsequent accumulation of reports of biomechanical failure, intense inflammation, infection, and extrusion related to Proplast temporomandibular joint implants, resulted in the removal of all forms of Proplast from American markets by the FDA in 1990.

References

1. Bucholz RW, Carlton A, Holmes RE. Hydroxyapatite and tricalcium phosphate bone graft substitutes. *Orthop Clin North Am*. 1987;18:323.
2. Burstein FD, Cohen SR, Hudgins R, et al. The use of hydroxyapatite cement in secondary craniofacial reconstruction. *Plast Reconstr Surg*. 1999;104:1270.
3. Breitbart AS, Staffenberg DA, Thorne CHM, et al. Tricalcium phosphate and osteogenin: a bioactive onlay bone graft substitute. *Plast Reconstr Surg*. 1995;96:699.
4. Gosain AK, PSEF DATA Committee. Bioactive glass for bone replacement in craniomaxillofacial reconstruction. *Plast Reconstr Surg*. 2004;114:590.
5. Manson PN, Crawley WA, Hoopes JE. Frontal cranioplasty: risk factors and choice of cranial vault reconstruction material. *Plast Reconstr Surg*. 1986;77:888.
6. Eppley BL, Kilgo M, Coleman JJ. Cranial reconstruction with computer-generated hard-tissue replacement patient-matched implants: indications, surgical techniques, and long-term follow-up. *Plast Reconstr Surg*. 2002;109:864.
7. Eppley BL, Morales L, Wood R, et al. Resorbable PLLA-PGA plate and screw fixation in pediatric craniofacial surgery: clinical experience in 1883 patients. *Plast Reconstr Surg*. 2004;114:850.
8. Mason JM, Breitbart AS, Barcia M, et al. Cartilage and bone regeneration using gene-enhanced tissue engineering. *Clin Orthop Rel Res*. 2000;379S:171.
9. Breitbart AS, Grande DA, Kessler R, et al. Tissue engineered bone repair of calvarial defects using cultured periosteal cells. *Plast Reconstr Surg*. 1998;101:567.
10. Yaremchuk MJ. Facial skeletal reconstruction using porous polyethylene implants. *Plast Reconstr Surg*. 2003;111:1818.
11. Schoenrock LD, Chernoff WG. Subcutaneous implantation of Gore-Tex for facial reconstruction. *Otolaryngol Clin North Am*. 1995;28(2):325.
12. Terino EO. AlloDerm acellular dermal graft. Applications in aesthetic soft-tissue augmentation. *Clin Plast Surg*. 2001;28:83.

CHAPTER 8 ■ PRINCIPLES OF MICROSURGERY

LOK HUEI YAP AND CHARLES E. BUTLER

Microsurgery refers to a set of surgical techniques performed beyond the limits of normal human eyesight. These procedures require magnification by either surgical loupes or an operating microscope. Contemporary procedures that use microsurgical techniques include nerve and blood vessel repairs and grafts, free tissue transfers, and limb replantation.

HISTORY

The first successful end-to-end anastomosis of the carotid arteries in sheep was reported in 1889 by Jassinowski, who used fine, curved needles and silk sutures. In 1897, Murphy reported an invagination method in which two double-ended silk sutures were used to intussuscept one vessel end into another, following which interrupted sutures were used to oversew the overlapping ends. This technique led to anastomotic narrowing and thrombosis in animal experiments, but was used clinically for human femoral artery repair.

Prior to the standardization of vascular repair techniques, there was controversy regarding whether to include the tunica intima vasorum in vascular sutures. Carrel, Burci, and Jassinowski favored excluding the intima, whereas Briau, Döfler, Jensen, and Höpfner recommended including the intima in anastomoses. Guthrie and Carrel examined various techniques for anastomoses and found that inclusion of the intima promoted "uniformly successful results," laying the foundations for standardization of anastomotic techniques (5,12).

The technique of first placing triangulating sutures to ensure equal traction on the blood vessels was first described by Carrel, who received the 1912 Nobel Prize in Medicine and Physiology for his work in this field.

In 1966, Buncke reported rabbit ear replantation with anastomosis of vessels approximately 1 mm in diameter. This microsurgical procedure was made possible by the use of fine instruments adapted from those used by watchmakers and jewelers, as well as by the development of fine sutures swaged on suitably fine needles (2).

Advances in magnification technology paralleled those in surgical technique and were essential to the evolution of modern microsurgical techniques. The first compound microscope was invented by Zacharias and Hans Janseen in 1950. Nylen introduced the *operating microscope* for otolaryngologic surgery. The term *microvascular surgery* was coined by Jacobson, who desired operating on small blood vessels under microscope magnification and demonstrated a 100% patency rate in vessels from 1.6 to 3.2 mm in diameter (5). Further developments included foot-operated microscope controls to free up the surgeon's hands; a beam-splitting device to allow the use of a second set of eyepieces for surgical assistance during procedures; optical zoom and independent focus controls; and cooler fiberoptics with a reduced likelihood of tissue desiccation and with improved signal transmission.

These technical advances, along with increased interest in and knowledge of fine vascular anatomy, have made available the wide variety of microsurgical reconstruction options included in the armamentarium of reconstructive surgeons today.

INDICATIONS FOR FREE TISSUE TRANSFERS

The *reconstructive ladder* algorithm for tissue reconstruction suggests that defects should be reconstructed with the least-invasive option available that will produce successful results, beginning with direct closure and increasing in complexity and potential morbidity to options such as free tissue transfers. Free tissue transfers are usually located at the "top" of the reconstructive ladder and are considered when local or regional tissues are insufficient or suboptimal for reconstruction. The unavailability of local or regional tissues may be a result of infection, inflammation, prior irradiation, insufficient volume or surface area, insufficient vascular pedicle length, and/or the unacceptability of donor site morbidity at that location. Free tissue transfers are also the most suitable option when highly vascularized tissue is required, when specialized tissues such as functional muscle are not available locally, or when specialized components such as vascularized bowel or bone are required. Table 8.1 outlines common indications for free flap reconstructions.

A detailed discussion of the factors involved in choosing a reconstruction method is beyond the scope of this chapter but is covered elsewhere in this book. The operating surgeon should ensure that the tissue chosen is of sufficient size to cover the defect and that the benefits of the procedure chosen outweigh any disadvantages. Other factors to consider include tissue characteristics such as size, color, and composition (e.g., skin, fascia, muscle, bone, and nerve), aesthetics, pedicle length, and potential vessel match in terms of length and size.

PATIENT EDUCATION

The surgeon should establish that the patient is medically prepared for the proposed procedure, which may be complex and lengthy. Microsurgical procedures are not specifically contraindicated in elderly patients provided they are in reasonable health. However, the surgeon should rule out the presence of significant cardiovascular, respiratory, hepatic, or renal dysfunction, and abnormal bleeding or clotting states.

The proposed procedure should be discussed at a level of detail suitable for the patient. This should include a discussion of the likely donor sites for the tissue transfer, the anticipated or potential morbidity, the expected intraoperative and

TABLE 8.1

COMMON INDICATION FOR FREE TISSUE TRANSFER IN RECONSTRUCTIVE SURGERY

Indication	Example
Obliteration or reduction of dead space	Reconstruction after extensive soft-tissue resection
Coverage of exposed bone and/or neurovascular tissue	Reconstruction of calvarial, thoracic, or lower-extremity defect
Volume and contour reconstruction	Reconstruction of the breast
Vascularized enteral conduits	Reconstruction of pharyngeal and esophageal defects
Composite reconstruction	Combined mandibular and floor-of-mouth reconstruction
Functional muscle reconstruction	Facial reanimation for paralysis
Reconstruction and/or replacement of appendages	Digit, penile, and limb reconstructions/replantation

postoperative course, possible donor and recipient site complications, the expected level of discomfort and scarring, and the expected postoperative recovery times needed to regain preoperative function and activity levels.

EQUIPMENT AND OPERATIVE PREPARATION

The correct instrument set should be available for the operating team, along with additional sets in case of accidental damage or contamination of the instruments during the procedure. A microsurgical instrument set includes fine jeweler forceps, vessel dilating forceps, straight and curved microsurgical scissors, and microsurgical needle holders. Heparinized saline solution is frequently used for irrigation of the vessel lumen.

The choice of magnifying equipment depends on individual surgeon preference. Surgical loupes, which typically range from ×3.5 to ×8.0 magnification, can be used for the fine dissection and preparation of vessels. Some surgeons also prefer to use loupes rather than operating microscopes for the vascular anastomoses (10). Advantages of the operating microscope are that it provides wide-field adjustable magnification and it allows significant depth-of-field perception. The microscope should have two eyepieces to allow the surgeon and assistant to operate simultaneously. The use of a video output device allows viewing of the operative field on a separate monitor and is helpful for the scrub team in following anastomotic activity.

The free tissue transfer procedure should be outlined preoperatively to the anesthetic and nursing teams, as well as to the ablative surgical team. This ensures that all parties are aware of the donor and recipient sites and helps to streamline operative activity. The need for use of, or avoidance of, anticoagulation and neuromuscular paralysis, as well as antibiotic prophylaxis, should be discussed with the anesthesiologist. Patient positioning, preparation, and the expected length of the procedure along with any resulting physiologic and anatomic risks should also be discussed. Intravenous and intra-arterial access should be planned in conjunction with the anesthetic and nursing teams to avoid interference with potential flap harvest and recipient sites.

The patient should be positioned for easy access to the flap harvest site and for optimal exposure of the primary surgical site. Dependent and pressure areas on the patient should be padded to avoid pressure damage, and the patient should be well secured on the operating table to allow limited change of position without the risk of a fall.

OPERATIVE TECHNIQUE

Once the recipient site is available (e.g., after tumor resection or debridement), the defect is evaluated, and the final decision regarding the type of reconstruction is made. Surgical templates can be helpful in determining the exact dimensions and shape of the defect, particularly if it has a complex three-dimensional shape.

The recipient vessels are evaluated prior to flap harvest. Factors to evaluate include the presence of vessels, their distance from the defect (pedicle length required), their patency and flow, and their condition (including previous radiation damage, atherosclerotic change, previous trauma, and infection). If the initial vessels considered are inadequate, alternative recipient vessels are sought. Vein grafts may be required to bridge the distance between donor and recipient vessels. Free tissue transfer requires a thorough understanding of the relevant donor and recipient site anatomy of the main arterial and venous supply, major vessel variations, important associated structures, and associated nerve supply. The pedicle dissection should be carried out under magnification and with care taken to avoid injury to the flap blood supply. The length of the pedicle required should be apparent from operative planning and intraoperative measurement. Ideally, the vessels chosen should be of similar diameter to avoid significant size mismatch. The vessels should be handled with care. It is important to minimize handling of the vessels. The vessels should be manipulated by holding the adventitial tissue on the outermost aspect of the vessel wall. It is equally important to avoid significant traction on vessels. Manipulation of the lumen should be minimized to avoid intimal damage.

The anastomoses should be carried out under magnification. The operating table height is adjusted so that the operative field is approximately level with the surgeons' elbows. The microscope setup is one of the most important aspects of an anastomosis. The height of the microscope should be adjusted so that the surgeons can avoid excessive flexion or extension of their cervical spines and ligamentous and muscular strain; the focal length of the objective lens should be adjusted to achieve this. Both eyepieces should be set to neutral optical correction or adjusted for the surgeons' vision if corrective lenses are normally used (1).

The recipient site should be positioned for optimal exposure. This includes retraction of skin flaps or tissue using retractors, tension sutures, or skin hooks. The orientation of the flap pedicle should be checked to ensure that the anastomosis will not be under excessive tension. The pedicle should also be free of acute bends or twists, both before and after completion of the anastomosis. To aid visualization, a small sheet of background material (plastic polymer) of a contrasting color can be placed under the vessels. If the operative field is deep, elevation can be achieved by placing surgical sponges at the base of the defect.

The vessels to be anastomosed are positioned to allow tension-free, surface-to-surface apposition. Once the pedicle length and the orientation of the donor and recipient vessels are decided, low-pressure microvascular clamps are applied for vascular control. Application of vessel clamps on the donor vessels can help eliminate oozing. Both sets of recipient vessels are checked for open branches near the anastomosis that need to be ligated. The cut edges of the vessels are checked for a clean, uniform edge and retrimmed if necessary to avoid stray tissue ends encroaching into the lumen; these can be foci for thrombosis formation. For an end-to-end anastomosis, both vessels are most commonly cut perpendicular to the vascular axis. An oblique cut results in a larger circumference and can be used to minimize vessel size mismatch when coapting vessels of different diameters.

The quality of the luminal intima is then inspected for irregularities such as thrombi, atherosclerotic plaques, and friable, calcified walls. Any debris detected should be gently irrigated away. If a satisfactory internal surface cannot be obtained by a combination of gentle irrigation, then the vessel should be cut back a suitable distance with care taken not to jeopardize the flap pedicle length. It is also important to ensure that the recipient vessels are out of any zone of injury or infection in order to avoid using inflamed vessel segments and thereby increasing the risk of postanastomotic thrombosis (4).

Once a satisfactory vessel segment is attained, adventitial cleaning is carried out with sharp curved microsurgical scissors (Fig. 8.1). It is important to avoid separation of the intima from

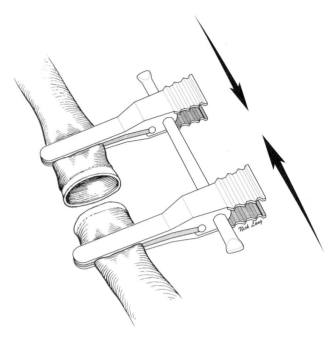

FIGURE 8.2. Use of double approximating microvascular clamps. The donor and recipient vessels are placed within the clamps, and the vessel ends are approximated along the direction of the arrows. This technique maintains the correct orientation of the vessels and facilitates suture placement. After the anterior suture line is complete, the clamps are turned over to allow access to the posterior suture line. (Visual Art © 2004 The University of Texas M. D. Anderson Cancer Center. Used with permission.)

the media in arteries, and to avoid excessive thinning of the vessel wall. Excessive stripping can result in a higher tear in the vessels during suture placement. Judicious tangential sharp excision is carried out for a distance of approximately 1 mm from the edge of each vessel. Some surgeons prefer to maintain luminal apposition by careful vessel positioning and the use of anastomotic traction sutures. Others prefer to use double vascular approximating clamps (Fig. 8.2) to maintain the ends of the vessels in apposition (1).

After adequate preparation, the vessels are aligned for suture placement. Fine, nonabsorbable sutures appropriate to the size and thickness of the vessels are used (most commonly 8-0, 9-0, or 10-0 nylon). Ideally, suture entry should be perpendicular to the vessel wall surface. Each bite should be a sufficient distance away from the edge so that the suture will not cut through the wall. These sutures should be placed an equal distance apart to distribute the tension evenly around the circumference of the anastomosis (1).

The method of suturing depends on personal preference (3,12). One popular method is to use two orientation sutures placed 180 degrees apart (Fig. 8.3A) or three orientation sutures placed 120 degrees apart (Fig. 8.3B). It has been suggested that it is easier to place the correct number of sutures between the orientation sutures when there are two, whereas the use of three orientation sutures may reduce the risk of including the opposite wall in a suture as this falls away from the anterior suture line with traction on the holding sutures.

The remainder of the sutures are then placed, usually beginning on the posterior wall, to facilitate visualization of the lumen, and ending on the anterior wall. These can be interrupted or continuous sutures. Interrupted sutures are preferred where the size match of the two vessel ends is less than ideal. Continuous (running) sutures require less knot tying, and the suture line tension can be distributed evenly between the orientation knots (Figs. 8.4 and 8.5). In practice, arterial anastomoses are

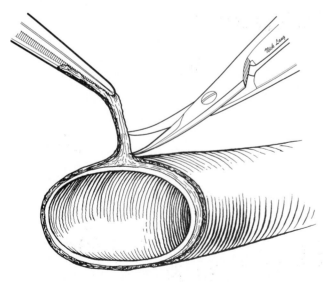

FIGURE 8.1. Donor and recipient vessel preparation. The excess adventitial tissue near the cut edge of the vessel is removed with dissecting scissors to prevent intrusion into the lumen during the anastomosis. Care should be taken to avoid excessive thinning, which can result in vessel tears during placement of sutures. (Visual Art © 2004 The University of Texas M. D. Anderson Cancer Center. Used with permission.)

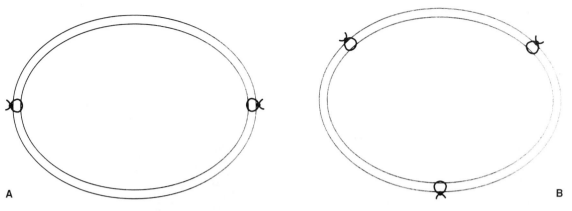

FIGURE 8.3. Orientation sutures. A: Bisecting interrupted sutures are placed 180 degrees apart, dividing the vessel circumference in half. This technique is particularly useful when there is vessel size mismatch. B: Triangulating interrupted sutures are placed 120 degrees apart, dividing the vessel circumference into thirds. This technique helps to prevent inadvertent inclusion of the opposite wall of the vessel in the remaining sutures; the surgeon applies gentle downward traction on the posterior orientation suture while the other two sutures are gently retracted upward and laterally during placement of the remaining anastomotic sutures. (Visual Art © 2004 The University of Texas M. D. Anderson Cancer Center. Used with permission.)

usually performed with interrupted sutures and venous anastomoses with continuous sutures. Several studies show no significant difference in thrombosis rates between the two suturing techniques (3,9,12).

Accidental penetration into or inclusion of the opposite wall (back wall) of a vessel in a suture is unacceptable and must be avoided by careful visualization and meticulous technique. This avoidance can be achieved by a combination of luminal irrigation to distend the vessel, particularly thin-walled veins, and ensuring that the vessel edges are everted. The tips of jeweler forceps can be placed just inside the vessel lumen to provide counterpressure to facilitate external to intraluminal passage of the needle (Fig. 8.6A) and against the adventitial surface of

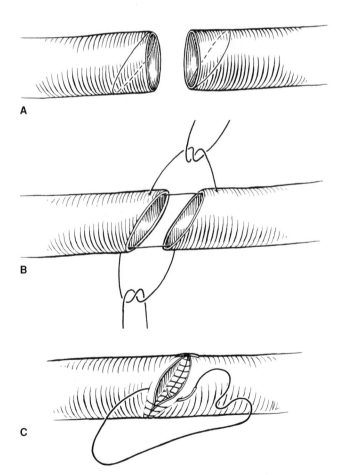

FIGURE 8.4. End-to-end anastomosis using running sutures. A: Donor and/or recipient vessel ends may be cut at an oblique angle to increase the circumference and facilitate suturing, particularly for small vessels. B and C: Interrupted traction sutures are placed at 180 degrees (shown) or 120 degrees (not shown) to orient the vessels and facilitate placement of the running sutures. (Visual Art © 2004 The University of Texas M. D. Anderson Cancer Center. Used with permission.)

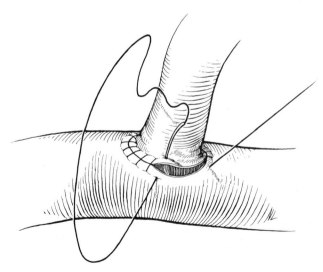

FIGURE 8.5. End-to-side anastomosis, using running sutures. An elliptical opening is created on the recipient vessel wall, and the end of the donor vessel is anastomosed to this opening. The end-to-side technique maintains distal flow in the recipient vessel and is frequently performed when there is donor and recipient vessel diameter mismatch. (Visual Art © 2004 The University of Texas M. D. Anderson Cancer Center. Used with permission.)

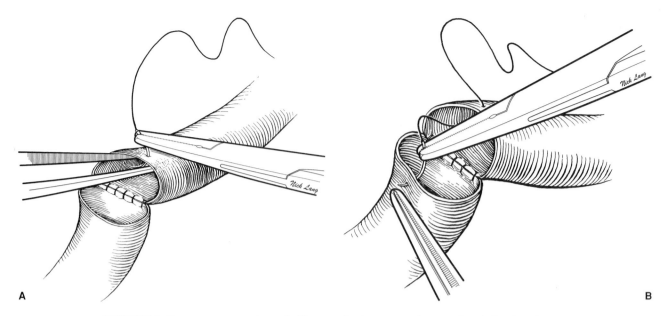

A   **B**

FIGURE 8.6. Forceps countertraction to facilitate needle placement and penetration. **A:** In selected cases, partially open blunt forceps tips may be placed into the lumen to evert the vessel wall, avoid inclusion of the back wall in sutures, and provide countertraction for needle penetration. Extreme care must be taken to avoid traumatizing the vessel intima; some microsurgeons avoid this technique for this reason. **B:** When passing the needle from inside the vessel lumen to outside the lumen, it is often useful to use the tips of the forceps to provide countertraction on the adventitial surface of the vessel to facilitate needle penetration. (Visual Art © 2004 The University of Texas M. D. Anderson Cancer Center. Used with permission.)

the vessel wall to facilitate intraluminal to external passage of the needle (Fig. 8.6B).

Square knots should be used whenever possible. For sutures under some tension, such as the initial orientation sutures, a surgeon's knot is frequently preferred. Three square throws are usually sufficient for interrupted suture knots. Ideally, sutures should be tied with a degree of tension sufficient to adequately coapt the vessel edges without causing excessive bunching. However, sutures that are tied too loosely may result in leakage at the anastomosis or cause thrombosis.

Nakayama introduced a vascular anastomotic coupling device, subsequently modified by Ostrup, consisting of polyethylene rings secured with steel pins (7). Use of such a device requires everted vessel walls and may not be possible with vessels that have a small diameter or atherosclerotic changes. Commercially available systems are available for vessels 1 to 4 mm in diameter. The patency rates achieved using anastomotic coupling devices are comparable to those using handsewn arterial anastomoses (7a). Figure 8.7 illustrates the technique for using an anastomotic coupling device.

Antispasmodic agents such as papaverine can be used throughout the dissection and anastomosis to reduce vasospasm. After the vascular clamps are released, the anastomosis is checked carefully for active leaks, which are managed by accurate placement of additional sutures. The entire pedicle is examined to ensure there is no tension, torsion, or bleeding from points on the flap or from vessel branches. The time at which flow is resumed is recorded and the flap ischemia time totaled.

A gentle Acland (vessel strip) test can be carried out near the venous anastomosis to confirm anastomotic patency (Fig. 8.8). Perfusion of the flap can be assessed by color, capillary refill time, tissue bleeding, and temperature assessment (6,12). A Doppler probe can be used to assess vascular flow within the pedicle and/or specific areas of the flap. These areas can be marked by a fine, nonabsorbable suture on the skin paddle for ease of location during postoperative monitoring.

POSTOPERATIVE MANAGEMENT

Anesthetic reversal should be gentle to avoid sudden changes in blood pressure, which may start unwanted bleeding. The patient should be kept warm, well hydrated, and pain free both during and after the procedure. The use of vasoconstrictive agents should be avoided. Blood pressure, oxygenation, ventilation, and fluid balance should be monitored carefully. The postoperative use of an anticoagulant agent such as dextran, heparin, or aspirin is dependent on surgeon preference (4). These are more often used only if there is a higher-than-normal risk of thrombosis, such as with small vessel caliber, poor vessel quality, friable vessel walls, previous radiation, or heavy smoking (3,8).

Experienced personnel are essential for monitoring the flap postoperatively. The gold standard for assessing viability of transferred tissue is clinical examination (6). Identification of a failing or insufficiently perfused flap can occasionally be challenging even for the experienced microsurgeon. **The threshold triggering re-exploration of a flap for suspected arterial or venous thrombosis should be extremely low as salvage rates are considerably greater with early identification and treatment.**

A number of clinical signs, when present either singly or in combination, suggest a perfusion problem. These include pale flap color, reduction in flap temperature, loss of capillary refill, and loss of flap turgor, all of which may indicate arterial insufficiency. Venous insufficiency, on the other hand, can result in a purple or blue hue in the flap, congestion, swelling, and rapid capillary refill in the early stages followed by eventual loss of capillary refill. There may be increased dark bleeding at the flap edges, hematoma formation, and eventual concomitant loss of arterial inflow.

A Doppler ultrasonic probe can be helpful for flap monitoring. One type of probe used is an external pencil probe, which is applied to the flap, often on the skin paddle over a cutaneous perforator location. For flaps in which no perforator

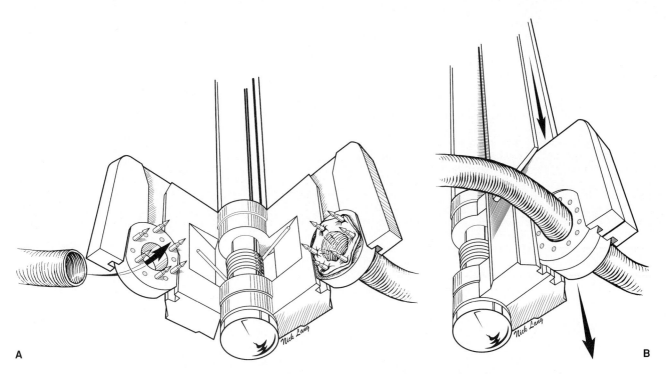

FIGURE 8.7. Use of the anastomotic coupling device (ACD). **A:** With the ACD's lateral wings open, each vessel is passed through a plastic ring, and the vessel walls are everted and impaled over pins mounted on the rings. **B:** After both vessels are mounted, the knob is turned to close the wings and secure the rings with the vessels in opposition. The rings are securely attached to each other by the pins of one ring interlocking with the opposite plastic ring. After the anastomosis, the coupled rings are released in the direction of the *arrow* by continuing to turn the knob. (Visual Art © 2004 The University of Texas M. D. Anderson Cancer Center. Used with permission.)

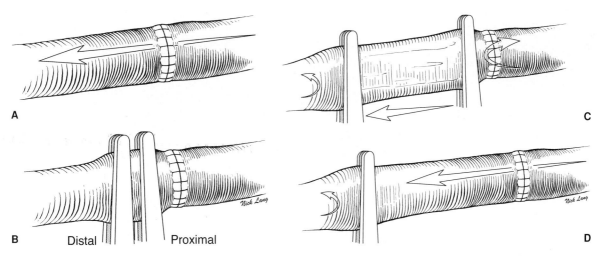

Distal   Proximal

FIGURE 8.8. Illustration of the Acland test to confirm antegrade vascular flow through the anastomosis. **A:** The direction of blood flow is indicated by the *arrow*. **B:** Two jeweler forceps are used to gently occlude the vessel distal to the venous anastomosis. **C:** Blood is milked out of the vessel between the two forceps by gently sliding the distal forceps along the vessel without injuring it. This results in a segment of collapsed vessel between the proximal and distal forceps. **D:** Releasing the proximal forceps results in filling of the collapsed vessel segment with antegrade flow if the anastomosis is patent. The distal forceps prevents retrograde filling of the collapsed segment. This test should be performed sparingly to minimize potential trauma to the vessel intima. (Visual Art © 2004 The University of Texas M. D. Anderson Cancer Center. Used with permission.)

signal is easily accessible (such as a buried flap), an implantable Doppler ultrasonic probe can be used. This consists of a small probe attached to a polymer sleeve that is placed around a pedicle vein and/or artery adjacent to the anastomosis, with a thin probe lead wire exiting through the incision (11). The lead wire easily detaches from the probe and is removed through the incision with gentle traction on the wire. Doppler signals have a characteristic pattern that can, with experience, be identified as arterial (pulsatile) or venous (undulating). A change in the character of the signals from strong to diminished or undetectable may indicate vascular occlusion. **Doppler monitoring is, however, subject to error, both false-positive and false-negative readings, and thus should always be used in conjunction with clinical assessments.**

The time between the clinical appreciation of a vascular problem in the flap and the return to the operating room for salvage is critical to the likelihood of flap salvage. Beyond a certain period, depending on flap type and clinical conditions, salvage of a compromised flap becomes impossible. It is therefore advisable to be overcautious rather than undercautious in assessing flaps, as the consequences of an undiagnosed problem may result in partial or complete loss of the flap (3).

CONCLUSION

The use of microvascular techniques has revolutionized reconstruction and expanded the range of options for reconstructing large anatomic defects in patients. Microsurgery is complex and technically demanding, but with careful preparation and proper execution, it can be beneficial to the patient and rewarding to the surgeon.

References

1. Acland RD. *Microsurgery: A Practice Manual.* St. Louis: Mosby; 1980.
2. Buncke HJ. Microsurgery-retrospective. *Clin Plast Surg.* 1986;13:315.
3. Chao JJ, Castello JR, English JM, et al. Microsurgery: free tissue transfer and replantation. *Sel Read Plast Surg.* 2000;9(11):1–32.
4. Johnson PC, Barker JH. Thrombosis and antithrombotic therapy in microvascular surgery. *Clin Plast Surg.* 1992;19:799.
5. Lee S, Frank DH, Choi SY. Historical review of small and microvascular vessel surgery. *Ann Plast Surg.* 1983;11:53.
6. Neligan PC. Monitoring techniques for the detection of flow failure in the postoperative period. *Microsurgery.* 1993;14:162.
7. Ostrup LT, Berggren A. The Unilink instrument system for fast and safe microvascular anastomosis. *Ann Plast Surg.* 1986;17:521.
7a. Yap LH, Butler CE. Venous thrombosis in coupled versus sutured microvascular anastomoses. *Ann Plast Surg,* 2006; in press.
8. Reus WF 3rd, Colen LB, Straker DJ. Tobacco smoking and complications in elective microsurgery. *Plast Reconstr Surg.* 1992;89:490.
9. Samaha FJ, Oliva A, Buncke GM, et al. A clinical study of end-to-end versus end-to-side techniques for microvascular anastomosis. *Plast Reconstr Surg.* 1997;99:1109.
10. Shenaq SM, Klebuc MJ, Vargo D. Free tissue transfer with the aid of loupe magnification: experience with 251 procedures. *Plast Reconstr Surg.* 1995;95:261.
11. Swartz WM, Izquierdo R, Miller MJ. Implantable venous Doppler microvascular monitoring laboratory investigation and clinical results. *Plast Reconstr Surg.* 1994;3:152.
12. Weiss DD, Pribaz JJ. Microsurgery. In: Achauer BM, Eriksson E, Guyuron B, et al., eds. *Plastic Surgery: Indications, Operations and Outcomes.* Vol 1. St. Louis: Mosby; 2000: 163–183.

CHAPTER 9 ■ MICROSURGICAL REPAIR OF PERIPHERAL NERVES AND NERVE GRAFTS

TERENCE M. MYCKATYN AND SUSAN E. MACKINNON

Peripheral nerve injuries must be appropriately managed to optimize motor and sensory recovery and to minimize pain. The surgeon must decide *if* and *when* to operate, and whether the goal should be the restoration of function or the resolution of pain. The latter is frequently equally or more debilitating than the functional loss. The management of peripheral nerve injuries has benefited from clinical experience gained in World War II, the evolution of microsurgical technique, improvements in surgical equipment, the development of novel agents to hasten neural regeneration, and the consistently advancing field of neuroscience.

In the normal nerve (Fig. 9.1), axons are either unmyelinated or myelinated. Unmyelinated axons are ensheathed by a Schwann cell-derived double basement membrane whereas myelinated axons are surrounded by a multilaminated, laminin-rich, myelin sheath. Individual nerve fibers are surrounded by the thin collagen fibers of the endoneurium. Fibers destined for a specific anatomic location are often grouped together in fascicles surrounded by perineurium. The connective tissue that surrounds the peripheral nerve is the epineurium. A thin layer of loose areolar tissue connects the epineurium to the surrounding structures and allows for the uninhibited excursion of nerves within the extremities. Bidirectional axonal transport within the nerve fiber is responsible for the structural support of the nerve and the delivery of neurotransmitters and trophic factors.

NERVE INJURY

Traumatized peripheral nerves are characterized by specific changes both proximal and distal to the site of injury. Proximally, axons retract a variable distance, and after a brief period of quiescence elongate as a hydralike regenerating unit in which a single parent axon gives rise to multiple daughter axons. In myelinated nerves, axons sprout at unsheathed gaps known as the nodes of Ranvier, and progress to their sensory or motor targets. Once a functional synapse is made, the remaining daughter axons degenerate, or are "pruned back." In the distal nerve segment, Schwann cells, fibroblasts, myocytes, and injured axons express a host of neurotrophic factors, including glial and brain-derived neurotrophic factors at discrete concentrations and time points as the degrading neural elements are phagocytosed in a process termed *wallerian degeneration*. Schwann cells assume a pro-regenerative phenotype instrumental in remyelinating and guiding regenerating axons to their appropriate targets along residual endoneurial tubes known as the bands of Bungner.

Neurotrophism, which literally means food for nerves, is the ability of neurotrophins secreted in an autocrine or paracrine fashion to enhance the elongation and maturation of nerve fibers. Functional recovery thus depends on the number of motor fibers correctly matched with motor endplates and the number of sensory fibers correctly matched with sensory receptors.

Experimental studies show that regenerating fibers can demonstrate both tissue and end-organ specificity (1,2). This process is called *neurotropism*. The preference of a nerve fiber to grow toward a nerve versus other tissue depends on a critical gap across which the fiber responds to the influences of the distal nerve. Current research suggests that the expression of various Schwann cell and myelin-associated glycoproteins may facilitate or impede the regeneration of damaged axons to their correct targets (3).

CLASSIFYING NERVE INJURIES (I TO VI)

The classification of nerve injuries, originally proposed by Seddon in 1947 and Sunderland in 1951, was subsequently expanded by Mackinnon to include a sixth category representing a mixed injury pattern (Fig. 9.2). The level and degree of injury are important in determining treatment. First-, second-, and third-degree injuries have the potential for recovery and for the most part do not require surgical intervention. A first-degree injury recovers function quickly (within 3 months). A second-degree injury recovers slowly (1 inch per month) but completely, whereas recovery after third degree injuries is slow and incomplete. Fourth- and fifth-degree injuries will not recover without surgical intervention. A sixth-degree injury shows a variable recovery.

First-degree injury (neurapraxia). A localized conduction block is produced that may result in segmental demyelination. Because the axons are not injured, regeneration is not required and remyelination and complete recovery occur within 12 weeks.

Second-degree injury (axonotmesis). Axonal injury occurs and the distal segment undergoes wallerian degeneration. Proximal nerve fibers will regenerate at a rate of 1 inch per month. By definition, the connective tissue layers are uninjured. Recovery will be complete unless the distance of the injury from the motor endplate results in such prolonged denervation of the receptor that motor recovery is adversely affected. The progress of regeneration can be followed by the advancing Tinel sign.

Third-degree injury. Wallerian degeneration is combined with some fibrosis of the endoneurium. Recovery will be incomplete because scar within the endoneurium may block or cause mismatching of regenerating fibers with the appropriate end organs. Surgery is indicated if the lesion localizes to a known area of entrapment where nerve regeneration is delayed. The recovery is uniformly better than that seen with a repair or graft unless it is associated with severe causalgia.

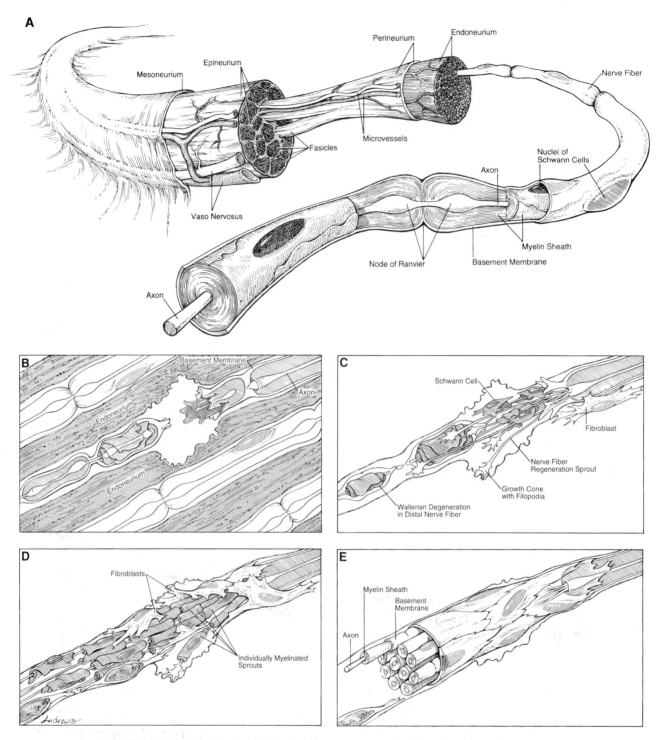

FIGURE 9.1. Nerve regeneration. **A:** The normal nerve consists of myelinated and unmyelinated axons. **B:** When a myelinated axon is injured, degeneration occurs distally and for a variable distance proximally. **C:** Multiple regenerating fibers sprout from the proximal axon forming a regenerating unit. A growth cone at the tip of each regenerating fiber samples the environment and advances the growth process distally. **D:** Schwann cells eventually myelinate the regenerating fibers. **E:** From a single nerve fiber, therefore, a regenerating unit is formed that contains several fibers, each capable of functional connections.

Fourth-degree injury. The nerve is in continuity but with complete scar block resulting from injury to the nerve. Regeneration will not occur unless the block is removed and the nerve is repaired or grafted.

Fifth-degree injury (neurotmesis). The nerve is completely divided and must be repaired before any regeneration can occur.

Sixth-degree injury. This represents a combination of any of the previous five levels of injury. Because of the longitudinal nature of crushing injuries, different levels of nerve injury can be seen at various locations along the nerve. This is the most challenging nerve injury for the surgeon as some fascicles will need to be protected and not "downgraded," whereas others will require surgical reconstruction.

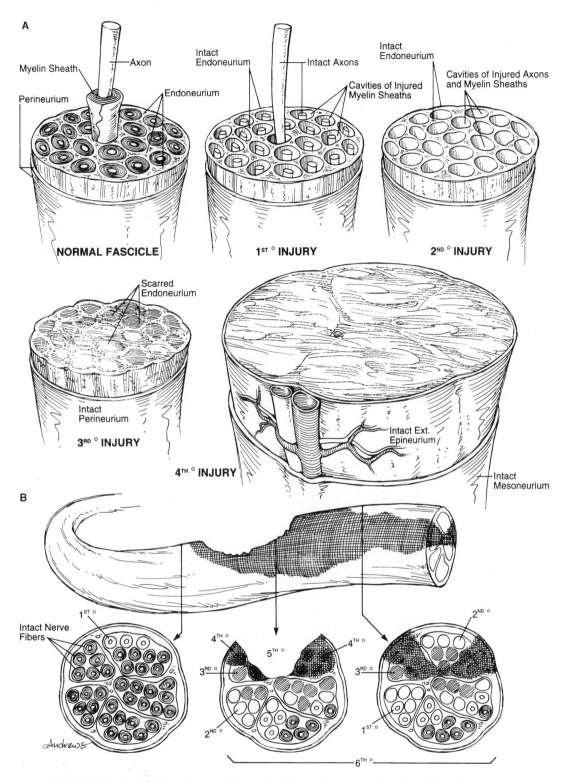

FIGURE 9.2. Classification of nerve injuries. **A:** Uninjured nerve consists of myelinated axons, surrounded by endoneurium, grouped into fascicles surrounded by perineum. The outer layer of the nerve is epineurium. In a first-degree injury, the axons are only demyelinated, whereas in a second-degree injury, the axons are injured and undergo degeneration. A third-degree injury includes damage to the axons, myelin, and endoneurium. A fourth-degree injury is a complete scar block that prevents any regeneration and a fifth-degree injury is a division of the nerve. **B:** The pattern of injury may vary from fascicle to fascicle along the nerve. This mixed pattern of injury is considered a sixth-degree injury.

TABLE 9.1

SENSORY TESTING

Sensory task	Pressure (constant touch)		Movement (moving touch)	
	Precision sensory grip		Tactile gnosis (object identification)	
Neurophysiologic correlate	Threshold	Innervation density	Threshold	Innervation density
Sensory test	Pressure perception	S2PD	Vibration perception	M2PD
				Ten Test
Testing instrument	Semmes-Weinstein	Disk-Criminator	Tuning fork	Disk-Criminator
Nerve fiber system	Monofilaments		Vibrometer	
	Slowly adapting		Quickly adapting	

M2PD, moving two-point discrimination; S2PD, static two-point discrimination.
Modified from Dellon AL. *Evaluation of Sensibility and Reeducation of Sensation in the Hand.* Baltimore: Williams & Wilkins, 1981.

Proper clinical assessment is paramount to development of a treatment plan. The extent of motor nerve injury is determined by an evaluation of weakness, loss of function, and atrophy. The extent of sensory nerve injury is determined by moving and static two-point discrimination, which are measurements of innervation density and the number of fibers innervating sensory end organs. Light moving touch, for example, evaluates the innervation of large A-β fibers and can be quickly screened with the valid and reliable "Ten Test" (4). Patients rank the quality of sensation in the affected digit compared with that in the normal contralateral digit using a scale from 0 to 10. Vibration instruments and Semmes-Weinstein monofilaments are also used as threshold tests to evaluate the performance level of nerve fibers and are more useful in evaluating chronic compressive neuropathies. Testing is also performed after nerve repair to assess the quality of nerve repair, determine the need for revision, and monitor recovery (Table 9.1).

PRINCIPLES OF NERVE REPAIR

Basic principles of nerve repair include the use of meticulous microsurgical techniques with adequate magnification, microsurgical instruments, and sutures. When the clinical and surgical conditions allow, a primary nerve repair is performed in a tension-free manner. To facilitate the repairs, the injured segments of the nerve can be mobilized, or in the case of the ulnar nerve at the elbow, transposed, to obtain length. Intrinsically, peripheral nerves do afford a limited degree of excursion as illustrated by the variable diameters of axons during axoplasmic transport. This property gives peripheral nerves a banded appearance by way of an optical phenomenon known as the bands of Fontana (5). These bands disappear when the nerve is compressed or stretched. **Extremes in the range of motion of joints in the vicinity of the repair and facilitation of an end-to-end repair with postural positioning of the extremity is discouraged. If a tension-free repair cannot be achieved, an interposition nerve graft is preferable with the limb in a neutral position.** In an effort to match sensory and motor modalities and to optimize the specificity of nerve regeneration, a grouped fascicular repair should be performed whenever the internal topography of the nerve is segregated into motor, sensory, or regional components. Otherwise an epineural repair is performed. Postoperative motor and sensory reeducation maximizes the surgical result.

FASCICULAR IDENTIFICATION

The object of peripheral nerve repair is to restore the continuity of motor and sensory fascicles in the proximal segment with the corresponding fascicles in the distal segment. The internal organization of nerves is different in the proximal extremity compared to the distal aspect of an extremity. Nerves in the proximal extremity are monofascicular, and each fascicle contains a mixture of motor and sensory fibers. There is considerable plexus formation between the fascicles, which decreases in the distal extremity. As nerves progress distally, they become polyfascicular and the fascicles are further differentiated into motor or sensory components (6,7). In the proximal segment of the nerve, motor fibers are distinguished from sensory fibers by knowledge of the internal topography, intraoperative stimulation, or "neurolysis with the eyes" (8). Using this technique, the distal stump of the injured nerve is dissected to discern motor from sensory fascicles. These fascicles are then visually traced back to the level of injury.

Knowledge of the usual internal topography of the peripheral nerves can direct proper alignment of fascicles at the time of nerve repair. For example, the fascicles of the ulnar nerve in the mid and distal forearm are divided into a dorsal sensory group, a volar sensory group, and a motor group. In the mid-forearm, the motor group is positioned between the ulnar dorsal sensory group and the radial volar sensory group (Fig. 9.3). The dorsal sensory group separates from the main ulnar nerve approximately 8 cm proximal to the wrist. The motor group remains ulnar to the volar sensory group until the Guyon's canal, at which time it passes dorsally and radially to become the deep motor branch to the intrinsic muscles. The size match between the motor and sensory groups at this level is approximately 2:3.

The median nerve topography is more complex because it contains more fascicles. In the forearm the anterior interosseous nerve is situated in the radial or posterior aspect of the median nerve as a distinct group. The distal internal topography of the median nerve approximates the distal anatomy; the motor fascicles to the thenar muscles are on the radial side and the sensory fibers to the third web space are on the ulnar side.

When repairing the radial nerve at or above the elbow, the priority is motor rather than sensory recovery (Fig. 9.4). The distal sensory fascicles should be identified and can be excluded from the repair, or harvested and used as a graft to repair the motor fibers. In a similar fashion, the sensory fibers of the peroneal nerve should be excluded from repair and

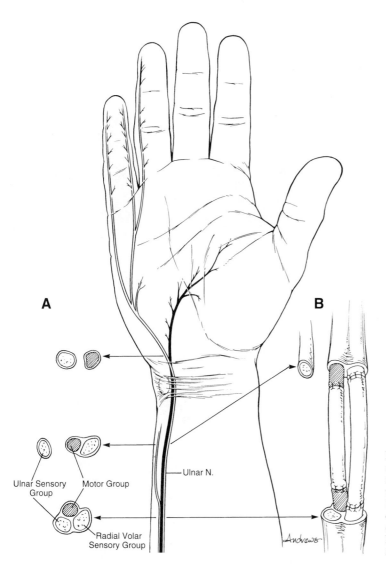

A

Ulnar Sensory
Group

Motor Group

Radial Volar
Sensory Group

Ulnar N.

B

Andrews

FIGURE 9.3. Ulnar nerve fascicular topography. **A:** At the mid-forearm the ulnar nerve is composed of three distinct fascicular groups. The dorsal sensory branch separates from the motor branch and the main sensory group. The motor branch remains ulnar to the sensory group until the Guyon canal, at which time it passes dorsally to the sensory branches of the little and ring fingers to innervate the intrinsic muscles. **B:** Knowledge of this topography can be used to accurately reconstruct distal forearm nerve injuries.

all efforts directed toward repairing the motor fibers to the anterior tibialis muscle (Fig. 9.4). The motor fibers to the anterior tibialis are located medially within the nerve as it crosses the knee and turns abruptly around the head of the fibula. Several histochemical techniques have been described that allow motor (acetylcholinesterase, choline acetyltransferase) or sensory (carbonic anhydrase) discrimination. However, these techniques require experienced histochemical personnel, are cumbersome, and are not universally available.

After the work of Sunderland, it was assumed that the motor and sensory fibers were diffusely scattered across the different fascicles and followed a tortuous course of plexus formation until they finally organized themselves into specific motor and sensory groups distally in the extremity (Fig. 9.5). Recent work contradicts this theory, showing that fibers destined for a specific territory organize themselves into distinct groups proximally within the nerve (6,9).

Fascicular identification also can be used to assist with nerve reconstruction after tumor extirpation (10). If it appears likely that a functioning nerve will have to be sacrificed during tumor extirpation, the individual fascicles proximal and distal to the resection site should be mapped. By performing direct nerve-to-nerve stimulation and recording, the proximal and distal corresponding fascicles can be identified.

After resection of the involved nerve, the proximal fascicles are repaired to their corresponding distal fascicles using nerve grafts.

TIMING OF NERVE REPAIR

The best results are obtained after immediate repair of a sharply transected nerve. The fascicular pattern and vascular landmarks guide the proper orientation of the nerve ends. Retraction and neuroma formation, which may result in the need for grafting, are avoided, and within the first 72 hours after injury, motor nerves in the distal nerve segment still respond to direct electrical stimulation because of the presence of residual neurotransmitters within the nerve terminals. If the nerve was injured by a crush, avulsion, or blast injury, however, the surgeon must be cognizant of nerve injury proximal and distal to the site of transection. In the acute setting, the extent of injury is difficult to determine even using the operating microscope. In this situation, the two nerve ends should be tacked together to prevent retraction and repair delayed for 3 weeks or until the wound permits. At the time of re-exploration, the extent of injury will be defined by neuroma and scar formation. The neuroma must be excised in a bread loaf fashion until a healthy

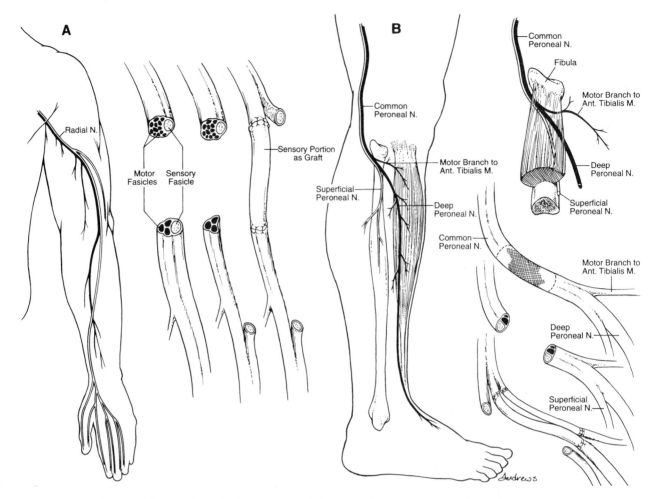

FIGURE 9.4. Radial nerve fascicular anatomy. **A:** In the radial nerve, the motor and sensory components are separated into discrete fascicles. Awake stimulation can be used to identify the motor and sensory components of the proximal nerve, whereas anatomic dissection is used to identify them distally. The sensory portion should be excluded from the repair and can be used as a source of donor graft material. If the sensory component cannot be separated from the distal stump because of plexus formation with the motor fascicles, it can be turned into the extensor carpi radialis brevis (ECRB) to neurotize this muscle. This ensures that regenerating motor fibers will not be lost in the sensory territory of the radial nerve. **B:** Foot dorsiflexion is the essential goal of peroneal nerve repair. Grafting may be limited to the motor branch of the anterior tibialis, which lies on the medial side of the nerve as it rounds the head of the fibula and travels transversely to reach the anterior tibialis. Again, the sensory portions of the nerve can be used as donor material.

fascicular pattern is seen proximally and distally. The resultant defect usually requires nerve grafting. Our current algorithms for the timing of nerve repair are shown in Figs. 9.6 and 9.7.

Clinical studies have not shown a clear superiority of fascicular repair over an epineural repair. If the internal topography of the nerve is known to be segregated in discrete motor/sensory groups, however, a grouped fascicular repair should have benefit over an epineural repair; otherwise the extra manipulation and suture material may actually decrease the functional results. Unless the surgeon is specifically trying to direct motor and sensory alignment because of a favorable internal topography, an epineural repair is standard. Bleeding from epineural vessels should be controlled with gentle pressure or fine bipolar coagulation under microscopic guidance. After transection of a nerve the individual fascicles tend to herniate out from the epineural sheath because of the normally high endoneurial fluid pressure. At the time of epineural repair, the fascicles may bend inward or outward, causing a misdirection of the regenerating fibers (Fig. 9.8). Appropriate trimming of the fascicles will allow them to lie end to end within the epineural sheath. The epineural sutures should be placed loosely so as not to cause

any additional bunching of the fascicles and so that the nerve can be realigned appropriately.

NERVE GRAFTS

During the primary repair of a nerve, the two ends of the nerve should lie in approximation without tension. If the repair will not hold with 9-0 suture, or if postural positioning is required, a nerve graft is preferable. One challenge with nerve grafting is to restore proper sensory/motor alignment. Often the internal topography of a nerve changes across a gap. The proximal nerve may contain mixed motor and sensory fascicles or a different number of fascicles compared to the distal nerve, and thus the alignment of the grafts cannot be specific. Proper orientation is aided by knowledge of the internal anatomy, distal dissection, and "neurolysis with the eyes." A second challenge is to maximize the number of axons that can traverse the nerve graft through both proximal and distal neurorrhaphy sites. To divert the maximal number of axons distally, nerve grafts are reversed in orientation. This maneuver is particularly

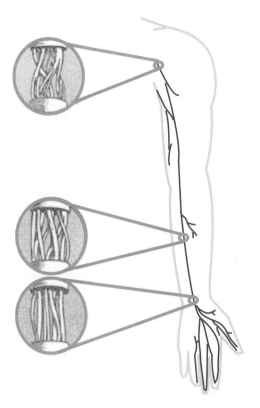

FIGURE 9.5. Nerve topography. Early surgeons believed that the fibers destined for a distinct fascicular group in the distal limb gradually came together as the plexus formation decreased. Recent work shows that fibers of a distinct fascicular group are actually located adjacent to each other, even in the proximal limb.

important when a long graft that possesses branches is noted. If the graft is placed anatomically, some regenerating axons travel along these branches instead of to the distal neurorrhaphy site. If the graft is reversed in orientation, it will funnel all regenerating axons distally.

When repairing long nerve defects the surgeon may wish to prioritize the functions of the nerve and consider excluding nonessential branches. In both the radial and peroneal nerves, the sensory components are expendable and the surgeon can concentrate on restoring the motor function. The sensory fascicles are identified by anatomic dissection distally and then separated from the main nerve by internal neurolysis. If necessary the sensory fascicles can be used as graft material.

NEUROMA IN CONTINUITY

A neuroma in continuity may arise after a partial nerve injury or a previous nerve repair in which portions of the nerve are functioning while other critical components are not. The surgeon must be careful not to downgrade the patient's function by sacrificing the functioning components in an attempt to repair the remainder of the nerve. Careful preoperative assessment will determine which fascicular components are functioning and should be preserved.

At the time of repair, the neuroma in continuity may involve the complete circumference of the nerve. Individual fascicles proximal and distal to the neuroma can be separated using a microneurolysis technique. A hand-held nerve stimulator or intraoperative nerve conduction testing is used to help identify functioning motor fascicles. If sensory fascicles are to be protected, intraoperative nerve conduction testing proximal and distal to the neuroma may be required.

Separating the functioning fascicles from within the neuroma should not be attempted as this internal neurolysis may cause additional injury to functioning components. In this situation, the neuroma possessing functioning fascicles should be preserved, whereas the nonfunctioning proximal and distal fascicles can be reconstructed with nerve grafts "black boxing" around the neuroma (Fig. 9.9). Expendable motor nerves that can be used as motor nerve grafts include the distal anterior interosseous nerve to the pronator quadratus, the obturator nerve branch to the gracilis, and thoracodorsal nerve branches to the latissimus dorsi. In fact, any nerve innervating a free muscle transfer could be used as a motor nerve graft.

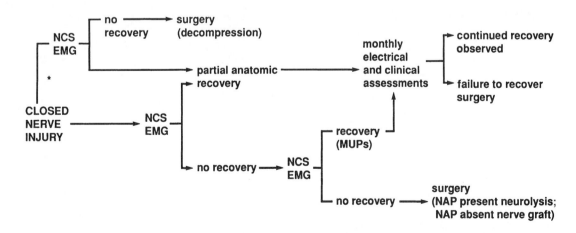

FIGURE 9.6. Algorithm for the management of closed nerve injuries.

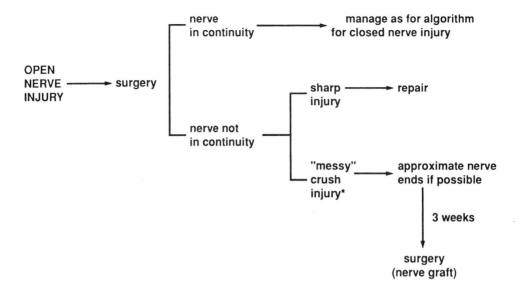

* **Surgeon uncertain as to proximal and distal extent of injury.**
† **As soon as soft tissue status permits.**

FIGURE 9.7. Algorithm for the management of open nerve injuries.

DONOR NERVE GRAFTS

The sural nerve in the adult can provide 30 to 40 cm of nerve graft. In 80% of dissections it is formed by a union of the medial sural cutaneous nerve and the peroneal communicating branch. When a large amount of graft material is needed, the communicating branch can contribute an additional 10 to 20 cm. The nerve is found adjacent to the lesser saphenous vein at the lateral malleolus and is usually harvested through a longitudinal incision to allow harvesting of both branches. The resultant area of numbness on the lateral side of the foot decreases in size over time. The disadvantages of the sural nerve are the separate distal donor site and the less-favorable neural-to-connective-tissue ratio as compared to upper extremity donor nerves.

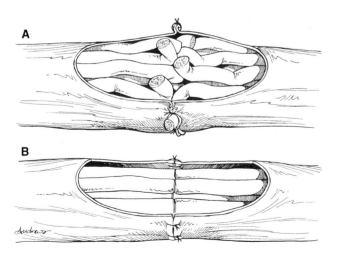

FIGURE 9.8. Nerve repair. A: In an epineural repair, the fascicles must be appropriately trimmed so that they do not buckle, which will result in misdirection of the regenerating fibers. Excessive tightening of the epineural sutures can also cause buckling of the fascicles. B: Well-performed nerve repairs will result in good alignment of fascicles without the need of fascicular sutures.

When a limited amount of graft material is required, the medial or lateral antebrachial cutaneous nerve can be harvested from the injured upper extremity. The lateral antebrachial cutaneous nerve is found adjacent to the cephalic vein along the ulnar border of the brachioradialis muscle. A maximum of 8 cm of nerve graft can be obtained and the loss of sensation is negligible as a result of the overlap in distribution by the radial sensory branch. The donor scar on the volar aspect of the forearm may be objectionable to some patients. The medial antebrachial cutaneous (MABC) nerve, found in the groove between the triceps and biceps muscles adjacent to the basilic vein, has a posterior and an anterior division. Harvesting of the anterior branch is preferred because this results in loss of sensation over the anterior aspect of the forearm, whereas loss of the posterior branch causes numbness over the elbow and the resting portion of the forearm. If necessary, up to 20 cm of nerve graft can be obtained with the MABC, and the donor scar on the medial side of the arm is more acceptable. Patients are instructed that an initial broad area of donor sensory loss will gradually (over 2 to 3 years) decrease in size.

Patients with complete median nerve sensory loss have loss of sensation in the first, second, and third web spaces. Because sensation is not critical in the third web space, the third web space nerve can be harvested to reconstruct the median nerve defect, avoiding any additional morbidity caused by nerve harvesting. The third web space nerve can be neurolysed from the main median nerve, providing up to 24 cm of nerve graft. In a similar manner the dorsal branch of the ulnar nerve can be harvested to reconstruct the ulnar nerve. Vascularized nerve grafts have a limited role in peripheral nerve reconstruction, and their use is typically limited to lengthy, large-caliber nerve grafts such as the ulnar nerve.

NERVE TRANSFERS

The use of nerve transfers has expanded over the last decade based on a more detailed knowledge of the intraneural topography and branching patterns of peripheral nerves in the upper and lower extremities. Nerve transfers are indicated in very

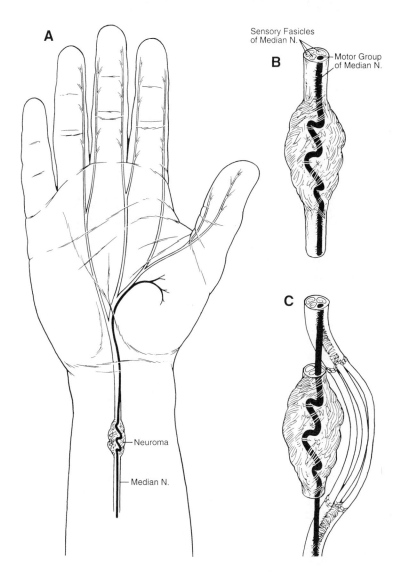

FIGURE 9.9. Neuroma in continuity. **A:** When reconstructing a neuroma in continuity with intact motor function, the motor fascicles through the neuroma must be preserved. **B:** Intraoperative nerve testing can identify the motor fascicles proximal and distal to the neuroma. **C:** The remaining sensory fibers are divided proximally and distally, then reconstructed with grafts bypassing the neuroma. Any attempt to dissect the motor fascicles out of the neuroma will only downgrade the function.

proximal peripheral nerve injuries or root avulsions where a proximal stump is unavailable for primary repair or grafting. Even when grafting is possible, the injury may be so proximal that a nerve transfer facilitates better reinnervation of motor endplates than does a nerve graft. Nerve transfers are also indicated to avoid operating in regions of severe scarring, when nerve injuries present in a delayed fashion, when partial nerve injuries present with a well-defined functional deficit, or when the level of injury is unclear such as in idiopathic neuritides or radiation-induced nerve injury.

Motor nerve transfers require an expendable donor motor nerve with a large number of pure motor axons that is located in close proximity to motor endplates, thus minimizing the distance and time regenerating axons need to travel to reinnervate their targets. It is also preferable that the donor nerve innervates a muscle that is synergistic with its target (8). The criteria for sensory nerve transfers include an expendable donor sensory nerve that innervates a noncritical sensory distribution, contains a large number of pure sensory axons, and is located near its sensory end organs.

The most common applications of motor nerve transfers include the restoration of elbow flexion, shoulder abduction, ulnar-innervated intrinsic hand function, forearm pronation, and radial nerve function (8). To restore elbow flexion, the medial pectoral, thoracodorsal, or intercostal nerves can be transferred to the musculocutaneous nerve. The flexor carpi

ulnaris branch of the ulnar nerve and the flexor carpi radialis branch of the median nerve can also be transferred to the biceps and brachialis branches of the musculocutaneous nerve to more specifically restore elbow flexion and limit donor nerve morbidity (Fig. 9.10). To restore shoulder abduction, the distal accessory nerve can be transferred to the suprascapular nerve, or the triceps branch of the radial nerve can be transferred to the axillary nerve. To restore intrinsic hand function, the distal anterior interosseous nerve can be transferred to the ulnar nerve. Transferring redundant fascicles of the flexor carpi ulnaris branches of the ulnar nerve to the median nerve-innervated pronator teres can restore forearm pronation. Alternatively, the flexor digitorum superficialis, or palmaris longus branches of the median nerve, can be transferred to its pronator branch. The radial nerve is most commonly reconstructed by transferring a redundant portion of the ulnar nerve supplying the flexor carpi ulnaris.

NERVE CONDUITS

Studies show that nerves will regenerate across a short nerve gap through various conduits, such as veins, pseudosheaths, and bioabsorbable tubes (5,9). The characteristics of the ideal nerve conduit include low antigenicity, availability, and biodegradability. Vein grafts have been used to reconstruct

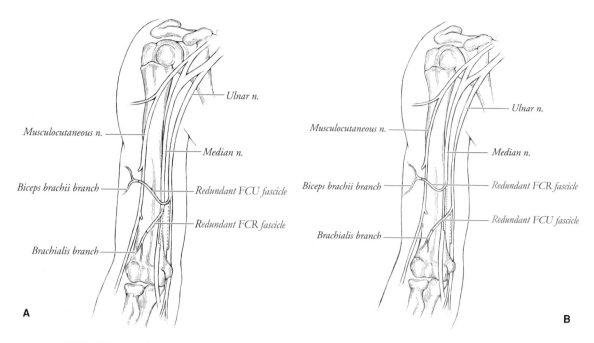

FIGURE 9.10. A double fascicular transfer for elbow flexion. **A:** Transfer of a redundant fascicle of the ulnar nerve to the biceps branch of the musculocutaneous nerve and a redundant fascicle of the median nerve to the brachialis branch of the musculocutaneous nerve. **B:** Transfer of a redundant fascicle of the median nerve to the biceps branch of the musculocutaneous nerve and a redundant fascicle of the ulnar nerve to the brachialis branch of the musculocutaneous nerve. FCR, flexor carpi radialis; FCU, flexor carpi ulnaris.

distal sensory nerve defects of less than 3 cm. Sensory results have been acceptable but not as good as conventional grafting. For this reason vein grafts are recommended only for reconstruction of noncritical nerve gaps of less than 3 cm.

Nerve regeneration across a 3-cm gap through a biodegradable polyglycolic nerve tube has been demonstrated in the primate model and in a clinical trial (7). Nerve regeneration was comparable to that across a standard nerve graft. The insertion of a short piece of nerve graft material into the center of the conduit will enhance regeneration by providing a local source of trophic factors. The ready availability of biodegradable synthetic grafts to span short nerve gaps would eliminate the morbidity associated with nerve graft harvest and would capitalize on the potential benefits of neurotropism in directing nerve regeneration. Synthetic nerve conduits are now available for reconstruction of small diameter nerves with a gap ≤3 cm, or with large diameter nerves with gaps ≤0.5 cm.

NERVE ALLOGRAFTS

Nerve allografts have demonstrated clinical usefulness in the setting of extensive peripheral nerve injuries where there is a paucity of donor nerve material. Because the nerve allograft serves as a scaffold that is repopulated by host axons and Schwann cells over time, its challenge to the immune system is of limited duration. The agent FK506 (tacrolimus) is most ideally suited for treating patients with peripheral nerve allografts based on its dual role as an immunosuppressive and neuroregenerative agent. By accelerating the rate at which axons traverse the nerve allograft, FK506 shortens the duration of immunosuppression and the period during which complications can develop. The optimal timing and dose of FK506 therapy has been identified in rodents, and a synergistic effect

with nerve allograft cold preservation, as well as an ability to rescue nerve allografts undergoing acute rejection, established. Based on these findings, FK506 is now the mainstay of clinical peripheral nerve allotransplantation.

Potential candidates for peripheral nerve allotransplantation receive nerve allografts from donors that have been screened for ABO blood-typing, HIV, and cytomegalovirus (CMV). These grafts are stored in University of Wisconsin cold storage solution at 41°F (5°C) for at least 7 days. This solution is supplemented with penicillin G, dexamethasone, and insulin. Immunosuppression of the nerve allograft recipient begins 3 to 5 days prior to nerve transplantation, and consists of FK506 whose dose is titrated to appropriate steady-state blood levels, azathioprine, and prednisone. The prednisone dose is tapered in the first 4 to 8 weeks after surgery. *Pneumocystis carinii* prophylaxis is performed at the time of immunosuppression to minimize opportunistic pulmonary infections. Immunosuppression continues for 6 months after a Tinel sign is noted to pass the last distal neurorrhaphy site and some functional recovery has occurred. Peripheral nerve allograft rejection resembles a superficial phlebitis with inflammation and tenderness, but is localized over the underlying nerve allograft and not a vein.

CONCLUSION

Nerve repair and grafting have benefited from the development of microsurgical techniques and advances in the neurosciences. State-of-the-art nerve repair not only requires precision techniques but additional measures to direct nerve regeneration to its original function. Although nerve grafting remains the standard for reconstruction of the nerve gap, synthetic conduits and allografts now play a limited role in the peripheral nerve surgeon's armamentarium.

References

1. Brushart TM, Seiler WD. Selective reinnervation of distal motor stumps by peripheral motor axons. *Exp Neurol*. 1987;97:289–300.
2. Strauch B, Lang A, Ferder M, et al. The ten test. *Plast Reconstr Surg*. 1997;99:1074–1078.
3. Jabaley ME, Wallace WH, Heckler FR. Internal topography of major nerves of the forearm and hand: a current view. *J Hand Surg [Am]*. 1980;5:1–18.
4. Torigoe K. [Stimulation and inhibition mechanisms in peripheral nerve regeneration]. *Kaibogaku Zasshi*. 1999;74:363–371.
5. Lee GW, Mackinnon SE, Brandt K, et al. A technique for nerve reconstruction following resection of soft-tissue sarcoma. *J Reconstr Microsurg*. 1993;9:139–144.
6. Williams HB, Jabaley ME. The importance of internal anatomy of the peripheral nerves to nerve repair in the forearm and hand. *Hand Clin*. 1986;2:689–707.
7. Dvali L, Mackinnon S. Nerve repair, grafting, and nerve transfers. *Clin Plast Surg*. 2003;30:203–221.
8. Hallin RG. Microneurography in relation to intraneural topography: somatotopic organisation of median nerve fascicles in humans. *J Neurol Neurosurg Psychiatry*. 1990;53:736–744.
9. Greenberg MM, Leitao C, Trogadis J, et al. Irregular geometries in normal unmyelinated axons: a 3D serial EM analysis. *J Neurocytol*. 1990;19:978–988.
10. Lundborg G, Dahlin LB, Danielsen N, et al. Tissue specificity in nerve regeneration. *Scand J Plast Reconstr Surg*. 1986;20:279–283.

CHAPTER 10 ■ TISSUE EXPANSION

BRUCE S. BAUER

Tissue expansion is a reliable method of providing additional cutaneous tissue, thereby optimizing contour and color match in a given reconstructive effort. The effects of expansion on skin, which include increased surface area and vascularity, allow coverage of a variety of complex wounds.

BACKGROUND

Although the genesis of modern-day tissue expansion is credited to innovators such as Radovan (1) and Austad (2), the technique takes some of its roots from early lessons in distraction osteogenesis. Bone traction with either internal or external devices at the turn of the 20th century, paved the way for the concept that mechanical stress on tissue could lead to lengthening. Putti extrapolated these ideas from bone to the surrounding soft tissue, by placing constant tension on a composite tissue to obtain soft-tissue lengthening. In the middle 1950s, Neumann (3) became the first surgeon to use an expansile implant when he used a latex balloon to enlarge periauricular skin for a traumatic ear deformity. Despite these early efforts, it was not until 20 years after Neumann's report that tissue expansion was revisited. Charles Radovan, a resident at Georgetown, reintroduced the concept of expansion when he inserted a contemporary device with an internally placed port (1). Shortly thereafter, Eric Austad produced a self-inflating device (2). In 1982, the first National Tissue Expansion Symposium was sponsored by Plastic Surgery Educational Foundation (PSEF), marking the recognition of a new advance and field in reconstructive surgery. Since that time expansion has been applied to a multitude of reconstructive problems with applications demonstrated in both regional expansion and expansion at distant sites for subsequent graft and flap transfer. Better understanding of expansion has allowed many modifications in flap design, increasing its worth as a reconstructive option (4).

PHYSIOLOGY

When a constant mechanical stress is applied to skin over time, two phenomena occur: **mechanical creep and biological creep**. The former is based on morphologic changes that occur on a cellular level in response to the applied stress—the cell is stretched. Disruption of gap junctions and increased tissue surface area then result in cell proliferation (biologic creep). Growth of the tissue by cell proliferation restores resting tension of the stretched tissue to baseline (5). The epidermis gets thicker with concurrent thinning of the dermis and alignment of collagen fibrils. These effects are maximized at 6 to 12 weeks postexpansion. On a molecular level, a panoply of growth factors—cytokines, hormones, adhesion molecules, cytoskeletal elements, and signal transduction proteins—are induced in response to expansion (6), confirming that tissue expansion is a dynamic process.

One feature that makes an expanded flap so reliable is its improved vascularity. Studies demonstrate that the vascularity of an expanded flap is superior to its nonexpanded counterpart in both number and caliber of vessels (7). Moreover, angiogenic factors, such as vascular endothelial growth factor (VEGF), are expressed on the surface of expanded tissue at a significantly higher level when compared to nonexpanded controls. This augmentation in blood flow is attributable to the capsule that forms around the expandable prosthesis. **Because of the similarity between expanded and delayed flaps in vessel caliber, tissue expansion is well regarded as a form of the delay phenomenon.** An expanded flap, therefore, is a delayed flap.

TYPES OF PROSTHESES

Several types of tissue expanders exist, based on shape, size, and type of filling valve. Expanders can be standard, customized, anatomic to the donor site (breast), or differential in fill volume to provide tapering of tissue. In terms of shape, they follow three basic patterns: round, rectangular, and crescent. The more commonly used include the round and rectangular types; crescent-shaped (and croissant) prostheses, originally developed to minimize dog-ears at the donor site, have fallen out of favor as it has been recognized that the added tissue gained with rectangular expanders may increase the choices possible for flap design (i.e., use of transposition flaps) (Fig. 10.1).

Expander volumes have a wide range and vary according to the anatomic site. Round expanders of 100 to 2,000 cm^3 and rectangular expanders of 100 to 1,000 cm^3 have been used (larger custom expanders are available). Saline is delivered in a controlled fashion via the valve port, which is either integrated into the prosthesis or connected to the device by silicone tubing of customized length. An integrated system offers the advantage of undermining a single pocket for expander placement, but also places the implant at risk of perforation by a misplaced needle. Internal remote ports remove the danger of perforation away from the prosthesis itself, but introduce the potential complications of overturn of the port, tube obstruction, and migration. To avoid these complications, the undermining for the port pocket is minimal, the port is placed over firm, supporting tissue, and if need be, the port position can be fixed with suture(s).

EXPANDED FLAP DESIGN

The design of an expanded flap is not a frivolous undertaking. **Consideration for the incisions, expander placement, flap movement in relation to the defect, and postoperative scars take appreciable preoperative planning and discussion with the patient and family.** In regards to donor site, one must match color, texture, and contour of the recipient site to

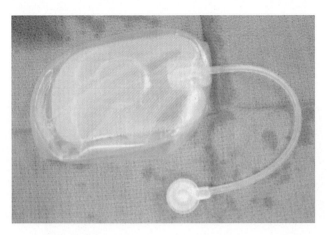

FIGURE 10.1. Tissue expander with rectangular shape, thicker base plate, tubing, and remote filling port.

maximize the aesthetic and functional outcome. The donor tissue must be free of infection, previous scars (or have stable scars), or trauma to prevent implant failure or extrusion. **If possible the expander is placed through an incision within the lesion to be excised.** Gentle handling of the resulting skin flaps is mandatory; rough, or aggressive, retraction or collision of the flaps with instruments can lead to skin edge necrosis. The port is placed over a region with firm skeletal support (e.g., rib or iliac crest or anterior thigh for trunk/abdominal tissue expansion) for ease of outpatient filling. Partial fill of the expander at the time of placement (usually to 10% to 20% of its listed volume), assures that the expander is properly positioned and without surface folds. Closed suction drains also serve to control potential dead space from wide undermining. In most cases, the expander pocket incisions are closed in watertight fashion with the judicious placement of 4-0 clear nylon (buried intradermal) followed by 4-0 black nylon (running continuous) sutures. Skin flaps are dressed nonadherently (bacitracin, Xeroform gauze), followed with soft padding (fluffs). Patients may be monitored overnight for pain control and flaps monitored for potential compromise or hematoma formation.

Serial expansion is started 7 to 10 days postinsertion, provided that the skin flaps are in excellent condition. After one or two postoperative visits for drain removal (postoperative days 3 to 10) and education, most pediatric patients go on a home expansion protocol, directed by parents or guardians. One study demonstrated that home expansion is just as safe as and equivalent to office expansion in the aspects of successful outcome (96% vs. 90%) (8). **Expansion should render the skin tense, but one should not expand until it is extremely painful to the patient or when skin compromise has occurred.** Both suggest excessive filling and must be corrected immediately. Families typically proceed with this home expansion protocol for 8 to 12 weeks prior to expander removal and reconstruction.

Although the early dogma of tissue expansion emphasized expansion as a means of generating large advancement flaps only, experience over the ensuing two decades demonstrates that expanded transposition and rotation flaps frequently are preferable for many reconstructions. Clearly, the increased vascular supply of the expanded flap places little limitation on the ingenuity of the surgeon in designing flaps unique to the varied recipient defects. Although requiring more planning and forethought, transposition of the flap provides greater versatility in flap design and range (4,9).

SCALP

Scalp reconstruction via tissue expansion has three general indications: large congenital nevi, scar and skin graft alopecia, and as an adjunct to craniofacial reconstruction (Fig. 10.2). Despite former thoughts that expansion may affect cranial vault morphology, CT scan examination of more than 20 infants in the early portion of my clinical practice found no distortion or untoward effects on cranial sutures. Temporary cranial molding occurs, but self-corrects within 3 to 4 months. For giant nevi, expanders are placed serially, with a larger expander placed after each stage to distribute the expansile forces evenly over the hair follicles. As previous studies showed, tissue expansion itself does not induce proliferation of hair follicles, but can double the size of the scalp without obvious alopecia. For expander placement, pocket dissection is performed in a subgaleal plane but staying above the periosteum. Flaps are designed with consideration of the major arteries to the scalp (superficial temporal, postauricular, and occipital arteries, and contributions from the supraorbital vessels). Finally, port placement in the preauricular region produces the least migration. Next to the breast, the scalp is the most frequently expanded region and the area with which most surgeons have familiarity. The ability to reconstruct areas of scar alopecia, resect and reconstruct large scalp lesions, and replace the defect with hair-bearing scalp makes it the reconstructive option of choice for many cases.

FOREHEAD

Expanded flap reconstruction of the forehead provides some of the most challenging cases, because of its potential morbidity and disfigurement of other upper facial structures (e.g., brow). One must have respect for the aesthetic subunits to avoid late complications (Fig. 10.3). Retrospective review of our clinical data revealed a 24% aesthetic complication rate in forehead tissue expansion, including brow asymmetry, brow ptosis, altered hair direction, and anterior hairline asymmetry (10). Over the years, certain guiding principles have been developed to minimize these late complications: (a) bilateral expansion of normal forehead tissue is often successful for midforehead lesions; (b) serial expansion of the forehead is often required for hemiforehead nevi; (c) supraorbital and temporal nevi are managed using a transposition of expanded normal skin medial to the nevus; (d) with minimal involvement of the temporal region, parietal expanded skin can be advanced to reconstitute the hairline; and (e) in cases of brow elevation, the abnormal brow can be returned to its preoperative position by interposing non–hair-bearing forehead skin.

FACE AND NECK

To achieve an optimal aesthetic and functional result in the facial and cervical regions, one must adhere to a subunit principle. This dictates expander placement and flap incisions so that the final result scars are hidden in natural creases (e.g., nasolabial fold). Just as undue tension on the upper facial structure (e.g., the brow and eyelid) can cause problems, tension on the lower face leads to lower-lip drooping and oral incompetence. **Advancement of cervical skin flaps cephalad to the cervicomandibular angle bears an increased risk of late complications.** Neale and associates report a 10% lower-eyelid ectropion rate and greater than 10% lower-lip deformity rate in this context (11). The increased use of expanded transposition and rotation flaps from the lateral cheek or neck/postauricular area minimizes this risk of these problems. Judicious flap design, use

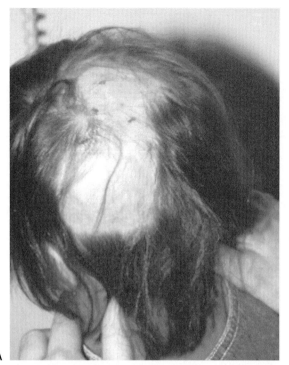

A

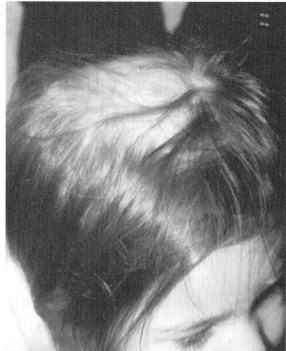

B

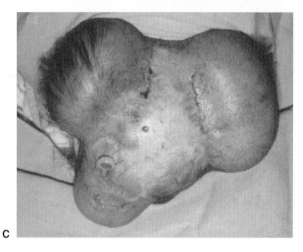

C

FIGURE 10.2. **A** and **B:** Posterior and anterior views of the scalp of a young child with cutis aplasia congenital, showing the areas of thin, unstable scar with associated alopecia. **C:** Posterior view of scalp with three expanders in place (one with injection port externalized) prior to excision of the scar and reconstruction of the scalp. *(Continued)*

of multiple prostheses and overexpansion are recommended to further minimize these complications.

Expansion is also extremely useful in enlarging donor sites for full-thickness skin grafts, which virtually eliminates the size of the graft as a limitation (12). Pre-expansion of donor sites allows larger full-thickness skin grafts to be harvested to resurface the periorbital and perioral area, as well as cover complete cheek or forehead aesthetic units when regional flap tissue is unavailable. Part of the expansion provides for the graft tissue and the remainder provides for primary closure of the donor site. The neck above the clavicle is the ideal donor site for grafts on the face because of excellent color and texture match. When expanded, these expanded full-thickness grafts have the same characteristics of their unexpanded counterparts in regard to durability, texture, minimal contraction, and growth.

TRUNK

Beyond its obvious usefulness in treatment of deformities and defects of the breast, tissue expansion has multiple applications on the trunk for treatment of giant nevi, vascular

malformations, and contour defects. Not unexpectedly, the lower abdomen is perhaps the most easily expanded site, and can be used for excision of adjacent lesions, as donor tissue for expanded free tissue transfer (13) (expanded transverse rectus abdominis musculocutaneous [TRAM] flaps where expansion is carried out to aid in donor-site closure), and as a donor site for large, expanded, full-thickness grafts (12). Expansion on the anterior trunk is limited in children by the need to avoid potential distortion of the breasts.

Expansion on the posterior trunk is the modality of choice for treatment of many giant nevi of the back and buttock area. Whether advancing skin caudally or cephalad, serial expansion is frequently required for excision of extensive lesions. Expansion can begin as early as 6 months of age for treatment of giant nevi in children, and is clearly easier in the earlier years than later in life. The lower back may be expanded to develop large transposition flaps for coverage of the buttock and the lower abdomen expanded to create similar flaps for coverage of the anterior thigh. Again, the use of large expanded transposition flaps has allowed the excision and reconstruction of giant nevi with fewer procedures and more aesthetic and functional positioning of the final scars (13).

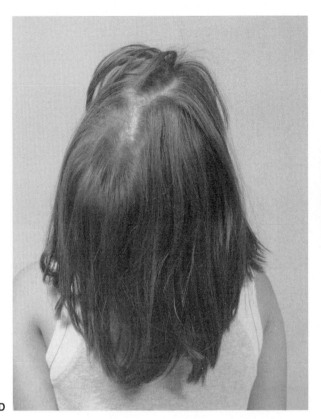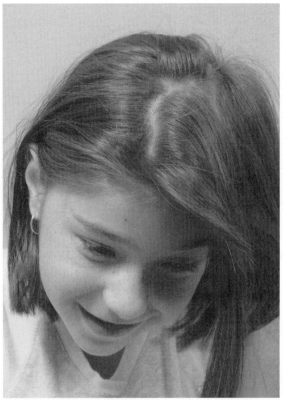

FIGURE 10.2. *(Continued)* **D** and **E:** Posterior and anterior views of reconstructed scalp with excellent hair coverage 3 years after the reconstruction.

BREAST

Expanders and expandable implants have found roles in breast surgery in postmastectomy reconstruction and habilitation of congenital anomalies (see Chapter 63).

Postmastectomy Reconstruction

Although autologous tissue reconstruction enjoys the limelight in postmastectomy breast reconstruction, expander–implant reconstruction is still performed and has some advantages. The relative ease and rapidity of subpectoral expander placement at the time of mastectomy has not been lost on general surgeons who have reported performing reconstructions in their literature over the last decade. Exchange of the implant for a permanent prosthesis can be combined with nipple–areola complex reconstruction and balancing procedures on the opposite breast. All donor-site morbidity is eliminated. Losken et al. confirmed these benefits in their retrospective report examining the number of surgeries needed to reconstruct the breast completely They report that fewer secondary procedures are necessary in expander–implant reconstructions than in TRAM reconstructions.

Expanders have been used as spacers during "delayed–primary" breast reconstruction. An expander is placed at the time of mastectomy to preserve the skin envelope while waiting for permanent sections to return. If no postmastectomy radiation is indicated, the planned reconstruction (either autologous or expander–implant) is completed rapidly. If radiation therapy ensues, the expander holds the original skin envelope until a delayed reconstruction can be performed. Theoretically, this strategy improves the outcome of delayed reconstruction by preserving the skin envelope and reducing the number of secondary procedures that would ensue after radiation of an autologous reconstruction.

Risks of expander–implant reconstruction of the breast are similar to the use of expanders in other parts of the body. To decrease the risk of expander exposure and ultimate implant capsule formation, the expander is generally placed beneath the pectoral muscle. Portions of the rectus abdominus and the serratus anterior muscles are recruited to cover the implant completely. This maneuver also improves the tactile quality of the reconstruction by placing a thicker soft-tissue envelope around the implant. Capsular contracture can be a challenging problem in the patient who requires radiation.

Tissue Expansion in Treatment of Congenital Breast Anomalies

Expanders can be helpful as "spacers" in the correction of congenital breast anomalies. Requests for breast habilitation come from patients with breast agenesis associated with Poland syndrome, idiopathic unilateral breast hypoplasia, and iatrogenic breast asymmetry as a consequence of juvenile breast bud damage. Traditional wisdom has been to wait for maturity prior to correcting breast asymmetries. This strategy assures that the surgeon knows what needs to be matched on the opposite side. Although this solution may have been acceptable previously, today's adolescent female has problems with changing in locker rooms, participating in sports activities, and wearing fashionable clothing. Questions of developing self-esteem, body image, and sexual identity further compound the issue of waiting. Expanders can function as an intermediate solution.

Many young women are happy with breast volume symmetry so that they appear normal in a bra. With this goal in mind,

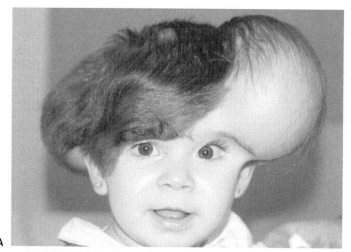
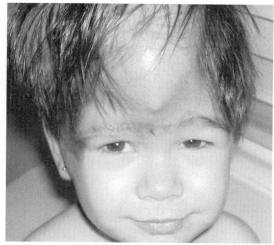
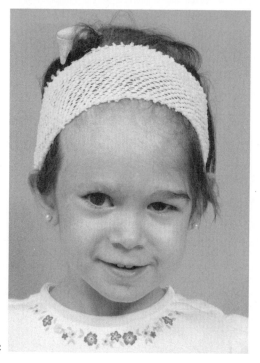

FIGURE 10.3. **A:** A 1.5-year-old child with giant nevus of forehead and scalp with expanders in place in preparation for excision of giant nevus and flap reconstruction. **B:** The first expansion allowed excision of the greater part of the nevus of the forehead. This figure demonstrates the second expander (partially expanded) used as a serial expansion of the forehead skin to allow excision of the remaining nevus. **C:** Reconstruction of full aesthetic unit of forehead and hairline 1 year after the second serial expansion of the forehead and scalp.

an expander can be placed as early as the opposite breast begins to develop and can be expanded over time. Aesthetic surgeons also use this trick to adjust breast size over time. Use of either an expander or an expander–implant in these cases may constitute an off-label use for these devices. Expanders are not constructed for prolonged use (i.e., over the 6 to 8 years of breast development). Postoperatively adjustable permanent implants are designed for longer-term use but are supposed to have their ports removed promptly after complete fill to prevent implant deflation. As such, a discussion of these possibilities needs to occur prior to placement. The postoperatively adjustable implants come in sizes, shapes, and volumes particularly suited to use in this situation. Depending on how much native breast exists, these expanders can be placed subglandularly or submuscularly.

Once the patient reaches maturity, the expander can be replaced with a permanent implant and balancing procedures to match breast shape can be performed on the opposite breast for "out-of-a-bra" symmetry. In the case of a patient with Poland syndrome with significant infraclavicular soft-tissue deficiency, a latissimus dorsi flap can be transferred or a custom permanent implant manufactured at the time of definitive reconstruction.

EXTREMITIES

Classically, the extremity as an anatomic site is viewed as an unfavorable donor for an expanded flap. **Complication rates in the limb were significantly higher than in nonlimb sites (47% versus 23%) in one study (14).** Casanova et al. found an overall 19.4% complication rate in their 10-year retrospective review of more than 200 cases, including a 15.5% major complication rate and a 4.9% failure rate (3,4). Despite these ominous reports, expansion in the lower limb is feasible, keeping in mind that remote incisions lead to lower infection, extrusion, and flap failure rates. Unstable, infected wounds are relative contraindications to tissue expansion in the extremity. Expanded free flaps (TRAM, scapular) are also powerful options to reconstruct large lower-extremity defects (Fig. 10.4).

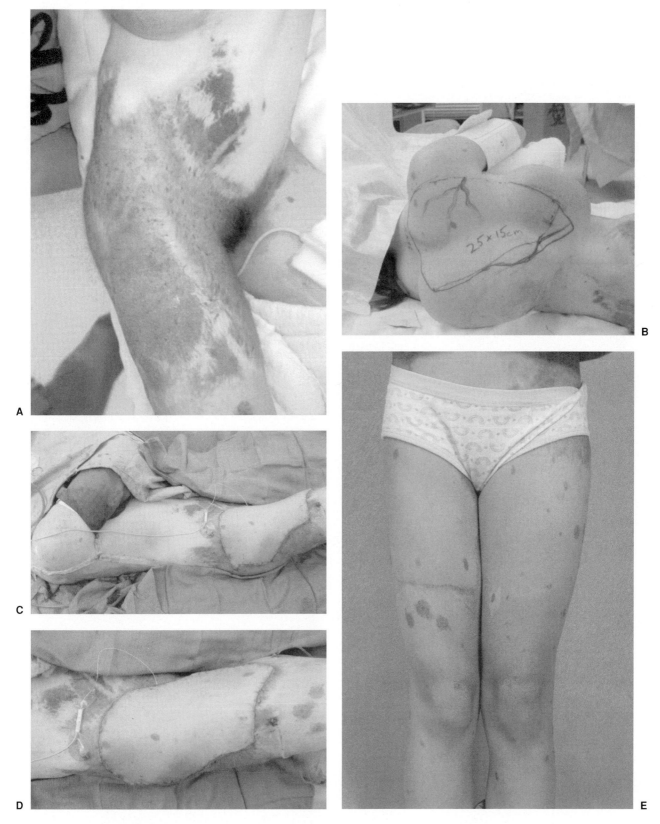

FIGURE 10.4. A: Anterolateral view of a 6-year-old child with giant nevus of lower abdomen, groin, and right thigh, with the plan to excise a large segment of the nevus of the anterior thigh and reconstruct it with an expanded free scapular–parascapular flap. No regional tissue is available to expand in the region of the thigh. **B:** Posterior view of expanders on back adjacent to the outlined free flap. Expanders are used to aid in closure of this large donor site. **C:** Lateral view of the child with the donor site closed and the free flap in place on the anterolateral thigh. **D:** Closer view of the 25×15-cm free flap in place on the thigh. **E:** Excellent color and contour match of the expanded flap on the right thigh at 9 months after reconstruction.

A useful algorithm for complex defects has been devised for upper limb reconstruction. Based on our experience, successful contour and color match of the upper extremity comes from approaching it in thirds (proximal arm to elbow; midforearm; and the hands, web spaces, and fingers), and from whether or not the lesion is circumferential or noncircumferential. For proximal noncircumferential defects, expanded transposition flaps from the back or shoulder serve the purpose well. If the lesion is large and circumferential, covering the majority of the proximal arm, expanded free TRAM flaps are the media of choice. Distally, for large, circumferential mid- or lower forearm lesions, expansion of the flank creates a pedicled carrier "sling" through which the forearm can be placed for 3 weeks prior to pedicle division. As previously reported, expanded full-thickness skin grafts from the abdomen or the groin remain the treatment of choice for reconstruction of fingers, webs, and hand.

COMPLICATIONS

Beyond the site-specific complications of tissue expansion mentioned above, general complications can be divided into major and minor categories. Major complications involve infection, implant exposure, and flap ischemia. Traditionally, it has been taught that early postoperative infections should be managed with expander removal and antibiotics; infections occurring late in the expansion course can sometimes be salvaged with antibiotics. Extrusions have been dealt with similarly. However, we have found that a prosthesis may be salvageable if it lies in a dependent position in relation to the open wound. Such extrusions are also managed conservatively, with local wound care and oral antibiotics. Under such conditions, most wounds achieve closure secondarily without consequence.

Minor complications with expansion include transient pain with expansion, seroma, dog ears at the donor site, and widening of scars. In one study, these minor untoward events collectively occurred at a rate as high as 17% of patients.

Acknowledgment

I would like to thank Dr. Russell R. Reid for his help with this chapter.

References

1. Radovan C. *Adjacent Flap Development Using Expandable Silastic Implants*. Paper presented at annual meeting of the American Society of Plastic and Reconstructive Surgeons, Boston, September, 1976.
2. Austad ED, Rose GL. A self-inflating tissue expander. *Plast Reconstr Surg.* 1982;70:588.
3. Neumann CG. The expansion of an area of skin by progressive distention of a subcutaneous balloon. *Plast Reconstr Surg.* 1957;19:124.
4. Bauer BS, Margulis A. The expanded transposition flap: shifting paradigms based on experience gained from two decades of pediatric tissue expansion. *Plast Reconstr Surg.* 2004;114:98–106.
5. DeFilippo RE, Atala A. Stretch and growth: the molecular and physiologic influences of tissue expansion. *Plast Reconstr Surg.* 2001;109(7):2450–2461.
6. Takei T, Mills I, Arai K, et al. Molecular basis for tissue expansion: clinical implications for the surgeon. *Plast Reconstr Surg.* 1998;102(1):247–258.
7. Cherry GW, Austad E, Pasyk K, et al. Increased survival and vascularity of random pattern skin flaps elevated in controlled, expanded skin. *Plast Reconstr Surg.* 1983;72:680.
8. Mohmand MH, Sterne GD, Gowar JP. Home inflation of tissue expanders: a safe and reliable alternative. *Br J Plast Surg.* 2001;54:610–614.
9. Bauer BS, Vicari FA and Richard ME. The role of tissue expansion in pediatric plastic surgery. *Clin Plast Surg.* 1990;17(1):101–113.
10. Bauer BS, Few JW, Chavez CD, et al. The role of tissue expansion in the management of large congenital pigmented nevi of the forehead in the pediatric patient. *Plast Reconstr Surg.* 2001;107(3):668–675.
11. Neale HW, Kurtzman LC, Goh KB, et al. Tissue expanders in the lower face and anterior neck in pediatric burn patients: limitations and pitfalls. *Plast Reconstr Surg.* 1993;91:624.
12. Bauer BS, Vicari F, Richard ME, et al. Expanded full thickness skin grafts in children: case selection, planning and management. *Plast Reconstr Surg.* 1993;92:59.
13. Bauer BS. Commentary on Gosain AK et al. Giant congenital nevi: a 20-year experience and an algorithm for their management. *Plast Reconstr Surg.* 2001;108:632–636.
14. Casanova D, Bali D, Bardot J, et al. Tissue expansion of the lower limb: complications in a cohort of 103 cases. *Br J Plast Surg.* 2001;54:310–316.
15. Margulis A, Bauer BS, Fine NA. Large and giant congenital pigmented nevi of the upper extremity: an algorithm to surgical management. *Ann Plast Surg.* 2004;52(2):158–167.

CHAPTER 11 ■ LOCAL ANESTHETICS

ALISA C. THORNE

The clinically useful local anesthetics are either amino amides or amino esters. These agents are effective when applied topically, injected subcutaneously, or injected in the area of major peripheral nerves.

MECHANISM OF ACTION

Local anesthetics cause a blockade in nerve condition. The local anesthetic diffuses passively through the neuronal cell membrane in the nonionic state, becomes charged, and blocks the sodium channel within the neuron. With sodium conductance inhibited, threshold potential is not reached and an action potential is not generated.

PHARMACOLOGY

The molecular structure of local anesthetic agents consists of an aromatic moiety at one end, an amine moiety at the other end, and an intermediate chain between. The latter contains either an amide or an ester linkage, allowing local anesthetics to be classified as either amides or esters. Commonly used esters are procaine (Novocain), chloroprocaine, tetracaine, and cocaine. Commonly used amides are lidocaine, mepivacaine, prilocaine, bupivacaine (Marcaine), and etidocaine. Differences in the metabolism of local anesthetics, their stability in solution, and differences in allergenicity are all related to the presence of an ester or amide linkage.

Metabolism

Esters undergo hydrolysis in the plasma by pseudo-cholinesterase, whereas the amides are metabolized in the liver. The rate of metabolism of local anesthetics is related to the number of additional carbon atoms on the aromatic or amine side of the molecule.

Stability in Solution

Esters are unstable in solution. Amides are stable in solution.

Allergenicity

Esters are also more likely to cause allergenic reactions than amides. A true allergic reaction to lidocaine is extremely rare, although many patients will state, incorrectly, that they have such an allergy.

Potency and Toxicity

Potency and toxicity are determined by the structure of the aromatic and the amine group.

ANESTHETIC PROFILE

The profile of a particular local anesthetic agent is related to its lipid solubility, protein binding, acid strength (pKa), and vasodilator activity.

Potency

Anesthetic potency is determined primarily by the degree of lipid solubility. The local anesthetic molecule must penetrate the nerve cell membrane to have an effect. In vitro, hydrophobicity alone determines the potency of a given local anesthetic. In clinical settings, however, other factors, such as vasodilatory activity and the tissue redistribution properties of the different local anesthetics, influence potency to some extent.

Onset of Action

The onset of action is primarily a result of the pKa, but the dose and the concentration are also factors. In vitro studies confirm the relationship between pKa of a local anesthetic compound and the onset of anesthesia. Lidocaine has a pKa of 7.4 and a more rapid onset of action than tetracaine, which has a pKa of 8.6.

Duration of Action

In the clinical arena, the duration of local anesthesia is principally influenced by the vasodilator effects of the individual drugs. With the exception of cocaine, all local anesthetics cause some degree of vasodilation. The greater the degree of vasodilation, the greater the amount of the drug that is absorbed by the vascular system, leaving less drug to act on the nerve cell. Therefore, the degree of vasodilation is inversely related to the duration of action. See the section Addition of Epinephrine.

Duration and Potency Summary

In summary, agents with low potency and short duration are procaine (Novocain) and chloroprocaine; agents with moderate potency and duration are lidocaine (Xylocaine), mepivacaine, and prilocaine; agents with a high potency and a long duration are tetracaine, bupivacaine (Marcaine), and etidocaine.

TABLE 11.1

DOSAGE AND DURATION CHARACTERISTICS OF THE LOCAL ANESTHETICS WHEN USED FOR MINOR NERVE BLOCKS (E.G., MEDIAN NERVE BLOCK AT THE WRIST)

Drug	Usual concentration (%)	Plain solutions			Epinephrine-containing solutions
		Usual volume (mL)	Dosage (mg)	Average duration (min)	Average duration (min)
Procaine Chloroprocaine Lidocaine	2	5–20	100–400	15–30	30–60
Mepivacaine Prilocaine	1	5–20	50–200	60–120	120–180
Bupivacaine	0.25	5–20	12.5–50	180–360	240–480
Etidocaine	0.5	5–20	25–100	120–240	180–420

Reprinted with permission from Strichartz, G. R., and Covino, B. G. Local Anesthetics. In R. D. Miller (ed.), *Anesthesia* (4th ed.), New York: Churchill Livingstone, 1994.

Effect of Total Dose

Other factors determine a local anesthetic agent's activity in the clinical setting. Total dose is probably the single most important factor in determining satisfactory local anesthesia. Also, as mentioned earlier under Onset of Action, the greater the dose, other factors being equal, the faster the onset of action.

Addition of Epinephrine

The addition of vasoconstrictors is another factor determining the performance of local anesthetic. Epinephrine markedly prolongs the duration of action of all local anesthetics when used for local infiltration or peripheral nerve blocks. By decreasing the rate of vascular absorption, vasoconstrictors cause a higher concentration of local anesthetic molecules to be available to act on the nerve cell membrane.

Epinephrine is frequently used in combination with local anesthetics at concentrations of 1:100,000 or 1:200,000. In fact, epinephrine is probably equally effective at much lower doses (1:1,000,000) and might decrease the danger of an intravascular injection.

Location of Injection

The anatomy of the site of injection also has a role in determining the activity of a local anesthetic. Intradermal injection allows for the most rapid onset of action but the shortest duration of these agents, whereas brachial plexus block injections yield some of the longest durations and slowest onsets of action seen with local anesthetics. Although intradermal injection provides the most rapid onset, it is more painful than subcutaneous injection.

PERIPHERAL NERVE BLOCKS

There are two general types of peripheral nerve blockade: major and minor. Blocks of individual nerves, such as radial nerve block, are referred to as minor, and blocks of two or more nerves or a plexus of nerves are called major nerve blocks. A wide variety of local anesthetics can be used for minor nerve blocks. The drug is usually selected based on the duration of anesthesia that is required. The duration of action of minor

nerve blockade is prolonged by the addition of epinephrine to the local anesthetic solution.

A commonly used major nerve block is the brachial plexus (or axillary) block. Although the onset of action for minor nerve blocks is generally rapid for all the local anesthetics, there are differences in onset between the various anesthetic agents when major nerve blocks are performed. Epinephrine, in general, will prolong the duration of brachial plexus blockade. The longer-acting local anesthetics do not demonstrate as much prolongation of action with epinephrine as do the shorter-acting agents. Tables 11.1 and 11.2 show the maximal dose, onset, and duration of action of the commonly used local anesthetics for minor and major nerve blocks.

TOPICAL ANESTHESIA

Topical anesthesia is increasingly important in pediatric intravenous insertion and is used by some surgeons to lessen the discomfort of injectables such as Restylane and Botox. These topical agents will provide dermal anesthesia if applied far enough in advance but do nothing to lessen the burning associated with subcutaneous injection.

Eutectic mixture of local anesthetics (EMLA) is a combination of 25 mg lidocaine and 50 mg prilocaine per gram of EMLA. L-M-X4 contains 4% lidocaine per gram. These formulations decrease pain secondary to intravenous insertion and also provide adequate analgesia for split-thickness skin graft harvesting. L-M-X4 may have a slightly faster onset but both preparations are best applied between 30 and 60 minutes prior to the procedure and are best covered with an occlusive dressing such as Tegaderm or OpSite.

Several other topical local anesthesia preparations are available that provide brief periods of anesthesia when they are applied to mucous membranes or abraded skin. The most common local anesthetic agents used topically are lidocaine, dibucaine, tetracaine, and benzocaine.

INFILTRATION OF LOCAL ANESTHETICS

The most common method of achieving local anesthesia for minor office procedures is infiltration anesthesia, in which the agent is injected into the operative site without selectively blocking a specific nerve. Any local anesthetic can be used for

DOSAGE AND DURATION CHARACTERISTICS OF THE LOCAL ANESTHETICS WHEN USED FOR MAJOR NERVE BLOCKS (E.G., AXILLARY BLOCK OF THE BRACHIAL PLEXUS)

Drug with epinephrine 1:200.000	Usual concentration (%)	Usual volume (mL)	Maximal dose (mg)	Usual onset (min)	Usual duration (min)
Lidocaine	1–1.5	30–50	500	10–20	120–240
Mepivacaine	1–1.5	30–50	500	10–20	180–300
Prilocaine	1–2	30–50	600	10–20	180–300
Bupivacaine	0.25–0.5	30–50	225	15–30	360–720
Etidocaine	0.5–1.0	30–50	400	10–20	360–720
Tetracaine	0.25–0.5	30–50	200	20–30	300–600

Reprinted with permission from Strichartz, G. R., and Covino, B. G. Local Anesthetics. In R. D. Miller (ed.), *Anesthesia* (4th ed.). New York: Churchill Livingstone, 1994.

infiltration except cocaine. Injection may be intradermal, subcutaneous, or both. Again, the duration of action will vary and the addition of epinephrine will prolong the duration of analgesia. Dilute anesthetic solutions are recommended for large areas to avoid toxicity. Infiltration of local anesthetic causes a painful, burning sensation. Injection into the dermis is the most painful and provides the fastest onset of action. Addition of sodium bicarbonate decreases the pain associated with infiltration. Table 11.3 shows the maximal dose and duration of local anesthetics when used for infiltration anesthesia. When maximal doses are employed, the onset is very rapid regardless of which agent is selected.

TOXICITY OF LOCAL ANESTHETICS

To avoid toxicity, local anesthetics must be administered within a safe dose range and in the correct anatomic location. **During local anesthesia, when toxic reactions occur, they are almost always the result of inadvertent intravascular injection or the administration of an excessively large dose.** Many patients report an "allergy" to local anesthesia that was probably actually symptoms related to an intravascular injection and probably related to the epinephrine rather than the local anesthetic. Every effort should be made to avoid intravascular injection. The syringe should always be aspirated before the local anesthetic is injected, regardless of the anatomic site of injection. Repeat aspirations should be made after injecting 2 to 3 mL of local anesthetic. If blood is seen in the syringe, the needle must be repositioned. **An intravascular injection of an epinephrine containing solution may produce a dangerously hypertensive response.**

As mentioned earlier, the addition of epinephrine to the anesthetic solution delays absorption and results in lower anesthetic blood levels, as well as a longer duration of the action. Epinephrine is especially useful when local anesthetic is being injected into highly vascular areas such as the face. It was previously believed that epinephrine should be omitted from anesthetic solutions injected in proximity to end arteries (e.g., fingers, toes, and penis) because of the danger of ischemic necrosis. Recent studies cast doubt on this dictum.

The toxicity of local anesthetic agents affects the central nervous system (CNS) and the cardiovascular system (CVS). CNS toxicity occurs at a lower dose range than does CVS toxicity. Whereas CNS toxicity is more common, CVS toxicity is more dangerous and more challenging to treat.

DOSAGE AND DURATION CHARACTERISTICS OF THE LOCAL ANESTHETICS WHEN USED FOR INFILTRATION ANESTHESIA (E.G., INFILTRATION AROUND THE PERIPHERY OF A SKIN LESION BEFORE EXCISION)

Drug	Plain solution			Epinephrine-containing solution		
	Concentration (%)	Max dose (mg)	Duration (min)	Max dose (mg)	Duration (min)	
Short duration						
Procaine						
Chloroprocaine	1.0–2.0	800	15–30	1,000	30–90	
Moderate duration						
Lidocaine	0.5–1.0	300	30–60	500	120–360	
Mepivacaine	0.5–1.0	300	45–90	500	120–360	
Prilocaine	0.5–1.0	500	30–90	600	120–360	
Long duration						
Bupivacaine	0.25–0.5	175	120–240	225	180–420	
Etidocaine	0.5–1.0	300	120–180	400	180–420	

Reprinted with permission from Strichartz, G. R., and Covine, B. G. Local Anesthetics. In R. D. Miller (ed.), *Anesthesia* (4th ed.). New York: Churchill Livingstone, 1994.

Local anesthetics freely cross the blood–brain barrier. The initial result of toxic levels of local anesthetics is depression of cortical inhibitory pathways, which allows excitatory pathway activity to be unopposed. When even higher blood levels are reached, generalized CNS depression occurs. Early signs of CNS toxicity include light-headedness, restlessness, tinnitus and other auditory or visual disturbances, slurred speech, tremors, metallic taste in the mouth, and numbness of the lips or tongue. If more local anesthesia is given, grand mal seizures may result. At even higher blood levels, loss of consciousness, apnea, and cardiovascular collapse are seen. If a large dose of local anesthetic is anticipated, pretreatment with a benzodiazepine may prevent toxicity. Diazepam doubles the seizure threshold for lidocaine.

CVS toxicity is the result of direct myocardial depression by the local anesthetic. A depressant effect on vascular smooth muscle, as well as on the conducting system, is seen. This effect is rarely observed in the clinical setting. Cardiac stimulation is the more common result of toxic levels of local anesthetics and is the result of an increase in CNS activity. CVS toxicity may present itself as a drop in blood pressure, an increase or decrease in heart rate, ventricular fibrillation, or cardiac arrest.

The inadvertent intravenous injection of bupivacaine (Marcaine) or etidocaine can result in severe cardiovascular compromise and collapse, frequently refractory to attempts at resuscitation. This is because of the high degree of tissue binding of these two local anesthetics. Consequently, bupivacaine (Marcaine) should probably not be used when an intravascular injection is likely. For example, it should probably not be used for subcutaneous injection prior to a facelift where large volumes of solution are injected in a vascular area. Also, the pregnant patient is more sensitive to CVS toxicity of bupivacaine (Marcaine) than is the nonpregnant patient.

TUMESCENT TECHNIQUE FOR LIPOSUCTION

Experience with the "tumescent technique" of local anesthesia infiltration casts doubt on previous "facts" regarding maximal local anesthetic dose. This technique involves the infiltration of large volumes of a dilute solution of lidocaine (0.1% or 0.05%) and epinephrine (1:500,000 to 1:1,000,000) into the subcutaneous adipose tissue prior to liposuction procedures. Studies demonstrate that doses up to 35 mg/kg lidocaine (five times the manufacturer's recommended dose) can be given safely. Serial serum lidocaine levels drawn postoperatively appear to verify the safety of this technique, which has been extended to other procedures such as abdominoplasty (see Chapter 53). The safety of this technique probably depends on the anatomy of the site of injection and the dilute nature of the solution injected. **The face is not the same as the body. Although the exact dose of lidocaine that can be used safely in the face has not been clarified, it is clear that doses such as 35 mg/kg, which are safe in the subcutaneous tissues of the trunk, are far too large for the face. Until a safe maximum dose is defined, surgeons are advised to use no more than the 7 mg/kg recommended by the manufacturer.**

TREATMENT OF LOCAL ANESTHETIC TOXICITY

The first step in the treatment of a patient who is convulsing as a consequence of local anesthetic toxicity is hyperventilation with an Ambu bag and face mask using 100% oxygen. Hypercarbia can worsen CNS toxicity. If the patient has a full stomach, an endotracheal tube should be placed as soon as possible to prevent aspiration. Hyperventilation may terminate the

seizure, but if it does not, diazepam, 0.1 mg/kg, or thiopental, 2 mg/kg, intravenously is usually effective.

In the patient who is hypotensive as a result of local anesthetic toxicity, the treatment is intravenous (IV) fluids, peripheral vasoconstrictors (e.g., phenylephrine), and Trendelenburg positioning. An inotropic agent (e.g., dopamine) may also be required. The patient in whom arrhythmias develop as a consequence of toxicity may be refractory to therapy. If the arrhythmia is causing the cardiac output to be significantly compromised, or if cardiac arrest occurs, a prolonged period of resuscitation may be necessary, as these conditions are known to resolve over time as redistribution of the local anesthetic occurs.

COCAINE

Cocaine is unique in that it has both local anesthetic and vasoconstrictive action. It has considerable potential for abuse and addiction. Over the past several decades, illegal use of cocaine has become epidemic. Cocaine is a crystalline, water-soluble powder (pKa 8.6) that is readily absorbed through mucous membranes. It undergoes hydrolysis by plasma pseudocholinesterase. A small percentage of cocaine is metabolized in the liver.

As with the other local anesthetics, the mechanism of action of cocaine involves inhibition of conduction in nerve fibers by blockade of sodium channels, which, in turn, prevents an action potential from being generated. Cocaine is the only local anesthetic that is a potent sympathomimetic. It blocks reuptake of norepinephrine and epinephrine, both in the central nervous system and systemically. Cocaine has multiple effects on the central nervous system, resulting in intense behavioral stimulation, euphoria, and arousal. The seizure threshold is initially raised, but is lowered with increasing dose, and seizures can result. The adrenergic effects of cocaine are responsible for the increased heart rate, hypertension, mydriasis, tremors, and perspiration seen with an overdose.

Traditionally, the most common clinical use of cocaine in plastic surgery is as a topical anesthetic and vasoconstrictor in rhinoplasty. It is no longer often used as other agents are safer, cheaper, and have less potential for abuse. **The addition of epinephrine to the topical cocaine may enhance vasoconstriction but is not safe.** The combination can cause dangerous arrhythmias. It is not even clear that adding epinephrine to topical cocaine enhances the operating conditions. Studies have not demonstrated a consistent benefit from adding epinephrine to either 10% cocaine or to lower concentrations of topical cocaine.

General anesthesia and topical cocaine are frequently used together, and there are multiple studies and case reports describing the complexity of drug interactions that occur. These reports offer conflicting views of the effect that cocaine has on anesthetic requirements as well as the effect of the combination of cocaine and varying anesthetics on their arrhythmogenic potential. Studies on the combination of cocaine and general anesthetics suggest that anxious or unpremeditated patients are more prone to arrhythmias and that cocaine should not be applied before induction or soon after induction, before the achievement of a deep level of anesthesia. In those patients in whom topical cocaine was used after induction, and after a deep level of anesthesia was achieved, there were no arrhythmias. Therefore, a patient's endogenous catecholamines are involved in these complex drug interactions.

There is also widespread agreement that ketamine significantly enhances the arrhythmogenicity of cocaine. Additionally, patients receiving monoamine oxidase (MAO) inhibitors are especially at risk for dangerous interactions with cocaine. Topical cocaine should be avoided unless the patient has been taken off the MAO inhibitor 2 weeks before the surgical procedure. Because of its sympathomimetic effects, cocaine also should be avoided in hypertensive patients. Unfortunately, individual response to cocaine varies. In some patients ventricular fibrillation and cardiac arrest can occur as a result of a dose as small as 0.4 mg/kg.

The safe maximum dose for nasally administered 4% cocaine solution is 1.5 mg/kg. Each drop of 4% cocaine solution has approximately 3 mg cocaine. Given the above disadvantages of cocaine, however, there may no longer be a good indication for its use.

Suggested Readings

Covino BG. Pharmacology of local anesthetic agents. *Ration Drug Ther.* 1987;21:1.

De Jong RH, Heavner JE. Diazepam prevents local anesthetic seizures. *Anesthesiology.* 1971;34:523.

Fleming JA, Byck R, Barash PG. Pharmacology and therapeutic applications of cocaine. *Anesthesiology.* 1990;73:518.

Hallen B, Uppfeldt M. Does lidocaine-prilocaine cream permit pain free insertion of IV catheters in children? *Anesthesiology.* 1982;57:340.

Kelton PL Jr. Local anesthetics, cocaine, and CPR. *Sel Read Plast Surg.* 1992;7(5):1.

Klein JA. Tumescent technique for regional anesthesia permits lidocaine doses of 35 mg/kg for liposuction. *J Dermatol Surg Oncol.* 1990;16:248.

Koehntop DE, Liao J-C, Van Bergen FH. Effects of pharmacologic alterations of adrenergic mechanisms by cocaine, tropolone, aminophylline, and ketamine on epinephrine-induced arrhythmias during halothane-nitrous oxide anesthesia. *Anesthesiology.* 1977;46:83.

Lynch C. Depression of myocardial contractility in vitro by bupivacaine, etidocaine, and lidocaine. *Anesth Analg.* 1986;65:551.

Ohlsen L, Englesson S, Evers H. An anaesthetic lidocaine/prilocaine cream (EMLA) for epicutaneous application tested for cutting split skin grafts. *Scand J Plast Reconstr Surg.* 1985;19:201.

Strichartz GR, Covino BG. Local anesthetics. In: Miller RD, ed. *Anesthesia.* 3rd ed. New York: Churchill Livingstone; 1990:437.

Swerdlow M, Jones R. The duration of action of bupivacaine, prilocaine and lignocaine. *Br J Anaesth.* 1970;42:335.

CHAPTER 12 ■ PRINCIPLES OF CRANIOFACIAL DISTRACTION

JOSEPH G. McCARTHY

Distraction osteogenesis is now an established therapeutic tool for the plastic surgeon, especially in the augmentation or enlargement of the craniofacial skeleton. It has the enormous advantage of eliminating the need for bone grafts and alloplastic materials.

The technique is unique in the armamentarium of the surgeon in that it applies gradual and incremental traction force/tension to surgically separated bony segments to produce additional bone. In essence, it releases inherent biologic forces to generate human tissues, that is, bone and the associated neuromuscular/soft-tissue complex. The technique could actually be called distraction histogenesis in that distraction of the skeleton also causes enlargement of the overlying or surrounding soft tissue.

HISTORY

The concept of skeletal molding or lengthening has, in reality, been practiced by various cultures for centuries. In certain African tribes, serial applications of metal necklaces at a young age result in elongation of the neck for aesthetic purposes. Other cultures have performed cranial molding with the application of helmets to the skulls of infants.

Early in the 20th century, Codivilla reported a technique involving an osteotomy of the femur and application of external traction to lengthen the lower extremity. A similar report was also provided by Abbot in 1927. However, the biologic principles were insufficiently studied; consequently, the devices were poorly designed, and infection, fibrous union, nerve palsy, and joint contractures resulted.

It remained for Ilizarov (1,2) to conduct the laboratory studies and popularize the concept of distraction osteogenesis in the long (endochondral) bones of the extremities for limb lengthening and for the closure of bony defects. McCarthy et al. at New York University (3–5) applied the technique to the bones (membranous) of the craniofacial skeleton in a series of canine mandible studies, and clinical craniofacial distraction was introduced in 1989.

At the present time, in addition to the use of distraction by orthopedic surgeons for defects of the long bones of the extremity, distraction has found even wider application in the craniofacial skeleton, for the correction of deficiencies of the mandible, maxilla, midface, zygomas, and cranial vault.

PRINCIPLES

The biologic concept of targeted bone growth/deposition is probably best demonstrated by cranial sutures. As the rapidly enlarging brain in the growing infant separates the individual cranial bones, the sutures react by depositing new bone. In this manner the cranial vault increases in surface area to provide a skeleton of adequate volume for the brain. Maxillary arch expansion by activation of a device placed across the palatine suture, as routinely practiced by orthodontists, is yet another example of distraction osteogenesis.

The concept is relatively simple.

1. The bone is separated into segments by either a full-thickness osteotomy or by a low-energy corticotomy (sparing the endosteum or marrow space). The location of the bony separation is termed the *distraction zone*.
2. Time is allowed (5 to 7 days) for reparative callus formation in the distraction zone (the *latency period*).
3. Gradual distraction forces are applied to separate the edges and elongate the intersegmentary callus under tension (the *activation period*).
   a. Rigidity of the distraction device is critical to maintain the intersegmentary gap tissues in a direction or vector parallel to the orientation of the device (the *vector of distraction*).
   b. A *rhythm* of 0.25 mm four times a day is preferable (0.5 mm twice a day is generally acceptable in a clinical setting).
4. At the end of activation, the external fixation must be maintained in position to allow consolidation of the newly formed bone (*distraction generate*). The *consolidation period* usually lasts approximately 8 weeks.

The three types of distraction osteogenesis are as follows (Fig. 12.1):

1. *Unifocal*—a single osteotomy with distraction forces applied by a device attached by screws on either side of the osteotomy;
2. *Bifocal*—one osteotomy with pins on either side of the osteotomy and defect and with a single spanning device encompassing the transport segment; and
3. *Trifocal*—two osteotomies used to fill a skeletal defect in a bidirectional manner.

The *transport segment* is delivered into the skeletal defect by forces applied by the distraction device. The leading edge of the segment has a fibrocartilage cap. Bone grafting is usually required after the transport segment has been finally "docked," the fibrocartilage tissue resected, and the defect replaced by the graft.

The most usual type of distraction is *transosteotomy* (or *transcorticotomy*) distraction. However, in very young patients, successful distraction can be performed across patent or open sutures (*trans-sutural* distraction). Palatal expansion with an orthodontic appliance is an example of the latter.

Distraction represents a unique form of fracture healing. In contrast to fracture healing that occurs via a cartilaginous intermediate, distraction of both the membranous bone of the craniofacial skeleton and the endochondral bone of the extremities occurs without a cartilaginous intermediate.

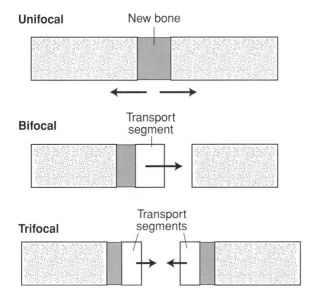

Unifocal

New bone

Bifocal

Transport segment

Trifocal

Transport segments

FIGURE 12.1. There are three types of distraction osteogenesis: unifocal, bifocal, and trifocal. The solid gray zone represents the newly generated bone at the osteotomy/corticotomy site. The *arrows* designate the direction of the distraction (strain) forces. The transport segments are white. (Adapted from Aro H. Biomechanics of distraction. In: McCarthy JG, ed. *Distraction of the Craniofacial Skeleton.* New York: Springer; 1999.)

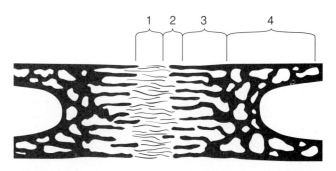

FIGURE 12.2. Schematic of the temporal stages of bone generation in unifocal distraction. (From Karp NS, McCarthy JG, Schreiber JS, et al. Membranous bone lengthening: a serial histologic study. *Ann Plast Surg.* 1992;29:2, with permission.)

In summary, the following four temporal zones are observed in the distraction gap (Fig. 12.2):

1. Fibrous central zone (mesenchymal proliferation)—longitudinally oriented fibrous bundles;
2. Transition zone—osteoid formation along the collagen bundles in the distraction gap;
3. Remodeling zone—the appearance of osteoclasts with remodeling of the newly formed bone; and
4. Mature bone zone.

Histologic Analysis

The histologic changes occurring in the distraction zone have been elucidated in animal experiments. A circumferential corticotomy was performed in the region of the angle of the mandible at a position posterior to the molars in a canine model (4). After the application of a distraction device, there was a *latency period* of 7 days. The device was activated at the *rate* and *rhythm* of 0.5 mm twice a day for a total of 20 mm (*activation period*). The distracted mandibles were harvested at several time points during the activation and consolidation periods, and subjected to histologic and microradiographic examination.

During the latency period (after osteotomy and before activation of the device) bone repair is similar to that observed after fracture healing—hematoma formation and the migration of inflammatory cells into the osseous gap. This is obviously a hypoxic zone of injury stimulating an angiogenic response and initiating the migration of primitive mesenchymal cells and the synthesis of collagen I matrix. Angiogenesis is definitely a precursor to evidence of osteogenic activity. Angiogenesis occurs on a collagen matrix.

Microscopic examination after activation of the distraction device demonstrates tapered cells, similar to fibroblasts, and new blood vessels, which form a fibrovascular matrix aligned longitudinally in the direction of the distraction vector. Osteoid synthesis and mineralization are not apparent until almost 14 days after the initiation of activation.

At approximately 3 weeks after activation, calcification of the linear-oriented collagen bundles is first noted, followed by the appearance of osteoblasts along the collagen bundles and the formation of bony spicules that extend from the edges of the osteotomy toward the central portion of the distraction zone. With progressive calcification of the generate, there is bony closure of the distraction defect. Continued remodeling of the newly formed bone, as evidenced by the appearance of osteoclasts, results in lamellar bone with marrow elements of adequate volume.

Biomolecular Analysis

The development of a laboratory rat model of mandibular distraction has permitted the study of a relatively large number of animals with the potential for detailed biomolecular analysis of the distraction zone (6). At the end of the latency and in the early activation periods, there is a metabolically active, heterogeneous cell population (endothelial cells, fibroblasts, and polymorphonuclear leukocytes) in the distraction zone, all associated with the presence of type I collagen bundles. The latter become organized and oriented as a fibrovascular bridge in a plane parallel to the distraction vector. The arrival of large osteoblasts at the edges of the osteotomized bone is associated with osteoid deposition along the collagen bundles; this is followed by mineralization of the generate in the distraction gap.

A marked increase in transforming growth factor-β_1 (TGF-β_1) is demonstrated as early as 3 days into the latency period; expression of this cytokine peaks during the late stages of the activation period (7). It returns to near-normal levels toward the end of the consolidation period. These findings imply a regulatory mechanism for TGF-β_1 in inducing collagen deposition and noncollagen extracellular matrix proteins involved in the mineralization and remodeling of bones. TGF-β_1 is also important in the activation of VEGF (vascular endothelial growth factor) and basic FGF (fibroblast growth factor). TGF-β_1 also plays a regulatory role in osteoblast migration, differentiation, and bone remodeling.

Although osteocalcin (a noncollagenous matrix protein) expression is decreased during the latency period, an increased expression is observed early in the activation period, and it is increased to normal levels by the end of the consolidation period. Osteocalcin plays an important role in mineralization and bone remodeling. The key quality of bone, that is, its rigidity or hardness, is attributable to the mineralization of the linear-oriented extracellular matrices.

A more complete understanding of the biomolecular regulation of distraction osteogenesis offers the possibility of future clinical manipulation of the distraction zone, for example, increasing the rate of activation and decreasing the length of the consolidation period. If the latter goals can be achieved, the length of the overall distraction treatment period would be significantly reduced.

Biomechanics

In distraction osteogenesis, the tensile forces delivered to the developing callus at the osteotomy site cause elongation of the callus. The mechanical environment in the distraction zone is determined by the following factors: the rigidity of the distraction device, the applied distraction forces, the inherent physiologic loading (muscle action), and the properties of all of the local soft tissues (8).

Tensile strain is defined as the amount of elongation as a fraction of the original bone length (9). At an activation rate of 1.0 mm per day and an osteotomy defect of 1.0 mm, the strain is 100% during the first day of activation. By activation day 10, when there is a 10-mm gap, the tensile strain has decreased to 10%. Because bone can tolerate only 1% to 2% of tensile strain ("ultimate tensile strain"), bone tissue cannot long survive a load exceeding more than 1% to 2% tensile strain. Consequently, bone formation is not observed in the distraction zone until approximately 4 weeks of activation, that is, that period when the tensile strength is at or below the ultimate tensile level.

The process by which mechanical forces are converted to cellular signals is termed *mechanical transduction* (9). A studied pathway is the integrin-mediated signal transduction cascade. In the rat mandibular model of distraction, the demonstration of immunolocalization of focal adhesion kinase and other molecular mediators supports the hypothesis that bone formation in mandibular distraction is regulated by mechanical forces, signaling integrin-mediated single-transduction pathways at the molecular level.

MANDIBLE DISTRACTION

The mandible was the obvious first choice for craniofacial distraction (5). It is an accessible, somewhat tubular, bone in which changes can be easily documented by radiography and measurement of occlusal changes. In addition, a clinical need existed for a therapeutic paradigm shift, especially in pediatric patients with deficiency of the mandibular ramus and life-threatening respiratory problems.

In contrast to classic mandibular osteotomies, distraction permits surgery at a younger age without the need for bone grafts, blood transfusions, and prolonged operations and hospital stays. There is also an associated expansion or lengthening of the overlying soft tissues and muscles. **The relapse rate is lower, as the bone is lengthened gradually at the rate of 1 mm per day, in contrast to an acute**

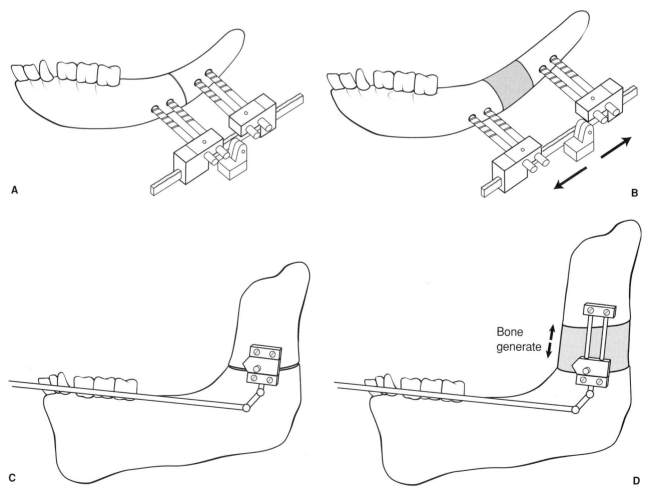

FIGURE 12.3. Mandibular distraction devices. **A** and **B:** Extraoral device illustrating bone generation at the osteotomy site. **C** and **D:** Intraoral or buried mandibular distraction device. (From Mathes SJ. *Plastic Surgery.* Philadelphia: Elsevier; 2005, with permission.)

intraoperative advancement against deficient and restrictive soft tissues.

A variety of mandibular distraction devices are available and the surgeon must chose between an external (extraoral) or buried (intraoral) device (Fig. 12.3). **In general, extraoral devices are associated with more successful and consistent outcomes.** They are especially indicated when the skeletal site for the osteotomy and pin insertions is diminutive in area and volume. A distinct disadvantage is that it leaves an external scar, which can be obvious and hypertrophic in a few patients.

Although intraoral or buried devices are associated with better scar formation, it is usually also necessary to place a transcutaneous scar for their insertion. Consequently, there is always a resulting scar. The actual progress of the activation cannot be observed externally, and in the infant in whom serial radiographs are not possible, there can be an undetected mechanical problem. Moreover, there is less flexibility in terms of device placement with the result that the optimal vector (10) cannot always be achieved and molding of the generate is also not possible. Intraoral devices are also *much more difficult* to remove, which is an underestimated disadvantage.

Technique

The mandible is approached by individual or combined *transcutaneous* (submandibular) or *intraoral* incisions.

The first decision is the choice of a *vector* (10). The *vertical vector* is defined as one at 90 degrees to the maxillary occlusal plane and is indicated when there is a vertical deficiency of the ramus (Fig. 12.4). In patients with severe micrognathia associated with deficiency of the mandibular body, the *horizontal vector* (parallel to the maxillary occlusal plane) is selected. The *oblique vector* is selected when there is a deficiency in both the vertical ramus and the horizontal body of the mandible.

The indications for mandibular distraction are functional and aesthetic. Distraction has revolutionized the treatment of the infant or young patient with sleep apnea and the associated alimentary problems of eating and swallowing. The technique can be employed in the neonate, and it has obviated the need for tracheostomy and its attendant problems. Moreover, it has permitted the decannulation of tracheotomies in infants and young children. Sleep apnea is also an unrecognized problem in the older patients, accounting for learning disabilities and behavioral problems. Mandibular distraction can have a positive impact on the quality of life of such children.

Mandibular distraction is also indicated for patients with facial dysmorphism in such conditions as craniofacial microsomia, developmental micrognathia, and Treacher Collins syndrome. Postablative mandibular defects and temporomandibular joint ankylosis are other conditions that can be treated by transport distraction. Alveolar ridge distraction is indicated to increase ridge volume for the insertion of dental implants or for orthodontic tooth movements.

Treatment Goals

Unlike most surgical procedures, the surgeon is intimately involved during the postoperative period. After the completion of the latency period, the surgeon and orthodontist oversee

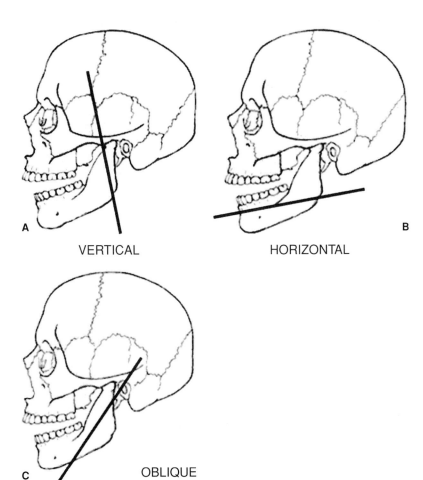

A   VERTICAL

B   HORIZONTAL

C   OBLIQUE

FIGURE 12.4. The vectors of mandibular distraction. (From Mathes SJ. *Plastic Surgery.* Philadelphia: Elsevier; 2005, with permission.)

device manipulation (activation). In addition to lengthening of the device and mandible, it may also be necessary to "mold the generate."

In unilateral mandibular distraction, as in the patient with unilateral craniofacial microsomia, the treatment end points are the movement of the chin to the contralateral side with lowering of the ipsilateral oral commissure, the inferior border of the mandible, and the occlusal plane to a level below that of the contralateral side. Such "overcorrection" is especially indicated in the growing child. In bilateral mandibular distraction,

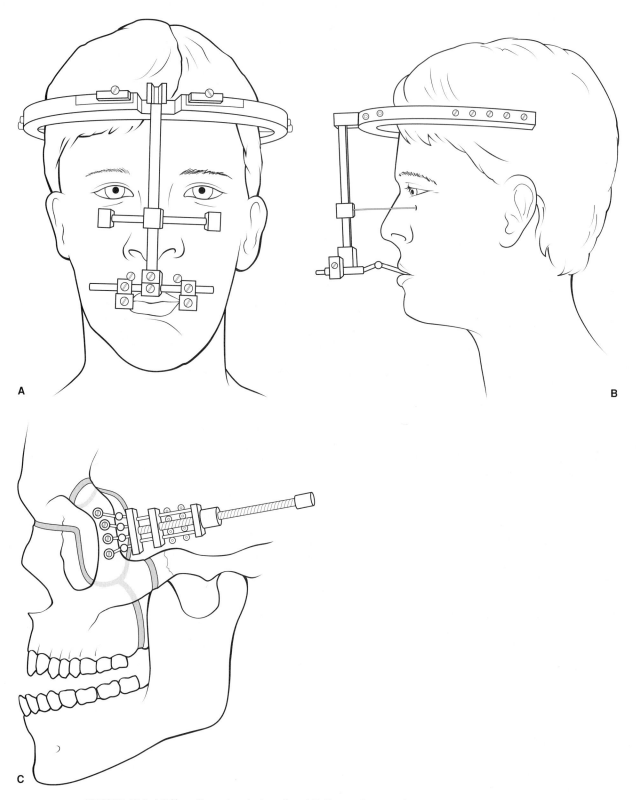

FIGURE 12.5. Midface distraction devices. **A** and **B:** External (RED) device. **C:** Buried device with an activation arm that penetrates the scalp. (From Mathes SJ. *Plastic Surgery*. Philadelphia: Elsevier; 2005, with permission.)

the treatment end points include the achievement of a slight anterior crossbite, especially in the growing child.

MAXILLARY DISTRACTION

Maxillary Le Fort I distraction is indicated for the correction of maxillary retrusion usually associated with cleft lip and palate patients and the maxillary deformity in craniofacial microsomia. The latter can be treated by combined maxillomandibular distraction.

The advantages of maxillary distraction are that it can be performed at a younger age, especially in the child with respiratory obstruction or a severe malocclusion (anterior crossbite) and midface retrusion that impact on psychosocial functioning. Because activation is at the rate of only 1 mm per day, and because the associated soft tissue is also being distracted, the relapse problems associated with a classic Le Fort I advancement in the patient with severe palatal scarring are reduced. **It should be emphasized, however, that a second maxillary advancement will most likely be required when the patient achieves craniofacial maturity at the age of 17 or 18 years.**

Several types of maxillary distraction devices are available. An external head frame rigid eiteral distractor (RED) provides relative stability and the ability to change the vector during activation (Fig. 12.5 A & B), but is somewhat cumbersome to wear; a variety of buried devices are also available.

A maxillary degloving incision is made and the osteotomy or corticotomy is carefully performed along the traditional Le Fort I lines with care being taken to avoid injury to unerupted maxillary teeth. A vector is usually chosen in a forward and downward direction.

The treatment's end point is a class II malocclusion or overjet in the growing child ("overcorrection"). The consolidation period is approximately 2 months.

MIDFACE DISTRACTION

The clinical technique of midface or subcranial Le Fort III distraction is based on laboratory studies (11). It has several advantages in that it avoids the need for bone grafts and the application of plates and screws. The length of the surgical procedure and the volume of blood transfusion are reduced, as is the length of the hospitalization. Moreover, the aesthetic results are superior to those of the traditional Le Fort III advancement with bone grafts because of more zygomatic projection and a lower relapse rate. Serial computerized tomography (CT) studies have demonstrated bone deposition along the entire Le Fort III osteotomy line.

Midface distraction is especially indicated in the syndromic craniofacial synostosis patient with exorbitism, malocclusion, sleep apnea, midface retrusion, and severe dysmorphism. Patients with orbitofacial clefts are also candidates. **When performed in a growing child, it must be emphasized to the family that a second midface procedure will be required when the child completes craniofacial skeletal growth in late adolescence.**

There are two types of available distraction devices: head frames and buried devices that can be directly applied to the craniofacial skeleton through a coronal incision (Fig. 12.5).

The osteotomy is performed through a coronal incision. In the establishment of the vector (device application and orientation), it is desirable to move the midface segment in an anterior direction. However, one should guard against closing the anterior open bite and increasing the vertical dimension of the orbit. Treatment end points *in the growing child* include overcorrec-

tion with a resulting overjet or class II occlusion and maximal zygomatic advancement.

FRONTOFACIAL (MONOBLOC) DISTRACTION

Frontofacial or monobloc distraction is similar to subcranial midface distraction except that the superior part of the orbits and frontal bones are distracted along with the midface fragment. It involves an intracranial procedure and collaboration with a neurosurgeon and is indicated in patients with severe exorbitism and the need for expansion of orbital volume, as well as in patients who require expansion of the cranial vault (anterior) for symptoms of increased intracrania pressure.

Because the process is gradual and the interface between the frontal bone and brain is not disturbed, there is no resulting intracranial dead space. This almost eliminates the risk of infection and cerebrospinal fluid leakage, common complications when monobloc osteotomies were performed without distraction.

CRANIAL DISTRACTION

Research studies (12) and clinical reports demonstrate that cranial bone distraction is also possible. It is a form of bifocal or trifocal distraction in that an osteotomized transport segment of cranial bone is moved into a cranial defect with bony generation in the donor defect.

FUTURE

The possibilities of craniofacial distraction are only beginning to be realized. It has been demonstrated that all components of the craniofacial skeleton—the mandible, maxilla, zygoma, orbits, and cranial bone—can be successfully distracted. As the devices are miniaturized and automated, it is possible that multiple bones can be individually distracted at the same time without the need for external devices. In the infant or young patient it may be possible to practice transutural distraction without the need for osteotomies. As the molecular biology of the distraction zone is more fully understood, the rate of activation may be increased beyond 1.0 mm per day and the consolidation period reduced far below the current requirement of 8 weeks, thereby significantly reducing the overall length of treatment.

References

1. Ilizarov G. The tension-stress effect on the genesis and growth of tissues: part I. The influence of stability of fixation and soft-tissue preservation. *Clin Orthop*. 1989;238:249.
2. Ilizarov G. The tension-stress effect on the genesis and growth of tissues: part II. The influence of the rate and frequency of distraction. *Clin Orthop*. 1989;239:236.
3. Karp NS, Thorne CH, McCarthy JG, et al. Bone lengthening in the craniofacial skeleton. *Ann Plast Surg*. 1990;24:231.
4. Karp NS, McCarthy JG, Schreiber JS, et al. Membranous bone lengthening: a serial histologic study. *Ann Plast Surg*. 1992;29:2.
5. McCarthy JG, Schreiber J, Karp NS, et al. Lengthening the human mandible by gradual distraction. *Plast Reconstr Surg*. 1992;89:1.
6. Rowe NM, Mehrara BJ, Dudziak MD, et al. Rat mandibular distraction osteogenesis: part I. Histologic and radiographic analysis. *Plast Reconstr Surg*. 1998;102:2022.

7. Mehrara BJ, Rowe NM, Steinbrech DS, et al. Rat mandibular distraction osteogenesis: part II. Molecular analysis of transforming growth factor beta-1 and osteocalcin gene expression. *Plast Reconstr Surg.* 1999;103:536.

8. Aro H. Biomechanics of distraction. In: McCarthy JG, ed. *Distraction of the Craniofacial Skeleton.* New York: Springer; 1999.

9. Yu JC, Fearon J, Havlik RJ, et al. Distraction osteogenesis of the craniofacial skeleton. *Plast Reconstr Surg.* 2004;114:1e.

10. Grayson BH, McCormick S, Santiago PE, et al. Vector of device placement and trajectory of mandibular distraction. *J Craniofac Surg.* 1997;8:473.

11. Staffenberg DA, Wood RJ, McCarthy JG, et al. Midface distraction advancements in the canine without osteotomies. *Ann Plast Surg.* 1995;34:512.

12. Bouletreau PJ, Warren SM, Paccione MF, et al. Transport distraction osteogenesis: a new method to heal calvarial defects. *Plast Reconstr Surg.* 2002;109:1074.

PART II ■ SKIN AND SOFT TISSUE

CHAPTER 13 ■ DERMATOLOGY FOR PLASTIC SURGEONS

ALFRED CULLIFORD IV AND ALEXES HAZEN

The skin, the largest "organ" in the body, performs numerous functions. It provides a barrier from the external world, protecting the body from temperature extremes, evaporative losses, minor trauma, and invasion by micro-organisms. The skin also provides sensibility.

The skin is derived from two embryologic layers—the ectoderm and the mesoderm. The epidermis, pilosebaceous and apocrine units, eccrine sweat glands, and nails are derived from the ectoderm. The neuroectoderm provides melanocytes, nerves, and specialized sensory receptors. The mesoderm gives rise to Langerhans cells, macrophages, mast cells, Merkel cells, fibroblasts, blood vessels, lymph vessels, and fat cells.

ANATOMY

The skin is comprised of two basic layers—the epidermis and the dermis. The epidermis is the outer layer containing four major cell types: keratinocytes, melanocytes, Langerhans cells, and Merkel cells. The stratified squamous, in turn, consists of five layers or strata: squamous corneum, s. lucidum, s. granulosum, s. spinosum, and s. basale (Fig. 13.1). The dermis is much thicker than the epidermis and is comparatively rich in noncellular connective tissue elements—collagen, elastin, and ground substance. The nerves, blood vessels, lymphatics, muscle fibers, pilosebaceous, and apocrine and eccrine units are within the dermis. The papillary dermis, so named because it abuts the epidermal papillae, contains fibroblasts, mast cells, histiocytes, Langerhans cells, and lymphocytes. The reticular dermis is deeper than the papillary dermis, is thicker than papillary dermis, and extends to the underlying fat. The reticular dermis contains loosely arranged elastin fibers interspersed with large collagen fibers.

BENIGN VERSUS MALIGNANT LESIONS

The plastic surgeon is often faced with distinguishing between benign and malignant lesions, and thus deciding when to biopsy, when to "observe," and when to reassure. Signs that should lead the physician to biopsy include crusting and bleeding, scaling, pain, increasing size, change in color, and surrounding inflammation. The most common malignant skin lesions are basal cell and squamous cell carcinomas, with basal cell carcinoma being the most common. Of particular challenge are pigmented skin lesions. **Although new techniques for diagnosis of melanoma (Fig. 13.2) are being developed, including computerized assessment of color variability and irregularity, the ABCDs (asymmetry, border irregularity, color variability, and diameter >8 mm) remain the most generally accepted criteria to indicate biopsy (Chapter 16).**

PIGMENTED LESIONS

Nevi

Nevi are categorized as intradermal, junctional, or compound, depending on where the nevus cells are in the dermis, at the dermoepidermal junction or both, respectively. Junctional nevi appear smooth and flat and have irregular pigment. They can occur anywhere on the body and occur most commonly in early adulthood, although they can arise at any age. Junctional nevi generally transform to compound nevi in adulthood. Intradermal nevi are more commonly known as "moles." They can appear anywhere on the body and are characteristically smooth, raised, flat, tan or pink, round or oval, and less than 6 mm in size.

Atypical Moles

Atypical moles (formerly known as dysplastic nevi) are acquired lesions that are often mistaken for melanoma (Fig. 13.3). Histologically, they are formed from a cluster of melanocytes. The lesions vary in color from brown to black to pink, typically are smooth, may have irregular borders, and may be scaly. Lesions are usually between 5 and 10 mm. Atypical moles are most often sporadic, although they can be familial. Lesions tend to occur in sun-exposed areas. The risk of melanoma is higher in patients who have atypical moles, and the risk increases as the number of atypical moles increases. Most patients have a few atypical moles, although **some** patients may have more than 100 atypical lesions. **These patients present a clinical challenge because atypical moles, by definition, are moles that have the appearance of melanomas. They require close follow-up with baseline total-body photography.** It is impractical and infeasible to biopsy all lesions in such patients. Removal of lesions is reserved for those that exhibit changes, emphasizing the importance of close follow-up. When surgery is warranted, excisional biopsies should be performed, with histologic confirmation of clear margins.

Other related pigmented lesions include *blue nevus* (Fig. 13.4), *ephelis* (Fig. 13.5), *solar lentigo* (Fig. 13.6), *congenital nevi* (Fig. 13.7), and *nevus of Ota*. Although there is a recognized malignant potential for a congenital nevus to transform to malignant melanoma, the true incidence varies widely in the literature (**Chapter 16**). Malignant degeneration of a blue nevus is rare and close observation is necessary. The nevus of Ota is totally benign, occurs in the distribution of the first and second branches of the trigeminal nerve, and management can use the Q-switched ruby, neodymium:yttrium-aluminum-garnet (Nd:YAG), or alexandrite lasers (**Chapter 20**). The other lesions are benign and may be excised (with a minimal area of surrounding tissue) for cosmetic purposes.

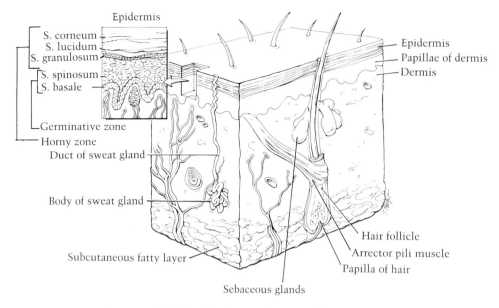

Epidermis

S. corneum
S. lucidum
S. granulosum
S. spinosum
S. basale
Germinative zone
Horny zone
Duct of sweat gland
Body of sweat gland
Subcutaneous fatty layer

Epidermis
Papillae of dermis
Dermis

Hair follicle
Arrector pili muscle
Papilla of hair
Sebaceous glands

FIGURE 13.1. Cross-section view of skin.

There are many different categorizations of benign, premalignant, and malignant skin tumors. A particularly useful categorization is to classify tumors according to their primary origin. Thus the tumors that originate from the epidermis are categorized together.

EPIDERMAL LESIONS

Seborrheic Keratosis

Seborrheic keratoses (SKs), also known as verruca senilis or pigmented papilloma, are extremely common and arise from the basal layer of the epidermis. They are composed of well-differentiated basal cells, and contain cystic "inclusions" of keratinous material called "horn cysts." Typically lesions exhibit hyperkeratosis, acanthosis, and papillomatosis. The growth and depth of pigmentation vary directly with exposure to sunlight. Microscopically, a benign epithelial proliferative process is seen. If left untreated, they will gradually enlarge and increase in thickness; there is no spontaneous involution. SKs are most commonly seen on the head, neck, and trunk after the fifth decade of life. They are often distinctly marked and have a **waxy,** stuck-on appearance. The surface is soft, verrucoid, often pedunculated and oily to the touch. They can vary in color from light tan to yellow, dark brown, and black. They range in size from 1 mm to 5 cm. No treatment is necessary but these lesions

are unsightly and patients frequently request removal for cosmetic purposes. Cutaneous malignancies (including small cell carcinoma [SCC], basal cell carcinoma [BCC], and melanoma) can develop within seborrheic keratoses. For typical SKs, shave techniques tend to be efficient and effective. Dermabrasion and cryotherapy can also be used. For larger lesions and pigmented lesions where the diagnosis is unclear, excisional biopsy may be performed.

Verruca Vulgaris

The common wart is an infection caused by the human papilloma virus; it is not a true neoplasm. It can be solitary or occur in clusters. Verruca most often occurs on the upper extremity, occasionally on the face, and is most common in children and young adults. The lesion has a characteristic scaly and rough appearance with variations and a cap of friable keratotic material. A lesion can persist for months to years, although most often is self-limited and resolves spontaneously. Histology shows hyperkeratosis and parakeratosis. Lesions arise from

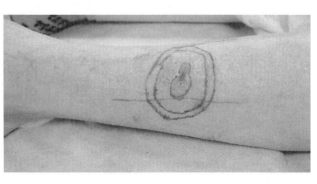

FIGURE 13.2. Melanoma of the lower extremity.

FIGURE 13.3. Atypical mole.

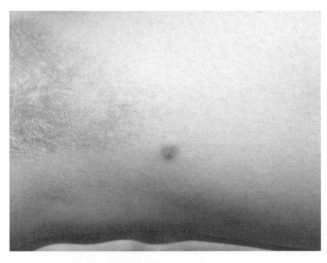

FIGURE 13.4. Blue nevus.

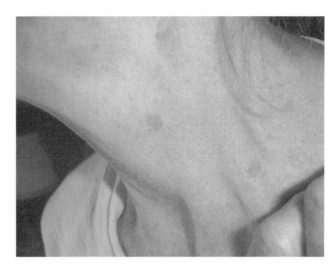

FIGURE 13.6. Solar lentigo.

the stratum granulosum of the epidermis. Various treatments are possible, including cryotherapy and chemical ablation, but multiple treatments may be necessary. Excision is reserved for a lesion that is painful or resists other treatment options.

Actinic Keratosis

Otherwise known as solar keratoses, actinic keratoses (AKs) occur on sun-exposed skin (Fig. 13.8). An aggressive form of AK called actinic cheilitis occurs on the lips. Fair-skinned individuals with blue or green eyes are at highest risk, and patients with immune compromise are also at risk. AKs represent the most common premalignant skin lesion. Despite the similarity of the name, AKs are totally distinct from seborrheic keratoses. Lesions are most often multiple and small (<1 mm) and appear as scaly patches. They are usually flat or slightly raised erythematous lesions with adherent epidermal scales. Histologically, AKs are characterized by dyskeratosis and atypia in the basal layer of the epidermis. Inflammation, hyperkeratosis, hyperchromasia, and nuclear pleomorphism are often seen. AKs may progress to squamous carcinoma, and **therefore require treat-**

ment. An estimated 5% to 20% of patients with these lesions will develop SCC.

Treatment involves monitoring closely and removal. Patients with multiple lesions and lesions with significant erythema should be biopsied. Multiple treatment modalities are effective in the treatment of AKs, including cryosurgery, typically with liquid nitrogen, electrodesiccation and curettage, topical treatments, and laser and surgical excision.

Many topical treatments are effective, including 5-fluorouracil (5-FU) cream, imiquimod 5% (Aldara), chemical peels using trichloroacetic acid (TCA) or phenol, and combination gel treatments using diclofenac and hyaluronic acid. **Aldara is popular for the treatment of AKs and viral infections. It can be administered three times a week for 8 to 12 weeks and works by stimulating an immune response.** 5-FU can be used in 5% (Efudex), 1% (Fluoroplex), and 0.5% (Carac) concentrations. Some patients experience sensitivity with 5-FU, resulting in significant erythema, scaling, and crusting; however, lower concentrations seem to be well tolerated by most patients. Laser resurfacing with a carbon dioxide laser or the YAG laser directed at the lesion can result in removing the epidermis, which can be effective in small areas, particularly on the lips. Loss of pigment is a sometimes unwelcome side effect

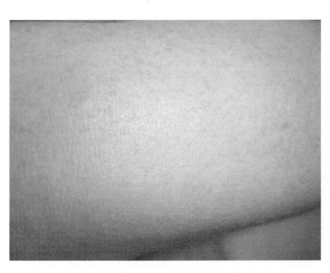

FIGURE 13.5. Ephelis.

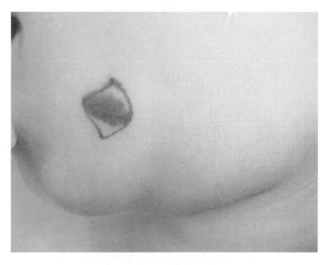

FIGURE 13.7. Congenital nevus.

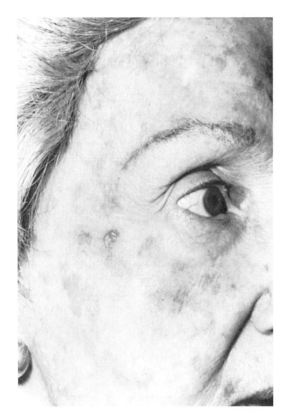

FIGURE 13.8. Actinic keratosis.

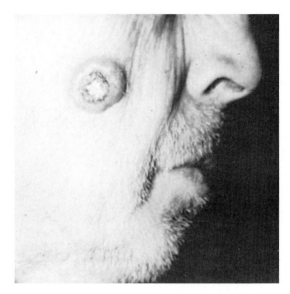

FIGURE 13.9. Keratoacanthoma.

of laser treatment. Photodynamic therapy (PDT) is a relatively new treatment that involves the application of a topical agent, such as 5-aminolevulinic acid, followed by exposure to strong light 24 hours later, which results in activating the acid and selective destruction of the actinic keratosis. PDT is quite effective for lesions on the face or scalp, although it has the unwanted and common side effect of localized swelling. Topical treatment may be preferred over surgical treatment in patients with multiple lesions in cosmetically sensitive areas.

Cutaneous Horn

The typical lesion appears as a well-circumscribed cone with hyperkeratotic features. Horns consist of a buildup of cornified material; thus their height comes to exceed their radius. Histologically, they resemble actinic keratoses and must be distinguished from squamous cell carcinoma. The treatment usually calls for excisional biopsy with careful pathologic evaluation of the base of the lesion.

Leukoplakia

This is a mucosal lesion that consists of a white plaque that exists on the stratified squamous epithelium and cannot be removed. The oral mucosa is the most common site of these lesions, although they also can occur on the mucosal surface of genitalia. Leukoplakia is often associated with chronic inflammation and irritation often associated with alcohol and tobacco consumption. Treatment of leukoplakia involves eliminating the irritant. **These lesions can degenerate into SCC. In cases where the lesions remain after the irritant has been removed, biopsy is indicated.**

Keratoacanthoma

Keratoacanthomas (KAs) are common lesions encountered by plastic surgeons. Most often they occur as solitary lesions on the head, neck, and sun-exposed regions of elderly patients. The lesion has a characteristic growth pattern that consists of a rapid growth phase followed, in some cases, by a spontaneous regression (Fig. 13.9). The lesion begins as a firm, dome-shaped nodule and grows to approximately 1 to 3 cm within a period of 6 to 8 weeks. Mature lesions become raised and have a prominent horn-filled central depression. Typically, these resolve over 6 months, but leave a small scar. Histologically, the mature lesion demonstrates a central crater filled with keratin and surrounded by thickened epidermis. **Because KAs are difficult to distinguish from SCCs, most clinicians excise lesions when the diagnosis is made.** Topical agents, such as 5-fluorouracil, are effective and are practical for use in patients with multiple lesions.

Bowen Disease

Bowen disease is cutaneous squamous cell carcinoma in situ and is characterized by a thickened, scaly, rough, red, patchlike, crusting, slow-growing lesion. Lesions can occur anywhere on the body, but are most often found on the trunk and extremities. Histologic examination demonstrates a thickened epidermis with an intact dermal–epidermal junction. Chronic exposure to arsenic has been implicated as a possible etiologic agent. If left untreated, Bowen disease may progress to invasive squamous cell carcinoma. Treatment by surgical excision is preferred over other techniques (such as dermabrasion). If a patient has multiple areas of Bowen disease, a visceral work-up is indicated.

Adnexal Tumors

The term *adnexal tumor* is a catch-all phrase that describes lesions in which the normal relationship between epithelial and stromal components of skin is altered. There may be preferential differentiation of sebaceous glands, hair follicles, or apocrine or eccrine sweat glands. Descriptive terms such as appendageal, organoid, and hamartomas are used interchangeably with the term adnexal tumor. They may be classified as

forms include comedones, inflammatory cysts, and seborrheic plaques. More severe forms can affect deeper tissue planes with subsequent inflammatory fluid collections that may ultimately become infected (cystic acne). Visible non–hair-bearing areas of the face are the most commonly affected sites. Drainage of infected pustules can treat lesions that exceed the local control measures previously instituted. In the past two decades there have been remarkable advances in the care of affected patients. Retinoic acid (applied topically) can have dramatic results when used appropriately. Retin-A and oral antibiotics (typically clindamycin) are effective treatments for both prevention and treatment of flare-ups. Antibiotic pads (benzoyl peroxide) and washes also have good results for acne. Permanent remission is frequently seen after cessation of the drug. Once the disease process has been controlled, attention can be focused on skin resurfacing. The most commonly used modalities are dermabrasion and laser resurfacing.

Acne rosacea is a spectrum of disorders affecting the forehead, glabella, malar region, nose, and chin, and has been described as having four stages by Rebora. The earliest stage is characterized by facial flushing, which represents increased vascularity. This, consequently, contributes to the second stage, where thickened skin erythema, and telangiectasias are seen. Formal *acne rosacea* follows, which is characterized by erythematous papules and pustules. *Rhinophyma* (Fig. 13.11) is the fourth and final stage and most frequently affects the nose, although involvement of other facial structures may occur. The nasal skin becomes erythematous with telangiectatic changes; over time, pits and scarring develop. Acne rosacea can be treated with oral antibiotics and retinoids (much like acne). Ideally, treatment will prevent the progression of acne rosacea to rhinophyma; however, some patients will require surgical treatment for rhinophyma. The basic principles of the surgical treatment of rhinophyma include skin excision followed by resurfacing. There are numerous techniques for removing the involved layers of skin. Simple sharp excision, dermabrasion, cryosurgery, and carbon dioxide laser are all reasonable options and can yield excellent results. Currently, the most common methods of treatment are scalpel excision and dermabrasion. Care must be taken not to remove the entire dermis, which will result in scarring. Following excision, contraction of the freshly epithelialized surface with further contribute to reduction in an often bulbous nose. Should full dermal excision be necessary, skin grafting is required.

Hydradenitis suppurativa is a chronic infection of the apocrine sweat glands, most frequently affecting the axilla, perineum, breast, and buttocks. It is most often seen in younger patients, particularly darker-skinned individuals. This is an unfortunate affliction that causes significant pain and suffering, conferring tremendous disability as a result. Affected tissues be-

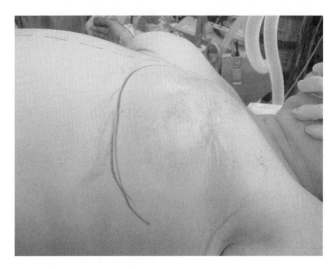

FIGURE 13.12. Radiation dermatitis of the breast.

come thick and fibrotic, have a "wooden" appearance, and frequently have chronic draining sinus tracts and deeper abscesses (Fig. 13.12). Oral and intravenous antibiotics are required for local control of infection, which are usually *Staphylococcus aureus* or *S. epidermidis*. Excision of all involved soft tissue is required. There are generally numerous microabscesses in these excisions, and the wound is frequently kept open and treated with dressing changes prior to definitive closure or coverage with a graft. Once the wound is clean, skin grafting can be performed. Healing by secondary intention is also a potential approach that yields good results.

Pyoderma gangrenosum is a pathologic term to describe the multiple superficial abscesses with significant ulceration and skin necrosis. Although lesions may become superinfected, the primary etiology is believed to be a necrotizing vasculitis with subsequent liquefaction necrosis of the skin. Any anatomic site can be affected, although it is frequently seen in the intertriginous folds of the body, especially in overweight patients. When lesions become infected, the patient may become septic and fatalities have occurred. Broad-spectrum antibiotics, hemodynamic support, and surgical debridement might be necessary in these cases. In nearly half of affected patients there is associated ulcerative colitis. Judicious debridement and carefully tailored antibiotic therapy may facilitate the use of local or systemic steroids to control the vasculitis.

BASAL CELL CARCINOMA

Basal cell carcinoma is the most common human malignancy worldwide. It accounts for more than 75% of skin cancers in the United States, affecting nearly 800,000 people yearly. Although the incidence has risen sharply over the last several decades, the average age of diagnosis has steadily decreased because of improved awareness and surveillance. The disease predominantly affects people with white skin, and the male-to-female ratio is 3:2.

Chronic exposure to sunlight is the principal cause of basal cell carcinomas, and thus lesions characteristically occur on exposed parts of the body—the face, ears, neck, scalp, shoulders, and back (Fig. 13.13). Other known etiologic factors include exposure to ultraviolet (both short and long rays) light, certain chemical carcinogens (arsenic and hydrocarbons), ionizing radiation, xeroderma pigmentosum, Bazex syndrome, Gorlin syndrome (basal cell nevus syndrome), chronic irritation or

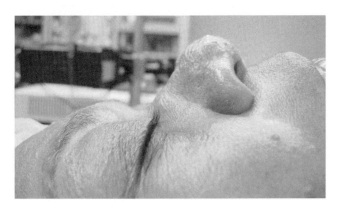

FIGURE 13.11. Rhinophyma.

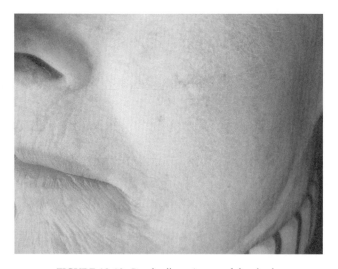

FIGURE 13.13. Basal cell carcinoma of the cheek.

ulceration, and human papillomavirus. Patients who are immunocompromised have an increased risk of developing this skin cancer.

Histologically, basal cell carcinomas arise from the basal layer of the epidermis. They classically have raised borders and a pearly central area with associated telangiectasias. They may appear scaly with areas of atrophy or scarring from chronic inflammation. BCC is classified by subtypes that exhibit more or less aggressive behavior. The subtypes are nodular, micronodular, superficial, pigmented, cystic, infiltrating, and morpheaform. The term *rodent ulcer* has been used to describe the **ulcerative** lesion, often the nodular subtype. The infiltrating and morpheaform subtypes are the most aggressive and often exhibit focal areas of tumor penetrating into local tissues. This pathologic finding makes these two subtypes the most locally aggressive, resulting in the highest rates of recurrence and positive margins among the various subtypes. The least aggressive are the nodular and superficial. The micronodular variant displays an intermediate level of aggressive biologic behavior.

Obtaining a histologic diagnosis may be achieved through a biopsy or after definitive surgical excision. Smaller lesions may be excised completely with no biopsy necessary, but larger ones often require tissue biopsy prior to final therapy. Different methods for obtaining tissue include a shave, punch, incisional, and excisional biopsies.

Treatment of basal cell cancers involves complete removal of the lesion, which may be accomplished by several methods. Cryotherapy is a technique that can be used when primary lesions are smaller than 2 cm. Although excellent results have been reported with this technique (>95% cure rate), there are potential shortcomings. Hypopigmentation, scarring, and inadvertent injury to local nerves are associated with this form of treatment. The technique is limited to the less aggressive subtypes, and is contraindicated in patients with cryoglobulinemia or in areas in which scar contracture may lead to an unacceptable functional or cosmetic result.

Electrodesiccation and curettage is a commonly employed treatment option for lesions that are less-well circumscribed. It may be used as a primary treatment modality with nodular subtypes of less than 2 cm and superficial variants of any size. Although cure rates in excess of 90% are reported, local recurrence is reported in 30% of lesions greater than 3 cm in diameter.

Radiotherapy may be used to treat patients with basal cell carcinoma, although overall cure rates may be low. It is generally reserved for patients who are deemed to be at high risk for

surgical complications. Topical chemotherapy (5-fluorouracil) may be used to treat nodular and superficial (least aggressive variants) subtypes; it is employed more often in treatment of premalignant lesions. Other less-traditional treatments include chemotherapeutic injection to tumor site and PDT.

Surgical excision of basal cell carcinoma results in a cure rate greater than 90%. As with other forms of treatment, the size, location, and histologic subtype contribute to overall prognosis. There is no uniform recommendation regarding the size of surgical margins; most surgeons will choose a margin of at least 3 to 5 mm for small, well-circumscribed lesions, and 1 cm or greater for larger, more aggressive variants of basal cell carcinoma. The margin simply has to be sufficient to be confirmed "negative" by histologic examination. Mohs micrographic surgery (Chapter 14) is the treatment of choice for lesions in difficult areas and recurrent lesions.

Gorlin syndrome, or basal cell nevus syndrome, is an autosomal dominant condition in which the patient develops multiple BCCs, along with odontogenic keratocysts, palmoplantar pitting, intracranial calcification, and rib anomalies. Treatment is close observation and judicious excision of suspicious lesions.

SQUAMOUS CELL CARCINOMA

Squamous cell carcinomas account for 20% of skin cancers in the United States. It affects approximately 200,000 people every year. Risk factors are similar to those of basal cell carcinoma, with exposure to sunlight the principal cause. Other known etiologic risk factors include ultraviolet light exposure, chemical carcinogens, chronic irritation, cigarette smoking, and infection with human papillomavirus.

Squamous cell carcinomas arise from basal keratinocytes of the skin. They migrate from the proliferating basal layer, and acquire the ability to undergo uncontrolled growth. Lesions are typically on exposed areas of skin and typically present with a firm nodular plaque on an erythematous base with raised borders (Fig. 13.14). An area of central ulceration may be

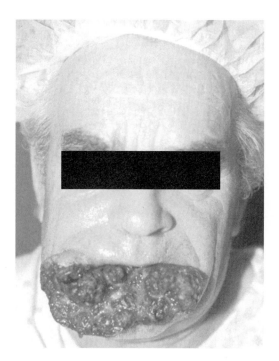

FIGURE 13.14. Squamous cell carcinoma.

present. Larger lesions may present with infection. Histologically, there are irregular nests of epidermal cells invading the dermal layer. As with other tumors, histologic grading relies on the degree of cellular differentiation. The better differentiated the lesion, the less invasive a growth pattern it displays, leading to an improved prognosis. Although uncommon, squamous cell carcinomas can metastasize to regional lymph nodes. Overall, this occurs in approximately 2% to 5% of cases. If lymph node spread has occurred, further metastatic sites include bone, brain, and lungs. **A Marjolin ulcer is a squamous cell carcinoma that has developed in an area of chronic inflammation and scarring, which carries a risk of metastasis of nearly 50%.**

Squamous cell carcinomas are generally treated with curettage and electrodesiccation, radiotherapy, or surgical excision. The same limitations of radiotherapy in treatment of basal cell carcinoma are applicable. Curettage may be used in treatment of lesions less than 2 cm in diameter with clear, well-defined borders. It should not be used for larger lesions. Mohs microsurgery technique may be used in challenging anatomic locations.

Surgical excision yields excellent results for small, well-differentiated lesions. As in BCC, there is no standard margin of resection. Larger lesions require larger margins. There is no way to know if a margin is adequate until histologic confirmation is made. This group of higher-risk tumors has an increased tendency to metastasize to regional lymph nodes. Lymphadenectomy is indicated for clinically palpable nodes or if biopsy of a lymph node is positive for malignancy. Radiotherapy is indicated in situations where disease is present in more than one lymph node, there are microscopic margins, there is perineural tumor involvement, or there are larger lesions. Close surveillance and clinical follow-up is mandatory, as the majority of patients who develop recurrence do so within 2 years of initial treatment.

SKIN PRODUCTS

Alpha-Hydroxy Acids

Alpha-hydroxy acids (AHAs) are organic carboxylic acids and the mildest peeling agents used. They improve fine lines and wrinkles, areas of sun damage, dry and scaly patches, acne scars, and acne rosacea. AHA peels are also sometimes used as pretreatment for stronger chemical peels such as TCA. AHAs are often combined in skin products such as creams and cleansing agents at lower concentrations than in peels, as part of a daily regimen. Glycolic, lactic, malic, citric, pyruvic, salicylic, and fruit acids chemically exfoliate the skin. Their action is thought to be at the layer of the stratum corneum resulting in increased cell turnover, although the precise mechanism is not well understood. The overall effect is increased thickness of the skin with greater collagen and mucopolysaccharide content, which makes skin look fresher, healthier, and smoother. Salicylic acid has been long used for the treatment of comedones. Except in rare cases, AHAs have virtually no long-term side effects, although the greater the dermal penetration, the greater the irritancy of the product. The benefits of AHAs are also limited.

Retinoids

Topical retinoids such as retinol are derivatives of vitamin A. Tretinoin (or Retin-A) and Retin-A Micro are also retinoids that are the most commonly used products for treatment and prevention of photoaged skin. They improve skin quality and texture by increasing cell turnover in the dermal layer of the skin. These improvements are likely a result of mediation of binding to retinoic acid receptors (RARs), which then can bind to specific genes. Retin-A is available in many formulations and strengths. Higher concentrations induce greater irritation. Renova is a combination of tretinoin 0.05% in a water-in-oil emulsion. This is thought to moisturize and thus reduce the incidence of dermatitis. Retin-A Micro is a gel formulation of tretinoin encapsulated in microspheres, which may result in slower delivery of the medication and thus decreased redness. Retin-A Micro (in 0.1% and 0.04% concentrations) was specifically designed for the treatment of acne, but also can be used for aging skin. Third-generation retinoids such as Differin and Galderma are made of adapalene gel and are approved for the treatment of acne; they have a smaller side-effect profile, with fewer reports of sensitivity. Tazarotene gel is a retinoid used for psoriasis and acne and thought to bind selectively to RARs. In aging, the process of cell turnover slows, the skin appears dull and thickened, pores can appear larger, and wrinkles develop. Increasing the cell turnover results in a smoother, healthier-looking skin, smaller pores, finer wrinkles, and decreased pigmentation, roughness, and sallowness. Although retinols are very effective, they have the common side effects of increased sun sensitivity and redness, called retinal dermatitis, which typically develop at 2 to 4 weeks of treatment and subsequently subside. Patients need to avoid sun exposure when being treated with retinoids. Clinicians use retinols in combination with bleaching agents (hydroquinones) for the treatment of hyperpigmentation.

Systemic Retinoids

Isotretinoin as a systemic formulation has primarily been used to treat acne and psoriasis, but has some usefulness in the treatment of photoaged skin. Women of child-bearing years need to be counseled carefully before embarking on the use of isotretinoin because of the birth defects associated with their use.

Vitamin A

Vitamin A, also known as retinol, is a precursor to retinoic acid. Although it can be effective in the treatment of photoaged skin, patients frequently do not tolerate the side effect of skin irritation, causing them to abandon treatment.

Furfuryladenine

This is a newer, less-prescribed agent, also known as kinetin (active ingredient in Kinerase). It acts on photoaged skin by slowing the aging process at the cellular level by altering the cell shape, changing the cytoskeleton structure, changing growth rates, and altering the synthesis and quantity of lipofuscin.

Vitamin C

Topical vitamin C, or ascorbic acid, is an antioxidant. It helps to regenerate vitamin E and inhibits lipid peroxidation. After UV exposure vitamin C stores become deleted, yet when vitamin C is used topically, it seems to have a protective effect against UVB rays. It is thought to improve skin quality and texture by increasing collagen turnover. Some studies suggest an impact on dermal fibroblasts proliferation and improved wound healing and scar formation. Many forms of vitamin C are unstable and thus easily degraded. L-Ascorbic acid is well absorbed by the skin and relatively stable, thus is an excellent topical formulation. The formulation and percentage of vitamin in the cream or gel is critical to its effectiveness, with the best results seen in 10% to 20% formulations. Vitamin C seems to have an effect on fine lines and wrinkles and to improve wound healing. It may also have an anti-inflammatory effect. Because some studies have shown that vitamin C improves the efficacy of bleaching agents on the skin, many clinicians use it in combination with bleaching agents.

Vitamin E

Vitamin E is widely thought to improve scars. Many people use it topically on healing scars with the belief that it will improve the color and texture of the scar. Vitamin E is a lipid-soluble antioxidant that can serve to reduce free radical production. Alpha-tocopherol is the biologically active form of vitamin E. It inhibits protein kinase C, which, in turn, inhibits collagenase production and collagen degradation. In theory, this leads to increased collagen and decreased aging in the skin; however, few studies exist that support this clinically. There may be a selective photoprotective effect with topical application of the active form of vitamin E and UVB exposure, but it is not clearly beneficial.

Bleaching Agents

Many formulations exist for the treatment of solar lentigos, melasma, and dyschromia. Hydroquinone is the most commonly used agent and produces a reversible depigmentation of the skin. The 4% formulation is frequently used with the best effect; however, combination products exist with lower concentrations. It can also be combined with hydrocortisone to reduce irritation seen with hydroquinone use. It often is also combined with sunscreen, an essential treatment in the effective improvement of pigmented areas of skin, and with vitamin C and lipid-soluble vitamin E, which are thought to improve the efficacy of the bleaching agents. Hydroquinone has the frequent side effect of local skin irritation and the uncommon, but devastating, side effect of exogenous ochronosis, the irreversible blue-black pigmentation of treated areas. Patients should always patch test prior to treatment. Patients can also have severe allergic reaction (hives, wheezing, and even anaphylaxis) to the product.

Kojic acid is an alternative to hydroquinone and can be used alone or in combination with hydroquinone or AHAs. It is derived from a Japanese mushroom and, like hydroquinone, is a tyrosinase inhibitor.

Sunscreen

If a physician could prescribe a single agent to treat photoaging, it should be sunscreen. Not only can sunscreen help prevent skin cancers, but the judicious use of sunscreen and limited exposure to the sun will reduce the development of unwanted pigmented areas of the skin, reduce the development of fine lines and wrinkles, and help slow the aging process of the skin. Sunscreens are typically either selective in their absorption of particular rays, or physical blocks that serve as a barrier that reflects or scatters radiation. The first sunscreens were developed in 1920s and were selective for UVB protection (the part that causes sunburn); they contained benzyl salicylate and benzyl cinnamate. UVB sunscreens tend to absorb the entire spectrum of UVB rays, whereas UVA sunscreens absorb selective shorter wavelengths. The main active ingredients in sunscreens that are selective for UVB rays are *p*-aminobenzoic acid (PABA) and derivatives thereof. UVA sunscreens contain benzophenones, dibenzoylmethanes, and anthranilates. The physical barrier creams contain titanium dioxide, micronized zinc oxide, micronized metallic oxide reflecting powders, and avobenzone (Parsol 1789). PABA and its derivatives were very common sunscreen ingredients in the 1950s and 1960s, but have recently fallen out of favor because they do not effectively absorb all wavelengths of UV light, are not water soluble, some people are allergic to the compounds, and they can cause yellow discoloration of fabric. Cinnamates are effective UVB blockers but have poor waterproofness, thus are used in combination with other agents. The FDA rates sunscreens for their effectiveness and their waterproofness. Agents available in Canada and Europe that seem to be quite effective are Mexoryl, which is a camphor-based lotion that produces a total physical block. A sun protection factor (SPF) of 20 means that it would take you 20 times longer to sunburn with the sunscreen than if you stayed in the sun with untreated skin. New FDA categories will soon be implemented that will describe sunscreen as 1 (minimal protection), 2 (moderate protection), and 3 (high sunburn protection; SPF of 30 or greater). A sunscreen or block should protect against both UVB and UVA rays.

Suggested Readings

Anthony ML. Surgical treatment of nonmelanoma skin cancer. *AORN J.* 2000;71(3):552–554.

Barrett TL, Greenway HT, Masullo V. Treatment of basal cell carcinoma and squamous cell carcinoma with perineural invasion. *Adv Dermatol.* 1993;8:277–304; discussion 305.

Bogdanov-Berezovsky A, Cohen A, Glesinger R. Clinical and pathological findings in reexcision of incompletely excised basal cell carcinomas. *Ann Plast Surg.* 2001;47(3):299–302.

Dixon AY, Lee SH, McGregor D. Factors predictive of recurrence of basal cell carcinoma. *Am J Dermatopathol.* 1989;11(3):222–232.

Fleming ID, Amonette R, Monaghan T. Principles of management of basal and squamous cell carcinoma of the skin. *Cancer.* 1995;75(2 suppl):699–704.

Friedman HI, Cooper PH, Waneho H. Prognostic and therapeutic use of microstaging of cutaneous squamous cell carcinoma of the trunk and extremities. *Cancer.* 1985;56(5):1099–1105.

Har-Shai Y, Hai N, Taran A. Sensitivity and positive predictive values of presurgical clinical diagnosis of excised benign and malignant skin tumors: a prospective study of 835 lesions in 778 patients. *Plast Reconstr Surg.* 2001;108(7):1982–1989.

Karagas MR, Stukel TA, Greenberg E. Risk of subsequent basal cell carcinoma and squamous cell carcinoma of the skin among patients with prior skin cancer. Skin Cancer Prevention Study Group. *JAMA.* 1992;267(24):3305–3310.

Kuflik EG, Gage AA. The five-year cure rate achieved by cryosurgery for skin cancer [see comments]. *J Am Acad Dermatol.* 1991;24(6 pt 1):1002–1004.

Lang PG Jr, Maize JC. Histologic evolution of recurrent basal cell carcinoma and treatment implications. *J Am Acad Dermatol.* 1986;14(2 pt 1):186–196.

Luce EA. Advanced and recurrent nonmelanoma skin cancer. *Clin Plast Surg.* 1997;24(4):731–745.

Marks R. The epidemiology of non-melanoma skin cancer: who, why and what can we do about it. *J Dermatol.* 1995;22(11):853–857.

Padgett J, Hendrix KJD Jr. Cutaneous malignancies and their management. *Otolaryngol Clin North Am.* 2001;34(3):523–553.

Preston DS, Stern RS. Nonmelanoma cancers of the skin [see comments]. *N Engl J Med.* 1992;327(23):1649–1662.

Rowe DE, Carroll RJ, Doy C. Prognostic factors for local recurrence, metastasis, and survival rates in squamous cell carcinoma of the skin, ear, and lip. Implications for treatment modality selection [see comments]. *J Am Acad Dermatol.* 1992;26(6):976–990.

Sexton M, Jones DB, Maloney M. Histologic pattern analysis of basal cell carcinoma. Study of a series of 1039 consecutive neoplasms. *J Am Acad Dermatol.* 1990;23(6 pt 1):1118–1126.

Stegman SJ. Basal cell carcinoma and squamous cell carcinoma. Recognition and treatment. *Med Clin North Am.* 1986;70(1):95–107.

Vuyk HD, Lohuis PJ. Mohs micrographic surgery for facial skin cancer. *Clin Otolaryngol Allied Sci.* 2001;26(4):265–273.

CHAPTER 14 ■ MOHS MICROGRAPHIC SURGERY

KAREN H. KIM AND ROY G. GERONEMUS

Mohs micrographic surgery (MMS) is a surgical technique that combines tumor extirpation and microscopic examination of tissue margins by the same surgeon. **Beveled excision and careful mapping of the peripheral and deep margins of horizontal frozen sections permit a comprehensive examination of all the borders of the excised tissue and ensure excellent cure rates, exceeding 98% for most skin cancers.** In addition to the high cure rate, Mohs surgery is a tissue-sparing procedure. The need for wide, extensive excision is reduced because of the precise control of tumor margins. This is an important advantage in cosmetically and functionally sensitive areas.

HISTORY

The Mohs technique is named after Dr. Frederic Edward Mohs, the inventor of the procedure. First introduced in 1936 at the University of Wisconsin, the procedure was initially met with much skepticism and resistance. Most of the early patients treated with Mohs surgery were patients with recurrent tumors who failed other treatments. In 1941, a physician with a mucoepidermoid carcinoma of the parotid gland was originally told that his tumor involved the facial nerve and it would have to be sacrificed. The patient was treated with the Mohs technique in an effort to surgically remove the tumor without losing the nerve. Preservation of the facial nerve was successful and there was no recurrence of the carcinoma after a 17-year follow-up. The success of this case proved to be a landmark in establishing the legitimacy and usefulness of the Mohs technique (1).

The original technique involved the topical application of 20% zinc chloride paste to malignant tissue for 12 to 24 hours, enabling tissue fixation in situ. This was followed by excision of the tumor and histologic examination of frozen horizontal sections. If a margin was positive, the tissue was fixed with zinc chloride paste for an additional 12 to 24 hours and the tissue was removed for microscopic examination. Hence, the term *Mohs chemosurgery* was invoked to convey in situ tissue preservation with zinc chloride. Tissue fixation with zinc chloride had its limitations, however: It was time-consuming, laborious, and very painful for patients. Dense inflammation from in situ fixation obscured tumor cells and made pathologic review of the tissue difficult. The intense inflammatory response caused by the chemical paste also prohibited immediate repair of the defect, and repairs were either delayed or left to heal by secondary intention. **In 1953, the technique was changed to incorporate fresh tissue rather than tissue fixed with zinc chloride, which eliminated these problems and reduced the total treatment time to 1 day.** There was also significantly less inflammation in the surrounding tissue, which reduced the overall surgical defect size and enabled immediate repair. Patients no longer required hospitalization between the stages of Mohs surgery and local anesthesia could be used, making this an ambulatory procedure. The Mohs procedure became a more practical and comfortable procedure. This "fresh-tissue technique" was later popularized by Drs. Theodore Tromovitch and Samuel Stegman in the early 1970s and is the standard practice today (2).

The term *Mohs micrographic surgery* encompasses the key features (Table 14.1) of the procedure: microscopic control of 100% of the tissue margin and meticulous cancer mapping of the excised specimen (3). Horizontal sectioning of the extirpated tumor in one plane (**as opposed to vertical sections of paraffin-embedded tissue after standard excision**) and detailed mapping enables the surgeon to have control of the entire tissue margin and re-excision of microscopic tumor extension.

INDICATIONS FOR MOHS MICROGRAPHIC SURGERY

Mohs micrographic surgery is an excellent technique for most cutaneous tumors of the face and body (Table 14.2). **It is the treatment of choice for primary skin malignancies such as basal cell carcinomas and squamous cell carcinomas that are recurrent, have aggressive features, or with ill-defined margins.** Skin tumors in areas that are at high risk for recurrence and deep extension, often called the *H-zone of the face*, should be treated with Mohs surgery. These areas correlate with embryonic fusion plates and include sites such as the inner canthus, nasolabial fold, nose, periorbital, temple, upper lip and periauricular regions, retroauricular, and chin. The ear also has a high rate of recurrence and is suitable for treatment with Mohs surgery.

Tumors measuring >2 cm in diameter have higher rates of recurrence. Mohs surgery is the treatment of choice for these tumors.

Recurrent tumors often have ill-defined margins given the presence of fibrosis from previous interventions. Tumors previously treated with other modalities, including radiation therapy, electrodesiccation and curettage, surgical excision, and cryotherapy, may have subclinical extension when they recur (4). Recurrence rates of previously treated tumors is 18% with excision, 10% with radiation therapy, 40% with electrodesiccation and curettage, and 12% with cryotherapy. **Mohs surgery yields the most favorable recurrence rate of 3.4% to 7.9%, establishing it as the treatment of choice for recurrent skin tumors** (5). For lesions in *cosmetically or functionally important areas* such as the nose, eyes, and lips, Mohs surgery is an excellent treatment choice because of the tissue-sparing advantage. The genitalia, digits, and the nipple area are locations with very little tissue laxity. Given the need for tissue preservation, Mohs surgery is the optimal treatment.

Cutaneous tumors occurring in immunosuppressed patients should also be treated with Mohs surgery, as these tumors

TABLE 14.1

KEY FEATURES OF MOHS MICROGRAPHIC SURGERY

Curettage
Beveled incision
Specimen orientation
Color coding and mapping
Specimen flattening
Horizontal frozen section
Histologic review by Mohs surgeon
Immediate repair

can behave aggressively. Two other groups that deserve special mention are patients with a genetic predisposition for developing multiple skin cancers, such as patients with basal cell nevus syndrome and patients with xeroderma pigmentosa. Mohs surgery is ideal because of its tissue-sparing capability and superb cure rates. Table 14.3 is a complete list of tumors treatable by Mohs surgery.

BASAL CELL CARCINOMA AND SQUAMOUS CELL CARCINOMA

Basal cell carcinoma (BCC) is the most commonly diagnosed skin cancer, representing 75% of all cutaneous malignancies. This is followed by squamous cell carcinoma (SCC), which represents 20% of all cutaneous malignancies. Mohs micrographic surgery is the treatment of choice for basal and squamous cell carcinomas that display aggressive histologic features and unfavorable location. Morpheaform, infiltrative, sclerosing, and basosquamous BCCs typically have ill-defined clinical margins and deep-tissue invasion, and tend to have higher rates of recurrence with treatment methods other than Mohs surgery. Large tumors, measuring >2 cm in diameter, also tend to behave more aggressively and have higher recurrence rates, and are better treated with Mohs surgery.

Tumors located on the ear, periauricular region, nose, temporal region, periocular region, melolabial sulcus, and upper lip

TABLE 14.2

INDICATIONS FOR MOHS MICROGRAPHIC SURGERY

Location
    Areas prone to recurrence: midface, ear, lip, nose, temple
    On or near a critical structure: eyes, lips, digits, genitalia
Recurrent tumors: basal cell carcinoma and squamous cell carcinoma
Large tumors (>2 cm)
Ill-defined tumor margins
Aggressive histology
    Basal cell carcinoma—morpheaform, infiltrative, basosquamous, perineural
    Squamous cell carcinoma—poorly differentiated, invasive, perineural
Special hosts
    Immunosuppressed patients
    Basal cell nevus syndrome patients
    Xeroderma pigmentosa patients

TABLE 14.3

TUMORS TREATED BY MOHS SURGERY

Basal cell carcinoma
Squamous cell carcinoma
    Keratoacanthoma
    Verrucous carcinoma
    Erythroplasia of Queyrat
    Bowen disease
Extramammary Paget disease
Melanoma in situ
Dermatofibrosarcoma protuberans
Atypical fibroxanthoma
Microcystic adnexal carcinoma
Sebaceous carcinoma
Cutaneous leiomyosarcoma
Malignant granular cell tumor
Merkel cell carcinoma
Eccrine/apocrine adenocarcinoma
Angiosarcoma
Trichilemmal carcinoma

(the H-zone) have higher recurrence rates and are cosmetically sensitive areas with a limited amount of surrounding tissue. Given these circumstances, such tumors are best treated with Mohs surgery. The nose is the most common site for BCC and is the site with the highest recurrence rate. In contrast to other treatment modalities, Mohs surgery has the highest cure rate (97% to 99%) for BCCs on the nose and is the optimal treatment method. Periauricular tumors are also best treated with Mohs surgery because of the high recurrence rate given the proclivity for cartilaginous spread or extension into the external auditory canal.

Unlike BCCs, which can recur but tend not to metastasize, **squamous cell carcinomas** have metastatic potential and therefore pose a more threatening problem. This emphasizes the need to use the optimal treatment modality with excellent cure rate. Complete removal of SCC is critical, because recurrent tumors are very difficult to treat and are associated with a 25% to 45% rate of metastasis. Mohs surgery has the highest cure rate (98%) in the treatment of SCCs (6).

SCCs on the scalp often extend widely beyond clinically obvious borders. Tissue inelasticity of the scalp can make subsequent repair challenging. Mohs surgery minimizes the defect size while maximizing cure rate. Mohs surgery is also an excellent option for SCCs involving the digits without bony involvement. Especially helpful in the periungual region, Mohs surgery can avoid the need for disfiguring, functionally compromising surgery or amputation.

SCCs exhibiting perineural involvement or malignancies arising from previous radiation, burn, or scar should be treated with Mohs surgery because of the infiltrative nature of the tumor and high risk of recurrence.

OTHER TUMORS TREATED BY MOHS MICROGRAPHIC SURGERY

Dermatofibrosarcoma protuberans is a fibrous tumor that tends to extend widely beyond clinical borders. Prior to the availability of Mohs surgery, treatment was fraught with high rates of recurrence. Mohs surgery has had tremendous success in the treatment of dermatofibrosarcoma protuberans, with a recurrence rate of only 1.6% seen in Mohs surgery-treated tumors, compared to a 20% recurrence rate with wide excision (7). Other fibrous tumors that have been successfully treated with Mohs surgery are atypical fibroxanthomas and their deeper counterpart, malignant fibrous histiocytoma.

Variants of SCCs that are suitable for Mohs surgery include verrucous carcinoma, Bowen disease, and erythroplasia of Queyrat.

Other tumors successfully treated with Mohs micrographic surgery are sebaceous carcinoma, which commonly occurs on the eyelid and has high rates of local recurrence and metastasis, and extramammary Paget disease, which often has subclinical extension.

Mohs surgery has also been used for the treatment of less-common cutaneous malignancies, including leiomyosarcoma, angiosarcoma, and liposarcoma. Microcystic adnexal carcinoma, or sclerosing sweat duct carcinoma, occurs on the upper lip or cheek and chin area, and tends to behave aggressively, invading deeply. It is also treated with Mohs surgery.

MELANOMA

The role of Mohs micrographic surgery in the treatment of melanoma is controversial and has been the subject of extensive discussion. The difficulty in identifying single atypical melanocytes in frozen section because of freeze artifact has prevented this technique from being used widely in invasive melanoma. However, some Mohs surgeons have applied the procedure to melanoma in situ and invasive melanoma (8). Immunohistochemical stains to label melanocytes have been used as an adjunct to improve the diagnostic accuracy of Mohs surgery with melanomas, especially in equivocal sections. Unfortunately, currently available stains have low sensitivity and prolong procedure time, without much discernible improvement over standard wide excision.

TECHNIQUE

Mohs surgery is performed in an outpatient setting under local anesthesia. All tumors are first biopsied for diagnostic confirmation. Depending on the lesion, additional studies may be obtained, including computed tomographic (CT) scans, magnetic resonance imaging (MRI), and radiographs, to evaluate for tumor invasion into bone or regional lymph node involvement. If the lesion is located in an area where a significant motor or sensory nerve may need to be sacrificed, this is discussed with

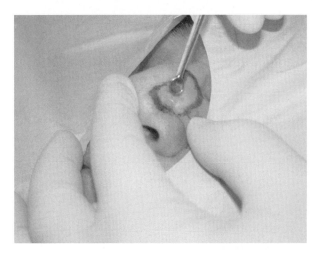

FIGURE 14.2. Curettage to delineate clinical borders.

the patient prior to surgery. Regional lymph node examination is performed as well.

When the patient presents for surgery, the tumor is identified and marked with a skin marker (Fig. 14.1). Mohs micrographic surgery is performed using standard surgical preparation of the skin with sterile instruments and drapes. The area is infiltrated with local anesthesia (usually lidocaine with epinephrine). The tumor is debulked and lateral margins are delineated with a sharp curette (Fig. 14.2). The tumor is cut via a tangential incision around the circumference of the lesion, with the scalpel held at a 45-degree angle to the skin (as opposed to the customary 90-degree angle) (Fig. 14.3). Approximately 2 mm of clinically normal skin is removed in the periphery. The deep margin is cut in a horizontal fashion, parallel to the surface of the skin. Prior to tissue removal, a thin cut is made on the specimen and the surrounding skin, for location identification in the event that additional tissue needs to be taken from a particular area. The tissue is removed and divided into smaller pieces.

Skin edges are painted with different colors corresponding to specific sites on the tumor map. Painting the edges also assures the histotechnician that the complete margin is being properly sectioned, as the color dye remains present during the processing and is readily identifiable on the glass slide. **Peripheral and deep skin edges are flattened such that specimen edges**

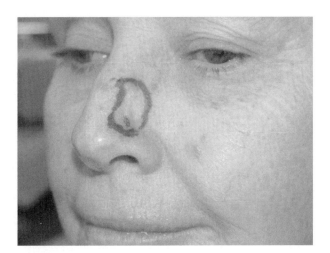

FIGURE 14.1. Preoperative view of recurrent basal cell carcinoma on the nose.

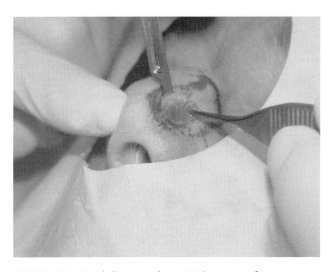

FIGURE 14.3. Beveled incision during Mohs surgery (first stage).

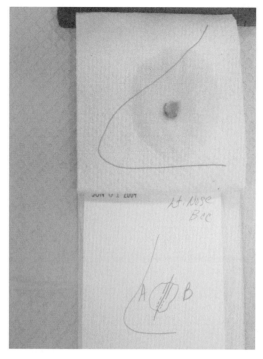

FIGURE 14.4. Excision of skin tumor placed on labeled paper towel, adjacent to tumor map.

are lying completely flat. This step is critical because it ensures complete margin assessment.

The surgical specimen is put on a cryostat object disk and fixed in optimal cutting temperature (OCT) embedding compound. A heat extractor can be applied to facilitate fixation. The tissue is flipped and pressure is applied to flatten the tissue such that the three-dimensional tissue becomes two-

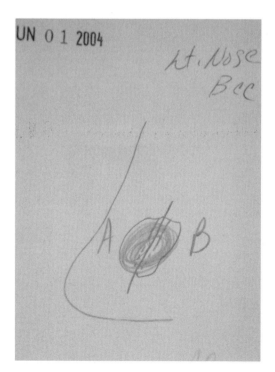

FIGURE 14.5. Areas of residual tumor marked on tumor map after microscopic examination.

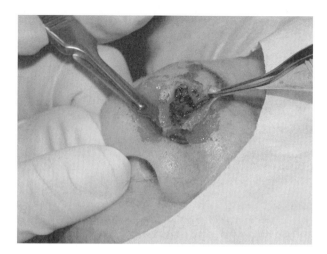

FIGURE 14.6. Additional tissue excision (second stage).

dimensional. The tissue is cut into 6- to 10-μm–thick sections in the cryostat. The sections are placed on a glass slide and stained with either hematoxylin and eosin or toluidine blue.

The Mohs surgeon reviews the histologic sections. If any tumor is identified on the slide, it is marked on the tumor map and that area is removed in the same manner (Figs. 14.4 and 14.5). Each time the surgeon repeats the process, it is an additional "stage" (Figs. 14.6 and 14.7). Once the tumor has been completely extirpated, reconstruction options are explored (Fig. 14.8).

Patients are informed that the procedure in its entirety may take anywhere from 1 to 4 hours, based on the size and depth of the tumor. The majority of time is attributed to tissue processing time. Tissue processing typically takes 20 to 40 minutes, depending on the size of the tissue and the skill of the laboratory technician.

The central tenet of Mohs micrographic surgery is that the Mohs surgeon handles the tissue personally, starting with the initial incision through the transfer of the tissue to the histotechnician. This quality assurance minimizes mistakes in labeling and orientation and ensures optimal results.

The laboratory for tissue processing is essential for Mohs surgery. It must be located on the premises to allow the Mohs surgeon and histotechnician to work together closely.

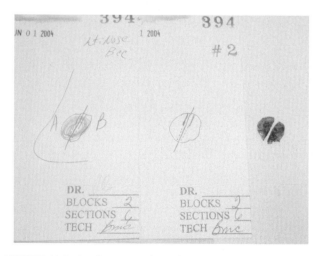

FIGURE 14.7. Another map is drawn based on excised tissue.

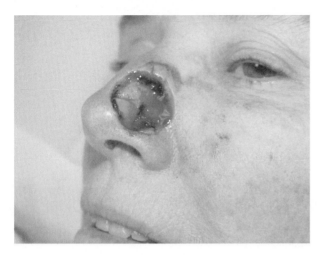

FIGURE 14.8. Final defect after margins are clear of tumor (after four stages).

A critical feature of Mohs surgery is the horizontal sections of the frozen tissue that is examined. This differs from **perpendicular vertical sections** that are obtained in standard surgical pathology laboratories. In routine paraffin-embedded slides, **vertical sections** are cut like slices of a bread loaf and representative slices from various sections throughout the specimen are examined to look for margin clearance. In Mohs surgery, horizontal sections enable microscopic examination of the entire deep and peripheral margins of the specimen in one continuous layer. So, theoretically, there is no skip area and the tissue margins are viewed in total.

CONCLUSION

Mohs micrographic surgeons are usually trained in approved 1- or 2-year fellowships under the auspices of the American College of Mohs Micrographic Surgery and Cutaneous Oncology. Fellows receive training in surgical technique, preparation and reading of horizontal frozen sections, and repair of post-surgical wounds. In the majority of cases, the Mohs surgeon repairs the defect immediately. When the defect is extensive or in specialized anatomic regions, the Mohs surgeon coordinates reconstruction with another surgical specialty, such as plastic surgery or oculoplastic surgery.

Mohs micrographic surgery has the highest cure rate among the various therapeutic modalities available for skin cancer treatment. The recurrence rate is 2% or less for primary skin cancers treated with Mohs surgery. Conservative removal of tissue can be performed without compromising the excellent cure rate (9). Management of complex skin cancers that might otherwise have required general anesthesia, the use of operating rooms, and potential hospitalization are obviated with Mohs surgery.

Given the ambulatory nature of the procedure and the low incidence of complications, Mohs surgery is a cost-effective technique when used appropriately (10, 11). Cost analysis comparing Mohs surgery with traditional surgical excision of facial and auricular nonmelanoma skin cancers demonstrates Mohs micrographic surgery to be cost comparable with traditional wide excision (12). Mohs surgery is also less expensive than traditional surgery performed in the office or in ambulatory surgery centers with frozen section margin control (13).

It is an enormous convenience for patients as well, because they can be assured when they leave the office postprocedure, they are tumor free and are able to resume their lifestyle immediately. The unique features of Mohs micrographic surgery make it the treatment of choice for most cutaneous malignancies.

References

1. Snow SN, Madjar DD. Mohs surgery in the management of cutaneous malignancies. *Clin Dermatol.* 2001;19:339–347.
2. Tromovitch TA, Stegman SJ. Microscopically controlled excision of skin tumors. *Arch Dermatol.* 1974;110:213–232.
3. Russell BA, Amonette RA, Swanson NA. Mohs micrographic surgery. In: Freedberg IM, Eisen AZ, Wolff KM, eds. *Fitzpatrick's Dermatology in General Medicine.* Vol. 2 5th ed. New York, McGraw-Hill; 1999.
4. Rowe DE, Carroll RJ, Day CL. Mohs surgery is the treatment of choice for recurrent (previously treated) basal cell carcinoma. *J Dermatol Surg Oncol.* 1989;15:424–431.
5. Mohs FE. *Chemosurgery and Microscopically Controlled Surgery for Skin Cancer.* Springfield, IL: Charles C Thomas; 1978.
6. Vuyk HD, Lohuis PJFM. Mohs micrographic surgery for facial skin cancer. *Clin Otolaryngol.* 2001;26:265–273.
7. Gloster HM, Harris KR, Roenigk RK. A comparison between Mohs micrographic surgery and wide excision for the treatment of dermatofibrosarcoma protuberans. *J Am Acad Dermatol.* 1996;35:82–87.
8. Beinart TN, Trotter MJ, Arlette JP. Treatment of cutaneous melanoma of the face by Mohs micrographic surgery. *J Cutan Med Surg.* 2003;7:25–30.
9. Swanson NA, Grekin RC, Baker SR. Mohs surgery: techniques, indications and applications in head and neck surgery. *Head Neck Surg.* 1983;6:683–692.
10. Cook JL, Perone JB. A prospective evaluation of the incidence of complications associated with Mohs micrographic surgery. *Arch Dermatol.* 2003;139:143–152.
11. Lang PG. The role of Mohs micrographic surgery in the management of skin cancer and a perspective on the management of the surgical defect. *Clin Plast Surg.* 2004;31:5–31.
12. Bialy TL, Whalen J, Veledar E, et al. Mohs micrographic surgery vs. traditional surgical excision: a cost comparison analysis.2004;140:736–742.
13. Cook J, Zitelli J. Mohs micrographic surgery: a cost analysis. *J Am Acad Dermatol.* 1998;39(5 Pt 1):698–703.

CHAPTER 15 ■ CONGENITAL MELANOCYTIC NEVI

JOHN N. JENSEN AND ARUN K. GOSAIN

DEFINITION

Nevus cells are distinguished from melanocytes by their lack of dendrites. Congenital nevi are theorized to represent a disruption of the normal growth, development, and migration of melanoblasts. Congenital melanocytic nevus (CMN) contains nevus cells and is present at birth or, in some cases, may appear within the first year of life. In the latter case, it is believed that the lesions are present at birth but do not become pigmented until the postnatal period. The lesions are thought to form between weeks 5 and 24 of gestation. Most are thought to be sporadic, but familial association is occasionally observed. Color ranges from light to dark brown, and may appear blue in more darkly pigmented individuals. Lesions are usually round or oval with well-defined borders, and vary considerably in size, pattern, and anatomic location. Although some may lesions have no raised qualities, most cause some degree of skin surface distortion. Small nevi are those <1.5 cm in diameter. **Giant nevi are variously defined as those requiring serial excision or tissue expansion for reconstruction, or, more commonly, >20 cm in greatest dimension in adulthood.** Because growth of these lesions is usually commensurate with overall growth, this corresponds roughly to a 9-cm scalp or a 6-cm trunk lesion in an infant (1). A more precise classification of giant CMN relates the lesion's size as compared to body surface area, with those occupying 2% or more body surface area considered to be giant. However, because it is more difficult to determine the size of a lesion relative to body surface area, the majority of authors report nevus size in terms of the greatest diameter of the lesion.

EPIDEMIOLOGY

Approximately 1% of the general population is thought to have CMN, most of which are of the small variety. The incidence of *large* (>10 cm) CMN is estimated at 1 in 20,000 livebirths (2). The very large "bathing trunk" examples are rarer still, occurring in approximately 1 in 500,000 live births.

HISTOLOGIC CHARACTERISTICS

Histologic features of large and small congenital melanocytic nevi include nests of nevomelanocytes at the epidermal–dermal junction or within the epidermis. In a large CMN, the morphology of nevus cells can vary and is usually more complex. The finding of nevocellular nests in the middle to deep reticular dermis is more characteristic of a congenital nevus than of the acquired variety, but no single feature is unique to either. Nevus cells present in structures deeper than the skin (e.g., bone, cranium, muscle) rarely occur except in very large congenital melanocytic nevi.

CLINICAL CHARACTERISTICS

The most common anatomic location for a large CMN is the trunk, followed in frequency by the legs, arms, and head and neck (3). Giant nevi often cross multiple anatomic zones, resulting in a more descriptive terminology to denote their pattern. Specific anatomic patterns of these lesions are observed; most notable are the "bathing trunks" and "glove-stocking" distributions. They often may appear with multiple smaller satellite lesions dispersed over the trunk, extremities, or head and neck. Often, the natural course of these lesions is to become less (or sometimes more) pigmented, and to develop hypertrichosis and a variegated texture, including nodularity. Figure 15.1 shows an infant who presented with a giant CMN in the bathing suit distribution.

The differential diagnosis for CMN includes other congenital pigmented lesions, such as epidermal nevus, nevus sebaceous, café-au-lait spot, and Mongolian spot.

Features that should prompt biopsy, if not complete early excision, include those suggestive of dysplasia or melanoma, such as ulceration, uneven pigmentation, a change in shape, and nodularity.

MALIGNANT TRANSFORMATION

The risk for malignant transformation of a CMN to melanoma was appreciated in the 19th century. Less than 0.5% of melanomas appear in preadolescent children, but 33% of those are thought to arise from CMN. There is some controversy regarding the risk of melanoma transformation. Previous attempts at quantification of the incidence of malignant transformation have been criticized, and newer studies question the existence of significant risk. Most experts believe that melanoma may arise directly from CMN (3–6). Some studies reported only extracutaneous melanoma in patients with CMN. No studies convincingly show that excision of large CMN effectively reduces the rate of malignant transformation to melanoma. This raises the question of the efficacy of prophylactic excision of CMN (7). Even those studies that cannot demonstrate a direct link between CMN and melanoma do recognize the possibility that melanoma originated in a lesion that was incompletely excised or in which the primary tumor was not clinically discovered. In the Swedish prospective trial in which no malignant transformation was proven, the incidence of CMN was reported as 0.2% (8). However, the rate of excision, especially of large (i.e., high-risk) lesions, was 40%, which might have affected the melanoma incidence. The slight variation in risk for melanoma between trials can be explained by several

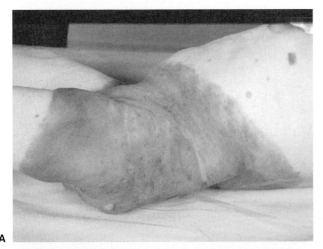

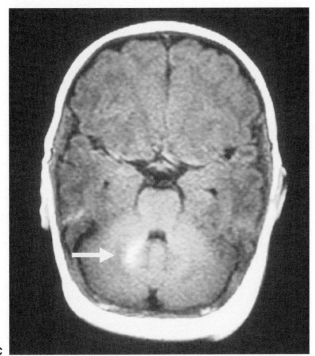

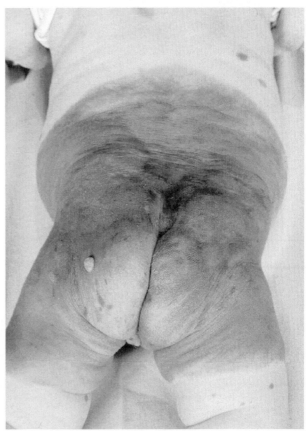

FIGURE 15.1. A, B: A 2-week-old female presented with a giant congenital melanocytic nevus in a bathing trunk distribution. Note that multiple satellite nevi are often associated with these lesions. There was a small area of ulceration within a portion of the nevus over the buttock. Clinical suspicion for congenital melanoma is an indication for early incisional biopsy prior to initiating more extensive reconstructive procedures. **C:** Risk factors in this patient were high for neurocutaneous melanosis: the presence of a large CMN overlying the posterior midline and multiple satellite nevi. A screening magnetic resonance imaging scan demonstrated a focus of neurocutaneous melanosis in the left occipital lobe (*arrow*) which was asymptomatic.

factors, including imprecise definition of "large" CMN, variable excision of primary lesions, and unclear histologic analysis of specimens (3). What is significant is the consistency with regard to risk between separate studies performed in different geographic areas by different groups (1,3–6).

When considering malignant transformation, it is essential to distinguish between small and large congenital melanocytic nevi. The lifetime risk for melanoma arising in small congenital melanocytic nevi is between 0% and 5%; the risk in large congenital melanocytic nevi is estimated to be between 5% and 10% (9). **In larger congenital melanocytic nevi, melanoma usually develops deep to the dermal–epidermal junction or occurs extracutaneously** (e.g., the central nervous system [CNS] or retroperitoneum), **is more difficult to detect, and usually (70%) occurs in the first decade of life.** This has obvious clinical implications; removal of large and giant congenital melanocytic nevi must be undertaken much earlier and the excision must be more aggressive than for small lesions.

When melanoma is reported, it tends to occur in the trunk (3) and head and neck; it has never been reported in satellite lesions. Clinically, malignant transformation may manifest as increasingly dark pigmentation, accelerated growth, a change in shape, the appearance of nodularity, pain, ulceration with or without bleeding, or pruritus. Unfortunately, many of these features are also common to the benign course of CMN. Transformation may occur later in life, and underscores the importance of long-term follow-up, even after surgical intervention.

In addition to melanoma, patients with large congenital melanocytic nevi are at increased risk to suffer from neurocutaneous melanocytosis, in which collections of melanocytes are present in the leptomeninges. Malignant transformation can also occur in neurocutaneous melanosis and result in primary central nervous system (CNS) melanoma. Even without malignant transformation, neurocutaneous melanosis can carry significant morbidity and mortality, often from seizures, hydrocephalus, and other signs of CNS irritation. Neurocutaneous melanosis may also present asymptomatically, as illustrated by the patient in Figure 15.1 whose presentation included a large CMN in the posterior midline with multiple satellite lesions (Fig. 15.1C). Magnetic resonance imaging (MRI) screening of the CNS early in life is recommended for those patients who are at high risk for malignant transformation, particularly when the presentation includes a large nevus in the posterior midline and/or multiple satellite nevi. The incidence of rhabdomyosarcoma is also increased in patients with large congenital melanocytic nevi.

In summary, all pigmented lesions have the potential to give rise to melanoma, and congenital melanocytic nevi are believed by most physicians to have a measurable risk for malignant transformation. The risk is thought to be related to the size of the lesion, but melanoma is also documented to have arisen from small congenital melanocytic nevi. Moreover, the larger the lesion, the more likely it is accompanied by greater depth into the dermis and subcutaneous tissue. Although malignant transformation to melanoma is rare, it is the essential concern in the management of these lesions.

MANAGEMENT

Many different treatment regimens have been advocated for CMN, including partial and complete excision, dermabrasion, chemical peel, and laser ablation. **The fundamental guiding principle is related to achieving a balance between treatment goals; namely, elimination (or at least reduction) of the risk for malignant transformation, preservation of function, and improved cosmesis.** Central to these considerations, in turn, is an understanding of the psychological impact caused both by the original appearance of the lesion and any functional or cosmetic impairment from therapeutic intervention.

Dermabrasion, chemical peels, and lasers have been reported as treatment for CMN (10). Cosmetic improvement usually is demonstrated in these reports, but none of these modalities is effective in the complete removal of nevus cells. In fact, at least one report suggests the possibility of a link between the kind of energy emitted by lasers and an increased metastatic potential in vitro (9). An additional criticism of these techniques is that lightening the nevus while selectively leaving unaffected nevus cells in the deeper layer of the dermis and subcutaneous tissue makes it more difficult to monitor the patient for clinical signs of malignant transformation of the remaining nevus cells.

To address the malignant potential, only complete excision of the nevus can be recommended as a solution. However, in some cases the nevus cells extend deeply into the subcutaneous tissue and the underlying muscle. Although it is not always possible to clear the peripheral surgical margins in all giant congenital melanocytic nevi, an effort should be made to clear the deep margin of nevus. If the deep margin of resection remains positive, it is impossible to monitor the behavior of residual nevus on a clinical basis following reconstruction. In more complex cases, anatomic structures that cannot be effectively reconstructed, like the perineum, may be involved and contribute to the difficulty. Moreover, even though some studies

report melanoma as arising from congenital melanocytic nevi, other studies demonstrate only extracutaneous melanoma. Surgical excision in these cases does not appear to lower the risk; in fact, **no study to date has objectively demonstrated that prophylactic excision lowers the risk for melanoma in these patients.** Conversely, an overall decline in melanoma risk from large congenital melanocytic nevi has been reported and may be partly a consequence of a greater acceptance of surgical excision of these lesions as newer techniques have been developed.

Several surgical algorithms have been reported (11,12). The mainstays of surgical management of CMN remain one-stage excision with primary closure, serial excision, tissue expansion, and excision with skin grafting. A combination of these techniques is often employed. Newer synthetic skin substitutes are being employed with success. Serial excision is preferable in most cases when complete excision can be accomplished in two stages or less. In cases of extensive nevi formation and limited normal donor skin for grafting, an option is to expand the donor skin prior to harvest.

A sensible approach is to consider the lesion or lesions within an anatomic context. In the scalp and face, multimodality treatment is often indicated. For example, tissue expansion is the first choice in hair-bearing scalp. Full-thickness skin grafts, however, are preferred for structures like the ear and eyelids, where serial excision would cause a deformity. Tissue expansion is associated with more morbidity and a higher failure rate in the extremities. For larger lesions distal to the knee or elbow, skin grafting is preferred in lesions not amenable to serial excision.

Finally, clinical surveillance remains an important treatment option, especially for lesions that are amenable to serial observation, are minimally disfiguring, or are such that ablative surgery would cause significant anatomic or functional disruption. Given the low risk for malignant transformation in CMN, it is difficult to justify potentially mutilating procedures for its excision. This is weighed against the risk of malignant transformation, and those patients who are probably at greatest risk (because they have large, thick, deeply textured lesions) are also the least likely to show signs that could allow early diagnosis of melanoma. Because sun exposure is thought to increase the risk for malignant transformation, strict sun avoidance should be advised as a prophylactic measure in these patients.

In summary, congenital pigmented nevi can be thought of as falling into two groups: large CMN and all others. Large CMN represent the greater risk for malignant transformation; require earlier, more aggressive intervention; and represent the most complex reconstructive challenges. A number of surgical techniques may be indicated and employed to reduce the risk for malignant transformation and to minimize functional and cosmetic deformity, while considering the psychological impact of intervention versus nonintervention. Should intervention be chosen, we recommend that the modality chosen not mask the clinician's ability to monitor any residual nevus for signs of malignant transformation. Until data contradict these principles, we recommend caution when treating CMN with laser, chemical peel, or dermabrasion. If surgical resection of CMN is chosen, particular effort should be made to achieve a clear, deep margin of resection so subsequent surgical reconstruction will not mask residual nevi.

References

1. Marghoob AA, Schoenbach SP, Kopf AW, et al. Large congenital melanocytic nevi and the risk for the development of melanoma: a prospective study. *Arch Dermatol.* 1996;132:170–175.
2. Castilla EE, da Graca Dutra M, Orioli-Parreiras IM. Epidemiology of

congenital pigmented nevi: incidence rates and relative frequencies. *Br J Dermatol.* 1981;104:307–315.

3. Egan CL Oliveria SA, Elenitsas R, et al. Cutaneous melanoma risk and phenotypic changes in large congenital nevi: a follow-up study of 46 patients. *J Am Acad Dermatol.* 1998;39:923–932.

4. Quaba AA, Wallace AF. The incidence of malignant melanoma (0 to 15 years of age) arising in "large" congenital nevocellular nevi. *Plast Reconstr Surg.* 1986;78(2):174–179.

5. Ruiz-Maldonado R, Tamayo L, Laterza AM, et al. Giant pigmented nevi: clinical, histopathologic, and therapeutic considerations. *J Pediatr.* 1992;120:906–911.

6. Swerdlow AJ, English JSC, Qiao Z. The risk of melanoma in patients with congenital nevi: a cohort study. *J Am Acad Dermatol.* 1995;32:595–599.

7. Watt AJ, Kotsis SV, Chung KC. Risk of melanoma arising in large congenital melanocytic nevi: a systematic review. *Plast Reconstr Surg.* 2004;113(7):1968–1974.

8. Berg P, Lindelöf B. Congenital nevocytic nevi: follow-up of a Swedish birth register sample regarding etiologic factors, discomfort, and removal rate. *Pediatr Dermatol.* 2002;19(4):293–297.

9. Burd A. Laser treatment of congenital melanocytic nevi [letter]. *Plast Reconstr Surg.* 2004;113(7):2232–2233.

10. Marghoob AA. Congenital melanocytic nevi: evaluation and management. *Dermatol Clin.* 2002;20:607–616.

11. Gur E, Zucker RM. Complex facial nevi: a surgical algorithm. *Plast Reconstr Surg.* 2000;106(1):25–35.

12. Gosain AK, Santoro TD, Larson DL, et al. Giant congenital nevi: a 20-year experience and an algorithm for their management. *Plast Reconstr Surg.* 2001;108(3):622–631.

CHAPTER 16 ■ MALIGNANT MELANOMA

CHRISTOPHER J. HUSSUSSIAN

Melanoma results from malignant transformation of the melanocyte, the pigment-producing cell of the body. As such, it can occur anywhere melanocytes are present, including skin, eye, and the mucous membranes of the upper digestive tract, sinuses, anus, and vagina. By far, the most common tissue in which melanomas arise is the skin. **The incidence of cutaneous melanoma in the United States has increased steadily over the last 50 years and is now 15 per 100,000.** It represents approximately 4% of all cancers and in 2005, it is estimated that 59,580 new cases of melanoma will be diagnosed, with 7,770 deaths (1). The incidence varies widely: In Australia it is 45 per 100,000, whereas in China it is <1 per 100,000. This is generally reflective of variation in genetic, phenotypic, and ultraviolet (UV) exposure risk factors.

Major risk factors include exposure to UV radiation and genetic predisposition. **The exposure risk primarily involves intermittent, damaging exposure to the sun such that history of a severe sunburn (blistering or pain for more than 2 days), even in youth, confers an approximately twofold increase in risk. Chronic occupational exposure confers less of a risk for development of melanoma and more of a risk for development of basal or squamous cell cancers.** Host-related risk factors include skin type, pigmentation, and hereditary susceptibility genes. The high-risk phenotypes include fair skin, blue eyes, red hair, and easy freckling. Mutations in two genes are associated with hereditary melanoma predisposition. These include p16 (INK4a) and CDK4, both of which are involved in the regulation of the retinoblastoma (Rb) cell-cycle pathway. In addition, activating mutations of a third gene, B-RAF, is associated with sporadic melanomas, indicating that the extracellular signaling pathway controlled by this gene is important in the development of melanomas. Although there is a genetic test for p16 mutations, it is not yet in widespread use.

The diagnosis of melanoma generally proceeds from biopsy of a clinically suspicious lesion. **Guidelines for recognition of a high-risk lesion have been codified as the well-known ABCDE criteria: Asymmetry, Border irregularity, Color variegation, Diameter >6 mm, and Evolution.** This schema is probably more useful for public awareness, as benign lesions often fulfill one or more of these criteria. Additionally, approximately 5% of melanomas are amelanotic (nonpigmented), and in the earliest stages of development, most melanomas are <6 mm in diameter. Lesions that demonstrate a history of recent change or bleeding or itching should especially be considered high risk. As even experienced clinicians can misjudge melanomas as benign, one should err on the side of biopsy for definitive histologic diagnosis. Biopsy technique is important as significant prognostic information is initially attained from the depth of the lesion. **Sampling error is reduced when *excisional* biopsy is performed. If this is not feasible because of the location or size of the lesion, it is acceptable to perform *incisional* or *punch* biopsy. Shave biopsies should *never* be performed on lesions suspected of being melanoma.**

Further staging work-up is relatively limited and is based on the results of the primary biopsy and presenting symptoms. Generally all patients with invasive melanoma are screened with chest radiography and serum lactic dehydrogenase (LDH). Patients with head or neck primary lesions who are candidates for sentinel node biopsy are additionally screened with a head and neck computerized tomography (CT) scan or a positron emission tomography (PET) scan. Patients with clinically positive nodes in the head or neck or groin are further staged with CT (head and neck or abdomen and pelvis). Patients who present with distant metastatic disease are staged with complete blood count (CBC); alkaline phosphatase; LDH; creatinine; CT of chest, abdomen, and pelvis; magnetic resonance imaging (MRI) of brain; and bone scan if symptomatic.

STAGING

A revised American Joint Committee on Cancer (AJCC) staging system for cutaneous melanoma was developed from analysis of 17,600 melanoma cases and published in August, 2001 (Tables 16.1 and 16.2) (2). The modified staging system makes several significant changes to TNM (tumor, node, metastasis) criteria based on risk analysis of these patients as well as evidence from the literature. Major changes include T classification breakpoints of whole-integer thickness (1 mm, 2 mm, 4 mm) to better correspond to clinical practice guidelines. In recognition of the prognostic significance of tumor ulceration, it is included as a factor in the T classification and the presence of ulceration upstages patients with stages I, II, and III disease. Clark level (Fig. 16.1) is now used only to subclassify T1 (≤1 mm) tumors. The number of metastatic lymph nodes is prognostically significant, replacing the use of gross dimension in the N classification, and new subclassifications that account for information gained from sentinel node biopsy are incorporated. Metastatic disease in lymph nodes detected after sentinel node biopsy and microscopic examination (subclassification "a") is distinguished from clinically detectable (subclassification "b") disease. Finally, the site of distant metastases and the presence of elevated LDH are used to subclassify M stage. The 5-year survival rates by stage are stage I, 92%; stage II, 68%; stage III, 45%, and stage IV, 10%.

SURGICAL MANAGEMENT

Wide Local Excision

After diagnosis, the primary treatment for virtually all melanomas is surgical. Surgical treatment of melanoma primarily concerns itself with wide excision of the primary tumor and removal of regional lymph nodes that are involved or at high risk for involvement. The advent of sentinel node biopsy and a trend toward decreasing the margin of wide local excision has dramatically altered the surgical approach to melanoma treatment over the last 10 to 15 years.

TABLE 16.1

MELANOMA TNM CLASSIFICATION

T classification	Thickness	Ulceration status
T1	1.0 mm	a: Without ulceration and level II/III b: With ulceration or level IV/V
T2	1.01–2.0 mm	a: Without ulceration b: With ulceration
T3	2.01–4.0 mm	a: Without ulceration b: With ulceration
T4	>4.0 mm	a: Without ulceration b: With ulceration

N classification	No. of metastatic nodes	Nodal metastatic mass
N1	1 node	a: Micrometastasis[a] b: Macrometastasis[b]
N2	2–3 nodes	a: Micrometastasis[a] b: Macrometastasis[b] c:
N3	In transit met(s)/satellite(s) without metastatic nodes or more metastatic nodes, or matted nodes, or in transit met(s)/satellite(s) with metastatic node(s)	

M classification	Site	Serum lactate dehydrogenase
M1a	Distant skin, subcutaneous, or nodal mets	Normal
M1b	Lung metastases	Normal
M1c	All other visceral metastases Any distant metastasis	Normal Elevated

[a]Micrometastases are diagnosed after sentinel or elective lymphadenectomy.
[b]Macrometastases are defined as clinically detectable nodal metastases confirmed by therapeutic lymphadenectomy or when nodal metastasis exhibits gross extracapsular extension.
Reproduced from Balch C, Buzaid A, Soong S-J, et al. Final version of the American Joint Committee on Cancer staging system for cutaneous melanoma. *J Clin Oncol.* 2001;19:3635, with permission.

It has long been recognized that a wide margin must be excised with the primary lesion in order to decrease the risk of local recurrence. Until relatively recently, this involved removal of 5 cm of normal-appearing skin around the lesion, as well as the soft tissue down to, and including, muscle fascia. The primary rationale for this approach was the observance of centrifugal lymphatic permeation of tumor emboli in some melanoma specimens. The origin of the wide excision guidelines is generally attributed to a 1907 study by Handley (3). Handley sought to apply to melanoma the evolving concept of the regional lymph nodes as a filter and temporary barrier to metastatic disease. Although his emphasis on the importance of the lymphatic system as the dominant mode of melanoma dissemination was correct, it is important to realize that his study involved the analysis of a single cadaveric specimen with very advanced melanoma. Additionally, Handley never advocated a 5-cm margin of skin, only a 5-cm margin of underlying fascia.

Despite a lack of definitive clinical data demonstrating its advantage, the 5-cm standard margin was the standard of care through most of the 20th century. It was not until the late 1970s that a series of retrospective reviews suggested that narrower margins do not lead to significantly higher mortality or local

recurrence rates. These initial studies led to several large, randomized trials that more definitively corroborated these findings.

The World Health Organization (WHO) melanoma program randomized patients with melanomas <2 mm thick to receive wide local excision with a 1- versus 3-cm margin (4). A total of 612 patients were enrolled, and the mean follow-up was 55 months. There were no significant differences in disease-free survival, overall survival, or the subsequent development of metastatic disease in either group. Only three patients developed local recurrence as a first relapse. All were in the 1-cm excision group and each had a primary lesion with a thickness >1 mm. **The authors concluded that for patients with primary lesions <1 mm, a 1-cm margin excision is safe and effective.** Although these investigators did not advocate a 1-cm margin for melanomas >2 mm, subsequent authors have noted that this approach may be appropriate if one is willing to accept a slightly higher local recurrence rate (3% vs. 0%) as overall survival is not affected.

The Intergroup Melanoma Trial randomized patients with melanomas between 1 and 4 mm thick to receive a wide local excision with a 2- versus 4-cm margin (5). A total of 486 patients were enrolled, and the median follow-up was 6 years.

TABLE 16.2

STAGE GROUPINGS FOR CUTANEOUS MELANOMA

	Clinical staging[a]			Pathologic staging[b]		
	T	N	M	T	N	M
0	Tis	N0	M0	Tis	N0	M0
IA	T1a	N0	M0	T1a	N0	M0
IB	T1b	N0	M0	T1b	N0	M0
	T2a	N0	M0	T2a	N0	M0
IIA	T2b	N0	M0	T2b	N0	M0
	T3a	N0	M0	T3a	N0	M0
IIB	T3b	N0	M0	T3b	N0	M0
	T4a	N0	M0	T4a	N0	M0
IIC	T4b	N0	M0	T4b	N0	M0
III[c]	Any T	N1	M0			
		N2				
		N3				
IIIA				T1–4a	N1a	M0
				T1–4a	N2a	M0
IIIB				T1–4b	N1a	M0
				T1–4b	N2a	M0
				T1–4a	N1b	M0
				T1–4a	N2b	M0
				T1–4a/b	N2c	M0
IIIC				T1–4b	N1b	M0
				T1–4b	N2b	M0
				Any T	N3	M0
IV	Any T	Any N	Any M1	Any T	Any N	Any M1

[a]Clinical staging includes microstaging of the primary melanoma and clinical/radiologic evaluation for metastases. By convention, it should be used after complete excision of the primary melanoma with clinical assessment for regional and distant metastases.
[b]Pathologic staging includes microstaging of the primary melanoma and pathologic information about the regional lymph nodes after partial or complete lymphadenectomy. Pathologic stage 0 or stage 1A patients are the exception; they do not require pathologic evaluation of their lymph nodes.
[c]There are no stage III subgroups for clinical staging.
Reproduced from Balch C, Buzaid A, Soong S-J, et al. Final version of the American Joint Committee on Cancer staging system for cutaneous melanoma. *J Clin Oncol.* 2001;19:3635, with permission.

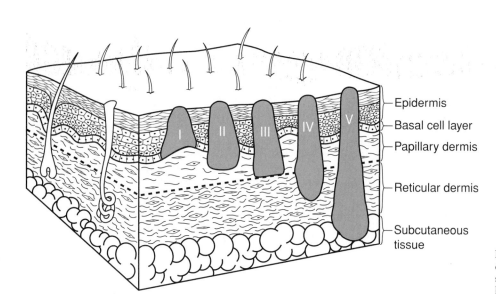

FIGURE 16.1. The Clark level is determined by the level of invasion relative to defined anatomic layers.

There were no significant differences in local recurrence, in-transit metastases, or 5-year survival. However, the narrower margins significantly reduced the need for skin grafting and shortened the hospital stay. **The authors concluded that for this group of patients, the margin of excision (1 to 4 mm in thickness) could be safely reduced to 2 cm.**

A more recent trial randomized 900 patients with melanomas >2 mm to receive 1- versus 3-cm margin wide local excisions (6). With a median follow-up of 60 months, there was a significantly higher locoregional recurrence (37% vs. 32%) and disease-specific mortality (28% vs. 23%) in the group with narrower margins. However, there are significant limitations in this study. Although the locoregional recurrence rate was higher, most of the difference results from a higher *nodal* recurrence rate in the narrow margin group; there was no difference in the *local* recurrence rate. With the advent of sentinel node biopsy subsequent to the inception of this trial, it is likely that nodal recurrences would be significantly reduced in both groups. In addition, although disease-specific survival was affected by the margin of excision, overall survival was unaffected. **The authors concluded that to optimize disease-specific survival, the use of a 1-cm margin should be avoided in patients with melanoma >2 mm.**

There are no randomized trials to guide treatment standards for patients with thick melanomas (>4 mm). In the absence of definitive safety data for narrower excisions in these patients, margins should be carefully considered and, in general, a wider margin should be used unless it unduly increases morbidity by affecting function or cosmesis. Conducting a randomized trial for patients with thick melanomas is difficult as they represent only approximately 10% of melanoma cases. A large retrospective review combining data from the M.D. Anderson and the Moffit Cancer Centers studied the effect of surgical margins (7). A total of 278 patients were studied and grouped into those who received less than versus those who received >2-cm margins. With a median follow-up of 27 months, the local recurrence rate was 12% for all patients. Interestingly, while positive nodal status, thicker lesions, and ulceration were significantly associated with a decreased overall survival, neither local recurrence nor excision margin affected disease-free or overall survival. This likely represents the increased incidence of distant metastatic disease at time of presentation in this group of patients. **Generally, a margin of 2 to 3 cm is recommended for patients with melanomas >4 mm in thickness.**

Excision margins for in situ melanomas are likewise poorly studied. Excision margins of 0.3 to 1 cm have yielded local recurrence rates of 6% to 20% in retrospective reviews (8,9). Most guidelines for treatment of in situ melanoma reference the National Institutes of Health (NIH). Consensus Statement on the diagnosis and treatment of early melanoma, which recommends margins of 0.5 cm (10). Although melanoma in situ theoretically should carry no risk of metastatic spread, recurrence can be invasive and, therefore, health threatening. In light of the paucity of data to support a 0.5-cm margin, it may be reasonable to use a larger excision if there is minimal impact on morbidity. Table 16.3 summarizes the current recommendations on wide local excision margins.

Subungual melanomas occur in an anatomically unique area. The skin of the matrix is so thin that the underlying phalanx should be considered as being involved. Consequently, wide excision should include amputation of the distal phalanx with enough dorsal skin to achieve adequate margin (1–2 cm). Generally, the remaining volar skin should be sufficient to close the stump (Fig. 16.2). Subungual melanomas comprise only 3% of all melanomas and have a 5-year survival rate of 40%. Likewise, the thin skin of the ear generally necessitates resection of the underlying cartilage and subsequent ear reconstruction. Most ear melanomas occur on the helix and the

TABLE 16.3

CURRENT RECOMMENDATIONS FOR MARGINS OF WIDE LOCAL EXCISION FOR MELANOMA

Thickness	Margin	Source (Ref. No.)
In situ	0.5 cm	10
<1 mm	1 cm	4, 10
1–2 mm	1–2 cm	4, 5
2–4 mm	2 cm	5, 6
>4 mm	2–3 cm	Retrospective data

ear reconstructed with chondrocutaneous advancement flaps. Some authors have reported success with skin-only resection and skin grafting. However, these have been limited case reports and at most this approach should be reserved for in situ melanomas.

Lymphadenectomy

Controversy has long existed regarding the appropriate treatment of the regional lymph nodes in melanoma. In 1907, Handley recommended removal of the regional lymph nodes. Others have recommended going further and resecting not only the primary lesion and draining lymph nodes but also the soft tissue carrying the lymphatic channels in an en bloc fashion. Although practitioners generally agree that removal of clinically involved lymph nodes is indicated, there is disagreement regarding excision of clinically uninvolved nodes (elective lymph node dissection [ELND]). The potential benefit of ELND is based on the dogma of sequential spread of metastatic disease to the regional lymph nodes prior to distant organs. Theoretically, if one can remove the lymph nodes early in the progression of disease, complete eradication is possible. Certainly there are anecdotal cases of long-term survivors following elective resection of affected regional lymph nodes, giving proof of concept to the potential for ELND to effect surgical cure. However, four large randomized clinical trials have failed to demonstrate any consistent survival advantage with addition of ELND.

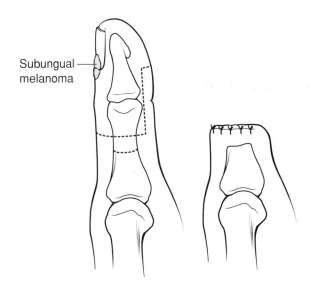

FIGURE 16.2. The typical level of amputation for treatment of a subungual melanoma.

The Intergroup Melanoma Surgical Trial (11) was designed to maximize the benefit of ELND. Patients with melanomas <1 mm were excluded because they were unlikely to have disease metastatic to the lymph nodes and patients with melanomas >4 mm were excluded because of the relatively high probability of distant metastatic disease. Because early studies of cutaneous lymph drainage patterns demonstrated a degree of unpredictability in choosing the draining lymph node basin, all patients with trunk melanomas underwent preoperative cutaneous lymphoscintigraphy. A total of 740 patients were randomized to receive ELND versus observation with an average follow-up of 7.4 years. There was no significant difference in survival for the patients as a group. However, when broken down into subgroups by post-hoc analysis, there was a significant survival advantage conferred by ELND in patients younger than 60 years of age and for tumors between 1 and 2 mm thick without ulceration. This analysis has been criticized as statistically unsound because these subgroups were not stratified at the start of the trial, making these results nondefinitive. **Nonetheless, in combination with the anecdotal evidence of long-term cure following ELND, these data suggest there may be survival advantage for ELND in certain subgroups of melanoma patients.** The question of patient selection remains unanswered but now may be irrelevant because of the advent of sentinel node biopsy. Some authors propose that sentinel node biopsy may improve survival by removing lymph node metastases at a very early stage and subsequently selecting patients who will benefit from completion lymphadenectomy.

Sentinel Node Biopsy

Sentinel node biopsy (SNB) is also known as sentinel or selective lymphadenectomy. The sentinel node is defined as the first node to receive lymph from a specific region of skin. The benefits of SNB are based on three assumptions: (a) lymphatic drainage is orderly and initially proceeds to one or two sentinel nodes; (b) the sentinel node(s) can be reliably identified and biopsied; and (c) lymphatic mets are detectable in the sentinel node(s) prior to dissemination elsewhere. The first two assumptions have been demonstrated through multiple, large, retrospective reviews at large cancer centers. The ability to identify and excise the sentinel node ranges from 93% to 100% in recent studies. Three large studies in which completion lymphadenectomy was performed following SNB demonstrated false-negative rates of 1.0% to 1.7%. **These data suggest that SNB is feasible and that the metastatic status of the sentinel node is predictive of the metastatic status of the rest of the basin.** The third assumption speaks to the ability of SNB to allow for surgical eradication of disease and to increase overall survival. Randomized trials are underway now to address this question.

Identification of the sentinel node is achieved with intraoperative lymphatic mapping, usually assisted by preoperative lymphoscintigraphy. In general, the mapping is carried out with injection of a radiocolloid intradermally at the site of the proposed excision. The radiocolloid rapidly enters the lymphatic system and a series of images is obtained to create a dynamic picture of the drainage pattern. As the agent encounters a lymph node, it is retained for a period of time, allowing for radiographic and subsequent intraoperative identification. Once definitive images are obtained, the skin over the identified nodes is marked and the images are sent along with the patient to the operating room. After induction of general anesthesia, isosulfan blue is injected intradermally at the site of the proposed excision. The isosulfan blue serves as a second and complementary identifying agent for intraoperative lymphatic mapping. Intraoperatively, two modalities are used to identify the sentinel node(s): (a) radiocolloid detection with a γ probe and (b) visual detection of the isosulfan blue. A limited inci-

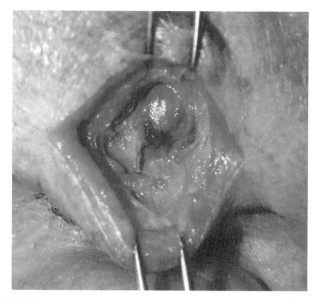

FIGURE 16.3. Sentinel Node Biopsy. Sentinel node biopsy generally involves a limited incision and dissection. Blue dye can be seen in the afferent lymph channel and a portion of the node.

sion and guided dissection allows for biopsy of the sentinel node with minimal morbidity (Fig. 16.3).

The exact technique of SNB varies between centers. Preoperative lymphoscintigraphy is not used for all patients at all centers. The lymphoscintigram is used to identify the draining nodal basin(s) and in-transit nodes. It is imperative to obtain preoperative lymphoscintigraphy in areas with a high likelihood of aberrant drainage patterns. These include the trunk where unpredictable drainage patterns can occur in 20% to 35% of cases and in-transit nodes are found 10% of the time. **In addition, head and neck lesions typically drain to multiple basins and are unpredictable in 60% of cases.** In contrast, extremity lesions generally drain to predicable basins (e.g., axillary, epitrochlear, inguinal, and popliteal) and drain to interval nodes only 5% to 10% of the time (Fig. 16.4). A secondary benefit to preoperative lymphoscintigraphy is confirmation of removal of all affected nodes. If more than one "hot" node is identified on lymphoscintigram, that represents the minimum number of sentinel nodes requiring biopsy. Because injection of the radiocolloid is necessary for intraoperative lymphatic mapping, there is little downside to obtaining preoperative lymphoscintigraphy and, in the author's practice, these scans are obtained on all patients undergoing SNB.

The choice of radiocolloid likewise varies between centers. Technetium-99m (^{99m}Tc) is preferred as the radioactive component because of its short half-life and γ-emitting properties. The ideal colloid would be taken up rapidly by draining lymphatic channels and then concentrated in the lymph node for an extended period of time to allow for imaging and excision. Human serum albumin is rapidly carried to the lymph nodes, but also rapidly passes through to secondary nodes. Trisulfide is used by some centers outside the United States but is not available here. Sulfur colloid (SC) concentrates in the lymph node but has a relatively large particle size and travels to the draining basin slowly. Filtering ^{99m}Tc-SC decreases the particle size and allows for travel to the draining basin in 1 to 2 hours. Therefore, filtered ^{99m}Tc-SC offers a good compromise between rapid accumulation and extended retention in the sentinel node(s).

In the author's practice, patients come to the nuclear medicine suite early on the day of surgery. They are injected

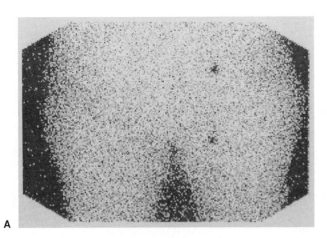
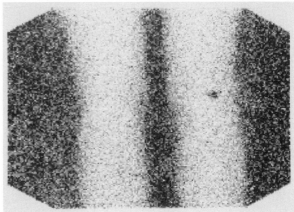

A   B

FIGURE 16.4. A: Lymphoscintigram. Lymphoscintigram demonstrating sentinel nodes in the femoral (superficial) and iliac (deep) basins. B: Lymphoscintigram demonstrating a sentinel node in the popliteal basin.

with 450 μ Ci of filtered ^{99m}Tc-SC at the proposed excision site and serial lymphoscintigrams are obtained starting at 15 minutes postinjection. All lymphatic basins at risk for metastatic spread, as well as all soft tissue at risk for in-transit mets and/or interval sentinel nodes, are monitored. After accumulation of radiocolloid, the skin over the sites is marked with permanent marker and the patient is sent to the operating room. The lymphoscintigram is reviewed in the preoperation holding area and the radiologist is contacted as necessary. After induction of general anesthesia and prior to surgical prepping, the proposed site of excision is intradermally injected with 0.5 to 1 mL of 1% isosulfan blue (Lymphazurin, United States Surgical). The area is massaged for 5 minutes and the patient is prepped and draped. This gives enough time (20 to 30 minutes) for travel of the isosulfan blue to the lymph nodes. Using a hand-held γ probe, the skin over the sentinel node(s) is scanned and incision(s) planned. The incision should fall along that which would be used in the event of eventual completion lymphadenectomy (i.e., inferior axillary hairline, inguinal crease), although the length should be limited to that necessary for access to the node(s). Nodes and lymphatic channels are localized by visualization of the blue dye and confirmation with the hand-held γ probe, although at times the blue dye is unreliable and, localization is accomplished with radioactivity detection alone. The sentinel node(s) are dissected intact and care is taken to tie or clip afferent and efferent lymph channels to avoid seroma. After node excision, its radioactivity is measured using the γ probe and the operative site rescanned. Background counts >10% of the resected node indicated the presence of another sentinel node. Sentinel node excision continues until the background is <10% of the most radioactive node removed. All sentinel nodes are sent to pathology for special processing, including serial sectioning and immunohistochemistry. The primary site is generally excised after removal of the sentinel node(s), although in cases where background radioactivity from the site interferes with lymph node localization, it can be excised prior to SNB. Drains are infrequently required and most patients are discharged on the same day.

Because of the high success rate at identification and excision of the sentinel node(s) and the minimal morbidity of the procedure, it has become a de facto standard of care for patients at high risk of nodal metastasis. The primary benefit of SNB is a highly accurate staging of the nodal basin. It is estimated that the serial sectioning and immunohistochemical staining possible by the submission of a limited amount of nodal material (as opposed to an entire nodal basin) allows for a 10-fold increase in sensitivity for detection of metastatic disease. **Nodal status is the single most important prognostic factor in melanoma staging, and sentinel node status can guide further treatment decisions.** A positive sentinel node upstages a patient to stage III and completion lymphadenectomy of the affected basin is indicated. In addition, these patients become candidates for interferon α-2b adjuvant therapy and/or entry into clinical trials. It should be remembered, however, that definitive data regarding the impact of SNB and ensuing treatments on overall survival awaits completion of ongoing clinical trials. In addition, although SNB is generally a low-morbidity procedure, complications such as wound infection, seroma, lymphocele, and injury to sensory or motor nerves have been reported.

Indications for SNB include (a) melanoma >1 mm, (b) melanoma >0.75 mm with ulceration or Clark level IV/V, and (c) melanoma specimens truncated at the base (because of inadequate biopsy) and therefore of unknown depth. Melanomas <0.75 mm rarely metastasize and are not currently considered for SNB. Using these criteria, approximately 20% of patients will have evidence of metastatic spread. Patients who have evidence of stage III disease, including clinical or radiologic adenopathy, satellitosis, or in-transit mets, do not need further staging with SNB and are instead offered lymph node dissection and/or wide excision of their locoregional disease. Relative contraindications include prior wide local excision and prior surgery to the regional basin or soft tissues between the primary site and regional basin. SNB in the head and neck area remains somewhat controversial because of the increased degree of difficulty (a result of the close proximity of the primary site and the draining basin) and the higher risk of nerve injury, as well as the increased difficulty of eventual lymphadenectomy as a consequence of scarring. Because the benefits of SNB in this area are presumably the same as in any other area of the body, patients with head or neck primaries are offered this approach. However, because of the increased difficulty, patients with indications for SNB in the head and neck undergo preoperative staging with PET/CT and definitive lymphadenectomy if adenopathy is detected.

Therapeutic Lymphadenectomy

Therapeutic lymphadenectomy is performed in the case of positive sentinel node, or clinically or radiographically detectable adenopathy. The goals are complete removal of the regional lymph nodes at risk. The contexts in which therapeutic lymphadenectomy may improve overall survival are not well defined. However, most practitioners agree that the benefits of removing affected nodes outweigh the risks, if only for palliation.

Therapeutic axillary lymphadenectomy for melanoma should result in complete lymphatic clearing of levels I to III. This can be facilitated by an S-shaped incision to expose the entire axilla and intraoperative arm abduction over the chest wall. If macroscopic or bulky disease is detected under the pectoralis minor, this muscle can be cut to improve exposure. Care is taken to preserve the following structures: pectoralis major muscle, axillary vein, brachial plexus, and the long thoracic, thoracodorsal, and medial pectoral nerves. Major complications include infection (7%), seroma (25%), and nerve dysfunction or pain (20%).

Therapeutic inguinal lymphadenectomy involves dissection of the superficial (inguinal) with or without the deep (ilioinguinal) nodes. Patients with disease detected in an inguinal node or with clinically detectable inguinal adenopathy undergo further staging with pelvic CT scan. Deep nodes are included when there exists a positive iliac sentinel node or iliac adenopathy is detected on CT scan. The incision is placed just inferior to and parallel to the groin crease with extensions onto the abdomen laterally or down the thigh medially if needed. The superficial nodes lie within the femoral triangle bounded by the inguinal ligament superiorly, the sartorius muscle laterally, and the adductor longus muscle medially. The femoral vessels, femoral nerve, and lateral femoral cutaneous nerve are identified and carefully preserved. The most superior node located at the femoral ring (Cloquet node) is identified and marked with a suture. If this node is involved with disease, most authors recommend iliac node dissection. Deep (iliac) nodes are dissected via a retroperitoneal approach with an incision in the external oblique fascia. Major complications include wound infection/healing (30% to 50%), seroma (25%), and lymphedema (25%). Because of the high rate of wound problems, most authors recommend sartorius muscle transposition at the time of node dissection to protect the femoral vessels.

Lymph nodes in the head and neck at risk for metastatic disease include those in the parotid, cervical (levels I through V), occipital, and postauricular basins. Lymph drainage patterns can be difficult to predict but, generally, lesions in the face and anterior scalp drain to the parotid and cervical levels I to IV. Lesions in the posterior scalp drain to cervical levels II to V, occipital, and postauricular basins. There is a wide coronal band where drainage can occur in anterior and posterior directions, and lesions near the midline can drain to either side. Choice of basins to dissect is made using location of lesion, adenopathy on preoperative imaging, or preoperative lymphoscintigram. In general, functional neck dissections preserving the sternocleidomastoid muscle, internal jugular vein, and spinal accessory nerve are performed.

TREATMENT OF ADVANCED MELANOMA

Local Recurrence

Local recurrence of melanoma can indicate an aggressive biology. Although recurrence rates are low (2% to 3%), the disease-specific mortality is as high as 80%. Recurrence is associated with increasing tumor thickness, presence of ulceration, and location on the foot, hand, scalp, or face. Local recurrence is differentiated from locoregional recurrence (satellitetosis or in-transit mets) by its location within 2 cm from the primary site of excision. Recurrence in an area discontinuous with the primary site likely has a worse prognosis than that occurring at the surgical margin. When possible, surgical excision with a generous (1- to 3-cm) margin is the recommended treatment. In cases of extremity melanomas, when surgical excision is not possible because of location, functional loss, or high tumor burden, isolated limb perfusion is an alternative form of therapy.

Isolated Limb Perfusion

Isolated limb perfusion (ILP) is a surgical procedure for regional delivery of chemotherapeutic agents to an extremity. It consists of vascular cannulation of an arm or leg and mechanical perfusion with blood containing high doses of agent. Because the vasculature of the limb is isolated from the rest of the body, the normal toxicity of the agents to visceral organs is minimized, allowing for otherwise lethal doses to be regionally administered. Although the use of a variety of agents has been described, the most common regimen used currently consists of melphalan with or without tumor necrosis factor. In addition, hyperthermia may be used to potentiate the effect.

Currently, there is no convincing data indicating a benefit in overall survival with ILP; consequently, its use in the adjuvant setting should be confined to clinical trials. The major role for ILP currently is for palliation of unresectable extremity disease. Because of the high risk of recurrence, patients with more than four recurrent lesions on a limb are also candidates for ILP. Systemic toxicity results from leakage of agent into the systemic circulation and includes nausea, vomiting, and neutropenia. Regional toxicity is more common, and includes erythema, blistering, edema, myopathy, neuropathy, arterial embolism, and deep vein thrombosis.

Chemotherapy

Despite intensive investigation, there are few agents that convincingly demonstrate improvement in overall survival in patients with systemic disease (12). In 1995, the FDA approved high-dose interferon (IFN) α-2b for the treatment of stage III and stage IIb melanoma. Despite controversy over its use, two randomized clinical trials do demonstrate significant, albeit modest, increases in relapse-free and overall survival. There are significant toxicities, including nausea/vomiting, malaise, hematopoietic suppression, liver toxicity, and neuropsychiatric effects (major depression, psychosis). Because the treatment regimen lasts for a year, patients need to be carefully selected based on age, performance status, and pre-existing medical conditions. Despite modest benefits and significant toxicity, IFN remains the only FDA-approved treatment for stage IIb–III melanoma and continues to play an important role in the overall treatment of these patients.

No systemic treatment has convincingly demonstrated a survival benefit for patients with stage IV melanoma. This includes single-agent and combination chemotherapy, interleukin (IL)-2, and biochemotherapy. In highly selected patients, high-dose IL-2 in combination with biochemotherapy can provide some clinical benefit in 10% to 20% of cases. Other agents include dacarbazine (DTIC), which received initial FDA approval in 1975 and remains the most common initial treatment for patients off protocol, although response is limited. Because of the limited efficacy of current chemotherapy regiments, patients with metastatic melanoma are encouraged to enter a clinical trial. Current investigational therapies include immune-based therapies, including vaccines and monoclonal antibodies. The most promising is the CancerVax vaccine developed by Morton et al., which is in phase III trials. Alternate treatment strategies involve therapy targeted at molecules important in melanoma tumorigenesis. These include Bay 43-9006 (targets B-Raf kinase, Bayer/Onyx), G3139 (targets Bcl-2, Genasense; Genta, Inc.), and R115777 (targets farnesyltransferase, Zarnestra; Johnson & Johnson).

Radiation

Melanoma is thought to be a particularly radioresistant cancer, thus the use of radiation for its treatment has been limited. However, a number of studies demonstrate that it can be useful in local control of disease (13). Unfortunately, there is a lack of large, randomized trials to guide treatment decisions, thus there are no uniform guidelines regarding its use. Although the use of radiation to treat melanoma has been reported in the primary, adjuvant, and elective settings, the most encouraging data come from studies of adjuvant therapy of head and neck nodal basins. Radiation seems to improve local control in the head and neck after surgical resection of lymph nodes, particularly in the presence of risk factors such as extracapsular extension, lymph nodes ≥ 3 cm, multiple nodal involvement, and recurrent disease after previous surgery. Improved local control at the primary site has also been documented for desmoplastic melanoma. Other relative indications include multifocal or recurrent disease, although this is probably best treated by isolated limb perfusion when occurring in an extremity. Additionally, its use in treatment of unresectable disease is indicated for palliation. Because of evidence that some melanoma cell lines are more sensitive to large doses of radiation per dose, hypofractionated delivery is generally used to treat melanoma when indicated. It should be remembered that findings in four randomized trials have failed to show a survival advantage with radiation treatment, thus it is primarily used to improve local control. Because of a lack of high-quality data documenting its efficacy, radiation should never be considered a viable alternative to surgical excision unless the disease is unresectable.

Surgical Excision of Distant Metastases

The clinical course of systemic melanoma is highly variable and difficult to predict. Slow-growing tumors may not cause life-threatening problems for years, and the presence of a small number of metastatic foci can cause a deteriorating quality of life. Although virtually all patients with systemic melanoma will eventually succumb to their disease, the goals of further surgery in these individuals should be relief of pain, wound hygiene, and, in some cases, prolongation of survival. Careful patient selection is required for surgery to be beneficial. Patients need to fully understand the goals of surgery and its limitations, as well as the risks involved.

The site of metastatic spread is important when considering metastectomy. Patients with complete resection of skin metas-

tases have a median survival of 24 to 30 months, and the procedures generally carry low morbidity rates. Consequently, patients with limited numbers of skin metastases as their only site of spread are generally good candidates for metastectomy. When such procedures can be done safely, excision of solitary lung or brain metastases can result in 18- and 12-month median survival, respectively. Surgical excision of these visceral mets can result in 5% to 20% long-term survival. On the other hand, patients with liver metastases have a worse prognosis with a median survival of 4 to 6 months, and the duration of palliation following resection is usually short. Symptomatic relief can result from cholecystectomy for localized gall bladder metastases, but these patients can be expected to succumb to their disease within 1 year. Because long-term survival is possible, an aggressive approach to surgical resection of melanoma metastases is warranted; however, this needs to be tempered with realistic goals, and extensive patient counseling is required to ascertain their understanding and participation.

References

1. Jemal Al A, , Murray T, Ward E, et al. Cancer statistics, 2005. *CA Cancer J Clin.* 2005;55:10.
2. Balch C, Buzaid A, Soong S-J, et al. Final version of the American Joint Committee on Cancer staging system for cutaneous melanoma. *J Clin Oncol.* 2001;19:3635.
3. Handley W. The pathology of melanocytic growths in relation to their operative treatment. *Lancet.* 1907;1:927.
4. Veronesi U, Cascinelli N, Adamus J, et al. Thin Stage I primary cutaneous malignant melanoma. Comparison of excision with margins of 1 or 3 cm. *N Engl J Med.* 1991;325:292.
5. Balch C, Urist M, Karakousis C, et al. Efficacy of 2-cm surgical margins for intermediate-thickness melanomas (1 to 4 mm). Results of a multi-institutional randomized surgical trial. *Ann Surg.* 1993;218:267.
6. Thomas J, Newton-Bishop J, A'Hern R, et al. Excision margins in high-risk malignant melanoma. *N Engl J Med.* 2004;350:757.
7. Heaton K, Sussman J, Gershenwald J, et al. Surgical margins and prognostic factors in patients with thick (>4 mm) primary melanoma. *Ann Surg Oncol.* 1998;5:322.
8. Osborne J, Hutchinson P. A follow-up study to investigate the efficacy of initial treatment of lentigo maligna with surgical excision. *Br J Plast Surg.* 2002;55:611.
9. Bartoli C, Bono A, Clemente C, et al. Clinical diagnosis and therapy of cutaneous melanoma in situ. *Cancer.* 1996;77:888.
10. Diagnosis and treatment of early melanoma. NIH Consensus Development Conference. *Consensus Statement.* 1992;10:1.
11. Balch C, Soong S-J, Bartolucci A, et al. Efficacy of an elective regional lymph node dissection of 1 to 4 mm thick melanomas for patients 60 years of age and younger. *Ann Surg.* 1996;224:255.
12. Linette G, Cornelius L, Hussussian C. Management of advanced melanoma. *Contemp Oncol.* 2003;15:1.
13. Ballo M, Ang K. Radiotherapy for cutaneous malignant melanoma: rationale and indications. *Oncology.* 2004;18:99.

CHAPTER 17 ■ THERMAL, CHEMICAL, AND ELECTRICAL INJURIES

MATTHEW B. KLEIN

Few areas of medicine are as challenging medically and surgically as burn care. Burn injuries affect the very young and the very old of both sexes. Burn injuries can vary from small wounds that can be easily managed in the outpatient clinic, to extensive injuries resulting in multiorgan system failure and a prolonged hospital course.

According to the National Institutes of General Medical Sciences, an estimated 1.1 million burn injuries require medical attention annually in the United States. Of those injured, about 50,000 require hospitalization and about 4,500 die annually from burn injuries. Survival following burn injury has significantly improved over the course of the 20th century. Improvements in resuscitation, the introduction of topical antimicrobial agents, and, most importantly, the practice of early burn wound excision have contributed to the improved outcome. However, extensive burn injuries remain potentially fatal.

BURN MANAGEMENT: OVERVIEW

Etiology

Burn injuries result from a variety of causes. Scald burns are the most common cause of burn injury in the civilian population. The depth of scald burn is related to the temperature of the liquid, the duration of exposure to the liquid (Table 17.1), and the viscosity of the liquid (there is usually prolonged contact with more viscous liquids). Scald burns will typically heal without the need for skin grafting. Grease burns, however, tend to result in deeper dermal burns and will occasionally require surgical management. Flame burns, the next most common cause of burn injury, typically result from house fires, campfires, and the burning of leaves or trash. If the patient's clothing catches fire, burns are usually full thickness. Flash burns also are quite common and typically result from ignition of propane or gasoline. Flash burns typically injure exposed skin (most commonly face and extremities) and usually result in partial-thickness burns. Contact burns occur from contact with woodstoves, hot metals, plastics, or coals. Contact burns are usually deep but limited in extent. In addition, burn injury can result from electrical and chemical agents.

Organization of Burn Care

The essence of successful burn care is the team. No individual is capable of meeting the many acute and long-term needs of the burn patient. Consequently, burn care is best delivered in a specialized burn center where experienced physicians, nurses, physical and occupational therapists, nutritionists, psychologists, and social workers can all participate in the care of the individual. With the exception of small burns, patients with burn injuries should be referred to a burn center. The American Burn Association (ABA) has established formal criteria for transfer to a burn center (Table 17.2). It is important to consider these as only guidelines. Patients who do not have a local physician comfortable caring for even a minor burn should be transferred to the nearest burn center.

Prior to the transfer of a patient to a burn center, specific steps are followed to ensure safe transport. Ideally, the burn center works in conjunction with the hospital's transfer center. The transfer center puts the referring physician in contact with the on-call burn surgeon. This communication is effective in clarifying the details of the injury and guiding the referring physician in the appropriate early management of the burn patient. Patients should be transported in warm, dry dressings to prevent hypothermia during transport. The application of topical agents is usually unnecessary because the wounds will require cleansing and assessment following arrival at the burn center.

The single most critical issue to address prior to patient transport, as in any trauma patient, is the airway. If the patient has signs and symptoms of inhalation injury or the circumstances of the burn raise the suspicion of inhalation injury (e.g., closed-space fire), then securing the airway prior to transport is recommended. Although intubation itself is not without risk—including a risk of inflicting an airway injury—it is far safer to err on the side of intubation than to lose an airway in transit. If carbon monoxide or cyanide inhalation is suspected, the patient should be placed on a 100% oxygen by face mask. In addition, intravenous access, Foley catheter placement, and initiation of fluid resuscitation should also occur prior to transport. Accurate assessment of burn size and depth (described below in Evaluation of the Burn Patient section) may be difficult for the emergency room physician inexperienced in managing burn patients. The accepting burn physician should assist the referring physician in determining whether resuscitation is necessary and how to calculate fluid requirements.

Evaluation of the Burn Patient

On arrival at the burn center, a thorough evaluation is performed and a treatment plan is developed. Burn patients are trauma patients, and they require evaluation in accordance with the Advanced Trauma Life Support (ATLS) protocol. Airway, breathing, and circulation are assessed immediately following burn injury. In addition to ensuring a patent airway, adequate breathing, and circulation, the presence of additional injuries—particularly life-threatening injuries—should be excluded.

A thorough history of the burn may provide important information that will affect management. Details related to the location of the injury (indoors vs. outdoors), type of liquid involved in a scald, duration of extraction from fire, as well as

TABLE 17.1

IMMERSION TIME TO PRODUCE FULL-THICKNESS BURNS

Time	Temperature (°F)
1 second	158
2 seconds	150
10 seconds	140
30 seconds	130
1 minute	127
10 minutes	120

details of the patient's other medical problems, are important elements of an adequate history.

The ABA transfer guidelines described above provide criteria for referral to a specialized burn center. The final decision to admit a patient to the burn center, however, is based on a number of factors. Critically ill patients and patients requiring volume resuscitation require admission. Consideration of the patient's home situation, including assistance with wound care and the patient's own compliance with wound care and therapy, is factored into the decision regarding admission. In addition, any child who has an injury that is suspicious for abuse

TABLE 17.2

BURN CENTER REFERRAL CRITERIA

The American Burn Association has identified the following injuries as those usually requiring a referral to a burn center. Patients with these burns should be treated in a specialized burn facility after initial assessment and treatment at an emergency department. Questions about specific patients can be resolved by confirmation with the burn center.

Second and third degree burns >10% body surface area (BSA) in patients <10 or >50 years old.

Second and third degree burns >20% BSA in other groups.

Second and third degree burns with serious threat of functional or cosmetic impairment that involve face, hands, feet, genitalia, perineum, and major joints.

Third degree burns >5% BSA in any age group.

Electrical burns, including lightening injury.

Chemical burns with serious threat of functional or cosmetic impairment.

Inhalation injury with burn injury.

Circumferential burns with burn injury.

Burn injury in patients with pre-existing medical disorders that could complicate management, prolong recovery, or affect mortality.

Any burn patient with concomitant trauma (for example fractures) in which the burn injury poses the greatest risk of morbidity or mortality. However, if the trauma poses the greater immediate risk, the patient may be treated in a trauma center initially until stable, before being transferred to a burn center. Physician judgment will be necessary in such situations, and should be in concert with the regional medical control plan and triage protocols.

Hospitals without qualified personnel or equipment for the care of children should transfer burned children to a burn center with these capabilities.

should be admitted to the hospital so that the appropriate social services agency can be contacted and the circumstances surrounding the injury investigated.

Adults with burn injuries greater than 15% to 20% should be admitted to an intensive care unit for adequate monitoring and infection control. Infants and children and elderly patients with less-extensive burn injuries should also be monitored in an intensive care setting. In addition, patients requiring close airway monitoring because of suspected inhalation injury or frequent neurovascular checks also should be placed in an intensive care unit setting.

Determination of Burn Extent

The extent and depth of burn wounds are established shortly following admission. There are several techniques used to calculate the total body surface area (TBSA) burned. **When calculating TBSA, only include those areas of partial- and full-thickness dermal injury. Superficial burns involving the epidermis only are not included in the calculation.** The *rule of nines* (Fig. 17.1) is the best-known method of estimating burn extent. However, it is important to note that the proportions of infants and children are different from those of adults. The heads of children tend to be proportionally greater than 9% TBSA, and the lower extremities tend to be proportionally less than 18%. In addition, it is important to explain to the inexperienced person that the percentage assigned to a body part represents a total area, so that a portion of an arm burn is only a portion of 9%. A second technique of estimating TBSA uses the patient's hand. The patient's hand represents approximately 1% TBSA and total burn size can be estimated by determining how much of the patient's (not the examiner's) hand area is burned. Lund and Browder charts are a more accurate method of assessing burn extent. They provide an age-based diagram to assist in more precisely calculating the burn size (Fig. 17.2).

Depth of Burn Injury

Thermal injury can injure the epidermis, a portion of or the entirety of the dermis, as well as subcutaneous tissue. The depth of the burn affects the healing of the wound, making assessment of burn depth important for appropriate wound management and, ultimately, the decision for operative intervention. The characteristics of superficial, partial-thickness, and full-thickness burns are described below and summarized in Table 17.3.

Superficial burns involve the epidermis only and are erythematous and painful. These burns typically heal within 3 to 5 days and are best treated with topical agents such as aloe lotion, which accelerate re-epithelialization and soothe the patient. In addition, oral analgesics can be helpful. Sunburns are the prototypical superficial burns.

Partial-thickness burns involve the entirety of the epidermis and a portion of the dermis. Partial-thickness burns are further divided into superficial and deep based on the depth of dermal injury. Superficial and deep partial-thickness burns differ in appearance, ability to heal, and potential need for excision and skin grafting. Superficial partial-thickness burns are typically pink, moist, and painful to the touch (Fig. 17.3). Water scald burns are the prototypical superficial partial-thickness wound. These burns typically heal within 2 weeks and generally do not result in scarring, but could result in alteration of pigmentation. These wounds are usually best treated with greasy gauze with antibiotic ointment.

Deep partial-thickness burns involve the entirety of the epidermis and extend into the reticular portion of the dermis. These burns are typically dry and mottled pink and white in appearance and have variable sensation. If protected from infection, deep partial-thickness burns will heal within 3 to 8 weeks, depending on the number of viable adnexal structures

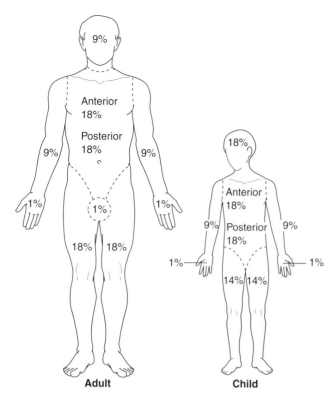

FIGURE 17.1. The Rule of Nines. This classic technique provides a facile method of estimating total body surface area burned. Because of differences in body proportions, the percentage for each body area are different in adults and children.

in the burn wound. However, they will typically heal with contraction, scarring, and possible contractures. **Therefore, if it appears that the wound will not be completely re-epithelialized in 3 weeks, operative excision and grafting is recommended.**

Full-thickness burns involve the epidermis and the entirety of the dermis. These wounds are brown-black, leathery, and insensate (Fig. 17.4). Occasionally, full-thickness burn wounds have a cherry-red color from fixed carboxyhemoglobin in the wound. These wounds can be differentiated from more superficial burns because they are usually insensate and do not blanch. Full-thickness burns are best treated by excision and grafting, unless they are quite small (size of a quarter).

Determination of burn depth is usually easy for superficial and very deep wounds. However, determining the depth of deep dermal burns and their healing potential can be more challenging. It often takes several days to determine which wounds will heal within 3 weeks and which would be better managed with excision and grafting. A variety of techniques have been described for precise determination of burn depth, including fluorescein dyes, ultrasound, laser Doppler, and magnetic resonance imaging. However, none of these methods have proved to be more reliable than the judgment of an experienced burn surgeon.

Initial Management

Intravenous Access

Intravenous access is important for patients who will require fluid resuscitation as well as for those patients who will require intravenous (IV) analgesia. Two peripheral IV lines are usually sufficient for patients with less than 30% burns. How-

ever, patients with larger burns or significant inhalation injury will require central line placement. Both peripheral and central lines can be placed through burned tissue when required. The burned area is prepared with topical antimicrobial solution as is done when preparing uninjured skin. Lines should be securely sutured in place, particularly over burned areas where the use of tape dressings is difficult. Typically, a triple lumen is adequate access because large volume fluid boluses are not a standard component of burn resuscitation. Furthermore, there is usually no need for a pulmonary artery catheter introducer because these catheters are of little benefit, and possibly detrimental, in the resuscitation of the burned patients. Arterial line placement is usually necessary in the patient who is intubated and is likely to remain intubated for several days. Again, placement of the arterial line through unburned tissue is preferred, but may not always be possible. If femoral arterial and venous lines are needed, one must be cognizant of the risk of both arterial and venous thrombosis. In addition, if the patient is awake and alert, it is difficult to sit upright and to ambulate with a groin catheter in place. Regardless of location, arterial and venous lines should be removed as soon as possible.

Escharotomy

An important component of early burn wound management is the determination of whether escharotomies are necessary. The leathery eschar of a full-thickness burn can form a constricting band that compromises limb perfusion or, in the case of the torso, ventilation. During fluid resuscitation the problem worsens. **In general, escharotomies are indicated for full-thickness circumferential burns of the extremity or for full-thickness burns of the chest wall when the eschar compromises thoracic cage excursion and, thus, ventilation of the patient.** Escharotomy can be performed at the bedside using a scalpel or electrocautery. Adequate release occurs when the eschar separates, perfusion improves and, on occasion, a popping sound is heard. Figure 17.5 shows the placement of escharotomy incisions. It is important to be aware of the position of superficial nerves when performing escharotomy. It is also important to be wary of the depth of escharotomy incision. **The incision should go through only eschar, not fascia. An escharotomy is not a fasciotomy.** Incisions that are too deep can unnecessarily expose vital underlying structures such as tendons, and also increase the chance of desiccation and death of otherwise healthy tissue.

Early management of tar burns and burns resulting from manufacture of methamphetamine require special mention. Tar in the mother pot is maintained at a temperature of 400°F to 500°F. Once the tar is applied it generally has cooled significantly but will still cause thermal injury. Tar burns from the mother pot are typically full-thickness burns, whereas cooler tar burns may result in partial- or deep partial-thickness injury. As the tar cools on the skin, it solidifies, thereby becoming difficult to remove (Fig. 17.6). Solvents such as petrolatum, petrolatum-based ointments, lanolin, and Medi-Sol (Orange-Sol, Gilbert, AZ) are useful for this purpose. For optimal effect, allow 10 to 15 minutes after solvent application before removal of the tar is attempted. The solvent may need to be reapplied to achieve complete removal.

Unfortunately, burn injuries resulting from the manufacture of methamphetamine are increasingly common. Methamphetamine injury can result in both flash and flame burns following explosion and in a severe inhalation injury. Anhydrous ammonia which is commonly used in the synthesis of methamphetamine, is a caustic agent that can lead to a devastating pulmonary injury. On admission, patients suspected of methamphetamine-related injuries should have a toxicology screen and should undergo decontamination to minimize the

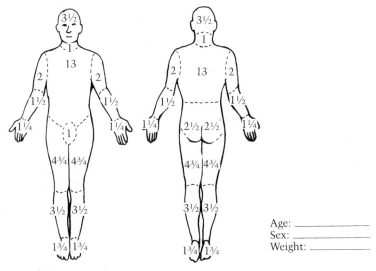

Age: _____
Sex: _____
Weight: _____

Area	Birth–1 yr	1–4 yr	5–9 yr	10–14 yr	15 yr	Adult	Partial thickness 2°	Full thickness 3°	Total
Head	19	17	13	11	9	7			
Neck	2	2	2	2	2	2			
Anterior trunk	13	13	13	13	13	13			
Posterior trunk	13	13	13	13	13	13			
Right buttock	2½	2½	2½	2½	2½	2½			
Left buttock	2½	2½	2½	2½	2½	2½			
Genitalia	1	1	1	1	1	1			
Right upper arm	4	4	4	4	4	4			
Left upper arm	4	4	4	4	4	4			
Right lower arm	3	3	3	3	3	3			
Left lower arm	3	3	3	3	3	3			
Right hand	2½	2½	2½	2½	2½	2½			
Left hand	2½	2½	2½	2½	2½	2½			
Right thigh	5½	6½	8	8½	9	9½			
Left thigh	5½	6½	8	8½	9	9½			
Right leg	5	5	5½	6	6½	7			
Left leg	5	5	5½	6	6½	8			
Right foot	3½	3½	3½	3½	3½	3½			
Left foot	3½	3½	3½	3½	3½	3½			
						Total			

FIGURE 17.2. The Lund and Browder chart. This chart provides a more precise estimate of burn TBSA for each body part based on the individual's age.

exposure of staff members to potentially toxic fumes. Burns associated with methamphetamine production have also been found to result in higher mortality levels.

Topical Wound Agents

Following admission to the burn center, the patient's wounds should be cleansed with soap and water. Loose tissue and blisters should be debrided. Body and facial hair should be shaved if involved in the area of a burn. Daily wound care should occur on a shower table with soap and tap water, or if the burn wound is small, at the patient's bedside following a shower. **The use of tanks for wound care is disfavored because of the risks of cross-contamination**.

Burn injury destroys the body's layer of protection from the environment, and dressings are needed to protect the body from infection and minimize evaporative heat loss from the body. The ideal dressing would be inexpensive, easy to use, require infrequent changes, and be comfortable. Although a number of topical agents are available for burn wound care, it is best to have a simple, well-reasoned wound care plan.

TABLE 17.3

BURN DEPTH CATEGORIES IN THE UNITED STATES

Burn degree	Cause	Surface appearance	Color	Pain level
First (superficial)	Flash flame, ultraviolet (sunburn)	Dry, no blisters, no or minimal edema	Erythematous	Painful
Second (partial thickness)	Contact with hot liquids or solids, flash flame to clothing, direct flame, chemical, ultraviolet	Moist blebs, blisters	Mottled white to pink, cherry red	Very painful
Third (full thickness)	Contact with hot liquids or solids, flame, chemical, electrical	Dry with leathery eschar until debridement; charred vessels visible under eschar	Mixed white, waxy, pearly; dark, khaki, mahogany; charred	Little or no pain; hair pulls out easily
Fourth (involves underlying structure)	Prolonged contact with flame, electrical	Same as third degree, possibly with exposed bone, muscle, or tendon	Same as third degree	Same as third degree

The choice of topical burn wound treatment is contingent on the depth of burn injury and the goals of management. Superficial burn wounds (such as sunburns) require soothing lotions such as aloe vera that expedite epithelial repair. Partial-thickness burn wounds need coverage with agents that keep the wound moist and provide antimicrobial protection. Deeper partial-thickness burn wounds should be covered with agents that protect the eschar from microbial colonization. Once the eschar has lifted, and the wound has begun to epithelialize, a dressing that optimizes epithelialization (e.g., greasy gauze and antibiotic ointment) should be used. Full-thickness burns should also be covered with a topical agent that protects the burn wound from getting infected until the time of burn excision.

It is important to emphasize that prophylactic systemic antibiotics have no role in the management of burn wounds. In fact, the use of prophylactic antibiotics increases the risk of opportunistic infection. Because burn eschar has no microcirculation, there is no mechanism for the local delivery of systemically administered antibiotics. Consequently, topical agents need to provide broad-spectrum antimicrobial coverage at the site of colonization—the eschar.

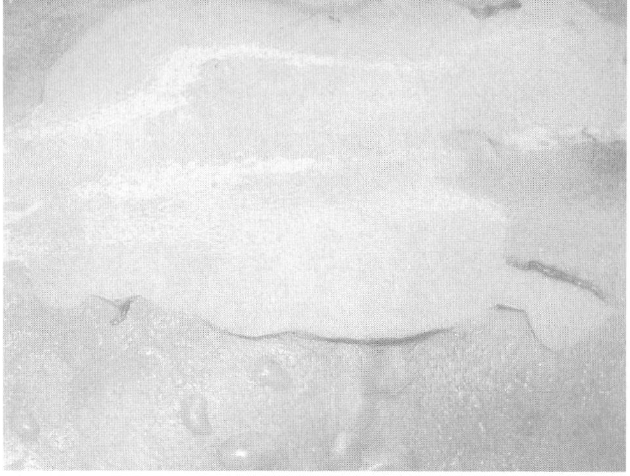

In the early postburn period, the dominant colonizing organisms are staphylococci and streptococci—typical skin flora. Over time, however, the burn wound becomes colonized with gram-negative organisms. Thus, topical antimicrobial agents used in early burn care should have broad-spectrum coverage to minimize colonization of the wound, but they need not be able to penetrate the burn eschar deeply.

Silver sulfadiazine is the most commonly used topical antimicrobial agent. Silver sulfadiazine has broad-spectrum antimicrobial coverage, with excellent staphylococcus and streptococcus coverage. **However, silver sulfadiazine does not penetrate an eschar and is therefore less useful in the management of an infected burn wound.** Wounds treated with silver sulfadiazine develop a yellowish-gray pseudoeschar that can be easily cleansed during daily wound care. Traditionally, the principal drawback of silver sulfadiazine was thought to be leukopenia. However, it is not clear whether the leukopenia

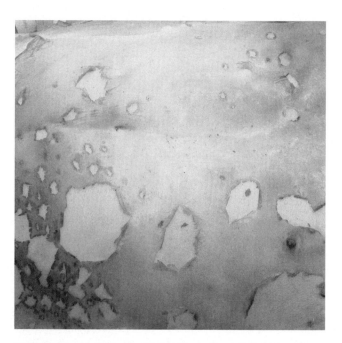

FIGURE 17.3. Superficial partial-thickness scald burn. These burns are typically moist, pink, and tender, and usually heal within 1 to 2 weeks.

FIGURE 17.4. Appearance of full-thickness burn. Full-thickness burn wounds have a dry, leathery appearance and can vary in color from brown to black to white. Full-thickness burns are insensate and will not blanch.

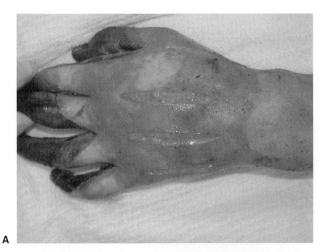

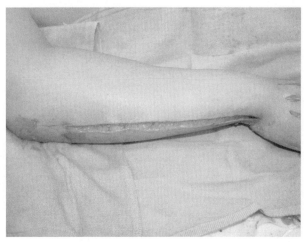

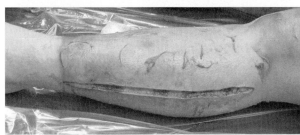

FIGURE 17.5. Escharotomy. The location of escharotomy incisions on the (**A**) upper extremity, (**B**) hand, and (**C**) lower extremity.

that occurs results from silver sulfadiazine toxicity or from the margination of leukocytes as part of the body's systemic inflammatory response to the burn injury. Regardless, the leukopenia is typically self-limited and, therefore, the silver sulfadiazine should not be discontinued. Patients with a documented sulfa allergy may or may not have a reaction to the silver sulfadiazine. If there is concern about an allergy, a small test patch of silver sulfadiazine can be applied. Typically, if there is an allergy, the silver sulfadiazine will cause irritation rather than be soothing, as is usually the case. In addition, a rash could signal a silver sulfadiazine allergy.

Mafenide is another commonly used antimicrobial agent. Mafenide is available as a cream and, more recently, a 5% solution. Mafenide, like silver sulfadiazine, has a broad antimi-

crobial spectrum, including gram-positive and gram-negative organisms. In addition, mafenide readily penetrates burn eschar, making it an excellent agent for treating burn wound infections. Mafenide is commonly used on the ears and the nose because of its ability to protect against suppurative chondritis; however, silver sulfadiazine appears to be equally effective in this setting. Because mafenide penetrates eschar well, twice-daily administration is typically necessary. Mafenide-soaked gauze can also be used as a dressing for skin grafts that have been placed over an infected or heavily colonized wound bed. **There are two well-recognized drawbacks of mafenide. Mafenide is a potent carbonic anhydrase inhibitor that can cause a metabolic acidosis, which can confound ventilator management. In addition, the application of mafenide can be painful, which may limit its use in partial-thickness burn wounds.**

Silver nitrate is another commonly used topical antimicrobial agent. Silver nitrate provides broad-spectrum coverage against gram-positive and gram-negative organisms. It is relatively painless on administration and needs to be applied every 4 hours to keep the dressings moist. Silver nitrate has two principal drawbacks. First, it stains everything it touches black, including linen, floors, walls, and staff's clothing. Second, because silver nitrate is prepared in water at a relatively hypotonic solution (0.5%), osmolar dilution can occur, resulting in hyponatremia and hypochloremia. Consequently, frequent electrolyte monitoring is needed. Rarely, silver nitrate can cause methemoglobinemia. If this occurs silver nitrate should be discontinued.

Bacitracin, neomycin, and polymyxin B ointments are all commonly used for coverage of superficial wounds, either alone or with petrolatum gauze to accelerate epithelialization. These ointments are also used routinely in the care of superficial face burns. Mupirocin is another topical agent that is effective in treating methicillin-resistant *Staphylococcus aureus* (MRSA). Mupirocin (Bactroban) should be used only when there is a culture-proven MRSA infection, to avoid the development of resistant infections.

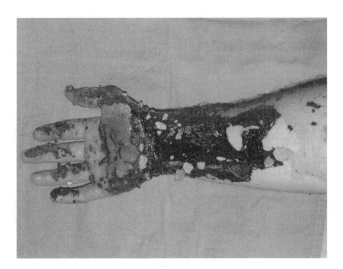

FIGURE 17.6. Once tar cools it adheres to the skin and can be removed by applying a solvent such as Medi-Sol.

Fluid Resuscitation

Significant burn injury not only results in local tissue injury, but initiates a systemwide response that can impact nearly every organ system. The release of inflammatory mediators (including histamine, prostaglandins, and cytokines) can lead to decreased cardiac output, increased vascular permeability, and alteration of cell membrane potential. In fact, for many decades there was believed to be a myocardial depressant factor that decreased the cardiac output in the first several days following burn injury. This decrease in cardiac function is likely caused by any number of cytokines. The purpose of fluid resuscitation is to provide adequate replacement for fluid lost through the skin and fluid lost into the interstitium from the systemic capillary leak that occurs as part of the body's inflammatory response. Therefore, significant volumes of intravenous fluid may be required to maintain adequate organ perfusion.

The realization of the importance of fluid resuscitation following burn injury in the early part of the 20th century was one of the most significant advances in burn care. Frank Underhill introduced the notion of burn shock and the need for resuscitation after studying the management of victims of the Rialto Theater fire in New Haven, Connecticut in 1921. Two decades later, following the Cocoanut Grove fire in Boston, the need for resuscitation was confirmed by the studies of Cope and Moore. The first formula for fluid resuscitation was developed a decade later by Evans, and this became the standard for fluid management for the 1950s and 1960s.

An understanding of burn shock physiology is essential to understanding the need for and the rationale for the various formulas that have been described for fluid resuscitation. Burn injury destroys the body's barrier to evaporative fluid losses and leads to increased cellular permeability in the area of the burn. In addition, in cases of larger burns (>20%) there is systemic response to injury that leads to capillary leakage throughout the body. In 1979, Arturson demonstrated that increased capillary permeability occurs both locally and systemically in burns greater than 25% (1), and Demling demonstrated that half of the fluid administered following 50% TBSA burns ends up in uninjured tissue (2). Therefore, burn resuscitation must not only account for the loss of fluid at the site of injury, but to the leak of fluid throughout the body. These losses are even greater if an inhalation injury is present because there will be increased fluid leak into the lungs as well as an increased release of systemic inflammatory mediators. Capillary leak usually persists through the first 8 to 12 hours following injury.

The use of formal fluid resuscitation is reserved for patients with burns involving more than 15% to 20% TBSA. Awake and alert patients with burns less than 20% TBSA should be allowed to resuscitate themselves orally as best as possible. A number of approaches using a number of different solutions have been proposed for intravenous fluid resuscitation.

Crystalloid

The Parkland formula, as described by Baxter, is still the most commonly used method for estimation of fluid requirements (Table 17.4). The formula (4 cc × weight in kilograms × %TBSA) provides an estimate of fluid required for 24 hours. The fluid administered should be lactated Ringer (LR) solution. LR is relatively hypotonic and contains sodium, potassium, calcium chloride, and lactate. Sodium chloride is not used because of the risk of inducing a hyperchloremic acidosis. Half the calculated fluid resuscitation should be administered over the first 8 hours, and the second half administered over the next 16 hours. Children who weigh less than 15 kg should also receive a maintenance IV rate with dextrose-containing solution because young children do not have adequate glycogen stores.

TABLE 17.4

THE PARKLAND FORMULA FOR FLUID RESUSCITATION

Formula: 4 cc/kg/%TBSA = total fluid to be administered in the first 24 hours
    50% of fluid should be given in the first 8 hours
    50% of fluid should be given in the next 16 hours
    Fluid should be lactated Ringer solution
Sample calculation: 70-kg person with a 50% TBSA burn
    4 × 70 × 50 = 14 L of fluid
    7 L in the first 8 hours (875 cc/hr)
    7L in the next 16 hours (437 cc/hr)
The formula is only a guideline. Fluid administration should be titrated to urine output of 30 cc/hr for adults and 1 cc/kg/hr for children.
    Pediatric patients weighing less than 15 kg should also receive maintenance fluid based on their weight.

It is important to remember that the formula provides merely an estimate of fluid requirements. Fluid should be titrated to achieve a urine output of 30 cc/hr in adults and 1 cc/kg/per hour in children. A Foley catheter should be used to accurately track urine output. If urine output is inadequate, the fluid rate should be increased; conversely if the urine output is greater than 30 cc/hr, the fluid rate should be decreased. Fluid boluses should only be used to treat hypotension, and should not be used to improve urine output. Patients with deeper, full-thickness burns and patients with inhalation injury tend to require higher volumes of resuscitation.

Colloid

Protein solutions have long been used in burn resuscitation and have been the subject of debate for decades. The use of colloid has the advantage of increasing intravascular oncotic pressure, which could minimize capillary leak and potentially draw fluid back intravascularly from the interstitial space. The Brooke and Evans formulas, developed during the 1950s and 1960s, both included the use of colloid in the first hours of resuscitation. **However, the use of colloid in the early postburn period can lead to the leakage of colloid into the interstitial space, which can aggravate tissue edema. Consequently, colloid is typically not used until 12 to 24 hours following burn injury, when the capillary leak has started to seal.**

Several different colloid formulations have been used. Albumin is the most oncotically active solution and does not carry a risk of disease transmission. Fresh-frozen plasma has also been used, but because this is a blood product, there is a risk, albeit small, of disease transmission. Dextran is a nonprotein colloid that has also been used in burn resuscitation. Dextran is available in both a low- and a high-molecular-weight form. Low-molecular-weight dextran (dextran 40) is more commonly used. Because dextran increases urine output with its osmotic effect, urine output may not be an accurate indicator of volume status. Additionally, dextran has been reported cause fatal allergic reactions in some patients.

Hypertonic Saline

Hypertonic saline solutions have been used for many years for burn resuscitation. Advocates of hypertonic saline argue that hypertonic solutions increase serum osmolarity and minimize the shift of water into the interstitium. This should theoretically maintain intravascular volume and minimize edema. However, this theory is not well substantiated in the literature. **Several** studies show similar resuscitation volumes and edema formation with either hypertonic or nonhypertonic solutions (3). The principal risk of hypertonic solutions is the development of hypernatremia.

Regardless of the type of resuscitation fluid used, urine output is the best indicator of resuscitation. Tachycardia is often present as a result of the body's systemic inflammatory response, pain, or agitation, and, therefore, should not be used as a barometer of volume status. The use of pulmonary artery catheter parameters to guide fluid resuscitation leads to overresuscitation. Serial lactates and hematocrits serve as secondary indicators of resuscitation so decisions regarding fluid administration and titration should be dictated by urine output. Poor urine output is likely the result of hypovolemia, and is therefore appropriately treated with increased fluid administration not diuretics or pressors.

The risks of underresuscitation—hypovolemia and worsening organ dysfunction—are well understood. More recently, the risks of overresuscitation are becoming clear. The need for intubation and prolonged ventilation, worse extremity edema that can extend the zone of burn injury, and the potential for extremity and abdominal compartment syndrome can all result from excessive fluid resuscitation.

Although there are several formulas to guide fluid resuscitation during the first 24 hours following burn injury, it is important to remember that patients may continue to have large fluid requirements for several days following injury. At the conclusion of the first 24 hours, fluids should not be discontinued; rather, continue to titrate fluids for a goal urine output of 30 cc/hr. Patients with large burns will have large volumes of insensible loses that require replacement with intravenous fluids.

Decision not to Resuscitate

Advances in burn care and fluid resuscitation, particularly the practice of early burn wound excision, have significantly increased survival following burn injury. However, there may be some cases of such extensive burn injury that the decision needs to be made whether or not efforts at resuscitation may be futile. This is a difficult decision. The decision is based on several factors, including an accurate assessment of the patient's injury, location of burns, depth of burns, presence of inhalation injury, the patient's age and comorbidities, and the typical mortality level based on these factors.

Several formulas have been described for estimating mortality, but none is perfect. Baux suggested that adding age and TBSA gives an estimate of mortality. Zawacki's description of the Z score is another formula that estimates mortality. The score is based on several factors, including extent of burn injury, extent of full-thickness burn injury, presence of inhalation, and age.

Part of the difficulty in determining survivability is that each burn is quite different. In addition, each patient is quite different. This is particularly true in older patients (≥65 years), because there is great heterogeneity in patients of the same age. Prior to making a decision regarding resuscitation, frank discussion with the patient's family, if possible, should occur. Members of the burn team—particularly the nurses caring for the patient—should be included in the discussion and comfortable with the sometimes very difficult decision not to resuscitate.

Patients who are awake and alert who are not candidates for resuscitation should also be involved in the process. These patients should be informed of the decision not to resuscitate and given the opportunity to talk with family members. Often patients with extensive full-thickness burns can be extubated and be awake and alert enough to have an opportunity to say goodbye to family members.

INHALATION INJURY

The inhalation of the products of combustion can lead to devastating pulmonary injury. Direct thermal injury to the lungs occurs rarely and usually only in the case of steam burns. Inhalation injury caused by products of combustion significantly increases burn mortality for a given percent skin burn. Carbon monoxide inhalation is particularly devastating because carbon monoxide will bind to hemoglobin and interfere with the delivery of oxygen.

Diagnosis of inhalation injury is best made by consideration of the circumstances surrounding the burn injury and findings on physical examination. Typically, patients who are trapped inside a burning room or house are at increased risk of inhalation injury because of prolonged exposure to smoke and products of production. Conversely, flash burns that occur outdoors will rarely result in inhalation injury. On physical examination, the presence of carbonaceous sputum, raw oral and nasal mucosa, and soot on the vocal cords (on laryngoscopy) all signify inhalation injury. In addition, patients may have a cough, hoarse voice, and difficulty breathing. The presence of singed nasal and facial hair may be suggestive of inhalation injury but, alone, is not diagnostic.

Evaluation of inhalation injury should include an arterial blood gas and carboxyhemoglobin level. Although an elevated carboxyhemoglobin is consistent with inhalation injury, patients who smoke cigarettes will have an elevated baseline carboxyhemoglobin, sometimes as high as 10. In addition, the carboxyhemoglobin level should be interpreted in light of the time since injury and the level of oxygen support the patient has received since the injury. The half-life of carboxyhemoglobin on 100% oxygen is 40 minutes, so a patient with a carboxyhemoglobin level of ten 40 minutes following injury may have had an initial level of 20.

Chest radiographs are of little usefulness in the evaluation of inhalation injury. Radionuclide studies have been used to diagnose inhalation injury but they might not add much more reliable diagnostic information beyond good clinical evaluation. Bronchoscopy can demonstrate mucosal inflammation in the upper airways, subglottic edema, and carbonaceous particles, and therefore can be useful in making the diagnosis of inhalation injury. However, the diagnosis can usually be made without the need for bronchoscopy.

Management of inhalation injury is usually supportive. Patients with signs and symptoms of inhalation injury may require intubation. In general, it is better to secure a patient's airway early in the postburn period, particularly if the patient will require large volumes of fluid resuscitation. In addition, if a patient is admitted with a suspected inhalation injury and has a worsening respiratory status, intubation should be promptly performed. Aggressive pulmonary toilet, bronchodilators, and clearing of secretions are all essential components of patient management. Steroids are not beneficial in the treatment of inhalation injury and the use of prophylactic antibiotics should be avoided. Radiographs may be useful following admission to evaluate possible pneumonia. Repeat bronchoscopy can be useful in obtaining sputum samples for culture and for assistance in suctioning sloughed mucosa that the patient is unable to clear. Patents who sustain inhalation injury are at increased risk for respiratory failure and subsequent infection.

Patients who develop signs of adult respiratory distress syndrome (ARDS) should be placed on low (protective) tidal volumes on the ventilator in order to protect the pulmonary parenchyma from additional damage. Typically, these lower tidal volumes result in hypercapnia, which should be permitted in order to protect the lungs.

The usefulness of hyperbaric oxygen for patients with elevated carboxyhemoglobin levels has long been debated. The potential benefit of hyperbaric oxygen is the rapid reduction of carbon monoxide levels with the potential to minimize potential neurologic sequelae of carbon monoxide poisoning. **Hyperbaric oxygen can reduce the half-life of carbon oxide from 40 minutes on 100% FiO$_2$ (fraction of inspired oxygen) to 20 minutes. However, hyperbaric oxygen is not without risk. Hyperbaric oxygen can cause pneumothorax and perforation of the tympanic membranes.** If the patient must be transported to another medical center for hyperbaric oxygen, it may be possible to effectively treat an elevated carboxyhemoglobin with 100% oxygen in the time it takes to transport the patient to the hyperbaric chamber. One must also carefully weigh the risks of placing a critically ill patient in a chamber where patient access might be limited. Any patient who is hemodynamically unstable, requiring aggressive resuscitation, and hypothermic should probably not be transported for hyperbaric oxygen.

PATIENT MANAGEMENT

Nutrition

Nutritional support is a cornerstone of burn patient management. Hypermetabolism and hypercatabolism both occur following burn injury. This increased metabolic rate begins immediately following injury and persists until complete wound coverage is achieved, which may take months. In addition, the nutritional requirements to heal burn wounds, skin grafts, and donor sites all increase the nutritional needs of the burn patient.

Feeds, whether oral or enteral, should be initiated as soon following admission as possible. Most patients with burns of under 20% TBSA can obtain enough calories on their own. However, patients with larger burns and patients who will be intubated for several days should have an enteral feeding tube placed on admission. Ileus following burn injury commonly occurs, and it may take days for the return of gastrointestinal function. However, ileus can be prevented by starting feeds in the immediate postinjury period. The burn team's dietician should be consulted to assist in determining nutritional needs, to provide monitoring of caloric intake, and to make appropriate adjustments to the patient's nutrition plan. Because of the high levels of narcotics patients receive, routine use of stool softeners should also begin on admission to prevent constipation and feed intolerance.

Parenteral nutrition is associated with higher rates of infection, attributable, in part, to the prolonged need for central venous access. Parenteral nutrition should only be used in cases when the patient has a prolonged paralytic ileus, pancreatitis, bowel obstruction, or other contraindication to enteral feeding.

Enteral feeds can be continued when the intubated patient is taken to the operating room unless the patient needs to be placed in the prone position. If the patient is not intubated and requires intubation for surgery, feeds should be discontinued 6 hours prior to surgery and restarted as soon as possible following the completion of surgery and extubation.

There are several equations for the estimation of caloric requirements. The two most commonly used formulas for calculating caloric requirements are the Curreri formula and the Harris-Benedict formula. The Curreri formula differs for children and adults as follows:

Adult: 25 kcal × weight (kg) + 40 kcal × %TBSA

Children: 60 kcal × weight (kg) + 35 kcal × %TBSA

The Harris-Benedict formula provides an estimate of basal energy expenditure (BEE):

Men: 66.5 + 13.8 × weight (kg) + 5 × height (cm)
− 6.76 × age (years)

Women: 65.5 + 9.6 × weight (kg) + 1.85 × height (cm)
− 4.68 × age (years)[4]

The calculated BEE is multiplied by an injury factor (typically 2.1 for patients with large burns) to provide an estimate of caloric requirements. Because the Curreri formula generally overestimates caloric requirements, particularly in the elderly, and the Harris-Benedict formula underestimates caloric requirements, an average of the two is often used. Indirect calorimetry using a metabolic chart can be used for patients on a ventilator. However, the calorimetric formula is less reliable at FiO$_2$ levels above 50%. The metabolic chart will provide an estimate of energy expenditure by measuring oxygen consumption and carbon dioxide production. In addition, a respiratory quotient can be calculated from these data that will provide information about whether the patient is being over- or underfed (4).

Protein requirements should also be calculated. Burn patients catabolize significant amounts of skeletal muscle and require protein replacement to maintain muscle mass and function and to provide building blocks for wound healing. **Patients with normal renal function should receive 2 g of protein per kilogram per day.** Supplemental vitamins and minerals should also be provided to optimize wound healing. Vitamins A and C, as well as zinc, have known benefits in wound healing, and the use of vitamin E, selenium, and iron supplements have also been described.

Regular nutrition monitoring, particularly for intensive care unit patients, should be performed weekly with C-reactive protein, albumin, prealbumin, and vitamin C levels, as well as a 24-hour total urea nitrogen. Calorie counts should be used to monitor the patient's oral intake and to help determine when enteral feeds can be safely weaned and ultimately discontinued.

Patient blood glucose levels should be closely monitored, particularly if the patient is in the intensive care unit. Enteral feeding, along with the body's systemic inflammatory response, can increase blood glucose levels. **The benefits of tight glucose control in a critically ill patient is well documented.** Sliding-scale insulin coverage should be initiated for all burn patients in the intensive care unit and there should be a low threshold for initiating an insulin drip, because this allows for tighter blood sugar control.

Gastrointestinal Prophylaxis

Stress ulcers (Curling ulcers) were once a common complication following severe burn injury. The development of prophylactic agents, including histamine receptor blockers, sucralfate, and protein pump inhibitors have minimized the incidence of stress ulcers. Perhaps the best protection against stress ulcers is feeding the patient. Feeding the stomach early in the hospital course minimizes post-traumatic gastric atony, provides continuous coating of the stomach, and is easier to place at the bedside than a duodenal tube. Stress ulcer prophylaxis is only necessary in those patients who are not taking oral diet or enteral feeds or in patients with previous history of peptic ulcer disease.

DEEP VENOUS THROMBOSIS

Patients who sustain burn injuries often have multiple risk factors for deep venous thrombosis. Injuries to an extremity as well as the occasional need for prolonged bedrest (particularly in the intubated patient) and indwelling catheters increase the risk of venous thrombosis. Consequently, deep venous thrombosis prophylaxis is required in burn patients who are hospitalized and unable to regularly ambulate. The use of sequential compression devices and antiembolism stockings may not be practical for use in patients with lower-extremity burns. These patients should receive subcutaneous heparin. Patients who develop sudden extremity swelling or acute hypoxia should be evaluated for deep venous thrombosis and pulmonary embolism. Duplex ultrasound imaging of both the upper and lower extremities is performed if the patient has burns to the upper extremities or subclavian intravenous lines. It is also important to be aware that pediatric patients can sustain deep venous thrombosis and pulmonary embolus. Therefore, deep venous thrombosis prophylaxis should be considered in the pediatric patient who is on prolonged bedrest.

Infection

Infection remains a significant risk following burn injury. Prolonged intensive care unit stay, prolonged periods of intubation and mechanical ventilation, and potential colonization of burn eschar contribute to the risk of infection. In addition, indwelling vascular and bladder catheters provide another source of invasive infection.

Burn patients are also functionally immunocompromised for a number of reasons. First, the skin, which serves as the principal barrier between an individual and the environment, is lost. Similarly, the mucosal barrier of the respiratory tract may also be injured. In addition, the cellular and humoral portions of the immune response are compromised following burn injury. Decreased production of antibodies, impaired chemotaxis, and phagocytosis all increase the risk of infection and decrease the body's ability to fight infection (5).

For many decades, patients who survived the first week following injury frequently succumbed to burn wound sepsis. Colonization of devitalized eschar would lead to bacterial invasion and, ultimately, to burn wound sepsis. The best treatment for burn wound sepsis is prevention. **The practice of early burn wound excision has significantly decreased the incidence of burn wound sepsis and improved survival.**

However, infection remains a reality in the management of the burn patient. The diagnosis and management of infection in the burn patient can be challenging. Fevers and leukocytosis can result from the systemic inflammatory response to burn injury and not necessarily infection. Thrombocytosis is also frequently observed in stable burn patients. Nearly all patients with greater than 15% TBSA burns are febrile within the first 72 hours following burn injury. Therefore, routine culture of these patients in this early time period is unnecessary. However, following the initial 72 to 96 hours, periodic cultures are important in making a diagnosis of infection. Temperature spikes warrant culturing of urine, sputum, blood, and central lines. In addition, any change in the patient's status including hypotension, altered mental status, intolerance of tube feeds, hyper- and hypoglycemia should raise the suspicion of infection.

Management of infections in burn patients must be culture-driven. Presumptive broad-spectrum antimicrobial coverage is fraught with potential complications, including breeding resistant organisms and increasing the risk of fungal infections. Selection of antibiotics should be based on culture results. In the case of suspected pneumonia, bronchoscopic samples may be helpful in differentiating pneumonia from airway colonization.

Although the most common sites of infection include the blood, urine, and lungs, patients with a prolonged intensive care unit course can also develop sinus infections, pancreatitis, cholecystitis, meningitis, and endocarditis. Thus, persistent fevers and signs of infection may require a more thorough evaluation beyond routine culture.

Pain Control

Pain management is an important factor in caring for the burn patient. Burn patients typically have two types of pain: background and procedural. Background pain is present on a daily basis with little variation. Procedural pain occurs during daily wound care and therapy. The best approach to pain management is to keep it simple. Polypharmacy can easily occur on a patient who is hospitalized for a long time and will make weaning the patient from the medications very difficult.

Narcotics are the most commonly used analgesics. Nonsteroidal medications are typically not used in patients who are going to undergo surgery because of the increased risk of bleeding. However, they may be useful following discharge and for the pain and muscle soreness associated with increasing range of motion and increasing activity level.

Background pain is best treated with longer-acting agents. Methadone can be used for patients who are going to have a long hospital course. Methadone has a half-life of 6 hours and can reduce the need for high doses of other agents. However, patients on methadone require a taper prior to discontinuation of the medication. Oxycodone or morphine can then be used for breakthrough pain. It is probably best to use only one of the two agents. If the patient is tolerating an oral diet, using an oral agent is probably better.

For procedural pain, shorter-acting agents are probably best because wound care is usually a short-duration activity. If the patient requires something stronger than oral analgesics, fentanyl is the agent of choice for procedural pain. Many patients may also benefit from low-dose benzodiazepines because wound care can be anxiety provoking for many patients. Again, the use of short-acting benzodiazepines is favorable.

Intubated patients are usually treated with morphine and Ativan—longer-acting agents—for background pain and sedation. Procedural pain is usually managed with fentanyl.

SURGICAL MANAGEMENT

Early burn excision and skin grafting is the standard of care for full-thickness burn wounds. The concept of early excision was popularized in the early 1970s by Janezovic (6). Traditionally, burn eschar was left on the wound, and the proteolytic enzymes produced by neutrophils and bacteria led to the separation and sloughing of the eschar. The underlying granulating wound was then skin grafted. It has become clear, however, that in cases of extensive burn injury, this delay in management results in more extensive bacterial colonization, and an increased likelihood of burn-wound sepsis, multiple organ failure, and, ultimately, death.

The benefits of early burn excision are clear and are well documented (7). **Early excision and grafting results in increased survival, decreased infection rates, and decreased length of hospital stay.** In addition, early removal of burn eschar also appears to decrease the risk of hypertrophic scarring.

If feasible, early staged excision should begin on post-burn day 3 for major burns that are clearly full thickness. Operations can be spaced 2 to 3 days apart until all eschar is removed and the burn wound covered. The interval days are to allow for stabilization and resuscitation of the patient. Debrided wounds can be temporarily covered with biologic dressings or cadaveric allograft until autogenous donor sites are available.

Techniques of Excision

The two techniques of burn-wound excision are tangential excision and fascial excision. Tangential excision is the sequential

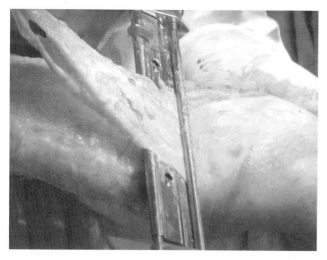

FIGURE 17.7. Tangential excision. Tangential excision is performed using a Watson (shown) or Goulian knife. Tissue is serially excised until viable, bleeding tissue, which can accept a graft, is reached.

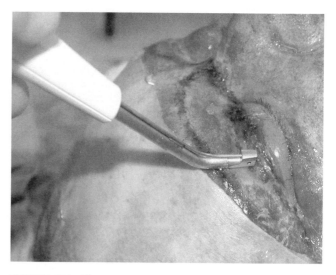

FIGURE 17.9. The VersaJet water dissector. This relatively new technology can be very useful for the excision of eyelid (shown), ear, and web space burns.

removal of layers of eschar and necrotic tissue until a layer of viable, bleeding tissue, which can support a skin graft, is reached. Tangential excision is carried out using a Watson or Goulian (Weck) knife (Fig. 17.7). The Watson knife has a dial to set the depth of excision and Goulian knives have guards of varying opening size to allow adjustment of excision depth. These settings and guards are only guides, and ultimate depth of excision is determined by the surgeon. There are two principal disadvantages of tangential excision. **First, when excising a large surface area there can be substantial blood loss; second, it may be difficult to accurately assess the viability of the excised wound bed.** This particularly can be a problem when excision is carried down to fat.

Fascial excision involves excision of the burned tissue and subcutaneous tissue down to the layer of the muscle fascia. Fascial excision can be carried out using electrocautery, which makes for a more hemostatic excision (Fig. 17.8). In addition, by carrying out excision through a well-defined anatomic plane, it is easier to control bleeding by identifying and ligating

larger vessels. However, in performing fascial excision, it is possible to excise viable subcutaneous tissue. Fascial excision also can result in an unsightly contour deformity and lymphedema of the excised extremities.

A newer device for burn excision is the water jet-powered VersaJet (Smith and Nephew, Largo, Florida). This device provides a relatively facile and precise tool for the excision of eschar and is particularly useful for excision of concave surfaces of the hand and feet, as well as for excision of the eyelids, ear, and nose (Fig. 17.9).

Regardless of which technique is used, extremity excisions should be performed under tourniquet control to minimize blood loss. In addition, suspension of upper and lower extremity from overhead hooks can facilitate excision and graft placement, particularly on the posterior aspect of the lower extremities. The risks of blood loss and probable need for transfusion should be clearly communicated to the anesthesia team prior to the start of excision. In addition, the operating room should be warmed and bear huggers should be used when possible to minimize hypothermia.

Adequate hemostasis is critical to minimizing hematoma formation and, ultimately, graft loss. Telfa pads (Kendall, Mansfield, MA) soaked in an epinephrine solution (1:10,000) are a mainstay of hemostasis, and are combined with topical pressure and cauterization when necessary. More recently, the use of tissue sealants such as Tisseel Fibrin Sealant (Baxter, Deerfield, IL) has gained popularity in assisting with hemostasis and with graft fixation.

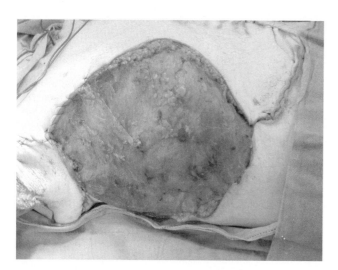

FIGURE 17.8. Full-thickness chest burn. This elderly patient had full-thickness burns to the chest, which were excised using a fascial excision. The edges of the wound were sutured to the pectoral fascia to minimize the step-off or ledge at the perimeter of the excision.

Technical Aspects of Skin Grafting

The process of engraftment is essentially that of revascularization of the graft. Initially the graft has no vascular connection with the recipient bed and survives through the process of diffusion of nutrients from the wound bed, a process known as plasma imbibition. Typically, the process of revascularization begins 48 hours after graft placement. The process of revascularization occurs by a combination of neovascularization (ingrowth of host vessels into the graft) and inosculation, the direct biologic anastomosis of cut ends of recipient vessels in the graft bed with those of the graft itself. Concomitant with revascularization of the graft is the organization phase, which describes the process by which the graft integrates with the wound bed (see Chapter 1).

Skin grafts are typically classified according to their thickness as either split (partial) thickness or full thickness, depending on whether they include the full thickness of dermis or just a portion of it. Split-thickness grafts are further classified into thin, intermediate, and thick, depending on the amount of dermis. The thinner a skin graft is, the more contraction that occurs at the recipient site following transplantation. Thicker grafts contract less at the recipient site, but leave a greater dermal deficit at the donor site, which will therefore take longer to heal and have an increased risk of hypertrophic scarring.

Skin grafts can also be meshed or unmeshed (sheet grafts). From an aesthetic viewpoint, sheet grafts are always superior to meshed grafts. It is best to perform sheet grafting over the face, hands, and forearms because these are exposed areas. In larger burns there is inadequate skin available to perform sheet grafting over all burned areas and the skin grafts need to be meshed. Skin grafts can be meshed 1:1, 2:1, 3:1, 4:1, and even 6:1. However, for practical and cosmetic purposes, mesh of 2:1 is the most commonly used. Meshing of skin grafts allows for the egress of fluid from the wound bed, which minimizes seroma and hematoma formation and therefore decreases the risk of graft loss. In addition, meshing a graft allows for expansion, which provides greater wound coverage.

Skin grafts can be affixed to the wound bed using a variety of techniques. Staples are the most commonly used and are probably the most expeditious way to secure grafts when a large area of the body is being covered. Suturing of grafts is particularly useful in children because absorbable sutures need not be removed. My burn center has had a great deal of success using Hypafix (Smith and Nephew, London, England), particularly for fixation of sheet grafts. Hypafix is an elastic adhesive dressing can be easily applied using Mastisol as an adhesive. The Hypafix remains in place and can only be removed by using Medisol. Fibrin glue and other tissue sealants have also been used to affix skin grafts to the wound bed.

There are numerous options for skin-graft dressings. Typically, the decision is guided by the type of graft—meshed or unmeshed—and the location of the graft.

A number of dressings can be used for meshed skin grafts. Wet dressings, consisting of antimicrobial solution (Sulfamylon) provide a moist environment to accelerate epithelialization of the interstices. Greasy gauze and Acticoat (Smith and Nephew, London, England) have also been used as dressings over meshed grafts. Acticoat is a relatively new antimicrobial dressing that consists of a polyethylene mesh impregnated with elemental silver. Silver provides antimicrobial activity by disrupting bacterial cellular respiration. Both greasy gauze and Acticoat are capable of providing a moist environment that accelerates closure of graft interstices. Bolsters of cotton or greasy gauze are needed when grafts are placed over areas of convexity or concavity.

Sheet grafts can be left open to the air to allow for monitoring or can be dressed with a nonadherent gauze. Typically, dressings over sheet grafts are removed on the day following skin grafting to allow for evacuation of seroma or hematoma that can occur. Facial skin grafts should similarly be covered with a nonadherent or greasy gauze, and we will commonly use a Jobst skin featureless face mask garment (Bielsdorf-Jobst, Rutherford College, NC) to minimize graft shearing.

The Vacuum Assisted Closure (V.A.C.) device (Kinetic Concepts, San Antonio, TX) is another option for skin graft coverage. The V.A.C. device is a negative pressure device that is able to prevent graft sheering and is particularly useful over areas of convexity or concavity. The V.A.C. device can be left in place over a skin graft for 5 days, and then can be easily removed at the bedside. Alternatively, an Unna boot dressing can be applied over grafts of the arm and leg. The Unna boot dressing provides vascular support and prevents graft shearing while allowing early mobilization.

Donor Site Selection and Care

Selection of donor sites is often dependent on the availability of unburned skin. For children, the buttock and scalp provide the most inconspicuous donor sites. Plasmalyte can be infused subcutaneously to facilitate graft harvest in these areas. When larger amounts of skin are needed, the thighs and back can be used.

The ideal donor-site dressing minimizes pain and infection, accelerates epithelialization, and is cost-effective. There are a number of donor-site dressings available, which may suggest that no perfect dressing exists. Greasy gauze and Acticoat are two commonly used donor-site dressings. They are applied at the time of surgery and left in place until epithelialization is complete, at which time, they can be easily removed. Alternatively, OpSite, a transparent polyvinyl adherent dressing, can be used. Although OpSite allows for observation of the underlying healing wound, the accumulation of fluid beneath the dressing can lead to leakage, which is both uncomfortable and disturbing to the patient. In addition, OpSite is not well suited for use over joint or convex surfaces. For children with buttock skin donor sites, Silvadene in the diaper works particularly well. The Silvadene can be replaced with each diaper change.

Management of Specific Areas

Face

Plastic surgeons who do not routinely care for burn patients may be called on to manage both acute and reconstructive facial burns. Few areas of burn care can be more challenging than the management of facial burns. The aesthetic and functional outcomes are critical to the daily life of the patient and are intimately related to feelings of self-esteem.

Management of facial burns begins at the time of admission. Many patients with facial burns sustain inhalation injuries and are intubated. The endotracheal tube should be secured in such a way as to minimize pressure necrosis of the lip. Patients who are going to be intubated for a long period of time may benefit from the wiring of the endotracheal tube to the teeth or to a segment of an arch bar that can be wired to the upper teeth. This provides a reliable and sturdy method for tube fixation and will minimize pressure on the lip. This will also allow for facile and secure positioning of the tube in the operating room (Fig. 17.10). Similarly, if a feeding tube is placed, care must be taken to minimize alar or columellar pressure necrosis.

All patients with periorbital burns should undergo an intraocular exam with a Wood lamp. If this exam is positive, an ophthalmologic consult is required. In addition, if the patient has a lagophthalmos it is important to keep the eyes well moisturized with ophthalmic ointment to prevent exposure keratitis. Tarsorrhaphy is rarely necessary in the early burn period.

The practice of excising facial burns has long been debated in the literature. The traditional method of facial burn management was to perform daily wound care until the face either healed or the underlying eschar lifted, leaving a granulating wound bed that could accept a skin graft. It is now clear that better outcomes are achieved if nonhealing areas are excised and then subsequently skin grafted. As in other parts of the body, it is generally easy to determine the healing capacity of shallow burns and deep burns. The burns of indeterminate depth pose a greater challenge.

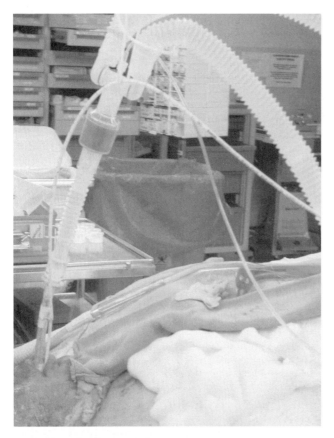

FIGURE 17.10. Securing of the endotracheal tube. The endotracheal tube can be secured to a segment of an arch bar and then suspended from the ceiling using a rope. This provides both stable fixation of the tube and complete access to the face for excision.

Over the past 25 years it has been our practice at the University of Washington to excise facial burns. Our protocol and results can be found in a recent publication (8). Patients who are admitted with facial burns undergo debridement of loose blisters and debris and then daily wound care. It is our practice to assess patients with facial burns at day 10, at which time it is usually clear which burns will heal within 3 weeks and which will not. Patients with burns that are thought unlikely to heal within 3 weeks are scheduled for excision and grafting. It is important to note that patients with full-thickness burns with clearly no healing potential should be operated on in the 7 to 10 days if the patient is stable and there are no other more urgent areas of excision.

Facial excision is typically carried out using Goulian knives. Traction sutures are frequently used on the upper and lower eyelids to aid in excision. More recently, the availability of the VersaJet water dissector has helped in excising areas with difficult contour, such as the eyelids and ears. Small areas of exposed cartilage of the ear should be excised and the skin closed primarily over the defect.

Sheet autograft should always be used for coverage of the face. The appearance of meshed grafts to the face is cosmetically unacceptable. The scalp is an excellent source of autograft, given the color match with the face. However, in the case of full-facial burns, scalp skin is usually inadequate and a different donor site is needed so there is uniformity in the coloring of the skin grafts. A face mask (such as a Jobst featureless face mask) should be placed in the operating room to help immobilize the skin grafts. Skin grafts should be inspected on the first postoperative day so any blebs or fluid collections that might impair graft take can be drained.

Neck

Excision and grafting of the neck can also be challenging. The key to management of the neck is to make every effort to minimize wound and graft contraction. Whenever possible, it is best to cover the neck with sheet grafts. The grafts should be placed with the neck in maximal hyperextension. For the first several days following graft placement, the neck should be immobilized in a splint. Once the grafts have taken, the patient should be started on aggressive range-of-motion exercises. Aggressive range-of-motion exercises are critical for patients who heal without grafting and for patients who undergo grafting. These exercises should continue for the several months it takes for the grafts to mature.

Hands

Hand burns occur from a variety of mechanisms. In the pediatric population, hand burns frequently occur as a result of contact with a fireplace or wood stove, or from grabbing a hot object. The palm has excellent healing capacity and these pediatric palm burns rarely require grafting. However, it is critical to emphasize to the patient's parents the importance of range-of-motion exercises. Stretching should be performed on a routine basis—either during diaper changes or feeding times, to minimize contractures of the palm and digits. In the case of deeper palm burns, nocturnal extension splints may be necessary. It is also important to emphasize to parents to let the child use his or her hands as soon following injury as possible and that bulky dressings that inhibit mobility should be minimized.

Similarly, adult hand burns often heal without the need for skin grafting. Patients should be encouraged to begin range-of-motion exercises as soon following burn injury as possible. Range-of-motion exercises reduce extremity edema and optimize the return of function once the skin wounds have healed. Static splinting is not recommended, unless the patient is intubated and unable to participate in therapy. If splinting is necessary, the wrist should be placed in mild extension, the metacarpophalangeal joints in 70 degrees to 90 degrees of flexion, and the interphalangeal joints in extension. Even in those instances, however, therapists should regularly range the extremities.

If it is clear that a burn wound will not heal within 3 weeks, the best treatment is excision and grafting. With few exceptions, burns of the hand should be grafted with sheet grafts. Hand excision, particularly of the web spaces and digits, can be challenging. Great care should be taken to not expose tendons. In addition, excision should occur under tourniquet control. If a burn is so deep that adequate excision would surely expose tendons, then flap coverage should be considered.

Following excision and grafting of the hand, splint immobilization should occur for at least 5 days afterwards. The wrist should be positioned in slight extension, the metacarpophalangeal joints should be placed in flexion, the interphalangeal joints in extension, and the thumb in abduction. Graft take should be assessed at postoperative day 5 and the decision for initiation of range-of-motion exercises should be made. Once graft healing is complete, compression gloves, which will minimize hand edema and possibly scar hypertrophy, should be worn.

Perineum

Scald burns remain the most common burns of the perineum, and they typically result from the spilling of hot beverages that are held between the legs while driving. These scald burns tend to heal within 1 to 2 weeks, and wound care and pain control are the mainstays of treatment. Full-thickness burns can occur as part of a larger flame burn, and the healing potential of these injuries can be more varied. It is not necessary to place a Foley catheter on all patients who sustain perineal burns. In fact, all patients should be given the option to void spontaneously; a catheter should be placed only if they have difficulty voiding. An external genital burn is unlikely to lead to urethral (internal) stenosis. Deep burns to the penis and scrotum should be given ample time to heal. In fact, the scrotum is rarely grafted because it can usually heal by contraction and not leave a noticeable scar. Patients who sustain full-thickness, charred burns of the genitals and who cannot have a Foley catheter placed, should be evaluated by urologists for placement of a suprapubic tube.

Lower Extremities

Of all the burns treated in the outpatient setting, patients with feet and leg burns tend to have the most difficulty. Edema can delay wound healing and increase patient discomfort. The key to treating lower-extremity burn wounds is to encourage the patient to ambulate, with the appropriate support of an Ace bandage or Tubigrip (ConvaTec, Princeton, NJ). Ambulating minimizes the pooling of blood in the distal aspect of the extremity and thereby decreases edema. In addition, the sooner the patient is able to ambulate, the sooner the patient will be able to resume a normal level of activities once the wounds heal. While not ambulating, leg elevation can help to minimize edema.

If leg or foot burns require excision and grafting, the postoperative physical therapy plan should be considered. Small burns of the leg and foot can be grafted and dressed with greasy gauze and then covered with an Unna boot dressing. The Unna boot dressing provides support and immobilization of the graft and allows for early mobilization. This is an excellent dressing for both adults and children. Patients with insensate feet are poor candidates for Unna boot dressings. Patients who require grafting both above and below the knee should be fitted with knee immobilizers postoperatively to maintain knee extension.

Outpatient Burn Management

Most burn patients will have some aspect of their care in the outpatient burn clinic. Again, a multidisciplinary approach in this setting is crucial to the success of outpatient burn-wound management. Experienced nurses, physical and occupational therapists, and psychologists all play an important role in patient management, even in the outpatient setting. Issues of range of motion, optimization of function, and the psychosocial aspects of reintegration into society all must be dealt with in the outpatient clinic. Prior to discharging a patient from the hospital to the clinic, a well-thought-out discharge plan should be established in conjunction with the clinic staff.

Some patients receive all of their care as an outpatient. Patients evaluated for the first time in the clinic need to have their wounds cleansed and debrided, after which a decision can be made regarding appropriate wound management. Patient education should focus on the wound-healing process, the risks of abnormal pigmentation, the risks of hypertrophic scarring, and the importance of range of motion. Burned extremities should not be immobilized. Patients should be encouraged to range injured extremities and to walk without the use of crutches and wheelchairs as soon as possible. Patients with burns to the plantar surface of their feet should similarly be encouraged to ambulate.

Issues related to returning to work also need to be addressed. Patients should be given a reasonable estimate of a return-to-work date so both the patient and the employer can prepare appropriately. When returning a patient to work, modified or part-time work may be required in order to allow the patient to regain the strength and endurance required to do their job.

Several other issues are particularly relevant to outpatient care. Newly healed burn wounds and donor sites are highly susceptible to blistering and to breakdown. The new epithelium lacks the connections to the underlying wound bed that prevent shearing. It can take as long a year for these critical basement membrane structures to be reconstituted. Blisters should be decompressed with a sterile pin, the epithelial layer can be left in place, and the area covered with a plastic bandage. Patients should be instructed to soak the plastic bandage prior to removal to protect against the adhesive causing further injury.

Protection from the sun is another important component of caring for the healed burn. Whether a wound has been skin grafted or healed by re-epithelialization, protection from the sun is critical. Newly healed wounds remain highly sensitive to the sun. In addition, sun exposure can increase the risk of hyperpigmentation of both grafted and nongrafted burn wounds. Patients should be encouraged to use sunscreen with a sun protection factor (SPF) of at least 15 as well as wear hats and protective clothing when outdoors. It is important to reinforce that sun-protective measures should be taken even on cloudy days.

Patients also frequently complain of pruritus of newly healed wounds. Moisturizer use is essential because newly grafted or healed wounds lack the glands that usually keep skin moist. Dry and scaly wounds are often itchy and feel tight, which can restrict range of motion. Frequent moisturizer application minimizes these symptoms. No special moisturizer is needed and patients often need to try several types to see which works best. We discourage the use of perfume- or alcohol-containing moisturizers because these can irritate newly healed wounds. Even with liberal use of moisturizers, pruritus remains a problem for many patients. The use of systemic antihistamines may be helpful in these cases.

The development of inclusion cysts is another problem commonly encountered in the clinic. Inclusion cysts can occur when skin grafts are placed over an excised wound bed that still contains a layer of dermis containing adnexal structures. Secretions from adnexal structures can accumulate beneath the graft to form inclusion cysts, which should be treated by unroofing the cyst with a sterile needle.

Chemical Injuries

Traditionally, chemical injuries are classified as either acid burns or alkali (base) burns. The severity of chemical injuries depends on the composition of the agent, concentration of the agent, and duration of contact with the agent. In general, alkaline burns cause more severe injury than acid burns because alkaline agents cause a liquefaction necrosis that allows the alkali to penetrate deeper, extending the area of injury. Chemical injuries are also classified according to their mechanism of tissue destruction: reduction, oxidation, corrosive agents, protoplasmic poisons, vesicants, and desiccants.

The first step in managing a chemical injury is removal of the inciting agent. Clothes, including shoes, that have been contaminated should be removed. Areas of affected skin should be copiously irrigated with water. Adequate irrigation can be verified by checking the skin pH. Burns from chemical powders are the one exception to the rule of water irrigation because the water can activate the chemical. The powder should first be dusted off, and then irrigation can take place. Neutralization of the inciting agent should never be attempted because this will produce an exothermic reaction that will superimpose a thermal injury on top of the chemical injury. Occasionally, the burned individual may not know specifically with which agent they were working and therefore it may be necessary to contact a plant manger or the manufacturer of the suspected inciting agent.

If ocular injury has occurred, the eyes should also be copiously irrigated. Eye wash stations should be located in most workplaces where chemicals are used. It is important that the eye be forced open to allow for adequate irrigation. An ophthalmologist should be consulted to assist in the management of these patients.

Certain chemical agents have specific treatments. Hydrofluoric acid requires specific mention. Hydrofluoric acid is commonly used in the glass and silicon chip industries, as well as in a number of industrial cleaning solutions. Hydrofluoric acid readily penetrates the skin and continues to injure tissue until it comes into a calcium source, likely bone. Given the ability of the fluoride ion to chelate calcium, patients with even small hydrofluoric acid burns are at risk for the development of hypocalcemia, which can be severe enough to have cardiac effects. In fact, hydrofluoric acid burns in excess of 10% can be fatal. The use of calcium is the most effective treatment agent. Calcium gluconate gel can be applied topically if the patient is treated rapidly enough; that is, before the hydrofluoric acid has penetrated the skin. Although direct injection of calcium gluconate into the burned area has long been advocated, this may not effectively neutralize the hydrofluoric acid and may cause skin necrosis. If copious irrigation and topical treatment with calcium has been ineffective, the patient should be treated with an intra-arterial infusion of calcium gluconate. Diminished pain is the hallmark of effective treatment. Patients with extensive hydrofluoric acid burns, and certainly patients with intra-arterial infusions, require close monitoring and should have frequent serum calcium checks.

Ingestion of chemically toxic agents can occur by children or by adults as part of a suicide gesture or attempt. Again, the principle of lavage to dilute the inciting agent is practiced. These injuries are typically managed by, or in conjunction with, gastroenterologists, pulmonary specialists, or general surgeons. Laryngoscopy and endoscopy should be performed to help define the extent of injury. Enteral feeding beyond the zone of injury is often necessary.

Electrical Injuries

Electrical injuries are potentially devastating events that result in damage to the skin as well as other tissues, including nerve, tendons, and bone. Electrical burns can take several forms, including injury from the electrical current itself, flash burns, flame burns, contact burns, or a combination thereof.

Traditionally, electrical injuries have been divided into low voltage (less than 1,000 volts) and high voltage (greater than 1,000 volts). The considerations and management issues between the two are often different. Following electrical injury the ATLS protocol is followed, and the patient's airway, breathing, and circulation are assessed. Once stabilized, the circumstances surrounding the injury, the voltage of the injuring current, the presence/absence of loss of consciousness and the existence of other associated injuries (e.g., fall from a cherry picker basket) are ascertained. Most importantly, it is determined if a cardiac or respiratory arrest occurred.

Evaluation in the emergency room includes a thorough physical examination, during which the percent TBSA is calculated (if there was a flame burn) and the neurovascular status of injured extremities is determined. In addition, all patients who sustain electrical injuries should have an electrocardiogram (ECG) in the emergency room.

Patients with a low-voltage injury who had no loss of consciousness and who have no dysrhythmia can be discharged home. The notable exception is a child who has an oral burn

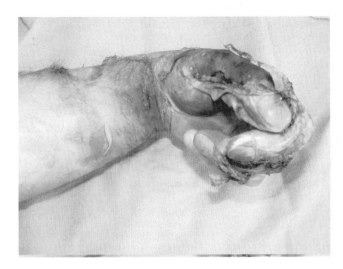

FIGURE 17.11. Electrical burn. This patient sustained a high-voltage electrical injury and presented with a contracted wrist and tight forearm compartment. He was taken emergently to the operating room for forearm fasciotomy and carpal tunnel release.

from biting an electrical cord. These patients require admission and monitoring for labial artery bleeding.

Management of patients with high-voltage injuries is dictated by the extent of injury, the presence of cutaneous burns, and the presence of myoglobinuria. There is no formula for fluid management of electrical burn patients per se. If there are extensive cutaneous burns, then the Parkland formula (Table 17.4) is applied and fluid administration is titrated to achieve a urine output of 30 mL/hr. If myoglobinuria is present, intravenous fluids should be titrated to a goal urine output of 100 mL/hr until the urine clears. Serial urine myoglobin checks are usually unnecessary, because treatment is initiated based on the presence of tea-colored urine and should be continued until the urine clears. If myoglobinuria persists despite fluid resuscitation, mannitol can be administered. Alkalinization of urine has also been advocated following electrical injury in order to prevent precipitation of myoglobin in the kidney tubules.

Patients who sustain high-voltage injuries are placed on a cardiac monitor for the first 24 hours following admission. This has been the traditional practice regardless of whether or not a dysrhythmia is present at the time of admission. There is no data substantiating routine monitoring of high-voltage injuries, and this is a practice that may change over time.

Early surgical management of electrical injuries should focus on the need for fasciotomy or compartment release. Peripheral neurovascular exams should be performed to monitor for signs of compartment syndrome. Some patients will present with a contracted upper limb and tight forearm compartments, and these patients should undergo immediate fasciotomy and carpal tunnel release (Fig. 17.11). Otherwise, progressive sensory and motor loss, as well as increased compartment pressures, should be indicators of the need for fasciotomy. Many surgeons believe that all patients should undergo immediate surgery for nerve decompression and debridement of necrotic tissue. On the one hand, carpal tunnel release and fasciotomy are relatively facile operations to perform and, if the patient derives even a small amount of benefit, the procedures may be worthwhile. On the other hand, the risks of the procedures, particularly if not necessary, can be significant. Exposure of the median nerve and forearm musculature increases the risk of tissue desiccation and necrosis.

It is often difficult to determine preoperatively who will benefit from the decompression procedures. Decreased sensation and motor function may represent a neurapraxia from direct current injury to the nerve. Mann et al. explored the issue of routine immediate decompression of high-voltage injuries (10). They concluded that a select group of patients require immediate decompression of the arm or hand or both to prevent additive injury from pressure. Clinical indications for this group of patients include progressive motor and sensory exam, severe pain, loss of arterial Doppler signal, and inadequate resuscitatation because of suspected ongoing myonecrosis. Patients with a fixed neurologic deficit typically do not benefit from decompression.

The ideal timing for tissue debridement has similarly been controversial. The ideal time to determine the presence of myonecrosis is typically 3 to 5 days following injury. Therefore, early debridement might not be sufficient because irreversibly injured tissue may not have demarcated. At 3 to 5 days, all unhealthy tissue can be debrided and definitive wound closure can be achieved. In cases of extensive limb injury, free tissue transfer might be necessary to provide wound coverage or to preserve limb length for optimal prosthesis fitting. In these cases, definitive wound closure can be performed at a second operation following wound debridement to allow for appropriate planning and patient counseling.

There are several long-term sequelae of electrical burns of which the patient and physician should be aware. Neurologic deficits, including peripheral and central nervous system disorders, can develop weeks to months following electrical injury. Consequently, all patients who sustain high-voltage electrical injuries should undergo a thorough neurologic evaluation at the time of admission and prior to hospital discharge. Cataracts can also occur following electrical injury. The exact mechanism is unknown, but all patients should undergo a baseline ophthalmologic examination following high-voltage electrical injury. A number of complications can also arise in the injured extremity, including heterotopic ossification, neuromas, phantom limb pain, and stump breakdown if the patient has undergone amputation.

Cold Injury

Exposure to extremes of cold (and wet) conditions can lead to cellular injury and death. Cell death and tissue necrosis occur from the formation of ice crystals within the cells and extracellular space, as well as from microvascular thrombosis. Cellular injury from ice crystal formation occurs during the period of cold exposure, whereas microvascular thrombosis is thought to occur during reperfusion when the affected limb is rewarmed. Similar to burn injury, frostbite injury is classified according to the depth of injury. Mild frostbite, also known as frost nip, is similar to a superficial burn injury, with tissue erythema, pain, and edema. Second-degree frostbite is marked by blistering and partial-thickness skin injury. Third-degree frostbite occurs when there is full-thickness necrosis of the skin, and fourth-degree frostbite occurs when there is full-thickness skin necrosis as well as necrosis of the underlying muscle and/or bone. Again, it is important to note that determination of the full depth of tissue injury is not possible until several weeks following injury.

The first step in management of frostbite is removal of all wet clothes, gloves, socks, and shoes. Patients should then be wrapped in warm blankets. Frostbite can also be associated with hypothermia. In these cases, care must be taken to rewarm the entire body. In cases of extreme hypothermia (less than 32°C) warming can be achieved with use of warm intravenous fluids, bladder irrigation with warm solutions, placement of peritoneal catheters and chest tubes through which warm fluids can be administered, and even, if available, cardiopulmonary bypass. Frostbitten extremities should be rapidly rewarmed in water that is 104°F (40°C). Typically, rewarming can be completed in 20 to 30 minutes. Adjunctive use of anti-inflammatory medications and anticoagulants has also been described.

Patience is required in determining which areas require debridement. There is an old adage that states "frostbite in January, amputate in July (11)." While this might be hyperbole, the concept of allowing tissue to fully demarcate is essential because it is difficult to determine which tissue may survive in the immediate postinjury period. Early debridement and amputation are necessary if soft-tissue infection occurs during the waiting period.

Skin Replacement

Early excision and skin grafting has become the standard of care for surgical management of the burn wound. However, in cases of extensive burn wounds the surface area burned may exceed the available donor sites. In these cases, burn wounds are excised and covered with biologic dressings until complete coverage with autografts can occur. These cases of extensive burn injury have demonstrated the need for a replacement for human skin. Efforts over the past two decades have focused on the development of a temporary and, ideally, permanent replacement to native human skin.

The relatively simple biology of the epidermis and the ability to culture and expand keratinocytes in the laboratory into a stratified layer of cells has allowed for the development of pure epidermal replacement. However, epidermal replacement alone ignores the fundamental importance of the dermis in providing the skin with its integrity and durability. The retarded formation of basement membrane structures using cultured epidermal autografts (CEAs) alone results in high rates of culture loss and high rates of infection. Although early reports in the literature documented successful coverage of more than 90% TBSA burns with cultures alone, today CEAs are rarely used alone.

Dermal replacement provides a more formidable challenge. The complex acellular dermal structure and the inability of dermis to regenerate have prevented the facile development of cultured dermis. A number of products have been developed over the past two decades that can serve as a dermal replacement in combination with a thin split-thickness autograft.

One of the pioneering attempts at dermal replacement was Integra (Integra Life Sciences, Plainsboro, NJ), initially developed by Burke and Yannas in the late 1970s. Integra is available today as a bilayer construct. The bottom layer consists of bovine collagen and chrondroitin-6-sulfate and the outer layer is a silastic membrane that serves as a temporary epidermal replacement. Integra is placed on a newly excised wound bed and fixed into place. The silastic layer remains in place until the dermal component vascularizes, which is typically 2 to 3 weeks. The patient is then taken back to the operating room, the silastic is removed, and a thin (0.006-in.) autograft is placed on top. The Integra neodermis serves as a scaffold for the ingrowth of tissue from the patient's wound bed (Fig. 17.12).

Integra has been used in the management of extensive burns, as well as for pediatric burns, with a great deal of success. In addition, there are several recent reports of Integra used in grafting of the face, small areas of exposed bone and tendon, as well as in secondary reconstruction. Integra can be placed on a freshly excised wound bed. It must be emphasized, however, that for Integra to vascularize completely, it must be applied to a viable, noninfected wound bed. In addition, meticulous surgical technique and appropriate postoperative care are critical for a successful outcome.

Another product marketed for dermal replacement is AlloDerm (LifeCell, Woodlands, TX), which is an acellular dermal matrix produced from human cadaveric skin. The cadaveric

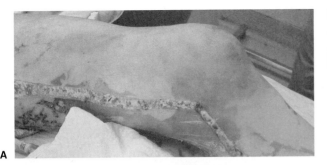

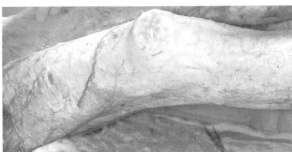

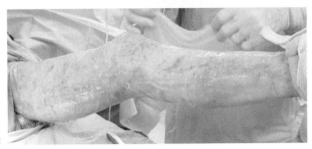

FIGURE 17.12. The use of Integra for burn wound coverage. **A:** Full-thickness burn wound prior to excision. **B:** Fascial excision of burn wound leaving a viable, well-vascularized wound bed. **C:** Application of Integra with silastic left in place.

skin is first stored in normal saline for 15 hours to remove the epidermal component. The cadaveric dermis is then incubated in sodium dodecyl sulfate to extract any remaining cellular components. The decellularized substrate is freeze dried and reconstituted by soaking it in crystalloid solution before use. AlloDerm can be used for immediate wound coverage in combination with a thin split-thickness autograft. Data from multicenter trials indicate that AlloDerm works best with thin (0.006 to 0.008-in.) autografts: The thicker the autograft, the lower the take rates (12). AlloDerm has also been used for abdominal wall reconstruction and for soft-tissue augmentation in the face.

A product known as TransCyte (Smith and Nephew, London, England)—formerly Dermagraft-TC—is approved by the U.S. Food and Drug Administration (FDA) as a temporary (as opposed to permanent) cover for full-thickness wounds after excision. TransCyte is produced by seeding neonatal fibroblasts isolated from foreskin onto Biobrane, a synthetic dressing consisting of silastic attached to a nylon mesh, which is coated with porcine peptides prepared from type I collagen. The silastic layer of Biobrane serves as a temporary impermeable barrier, whereas the fibroblast-impregnated nylon mesh serves as a dermal component. TransCyte is placed on an excised wound bed; when clinically indicated, it is removed and replaced with split-thickness autograft. TransCyte is statistically equivalent to cryopreserved human allograft skin with respect to adherence to the wound bed, fluid accumulation, and ease of removal. It has also been used as a dressing for partial-thickness wounds, including donor sites.

Dermagraft (Smith and Nephew, London, England), in contrast, is employed as a permanent dermal replacement. Dermagraft consists of human neonatal fibroblasts seeded onto an absorbable polyglactin mesh scaffold, which is intended to mimic the native dermal architecture. It is approved by the FDA for treatment of venous stasis ulcers, but it was developed for coverage of excised burn wounds in conjunction with a split-thickness autograft.

Although a permanent off-the-shelf skin replacement has yet to be developed, the available products have already significantly influenced the management of burn wounds. In addition, the shortcomings of each product has improved our understanding of skin biology and physiology, and confirmed the importance of both the epidermis and the dermis in the structure and function of skin.

LATE EFFECTS OF BURN INJURY

Hypertrophic Scarring

Hypertrophic scarring is one of the most distressing outcomes of burn injury. Hypertrophic scars can be both unsightly as well as painful and pruritic. Hypertrophic scarring can occur in grafted wounds and unexcised wounds that take longer than 2 to 3 weeks to heal (Chapter 18). Patients with pigmented skin tend to be at a higher risk for the development of hypertrophic scarring. The biologic and molecular basis of hypertrophic scarring is not well understood, limiting our ability to prevent hypertrophic scarring. However, several strategies exist to prevent or minimize hypertrophic scarring. Pressure garments are commonly used over areas that have been grafted or have taken longer than 3 weeks to heal. No study has clearly demonstrated that garments prevent hypertrophic scarring, but the elastic support of the garments can help symptoms of throbbing and pruritus. Silicone has similarly been advocated for the treatment and prevention of hypertrophic scarring. There are several theories as to how and why silicone works, but there is no well-accepted explanation. Steroid injection has also been used to minimize the symptoms associated with hypertrophic scarring.

Marjolin's Ulcer

Marjolin's ulcer is one of the most dreaded long-term complications of a burn wound. Marjolin's ulcer is the malignant degeneration of a chronic wound or a wound that took months or years to heal. The tumor can occur decades following injury. Typically, these tumors are aggressive and occur in areas that were not skin grafted. The presence of an ulceration in a previously healed burn wound should raise the suspicion of malignancy and warrants biopsy and appropriate evaluation.

Heterotopic Ossification

Heterotopic ossification results from the deposition of calcium in the soft tissue around joints. These calcium deposits block normal joint functioning. Heterotopic ossification most commonly affects the elbow and shoulder joints and occurs 1 to 3 months following injury. Patients who develop heterotopic ossification have increased pain and decreased range of motion of the affected joint. Radiographs demonstrate calcium in the soft tissue. Although several medical treatments have been described, few have proven effective. Surgical management involves direct excision of the heterotopic bone and is usually best carried out once complete wound coverage has been achieved.

Rehabilitation

Patients who sustain major burn injuries and require a prolonged hospital course often require a period of inpatient rehabilitation following discharge from the hospital. In reality, rehabilitation begins in the early postburn period. Careful attention to appropriate splinting, range-of-motion exercises, and even aspects of surgical management all impact long-term rehabilitation potential.

Many burn centers have their own rehabilitation units, which facilitate a smooth transition from acute care to rehabilitation. Clearly, a structured rehabilitation plan is necessary, incorporating physical and occupational therapy needs, nutritional needs, as well as psychosocial issues, which will be crucial to reintegration into society. Many patients will have ongoing wound care requirements and still be on narcotics, from which they will need to be weaned during the rehabilitation stay.

Patients who live far from the burn center may prefer to be at a rehabilitation facility closer to home. Careful planning is required to ensure that patient needs in all aspects of rehabilitation can be met before selecting a facility. Many therapists and rehabilitation physicians have little experience in the specialized needs of the burn patient, particularly in issues related to wound care and scar management.

FUTURE HORIZONS

The management of burn injuries has evolved over the past several decades. Burn resuscitation fluids, topical antimicrobial agents, and early burn wound excision have all significantly increased survival following burn injury. However, there is still room for improvement in several areas of burn care. With the increased specialization of critical care medicine, many aspects of acute burn care are evolving. The use of plasmapheresis in patients who are failing resuscitation is being used at several centers. There are also reports of the benefits of high-frequency oscillatory ventilators for patients with severe inhalation injury and ARDS. In addition, the potential protective effects of high doses of vitamins C and E following major burn injury are also being investigated.

Advances in burn wound management are also on the horizon. There has been a proliferation of silver-impregnated dressings that purportedly provide enhanced antimicrobial protection. The skin replacement technologies introduced over the past two decades have positively impacted burn care, yet much additional research will be needed in order to achieve an off-the-shelf skin replacement. Virtual reality is being used to minimize pain during wound care and to increase patient compliance with range-of-motion exercises.

CONCLUSION

Despite all the advances in burn care over the past century and the exciting prospects on the horizon, the core of burn care remains the burn team. As each aspect of burn care becomes increasingly complex, with increasingly specialized fields of knowledge, the importance of a team of experts becomes even more critical to successful care. Plastic surgeons must always be an integral member of that team.

References

1. Arturson G. microvascular permeability to macromolecules in thermal injury. *Acta Physiol Scand Suppl.* 1979;463:111.
2. Demling RH, Mazess RB, Witt TM, et al. The study of burn wound edema using dichromatic absorptiometry. *J Trauma.* 1978;18:124.
3. Gunn ML, Hansbrough JF, Davis JW, et al. Prospective randomized trial of hypertonic sodium lactate versus lactated Ringer's solution for burn shock resuscitation. *J Trauma.* 1989;29:1261.
4. Saffle J, Hildreth M. Metabolic support of the burn patient. In: Herndon D, ed. *Total Burn Care*, 2nd ed. New York: WB Saunders, 2002;271.
5. Barlow Y. T lymphocytes and immunosuppression in the burned patient: a review. *J Burn Care Rehabil.* 1990;20:487.
6. Janzekovic Z. A new concept in the early excision and immediate grafting of burns. *J Trauma.* 1970;10:1103.
7. Heimbach D. Early burn excision and grafting. *Surg Clin North Am.* 1987;67:93.
8. Sutcliffe J, Duin N. *A History of Medicine.* New York: Barnes and Noble Books, 1992.
9. Cole JK, Engrav LH, Heimbach DM, et al. Early excision and grafting of face and neck burns in patients over 20 years. *Plast Reconstr Surg.* 2002;109:1266.
10. Mann R, Gibran N, Engrav L, et al. Is immediate decompression of high voltage electrical injuries to the upper extremity always necessary? *J Trauma.* 1996;40:584.
11. Erikson U, Ponten B. The possible value of arteriography supplemented by a vasodilator agent in the early assessment of tissue viability in frostbite. *Injury.* 1974;6:150.
12. Lattari B, Jones LM, Varcelotti JR, et al. The use of a permanent dermal allograft in full thickness burns of the hand and foot: a report of three cases. *J Burn Care Rehabil.* 1997;18:147.

Suggested Readings

Luce EA. Burn care and management. *Clin Plast Surg.* 2000;27:1.
Fraulin FO, Illmayer SJ, Tredget EE. Assessment of cosmetic and functional results of conservative versus surgical management of facial burns. *J Burn Care Rehabil.* 1996;17:19.
Heimbach DM, Engrav LH. *Surgical Management of the Burn Wound.* New York: Raven Press, 1984.
Herndon D. *Total Burn Care.* New York: W.B. Saunders, 2002.
Hunt JL, Purdue GF, Spicer T, et al. Face burn reconstruction—does early excision and autografting improve aesthetic appearance? *Burns Incl Therm Inj.* 1987;13:39.
Jonsson CE, Dalsgaard CJ. Early excision and skin grafting of selected burns of the face and neck. *Plast Reconstr Surg.* 1988;88:83.
Practice guidelines for burn care. *J Burn Care Rehabil.* 2001.
Van den Berghe G, Wouters P, Weekers F, et al. Intensive insulin therapy in critically ill patients. *N Engl J Med.* 2001;345:1359.

CHAPTER 18 ■ PRINCIPLES OF BURN RECONSTRUCTION

MATTHIAS B. DONELAN

Reconstructive surgery following burn injury involves almost all aspects of plastic surgery. The patient population includes children and adults. All areas of the body can be involved. Deep structures can be injured either acutely or secondarily. Satisfactory outcomes require correction of both functional and aesthetic deformities. Yet, at the same time, the reconstruction of burn deformities requires a unique perspective and an emphasis on certain fundamentals and techniques that make it a specialized area of reconstructive surgery. The surgeon must thoroughly understand the processes of wound healing and contraction. The effect of time on the maturation of scars is of pivotal importance and requires patience and judgment on the part of the surgeon and patient. Correct timing of surgery is essential. Multiple operations are the rule and frequently take place over a period of many years. Donor sites are frequently compromised. Successful surgical outcomes require a well-functioning support system, including nurses, therapists, psychosocial practitioners, and, hopefully, a supportive family. All of these factors affect the outcome of surgery.

Burn injuries obviously vary greatly in severity and extent. Yet virtually all postburn deformities have similar components that must be addressed for reconstructive surgery to be successful. This chapter provides a strategic approach to burn reconstruction based on surgical principles particularly relevant to this field that will help in the analysis, management, and surgical treatment of this large and challenging group of patients.

GENERAL CONCEPTS

Over the past 50 years, primary excision and grafting of deep second-degree and full-thickness burns has become the standard of care in the United States and in most developed countries (1,2). Early excision and grafting has decreased the mortality and morbidity of acute burn injuries (3). The duration of acute hospitalization has been greatly reduced. Early excision and grafting has also decreased the frequency and severity of contractures and hypertrophic scarring; occasionally, however, one still encounters patients who were treated "expectantly" with late grafting and disastrous results (Fig. 18.1).

All burns of the second or third degree result in open wounds. Open wounds heal by contraction and epithelialization. Contraction may be decreased by early excision and grafting, but it is always present to some degree. Contraction leads to tension, and tension is one of the principal causes of hypertrophic scarring and unfavorable scarring in general. Understanding the role of tension in the evolution of postburn deformities is essential for their successful treatment.

Burn reconstruction is fundamentally about the release of contractures and the correction of contour abnormalities. It should not be focused on the excision of burn scars. Scar excision is an oxymoron. A scar can only be traded for another scar of a different variety. When the fundamental problem is that of inadequate skin and soft tissue, further excision of "scars" can easily add to the clinical problem. Well-healed burn scars, if given enough time to mature, are often an excellent example of nature's camouflage. The subtle and gradual transition from unburned skin to scar helps the deformity to blend into its surroundings. A burn scar that is conspicuous at 1 year because of hypertrophy, contracture, and erythema, can become inconspicuous with further maturation. Healed second-degree burn deformities under tension with resulting hypertrophy are unsightly. With time and relief of tension they will greatly improve. Premature early excision of such scars with primary closure frequently results in a wide iatrogenic scar, which then becomes a more obvious permanent deformity. Lacking camouflage, the surgical scar can be more noticeable than the burn scar and increased tension from the excision can create contour deformities. Excision and primary closure of burn scars should be limited and reserved for small scars in conspicuous locations that will allow a favorably oriented closure.

Although counterintuitive, it is helpful to learn to love burn scars. After all, without scarring, healing cannot occur, so scars are our friends. For successful burn reconstruction, one must learn to appreciate them and understand their behavior. Scars under tension are angry and respond with erythema, hypertrophy, pruritus, pain, and tenderness. Relaxed scars are happy scars. They respond by flattening, softening, and becoming pale and asymptomatic. Directing reconstructive surgery towards relieving tension is practical, achievable, and can result in great improvement. Ill-advised attempts to excise scars can be simplistic and are potentially harmful. Burn reconstruction must always strive to make the patient clearly better, not just different from normal in a different way.

Contracture releases can be carried out with local tissue rearrangement such as Z-plasties or transposition flaps or they can be carried out by releases and skin grafting of the resulting defects. Releases can be performed by either incising scars or excising scars. Release by incision takes advantage of the healing that has already occurred and because of the relief of tension, it will usually improve the appearance and quality of the tissue that is retained. Mature scars and grafts are a known commodity and will not contract significantly after release. New grafts are less predictable. Incisional releases also obviously create a smaller defect and, therefore, conserve donor sites. When the contracted tissue is of unacceptable quality, or too irregular, excision of scars should be done to give the best result (Fig. 18.2). In most cases, however, it is better to work with the grafts and scars that are already present than to excise them. Grafts can either be split-thickness skin grafts or full-thickness skin grafts. Releases can also be carried out and the resulting defects closed with distant flaps transferred with either traditional or microsurgical techniques. The choice of the appropriate intervention and the timing of reconstructive surgery are the essential ingredients that result in either successful or unsuccessful burn reconstruction.

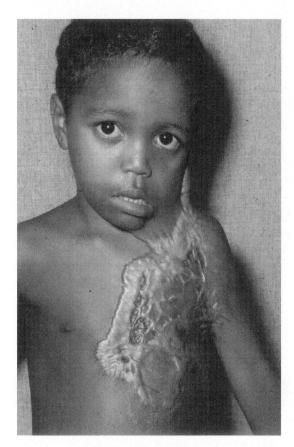

FIGURE 18.1. Late grafting. A 4-year-old boy from Central America treated with months of dressings and late grafting, resulting in severe contractures.

TIMING OF RECONSTRUCTIVE SURGERY

Patients with postburn deformities typically present to the plastic surgeon in one of three ways. The ideal circumstance is when the plastic surgeon is involved in the patient's care from the time of the acute injury. The involvement may either be as the treating physician or as a consultant and occasional participant in the patient's acute care. It is a truism that the reconstruction of burn deformities begins with the acute care. Plastic surgical consultation can help prevent secondary deformities by initiating appropriate acute surgical intervention. It can also enhance outcomes by helping in aesthetic decisions such as skin graft donor-site conservation. The second group of patients are those who only recently received their acute burn care at another facility and then come to the plastic surgeon for another opinion. The third group of patients are those who sustained their acute burn injury in the past and now present with mature scars and grafts and established burn deformities.

The timing of burn reconstruction falls into three distinct phases: acute, intermediate, and late. As a general rule, burn reconstruction is best delayed until all wounds are closed, inflammation has subsided, and scars and grafts are mature and soft. Acute reconstructive intervention is required during the early months following burn injury when urgent procedures are necessary to facilitate patient care, to close complex wounds such as open joints, or to prevent acute contractures from causing irreversible secondary damage. Examples of indications for acute surgical intervention are eyelid contractures with exposure keratitis, cervical contractures causing airway issues, and

"fourth-degree burns," such as in electrical injuries, where acute flap coverage is required.

The intermediate phase of burn reconstruction is best described as scar manipulation designed to favorably influence the healing process. After a patient's wounds have closed, physical and occupational therapy must continue to correct or prevent contractures, as well as enhance scar maturation with the use of pressure garments, silicone gels, and massage. The efficacy of such treatments has been demonstrated over many years (4,5). Enthusiastic support of these ancillary measures by the plastic surgeon and the entire burn team can be very helpful in maximizing patient compliance. The length of time required to reach the end point of burn scar maturation is considerably longer than is generally appreciated. Scars that are thick, raised, and erythematous at 1 year or longer, will improve dramatically if given significantly more time, often several years. When tension is present, scars never heal well. Judicious surgical intervention to relieve tension during this period can positively influence scar maturation. A longitudinal scar across the antecubital space subjected to constant tension and relaxation will remain contracted and hypertrophic despite pressure, silicone, massage, and splinting, and may result in ulceration or "spontaneous release." Relieving tension by either carrying out Z-plasties within the scarred tissue or performing a release and graft can help the entire scar to improve after the tension has been eliminated. Hypertrophic scars are common in healed second-degree burns under tension. When the tension is relieved, the subsequent improvement in appearance and elasticity is often remarkable.

Steroids are effective in diminishing and softening hypertrophic scars. They must be used carefully because of potential problems with atrophy of the scar and the underlying subcutaneous tissue. Topical steroids are helpful. Steroid injections are powerful. Their use should be limited to situations where time, pressure, silicone therapy, and massage are ineffective and surgery is not an option, for example, isolated hypertrophy without tension such as on the face or shoulders. A solution of triamcinolone (10 mg/mL mixed half and half with 1% Xylocaine with epinephrine) administered by intralesional injection with a glass tuberculin (TB) syringe, never more frequently than once a month, is efficacious in decreasing hypertrophy and preventing undesirable side effects.

Intermediate-phase scar manipulation is of particular benefit in the management of facial burn deformities. This is an area where treatment is evolving and there is considerable potential for improvement using multiple modalities. Computer-generated clear face masks with silicone lining are expensive but efficacious and well tolerated by patients. Relief of tension on facial scars by eliminating extrinsic contractures from the neck, as well as from the inconspicuous periphery of the face by release and grafting or Z-plasties, can be exceedingly beneficial to the healing of facial burns. The pulsed dye laser is effective in decreasing facial erythema when used in this intermediate phase and seems to result in more favorable long-term scar maturation. Z-plasties within the hypertrophic scar to decrease tension and more favorably align scars can achieve dramatic results over time (Fig. 18.3).

Late-phase reconstructive surgery includes all postburn deformities that are essentially stable and consist of mature scars and grafts. It is not uncommon in this group of patients for hypertrophic scars to present with areas of open ulceration. This is almost always caused by chronic tension. The resulting ischemia in the scar causes unstable epidermal coverage. Operations directed at relief of the tension will usually cure the chronic open wounds.

The transition from acute burn injury to the late phase of reconstructive surgery can be prolonged and is unique for each patient. The experience, judgment, and expertise of the plastic surgeon are extremely important during this period. It is

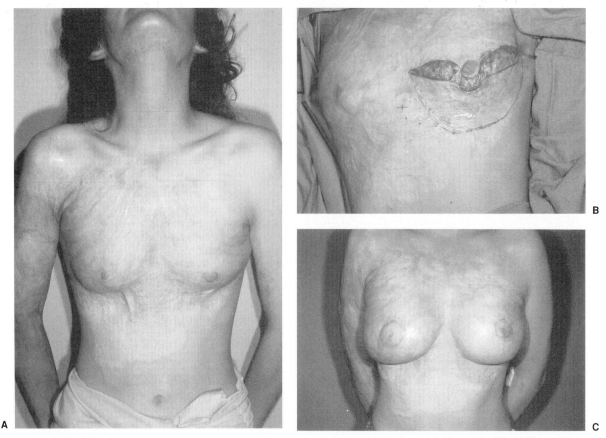

FIGURE 18.2. Excisional release. **A:** A 15-year-old girl with bilateral lower-pole breast contractures. **B:** Excisional release of the lower half of the breasts with split-thickness skin grafting allowed the compressed breast tissue to expand and assume its normal shape. **C:** Breast augmentation and nipple areola complex reconstruction achieved a satisfactory aesthetic outcome.

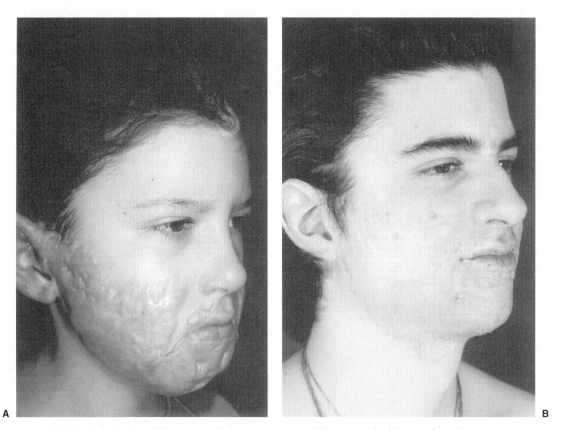

FIGURE 18.3. Multimodal scar manipulation. **A:** An 8-year-old boy 6 months following flame burn injury with diffuse facial hypertrophic scarring and contractures. **B:** Ten years later following pressure, massage, steroid injections, and multiple Z-plasties within the scar tissue, the hypertrophy has resolved. The depth of the burn is indicated by the absence of beard growth.

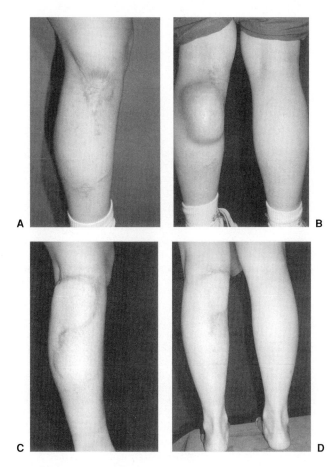

FIGURE 18.4. Iatrogenic deformity. **A:** A 13-year-old girl with hypertrophic, contracted, medial popliteal scar 1 year following burn injury. **B:** Tissue expander in place prior to scar excision and flap rotation. **C** and **D:** Postoperative result of scar excision shows a conspicuous surgical scar, and abnormal leg contour with compression of the calf. The flap fills and deforms the medial popliteal concavity.

common after the acute phase of a burn injury is over for the patient and the patient's family to desire expeditious reconstructive surgery. Patients would like their scars to be "removed" and they want to "get on with their lives." Most of the time, this is not in the patient's best interest. As mentioned before, the amount of time that is required for burn scars to reach their final state of maturation is not generally appreciated. If the prolonged process of scar maturation is allowed to occur, particularly when aided by appropriate help from the surgeon and therapists, hypertrophic, contracted, and conspicuous scars that are problematic at 1 year or longer can improve greatly with more time. Because of the gradual and subtle transition from unburned skin to burn scar, mature scars are usually less conspicuous than would be the surgical scars resulting from excision and primary closure. Education of the patient and the patient's family is essential in order to help guide them to the best possible outcome. The desire for "excision" can lead to iatrogenic deformities such as shown in Figure 18.4. This unfortunate result could have been completely avoided with more time and Z-plasties performed within the maturing hypertrophic scar tissue.

Reconstructive Plan

A prospective plan for reconstructive surgery should be worked out either with the patient and the patient's family during the

intermediate phase following an acute burn or at the time of consultation with a new patient who has established postburn deformities. Planning the reconstructive sequence is helpful to the patient, the family, and the surgeon. Because the patient's priorities may be different from the surgeon's, education, careful consultation, and mutual agreement are of extreme importance. Operations to improve essential function are the initial priority, but appearance, particularly of the face and hands, should always be a consideration. All reconstructive procedures should try to improve both the function and appearance of the operated area as much as possible. The planning process gives the patients perspective and helps them develop a positive attitude as they look forward to significant improvement in the future. Enthusiasm and optimism on the part of the surgeon and the entire reconstructive team is essential. Including the patient's family in these discussions is important. A strong support system is necessary for what is often a long and arduous process.

Fundamentals

Several basic concepts and techniques are worth reviewing in the context of burn reconstruction.

Contractures

Burns cause tissue loss, wounds heal with contraction, and contractures result. Contractures can be either intrinsic or extrinsic. Intrinsic contractures result from injury or loss of tissue in the affected area, causing subsequent distortion and deformity of the part. Extrinsic contractures occur when tissue loss at a distance from an affected area creates tension that distorts the structure. Eyelid ectropion, for example, can result from either intrinsic or extrinsic contractures. Although this concept is obvious and well known, the frequency with which it is ignored in burn reconstruction is astounding. Contracture deformities must be carefully evaluated and an accurate diagnosis made. Corrective measures can then be directed at the cause. There is very rarely any indication for release and graft or Z-plasty in unburned skin because of a deformity resulting from an extrinsic contracture.

Tension

For scars to mature as well as possible, tension must be eliminated. Tension deforms normal body contours, and the resulting abnormal shape draws attention to the injured area. Relief of tension and restoration of normal contour by either release and grafting or Z-plasties is perhaps the most basic fundamental of all burn reconstruction. The amount of tension in the skin following a burn injury is often not obvious, particularly to inexperienced surgeons. When releases are carried out and defects are created, the amount of tissue required to close the open defects can be surprising.

Donor Sites

Donor site availability is often problematic in burn reconstruction. Severe burns are usually extensive, and successful reconstruction requires careful allocation of donor-site material. Split-thickness grafts from the buttocks, thighs, and postaxial trunk are best used for contracture releases of the trunk and extremities. Full-thickness skin grafts from the retroauricular area, cervicopectoral area, and the upper inner arms, are best reserved for head and neck reconstruction. The lower abdomen and groin are excellent donor sites for full-thickness grafts, usually allowing primary closure of the donor site. Full-thickness skin grafts from these areas tend to have a yellowish hue in

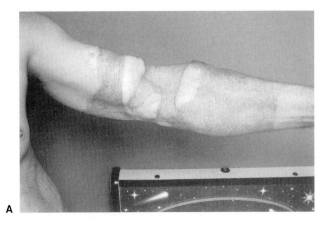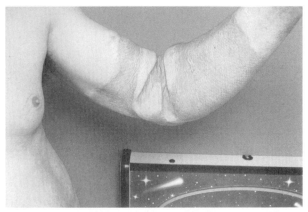

FIGURE 18.5. Failure to limit release to superficial tissue. **A:** Incisional release in the antecubital space violated the subcutaneous fat creating a severe contour deformity. **B:** With elbow flexion, the depression and skin prolapse is a conspicuous iatrogenic deformity.

fair-skinned patients, which is a disadvantage for facial reconstruction.

Release and Grafting

Nothing could be simpler than the concept of a surgical release and graft. Attention to detail is important, however, to obtain the best result. Burn contractures are usually limited to the superficial scars or grafts and a thin layer of fibrous connective tissue just beneath the skin surface. The underlying structures, such as subcutaneous fat, breast gland, and orbicularis muscle, are merely compressed and displaced. Releasing incisions or excisions should be limited whenever possible to the superficial scarred tissues alone. When this is done, normal contour is restored as the deep tissues unfurl, expand, and return to their normal shape (Fig. 18.2). Failure to limit the release to the superficial scar causes iatrogenic contour deformities that are often impossible to correct (Fig. 18.5). Releases should always try to overcorrect the contracture deformity and grafts should be sutured in with a bolster dressing. Placing fishtail darts at the ends of the releasing incisions adds additional skin and helps to prevent recurrent contracture by creating W-plasties at the ends of the graft. Postoperative management of grafts with pressure and conformers is essential to minimize graft contracture and wrinkling. The raised edges of the grafts that result from overcorrection and the tie-over dressing will virtually always flatten. If not, they can easily be excised or revised.

Z-plasty

The Z-plasty operation is an essential and powerful tool in the surgeon's armamentarium for burn reconstruction. For more than 150 years, the Z-plasty has been used for its ability to lengthen linear scars by recruiting relatively lax adjacent

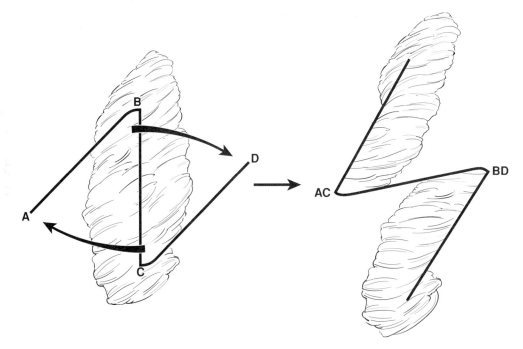

FIGURE 18.6. Z-plasty. Transposing the flaps of a Z-plasty lengthens the central limb and also narrows the involved scar by the medial transposition of the flaps. The flap tips should be incised perpendicular to the central limb for a short distance to supply more tissue and enhance the blood supply. Following transposition, the more irregular borders help to camouflage the scar.

lateral tissue. The Z-plasty, however, is much more than a simple geometrical exercise in lengthening a linear scar. When executed properly, it causes a profound beneficial effect on the physiology of scar tissue (6). Burn scar contractures are frequently diffuse, and excision is neither practical nor desirable. When a Z-plasty is performed properly, recruiting lateral tissue, two goals are accomplished. The central limb is lengthened, decreasing longitudinal tension on the scar, and the width of the scarred area is decreased by the medial transposition of the lateral flaps (Fig. 18.6). The narrowing of scars by Z-plasty revision can be very effective. A 60-degree Z-plasty lengthens a scar by 75% while narrowing it by approximately 30%. The Z-plasty also adds to scar camouflage by making the borders more irregular. For a Z-plasty to lengthen a burn scar and restore elasticity, the lateral limbs must extend beyond the margins of the scar. After a successful Z-plasty, the hypertrophic scar resolves, becomes more elastic, and it also has been narrowed by the procedure. The physiology of this phenomenon is related to the immediate and ongoing remodeling of collagen that occurs in hypertrophic scars following the relief of tension (7). Hypertrophic scar remodeling also takes place

when tension is relieved by release and graft, but the use of the Z-plasty is simple, elegant, and powerful. As John Stage Davis said, "It is difficult to realize how much permanent relaxation can be secured by the use of scar infiltrated tissue in this type of incision until one is familiar with the procedure and its possibilities. In addition, the improvements in the appearance of scars following Z-plasty revision is often dramatic" (6). When the Z-plasty flaps are incised, the tips should be cut perpendicular to the central limb for a short distance as shown in Figure 18.6. This adds additional tissue to the flap tips and improves blood supply.

Wherever burn scar crosses a concave surface, there is a tendency for the scar to contract, hypertrophy, and "bowstring." Z-plasty can alleviate this frequently occurring problem. The Z-plasty can also be used at the same time to enhance contour by appropriately designing the flaps. A Z-plasty release should be designed so that, following the transposition of flaps, the tight transverse limb of the Z-plasty is located where a normal concavity would occur. For example, the Z-plasties shown in Figure 18.7 both release contractures and are used to emphasize jawline definition. The axilla, antecubital space,

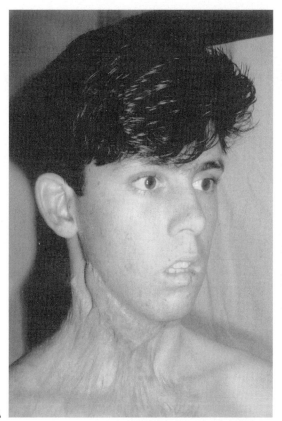

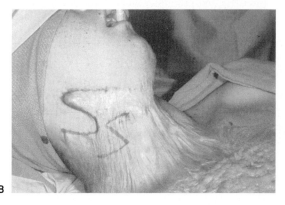

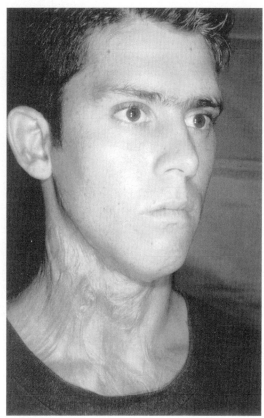

FIGURE 18.7. Z-plasty to increase jawline definition. A: Hypertrophic contracted neck scars create an extrinsic contracture deforming the lower eyelid, oral commissure, and the jawline. B: Z-plasty design incorporates the scarred tissues in the flaps. C: Four years following Z-plasties the facial deformities are corrected and the scar is flat, soft, and asymptomatic.

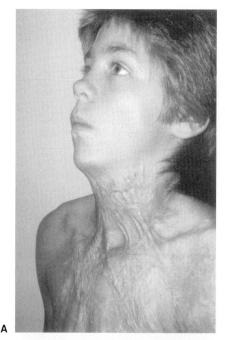

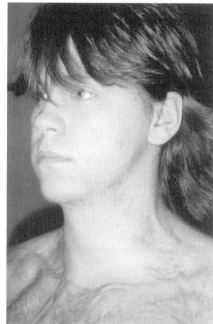

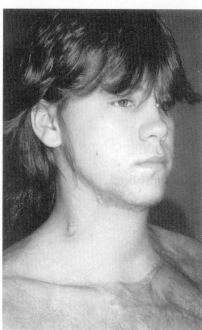

FIGURE 18.8. Correction of cervical contracture using regional flap. **A:** Recurrent anterior cervical contracture in a 17-year-old boy following split-thickness skin grafting. **B** and **C:** Transposition flap from the unburned right cervicopectoral area restores normal function and appearance.

and popliteal space are frequent sites of hypertrophic scar contracture with bowstringing and are often suitable for treatment with Z-plasty. The medial popliteal scar in Figure 18.4 could easily have been corrected with one or two Z-plasties within the scar, releasing the contracture, improving the appearance to the scar, and restoring the normal concave contour. Linear hypertrophic scar contractures are seen less frequently across extensor surfaces. The two exceptions are the wrist and anterior ankle because of their ability to dorsiflex.

Grafts

Skin grafts are pivotal in burn reconstruction. A few generalizations about their characteristics may be helpful. Split-thickness skin grafts contract more than full-thickness skin grafts, have more propensity to wrinkle, and always remain shiny with

a "glossy finish" look. Thick split-thickness skin grafts contract less and provide a more durable skin coverage, but do not possess elastic properties. Meshed split-thickness grafts are rarely indicated in burn reconstruction surgery. The meshed pattern is permanently retained and has an unattractive "reptilian" appearance. Hyperpigmentation of grafts is a frequent problem in dark-skinned patients, particularly those of African descent.

Full-thickness skin grafts are reliable workhorses in facial burn reconstruction. The use of full-thickness skin grafts in other areas of burn reconstruction should be carefully considered on an individual basis. Full-thickness grafts are elastic, contract less, have a "matte finish" like normal skin, and create a durable, resilient, skin surface. Full-thickness grafts, however, require a well-vascularized bed, primary closure or grafting of the donor site, and are best reserved for reconstruction of the

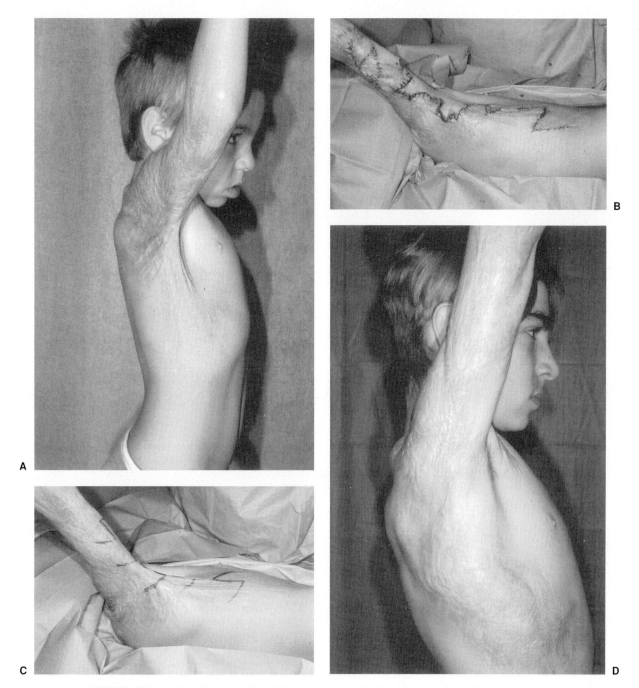

FIGURE 18.9. Multiple Z-plasties for axillary contracture. **A:** Extensive posterior axillary contracture with hypertrophic scarring. **B** and **C:** Multiple Z-plasties and local flaps in series easily release the contracture. **D:** Eight years later complete release has been maintained, the scars are flat and soft, and the contours are normal.

head and neck or the hand. Composite grafts from the ear are useful for complex facial burn reconstruction, but should only be used when there is adequate blood supply in the recipient bed.

Flaps

Flaps, with or without tissue expansion, are useful for burn reconstruction. They are mandatory for complex defects such as open joints or exposed vessels, or to provide tissue coverage that allows for later complex reconstruction, such as tendon or nerve grafting in the hand. Large flaps involve a

considerable tradeoff because of their donor-site morbidity. Their elasticity and minimal contracture, as well as excellent color and texture match, make them an excellent option when available for the correction of cervical contractures (Fig. 18.8). Flaps are frequently recommended in the literature for axillary contractures. The normal axilla is concave and lined with exquisitely thin skin. This allows the arm to rest comfortably at the side. Transposition of flaps into the axilla can effectively release contractures, but can also create terrible contour deformities. When potential flap tissue is available, either posterior or anterior to the axilla, multiple Z-plasties in series can usually release axillary contractures and preserve or restore

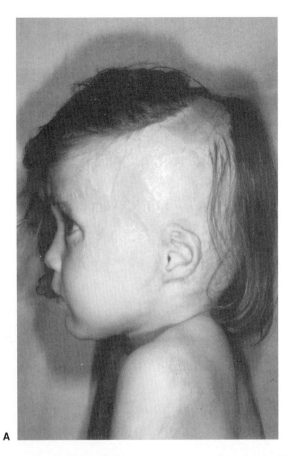
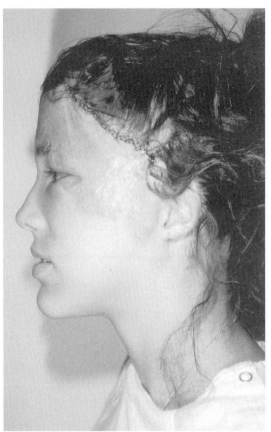

A   B

FIGURE 18.10. Tissue expansion. A: A 7-year-old girl with extensive alopecia involving the vertex, parietal, and occipital areas of the scalp. B: Ten years later following two tissue expansions, alopecia has been eliminated and a normal temporal hairline and sideburn restored.

normal contour (Fig. 18.9). When diffuse axillary scarring is present, release and graft is the best option, even though it requires postoperative splinting and often more than one intervention.

Tissue Expansion

Tissue expanders have transformed the treatment of postburn alopecia. Bald areas of 50% of the scalp or more can be successfully reconstructed, frequently requiring more than one expansion. Although there is conflicting data in the literature regarding complications, in general the scalp is a privileged site for tissue expansion (8,9). The scalp is an ideal site for tissue expansion because of its blood supply, convex shape, and the unyielding skull against which to expand (Fig. 18.10). The use of tissue expansion in other areas of burn reconstruction is more problematic. Because the underlying theme of almost all burn deformities is tension and tissue deficiency, stretching adjacent tissue in order to carry out scar excision can result in increased tension and iatrogenic contour abnormalities (Fig. 18.4). The complication rate of tissue expansion in burn patients is high, particularly in the extremities, reaching 25% to 50% in some reports (10). After alopecia, the most common use of tissue expansion is probably in the reconstruction of facial burn deformities. Care must be taken when advancing or transposing expanded flaps from the cervicopectoral area to the face. It is easy to create extrinsic contractures with a downward vector resulting in a "sad" facial appearance that is distressing to patients. Contour deformities can also be created in the neck with loss of jawline definition.

Evaluation and Treatment

Successful burn reconstruction requires perspective, patience, a thorough understanding of the problem and judicious application of the fundamentals of burn reconstruction. As noted previously, burn reconstruction is primarily about the release of contractures and the correction of contour abnormalities. When contractures have a predominantly linear component and there is a relative excess of vascular, elastic tissue lateral to the contracture, the Z-plasty is simple, reliable, and has the least morbidity. Z-plasty minimizes the need for most postoperative therapy, including pressure garments, and the benefit of the procedure is prolonged. The relaxed scar tissue will continue to soften, flatten, and loosen for many months to years after the operation is performed. Z-plasties can be used on the narrower, linear, components of diffuse areas of hypertrophic scarring to separate islands of scar and restore elasticity. Contour abnormalities can be corrected at the same time. The relief of tension leads to improved maturation. Following the benefit of initial scar revision, repeat surgery can be carried out 1 or 2 years later. Typically, this secondary surgery is directed toward scars that previously were not conspicuous or symptomatic but have become so after the treated scars flattened, softened, and become less noticeable. It is often remarkable how much improvement in appearance, contour, and softness can be accomplished by such Z-plasties. Patients are almost always pleased with the outcome and frequently ask for subsequent similar procedures, a true indication of successful surgery (Fig. 18.11).

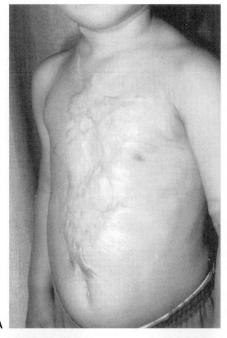
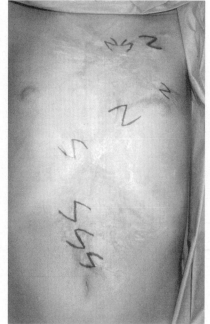
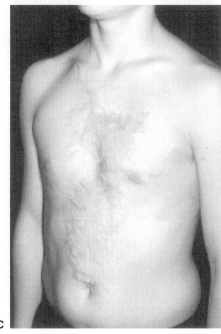

FIGURE 18.11. Effect of Z-plasties on hypertrophic scars. **A:** Diffuse hypertrophic scarring of the anterior chest and abdomen in an 8-year-old boy with deformity of the normal contours. **B:** Broad areas of scar were separated with multiple Z-plasties on two separate occasions as noted in the text. **C:** Ten years later, after two Z-plasty procedures, the scars are flat, soft, and elastic. The normal chest and abdominal contours have been restored.

When contracted scars or grafts are diffuse and Z-plasty or other local flap rearrangement is not possible, then release and split-thickness skin grafting is usually the best option to correct contractures. Care must be taken to preserve and restore normal tissue contours when releases are carried out to prevent unsightly iatrogenic contour abnormalities.

Flaps are excellent for cervical contractures when available (Fig. 18.8). Otherwise, release and split-thickness skin grafting is usually the best option for the neck, although this requires meticulous postoperative management and often more than one release and graft (11). Microvascular free tissue transfer has been advocated for anterior neck contractures but its use has been limited because of complexity and morbidity.

Tissue expansion is the ideal treatment for postburn alopecia. Even when the area of alopecia is relatively small, scalp expansion should be considered. Excision and direct closure of scalp alopecia usually results in a straight-line scar under tension that tends to widen and become conspicuous over time. Tissue expansion allows the closure to be carried out without tension, incorporating interdigitating local flaps and Z-plasties that obscure the scar and prevent widening. Whenever possible, the use of a single large expander is desirable, even if that requires expansion of some areas of alopecia. The larger the expander, the less separation of hair follicles occurs. When expansion is accomplished with a single large expander placed through a single small incision, manipulation of the scalp at the time of alopecia excision is facilitated because incisional scars are less likely to complicate the design of the best possible flaps for closure.

Facial burn reconstruction is complicated and can seem to be overwhelming in severe cases. The importance of time and allowing for maximal scar maturation to occur, along with the use of ancillary techniques such as pressure, silicone gel,

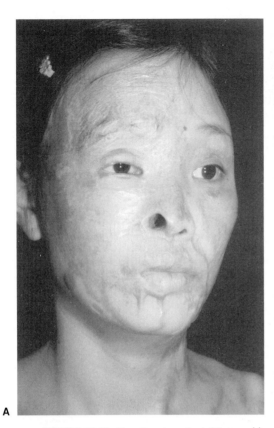
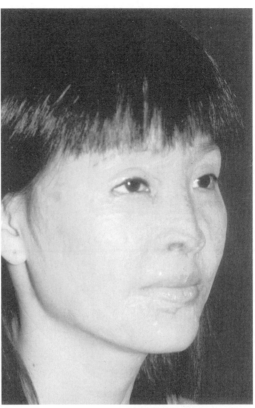

A

B

FIGURE 18.12. Type I patient. A: A 24-year-old woman following extensive acid burns to the face. B: Nasal reconstruction was performed with turn down flaps and split-thickness skin grafting. Four facial scar revisions with Z-plasties and local flaps were carried out over a 3-year period.

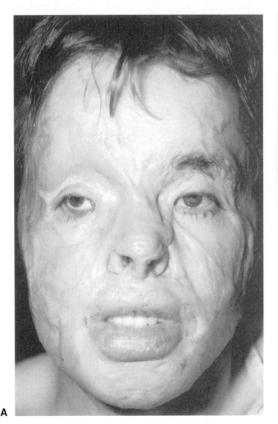
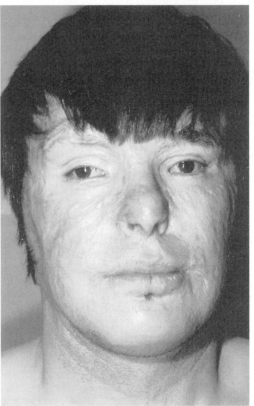

A

B

FIGURE 18.13. Type II patient. A: A 30-year-old male fireman following a severe facial burn with facial burn stigmata. B: Eight years later following extensive reconstructive surgery with full-thickness grafts, composite grafts, and multiple scar revisions.

TABLE 18.1

FACIAL BURN CATEGORIES

Type	Description
I	Essentially normal faces with focal or diffuse burn scarring with or without contractures
II	Panfacial burn deformities with some or all of the stigmata of facial burns (see Table 18.2)

TABLE 18.2

STIGMATA OF FACIAL BURNS

Lower eyelid ectropion
Short nose with ala flaring
Short retruded upper lip
Lower lip eversion
Lower lip inferior displacement
Flat facial features
Loss of jawline definition

steroids, judicious surgical intervention, and the use of the laser for erythema cannot be overemphasized.

It can be helpful to think of patients with facial burn deformities as falling into two fundamentally different categories as described in Table 18.1. Type I deformities consist of essentially normal faces that have focal tissue loss or diffuse burn scarring with or without associated contractures. Type II deformities make up a much smaller number of patients who have "panfacial" burn deformities consisting of what can be referred to as facial burn stigmata. Table 18.2 lists the stigmata of facial burns, which include lower eyelid ectropion, shortening of the nose with ala flaring, a short retruded upper lip, lower lip eversion, inferior displacement of the lower lip, flattening of facial features, and loss of jawline definition. The surgical goals when treating type I deformities should be different from those appropriate for treating type II deformities.

Type I patients have essentially normal faces and surgical intervention should not adversely affect overall facial appearance. The surgeon must not fall into the trap of compromising normal features and contours to "excise scars." Iatrogenic deformities create an abnormal look and can easily become grotesque. A normal-looking face with scars is more attractive than an even slightly grotesque face with fewer scars. Surgery should only be performed when it is reasonably certain it will make the patient definitely better, not just deformed in a different way. Scar revision with Z-plasties and local flaps is usually the best option for type I patients (Fig. 18.12). Full-thickness skin grafts from the most appropriate available donor sites are excellent for focal contractures. All human appearance is a mosaic to some degree and mosaic faces with normal movement and expression look much better in real life than they do in images. The pulsed dye laser is helpful in decreasing erythema.

Type II patients present a completely different clinical situation. The surgical goals for these patients should be the restoration of normal facial proportion and the return to normal of the position and shape of facial features. When normal facial proportion has been restored and facial features have been returned to their normal location and shape without tension, it is remarkable how much improvement in appearance can be accomplished in even severe facial burns (Fig. 18.13).

Cosmetics are effective in covering or minimizing abnormalities of color and texture in all body areas, but their application requires skill and commitment, and their use is usually limited to the face. Many female patients become exceedingly adept at cosmetic camouflage. Male patients are less likely to take advantage of this opportunity to minimize their deformity.

CONCLUSION

Advances in the care of acutely burned patients have created a challenge and an opportunity. More patients survive today with extensive areas of healed burn scar and graft. But this increased challenge provides great opportunity for plastic surgery. Although much gloom and doom tends to surround the acute care and reconstruction of burn patients, nothing could be further from the truth. Other than the burn scars and contractures, these patients are usually completely healthy, and successful reconstructive surgery can often restore them to a happy and productive life. Large series have shown excellent long-term outcomes in even extensively injured patients when compared with normal controls (12). Patience, persistence, and determination are essential to accomplish successful reconstruction. The skillful application of basic surgical techniques to the reconstruction of postburn deformities can be gratifying to patients and surgeons alike. The ultimate principle of burn reconstruction is learning to understand, appreciate, and favorably influence the processes of wound healing and scar maturation.

References

1. Cope O, Langohr JL, Moore FD, et al. Expeditious care of full thickness burn wounds by surgical excision and grafting. *Ann Surg.* 1947;125:1.
2. Janzekovic A. A new concept in early excision and immediate grafting of burns. *J Trauma.* 1970;10:1103.
3. Burke J, Bondoc CC, Quinby WC. Primary burn excision and immediate grafting: a method for shortening illness. *J Trauma.* 1974;14:389.
4. Larson D, Abston S, Evans DB, et al. Techniques for decreasing scar formation and contractures in the burn patient. *J Trauma.* 1971;11:807.
5. Ahn S, Monafo WW, Mustoe TA. Topical silicone gel: a new treatment for hypertrophic scars. *Surgery.* 1989;106:781.
6. Davis J. The relaxation of scar contractures by means of the Z-, or reversed Z-type incision: stressing the use of scar infiltrated tissues. *Ann Surg.* 1931;94:871.
7. Longacre J, Berry HK, Basom CR, et al. The effects of Z-plasty on hypertrophic scars. *Scand Plast Reconstr Surg.* 1976;10:113.
8. Neale H, High RM, Billmore DA, et al. Complications of controlled tissue expansion in the pediatric burn patient. *Plast Reconstr Surg.* 1988;82(5):840.
9. Pisarski G, Mertens D, Warden GD, et al. Tissue expander complications in the pediatric burn patient. *Plast Reconstr Surg.* 1998;102:1008.
10. Friedman R, Ingram AE, Rohrich RJ, et al. Risk factors for complications in pediatric tissue expansion. *Plast Reconstr Surg.* 1996;98:1242.
11. Cronin T. The use of a molded splint to prevent contracture after split-skin grafting on the neck. *Plast Reconstr Surg.* 1961;27:7.
12. Sheridan R, Hinson MI, Liang MH, et al. Long-term outcome of children surviving massive burns. *JAMA.* 2000;283:69.

CHAPTER 19 ■ RADIATION AND RADIATION INJURIES

JAMES KNOETGEN, III, SALVATORE C. LETTIERI, AND P. G. ARNOLD

Roentgen's 1895 discovery of x-rays was closely followed by the introduction of radiation therapy for the treatment of a variety of cancers and other disease processes. Although radiation therapy provides both diagnostic and therapeutic benefits, the resulting changes to exposed tissues can pose wound-healing problems and reconstructive dilemmas to the plastic surgeon. This chapter explains the basics of radiation therapy and discusses the radiation wound issues that are most commonly faced by the plastic surgeon, providing specific emphasis on the unique problems posed by various anatomic locations.

Radiation refers to the high-energy particles (α-particles, β-particles, neutrons) and electromagnetic waves (x-rays, γ rays) that are emitted by radioactive substances (uranium, radon, etc). α-Particles are large, positively charged, helium nuclei. Radium and radioactive isotopes can be consumed orally or intravenously to emit α-particles into surrounding tissues. β-Particles are small, negatively charged electrons and are used in electron-beam therapy (e.g., treatment of mycosis fungoides), and can penetrate up to 1 cm of tissue. γ-Rays are uncharged photons produced by the natural decay of radioactive materials (radium, cobalt 60, etc.) and can penetrate into deep tissues. Roentgen rays (x-rays) are similar to γ-rays, except they are artificially emitted from tungsten when bombarded with electrons.

Radiation doses are measured in a variety of units, and these units measure the energy absorbed from a radiation source per unit mass of tissue. The units include the roentgen (R), the gray (Gy), the rad, and the sievert (Sv). The sievert is equal to the gray except that it is adjusted to take into account the biologic effects of different types of radiation. **In current nomenclature, the Gy has replaced the rad, so that 1 Gy = 100 rad, or 1 rad = 100 centigray (cGy).**

The two main forms of radiation exposure are irradiation and contamination. Irradiation refers to radiation waves that pass directly through the human body, whereas contamination is contact with and retention of radioactive material. Contamination is usually the result of an industrial accident. The plastic surgeon is most concerned with irradiation as opposed to contamination as current regulations have made industrial accidents and exposures very rare.

Irradiation is a local therapy applied to a specific body site containing a tumor or disease process, or to draining lymph node beds thought to contain or potentially contain microscopic or gross disease. Large tumors may be treated preoperatively with radiation therapy (induction therapy) to decrease the tumor burden prior to surgery. Adjuvant radiation therapy is performed in addition to the surgical extirpation with the goal of treating the tumor's resection bed and regional lymph nodes in patients with specific clinical scenarios, such as large tumors, recurrent tumors, extracapsular lymph node involvement, and positive resection margins. **The potential advantage of radiation therapy over surgery is local treatment of disease** with preservation of surrounding uninvolved structures. Disadvantages include the length of treatment, the need for access to appropriate facilities and equipment, and the potential additive and chronic effects of radiation therapy.

DELIVERY OF RADIATION THERAPY

Radiation therapy is delivered via external or internal routes. The delivery technique most commonly used is external beam radiotherapy, which originates from a source external to the patient, a linear accelerator (LINAC). A variety of radiation beams can be delivered in this manner, such as low-energy radiation beams from a cobalt source in a cobalt machine. Other atomic particles, such as neutrons, are also delivered via this mechanism. This technique allows daily fractionated delivery of radiation over a several-week course. External-beam therapy can be delivered as an independent treatment preoperatively, intraoperatively, or postoperatively.

Delivery of radiation from within the patient's body is termed *brachytherapy*. Radioactive sources are inserted into the patient for temporary or permanent irradiation. This technique allows for continual treatment of the tumor with radiation over a course that usually lasts several days. Its advantages include decreased treatment time and greater ability to spare uninvolved local tissues. Brachytherapy may also be indicated in patients who have been previously irradiated and are therefore no longer candidates for external beam therapy because they have already received the maximum recommended dose for the specific anatomic area.

RADIATION DAMAGE

Regardless of delivery technique, radiation therapy works by damaging the targeted cells through complicated intracellular processes that continue to be studied to this day. The interaction of radiation with water molecules within the cell creates free radicals that cause direct cellular damage. A range of biochemical lesions occur within DNA following exposure to radiation, and can result in two different modes of cell death: mitotic (clonogenic) cell death, and apoptosis. The biochemical lesion most often associated with cell death is a double-stranded break of nuclear DNA (1).

Irradiated tissues suffer both early and late effects. Early effects occur during the first few weeks following therapy and are usually self limited. They result from damage to rapidly proliferating tissues, such as mucosa and skin. Erythema and skin hyperpigmentation are the most common problems and these are treated expectantly with moisturizers and local wound care. Dry desquamation occurs after low to moderate doses of radiation, whereas higher doses result in moist desquamation. At the tissue level, stasis and occlusion of small vessels occurs, with a consequent decrease in wound tensile strength. Fibroblast proliferation is inhibited, and may result in permanent damage to fibroblasts. This creates irreversible injury to the skin, which may be progressive. Although the plastic surgeon is often not required to treat early radiation injuries, chronic injuries frequently require the plastic surgeon's attention.

Late, or chronic, radiation effects can manifest anytime after therapy, from weeks to years to decades after treatment. Although acute effects are uncomfortable and bothersome to the patient, they are generally self-limited and resolve with minimal treatment and local wound care. **Chronic effects, however, can be progressive, disabling, cumulative, permanent, and even life-threatening.** Late injuries include, but are not limited to, tissue fibrosis, telangiectasias, delayed wound healing, lymphedema (as the result of cutaneous lymphatic obstruction), ulceration, infection, alopecia, malignant transformation, mammary hypoplasia, xerostomia, osteoradionecrosis, and endarteritis. Long-term effects of radiation therapy also include constrictive microangiopathic changes to small and medium sized vessels (2), which is very important when performing reconstructions with pedicled and free flaps.

GENERAL PRINCIPLES OF TREATING IRRADIATED WOUNDS

In most circumstances, a radiated wound will not heal as well as a nonirradiated wound. Consequently, plastic surgeons are often consulted for the wound closure of these patients (Fig. 19.1). The plastic surgeon is generally called on to care for two different populations of irradiated patients. The first population is those who have not yet received irradiation but who will receive radiation therapy intraoperatively or postoperatively. This is often seen in the immediate breast-reconstruction patient who is undergoing mastectomy and potential postoperative radiation therapy and in the sarcoma patient under-

going extirpation with intraoperative radiation therapy. Also, bronchial stumps can be reinforced when a completion pneumonectomy is anticipated, usually with intrathoracic transposition of a serratus muscle flap (3).

The second population includes patients who have already received radiation therapy and now have a recurrent or new tumor, or a radiation wound with exposure of vital or significant structures such as bone, vital organs, or neurovascular bundles. This patient requires tumor extirpation or wound debridement followed by reconstruction. The patient's treatment varies depending on which of these categories the patient falls into, the depth of the injury and tissues involved, and which specific anatomic area is affected.

Intraoperative radiation therapy is occasionally used in the treatment of sarcomas, pelvic tumors, and other malignancies. Plastic surgeons are often consulted for the closure of these wounds. In this situation, the reconstructive ladder is applicable, and if enough well-vascularized soft tissue is present, a primary layered closure can be attempted. Many of these wounds will heal well even though they have received intraoperative radiation therapy. However, if bone, prosthetic material, or neurovascular bundles are exposed, coverage with a well-vascularized flap is indicated to protect these structures. Likewise, if the wound lacks adequate soft-tissue coverage, a vascularized flap should be used to create a stable reconstruction.

When confronted with a wound that has late radiation changes, the plastic surgeon's first step is to rule out the presence of a recurrent or new tumor (possibly radiation induced). Diagnosis is often assisted by standard radiographs, computerized tomography (CT), and magnetic resonance imaging (MRI) scans, and confirmed with a tissue biopsy. If tumor is present, a full work-up and evaluation by the appropriate extirpative surgeon is required. After tumor extirpation is complete, reconstructive efforts of the resulting defect are then initiated.

If tumor is not present, the most critical first step in management of irradiated wounds is complete resection and debridement of all nonviable irradiated tissues and foreign bodies (sternal wires, previous sutures, etc.) (4). Primary closure or skin grafting of the irradiated wound may fail because of the poor

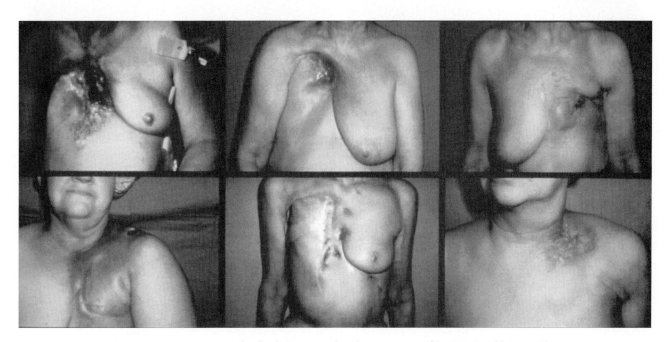

FIGURE 19.1. A to F: A sample of radiation wounds. (Photos courtesy of Dr. P.G. Arnold, Mayo Clinic, Rochester, MN.)

vascularity and fibrosis of the wound bed. Likewise, muscle flaps transposed into a poorly vascularized irradiated wound bed may not heal well. So it is imperative that the plastic surgeon first establish a clean wound with well-vascularized edges before proceeding with reconstruction. This is often accomplished in multiple debridements rather than a single operative endeavor, as the **extent of radiation injury often exceeds what grossly appears to be the boundary of damaged tissue.** The main cause of recurrent infections, sinus tracts, and wound healing problems is retention of nonviable materials such as foreign bodies, bone, or cartilage secondary to inadequate debridement.

If at the time of wound closure the nonirradiated tissue, such as omentum, is larger than the initial defect created by the debridement, then more of the radiated tissue can be removed, thus improving the chance of a well-healed wound. The "extra" omentum may also be placed beneath the remaining radiated skin thus reconstructing the missing or fibrotic subcutaneous tissue that was lost secondary to the radiation. This brings in additional blood supply to this skin, increases its "mobility," and vastly improves mobility of surrounding tissue to correct the situation where, for example, the skin was previously very thin and tightly adherent to the chest wall. Patients always appreciate this change toward normal. If the radiated tissue does not survive, the viable well-vascularized tissue (omentum) deep to it can be skin grafted.

When incising severely irradiated tissue, a defect much larger than anticipated is often created. This is because the irradiated tissue is often tight and creates a constricted skin envelope. When incised, the wound edges will often retract and create a larger defect than expected (Fig. 19.2B). This is an important concept to understand when planning the reconstruction, as one may need more nonirradiated tissue for reconstruction than originally estimated.

Once debridement is complete, stable wound closure is obtained. Thorough preoperative planning and a systematic approach to reconstruction of irradiated defects are needed. Reconstruction usually includes transposition of a well-vascularized nonirradiated soft-tissue flap into the wound bed. Reconstruction of these defects is often challenging and associated with relatively high complication rates. When planning the reconstruction, the plastic surgeon must choose which soft-tissue flap will best obtain a healed wound and maximize preservation of function. It is generally accepted that when performing a reconstruction, irradiated muscles should be avoided if possible, as this may result in partial or complete muscle necrosis (5). The transfer of a muscle whose pedicle has been irradiated may also be associated with a higher complication rate (6). If a well-vascularized muscle flap or the greater omentum is not available, a free tissue transfer may be required.

Another basic tenet of reconstructing irradiated wounds is that the first-line choice is either a muscle flap or the greater omentum. Although reconstruction of irradiated wounds with fascial or fasciocutaneous flaps has been reported, it is generally accepted that muscle flaps and the greater omentum have a better blood supply and, therefore, have a better chance of healing without complications. The remainder of this chapter addresses the pertinent issues of irradiated wound treatment by anatomic area.

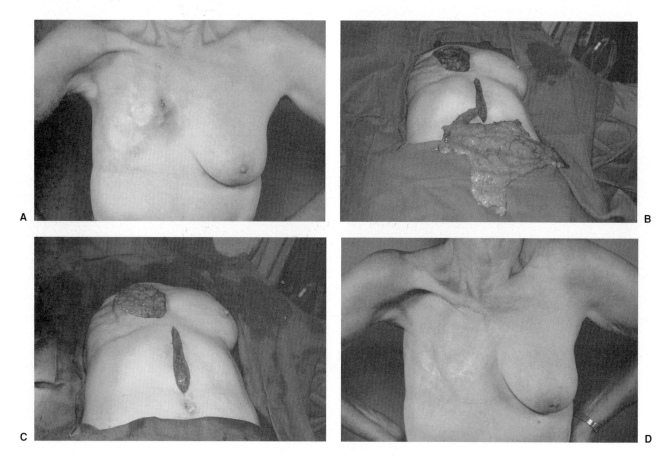

FIGURE 19.2. A to D: A patient with a radiation wound of the chest wall, reconstructed with a pedicled greater omentum flap. (Photo courtesy of Dr. P.G. Arnold, Mayo Clinic, Rochester, MN.)

Skin

Nonmelanoma skin malignancies can be treated with approximately a 90% cure rate with irradiation (see Chapter 13). Compared with extirpation, the radiation therapy option requires both prolonged therapy and access to radiation therapy facilities. Long-term complications, such as fibrosis, ulceration, ectropion, osteitis, and chondritis, make this treatment option less desirable. Consequently, it is generally reserved for patients who are not surgical candidates.

Low-dose radiation therapy can also be used postoperatively in the treatment of keloids and hypertrophic scars. This technique takes advantage of fibroblast inhibition caused by ionizing radiation. Radiation therapy is part of a multimodal approach to keloid treatment in some institutions.

Extremities

Soft-tissue sarcomas of the extremities can be aggressive tumors involving multiple structures and tissue planes. Surgical extirpation is often combined with intraoperative or postoperative radiation therapy, either external-beam or brachytherapy. Consequently, treatment of these patients requires a multidisciplinary approach, often involving surgical oncologists, vascular surgeons, orthopedic surgeons, radiation oncologists, plastic surgeons, and others. The goal is to obtain locoregional tumor control while simultaneously attempting limb salvage and maximal preservation of limb function. Patients may have received irradiation before extirpation, which is important in the planning of the radiation therapy (i.e., the patient may require brachytherapy as opposed to external-beam therapy or a modification of the external-beam dose). The sequence is especially important to the plastic surgeon and the planning of wound closure and reconstruction.

Wide local tumor resections of the extremity often result in large soft-tissue defects, as well as osseous defects. Osseous defects require orthopedic reconstruction with prosthetic materials, total arthroplasties, or bone grafts. All bone, tendons, prosthetic materials, and neurovascular bundles must be covered with well-vascularized viable tissue in order to obtain stable soft-tissue reconstruction and a healed wound. The addition of radiation therapy to the tumor bed, including all previous irradiation, must be considered when planning reconstruction.

The goal of soft-tissue reconstruction is to obtain stable coverage of all vital structures. Although the "reconstructive ladder" generally proceeds from primary wound closure through skin grafting, local flaps, regional flaps, and free microvascular flaps, occasionally, in complicated circumstances, such as patients who have received radiation therapy, the "reconstructive elevator" must be employed to ensure wound healing. In other words, it may be prudent to bypass one or more of the standard rungs of the reconstructive ladder to arrive at a more stable construct. For example, a defect in the medial thigh created by resection of a liposarcoma and irradiation that would normally be treated with primary closure may benefit from coverage with a pedicled musculocutaneous flap, especially if the femoral vessels are exposed. A soft-tissue defect over the knee may not be amenable to coverage with a gastrocnemius muscle flap if this muscle was within the field of previous irradiation and is fibrotic, and thus may be better treated with a free muscle flap.

Obliteration of a soft-tissue defect is not the only goal when reconstructing these wounds. Preserving and maintaining maximal function also is important. When critical muscles or large muscle masses are resected and/or irradiated, it is often advantageous to perform a neurotized muscle reconstruction. This can often give patients at least partial function of a joint or limb. The development and refinement in the use of pedicled and free muscle, bone, and fasciocutaneous flaps has increased the plastic surgeon's ability to obtain stable wound closures in these complex clinical situations of the extremity that previously required amputation.

Breast

The breast is undoubtedly the anatomic structure most frequently cared for by the plastic surgeon that has the potential to be irradiated. Breast reconstructions using autologous or prosthetic materials are commonly performed by plastic surgeons. These reconstructions can be made more complicated if the treatment plan includes radiation therapy. The plastic surgeon generally encounters two breast patient populations: (a) the patient who has already received radiation therapy to the breast(s) for the treatment of a previous malignancy and is now in need of further extirpation and/or reconstruction, and (b) the patient who is undergoing mastectomy and may need to receive postoperative radiation therapy, usually because of tumor size or nodal involvement.

The first clinical scenario requires the plastic surgeon to perform a breast reconstruction in an irradiated field. The surgeon must first evaluate the breasts and assess the degree of radiation damage. The patient should be examined for erythema, hyperpigmentation, and the degree of fibrosis of the breast and surrounding tissues and skin. **A basic tenet of reconstructing the irradiated breast is that delivery of well-vascularized tissue via autogenous reconstruction will yield a better result than prosthetic implants alone.** Reconstruction with tissue expansion and implants has been demonstrated to yield a higher rate of wound-healing problems and implant exposure, as well as a higher incidence of Baker III and IV capsular contracture (7,8). Reconstruction with autogenous tissue, usually via pedicled or free transverse rectus abdominis musculocutaneous (TRAM) flaps or a latissimus dorsi muscle flap with an expander/implant (see Chapter 65), will often yield a superior result. If autologous breast reconstruction is not an option, some surgeons advocate immediate insertion of a breast tissue expander/implant at the time of mastectomy with completion of expansion prior to irradiation (9), although this is a controversial opinion and not widely accepted. An alternative technique employs placement of a tissue expander before radiation therapy to create and maintain a soft-tissue envelope for a later reconstruction that includes autologous tissue, with or without an implant.

A critical issue that requires consideration when performing autologous breast reconstruction is the quality of irradiated vessels within pedicled flaps (internal mammary vessels in TRAM flaps and the thoracodorsal vessels in latissimus dorsi muscle flaps), and the quality of irradiated recipient vessels in autologous reconstruction with free flaps (TRAM, deep inferior epigastric perforator [DIEP], superior gluteal artery perforator [S-GAP], etc.). **When the pedicle is exposed to radiation preoperatively, pedicled TRAM flaps have a higher incidence of both skin and flap necrosis** (6), and an increased incidence of pedicled TRAM flap failure (10). When performing a pedicled TRAM flap with irradiated vessels, decreased complications in this group may be achieved with a flap delay, a bipedicled TRAM flap, or by turbocharging the flap (although turbocharging pedicled flaps is a controversial subject).

The alternative is a free tissue reconstruction using a flap that has not been irradiated. When performing a free tissue transfer for breast reconstruction, the surgeon must inspect the quality of the irradiated recipient vessels. Significant scarring and fibrosis surrounding the vessels and radiation damage to the lumen of the recipient vessels can increase the chance of a failed free tissue transfer. Radiation therapy can result in constrictive microangiopathic changes to small- and medium-size vessels, as well as inhibition of fibroblast function, which can increase the risk of anastomotic failure (2).

Occasionally, at the time of mastectomy, the need for postoperative irradiation is uncertain. In this setting, the plastic surgeon must decide whether to perform immediate reconstruction or delay reconstruction until after the potential radiation therapy is completed. Most plastic surgeons agree that superior outcomes are achieved with a delayed autologous reconstruction, rather than with an immediate reconstruction and postoperative radiation of the flap (11,12). Consequently, it is prudent to delay reconstruction until the final decision about postoperative irradiation is made.

Head and Neck

Because head and neck malignancies are frequently aggressive with high recurrence rates, treatment requires both surgical extirpation and radiation therapy. Surgical extirpation often results in large defects with exposure of vital structures that require complicated soft-tissue and/or osseous reconstruction. Reconstruction of these defects is often quite challenging, and is made more difficult if the irradiated tissues are fibrotic and if the vessels are damaged. Osteoradionecrosis of the mandible and maxilla is a complication occasionally seen after radiation therapy that requires resection/debridement of affected tissue followed by osseous reconstruction.

Although these defects were traditionally reconstructed with local and regional flaps, free tissue transfer is now the standard reconstruction technique. Historically, the pectoralis major muscle flap has been used for soft-tissue coverage of neck defects. However, this flap is limited by its bulkiness, the difficult arc of rotation, and its limited extension into the oral region. Free tissue transfer allows well-vascularized, nonradiated tissues from a distant site to be used for reconstruction of the radiated defect. Because of the vital structures located in the head and neck region, it is imperative to obtain a stable closure with viable flaps. Success is measured not only by the cure or control of the tumor, but also by wound healing and preservation of function.

Full-thickness defects of the head and neck region require reconstruction of several layers, including the intraoral lining, osseous reconstruction of the mandible or maxilla, and soft-tissue/skin coverage. Partial-thickness defects may only require intraoral lining or soft-tissue coverage. Usually, local flaps are not readily usable, except, perhaps, for a temporalis muscle flap to obliterate the maxillary sinus or the palate region. Free tissue transfer is usually preferred, especially in irradiated defects. The types of free tissue transfers often used include a thin fasciocutaneous flap (radial forearm flap), or intermediate-thickness flap (scapula or parascapular flap), or variable-thickness flap (anterolateral thigh flap). Muscle flaps (rectus abdominus or latissimus dorsi) can also be used. The omentum is excellent as a "carrier" for bone and skin grafts but offers no structural strength.

Generally, vessels in the neck are readily available and of adequate caliber. However, even if the vessel caliber is adequate, irradiated vessels may be more difficult to dissect and use for microanastomosis because of local fibrosis and radiation injury to the vessels. Local fibrosis makes the dissection difficult, as the soft-tissue planes that are ordinarily present may be unidentifiable. Consequently, thoughtful preoperative planning with a "plan A" and at least one "plan B" is necessary before undertaking the surgery. If the radiated vessels are deemed unsatisfactory for microvascular anastomosis, the surgeon should be prepared to find vessels in other areas of the neck, such as the contralateral side or the supraclavicular region. This is performed with vein grafts, so it is important to warn patients preoperatively about the potential need for

surgery to other parts of their body. **Although vein grafting generally increases microanastomotic failure rates, vein grafting into an area that is easily dissected with a technically easier anastomosis is better than a difficult anastomosis to poor vessels without a vein graft.**

Quite often, vein grafts are necessary for coverage of irradiated scalp defects. Many surgeons prefer to use the larger arteries and veins in the neck in lieu of smaller vessels near the scalp, such as the superficial temporal artery. Although several authors have been successful with the superficial temporal artery, it is generally accepted that the neck vessels are easier to work with and have less chance of causing anastomotic problems.

The timing of reconstruction in reference to the delivery of radiation also needs to be taken into consideration. Induction radiation therapy, used to downstage (shrink) tumors preoperatively, tends to create more bleeding and inflammation in the affected area. Although the irradiated vessels may be adequate for use, the dissection may be tenuous because of the inflammation. Chronic radiation injury, however, tends to have more fibrosis in the affected area, as well as thickening of the tissue planes and absence of standard anatomic landmarks, which makes dissection slow and difficult.

Patients who will be having postoperative irradiation do not have these problems and will have unoperated tissues and virgin surgical planes. In fact, after the neck dissection is performed, the vessels are exposed and often prepared for use. It is often prudent to recommend to the extirpative surgeon that an adequate length be left on the vessels that are ligated and resected during the dissection, so as to have a cuff for anastomosis, rather than ligating the branch flush with the larger vessel from which it arises.

Osseous reconstructions of the head and neck offer additional reconstructive challenges. Mandible resections are usually reconstructed with the fibula free tissue transfer to deliver well-vascularized nonirradiated tissue to the irradiated wound bed. Generally, a complex full-thickness defect with defects of the bone and intraoral lining are best served by a vascularized bone flap. In the absence of any viable alternatives for vascularized bone graft, a free tissue transfer with a nonvascularized bone graft could then be used. This is *not* an ideal option considering the adjunctive radiation that is often administered postoperatively. **Although some authors report successes with bone grafting or a cancellous "tray," these reconstructions need to be performed within a well-vascularized bed and thus are not often indicated in irradiated wounds.**

An uncommon, yet potentially lethal, complication of radiation therapy to the head and neck is an infection that leads to wound dehiscence and exposure of the vessels. This can result in vessel rupture or anastomotic leak, which can be lethal given the large size of these blood vessels. In the absence of irradiation to the neck, incorporation of the vessels and soft-tissue flap into the surrounding wound bed usually occurs and establishes stable coverage of the vessels, making this complication rare in the nonirradiated patient. Previous irradiation, however, impairs the progress of soft-tissue incorporation and therefore increases the risk of exposure.

Chest

Radiation therapy to the chest wall is used in the treatment of lymphomas, large chest wall or pulmonary tumors, and for recurrent malignancies after previous resections. Postradiation complications in this patient population include radiation ulcers, infected wounds, persistent or recurrent tumors, and cardiac and pulmonary disorders. As the thoracic cavity houses a variety of vital organs, radiation damage to the chest wall can create a potentially lethal clinical scenario requiring immediate attention from the cardiothoracic surgeon as well as the plastic surgeon. These patients are often quite ill, requiring prolonged stays in the intensive care unit and a multidisciplinary team approach.

The first step in evaluating a patient with one of these problems is to rule out the presence of new or recurrent tumor. This work-up includes standard imaging studies such as chest radiograph, CT, or MRI, and possibly bronchoscopy. After the extent of tumor involvement is determined, it must be completely resected with negative pathologic margins before reconstructive options are considered. If tumor is not present, then the radiation ulcer or infected wound must be thoroughly debrided, and all fibrotic radiated tissue and foreign bodies must be resected. Many chronic sinus tracts in the chest wall can be traced to a sternal wire, retained suture, or persistent infected cartilage. Debridements are often performed in multiple serial procedures, as it is often difficult to judge the extent of remaining nonviable tissue after only one procedure. As occurs in other anatomic areas, the extent of radiation injury often exceeds what initially appear to be the boundaries of damaged tissue.

After resection and debridement is complete, the wound must be evaluated to determine if it is a partial- or full-thickness defect. Because the chest wall is a relatively thin structure, most chest wall defects following thorough debridement are full thickness and will require chest wall reconstruction prior to soft-tissue coverage. Chest wall reconstruction is performed by either the thoracic surgeon or plastic surgeon experienced in chest wall reconstructions. Prosthetic material, such as Gore-Tex (W.F. Gore, Phoenix, AZ) sheeting or Prolene (Ethicon, Sommerville, NJ) mesh, is employed for this reconstruction, if the wound permits. The goal is to obtain an airtight seal at the time of closure so as to maintain appropriate intrathoracic negative pressure for respiration. The prosthetic material is then covered with a viable soft-tissue flap, usually a musculocutaneous flap or a muscle flap with a skin graft. Flaps frequently used for chest wall reconstruction include one or both of the pectoralis major muscles, latissimus dorsi muscles ($\pm$ the serratus anterior muscle), and rectus abdominis muscles, as well as the greater omentum (4).

Advantages of the pedicled greater omental flap are its large surface area and excellent vascularity. Complete debridement of irradiated chest wounds often results in large irregular defects, and the omentum tends to cover these defects nicely as it can be molded into irregular defects quite easily (Fig. 19.2). Many radiated wounds result in partial-thickness chest wall defects when there is no recurrent tumor present. There may be a full-thickness resection, but even then the lung may be adherent to the pleura secondary to the previous radiation and/or inflammation. In either case, the omentum with a skin graft is adequate, and underlying foreign bodies in the form of meshes can be avoided in contaminated wounds, thus taking advantage of this postradiation fibrosis.

The omentum is procured through an upper midline laparotomy incision, mobilized, and usually based on the usually dominant right gastroepiploic vessels (85% to 95% of cases). Skin grafting is generally performed in a delayed fashion after a few days of dressing changes and one is sure that all of the transposed omentum is well vascularized. This gives the plastic surgeon time to observe the omental flap; debride any nonviable portions, and re-advance or redistribute the pliable omentum as necessary. Disadvantages of the omentum are similarly the lack of structural strength. It is simply a vascularized "carrier" for skin in this case. There is also the addition of an upper midline laparotomy and violation of a second body cavity, but its large size, malleability, vascularity, and acceptable donor defect make it an attractive option. The omentum can also be used for lower back closures by tunneling it through the retroperitoneum and paraspinous muscles.

There are very special situations in patients with problematic radiated wounds of the chest that may involve disruption of the aerodigestive tract or the heart with the great vessels. These have been dealt with on some occasions with intrathoracic muscle flaps (3).

Because of the abundance of local pedicled muscles and the greater omentum, free tissue transfer is often not needed for a standard chest wall reconstruction. However, the radiated patient may not have adequate local muscles because of multiple surgeries and debridements and radiation damage to the muscles and vessels. Transposition of irradiated muscles can result in partial or total necrosis (5). If the greater omentum is not available, a free tissue transfer may be required in these extreme situations (13).

As in the treatment of all radiation wounds, the key to obtaining a well-healed chest wall reconstruction relies on adequate initial debridement of all nonviable irradiated tissues. Only then should attempts at chest wall and soft-tissue reconstruction be attempted.

Perineum

Gynecologic malignancies occasionally require extensive perineal resections and/or pelvic exenterations. These tumors will often be treated with radiation therapy as well and the resulting perineal wound is usually not amenable to primary closure. Similar perineal defects are created after abdominoperineal resections for anal, recurrent, or low rectal tumors. When combined with radiation therapy, these wounds often heal poorly. The addition of a well-vascularized soft-tissue flap is therefore warranted. Reconstructive options include a pedicled rectus abdominis musculocutaneous flap, which is often the flap of choice. If not available, other options include the use of thigh muscles (rectus femoris, gracilis) and fasciocutaneous flaps (anterolateral thigh flap).

The greater omentum has been used for decades to treat the chronic vesicovaginal fistula and to fill the severely irradiated pelvis with well vascularized tissue (14,15). It can also be employed to support a primary closure or, if no other options are available, it can be used alone with a skin graft (although the omentum is sometimes resected by the extirpative surgeon in cases of gynecologic malignancies).

The aforementioned muscle flaps can also be used to reconstruct the vagina, in addition to filling the dependent pelvic defect. In the male, a musculocutaneous flap can serve the purpose of obtaining a healed perineal wound and filling the most dependent portion of the pelvic defect to promote wound healing, prevent evisceration, and attempt to prevent adhesions deep in the pelvis.

CONCLUSION

Although radiation therapy has many benefits, late changes following irradiation have been well described and offer the plastic surgeon many reconstructive challenges. **Each anatomic location offers unique problems to the plastic surgeon. But the basic tenets of treating irradiated wounds are the same, regardless of anatomic location, and they are as follows:**

1. **Establish a diagnosis (rule out malignancy, determine the extent of tissue damage, etc.)**
2. **If tumor is present, perform the appropriate work-up and treatment.**
3. **Thoroughly debride the radiated wound of all nonviable tissue and foreign bodies and plan to transfer as much tissue as possible to permit resection of even *more* of the periphery in questionable wounds.**

4. After adequate debridement has been obtained, usually in stages, reconstruct osseous defects with vascularized bone and soft-tissue defects with well-vascularized, nonirradiated soft tissue. All neurovascular bundles, bone, tendon, prosthetic material, etc., must be covered with well-vascularized soft tissue.

5. In the case of pedicled flaps, it is better to base a flap on a nonirradiated pedicle; in the case of free tissue transfer, it is best to use nonirradiated recipient vessels.

6. Reconstruction of these defects is challenging and fraught with high complication rates, so always have a "plan B" in mind and anticipate complications.

References

1. Ross GM. Induction of cell death by radiotherapy. *Endocr Relat Cancer.* 1999;6:41.
2. Fajardo LF, Berthrong M. Vascular lesions following radiation. *Pathol Ann.* 1988;23:297.
3. Arnold PG, Pairolero PC. Intrathoracic muscle flaps. An account of their use in the management of 100 consecutive patients. *Ann Surg.* 1990;211(6):656.
4. Arnold PG, Pairolero PC. Chest wall reconstruction: an account of 500 consecutive patients. *Plast Reconstr Surg.* 1996;98:5.
5. Arnold PG, Lovich SF, Pairolero PC. Muscle flaps in irradiated wounds: an account of 100 consecutive cases. *Plast Reconstr Surg.* 1994;93:324.
6. Jones G, Nahai F. Management of complex wounds. *Curr Probl Surg.* 1998;35:194.
7. Evans RD, Schusterman MA, Kroll SS, et al. Reconstruction and the radiated breast: is there a role for implants? *Plast Reconstr Surg.* 1995;96(5):1111.
8. Forman DC, Chiu J, Restifo RJ, et al. Breast reconstruction in previously irradiated patients using tissue expanders and implants: a potentially unfavorable result. *Ann Plast Surg.* 1998;40:360.
9. McCarthy CM, Pusic AL, Disa J, et al. Unilateral postoperative chest wall radiotherapy in bilateral tissue expander/implant reconstruction patients: a prospective outcomes analysis. *Plast Reconstr Surg.* 2005;116(6):1642.
10. Hartrampf CR Jr, Bennett GK. Autogenous tissue reconstruction in the mastectomy patient: a critical review of 300 patients. *Ann Surg.* 1987;205:508.
11. Tran NV, Evans GR, Kroll SS, et al. Postoperative adjuvant irradiation: effects on transverse rectus abdominis muscle flap breast reconstruction. *Plast Reconstr Surg.* 2000;106:313.
12. Spear SL, Ducic I, Low M, et al. The effect of radiation on pedicled TRAM flap breast reconstruction: outcomes and implications. *Plast Reconstr Surg.* 2005;115(1):84.
13. Cordeiro PG, Santamaria E, Hidalgo D. The role of microsurgery in reconstruction of oncologic chest wall defects. *Plast Reconstr Surg.* 2001;108(7):1924.
14. Turner-Warwick RT, Wynne EJ, Handley-Ashken M. The use of the omental pedicle graft in the repair and reconstruction of the urinary tract. *Br J Surg.* 1967;54(10):849.
15. Turner-Warwick RT, Chapple C. The value and principles of omentoplasty and omental inter-position. In: Turner Warwick RT, Chapple C, eds. *Functional Reconstruction of the Urinary Tract and Gynaeco-Urology: An Exposition of Functional Principles and Surgical Procedures.* Oxford, UK: Blackwell; 2001:155.

CHAPTER 20 ■ LASERS IN PLASTIC SURGERY

DAVID W. LOW

The public is fascinated by high technology, and laser therapy has been, and continues to be, at least partially misrepresented as "state-of-the-art" treatment for a variety of conditions, most of them cosmetic in nature. **Often described as painless, and exaggerated as producing perfect results, lasers have been misused as a marketing tool to lure patients away from conventional low-tech techniques that can often produce equivalent results at significantly lower cost.** On the other hand, some conditions, such as port-wine stains, are best treated by laser, and the standard of care demands familiarity with this treatment modality.

The modern plastic surgeon faces the dilemma of trying to sort out which lasers are best for which conditions, which manufacturers' claims are realistic or incredible, and, ultimately, which lasers are the safest investment in a rapidly changing world of high-tech solutions to a variety of reconstructive and cosmetic problems.

This chapter is a basic introduction to laser technology, laser tissue interactions, and examples of what conditions are appropriate for laser treatment with currently available laser technology. Laser safety, discussed at the end of the chapter, is an important consideration for both the patient and the treating physician.

LASER PHYSICS

How Laser Light Is Produced

Leonard "Bones" McCoy, chief medical officer of the television show *Star Trek*'s *USS Enterprise* would have been quick to concede that he was a doctor, not physicist. Fortunately for the 21st-century physician, only a basic understanding of light energy is necessary to understand lasers. Light energy can be described as either a series of particles (photons) or as a wave phenomenon. **The color of light is determined by the distance between two successive waves (the wavelength, usually measured in nanometers).** The speed of light is always 186,000 miles per second, or nearly 300,000,000 meters per second.

A molecule or atom in its resting state is composed of a nucleus and circulating electrons. If energy is added to the system, the electrons become excited and circulate at a higher orbit. Eventually an excited electron will fall back to its resting orbit, releasing a specific packet of energy—a photon. A photon has a wavelength specific to that molecule. Because some molecules have more than one excited orbit, the light emitted may have more than one wavelength. If a photon collides with an excited electron, that electron falls back to its resting orbit, releasing another photon. The two photons are *in phase*, meaning their wave patterns are synchronized and reinforce each other. As these photons hit other excited electrons, more photons are released and the light energy increases (Fig. 20.1).

A laser tube has a mirror at each end and contains a solid, liquid, or gas medium whose electrons are in a resting state. As energy is added to the system, the majority of the electrons become excited (*population inversion*) and begin releasing photons. Only those photons that hit the mirrors directly are reflected back into the lasing medium, creating an increasing number of photons that travel back and forth between the mirrors, parallel to the tube. Because the photons are in phase, the intensity of the light increases in the tube. **This phenomenon has been described as *light amplification by the stimulated emission of radiation*, or the more familiar term *LASER*.** To allow light to escape from the tube, one mirror is only partially reflecting. The emitted light is *coherent*; that is, it is in phase, parallel, and in most cases monochromatic. In contrast, incandescent light is *noncoherent*, meaning it has many wavelengths and is not parallel.

Light energy can be visible or invisible depending on its wavelength. The spectrum of electromagnetic radiation ranges from long radio waves (wavelength >10 cm) to extremely short γ rays ($<10^{-11}$ m). The entire spectrum includes radio, microwave, infrared, visible (400 to 700 nm), ultraviolet, X-ray, and γ rays.

Types of Lasers

The laser tube contains either a gas, liquid, or solid lasing medium (Table 20.1). New lasers are constantly being invented and promoted to the medical community. The first laser used a synthetic ruby rod (1960). Other solid lasers include copper vapor and yttrium aluminum garnet (YAG). The YAG crystal contains either neodymium or erbium ions, each with its own specific wavelength and tissue interactions. In a dye laser, the medium is a solution of a fluorescent dye in a solvent such as methanol. Organic rhodamine dye is used in the yellow dye laser and, although the earlier dye lasers had adjustable (tunable) wavelengths ranging from yellow to red, currently available dye lasers offer single wavelength light energy. In a helium-neon laser, it is a mixture of the gases helium and neon. In a diode laser, it is a thin layer of semiconductor material sandwiched between other semiconductor layers. Excimer lasers (the name is derived from the terms *excited* and *dimers*) use reactive gases, such as chlorine and fluorine, mixed with inert gases such as argon, krypton, and xenon. When electrically stimulated, a pseudomolecule (dimer) produces light in the ultraviolet range.

Laser–Tissue Interactions

When the laser strikes an object, a variety of desirable and undesirable effects result as the light is *reflected, scattered, transmitted*, or *absorbed*. A series of reflecting mirrors directs CO_2

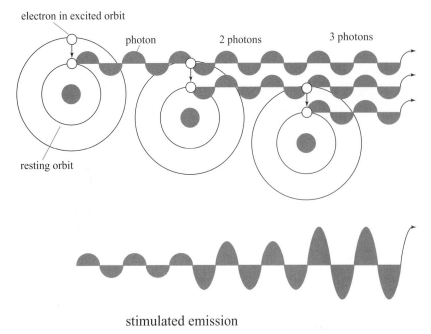

electron in excited orbit

photon   2 photons   3 photons

resting orbit

stimulated emission

FIGURE 20.1. Photons. A photon is released when an excited electron falls back into its resting orbit. If the photon strikes another excited electron, a second photon is released. The stimulated emission of multiple photons produces light of increasing intensity.

laser light to the handpiece, but reflected CO_2 light off of a shiny surgical instrument is hazardous. The risk of inadvertent light reflection can be reduced by using ebonized instruments. The dull finish scatters laser light, diffusing the concentrated energy beam. Glass and clear liquids will transmit some types of laser light, allowing photocoagulation through glass slides, the vitreous of the eye, and through water. Some lasers will also pass through the epidermis, allowing the energy to reach dermal vessels and pigment without disrupting the epidermal layer. **It is the absorbed light that causes desirable or undesirable biologic effects. Except for the excimer lasers, which break chemical bonds, most laser energy is converted to thermal (heat) energy.** Depending on the rate of tissue heating, surgical effects include *welding, coagulation, protein denaturation, dessication,* and *vaporization.* Some lasers will indiscriminately target living tissue, whereas other lasers will semiselectively target a specific chromophore such as oxyhemoglobin. *Selective photothermolysis* describes the ability of lasers to target dermal blood vessels without harming the surrounding dermis or the

overlying epidermis as the oxyhemoglobin in the blood absorbs the light energy. It is generally safer to deliver cutaneous laser light in pulses rather than as a continuous beam, as the interval between pulses allows the tissue to cool before the heat is transferred to the surrounding dermis. Pulsed lasers respect the *thermal relaxation time* of dermal vessels (the time to dissipate the heat absorbed during a laser pulse).

Ablative Lasers

Lasers that nonspecifically destroy tissue can be used to remove skin lesions or layers of skin, usually with minimal blood loss because the dermal vessels are coagulated as the tissue is vaporized. CO_2 laser light is absorbed by intracellular water, which vaporizes tissue as the water turns to steam.

Vascular Lesion Lasers

Oxyhemoglobin absorbs green and yellow light, spawning a variety of lasers appropriate for treating dermal vessels.

TABLE 20.1

LASERS WITH PLASTIC SURGERY APPLICATIONS

	Name	Wavelength (nm)	Target chromophore
Solid	Ruby	694	Melanin, tattoo pigment
	Neodymium:YAG	1064	Pigment
	KTP (potassium titanyl phosphate)	532	Oxyhemoglobin, melanin
	Erbium:YAG	2940	Water
	Diode	800	Melanin (oxyhemoglobin)
	Alexandrite	755	Melanin, tattoo pigment
	Copper vapor	578	Oxyhemoglobin
Liquid	Yellow dye	585	Oxyhemoglobin
	Yellow dye	595	Oxyhemoglobin
	Green dye	510	Melanin
Gas	Argon	488, 514	Oxyhemoglobin, melanin
	Helium:Neon	633	
	Carbon dioxide	10,600	Water
	Excimer	Ultraviolet	Breaks chemical bonds

Historically the argon (blue/green) laser was the first clinically useful laser, but yellow light has become the preferred color (oxyhemoglobin absorption peaks at 577 nm yellow light), with the pulsed yellow dye laser (intentionally adjusted to 585 nm and 595 nm for greater dermal penetration) the most popular type. The high-energy/short-duration pulse causes vascular disruption as the blood rapidly heats up and expands. The KTP laser (532 nm; green light) also targets oxyhemoglobin, but the pulses are much longer in duration, and tend to coagulate rather than disrupt vessels.

Pigmented Lesion Lasers

Pigmented lesion lasers target melanin. Benign pigmented lesions, such as lentigines, café-au-lait spots, melasma, and nevi of Ota or Ito, may improve with a series of laser treatments. Congenital nevi will also lighten with laser therapy, but this use of laser is controversial. Although it is unlikely that laser will increase the risk of malignant transformation, it may delay the diagnosis of a changing nevus by masking the color change associated with a melanoma.

Photodynamic Therapy

The use of light-activated drugs to treat acne and other skin conditions currently is best represented by Levulan (topical 5-aminolevulinic acid; DUSA Pharmaceuticals). The compound is metabolized by sebaceous glands into porphyrins. The acne bacteria itself also produces porphyrin, and the use of blue, green, or red light stimulates the production of oxygen free radicals that destroy the bacteria and suppress sebaceous gland activity. Levulan photodynamic therapy has also been used for actinic keratoses and may be useful for treating sebaceous nevi (1,2).

Nonlaser Phototherapy

Intense pulsed light is not actually laser light. Xenon flashlamps generate multiwavelength noncoherent light that is partially modulated by a series of filters. Intense pulsed light is used for sun-related pigmentary changes, telangiectasias, and for hair removal.

Radiofrequency uses radio waves to heat the collagen of the dermis and subdermis. It is thought to cause collagen contraction and stimulation of new collagen production. It has been promoted as a noninvasive, nonablative treatment for skin laxity. Marketed as a "nonsurgical facelift," current results are far less impressive and less predictable than surgical skin tightening. Time and experience will determine proper patient selection and realistic expectations with this new technology.

SPECIFIC LASER TREATMENTS

Table 20.2 lists clinically useful lasers and other phototherapy devices.

Vascular Lesions

Hemangiomas

Hemangiomas are the most common benign tumor of infancy, and at least 60% occur in the head and neck region (see Chapter 22). Although an estimated 70% of hemangiomas regress satisfactorily, 30% of patients have cosmetically significant deformities. Parents eagerly seek treatment options on a proactive basis, and the laser is a potentially useful option in several settings. The pulsed yellow dye laser may be useful for very early hemangiomas, ulcerated hemangiomas, and regressed he-

TABLE 20.2

CLINICALLY USEFUL LASERS AND OTHER PHOTOTHERAPY DEVICES

Vascular lesions	Yellow dye
	KTP
	Nd:YAG
	Copper vapor
	Intense pulsed light
Skin resurfacing	Carbon dioxide
	Erbium:YAG
	Radiofrequency
Benign lesions, pigmented	Intense pulsed light
	Diode
	Ruby
Benign lesions, cutaneous	Carbon dioxide
Hair removal	Alexandrite
	Diode
	Neodymium:YAG
	Ruby
	Intense pulsed light
Tattoo removal	Ruby
	Alexandrite
	Neodymium:YAG

mangiomas that still contain vascular pigmentation or visible ectatic vessels. The laser only penetrates about 1 mm into the skin, making it most effective for small, flat hemangiomas. Parents should be advised that multiple laser treatments may be necessary every 2 to 4 weeks, as hemangiomas often exhibit temporary regression followed by rebound growth. Laser therapy can be discontinued when the hemangioma finally enters a permanent state of regression. Topical application of anesthetic cream may be desirable to reduce both patient and parent discomfort. **Laser treatments are ineffective for already bulky or subcutaneous hemangiomas, as the light will not penetrate deeply enough to produce a noticeable improvement.**

Ulcerated hemangiomas can be excruciatingly painful, especially when located in the perineal region. There has been some success with pulsed yellow dye laser treatment of these hemangiomas, with some babies showing significant pain relief within 24 to 48 hours, probably as a result of coagulation of the sensitive nerve endings within the wound. Faster healing has also been reported, although the mechanism for this observation is unclear. Perhaps the laser induces some regression of the hemangioma, or wound care is facilitated once the area becomes less sensitive, allowing for more rapid re-epithelialization.

Lastly, hemangiomas that have regressed well enough to avoid the need for surgical excision may have residual ectatic vessels that will improve with pulsed dye laser therapy (Fig. 20.2). Larger telangiectasias may also respond to simultaneous sclerotherapy and laser treatment. Endothelial injury from the sclerosant followed by laser photocoagulation of the vessels may have a synergistic benefit in removing these residual vessels.

Capillary Vascular Malformations

Port-wine stains tend to darken with age as the dilated dermal capillaries and venules enlarge with time. The involved area may also show textural changes and soft-tissue hypertrophy, and hyperplastic vascular nodules (pyogenic granulomas) may develop, with problematic bleeding. The pulsed dye laser (585 or 595 nm) is the treatment of choice. Children respond better than teenagers and adults, and treatment can be offered beginning in infancy. **Parents should be advised that multiple (at**

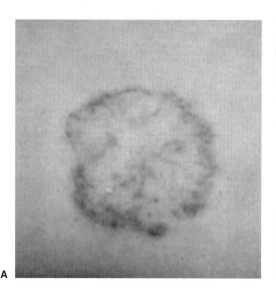
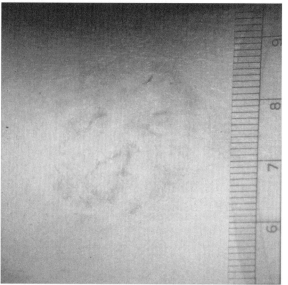

FIGURE 20.2. A: Hemangiomas. Hemangiomas may leave residual ectatic vessels, similar to telangiectasias and spiders veins. Laser treatment is usually reserved for hemangiomas that have not fully regressed by age 5 years, but can be given at an earlier age in an attempt to speed natural involution. **B:** Pulsed dye lasers and other vascular lesion lasers may significantly lighten the residual vascular pigmentation. Multiple laser sessions may be necessary for optimal results.

least six to eight) treatments are recommended for cumulative benefit, and that it is extremely rare for any capillary vascular malformation to completely disappear. Associated bruising from the laser lasts for about 2 weeks, and gradual lightening of the vascular pigmentation may continue for at least 2 months. Patients can be treated every 2 to 3 months. Although topical anesthetic cream can be very useful on the trunk and extremities, and for small areas of the face, most children with large, facial port-wine stains will be better treated under a general anesthetic (Fig. 20.3). Metal eye shields are available for periorbital laser therapy, and placement directly on the globe allows laser treatment of the eyelid skin. The eyelashes and eyebrows can be shielded by strategic placement of the wrapper of an alcohol wipe, to avoid undesirable singeing of the hairs.

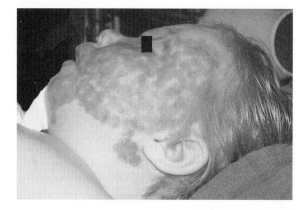

FIGURE 20.3. Port-wine stains. The pulsed yellow dye laser remains the laser of choice for pediatric capillary vascular malformations (port-wine stains), and parents should be advised of significant temporary bruising that will occur, as in this child immediately after laser treatment. Although anesthetic creams and cooling devices dramatically decrease the discomfort associated with laser treatment, general anesthesia may be preferable in the setting of large facial malformations.

Venous Malformations

Venous malformations consist of dilated clusters of varicose veins, and treatment options include laser photocoagulation, sclerotherapy, and surgical debulking. Small superficial veins may improve with pulsed dye laser therapy, but usually the energy pulse is too brief and the vessels are too large to show significant benefit. Longer energy delivery with a continuous wave laser, such as the KTP or neodymium:YAG laser, can result in significant heat absorption and vascular destruction, with a significant shrinkage in the size of the malformation. In this setting, although the target chromophore is still oxyhemoglobin, the prolonged energy delivery probably achieves its effect by nonspecific heat delivery to all tissue in the area, and the risk of postlaser scarring is higher. For this reason, the lips and oral mucosa are more forgiving areas when continuous laser energy is used. For other areas of the body, or if the physician wants to avoid excessive energy delivery to the surface layer, the fiberoptic tip can be passed intralesionally for deep coagulation. With the KTP laser, the glass tip can be placed directly on the mucosa, and a brief pulse will create a small hole through which the laser can be passed transmucosally to the heart of the malformation. In other areas, a large-gauge hypodermic needle can be used to penetrate and protect the skin while passing the laser fiber (Fig. 20.4). The physician must understand that this technique is highly operator dependent and somewhat blind. A high level of concentration is necessary, with constant verification of the location of the tip of the fiber by palpation or transillumination of the light, to decrease the risk of lasing too superficially or perforating the overlying intact skin (3).

Large venous malformations can by debulked by standard surgical techniques or by using the fiber of a KTP or neodymium:YAG laser as a contact-tip laser scalpel.

Lymphatic Malformations

Cutaneous vesicles resembling tiny water blisters represent the dermal component of a lymphatic malformation, which is usually associated with a more extensive subcutaneous

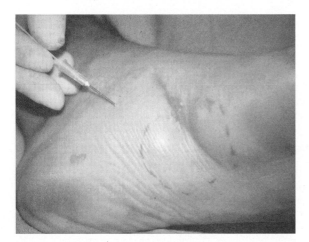

FIGURE 20.4. Venous malformations. Venous malformations can be photocoagulated using a laser fiber passed percutaneously through a hypodermic needle.

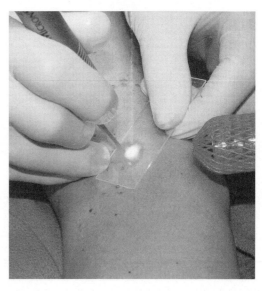

FIGURE 20.5. Venolymphatic malformations. Venolymphatic malformations often have cutaneous involvement characterized by dermal lymphatic vesicles and crusting scabs (angiokeratomas). Bleeding lesions can be compressed with a glass slide and coagulated with a vascular lesion laser such as the KTP laser.

component. Problematic lymphatic oozing from ulcerated vesicles can be palliatively treated with the CO_2 laser, which is absorbed by water. The heat of the absorbed laser energy may cause a desirable fibrosis of the dermis at the site of leaking lymphatic cisterns, in a sense "capping the well." The treatment is palliative rather than curative, but can be easily repeated for unresectable lesions.

Venolymphatic Malformations

Similar to lymphatic malformations, but associated with an additional venous component, the cutaneous component may present as tiny purple vesicles or crusting scabs (angiokeratomas). This is commonly seen in Klippel-Trenaunay syndrome (patchy capillary malformation with an underlying venolymphatic malformation and hypertrophy of the involved extremity). Because the vesicles tend to be more responsive to coagulation by a continuous rather than a pulsed laser, the KTP laser is more effective than the pulsed yellow dye laser. Crusting lesions can be tangentially shaved, then compressed with a glass slide to control bleeding while being lased (Fig. 20.5). Longstanding large crusted lesions may be more efficiently excised and oversewn. Because the cutaneous lesions overlie a much more extensive subcutaneous component, treatment is purely palliative and reoccurrence is to be expected.

Telangiectasias and Rosacea

Commonly called "broken blood vessels" by the lay public, telangiectasias represent undulating dilated dermal vessels that course through the dermal layer. They appear discontinuous because they are visible near the surface, and then disappear as they dive into the deeper dermis. Associated with accumulated ultraviolet (UV) damage or rosacea, they respond to a variety of vascular lesion lasers [4]. Smaller telangiectasias also respond to intense pulsed light therapy. Multiple treatment sessions are necessary for optimal results, and adult patients should be aware of the significant prolonged bruising (2 to 3 weeks) that can be associated with certain lasers and laser settings.

Pyogenic Granulomas

Pyogenic granulomas are shiny nodules of proliferative vascular tissue covered by a fragile epidermal layer (lobular capillary hemangioma) that have an annoying propensity to bleed when ulcerated. Commonly occurring in children and in pregnant

women, they can occur at any age, and may be the result of minor trauma. Although surgical excision is curative, tangential shave excision followed by laser photocoagulation of the dermal base often leaves an inconspicuous scar. A glass slide can be used to compress the bleeding base, and a continuous laser, such as the KTP laser, will pass through the glass and coagulate the residual proliferative lesion [5]. Although the pulsed dye laser alone has been reported as a treatment option, multiple laser sessions may be necessary for large lesions, and no specimen is available for pathologic confirmation.

Spider Angiomas

These superficial vascular lesions are characterized by a central feeding arteriole and radiating branches. Compression of the skin blanches the lesion, which will readily reappear at the center and expand outward after the pressure is released. Although small angiomas can be successfully treated by destroying the central feeding vessel by electric cautery, longstanding angiomas often have a persistent peripheral blush. The pulsed yellow dye laser is an excellent way to coagulate the entire lesion. The central feeding vessel may require a series of stacked pulses to destroy it, and it should appear black at the end of the treatment session. Patients should be aware that reoccurrence may require more than one treatment.

Cherry Angiomas

Also known as senile angiomas, these superficial macular or papular cherry-colored nodules are commonly seen on adult skin. They may range in size from punctuate lesions to several millimeters. Any of the vascular lesion lasers can be used to destroy them.

Spider Veins and Varicose Veins

Dilated leg spider veins may respond to a variety of lasers, but it is usually most efficient to remove the larger varicose veins first. Traditionally, a varicose greater saphenous vein is best treated by stripping and ligation whereas other varicose veins and large spider veins respond to sclerotherapy. There are recent reports of endovenous laser therapy using an

810-nm diode laser with a bare fiber for varicose veins. Short-term follow up is comparable in success to venous stripping and ligation, but the procedure is too recent to determine its efficacy over long-term results (6).

Pulsed dye laser (595 nm) or diode laser (800 nm) light will penetrate into the deep dermis to treat residual spiders veins as well as the peripheral blush that is often seen after sclerosis of the larger vessels. Laser treatment requires photocoagulation along the entire course of the vessel for best results, which is why patients with extensive spiders veins may be more efficiently treated initially by sclerotherapy.

Adenoma Sebaceum and Tuberous Sclerosis

Patients with tuberous sclerosis will develop firm pink nodules in a butterfly pattern across their cheeks and nose, with additional involvement of their chins and foreheads. Neither adenomatous nor sebaceous, these lesions are more accurately called angiofibromas. Although theoretically photocoagulation with a vascular lesion laser should improve these dermal lesions, vaporization with a defocused CO_2 laser appears to be much more efficient and effective in improving the skin surface contour. The heat of the laser coagulates the exposed dermis, making the procedure virtually bloodless, in contrast to dermabrasion or shave excision. Retreatment for recurrent nodules is common and easily repeated.

Pigmented Lesions

Because melanin absorbs light in the ultraviolet to near infrared range, a wide variety of lasers have been used to target benign melanocytic lesions. Blue, green, red, and infrared wavelengths have been used. Although, historically, continuous wave lasers, such as argon lasers, were initially useful, pulsed lasers are safer and less likely to cause scarring. Shorter wavelengths will treat epidermal pigmentation, whereas longer wavelengths are more effective for dermal pigmentation (7). Epidermal lesions such as freckles (ephelides), solar lentigines, and labial melanocytic macules may respond to green pulsed dye (510 nm), KTP, and frequency-doubled YAG laser (532 nm), while deeper dermal pigmented lesions such as café-au-lait spots, nevi of Ota (melanocytic pigmentation in the V1 and V2 distribution), and nevi of Ito (shoulder or upper arm distribution) may respond to longer wavelength ruby (694 nm), alexandrite (755 nm), and diode (800 nm) lasers.

Skin Lesions

Neurofibromatosis

Large plexiform neurofibromas should be excised or debulked by standard surgical techniques, but patients who request removal of hundreds of small neurofibromas may be well served by CO_2 laser destruction or excision. In a slightly defocused mode, the laser can vaporize and coagulate small neurofibromas. Large sessile or pedunculated neurofibromas can be readily excised with minimal bleeding by vaporizing a ring of skin around the base of the lesions with a focused beam, then amputating the subcutaneous tumor with a defocused beam to achieve better coagulation. Small excision ulcers can be left to heal spontaneously, while larger wounds can be loosely closed with a couple of monofilament sutures. Patients should be reminded the treatment is palliative.

Syringomas and Cylindromas

Syringomas are benign tumors of eccrine origin, most commonly found in the periorbital area. CO_2 laser vaporization results in rapid obliteration of these lesions, often without recurrence. Cylindromas are nodular dermal benign tumors thought to be of primitive sweat gland origin; an autosomal dominant inheritance pattern is associated with multiple cylindromas. Large disfiguring nodules involving the face and scalp (so-called turban tumor) can be excised or vaporized with the CO_2 laser to reduce associated operative blood loss. The procedure is only palliative.

Actinic Keratosis

Patients with extensive actinic changes of their facial skin or lower lip are candidates for laser skin resurfacing. This may be better tolerated than topical 5-fluorouracil therapy or a surgical lower-lip vermilion shave. The CO_2 laser can readily vaporize the epidermis and papillary dermis, allowing the regeneration of healthier skin. The laser will also readily vaporize the vermilion of the lower lip, which heals remarkably well in 2 to 3 weeks. Although painful until the vermilion mucosa regenerates, it avoids the need for a mucosal advancement flap.

Verruca Vulgaris

Wart removal consists of a long list of treatment modalities with variable rates of success, and most surgical strategies involve reduction of the viral burden by excision or destruction of the affected skin. The CO_2 laser is most commonly used to vaporize the involved area, particularly when there are multiple lesions that may make surgical excision difficult or undesirable. To reduce the risk of viral transmission to medical personnel, it is advisable to sharply excise the bulk of the lesion, and then vaporize the base. A viral mask for all participants (including the patient) and use of a plume evacuator is mandatory to minimize the possibility of inoculation of the bronchial tree. For small warts, some success has also been associated with the pulsed dye laser. Presumably energy delivery to the dermis layer either sterilizes it or makes the local environment inhospitable for the wart virus.

Sebaceous Nevi (Nevus Sebaceus of Jadassohn)

This congenital nevus is usually excised when it is located in the hair-bearing scalp because of the 15% risk of basal cell transformation in adulthood. Additionally, the nevus is characteristically non–hair-bearing, and it may become more cosmetically annoying during puberty with stimulation of the sebaceous glands. However, sebaceous nevi on the face may leave a cosmetically disfiguring scar if excised. Superficial laser vaporization with the CO_2 laser may offer surface textural improvement. More recently, the use of photodynamic therapy with Levulan (topical 5-aminolevulinic acid) and laser activation has been shown to suppress sebaceous gland activity in acne, and may have applicability in suppression of sebaceous nevi (2).

Epidermal Nevi

Epidermal nevi, while possessing no significant malignant risk, can cause severe disfigurement as the nevi thicken and create a verrucous surface texture. Palliative options include tangential shave excision, dermabrasion, and full-thickness excision, but CO_2 laser vaporization may provide a fast and clean way to improve the surface texture with minimal bleeding. For relatively thin but raised epidermal nevi, the laser appears to vaporize the nevus along a clean and consistent dermal plane. Thicker nevi may require multiple laser passes, and extensively verrucous lesions seem to lack a clear cleavage plane with less satisfying surface uniformity. Wounds are covered with topical antibiotic ointment and are left to re-epithelialize. Patients must understand that this treatment is usually not curative and future treatment sessions may be desirable for recurrent skin thickening.

Cosmetic Conditions

Wrinkles

Wrinkles (or rhytids) are also discussed in Chapter 44. The cosmetic and financial benefits of the CO_2 laser drew many plastic surgeons into the field of laser surgery for the first time, and it was instrumental in the development of comprehensive skin care programs to provide preoperative preparation and postoperative management of patients undergoing laser skin resurfacing. **Although dermabrasion and chemical peels can often achieve the same results at significantly lower cost, the public's fascination with high-tech therapy created a high demand for lasers, and equally high expectations of wrinkle removal and skin tightening.** While all three methods remove epidermis and papillary dermis, stimulating formation of new collagen and rejuvenated superficial skin layers, the dermal contraction visible with multiple laser passes suggested that the skin was actually tightening as the dermal collagen contracted because of the heat generated by the laser. **Much of the immediate effect is more likely a result of the water evaporation caused by the laser, and the ultimate effect is similar to the healing response to dermabrasion or acid penetration.** However, one advantage to laser skin resurfacing is that the treatment is almost blood-free, because the heat of the laser coagulates the dermal vessels. This permits accurate assessment of the depth of penetration as the pink papillary dermis eventually gives way to a yellow "chamois" reticular dermis, which is the end point of therapy. Additionally, the laser handpiece may offer more uniform skin ablation compared with a dermabrasion burr or topically applied acid.

Pre-treatment with 1 month of retinoic acid and hydroquinone bleaching cream is common, supposedly to stimulate faster healing and avoid postlaser hyperpigmentation. It is also common to prophylax against a herpes infection with peri-operative antiviral medication such as Valtrex (valacyclovir, GlaxoSmithKline) when treating the perioral area, to avoid potentially significant scarring.

The skin takes about 2 weeks to re-epithelialize and erythema may persist for many months following CO_2 laser skin resurfacing. Patients should be advised that complete wrinkle removal is not possible, but wrinkle softening is a realistic goal (Fig. 20.6).

Erbium:YAG laser light has an even greater affinity for water, thus the depth of penetration is even more shallow than with the CO_2 laser. The short-pulse erbium:YAG laser was initially promoted as superior to the CO_2 laser because of faster healing and less postoperative erythema. However, the results were generally less impressive because of the reduced penetration. More aggressive use of the erbium:YAG laser with longer pulses can achieve results comparable to the CO_2 laser (8).

Patients are more reluctant to endure the prolonged recovery time associated with ablative laser skin resurfacing, and the new generation of nonablative lasers has encouraged many patients to accept a lesser result in exchange for decreased downtime. Resurfacing techniques are covered in more detail in Chapter 44.

Acne Scars and Active Acne

The treatment of active acne by lasers is generally confined to the field of dermatology, and reports of significant improvement with Levulan and photodynamic therapy, and with blue light therapy are related to destruction of Propiorbacterium acne (p. acne).

Lentigines

Benign pigmented lesions associated with sun exposure and freckles will respond to a wide range of wavelengths. Green light lasers (510 nm pulsed dye laser; 532 nm KTP laser), diode lasers (800 nm), and nonlaser intense pulsed light will

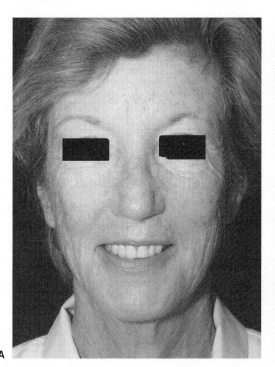
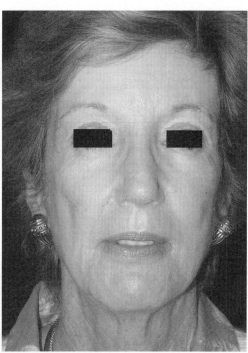

FIGURE 20.6. A, B: Laser skin resurfacing. Significant photodamage can be improved with laser skin resurfacing. The carbon dioxide laser removes the epidermis and papillary dermis, resulting in pigmentary and textural improvement. Wrinkles and actinic changes can be dramatically improved, but at the cost of a significant recovery period.

lighten melanocytic pigmentation. These lasers will also lighten melanocytic nevi, and clinical discretion must always be exercised when deciding which lesions can be safely lased and which deserve biopsy prior to laser treatment.

Hair Removal

The basic principle of laser hair removal is to use light energy to destroy the hair root for permanent hair reduction (9). This requires a deeply penetrating wavelength that must reach the dermal papilla without adversely destroying the surrounding dermis. **Most hair-removal lasers target melanin, and deeply penetrating lasers such as the diode (800 nm), alexandrite (755 nm), and YAG (1064 nm) lasers are most effective on patients with dark hair and fair skin.** Patients with light or gray hair are poor candidates for these lasers, even with efforts to darken the hairs with carbon particles. Intense pulsed light, with its range of wavelengths (510 to 1200 nm) has been promoted as a useful method of hair reduction for patients with fair hair (10).

Patients should be advised that multiple treatment sessions are the routine, and that hair removal is not necessarily permanent. Hair reduction and delayed hair regrowth are more realistic goals than complete hair removal.

Tattoo Removal

Tattoos are created by pigment or foreign matter that is imbedded in the dermis layer of the skin, intentionally in the case of decorative tattoos, therapeutically in the case of radiation marking or nipple/and areola reconstruction, and traumatically in the case of road rash. Historically, the tattoos have been removed by abrasion of the skin, until the deepest pigment has been removed. This routinely leaves shiny, atrophic scars at best, and hypertrophic or keloid scars in unfavorable areas. **The CO_2 laser is simply a high-tech method of dermabrasion, and offers little advantage over mechanical dermabrasion.** The advent of Q-switched ruby, YAG, and alexandrite lasers offers the possibility of tattoo removal without clinically apparent scarring. Pigment granules are fragmented into smaller particles that are phagocytized by macrophages.

Black ink is the most common color in tattoos, followed by blue, green, red, yellow, and orange. Additional colors, such as pink, brown, purple, and fluorescent colors, make tattoo removal by a single laser more difficult, as a particular color may reflect rather than absorb the laser light. For example, red tattoos will reflect ruby laser light (694 nm) but will absorb wavelengths below 575 nm. The Q-switched YAG laser (1064 nm) has a frequency-doubling KTP crystal, which emits green light at 532 nm, thereby making it effective for red tattoos.

Black and blue ink is well-absorbed at all wavelengths, and is effectively treated by the ruby, YAG, and alexandrite laser. The alexandrite laser is also good for green pigment. The 510-nm flashlamp-pulsed dye laser was originally developed to treat melanocytic lesions, but the short-pulse width (300 nanoseconds) has the capability to fragment pigment granules, and is effective for red, purple, orange, and yellow pigments.

Patients should be advised that multiple treatment sessions are necessary, scarring may occur, colors may not lighten sufficiently, and colors that contain iron oxide pigments (such as flesh tones) might paradoxically darken to black as a result of the extreme temperatures generated by the Q-switched lasers (11). Additionally, gunpowder tattoos may ignite when subjected to the extremely high temperatures of the Q-switched lasers, resulting in thermal burns.

LASER SAFETY

All surgical lasers are considered to be class IV devices—high-power lasers that are hazardous to view under any condition (directly or diffusely scattered), and which are a potential fire and skin hazard (12). The American National Standards Institute requires the laser key to be stored separately from the laser to prevent unauthorized use.

Patients and all personnel present must wear wavelength-specific safety goggles. There should be a limited number of entrances to the laser suite, each marked clearly with a laser warning sign. An extra pair of safety goggles should be left outside the door in areas of high traffic, such as an operating room. Treatment around the eyes may require using corneal eye shields. The patient should be further protected with wet drapes or crumpled aluminum foil (to reduce the risk of reflected laser light) when using the CO_2 laser. A laser-safe endotracheal tube should be used when lasing in or around the oral cavity. The lowest possible fraction of inspired oxygen (FiO_2) should be used to decrease the risk of an inhalation or flash burn. Exhaled oxygen can ignite singed nasal or lip hairs when using the CO_2, pulsed yellow dye, or hair-removal lasers in the setting of enriched oxygen delivery.

Lasers that create significant laser plume, such as the CO_2 laser, should be used with a plume evacuator to prevent potential transmission of live virus particles into the airway of treating personnel. When lasing warts, a viral mask is also highly recommended in addition to the plume evacuator, and the potential viral contamination can be reduced by shaving the bulk of the wart prior to laser vaporization of the base.

Lastly use of an expensive laser to treat conditions outside its capabilities, or exaggeration or falsification of the treatment outcome for monetary gain is unethical and medicolegally dangerous. Patients should have a realistic understanding of the expected results and the risk of treatment, as well as other treatment options.

References

1. Gold MH, Goldman MP. 5-aminolevulinic acid photodynamic therapy: where we have been and where we are going. *Dermatol Surg.* 2004;30(8):1077–1084.
2. Dierickx CC, Goldenhersh M, Dwyer P, et al. Photodynamic therapy for nevus sebaceus with topical delta-aminolevulinic acid. *Arch Dermatol.* 1999;135(6):637–640.
3. Low DW. Management of adult facial vascular anomalies. *Facial Plast Surg.* 2003;19(1):113–130.
4. Tan ST, Bialostocki A, Armstrong JR. Pulsed dye laser therapy for rosacea. *Br J Plast Surg.* 2004;57(4):303–310.
5. Kirschner RE, Low DW. Treatment of pyogenic granuloma by shave excision and laser photocoagulation. *Plast Reconstr Surg.* 1999;104(5):1346–1349.
6. Feied C, Min R, Hashemiyoon RB. Varicose vein treatment with endovenous laser therapy. Available at http://www.emedicine.com/derm/topic750.htm.
7. Grossman MC, Kauvar ANB, Geronemus RG. Cutaneous laser surgery. In: Aston SJ, Beasley RW, Thorne CHM, eds. *Grabb and Smith's Plastic Surgery.* 5th ed. Philadelphia: Lippincott-Raven; 1997.
8. Koch RJ. Laser skin resurfacing. *Otolaryngol Clin North Am.* 2002;35(1):119–133.
9. Sadick NS. Laser hair removal. *Facial Plast Surg Clin North Am.* 2004;12(2):191–200.
10. Dierickx CC. Hair removal by lasers and intense pulsed light sources. *Semin Cutan Med Surg.* 2000;19(4):267–275.
11. Kilmer S. Tattoo lasers. Available at http://www.emedicine.com/derm/topic563.htm.
12. Goldwasser SM. Lasers: safety, diode lasers, helium neon lasers, drive, info, parts—a practical guide for experimenters and hobbyists. 1997. Available at file://C: \ DOCUME~1 \ Dad \ LOCALS~1 \ Temp \ triJNOPLhtm.

PART III ■ CONGENITAL ANOMALIES AND PEDIATRIC PLASTIC SURGERY

CHAPTER 21 ■ EMBRYOLOGY OF THE HEAD AND NECK

ARUN K. GOSAIN AND RANDALL NACAMULI

There are a number of excellent references that describe the embryology of the head and neck in a clinically oriented fashion (1–3). Unfortunately, the average plastic surgeon has a poor understanding of head and neck embryology, and the development of the head and neck in the embryo is often thought of as esoteric and remote from clinical practice. However, an understanding of these concepts gives a rationale to the function of the cranial nerves, principles of craniofacial form, and anomalies of the head and neck that result from aberrations in their development. This chapter collates the established medical references regarding head and neck embryology and presents the essential information as simply as possible so that head and neck embryology can be better used to solve problems that may be encountered in the practice of plastic surgery.

EARLY EMBRYONIC DEVELOPMENT

The cranial end of the human embryo undergoes precocious development beginning in the middle of the third week, at which time the three germ layers in the cranial part of the embryo begin their specific development. This precocious development of the cranial portion of the embryo results in the head constituting nearly 50% of total body length from the fourth to eighth weeks of development. Subsequent development results in the head forming 25% of the body length at birth, but only 6% to 8% of total body length in adulthood. During the fourth week of development, the cranial region of the human embryo resembles a fish embryo at a comparable stage. The term *branchial* is often used to describe the embryonic arches; the root *branchia* is derived from the Greek term for "gill." In fish and amphibians, the branchial apparatus forms a system of gills for gas exchange between water and the organism's blood. While the branchial arches support the gills in lower forms of life, in human embryos the branchial arches develop but no gills form. Consequently, some authors prefer the term *pharyngeal arches,* rather than *branchial arches,* to describe the human embryo. However, the recommendation of Nomina Embryologica (4) is that the term *branchial arch* be used for the human embryo, and the terms in this chapter are consistent with that recommendation.

The three primary germ layers, consisting of ectoderm, mesoderm, and endoderm, serve as a basis for differentiation of the tissues and organs within the developing embryo. The ectoderm gives rise to the cutaneous and neural systems, differentiating into these elements at 20 days. The epidermalizing and neuralizing influences interact along an interface at the crest of the neural fold termed the *neural crest* (Fig. 21.1). Neural crest cells are unique in that, despite their ectodermal origin, they consist of pleopotential ectomesenchymal tissue comparable to the three primary germ layers. Neural crest cells migrate intramesodermally and along cleavage planes between the germ layers. During migration the neural crest cells divide and subsequently differentiate into their final cell type on reaching their predetermined destination. Neural crest derivatives include connective tissue, muscle tissue, nervous tissue, endocrine tissue, and pigment cells.

BRANCHIAL APPARATUS

Early in the fourth week, branchial arches begin to develop from the connective and muscle tissue elements of the neural crest. Differentiation of those neural crest cells that migrate ventrally and caudally is induced by contact with the pharyngeal endoderm. The pharyngeal endoderm and initial mesodermal core surround the six aortic arch arteries. Contact between the pharyngeal endoderm and migrating neural crest cells results in a series of mesenchymal swellings that constitute the branchial arches. The initial mesodermal core of each arch gives rise to muscle myoblasts, while the neural crest cells give rise to skeletal and connective tissues. The paired branchial arches decrease in size from cranial to caudal, with each pair merging midventrally to form "collars" in the cervical region. By the end of the fourth week, the three cranial arches, numbered 1 through 3, are clearly identified on the external aspect of the embryo (Fig. 21.2A). The fourth arch is less distinct but can often be recognized. Although the fifth branchial arch is usually absent, a rudimentary structure may be present with no cartilaginous components. The limits of the sixth branchial arch cannot be defined by external markings, but its derivatives can be clearly traced (Table 21.1).

Each branchial arch contains four essential tissue components (Fig. 21.2C):

1. Cartilage: This is a central rod that gives origin to bony, cartilaginous, and ligamentous structures. It is noteworthy that not all bones that originate from a given arch arise from endochondral ossification of its cartilage precursor. For example, the body and ramus of the mandible, which are derivatives of the first arch, do not form from endochondral ossification of the first arch (Meckel) cartilage, but from direct membranous ossification of the first arch dermal mesenchyme.
2. Aortic arch artery: These arteries course through the pharynx, joining the heart, which is ventrally located, to the aorta, which is dorsally located (Fig. 21.2B).
3. Nerve: These comprise both sensory and motor fibers from the respective cranial nerves.
4. Muscle.

Although anatomically two muscles may be intimately associated in the adult human, innervation may be different; innervation is determined by the embryonic origin of the muscles.

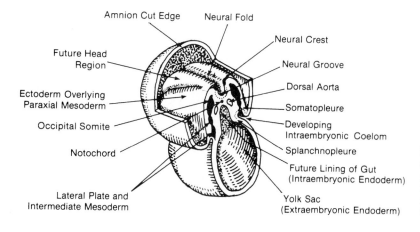

FIGURE 21.1. Transverse section through 20-day-old embryo depicting neural folds and neural crest formation. (Reproduced with permission from Sperber GH. *Craniofacial Embryology,* 4th ed. London: Wright; 1989:19. © 1996 Butterworth Heinemann Publishing Co.)

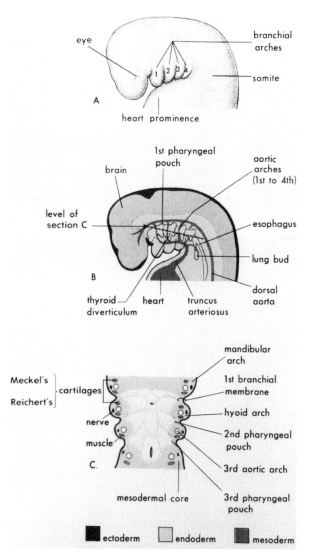

FIGURE 21.2. A: Drawing of the head and neck region of a human embryo (about 28 days), illustrating the branchial apparatus. **B:** Drawing shows the pharyngeal pouches and the aortic arches. **C:** Horizontal section through the embryo showing the floor of the primitive pharynx and illustrating the germ layer of origin of the branchial arch components. (Reproduced with permission from Moore KL, ed. *The Developing Human,* 4th ed. Philadelphia: Saunders; 1988:172.)

Muscles may migrate from their sites of origin, but the original nerve supply to these muscles is maintained during migration. Innervation of the tensor veli palatini and levator veli palatini muscles of the soft palate illustrate this point. Although these are adjacent muscles and they are functionally tethered to one another in patients with cleft palate through the aponeurosis of the tensor tendon (5), the muscles originate from different branchial arches and therefore have different patterns of innervation. The tensor veli palatini arises from the first branchial arch and is innervated by the trigeminal nerve, and the levator veli palatini originates from the fourth branchial arch and is innervated by the superior laryngeal branch of the vagus nerve. Not only does innervation of a muscle reflect its branchial arch of origin, but muscle development and innervation within the branchial arches are closely linked. Nerve fibers enter the mesoderm of the branchial arches and initiate muscle development in the mesoderm. This may explain the observation that in conditions such as Möbius syndrome, in which the facial nerve fails to innervate certain facial muscles, negligible development is noted within the effective muscles (6). Presumably, these muscles lacked the stimulus to develop from arch mesoderm.

The branchial arches are separated by a series of clefts, which are termed *branchial grooves* on their external aspect and *pharyngeal pouches* on their internal aspect (Fig. 21.3A). The lining of the branchial grooves is the surface ectoderm, and the lining of the pharyngeal pouches is the foregut endoderm. The branchial grooves and pharyngeal pouches are separated by a layer of mesodermal mesenchyme, and are numbered to correspond to the arch located immediately cephalad to them. With the exception of the dorsal end of the first branchial groove, all remaining branchial grooves are obliterated during embryonic development. The dorsal end of the first branchial groove deepens to form the external acoustic meatus (Figs. 21.3B, C, and 21.4). The membrane in the depth of the groove forms the tympanic membrane, consisting of ectoderm on its external surface, endoderm on its internal surface, and mesoderm in between.

The second, third, and fourth branchial grooves are obliterated within the cervical sinus, which develops as a result of caudal overgrowth of the second branchial arch. The cervical sinus appears as an ectodermal depression caudal to the third branchial arch. During the fifth week the second branchial arch overgrows the caudal arches, leaving a small opening into the cervical sinus (Fig. 21.5C, D). With continued growth of the second branchial arch structures, the opening into the cervical sinus seals during the sixth week (Fig. 21.5E, F). The second to fourth branchial grooves and the cervical sinus are obliterated by the end of the seventh week, producing a neck with a smooth contour.

Incomplete obliteration of the second, third, or fourth branchial grooves can result in a branchial fistula, sinus, or

TABLE 21.1

BRANCHIAL ARCH DERIVATIVES

Arch	Arch artery	Nerve	Muscles	Cartilage precursors	Skeletal elements	Ligaments	Endodermal pouch
First (mandibular)	Terminal branch of maxillary artery, portion of external carotid artery	Trigeminal[a] (CN V)	Muscles of mastication,[b] anterior belly of digastric, mylohyoid, tensor tympani tensor veli palatini	Maxillary (quadrate) cartilage[c]	→ Greater wing of the sphenoid bone, incus		(D) Auditory tube and middle ear cavity form the tubotympanic recess
				Maxillary prominence[d]	→ Maxilla, zygoma temporal bone (squamous portion)		(V) Obliterated by tongue
				Mandibular (Meckel) cartilage[c]	→ Malleus, mandibular condyles	Anterior ligament of malleus, spheno-mandibular ligament	
				Mandibular prominence[d]	→ Body and ramus of mandible		
Second (hyoid)	Stapedial artery (embryonic). cortico-tympanic artery (adult)	Facial[e] (CN VII)	Muscles of facial expression,[f] posterior belly of digastric, stylohyoid, stapedius	Reichert's cartilage	Stapes, styloid process, lesser cornu of hyoid, upper part of body of the hyoid bone	Stylohyoid ligament	(D) Palatine tonsillar fossa
							(V) Obliterated by tongue
Third	Proximal portion of internal carotid artery, small portion of common carotid artery	Glosso-pharyngeal[g] (CN IX)	Stylopharyngeus	Third arch cartilage	Greater cornu of hyoid, lower part of the hyoid bone		(D) Inferior parathyroid III
							(V) Thymus
Fourth	Arch of aorta (left arch), innominate and right subclavian arteries (right arch), distal part of pulmonary arteries	Superior laryngeal branch of vagus (CN X)	Constrictors of pharynx, cricothyroid, levator veli palatini, palatoglossus[h]	Fourth arch cartilage	Laryngeal cartilages[i]		(D) Superior parathyroid IV
							(V) Lateral thyroid, Vestigial thymus
Fifth and sixth[i]	Proximal part of pulmonary arteries, ductus arteriosus (left arch)	Recurrent laryngeal branch of vagus (CN X)	Intrinsic muscles of larynx (except cricothyroid), striated muscles of esophagus	Sixth arch cartilage	Laryngeal cartilages[i]		5th-Ultimobranchial body or cyst, calcitonin "C" cells
							6th-None

D, dorsal, and V, ventral endodermal pouch derivatives.

[a] Sensory fibers are supplied by all 3 divisions: motor fibers are supplied by the mandibular division.

[b] Temporalis, masseter, medial, and lateral pterygoids.

[c] Skeletal structures consist of endochondral bone, derived from endochondral ossification of cartilaginous precursors.

[d] Skeletal structures consist of membranous bone, derived from direct ossification of arch dermal mesenchyme

[e] Sensory fibers innervate the anterior two-thirds of the tongue.

[f] These muscles include the buccinator, auricularis, fronto-occipitalis, platysma, orbicularis oculi, and orbicularis oris.

[g] Sensory fibers innervate the posterior one-third of the tongue.

[h] Palatopharyngeus and palatoglossus muscles are supplied by the cranial part of CN XI through pharyngeal branch of CN X via pharyngeal plexus.

[i] Thyroid, cuneiform, cricoid, arytenoid, and corniculate cartilages. These form the cartilages of the larynx.

[j] The fifth branchial arch is usually absent. If the arch is present, it is rudimentary with no cartilaginous components.

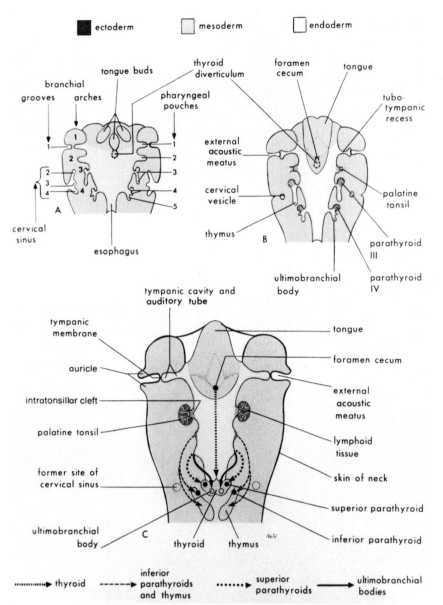

FIGURE 21.3. Schematic horizontal sections at the level shown in Figure 21.5A, illustrating the adult derivatives of the pharyngeal pouches. A: Five weeks. B: Six weeks. C: Seven weeks. Note that the second branchial arch grows over the third and fourth arches, thereby burying the second, third, and fourth branchial grooves in a cervical sinus. Note the migration of the thymus, parathyroid, and thyroid glands into the neck. (Reproduced with permission from Moore KL, ed. *The Developing Human*, 4th ed. Philadelphia: Saunders; 1988:178.)

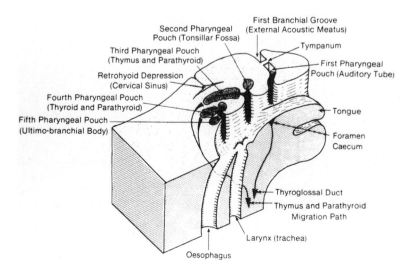

FIGURE 21.4. Schematic of pharyngeal pouch derivatives and their migration paths. (Reproduced with permission from Sperber GH. *Craniofacial Embryology*, 4th ed. London: Wright; 1989:70. © 1996 Butterworth Heinemann Publishing Co.)

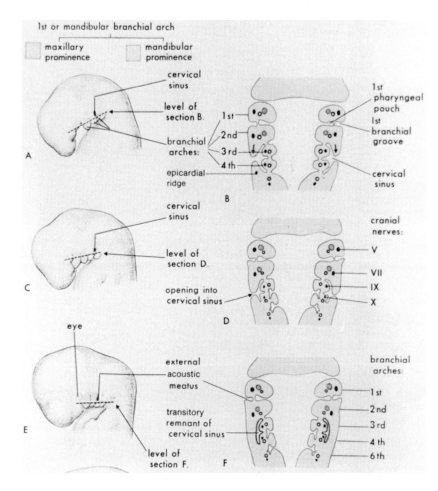

FIGURE 21.5. **A:** Lateral view of the head and neck region of an embryo (about 32 days), showing the branchial arches and the cervical sinus. **B:** Diagrammatic horizontal section through the embryo illustrating the growth of the second branchial arch over the third and fourth arches. **C:** An embryo (about 33 days). **D:** Horizontal section through the embryo, illustrating early closure of the cervical sinus. **E:** An embryo (about 41 days). **F:** Horizontal section through the embryo, showing the transitory cystic remnant of the cervical sinus. (Reproduced with permission from Moore KL, ed. *The Developing Human*, 4th ed. Philadelphia: Saunders; 1988:174.)

cyst, depending on whether the abnormal communication extends completely into the pharynx, ends in a blind sac, or is sealed off within the neck, respectively. Incomplete obliteration is most likely to occur with the second branchial groove, making this the most common source for a fistula, sinus, or cyst. Lining of the abnormal tract or cyst is ciliated or columnar if derived from endoderm of the pharyngeal pouch, or squamous if derived from ectoderm of the branchial groove.

The form and function of the head and neck are determined both by the site of origin of structures from the branchial apparatus and by migration of these structures to their final location. The parathyroid glands illustrate this relationship, as the inferior glands (parathyroid III) form from the dorsal endoderm of the third pharyngeal pouch, and the superior glands (parathyroid IV) form from the dorsal endoderm of the fourth pharyngeal pouch (Figs. 21.3B, C, and 21.4). The parathyroid derivatives of the third pharyngeal pouch migrate further caudally to a final destination located inferior to the parathyroid derivatives of the fourth pharyngeal pouch. Parathyroid III may migrate even further caudally into the upper mediastinum to remain with the thymus, also of third pharyngeal pouch origin. Conversely, congenital absence of the derivatives of the third pharyngeal pouch (thymus and parathyroid glands) can be seen in DiGeorge syndrome, resulting in hypocalcemia and defective cell-mediated immunity in association with other anomalies (6).

Table 21.1 lists the specific derivatives of the branchial arches and the corresponding endodermal (pharyngeal) pouches. We discuss these derivatives further with respect to the specific organ systems with which they are involved.

FACIAL DEVELOPMENT

The branchial arches are largely responsible for the formation of the face, neck, nasal cavities, mouth, larynx, and pharynx. The first branchial arch contributes to the maxillary and mandibular prominences and the anterior portion of the auricle. The paired maxillary and mandibular prominences derived from the first arch form the lateral and caudal borders of the stomodeum (primitive mouth), respectively (Fig. 21.6A, B). The frontonasal prominence, a central process formed by the proliferation of the mesenchyme ventral to the forebrain, forms the cranial boundary of the stomodeum. Although the frontonasal prominence is not a branchial arch derivative, it merges with first arch derivatives to form an integral part of facial development. These five facial prominences (two paired and one unpaired) bordering the stomodeum are responsible for the development of adult facial features (Fig. 21.6E). The quadrate cartilage within the maxillary prominence forms the incus and the greater wing of the sphenoid bone, while the maxilla, zygoma, and squamous portion of the temporal bone form from membranous ossification within the maxillary prominence. Similarly, the Meckel cartilage within the mandibular prominence forms the malleolus and provides a template for development of the mandible. However, only the mandibular condyles develop from endochondral ossification of the Meckel cartilage. The remainder of the cartilage precursor to the mandible serves only as a template for ossification, and is obliterated when the body and ramus of the mandible develop from membranous ossification within the mandibular prominences.

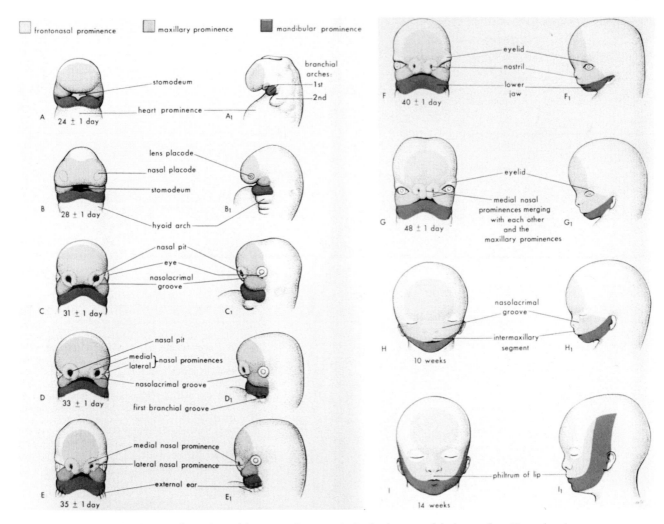

FIGURE 21.6. Illustrations of the progressive stages in the development of the human face. (Reproduced with permission from Moore KL, ed. *The Developing Human*, 4th ed. Philadelphia: Saunders; 1988:190.)

Although the five facial prominences that border the stomodeum are separated externally by grooves, the mesenchyme of all five is continuous. As a consequence, mesenchymal migration can occur freely between the facial prominences. Facial development largely occurs between the fourth and eighth weeks, and the face has a clearly human appearance by age 10 weeks (Fig. 21.6H). Bilateral thickenings of the surface ectoderm, called nasal placodes, develop at the inferior, lateral aspect of the frontonasal prominence by the end of the fourth week (Fig. 21.6B). With further elevation of the margins of the nasal placodes the sides develop into the medial and lateral nasal prominences, respectively, while the depressed central region of the placodes develops into the nasal pit (Fig. 21.6C, D). The nasal pits, initially in contact with the stomodeum, are precursors of the nares. The paired maxillary prominences continue to migrate medially, also affecting medial migration of the medial and lateral nasal prominences. Fusion of the medial nasal, lateral nasal, and maxillary prominences produces continuity between the nose, the upper lip, and the palate (Fig. 21.7).

Fusion of the medial nasal and maxillary prominences results in separation of the nasal pits from the stomodeum and subsequent separation of the oral and nasal cavities. Merging of the medial nasal prominences forms the philtrum and Cupid's bow region of the upper lip, the nasal tip, the premaxilla and primary palate, and the nasal septum (Figs. 21.6G, H, and 21.8B). The lateral nasal prominences form the nasal alae. The nasolacrimal groove develops as a furrow separating

the lateral nasal prominence from the maxillary prominence (Fig. 21.6C, D). Rods of epithelial cells sink into the subjacent mesenchyme to line this groove, which extends from the medial aspect of the developing conjunctival sacs to the external nares. The resultant nasolacrimal duct becomes patent only after birth. Lack of fusion of the lateral nasal and maxillary prominences results in an oblique facial cleft (Fig. 21.9C) or a persistent furrow that tracks the nasolacrimal groove. This is referred to as a number 3 cleft by the Tessier classification (7).

Adult facial form is largely a result of the development of the five facial prominences (Fig. 21.6H, I). Merging of the paired mandibular prominences produces the lower jaw, lower lip, lower cheek, and chin regions of the face. These are the first parts of the face to take on definitive form. The maxillary prominence accounts for the major portion of the upper lip (excluding the philtrum) and the upper cheek regions. The frontonasal prominence forms the forehead and nasal dorsum and the derivatives of the medial and lateral nasal prominences previously discussed.

A unilateral cleft lip results from failure of fusion of the medial nasal prominence and maxillary prominence on one side (Fig. 21.9A). A bilateral cleft lip results from failure of fusion of the merged medial nasal prominences with the maxillary prominence on either side (Fig. 21.9B). As a result, the merged medial nasal prominences (globular process) are often quite prominent, as they are not restrained by attachment to the maxillary prominences laterally. This is manifest at birth, as

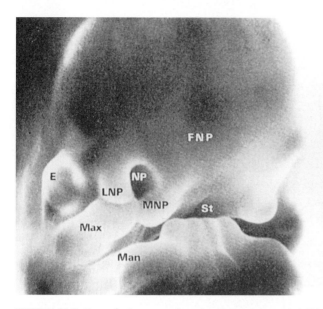

FIGURE 21.7. Face of a human embryo in a late somite period (30–32 days). The frontonasal prominence (*FNP*) projects the medial nasal (*MNP*) and lateral nasal (*LNP*) prominences on each side, surrounding the nasal placode. The eye (*E*) is seen in its lateral position. The maxillary prominence (*Max*) forms the superolateral boundary of the stomodeum (*St*), and the mandibular prominence (*Man*) forms the lower boundary. (Reproduced with permission from Sperber GH. *Craniofacial Embryology*, 4th ed. London: Wright; 1989:38. © 1996 Butterworth Heinemann Publishing Co.)

in a patient with a complete bilateral cleft lip and anterior overprojection of the premaxilla and prolabium.

Laterally, the maxillary and mandibular prominences join at the lateral commissure of the mouth. Failure of union of these prominences produces macrostomia, as a result of a cleft of the lateral commissure (Fig. 21.9F). This is a number 7 facial cleft by the Tessier classification (7). Another rare facial cleft is a median cleft lip (Fig. 21.9D), which is caused by incomplete merging of the medial nasal prominences in the midline and is usually associated with deep midline furrowing of the nose, resulting in various degrees of nasal bifidity. This condition is also described as a number 0 cleft by the Tessier classification (7). Failure of the mandibular prominences to unite in the midline produces a central defect of the lower lip and chin (Fig. 21.9E), which is referred to as a number 30 cleft by the Tessier classification (7).

Early development of the eyes is reminiscent of that of the nose. The eyes begin as bilateral lens placodes at the lateral aspect of the frontonasal prominence (Fig. 21.6B, C). Differentiation of the lens placodes is induced by the optic stalks, or neural connections to the forebrain. Invagination of the lens placodes leads to formation of the optic vesicles. The optic stalks become the optic nerves, the lens placodes become the lenses by way of lens vesicles, and the optic vesicles become the optic cups. Cells of neural crest origin surround the optic cups to form the sclera and choroid over the cups, the ciliary bodies at the margins of the cups, and the cornea over the lenses. From the fifth to ninth weeks, there is significant medial migration of the eyes, with slower medial migration thereafter. The eyelids are formed in the eighth week by folds of surface ectoderm that overgrow the eyes.

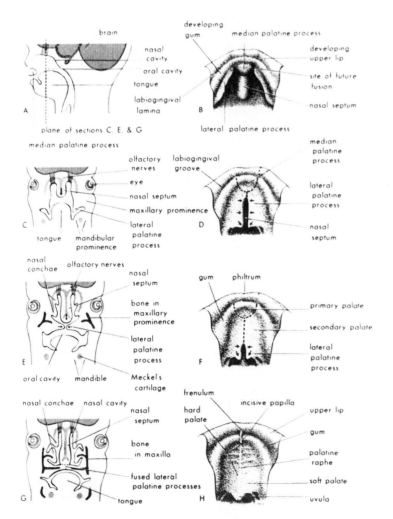

FIGURE 21.8. A: Sketch of a sagittal section of the embryonic head at the end of the sixth week showing the median palatine process, or primary palate. **B, D, F,** and **H:** Drawings of the roof of the mouth from the sixth to twelfth weeks illustrating development of the palate. The *broken lines* in (**D**) and (**F**) indicate sites of fusion of the palatine processes. The *arrows* indicate medial and posterior growth of the lateral palatine processes. **C, E,** and **G:** Drawings of frontal sections of the head illustrating fusion of the lateral palatine processes with each other and the nasal septum, and separation of the nasal and oral cavities. (Reproduced with permission from Moore KL, ed. *The Developing Human*, 4th ed. Philadelphia: Saunders; 1988:196.)

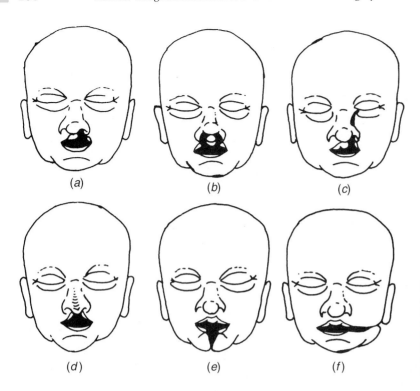

FIGURE 21.9. Defects of orofacial development. **A:** Unilateral cleft lip. **B:** Bilateral cleft lip. **C:** Oblique facial cleft and cleft lip. **D:** Median cleft lip and nasal defect. **E:** Median mandibular cleft. **F:** Unilateral macrostomia. (Reproduced with permission from Sperber GH. *Craniofacial Embryology*, 4th ed. London: Wright; 1989:53. © 1996 Butterworth Heinemann Publishing Co.)

THE PALATE

The palate represents both the frontonasal and maxillary prominences, with the interface between the two becoming the junction between the primary and secondary palates. The median palatine process is derived from the frontonasal prominence and is formed from the merging of the medial nasal prominences (Fig. 21.8B). The lateral palatine processes are derived from the maxillary prominences. All three elements are initially widely separated because of the vertical orientation of the lateral palatine processes, which are located on either side of the tongue (Fig. 21.8B, C). During the eighth week, the orientation of the lateral palatine processes alters from vertical to horizontal to initiate their fusion. This transition occurs within hours, although the exact mechanism for the transition is not well understood. During this process the mandible becomes more prognathic, thereby allowing more room for partitioning of the oronasal chambers without interference by the tongue. The medial edge epithelium of the palatal shelves degenerates in a process referred to as "programmed cell death," permitting mesenchymal coalescence of the palatal shelves. However, the epithelium of the oral and nasal surfaces of the palatal shelves remains intact during this process (Fig. 21.8C–F). Fusion then occurs between the lateral palatine processes and the median palatine process. The nasal septum, a downgrowth from the merged medial nasal prominences, also fuses with the developing palate at its nasal surface (Fig. 21.8E, G). The median palatine process subsequently gives rise to the premaxillary portion of the maxilla and forms the primary palate; the lateral palatine processes give rise to the secondary palate. Ossification occurs in the primary palate and the anterior portion of the secondary palate to form the hard palate, while the posterior portion of the secondary palate does not undergo ossification and remains the soft palate. A palatine raphe can be identified in the adult soft palate, indicating the line of fusion of the lateral palatine processes (Fig. 21.8H).

The embryologic basis of cleft palate is failure of the mesenchymal masses derived either from the maxillary prominences (i.e., the lateral palatine processes) or from the medial nasal prominences (i.e., either the median palatine process or the nasal septum) to meet and fuse with each other. The types of clefts seen in clinical practice help one to better understand the embryologic development of the palate. Clefts of the primary palate occur anterior to the incisive foramen and result from failure of the mesenchymal masses in the lateral palatine processes to fuse with those in the median palatine process. Clefts of the secondary palate occur posterior to the incisive foramen, and result from failure of the mesenchymal masses in the lateral palatine processes to fuse with each other and with the nasal septum. Clefting of either the primary or secondary palate can be complete or incomplete, depending on the degree of fusion that occurred during embryonic development.

Although numerous theories have been proposed for the etiology of clefting, it is believed that delay in elevation of the palatal shelves from vertical to horizontal is part of the underlying mechanism. Pierre Robin sequence, consisting of micrognathia, glossoptosis, and cleft palate, is an excellent illustration of the mechanism thought to occur between the tongue and the palatal shelves. With severe micrognathia, the tongue occupies a relatively greater proportion of the developing oropharynx, resulting in glossoptosis relative to the position of the small mandible. The vertically oriented palatal shelves, located on either side of the tongue (Fig. 21.8C), may be delayed in their transition to a horizontal position during the eighth week of development because of mechanical interference from the tongue. For this reason, Pierre Robin is described as a *sequence* and not a *syndrome*, as it is attributed to the sequence of events that occur during embryonic development (1).

In addition to overt clefts of the palate, anomalies of mesenchymal merging of the palatal shelves can result in a variety of other anomalies. While fusion of the palatal shelves occurs following programmed cell death of the epithelial lining specifically located over their medial edge, there may be cystic degeneration of the epithelial remnants, producing midline palatal microcysts. These are known as Epstein pearls, which are commonly located along the median raphe of the hard palate and at the junction of the hard and soft palates. A nasopalatine duct cyst may occur in the region of the incisive foramen, representing a region of epithelial entrapment at the junction of the developing primary and secondary palates. Although cysts in the soft palate region are rare, submucosal palatal clefts can occur when there is an imperfect muscle union across the velum but an intact mucosal surface (1). Abnormal muscular anatomy may be associated with abnormal velopharyngeal function and subsequent velopharyngeal insufficiency, resulting in hypernasal speech.

THE THYROID GLAND

The thyroid gland produces hormones that function to control body metabolism. It is the first endocrine gland to appear and begins to develop between the fourth and fifth week of fetal life. The thyroid diverticulum develops from an endodermal proliferation of the foramen cecum on the tongue (Figs. 21.3B, C, and 21.4). This diverticulum descends through the neck in front of the hyoid bone and laryngeal cartilages, connected by the thyroglossal duct to the foramen cecum. By the seventh week the diverticulum reaches its final position, distal to the cricoid cartilage, and solidifies to form the two lobes of the thyroid gland. The right and left lateral lobes are connected by an isthmus that lies in front of the trachea at the level of the second and third tracheal rings. The thyroglossal duct has usually degenerated by the seventh week as well. The thyroid becomes functional at the end of the third fetal month, aiding in the control of metabolism by producing the hormones thyroxine and triiodothyronine.

A thyroglossal duct cyst may form anywhere along the path of the thyroid gland as it descends. The duct ordinarily degenerates and disappears but may persist and form a cyst. Approximately 50% of the cysts that form are located inferior to the body of the hyoid bone, but they may also be found at the base of the tongue. A thyroglossal duct cyst usually presents as a painless enlarging midline neck mass. In some instances, the cyst may rupture following an infection and create an opening in the skin termed a thyroglossal duct sinus or fistula. These fistulas may also be present at birth. Accessory or aberrant thyroid tissue may remain as a remnant of the thyroglossal duct. This persistent tissue may be functional but is usually not of clinical significance. Rarely, the thyroid tissue may remain undescended at the foramen cecum, resulting in a lingual thyroid. In about half the population, thyroid tissue persists at the inferior end of the thyroglossal duct, resulting in a pyramidal lobe of the thyroid gland. This lobe may have persistent attachment to the hyoid bone.

THE TONGUE

During the fourth week, the median tongue bud (tuberculum impar) elevates from the floor of the primitive pharynx. Two distal tongue buds (lateral lingual swellings) grow over the tuberculum impar to form the anterior two-thirds (oral part) of the tongue (Fig. 21.10). These median and lateral swellings originate from the mesenchyme of the first branchial arch and are supplied by the lingual nerve, a branch of the mandibular division of the trigeminal nerve. The site of fusion of the distal tongue buds can be identified externally by the medium septum of the tongue.

The second, third, and fourth branchial arches contribute to the development of the posterior one-third (pharyngeal part) of the tongue. The hypobranchial eminence (third and fourth arches) grows over the copula (second arch) as the tongue develops. The copula soon disappears as the hypobranchial eminence completely covers it. The glossopharyngeal nerve (third branchial arch) and the superior laryngeal branch of the vagus nerve (fourth branchial arch) supply the sensory innervation to this part of the tongue. The facial nerve (second branchial arch)

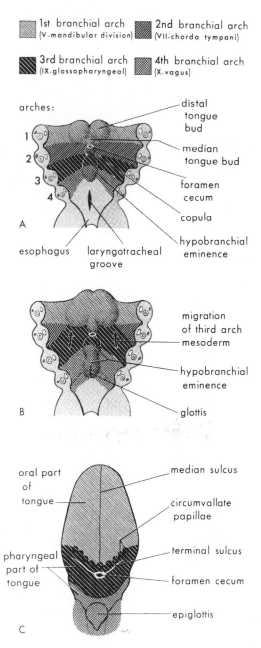

FIGURE 21.10. A and B: Schematic horizontal sections through the pharynx at the level seen in Figure 21.5A, showing successive stages in the development of the tongue during the fourth and fifth weeks. C: Adult tongue showing the branchial arch derivation of the nerve supply of its mucosa. (Reproduced with permission from Moore KL, ed. *The Developing Human*, 4th ed. Philadelphia: Saunders; 1988:187.)

does not provide sensory innervation to the posterior one-third of the tongue, because it is overgrown by the third arch. The anterior two-thirds of the tongue is separated from the posterior one-third of the tongue by a V-shaped groove, the terminal sulcus.

The hypoglossal nerve innervates all muscles of the tongue except for the palatoglossus. The latter muscle is innervated by the vagus nerve. Myoblasts from the myotome regions of the occipital somites form most of the tongue muscles, while the branchial arch mesenchyme forms the blood vessels, lymphatics, and connective tissue of the tongue.

Congenital malformations of the tongue are rare, but may include cysts (thyroglossal duct remnants), fistulas (persistent thyroglossal duct that opens through the foramen cecum), macroglossia, microglossia, cleft or bifid tongue (incomplete fusion of the distal tongue buds), and ankyloglossia. In ankyloglossia, also known as tongue-tie, the frenulum extends to the tip of the tongue and prevents free movement.

THE NASAL CAVITIES

During the sixth week of development, the nasal pits form from the nasal placodes (Fig. 21.6B–D). The nasal pits deepen as a result of the formation of the medial and lateral nasal prominences, eventually forming nasal sacs. The nasal sacs are initially separated from the oral cavity by the oronasal membrane. Once this membrane ruptures, the oral and nasal cavities communicate via the primitive choanae (foramina). These foramina initially lie behind the primary palate, then shift posteriorly to the junction of the nasal cavity and pharynx after the formation of the secondary palate. The fusion of the lateral palatine processes and the nasal septum are responsible for this final location of the choanae.

Elevations of the lateral walls of each nasal cavity form the superior, middle, and inferior conchae. Olfactory epithelium develops from the ectoderm in the roof of each nasal cavity. Diverticula of the lateral walls of the nasal cavities form the paranasal air sinuses. These expansions of the nasal cavities extend into the sphenoid, ethmoid, frontal, and maxillary bones. The maxillary and ethmoid sinuses develop during the third and fifth months of fetal life, respectively. The sphenoid sinus appears during the fifth month of postnatal life, and the frontal sinuses develop between the fifth and sixth years of childhood. Complete development of all sinuses is achieved by adolescence, contributing to the shape of the face and adding resonance to the voice during puberty.

THE EXTERNAL EAR

The external ear represents the interface between the first and second branchial arches. The auricle develops as a series of six swellings or hillocks on either side of the dorsal aspect of the first branchial groove. The anterior three hillocks develop from the first branchial (mandibular) arch, and the posterior three hillocks develop from the second branchial (hyoid) arch (Fig. 21.11). By the end of the eighth week, the auricle assumes its characteristic shape following differential growth and fusion of the hillocks (Fig. 21.12). The external acoustic meatus develops from the dorsal aspect of the cleft between the first and second branchial arches, or the first branchial groove. Although the auricle and external acoustic meatus begin in the cervical region, they migrate cranially to reach their normal location. For this reason, patients with microtia or partial arrest in auricular development may have a caudally placed ear with respect to the contralateral normal ear.

DEVELOPMENTAL BIOLOGY OF THE HEAD AND NECK

Cellular Origin of Tissues: The Neural Crest and Cephalic Mesoderm

As the embryoblast grows, it divides into two, then three, layers. This process of gastrulation ultimately results in the formation of three primary germ layers (ectoderm, mesoderm, and endoderm) by the third week. At the cellular level, craniofacial tissues are derived from two broad-based lineages, the neural crest and the cephalic mesoderm (8). Craniofacial morphogen-

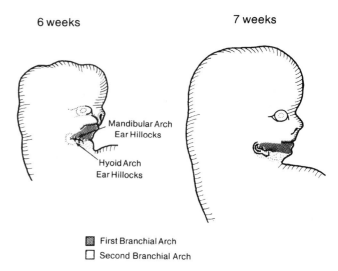

FIGURE 21.11. Auricle development from the first two branchial arches. (Reproduced with permission from Sperber GH. *Craniofacial Embryology*, 4th ed. London: Wright; 1989:208. © 1996 Butterworth Heinemann Publishing Co.)

esis is uniquely characterized by the massive relocation of cells, caused by both active cell migration and passive displacement.

After specification and patterning of the neural plate, the tissue begins to invaginate and roll up to form the neural tube. This occurs through a complex morphogenetic process in which the notochordal process underlying the ectoderm is a source of signals that specifies neural character in the ectoderm, and thus delineates it from nonneural ectoderm. Just prior to fusion a population of cells, known as the neural crest, is generated from the area of the neural folds. These cells give rise to the majority of neural, odontogenic, and skeletogenic tissues

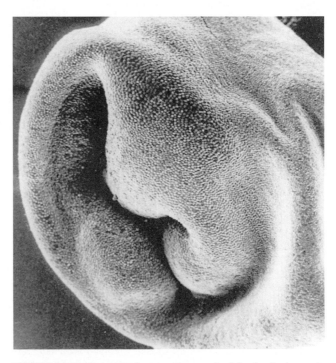

FIGURE 21.12. Scanning electron micrograph of the developing auricle of a human embryo at 8 weeks in utero. (By courtesy of Drs. K. K. Sulik and G. C. Schoenwolf. Reproduced with permission from Sperber GH. *Craniofacial Embryology*, 4th ed. London: Wright; 1989:209. © 1996 Butterworth Heinemann Publishing Co.)

of the head. Cranial neural crest cells give rise to a wide variety of neuronal and nonneuronal tissues, including ganglia of the dorsal root, the autonomic nervous system, and the cranial nerves, as well as the meninges, pigment cells, and the adrenal medulla.

Some of the molecular signals that instigate neural crest formation have been identified, and include secreted proteins in the Wnt and bone morphogenetic protein (BMP) families. Wnts induce BMPs in the dorsal neural tube, which promotes neural crest induction. The ability of Wnts to stimulate neural crest cell formation from naïve tissues raises the possibility that Wnt proteins may one day be used to induce the regeneration of cranial neural crest tissues. Newer studies help describe how cranial neural crest cells migrate from the dorsal part of the neural tube to the facial primordia. By transplanting quail neural crest into a chick host embryo, investigators were able to identify the migratory paths of subpopulations of the cranial neural crest. Now, innovative visualization techniques can provide a bird's-eye view of the migratory route of neural crest cells (9).

Interruption in Development of the Neural Crest and Cephalic Mesoderm

A plethora of craniofacial malformations are the consequence of inaccurate or interrupted migration of the neural crest cells. For example, genetic syndromes associated with aberrant neural crest migration include the DiGeorge, velocardiofacial, and the pharyngeal arch syndromes. Teratogens such as retinoic acid and alcohol also affect neural crest migration, causing well-documented craniofacial defects. Signals encountered by neural crest cells during their migration to the facial primordia can further alter development. These signals may be secreted from adjacent epithelia. Ephrins and the Eph receptors and semaphorin III–collapsin I appear to serve as migratory guidance cues. One feature shared by these molecules is their well-documented role in axon path finding, suggesting that a common molecular mechanism coordinates the directed migration of multiple cell types.

Incomplete fusion of the neural tube can cause a host of fetal and postnatal defects, ranging from spina bifida (incomplete fusion in the caudal end of the neural tube) to anencephaly (lack of fusion of the anterior neuropore). Holoprosencephaly is the most common structural malformation of the forebrain in humans, occurring in an astonishing 1 in 250 human abortuses and in 1 in 10–20,000 livebirths (10). The etiology of holoprosencephaly is heterogeneous. Mutations in Sonic hedgehog (*Shh*), *Zic2*, *Six3*, and *Tgif* are associated with human holoprosencephaly. Fetal exposure to a variety of environmental agents can also elicit holoprosencephaly-like defects.

One signal emanating from the endoderm is the secreted protein Cerberus (11). which has a unique role in governing head development. The Cerberus protein acts in part through its ability to regulate the expression of at least two homeodomain-containing transcription factors, Otx2 and Lim1, both of which are essential for forebrain and midbrain development. In the absence of Cerberus, rostral head development is severely compromised; likewise, the loss of its downstream targets Otx2 and Lim1 are associated with craniofacial malformations and the complete absence of head structures, respectively. These types of studies indicate the critical nature of signals emanating from endoderm during early head development.

Development of the Palate

Despite the difference in the shape of the median nasal–frontonasal processes in avians, rodents, and humans, the expression of genes such as fibroblast growth factor 8 (*Fgf8*),

Shh, *Bmp2*, and *Bmp4* are strikingly equivalent in these different species. In humans, the development of the median nasal process more closely resembles that of the mouse, although the fissure in the median nasal process is not as deep. In humans, this fissure is represented as the philtrum of the lip. The secondary palatal shelves appear to fuse by the process of epithelial–mesenchymal transformation, although some earlier reports suggest that apoptosis plays a predominant role.

Using a combination of experimental and genetic approaches, researchers are discovering the specific signaling events and cellular processes that often go awry in cases of craniofacial clefting. For example, polymorphisms in transforming growth factor-α (TGF-α), an epidermal growth factor receptor (EGFR) ligand synthesized by facial epithelia, are also be involved in isolated cases of cleft lip. *Egfr*$^{-/-}$ mice have midline defects that produce an elongated primary palate, micrognathia, and a high incidence of cleft palate (12). In vitro experiments suggest that a delay in epithelial degeneration occurs in the absence of EGFR signaling. The secretion of matrix metalloproteinases (MMPs) is also diminished in *Egfr*$^{-/-}$ explants, consistent with the ability of epidermal growth factor (EGF) to increase MMP secretion in other in vitro models. These experimental and genetic results indicate that the role of EGFR signaling in craniofacial development is mediated, at least in part, through regulation of an MMP. In addition, some cases of human cleft palate have been associated with the polymorphisms in the gene for TGF-α, an EGFR ligand.

TGF-β Signaling and Cranial Neural Crest Cell Differentiation

TGF-β signaling regulates the fate of the medial edge epithelium during palatal fusion and postnatal cranial suture closure (13). The IIR receptor to TGF-β (*Tgfbr2*) plays a crucial role in TGF-β signaling. Mice with *Tgfbr2* conditional gene ablation in the cranial neural crest have complete cleft secondary palate and calvaria agenesis. In mice, TGF-β$_3$ is essential for fusion between palatal shelves, because homozygous null TGF-β$_3$ newborns exhibit a cleft secondary palate without other craniofacial abnormalities. In the TGF-β$_3$ null mutants, the palatal shelves appear to approximate, but mesenchymal confluence does not occur.

Development of the Calvaria

Of the multitude of genes involved in the orchestration of bone formation, the most central is the transcription factor *Runx2/Cbfa1*. *Runx2* can be considered the "master switch" of osteoblast biology, and directly turns on many genes required for the deposition and mineralization of osteoblast extracellular matrix, including collagen I, osteopontin, and osteocalcin. In *Runx2*$^{-/-}$ mice, there is absence of formation of the appendicular and axial skeleton as a consequence of failure of osteoblast differentiation. Interestingly, mice that are *Runx2*$^{-/+}$ have a phenotype that resembles the human disease cleidocranial dysplasia, which is characterized by deficiencies in intramembranous bone formation, including wide, patent fontanels and hypoplasia of the clavicles.

A genetic approach in mice has provided convincing data about the cellular origins of the cranial skeleton. Investigators took advantage of the fact that the gene *Wnt1* is expressed in the neural crest cells. By placing the *Wnt1* promoter upstream of a *Cre* gene and crossing the mice with a reporter line, they succeeded in generating mice in which the neural crest cells were indelibly labeled with a reporter gene. This technique permitted scientists to follow the fate of the labeled neural crest cells throughout the lifetime of the animal. These studies suggested that the frontal and squamosal bones are of cranial neural crest origin. The parietal bone is derived from paraxial mesoderm, and the occipital bone is derived from both. These cells form bone through both endochondral and intramembranous ossification.

It was previously thought that the dividing line between mesoderm and neural crest had significance for the development and the repair of the cranial skeleton. More recent experimental results suggest that this is unlikely, because neural crest cells seem to be capable of responding to the same cues that promote skeletogenesis in mesoderm. These data underscore the plasticity of cranial neural crest and raise the question of whether mesoderm and neural crest make osseous tissue using the same molecular pathways. Recent data from analyses of mice carrying mutations in the transcription factor *Twist* may provide insight in this question. Mice heterozygous for a mutation in *Twist* survive to adulthood, but have a craniosynostotic phenotype similar to their human counterparts. The *Twist*$^{+/-}$ skull bone defect is caused by the inappropriate intermixing of neural crest-derived cells in the frontal bone with mesoderm-derived cells in the parietal bones. This is of clinical relevance because humans with the same mutations exhibit nearly identical skeletal defects. The majority of studies investigating the developmental biology of sutures in the craniofacial skeleton have focused on either cranial sutures or palatal development. TGF-β and the transcription factor Msx2 were found to be present in frontonasal sutures, similar to cranial sutures, but are differentially expressed over time. In a rat model, messenger ribonucleic acid (mRNA) levels for both genes were elevated during the period of suture morphogenesis and during active bone growth from the sutures in the early postnatal period. The authors concluded that the frontonasal sutures develop slightly later than cranial sutures and show increased complexity over time when compared to cranial sutures.

Recent studies investigating development of the calvaria suggest that a gradient of growth and/or other regulatory factors is created by the osteogenic fronts, suture mesenchyme, and dura mater (14). Studies in mice suggest that although the expression pattern of genes associated with the differentiation of osteoblasts is similar in the osteogenic fronts of patent and physiologically fusing sutures, genes implicated in the regulation of osteogenesis, such as fibroblast growth factor (FGF)-2 and BMP antagonists, are differentially regulated (15). This would imply that the maintenance of suture patency is partly a result of balancing the differentiation and proliferation of precursor cells in the suture mesenchyme. Many of the mutations associated with the syndromic craniosynostoses occur in genes implicated in the control of proliferation and differentiation in osteoblasts. For example, patients with Boston-type craniosynostosis have a point mutation in *Msx2*, a transcription factor that may regulate differentiation of preosteoblasts. Similarly, patients with Saethre-Chotzen craniosynostosis have mutations in the transcription factor *Twist*, a negative regulator of osteoblast proliferation.

References

1. Johnston MC, Sulik KK. Embryology of the head and neck. In: Serafin D, Georgiade NG, eds. *Pediatric Plastic Surgery*. St. Louis: Mosby; 1984: 184–215.
2. Moore KL. The branchial apparatus and the head and neck. In: Moore KL, ed. *The Developing Human*, 4th ed. Philadelphia: WB Saunders; 1988: 170–206.
3. Sperber GH. *Craniofacial Embryology*. 4th ed. London: Wright; 1989.
4. Nomina Embryologica. 3rd ed. In: *Nomina Anatomica*, 6th ed. Edinburgh: Churchill Livingstone; 1989.
5. Kriens O. Anatomy of the cleft palate. In: Bardach J, Morris HL, eds. *Multidisciplinary Management of Cleft Lip and Palate*. Philadelphia: WB Saunders; 1990: 292–295.
6. Gorlin RJ, Cohen MM Jr, Levin LS, eds. *Syndromes of the Head and Neck,*. 3rd ed. New York: Oxford University Press; 1990: 663–705.
7. Tessier P. Anatomical classification of facial, craniofacial, and laterofacial clefts. *J Maxillofac Surg*. 1976;4:69.
8. Helms JA, Schneider RA. Cranial skeletal biology. *Nature*. 2003;423(6937): 326–331.
9. Birgbauer E, Sechrist J, Bronner-Fraser M, et al. Rhombomeric origin and rostrocaudal reassortment of neural crest cells revealed by intravital microscopy. *Development*. 1995;121(4):935–945.
10. Muenke M, Beachy PA. Genetics of ventral forebrain development and holoprosencephaly. *Curr Opin Genet Dev*. 2000;103:262–269.
11. Piccolo S, Agius E, Leyns L, et al. The head inducer Cerberus is a multifunctional antagonist of Nodal, BMP and Wnt signals. *Nature*. 1999;397(6721): 707–710.
12. Miettinen PJ, Chin JR, Shum L, et al. Epidermal growth factor receptor function is necessary for normal craniofacial development and palate closure. *Nat Genet*. 1999;221:69–73.
13. Pelton RW, Hogan BL, Miller DA, et al. Differential expression of genes encoding TGFs beta 1, beta 2, and beta 3 during murine palate formation. *Dev Biol*. 1990;141:456–460.
14. Opperman LA, Sweeney TM, Redmon J, et al. Tissue interactions with underlying dura mater inhibit osseous obliteration of developing cranial sutures. *Dev Dyn*. 1993;1984:312–322.
15. Warren SM, Brunet LJ, Harland RM, et al. The BMP antagonist noggin regulates cranial suture fusion. *Nature*. 2003;422(6932):625–629.

CHAPTER 22 ■ VASCULAR ANOMALIES

JOHN B. MULLIKEN

NOMENCLATURE AND NOSOLOGY

Vascular anomalies all look similar: flat or raised and in various shades of blue, pink, purple, or red. For centuries, vascular nevi were called by vernacular terms for colored edibles, based on the folk belief that a pregnant mother's emotions could imprint her fetus. Physicians began designating vascular birthmarks *angiomas* after the advent of histopathology in the mid-19th century. Over the next 100 years, the descriptive and histologic terms became hopelessly jumbled, impeding development in the field. Accurate diagnosis and appropriate management of vascular anomalies required a new nosology.

Effective classification of disease begins with proper definition of terms. The Greek nominative suffix *-oma* means "swelling" or "tumor;" however, in modern usage, it denotes a lesion characterized by hyperplasia. This semantic refinement was the key to a binary classification of vascular anomalies as *hemangiomas* or *malformations*. This biologic system has been corroborated by clinical experience, and by radiologic and immunohistochemical studies. It has the imprimatur of the International Society for the Study of Vascular Anomalies (ISSVA) after a minor revision to include all vascular neoplasms (Table 22.1).

The term *hemangioma* refers to the common tumor of infancy that exhibits rapid postnatal growth and slow regression during childhood. The more precise designation is *infantile* hemangioma, so as not to cause confusion with uncommon vascular tumors that arise in late childhood and adulthood that are designated "hemangioma" or hemangioendothelioma. **Vascular malformations are comprised of abnormally formed channels that are lined by quiescent endothelium. Although congenital, they are not always obvious at birth. They never regress and often expand.** Vascular malformations are subcategorized according to channel morphology and rheology: *slow-flow* for capillary, lymphatic, and venous anomalies, and *fast-flow* for arterial and arteriovenous anomalies (Table 22.1). Combined vascular malformations are associated with soft tissue and skeletal overgrowth and most are known by eponyms (Table 22.3).

Accurate diagnosis is possible for most vascular anomalies by correlating history and physical examination. Deep subcutaneous, intramuscular, or visceral lesions can be ambiguous, and in these instances, radiologic evaluation is indicated. Imaging also confirms whether a vascular malformation is slow-flow or fast-flow, and documents the extent of anatomic involvement. Biopsy of a vascular lesion is necessary whenever there is any suspicion of malignancy.

INFANTILE HEMANGIOMA

Pathogenesis

Proliferating Phase

The growing infantile hemangioma is composed of plump, rapidly dividing endothelial cells and pericytes that form tightly packed sinusoidal channels. Immunohistochemical cellular markers elucidate the clinical phases of the hemangioma's life cycle (1). Even at this early stage, endothelial cells express phenotypic markers of maturity and cell-specific adhesion molecules. Upregulated angiogenesis is documented by expression of proliferating cell nuclear antigen, mediated, in part, by two angiogenic peptides, vascular endothelial growth factor (VEGF) and basic fibroblast growth factor (bFGF). Enzymes involved in the remodeling of extracellular matrix are also present, suggesting that breakdown of collagen is necessary to provide space for the growing capillaries. Erythrocyte-type glucose transporter protein-1 (GLUT1) is immunopositive throughout the life cycle and negative in most other vascular tumors and vascular malformations (2).

Involuting Phase

Regression is characterized by gradually diminishing endothelial activity and luminal enlargement. Endothelial cells degenerate; apoptosis begins before 1 year and reaches an apogee in 2-year-old specimens. There is progressive deposition of perivascular and interlocular/intralobular fibrous tissue, an influx of stromal cells (including mast cells, fibroblasts, and macrophages), and emergence of tissue inhibitor of metalloproteinase (TIMP)-1, a suppressor of new blood vessel formation (1).

Although mast cells appear in the late proliferative phase, they are more prominently seen during the involuting phase, interacting with macrophages, fibroblasts, and other cell types. Mast cells could secrete modulators that downregulate endothelial turnover.

Involuted Phase

At the end of a hemangioma's life cycle, all that remains are a few capillarylike vessels and draining veins. Multilaminated basement membranes, an ultrastructural hallmark of the proliferative phase, persist around the tiny vessels. The once highly cellular parenchyma is replaced by loose fibrofatty tissue intermingled with dense collagen and reticular fibers.

TABLE 22.1

ISSAV CLASSIFICATION OF VASCULAR ANOMALIES

Tumors	Malformations
Hemangioma	*Slow-flow*
Hemangioendotheliomas	Capillary
Angiosarcoma	Lymphatic
Miscellaneous	Venous
	Fast-flow
	Arterial
	Combined

Etiology

Histology and immunohistochemical staining demonstrate the biochemical happenings in the life cycle of infantile hemangioma, but tell us little about what initiated the cascade of events. The presence of GLUT1 (and other placenta-associated antigens) suggested that hemangioma might originate by embolized placental cells or involve an immunophenotypic alteration in primitive cells forming the tumor (2). There is evidence that hemangioma-genesis begins as a somatic mutation in a single endothelial cell, leading to clonal expansion (3). Antigen-specific staining reveals the presence of endothelial progenitor cells in early proliferating hemangiomas, but their origin remains to be determined. The possibility of a germline mutation is suggested by kindreds that show hereditary transmission of hemangioma.

Clinical Features

Hemangioma appears in neonatalhood, usually within the first 2 weeks. Deep subcutaneous tumors or visceral hemangioma(s) may not manifest until 2 to 3 months of life. Approximately 30% to 40% of hemangiomas are nascent at birth, presenting as a premonitory cutaneous mark—a barely visible pale area, telangiectatic, or macular red stain, or an ecchymotic spot. *Congenital hemangioma* is a rare variant that grows in utero and presents completely formed at birth.

Approximately 80% of hemangiomas are solitary; 20% are multifocal. Hemangioma is more common in females than males (3–5:1). The incidence is 10% to 12% in white infants and 23% in preterm infants who weigh <1,000 g. The frequency is lower in dark-skinned infants.

Proliferating Phase

Hemangioma grow rapidly during the first 6 to 8 months of infancy (Fig. 22.1). As the tumor permeates superficial dermis, the skin becomes raised, bosselated, and a vivid crimson color. If the tumor proliferates in the lower dermis and subcutis, the overlying skin may be only slightly raised and of a bluish hue. Local draining veins are usually present, typically in a radial pattern. The old adjectives "cavernous" for a deep hemangioma and "capillary" for a superficial lesion are confusing and should be discarded. There is no such entity as "cavernous hemangioma"; either the lesion is a deep infantile hemangioma or a mislabeled venous malformation.

Involuting Phase

Hemangioma reaches its peak before the first year; and for a time thereafter, growth is proportionate to that of the child. The first signs of the involuting phase appear as the crimson color fades to a dull purplish hue, the skin gradually pales, a patchy grey mantle forms, and the tumor feels less tense. **The involuting phase continues until the child is 5 to 10 years of age.** Usually the last traces of color disappear by 5 to 7 years of life.

Involuted Phase

Regression is complete in 50% of children by age 5 years and in 70% by age 7 years, with continued improvement until age 10 to 12 years. Nearly normal skin is restored in approximately 50% of children; otherwise there is a cutaneous blemish, either telangiectasias, crepelike laxity, yellowish hypoelastic patches, scarring (if ulceration occurred during the proliferating phase), or a fibrofatty residuum. Even extensive and bulky cutaneous hemangioma can regress totally. Conversely, a flat, superficial dermal hemangioma can permanently alter skin texture.

Skeletal Alterations

Hemangiomas, unlike vascular malformations, rarely cause bony distortion or hypertrophy. A large facial hemangioma can cause cartilaginous/bony overgrowth, presumably secondary to increased blood flow, or a localized mass effect on the facial skeleton. Axial skeletal overgrowth of an extremity is rare, but does occur with an extensive (reticular) hemangioma with arteriovenous shunting.

Congenital Hemangioma

Prenatal ultrasonography may reveal a solid cutaneous vascular tumor or intrahepatic tumor, either of which can cause

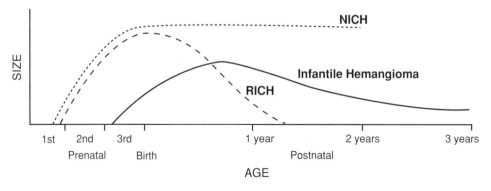

FIGURE 22.1. Natural history of infantile hemangioma, rapidly involuting congenital hemangioma (*RICH*), and noninvoluting congenital hemangioma (*NICH*).

cardiac overload and hydrops fetalis. These rare tumors present fully grown at birth as a *congenital hemangioma*, but they do not undergo the rapid neonatal proliferation, expected of common infantile hemangioma. There are two types: rapidly involuting congenital hemangioma (RICH) and noninvoluting congenital hemangioma (NICH). They are similar in appearance, location, and size, have the same sex ratio, and their radiologic and histologic features overlap those of infantile hemangioma (4). Curiously, both tumors are negative for GLUT1 immunostaining. RICH is a solitary raised, gray or violaceous tumor with ectasia, radial veins, central telangiectasias, and a pale surrounding halo. There can be sufficient shunting to cause high-output congestive cardiac failure. RICH's defining feature is accelerated regression, usually obvious within a few weeks after birth, and complete by 6 to 14 months of age. NICH is a well-circumscribed, plaquelike tumor with a pink, blue, or purple hue, central coarse telangiectasia, and a pale rim. In contrast, NICH grows proportionately to the child and remains unchanged, including fast-flow by Doppler examination (Fig. 22.1). There are rare instances of coexistence of either RICH or NICH in a child with infantile hemangioma, and also instances in which RICH ceases to regress and assumes the likeness of NICH.

Differential Diagnosis

Not All Hemangiomas Look Like Strawberries

A deep (subcutaneous) hemangioma, particularly in the neck or trunk, can be mistaken for a lymphatic malformation. Ultrasonography or magnetic resonance imaging (MRI) confirms the diagnosis. Infantile hemangioma can also imitate a capillary malformation (port-wine stain), especially in an extremity; however, its neoplastic nature is betrayed by fine telangiectasias, minor swelling, and prominent draining veins. RICH and NICH can be mistaken for arteriovenous malformation because of prominent fast-flow.

Not All Strawberries Are Hemangiomas

Pyogenic granuloma is frequently confused with hemangioma. These common tumors typically arise in the central face, they are small (average diameter, 6.5 mm), and rarely appear before 6 months of age (mean age, 6.7 years). Usually there is no history or preexisting dermatologic condition (although these lesions often occur in areas of capillary malformation). Pyogenic granuloma grows rapidly, erupting through the skin and forming a stalk or pedicle. Epidermal breakdown and crusting are common; recurrent bleeding (often copious) initiates the first visit to a physician or emergency room.

Other infantile tumors that can be mistaken for hemangioma include kaposiform hemangioendothelioma, tufted angioma ("angioblastoma of Nakagawa"), myofibromatosis ("infantile hemangiopericytoma"), and fibrosarcoma.

Cutaneous–Visceral Hemangiomatosis

If there are multiple cutaneous hemangiomas (estimated to be more than five lesions), the child is at risk for harboring visceral, particularly intrahepatic, hemangiomas. These infants can present from birth to 16 weeks of age with a triad of congestive heart failure, hepatomegaly, and anemia. The multifocal cutaneous lesions are typically small (<3–5 mm diameter), dark red in color, and dome-shaped, although more banal hemangiomas also occur. Multiple hemangiomas also implies the possibility of widespread involvement in other organs (*generalized hemangiomatosis*), such as the central nervous system and gastrointestinal tract. Thyroid-stimulating hormone (TSH) levels should be monitored in any infant with a large or extensive

hemangioma, as severe hypothyroidism is caused by production of type 3 iodothyronine deiodinase by the tumor.

Radiologic Characteristics

Ultrasonography of a proliferating-phase hemangioma demonstrates a remarkable shunting pattern, consisting of decreased arterial resistance and increased venous velocity. Even an experienced ultrasonographer can have difficulty distinguishing a young hemangioma from an arteriovenous malformation because both are rheologically fast-flow. MRI with contrast is the gold standard, but requires sedation or general anesthesia if the child is younger than 6 years old. MRI reveals parenchymatous (solid) tissue of intermediate intensity on T1-weighted spin-echo images and moderate hyperintensity on T2-weighted spin-echo images. Prominent flow-voids are located around and within the tumor, indicating rapid flow in feeding arteries and dilated draining veins. At some time in the late involuting phase, hemangioma becomes a slow-flow lesion, often with prominent fatty parenchyma.

Associated Malformative Anomalies

There are curious instances in which a facial hemangioma occurs with malformative anomalies. The acronym for these associations is PHACES (P = Dandy-Walker or other cystic malformations in the posterior cranial fossa; H = large, often plaquelike, facial hemangioma; C = cardiac defects; E = eye anomalies; S = sternal cleft) (5). Lumbosacral hemangioma also presents in association with occult spinal dysraphism (lipomeningocele, tethered cord, and diastematomyelia). Diffuse hemangioma of the perineum and lower limb is also seen with urogenital and anorectal anomalies.

Kasabach-Merritt Phenomenon

The common infantile hemangioma does not cause a bleeding disorder. Kasabach-Merritt phenomenon occurs with uncommon and more invasive vascular tumors, particularly kaposiform hemangioendothelioma and, less frequently, tufted angioma (6). Typical locations are the trunk, shoulder, thigh, and retroperitoneum. The skin is deep red-purple, tense, and shiny (edematous). Petechiae and ecchymoses overlie and are adjacent to the tumor. Platelet-trapping is the primary process. Thrombocytopenia is profound, typically less than $10,000/mm^3$; the prothrombin time (PT) and activated partial thromboplastin time (aPTT) are normal or minimally elevated. Hypofibrinogenemia and fibrinolysis are secondary. The infant with Kasabach-Merritt thrombocytopenia is at risk for intracranial, pleural-pulmonic, intraperitoneal, and gastrointestinal hemorrhage. Biopsy is not indicated; MRI confirms the clinical and hematologic diagnosis.

Management

Observation

Most infantile hemangiomas do not require consultation by a specialist. These small harmless tumors can be allowed to proliferate and involute under the watchful eye of a pediatrician because they will leave normal or slightly blemished skin. An infant with a hemangioma usually is referred because there is an indication for therapy. The consulting physician must fully appreciate the parent's anguish, for their once perfect child has a rapidly growing tumor. Even if the proper decision is not to intervene, this does not mean that nothing should be done. Parents deserve a thorough explanation of the hemangioma's natural history; photographs are used to illustrate this evolution. Scheduled follow-up visits are essential. Parents need repeated assurance regarding the benign nature of hemangioma and the anticipated outcome after spontaneous involution or intervention. More frequent visits are necessary whenever a hemangioma is large, ulcerated, multiple, or located in an anatomically critical area. For example, the typical nasal-tip hemangioma is usually small in volume and rarely compromises the airway, but produces major distress for the parents. As for other highly visible hemangiomas, parents relate stories of unsolicited comments by callous strangers. The physician must be alert to the parents' difficulties in dealing with these situations, spend sufficient time with the family, and always be available for questions. If the physician fails to gain the parents' confidence, they will go elsewhere for help.

Local Treatment for Ulceration and Bleeding

Spontaneous epithelial breakdown and ulceration occurs in 5% of all cutaneous hemangiomas, more commonly in the lip or anogenital area. Treatment is daily application of a topical antibiotic or hydrocolloid dressing. Viscous lidocaine (2.5%) helps to control pain. If there is superficial eschar, debridement or dressings are needed. An ulcerated hemangioma often does not re-epithelialize for weeks. There are reports that pulsed dye laser treatment relieves pain and accelerates healing; however, photocoagulation can also make ulceration worse. Punctate bleeding from a bosselated hemangioma is a rare occurrence and can be frightening to the parents. They should be instructed how to compress the area with a clean pad and to hold the pressure for 10 minutes by the clock. Rarely is it necessary to place a mattress suture to control a local bleeding site.

Pharmacologic Therapy

Approximately 10% of hemangiomas cause complications such as major ulceration/destruction, distortion of involved tissues, and obstruction of a vital structure. Spontaneous ulceration of the involved skin may extend to deeper tissues, causing partial loss of a structure, such as the eyelid, nose, lip, or pinna. Large facial tumors grow to expand skin and distort normal anatomic features. An orbitopalpebral hemangioma can block the visual axis and cause deprivational amblyopia. Even a small hemangioma in the upper eyelid can distort the growing cornea, producing astigmatic amblyopia. Subglottic hemangioma presents insidiously as biphasic stridor at 6 to 8 weeks, often, but not always, in the presence of cervicofacial hemangioma ("beard distribution"). Perhaps 1% of all hemangiomas cause life-threatening complications, such as diversion of sufficient blood flow to produce high-output cardiac failure. This is most likely with intrahepatic hemangioma, but also can occur with a large or extensive cutaneous tumor. Gastrointestinal hemangiomas can present with minor to major bleeding.

Pharmacologic treatment is indicated for problematic and endangering hemangiomas. There is a recent trend to also consider antiangiogenic therapy for less-threatening tumors that cause only cutaneous expansion that is likely to result in permanent alteration of skin or fibrofatty residuum.

Corticosteroid. Well-localized cutaneous hemangioma (<2.5 cm diameter) is treated with intralesional corticosteroid. Triamcinolone (25 mg/mL) is injected slowly at low pressure, (3-mL syringe, 30-gauge needle), placing no more than 3 to 5 mg/kg per procedure. Usually three to five injections are needed, given at 6- to 8-week intervals. The response rate is similar to that for systemic corticosteroid. There is increasing reluctance to inject an eyelid hemangioma with corticosteroid because of the risk of embolic occlusion of the retinal artery.

Systemic corticosteroid remains the first-line therapy for large, endangering, or life-threatening hemangioma. Oral prednisolone 2 to 3 mg/kg/day is given as a single morning dose for 4 to 6 weeks; thereafter the dosage is tapered slowly over several months and discontinued by 10 to 11 months of age. Corticosteroid causes gastric irritation so H_2 receptor inhibitor is also given. A sensitive hemangioma exhibits signs of responsiveness within several days to 1 week. For an acute situation, for example, a threatened upper airway or visual field, an equivalent dose of intravenous corticosteroid gives a more rapid change in a sensitive tumor. **With oral, parenteral, or intralesional corticosteroid, the overall response rate is approximately 85%, either accelerated regression or stabilization of growth (1).** Corticosteroid should be discontinued if there is no effect such as lightening of color, softening, or diminished growth. Rebound growth can occur if the drug level is lowered too rapidly. Live vaccines are withheld during therapy. Cushingoid facies occurs in virtually all treated infants; one-third exhibit temporary diminished rate of gain of length and weight that returns to normal after discontinuing the drug (7). Rare complications include myopathy, cardiomyopathy, premature thelarche, and hirsutism.

Interferon α-2a. Recombinant interferon (IFN) α-2a or 2b is a second-line agent for endangering and life-threatening hemangiomas. Indications for its use are (a) failure to respond to corticosteroid; (b) contraindications to prolonged parenteral corticosteroid; (c) complications of corticosteroid; or (d) parental refusal of corticosteroid. Corticosteroids and IFN should not be coadministered in therapeutic dosage; corticosteroids should be tapered quickly on initiation of IFN. There is no evidence for drug synergism. The empiric dose is 2 to 3 mU/m², injected subcutaneously daily. IFN dosage is titrated as the infant gains weight; otherwise regrowth can occur. The rate of response is >80%; usually 6 to 10 months of sustained therapy is required (1).

IFN is effective therapy for tumors that cause Kasabach-Merritt phenomenon. There are two caveats in managing this coagulopathy: (a) Do not transfuse platelets unless there is evidence of active bleeding or unless a surgical procedure (such as placement of a long-line) is indicated, and (b) do not give heparin because it can stimulate tumor growth and aggravate platelet trapping (6).

The infant given IFN usually has a fever for the first 1 to 2 weeks; pretreatment with acetaminophen 1 to 2 hours prior to injection dampens the febrile response. IFN causes reversible toxicoses of up to fivefold induction in liver transaminase, transient neutropenia, and anemia. Neutropenia is ascribed to "margination," not to suppression of bone marrow, and resolves on continued treatment. Infants on IFN grow and gain weight in a normal fashion. **The most worrisome possible long-term adverse reaction is spastic diplegia, which usually improves following prompt termination of therapy.** Children receiving IFN require periodic neurologic and developmental assessment.

Chemotherapy

Vincristine is another second-line for a problematic hemangioma in an infant who fails to respond to corticosteroid, cannot be weaned from corticosteroid, or has a serious complication of corticosteroid. It is also effective therapy for kaposiform hemangioendothelioma (with thrombocytopenia) and for other hemangioendotheliomas. Vinca alkaloid must be administered through a central intravenous line; the response rate is >80%. Side effects are peripheral neuropathy, constipation, minor hair loss, and sepsis and other complications related to the central line. Cyclophosphamide is rarely given for a benign vascular tumor because of its toxicity including the risk for late development of malignancy.

Laser Therapy

There is a common belief that "laser surgery," if used early for nascent hemangioma, will halt the spread of the tumor and prevent subsequent complications. The flashlamp pulsed-dye laser penetrates only 0.75 to 1.2 mm (577–585 nm) into the dermis. **Laser photocoagulation can lighten the involved skin; however, there is no evidence that even repeated application either diminishes bulk or accelerates involution of the deep portion of the hemangioma.** Although some hemangiomas only grow in the superficial dermis, these are the very tumors that do not cause problems and regress to leave nearly normal skin. Overzealous use of laser can result in ulceration, hypopigmentation, second-degree skin loss, and consequent scarring. There is an unequivocal role for laser photocoagulation of tiny telangiectasias that often remain in the involuted phase.

Surgical Management

A growing hemangioma can be likened to a tissue expander that provides extra skin. Consider circular excision and purse-string closure as the primary initial technique; this yields the smallest possible scar (8). Transverse lenticular excision is applicable in certain locations, such as eyelids, lip, and neck, or as the final stage after circular excision.

Infancy (Proliferating Phase). Indications for resection of a well-localized tumor in the first year are (a) obstruction, usually a tumor in the upper eyelid or subglottis; (b) deformation, for example, periorbital tumor causing amblyopia, retroauricular hemangioma causing a prominent ear; (c) bleeding; (d) ulceration unresponsive to topical, intralesional, or systemic therapy; and (e) predictable scar or hair loss, particularly if the infant must undergo a general anesthetic for another reason.

Early Childhood (Involuting Phase). Indications for removal prior to entering school are (a) resection is inevitable, for example, postulcerative scarring, unalterably expanded skin, or high probability of fibrofatty residuum; (b) same scar length/appearance if excision were postponed; (c) scar easily hidden in relaxed cutaneous tension lines or a border of a facial esthetic unit; and (d) necessity for staged resection or reconstruction. Children at this age rarely have low self-esteem. The excisional scar must be weighed against the degree of the child's (not the parents') emotional distress. Hemangioma in the nasal tip is a psychologically sensitive location. A useful stratagem is to debulk the tumor through unilateral or bilateral rim incisions to allow the nasal skin to contract. An open rhinoplasty approach is used if two-dimensional skin excision is necessary. Appose the splayed genua and avoid overaggressive removal of skin and fibrofatty tissue for fear of causing a blunted tip or nostril–tip disproportion. Protuberant involuting labial hemangioma is a common problem, requiring that mucosa be excised transversely; vermilion-cutaneous excision should be postponed; and vertical cutaneous resection should be avoided if possible.

Late Childhood (Involuted Phase). Resection of an involuted hemangioma is usually undertaken for (a) damaged skin; (b) abnormal contour (fibrofatty residuum); (c) distortion or destruction of an anatomic structure; or (d) because staged removal or reconstruction is necessary.

VASCULAR MALFORMATIONS

Clinical, Histologic, and Rheologic Categories

Vascular malformations are categorized by the predominant channel type and rheologic characteristics: *slow-flow* for capillary (CM) and telangiectasias, lymphatic (LM), and venous (VM) malformations, and *fast-flow* for arterial and arteriovenous malformations (Table 22.1). Each of the four major categories of vascular malformation has a particular histopathologic appearance and all are lined by quiescent endothelium.

CM comprises regular, ectatic, thin-walled capillary-to-venular-sized channels located in the papillary and upper reticular dermis. There is a deficiency of perivascular neural elements, which might account for the altered neural modulation of vascular tone and progressive ectasia. LM has walls of variable thickness comprised of both striated and smooth muscle, and nodular collections of lymphocytes in the connective tissue stroma. VM comprises thin-walled vascular spaces surrounded by abnormally formed layers of smooth muscle, often in clumps. The dysplastic venous networks drain to adjacent veins, many of which are varicose and lack valves. Pale acidophilic fluid is typically seen within the channels and sacs of a LM, whereas blood, fresh and organizing thrombi, and phleboliths characterize a VM. Arteriovenous malformation (AVM) comprises thickened fibromuscular walls, fragmented elastic lamina, and fibrotic stroma. The veins in an immature AVM are "arterialized" (reactive muscular hyperplasia), whereas in a mature AVM, the veins evidence degenerative fibrosis and muscular atrophy.

Molecular Genetics

Vascular malformations are caused by abnormal signaling processes that regulate the proliferation and apoptosis, differentiation, maturation, and adhesion of vascular cells (endothelium cells, smooth muscle cells, and pericytes) (9). Most vascular malformations are sporadic (nonfamilial), but some are inheritable in a mendelian autosomal dominant pattern. The causative genes for several familial vascular disorders have been identified, thereby opening the door to understanding basic mechanisms.

CM in the nuchal region is often familial, but of minor pathologic interest. A distinctive inheritable condition called capillary malformation–arteriovenous malformation (CM-AVM) is characterized by tiny ovoid vascular stains and sometimes by AVM. The causative genes are known for congenital lymphedema (Milroy disease), lymphedema-distichiasis syndrome, and hypotrichosis-lymphedema telangiectasia. Solitary VM is most likely sporadic, but multiple venous lesions suggest autosomal dominant or paradominant inheritance, the most common being glomuvenous malformation (GVM; "glomangiomatosis"). Cerebral cavernous venous malformations are inheritable; approximately 12% of affected patients have cutaneous and intramuscular venous lesions. Multiple lesions characterize familial cutaneous–mucosal venous malformation caused by two mutations in the gene coding for an endothelial receptor. Hereditary hemorrhagic telangiectasia (HHT; Rendu-Osler-Weber disease) is a genetically heterogeneous disorder caused by mutations in three genes that are involved in the transforming growth factor-β (TGF-β) signalling pathway (Table 22.2).

Radiologic Imaging

Radiologic techniques are used to determine the rheologic nature and anatomic extent of the malformations. Interpretation of these images requires a radiologist who is knowledgeable in the field of vascular anomalies.

Ultrasonography is the simplest and most cost-effective imaging modality. Ultrasonography and color Doppler study differentiate slow-flow from fast-flow anomalies, and a discrete tumoral mass from the anomalous channels of a vascular

TABLE 22.2

SUBCATEGORIES OF VASCULAR MALFORMATIONS

Slow-flow	Fast-flow
Capillary (CM)	Arterial (AM):aneurysm, coarctation, ectasia, stenosis
Sturge-Weber syndrome	Arteriovenous fistulae (AVF)
Cutis marmorata telangiectasia congenita	Arteriovenous malformation (AVM)
Macrocephaly-cutis marmorata	
Capillary malformation-arteriovenous malformation (CM-AVM) [*RASA1*]	
Telangiectasias	
Hereditary hemorrhagic telangiectasia (HHT) [*endoglin, activin, SMAD4*]	
Lymphatic (LM)	
Macrocystic/microcystic	
Generalized (multifocal)	
Milroy lymphedema [*VEGFR3*]	
Lymphedemia-distichiasis [*FOXC2*]	
Hypotrichosis-lymphedema-telangiectasia [*SOX18*]	
Venous (VM)	
Sporadic	
Cerebral cavernous malformation [*KRIT1*]	
Glomuvenous (GVM) [*glomulin*]	
Cutaneous-mucosal (CMVM) [*TIE2*]	
Blue rubber bleb nevus syndrome	

*Causative gene [ ]

malformation. A major drawback is that ultrasonography is highly operator-dependent and it is limited in delineation of size of the anomaly and its relationship to adjacent structures.

MRI with contrast (gadolinium) gives the most informative portrayal of abnormal channels, flow characteristics, and extent of involvement in tissue planes. CM is not seen by MRI, except as minor cutaneous thickening. VM gives high signal intensity on T2-weighted images, brighter than fatty tissue. Phleboliths are pathognomonic for a venous anomaly and seen as discrete round signal voids on T1- and T2-weighted spin-echo and gradient images. It is difficult to distinguish LM from VM or lymphaticovenous malformation (LVM); these are better delineated by administration of intravenous gadolinium and repetition of the T1-weighted sequences. VM enhances inhomogeneously, whereas LM shows either rim enhancement or no enhancement. AVM demonstrates a myriad of flow-voids in all sequences, high-flow vessels on gradient sequences, contrast enhancement with gadolinium sequences, and usually no discrete parenchymatous signal abnormality. Magnetic resonance angiography (MRA) and magnetic resonance venography (MRV) delineate major vascular channels without injection of contrast medium. These techniques are useful for confirming the fast-flow nature of AVM and for demonstrating abnormalities of major veins in patients with complex-combined vascular anomalies.

Contrast-enhanced computed tomography (CT) also accurately differentiates lymphatic, venous, and lymphaticovenous malformations. Phleboliths are more clearly shown on CT than MRI. CT retains a primary place in evaluation of intraosseous vascular malformations and secondary bony changes.

Arteriography, the most invasive technique, is rarely done for diagnostic purposes. It is used in conjunction with superselective embolization as the primary treatment for arteriovenous fistula (AVF), as palliation for AVM, and in preparation for surgical extirpation. Venous angiography (phlebography) is used for imaging and treatment of certain venous anomalies of the limbs. Slow-flow malformations are best evaluated during sclerotherapy by angiographic filming after direct cannulation and injection of the lesion.

Capillary Malformation

CM is a macular, red, vascular stain that presents at birth and persists throughout life. CM can be localized or extensive, on the face, trunk, or limbs. CM must be differentiated from the common fading macular stains (*naevus flammeus neonatorum*) that occur in 50% of neonates, and which are typically located on the glabella, eyelids, nose, upper lip ("angel kiss"), and nuchal area ("stork bite"). **Most CMs are harmless cutaneous birthmarks, but some are red flags that signal underlying abnormalities.**

Sturge-Weber syndrome comprises facial CM in association with ipsilateral leptomeningeal and ocular vascular anomalies. The capillary stain involves the ophthalmic (V1) trigeminal dermatome, whereas patients with either maxillary (V2) or mandibular (V3) involvement are at low risk for having the disorder. The leptomeningeal vascular abnormalities can cause seizures, contralateral hemiplegia, and variable developmental delay of motor and cognitive skills. MRI with contrast (gadolinium) is more sensitive than CT in revealing pial vascular abnormalities (CM, VM, AVF, and AVM), cerebral atrophy, and prominent cortical sulci. Gyriform calcifications of the outer layers of the cerebral cortex occur later, typically in the temporal and occipital lobes; these changes are probably secondary to the anomalous circulation. Funduscopic examination and tonometry should be done biannually for 1–3 years then yearly thereafter. Children who evidence ipsilateral increased choroidal vascularity are at risk for retinal detachment, glaucoma, and blindness, especially if the CM involves both V1 and V2 neurosensory areas.

Facial CMs are prone to darken in color and to develop fibrovascular changes. Thickened purple nodules manifest in adulthood; pyogenic granuloma can appear at any age. Curiously, these changes occur rarely in CM of the trunk or limbs. Facial CM is sometimes associated with hypertrophy of soft tissues and underlying skeleton. Lips and gums enlarge in the areas of capillary staining. Maxillary or mandibular overgrowth causes skeletal asymmetry and malocclusion. Extensive CM of a limb can be solitary or part of combined anomalies, such as Klippel-Trenaunay, Parkes Weber, or Sturge-Weber syndromes. **CM in a limb often is associated with axial and transverse hypertrophy.**

Midline cephalic CM may indicate an underlying occipital encephalocele, and a dorsal CM can signal underlying cervical or lumbosacral spinal dysraphism. Capillary malformation combined with pigmented nevus (more common in dark-skinned infants) is called *phakomatosis pigmentovascularis* and suggests a common defect in migration of neural crest cells.

Treatment

CM is treated by flashlamp pulsed-dye laser; the results are better if initiated in infancy and childhood. Significant lightening occurs in 70% to 80% of patients; laser therapy is often prolonged and repetitive. Outcome is better on the lateral facial area than on the central face or the trunk and limbs.

Soft-tissue and skeletal hypertrophy require surgical strategies such as contour resection for macrocheilia and orthognathic procedures for asymmetric vertical maxillary excess or for mandibular prognathism. Excision of localized fibrovascular nodules is easily accomplished. In rare instances, it is necessary to excise a thickened CM in an entire facial aesthetic unit and resurface with a skin graft.

Cutis Marmorata Telangiectatica Congenita

This distinctive condition presents as a congenital, reticulated, serpiginous, depressed, blue-violet, cutaneous vascular network, most commonly on the lower extremity and trunk. The lesions occur in either a localized or segmental distribution; rarely are they generalized. There can be ulceration and atrophy of the involved skin. Biopsy reveals dilated dermal capillaries and veins, and sometimes thin-walled, venous lakes in the subcutis. The lesions improve, particularly during the first year of life; however, cutaneous atrophy, vascular staining, and venous ectasia persist. This disorder should be differentiated from an accentuated pattern of normal cutaneous vascularity called *cutis marmorata* or *livedo reticularis*. The literature is replete with many, often dire, associated anomalies; most, however, are coincidental or examples of mistaken identity. Cutis marmorata telangiectatica congenita is a benign condition.

Macrocephaly-Cutis Marmorata Syndrome

This specific disorder, unfortunately, shares the label cutis marmorata. Its features include macrosomia, macrocephaly, nonobstructive hydrocephalus, hyperelastic skin, joint laxity, craniofacial and limb asymmetry, and syndactyly. The CM is patchy and reticulate, and is distributed on the central face, and often on the trunk. These patients are at high risk for neurologic problems and cardiac arrhythmias.

Telangiectasias

Spider Telangiectasia

These acquired vascular marks commonly occur in children on the dorsum of the hands, forearms, and face. In adults, they appear, in decreasing order of frequency, on the face, neck, thorax, and arms. Similar lesions occur during pregnancy and usually disappear during the early puerperium. Pulsed-dye laser photocoagulation is effective.

Generalized Essential Telangiectasia

This acquired lesion occurs almost exclusively in adult women. The primary lesions are pin-sized, red-purple vascular puncta, appearing in groups, usually in the lower extremities. The lesions extend proximally, and, over years, form gyrate or matted sheets of telangiectases. *Unilateral nevoid telangiectasia* is related condition associated with increased levels of estrogen during puberty, pregnancy, and in patients with alcoholic cirrhosis. Flashlamp pulsed-dye laser therapy is relatively effective for both conditions.

Hereditary Hemorrhagic Telangiectasia

The prevalence of HHT is 1 to 2 per 100,000 live births. HHT is a group of autosomal disorders of similar phenotype, caused by at least three known genes—*endoglin, activin,* and *SMAD4*—and characterized by multisystem vascular anomalies and recurrent hemorrhage. The homozygous form is probably lethal. The characteristic lesions are discrete, spiderlike, bright red maculopapules, typically with a diameter of 1 to 4 mm, located on the face tongue, lips, nasal and oral mucous membranes, conjunctiva, palmar aspect of the fingers, and nail beds. Lesions also occur on internal mucosal surfaces and in viscera. Although the telangiectasias can appear in childhood, they usually emerge after puberty and increase in number with age. Epistaxis is the most common manifestation. Other presenting signs are hematemesis, hematuria, or melena. Bleeding in the central nervous system can cause neurologic symptoms. HHT patients can develop AVMs, particularly in the lungs, brain, spinal cord, and liver. Arteriovenous shunting can lead to pulmonary hypertension. Septic emboli from pulmonary AVMs commonly cause intracranial abscess.

Lymphatic Malformations

LM comprises anomalous channels, vesicles, or pouches filled with lymphatic fluid. An LM can be described as *microcystic, macrocystic,* or *combined (micro-macrocystic)* (**the old terms are *lymphangioma* for microcystic LM and *cystic hygroma* for macrocystic LM). LM never regresses; it expands or contracts depending on the ebb and flow of lymphatic fluid and the occurrence of inflammation and intralesional bleeding.** There are extremely rare examples of rapid, spontaneous deflation of macrocystic posterior cervical lesions. Most LMs are evident at birth or detected before 2 years of age. Although they can suddenly manifest in an older child, they rarely manifest in adolescence. Prenatal ultrasonography can detect macrocystic LM as early as the late first trimester of pregnancy.

Anomalous dilated lymphatics in the skin or mucosa present as vesicles and intravesicular bleeding evidenced as tiny, dark-red, dome-shaped nodules. LMs in the cheek, forehead, and orbit are frequently combined micro-macrocystic. They cause facial asymmetry, ocular proptosis, and distortion of features. **Soft-tissue and bony hypertrophy is characteristic. LM is the most common cause for macrocheilia, macroglossia, macrotia, and macromala.** Overgrowth in the body of the mandible manifests malocclusion, typically anterior open bite, and class III occlusion (10). A bulky tongue, covered with vesicles, impairs speech and is complicated by recurrent infection, swelling, bleeding, poor dental hygiene, and caries. In the cervicofacial region, micro-macrocystic LM can cause airway obstruction, sometimes necessitating tracheostomy. Cervicoaxillary LM commonly involves the thorax and mediastinum, causing recurrent pleural and pericardial effusion. Extensive LM in an extremity is associated with lymphedema. Pelvic LM manifests with perineal lymphangiectasias. Visceral LM (old term, *lymphangiomatosis*) can result in hypoalbuminemia secondary to protein-losing enteropathy. Generalized LM denotes skeletal involvement, typically ribs, vertebrae, scapula, and long bones.

Treatment

Intralesional bleeding or cellulitis causes sudden enlargement. Pain medication, rest, and time is all that is needed for intralesional bleeding. Any systemic viral or bacterial infection can cause a LM to "flare up." Nonsteroidal anti-inflammatory drugs can be useful during these episodes. Bacterial cellulitis of the LM itself requires immediate antibiotic therapy. Sometimes prolonged intravenous administration is necessary; septicemia is life-threatening. **Sclerotherapy has assumed a major role in the management of LM**. Large cysts can be treated with aspiration of lymphatic fluid and instillation of sclerosing agents, such as absolute ethanol, doxycycline, sodium tetradecyl sulfate, or OK-432 (a killed strain of group-A streptococcus).

Surgical resection is the only way to potentially cure LM. Operative guidelines include focusing on a defined anatomic region, limiting acceptable blood loss, performing as thorough a resection as possible given anatomic restrictions, and not prescribing the duration of the procedure. Postoperative problems include cellulitis, hematoma, and prolonged drainage. Total resection is usually not possible. Remaining transected lymphatic channels can regenerate forming vesicles in the operative scar and a soft-tissue mass. Osteotomy/ostectomy is indicated for an abnormal maxillary–mandibular relationship associated with cervicofacial LM (10). Cutaneous LM (*lymphangioma circumscriptum*) requires resection to deep fascia and, usually, closure of the defect with a split-thickness skin graft.

Venous Malformations

VMs are present at birth, although not always evident. They are bluish, soft, and compressible, and manifest in many forms. VMs are localized or extensive within an anatomic region, and are typically located on face, limbs, or trunk. VMs also can occur in the oronasopharynx, genitalia, bladder, brain, spinal cord, liver, spleen, lungs, skeletal muscles, and bones. **In these locations, VM is often incorrectly called *cavernous hemangioma*. VM swells when dependent.** Patients often complain of pain and stiffness in the affected area, especially on awakening in the morning. Episodic thrombosis occurs; phleboliths can appear as early as 2 years of age. VM grows proportionately to the child, expands slowly, and often enlarges during puberty.

A VM usually is a solitary lesion; multiple cutaneous or visceral lesions can occur, suggesting the possibility of inheritance. GVM ("familial glomangiomas") is a relatively common autosomal dominant syndrome of high penetrance, consisting of multiple, often tender, blue nodular or plaquelike venous anomalies occurring anywhere on the skin. Histologically, these lesions differ from typical VM by the presence of numerous glomus cells lining the ectatic venous channels. *Familial cutaneous–mucosal venous malformation* is another autosomal dominant condition presenting with tiny-to-several

centimeter-sized dome-shaped lesions or dilations of major veins. *Blue rubber bleb nevus* is a sporadic disorder with cutaneous and visceral VM. The skin lesions are soft, blue, and nodular; they can occur anywhere, but are typically located on the hands and feet. The gastrointestinal lesions are sessile (submucosal) or polypoid; located in the esophagus, stomach, small and large bowel, and mesentery, they are best seen by endoscopy rather than by MRI, radionuclide scan, or arteriography. Recurrent intestinal bleeding can be severe, requiring repeated transfusion (Table 22.2).

Craniofacial VM is usually unilateral and often causes facial asymmetry and progressive distortion of features. Intraorbital VM induces expansion of the orbital cavity and may communicate through the sphenomaxillary fissure with VM in the infratemporal fossa and cheek. The result can be enophthalmos when the patient stands and exophthalmos when the head is dependent. Buccal VM typically involves the tongue, palate, and oropharynx. Intraoral VM can impair speech and typically causes dental malalignment and open-bite deformity. Pharyngeal and laryngeal VM commonly progress to cause obstructive sleep apnea. VM in an extremity can involve skin only, or extend into muscles, joints, and bone. An extremity VM rarely causes length discrepancy, although lower limb lesions can cause slight undergrowth because of disuse. Limb VM sometimes causes structural weakening of the bony shaft and pathologic fracture. Synovial VM in the knee often causes episodic attacks of joint pain as a result of bloody effusion leading to destruction of articular cartilage. Hemarthrosis is particularly troublesome in children with VM-associated coagulopathy.

MRI is the most informative radiologic technique: VM exhibits a a brighter signal than fat on T2-weighted sequences. **A coagulation profile should be done on any child with a large VM. There is usually localized intravascular coagulopathy (LIC) and these patients are at risk for disseminated intravascular coagulopathy (DIC) following trauma or therapeutic intervention. This coagulopathy is wholly different from** Kasabach-Merritt phenomenon. Platelets are minimally diminished, in the 100 to 150,000/mm^3 range; usually PT and aPTT are normal, fibrinogen is low (150–200 mg/100 mL), and there are increased fibrin split-products or D-dimer.

Treatment

Therapy is indicated for either appearance or functional problems (11). Small cutaneous VMs are sclerosed with 1% sodium tetradecyl sulfate. A large cutaneous or intramuscular VM requires general anesthesia and real-time fluoroscopic monitoring during sclerotherapy. **Absolute ethanol is the most effective agent, but should not be used near important nerves; otherwise, 3% sodium tetradecyl sulfate is used.** Sclerotherapy of a major VM is dangerous and must be done by a skilled and experienced interventional radiologist. Compression and other maneuvers prevent passage of the sclerosing agent into the systemic circulation. Local complications include blistering, full-thickness necrosis, and neural deficits. Systemic complications are reported, such as renal toxicity and cardiac arrest. Multiple sclerotherapeutic sessions are required, often at several monthly intervals. Venous anomalies have a propensity to recanalize and reexpand. **Surgical resection is considered after completion of sclerotherapy in an effort to reduce tissue mass for functional or cosmetic indications.** Malocclusion requires orthodontic management and, if necessary, orthognathic procedures after eruption of the secondary teeth. If there is an abnormal coagulative profile, preoperative anticoagulation is necessary.

Elastic support stockings are indispensable for management of VM in the extremity. Low-dose aspirin (80 mg q.d. or q.o.d.)

minimizes the occurrence of episodic, painful phlebothrombosis.

Subtotal (contour) resection is useful for VM of the hand or foot, particularly in the digits. Intramuscular VM in the thigh or calf can diminish function requiring resection. VMs in the gastrointestinal tract are managed by banding via the endoscope, sclerotherapy, and bowel resection.

Arteriovenous Malformations

Pure arterial malformation (AM), such as aneurysm, stenosis, and ectasia, can occur as an isolated lesion or in conjunction with AVM. The epicenter of an AVM is called the *nidus* and consists of arterial feeders, micro- and macroarteriovenous fistulas (AVFs), and ectatic veins. AVMs are present at birth, most are seen during infancy, but are underappreciated. Intracranial AVM is more common than extracranial AVM, followed, in frequency of location by limbs, trunk, and viscera.

The blush of an AVM can be mistaken for hemangioma or port-wine stain. Puberty and trauma appear to trigger expansion. The skin becomes a red or violaceous color, a mass appears beneath the vascular stain, and there is local warmth, a thrill, and a bruit. Whatever the site of an AVM, the eventual consequences are ischemic changes, ulceration, intractable pain, and intermittent bleeding. Pseudo-Kaposi sarcomatous cutaneous changes, scaling violaceous plaques, commonly occur in association with AVM in the lower limb. An extensive AVM, usually involving an entire extremity or the pelvis, can cause increased cardiac output. The natural history of AVM is documented by a clinical staging system introduced by Schobinger (12):

Stage I (Quiescence): Pink-blush stain, warmth, and AV shunting by continous Doppler or 20-MHz color Doppler

Stage II (Expansion): Same as stage I, plus enlargement, pulsations, thrill, bruit, and tottuous/tense veins

Stage III (Destruction): Same as above, plus dystrophic changes, ulceration, bleeding persistent pain, and expansion/destruction

Stage IV (Decompensation): Same as stage II, plus cardiac failure

Pulsed Doppler documents arterial output (compared to the normal side) and can be used to follow the progression of an AVM. MRI best demonstrates the extent of the malformation. Superselective angiography is unnecessary until intervention is considered.

Treatment

AVM is usually quiescent during infancy and childhood. Once the diagnostic evaluation is complete, the child is carefully followed. Early embolic/surgical management for Stages I and II AVM is debatable, but should be considered if resection is easily achievable and reconstruction does not disfigure. **Usually AVM is treated whenever endangering signs and symptoms arise, such as ischemic pain, recalcitrant ulceration, bleeding, or increased cardiac output (Schobinger Stages III and IV),** occurs.

Ligation or proximal embolization of arterial feeding vessels must never be done! This causes rapid recruitment of nearby arterial vessels to supply the nidus. Furthermore, arterial ligation limits access for therapeutic embolization. Angiography precedes radiologic or surgical intervention. Superselective arterial embolization is palliative for pain, bleeding, or cardiac failure, particularly in those instances where the AVM is out-of-bounds for resection. Embolization temporarily controls an AVM, but cannot cure an AVM, unlike a single direct arteriovenous fistula. **Arterial embolization is done to temporarily occlude the nidus in preparation for resection 24 to 72 hours** later. Direct puncture of the nidus, in conjunction with local arterial and venous compression, is necessary if the arteries are tortuous, or if there has been previous arterial ligation. Embolization or sclerotherapy minimizes intraoperative bleeding but does not diminish the limits of resection. The nidus and usually the overlying skin must be widely resected. The overlying skin can be preserved if it appears normal; however, if it is deeply stained and retained, recurrence is to be expected. Wound coverage is preferably done following resection. Microsurgical free flap transfer may be needed for reconstruction. After combined embolization–resection, the patient must be followed for years by clinical examination, ultrasonography, and/or MRI. The goal is to control AVM; cure is usually not possible (12).

Combined Vascular Malformations

Complex-combined vascular malformations can be slow-flow or fast-flow; many are remembered by eponyms and exhibit overgrowth (Table 22.3). These proper names probably should be relinquished because they are often misused, misleading, and indicate nothing of pathogenesis.

Slow-Flow Combined Malformations

Klippel-Trenaunay syndrome is a well-worn eponym for a combined capillary-lymphaticovenous malformation (CLVM) associated with soft-tissue/skeletal hypertrophy in one or more limbs. The CMs are multiple, often in a patchy geographic pattern, usually studded with hemolymphatic vesicles (CLM), and typically located on the anterolateral aspect of the thigh, buttock, or trunk. The anomalous veins are prominent laterally because of insufficient to absent valves; deep venous anomalies also occur. Lymphatic hypoplasia or localized lymphatic anomalies are primary defects. Limb hypertrophy can be minor to grotesque; some patients with classic CLVM have a short or hypotrophic limb. Often there is lipomatous dorsal swelling and digital overgrowth on the opposite foot.

Proteus syndrome is a sporadic disorder characterized by connective tissue nevi, lipomas, several unusual tumors, disproportionate skeletal growth, in addition to ocular, pulmonary, and renal abnormalities. Asymmetrical growth and soft-tissue changes are not present at birth; they evolve later, which serves to differentiate Proteus syndrome from Klippel-Trenaunay syndrome. Vascular anomalies (CM, VM, LM or combined forms) can occur, randomly distributed on the trunk and limbs. Proteus syndrome is thought to be caused by a dominant lethal gene that survives by somatic mosaicism.

Maffucci syndrome denotes the coexistence of exophytic venous anomalies with bony exostoses and enchondromatoses. These features usually do not manifest until early to mid-childhood. Enchondromas are discovered first, typically

TABLE 22.3

COMBINED VASCULAR MALFORMATION-OVERGROWTH SYNDROMES

Slow-flow	Fast-flow
Klippel-Trenaunay syndrome (CLVM)	Parkes-Weber syndrome (CAVM)(CLAVM)
Proteus syndrome (CM)(LM)(VM)	Bannayan-Riley-Ruvalcaba syndrome (AVM) [*PTEN*]
Maffucci syndrome (VM), enchondromas	

located in the metaphysis and epiphysis of the long bones. The venous lesions typically appear around 4 to 5 years of age as firm, dome-like, bluish spots, usually on a finger or toe. Venous anomalies also present in bones (particularly the limbs), leptomeninges, or gastrointestinal tract. Malignant degeneration, usually chondrosarcoma and other nonskeletal neoplasms, occurs in 20% to 40% of patients.

Fast-Flow Combined Malformations

Parkes-Weber syndrome, Capillary arterial venous malformation, Capillary lymphatic arterial venous malformation (CAVM, CLAVM) presents at birth with cutaneous warmth, bruit, and thrill in a limb and proximal trunk. The lower limb is more often affected than the upper limb. There is a geographic pink, macular stain and generalized enlargement. There may be lymphatic anomalies, either lymphedema or localized lesions. MRI in young children often reveals only diffuse hypervascularity of enlarged muscles and bones. MRA and MRV show generalized arterial and venous dilatation. Arteriography demonstrates microscopic AV fistulae throughout the affected limb, particularly near the joints.

Bannayan-Riley-Ruvalcaba syndrome is characterized by delayed motor and speech development, proximal myopathy, macrocephaly, pigmental penile macules, ileal and colonic hamartomatous polyps, subcutaneous lipomas, and Hashimoto thyroiditis. Vascular anomalies appear in wide spectrum from small nodular cutaneous lesions, intramuscular, intraosseous, and intracranial lesions to extensive AVM. Bannayan-Riley-Ruvalcaba syndrome is an autosomal dominant disorder, allelic with Cowden syndrome, and caused by mutations in *PTEN*, a tumor-suppressor gene. There is phenotypic overlapping, and patients with either syndrome are at risk for developing benign and malignant neoplasms.

Treatment of Combined Vascular Malformations

Leg length is radiologically measured by age 2 years. If the discrepancy is more than 1.5 cm, a shoe-lift is needed to prevent secondary scoliosis and limping. For fast-flow combined anomalies, ultrasonography and color Doppler evaluation of limb arterial and venous vessels is indicated when the child is 3 or 4 years old or is symptomatic. Superselective embolization is indicated for pain, ischemia, or ulceration.

Management is fundamentally conservative. Elastic compressive stockings are recommended for slow-flow anomalies with venous insufficiency and a functioning deep system. Superficial varicose veins are rarely treated unless they are grossly incompetent, the deep system is functional, and the patient has significant symptoms such as leg fatigue, heaviness, or inability to wear shoes because of enlarged dorsal veins. In selected patient, sclerotherapy is used to obliterate incompetent superficial veins and to shrink focal VMs or lymphatic cysts.

Staged contour resection or selective amputation is necessary for grotesque hypertrophy of the foot that prevents fitting of shoes or interferes with ambulation. It is unnecessary to correct for length differential in the upper limb; percutaneous epiphysiodesis is needed if the difference is 2 cm or more.

Circumferential thoracic CLVM is resected in stages. Postoperative healing is often problematic after resection of CLVM in any location. Episodic bleeding from the capillary-lymphatic (CLM) cutaneous vesicles is annoying. Elastic support helps by compressing the dilated underlying veins and provides protection from abrasion of the skin. Injection of the vesicles with alcohol or 1% sodium tetradecyl sulfate is effective. If bleeding persists, excision of the vascular plaque and replacement with a split-thickness skin graft gives long-term control.

VASCULAR ANOMALIES CENTERS

Children with vascular anomalies often become medical nomads. Parents take the child from one physician to another because no one seems to understand the condition. Because no single specialist has the knowledge and expertise to treat the wide variety of these disorders, major referral hospitals have organized vascular anomalies teams. Cyber-savvy parents can easily find these centers. Members of the team may differ, depending on local interest, expertise, and enthusiasm. Patients with vascular anomalies rarely engender conflicts over turf. Because the problems often seem insolvable, most physicians are all too happy to send the patient for consultation. A vascular anomalies team serves as a focus for accurate diagnosis, appropriate management, and clinical and basic research in this truly interdisciplinary field.

References

1. Mulliken JB, Fishman SJ, Burrows PE. Vascular anomalies. *Curr Prob Surg.* 2000;37:517.
2. North PE, Waner M, Mizeracki A, et al. A unique microvascular phenotype shared by juvenile hemangiomas and human placenta. *Arch Dermatol.* 2001;137:559.
3. Boye E, Yu Y, Paranya G, et al. Clonality and altered behavior of endothelial cells from hemangiomas. *J Clin Invest.* 2001;107:745.
4. Berenguer B, Mulliken JB, Enjolras O, et al. Rapidly involuting congenital hemangioma: clinical and histopathologic features. *Pediatr Dev Pathol.* 2003;6:495.
5. Metry DW, Dowd CF, Barkovich AJ, et al. The many faces of PHACE syndrome. *J Pediatr.* 2001;139:117.
6. Mulliken JB, Anupindi S, Ezekowitz RAB, et al. Case records of the Massachusetts General Hospital. Case 13-2004: a newborn girl with a large cutaneous lesion, thrombocytopenia, and anemia. *N Engl J Med.* 2004;350:1764.
7. Boon LM, MacDonald DM, Mulliken JB. Complications of systemic corticosteroid therapy for problematic hemangiomas. *Plast Reconstr Surg.* 1999;104:1616.
8. Mulliken JB, Rogers GF, Marler JJ. Circular excision of hemangioma and purse-string closure—the smallest possible scar. *Plast Reconstr Surg.* 2002;109:1544.
9. Vikkula M, Boon LM, Mulliken JB. Molecular genetics of vascular malformations. *Matrix Biol* 2001;20:327.
10. Padwa BL, Hayward PG, Ferraro NF, et al. Cervicofacial lymphatic malformation: clinical course, surgical intervention, and pathogenesis of skeletal hypertrophy. *Plast Reconstr Surg.* 1995;95:951.
11. Berenguer B, Burrows PE, Zurakowski D, et al. Sclerotherapy of craniofacial venous malformations: complications and outcome. *Plast Reconstr Surg.* 1999;104:1.
12. Kohout MP, Hansen M, Pribaz JJ, et al. Arteriovenous malformations of the head and neck: natural history and management. *Plast Reconstr Surg.* 1998;102:643.

CHAPTER 23 ■ CLEFT LIP AND PALATE

RICHARD A. HOPPER, COURT CUTTING, AND BARRY GRAYSON

Cleft lip and palate are the most common congenital craniofacial anomalies treated by plastic surgeons. Successful treatment of these children requires technical skill, in-depth knowledge of the abnormal anatomy, and appreciation of three-dimensional facial aesthetics. Cleft care requires that the plastic surgeon be a member of a collaborative multidisciplinary team. Through close self-scrutiny, disciplined evaluation of the results, and a great deal of imagination, a number of plastic surgeons continue to advance cleft care, seeing as many challenges ahead as they encountered at the beginning of their careers.

EPIDEMIOLOGY AND ETIOPATHOGENESIS

Among the cleft lip and palate population, the most common diagnosis is cleft lip and palate at 46%, followed by isolated cleft palate at 33%, then isolated cleft lip at 21%. The majority of bilateral cleft lips (86%) and unilateral cleft lips (68%) are associated with a cleft palate. Unilateral clefts are nine times as common as bilateral clefts, and occur twice as frequently on the left side than on the right. Males are predominant in the cleft lip and palate population, whereas isolated cleft palate occurs more commonly in females. In the white population, cleft lip with or without cleft palate occurs in approximately 1 in 1,000 live births. These entities are twice as common in the Asian population, and approximately half as common in African Americans. This racial heterogeneity is not observed for isolated cleft palate, which has an overall incidence of 0.5 per 1,000 live births.

Both environmental teratogens and genetic factors are implicated in the genesis of cleft lip and palate. Intrauterine exposure to the anticonvulsant phenytoin is associated with a 10-fold increase in the incidence of cleft lip. Maternal smoking during pregnancy doubles the incidence of cleft lip. Other teratogens, such as alcohol, anticonvulsants, and retinoic acid, are associated with malformation patterns that include cleft lip and palate, but have not been directly related to isolated clefts.

Genetic abnormalities can result in syndromes that include clefts of the primary or secondary palates among the developmental fields affected. More than 40% of isolated cleft palates are part of malformation syndromes, compared to less than 15% of cleft lip and palate cases. The most common syndrome associated with cleft lip and palate is van der Woude syndrome with or without lower lip pits or blind sinuses. Microdeletions of chromosome 22q resulting in velocardiofacial, DiGeorge, or conotruncal anomaly syndromes are the most common diagnoses associated with isolated cleft palate. Although there is a recognized genetic component to nonsyndromic cleft lip and/or palate, it appears to be multifactorial. Among other recent studies, a meta-analysis of 13 genome scans by Marazita et al. (2004) revealed multiple cleft lip/palate genes on 16 chromosomal regions.

Parents with a child with a nonsyndromic cleft, or a family history of clefting, often ask about their risk of clefts in subsequent pregnancies. The risk depends on whether the proband has a cleft lip alone (CL), cleft lip with cleft palate (CLP), or a cleft palate alone (CP). If the family has one affected child or parent with CLP, the risk of the child of the next pregnancy having CLP is 4%. If two previous children have CLP, the risk increases to 9%, and if one parent and one child were previously affected, the risk to children of subsequent pregnancies is 17%. For families with a history of CP, the risk of CP to children of subsequent pregnancies is 2% if one previously affected child, 1% if two children were previously affected, 6% if one parent has CP, and 15% if one parent and one previous child have CP.

MULTIDISCIPLINARY CLEFT CARE

Individuals born with cleft lip and or palate require coordinated care from multiple specialties to optimize treatment outcome. The ideal is in a center with a multidisciplinary cleft team, dedicated to treating cleft-related issues from birth to adulthood. Typical members of a cleft team include an audiologist, dentist, geneticist, nurse, nutritionist/dietitian, oral surgeon, orthodontist, otolaryngologist, pediatrician, plastic surgeon, psychologist, social worker, and speech pathologist.

The emphasis is on coordination to minimize the number of surgeries performed while maximizing the benefit to the patient. Although the number of surgical procedures required prior to adulthood has decreased with improved techniques, care of a child with a cleft still requires a complex lengthy surgical treatment plan (Table 23.1). The goal of cleft care is to eliminate as many steps in the treatment plan as possible by optimizing the outcome and benefit of each essential intervention. Recent advances in presurgical orthopedics, such as nasoalveolar molding and gingivoperiosteoplasty, are examples of optimization of early intervention with the goal of minimizing secondary surgeries and eliminating previously essential steps such as secondary alveolar bone grafting and rhinoplasty.

SURGICAL EVALUATION AND CLASSIFICATION

Ideally, the newborn infant with a cleft is evaluated by the cleft team in the first weeks of life. The increasing number of clefts detected by prenatal imaging allows early preparation of the family and introduction to the treatment plan. Patients with cleft lip and/or palate are not a homogenous group. As mentioned above, they can be divided into CL, CP, and CLP; however, the surgical treatment plan requires a more complex classification scheme. The cleft lip deformity is typically divided into unilateral or bilateral, and then subdivided into complete, incomplete, or microform. The width of the cleft deformity and the degree of alveolar arch collapse also play a part in surgical planning, as these directly relate to the degree of associated nasal deformity and the tension and difficulty of the

TABLE 23.1

SURGICAL TREATMENT OF A CLEFT LIP AND PALATE BY AGE

Age	Treatment	Cleft team members
Prenatal	Prenatal imaging, diagnosis, and counseling	Multidisciplinary
Newborn[a]	Feeding assessment, medical assessment, genetic counseling, treatment information	Multidisciplinary
0–3 months	Presurgical orthopedics	Orthodontist, plastic surgeon
3 months (or after presurgical orthopedics)[a]	Primary cleft lip repair and tip rhinoplasty ± gingivoperiosteoplasty	Plastic surgeon
12 months (delayed if airway or medical concerns)[a]	Primary cleft palate repair with intravelar veloplasty ± bilateral myringotomy and tubes	Plastic surgeon, otolaryngologist
Diagnosis of velopharyngeal insufficiency (3–4 years)	Secondary palate lengthening or pharyngoplasty, speech obturator	Speech pathologist, plastic surgeon, otolaryngologist, orthodontist
School-age years	Treatment of secondary lip and nasal deformities	Plastic surgeon
7–9 years (mixed dentition)[b]	Secondary alveolar bone graft	Orthodontist, plastic surgeon, oral surgeon
Postalveolar graft[a]	Presurgical orthodontics	Orthodontist
Puberty	Definitive open rhinoplasty	Plastic surgeon
Skeletal maturity	LeFort I ± mandible orthognathic surgery	Plastic surgeon, oral surgeon

[a]Essential treatments of cleft lip and palate deformity.
[b]Required if gingivoperiosteoplasty is not done or is unsuccessful.

repair. The associated nasal deformity is similarly categorized as mild, moderate, or severe. Mild nasal deformity is characterized by a lateral displacement of the alar base but normal alar contour, minimal columella shortening, and normal dome projection. Moderate nasal deformity has lateral and posterior displacement of the alar base, columella deficiency, and a depressed dome. Severe nasal deformity has an underprojecting alar dome with complete collapse of the lower lateral cartilage and a severe deficiency of columella height. Severe nasal deformities often have a reversed curvature to the alar rim. The nasal deformity is secondary to a three-dimensional distortion of the lower lateral cartilage, described by some as the "tilted tripod." It is not caused by hypoplasia or deficiency of the cartilage itself.

If a cleft palate is present, it is surgically classified as unilateral, bilateral, or submucous. The width of the cleft is noted as it affects the difficulty of closure.

Although most surgeons use the descriptive classification of cleft deformities during the initial assessment of a patient, other classification systems are often used for outcome research and record keeping. Kernahan and Stark's "stripped Y" diagrammatic classification scheme and its modifications continue to be used in many cleft centers. It recognizes the embryologic division of the primary (lip and alveolus) and secondary palates at the incisive foramen. Otto Kriens presented a palindromic acronym organization of cleft deformities. The acronym LAHSHAL denotes the bilateral anatomy of lip (*L*), alveolus (*A*), hard (*H*) and soft (*S*) palates, by convention from right to left. Lowercase letters represent incomplete clefts of the structure; a period denotes no cleft. A bilateral cleft lip

with a complete unilateral cleft of the secondary palate, with incomplete clefting of the lip and alveolus on one side would be represented as LAHSal. This system is currently used for the outcomes registry of the American Cleft Palate and Craniofacial Association.

Microform Cleft Lip

The microform cleft (Fig. 23.1A) is characterized by a furrow or scar transgressing the vertical length of the lip, a vermilion notch, imperfections in the white roll, and varying degrees of vertical lip shortness. Nasal deformity may be present and is sometimes more extensive than the associated lip problem. Surgery is generally indicated but is approached cautiously to avoid a surgical deformity worse than the congenital defect. If there is isolated disruption of the orbicularis oris sphincter, it can be repaired through an intraoral approach.

Unilateral Incomplete Cleft Lip

Unilateral incomplete clefts (Fig. 23.1B) are characterized by varying degrees of vertical separation of the lip, but they all have in common an intact nasal sill, or Simonart band. They require the same surgical technique as a complete cleft lip in order to restore normal nasal and lip anatomy, although the degree of dissection can be tailored to the magnitude of the deformity. As with complete clefts, the best time to address

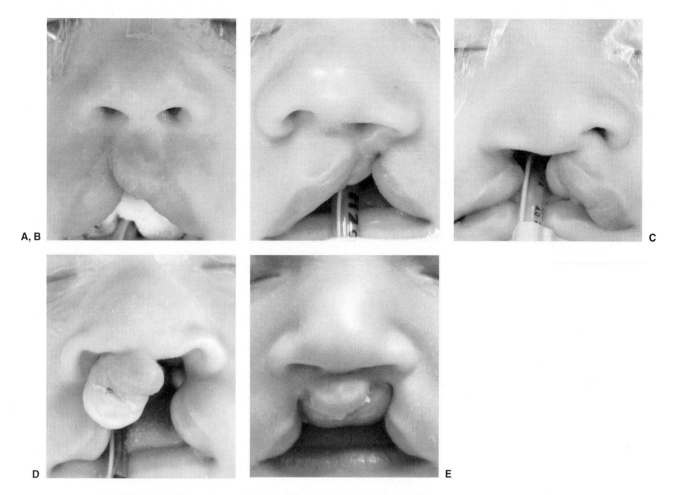

FIGURE 23.1. The spectrum of cleft lip deformities. **A:** Microform cleft lip. **B:** Unilateral incomplete cleft lip. **C:** Unilateral complete cleft lip. **D:** Bilateral complete cleft lip. **E:** Bilateral incomplete cleft lip.

the associated nasal deformity is at the time of the primary lip repair.

Unilateral Complete Cleft Lip

Unilateral complete clefts (Fig. 23.1C) are characterized by disruption of the lip, nostril sill, and alveolus (complete primary palate). Unlike the incomplete cleft lip there is no Simonart band connecting the alar base to the footplates of the lower lateral cartilages of the nose; consequently, the abnormal attachments of the orbicularis oris muscles on either side of the cleft cause a variable degree of collapse of the lower lateral cartilage framework and an associated increased nasal deformity. The critical factors for evaluating unilateral complete clefts are the position of the lesser and greater alveolar segments, the vertical height of the lateral lip element, and the degree of associated nasal deformity. The alveolar (maxillary) segments assume one of four positions: (a) narrow–no collapse; (b) narrow–collapse; (c) wide–no collapse; (d) wide–collapse. "Wide" is determined by an alveolus position lateral to the desired alar base position (i.e., with lip closure the alar base is sitting in the cleft). "Collapse" refers to a palatal displacement of the lateral maxillary segment as predicated by the arch configuration of the medial, noncleft dental ridge.

Clefts characterized as "narrow–no collapse" with minimal nasal deformity are treated with presurgical taping to prevent widening of the cleft with growth and feeding, prior to a primary cleft lip repair with primary tip rhinoplasty. If a gingivoperiosteoplasty is to be performed at the same time, a molding plate can be used to optimize contact of the opposing alveolar ridges. Clefts characterized as "narrow–collapse" or "wide–collapse" benefit from presurgical molding to create the desired arch form, alveolar contact, and nasal anatomy at the time of surgery. Clefts characterized as "wide–collapse" or "wide–no collapse" must be assessed closely by the dental members of the cleft team. If they feel that these cases are deficient in arch mesenchyme, presurgical orthopedics is used to align the arch segments by correcting the collapse, but not to close the alveolar cleft since this will result in a constricted arch. External taping can be used to correct the alar base position over the maintained arch form. The use of presurgical orthopedics or aggressive presurgical taping has eliminated the need for preliminary lip adhesion surgery at most centers. The primary benefit of a balanced noncollapsed arch configuration at the time of primary lip repair is the decreased tension on the lip repair and the secondary benefits to the nasal anatomy by providing a stable skeletal base.

Complete Bilateral Cleft Lip

The most obvious aspect of a complete bilateral cleft is the protruding premaxilla (Fig. 23.1D). Because of the lack of connection of the premaxilla with the lateral palatal shelves, the premaxilla has not been "reined back" into alignment with the lateral arch segments during fetal development. At the time of birth, the premaxilla protrudes on a vomerine stem.

Uncontrolled growth at the premaxillary suture results in over-projection of the premaxilla, with or without rotation and angulation of the segment. Just as the premaxilla is not reined back by the lateral palatal shelves, the lateral palatal shelves are not pulled forward by their attachment to the premaxilla. Without the intervening premaxilla to maintain arch width, the lateral palatal shelves collapse toward the midline. The severity of this disruption of arch morphology varies, and will dictate the tension on the repair, the degree of dissection required, and, ultimately, the final aesthetic result unless it is corrected with presurgical orthopedics.

The anterior nasal spine is poorly formed or absent in the bilateral cleft lip deformity, resulting in a retruded area under the base of the septal cartilage and recession of the footplates of the medial crura. The footplates of the lower lateral cartilages are displaced posteriorly and laterally, which in turn pulls the normal junction (genu) of the medial and lateral crura apart resulting in a broad, flat nasal tip. The recession of the medial crural footplates, along with lateralization of the domes, and deficient skin, produces the typical "absent columella." The most anterior and inferior extent of the frontonasal process, which normally contributes to the skin between the philtral columns of the lip, forms a wide, short disk, called a prolabium, that appears to hang directly from the nasal tip skin. In conventional techniques, linear distance from the inferior tip of the prolabium up to the nasal tip is inadequate to reconstruct both central upper lip and columellar length. This vertically limited tissue is used to create the central lip element at the cost of inadequate columella length and tip projection. A major benefit of nasoalveolar molding (NAM) is the ability to presurgically lengthen both the columella skin and the prolabium, creating enough skin to reconstruct the central lip length without compromising nasal tip projection.

Incomplete Bilateral Cleft Lip

Occasionally, bilateral clefts are incomplete with a near-normal nose, a normally positioned premaxilla, Simonart bands across the nasal floors, and clefts involving only the lip (Fig. 23.1E). In such circumstances, a rotation-advancement approach, or a triangular flap approach similar to that used in unilateral repairs, can be used either in a single-stage or a two-stage operation. In two-stage repairs one side is closed first, allowed to heal, and then the other side is repaired a short time later. Symmetry is difficult to achieve with a staged approach, and we prefer a single-stage procedure with a bilateral straight-line technique as described later in the chapter. More patients have complete clefts on one side and incomplete clefts on the other. These cases have both the nasal deformity of a unilateral complete cleft lip and the paucity of lip tissue of a bilateral cleft. If there is a discrepancy in columella height between the two sides, we will consider a rotation-advancement repair on the complete side to increase columella and a straight-line closure on the incomplete side.

Cleft Lip and Palate

The primary palate consists of the lip, alveolus, and anterior palate back to the incisive foramen. The secondary palate consists of the hard and soft palates from the incisive foramen back to the uvula. The presence of a cleft palate introduces feeding difficulties, concerns regarding speech development, and the possibility of impaired facial growth. The width of a primary palate cleft and the degree of collapse are typically increased in the presence of a cleft of the secondary palate. The family is counseled about the anticipated increased number of surgical operations that will be required if a cleft palate is present:

primary cleft palate repair with intravelar veloplasty; possible secondary surgery on the palatopharyngeal muscle sling, such as a sphincteroplasty or pharyngeal flap; and possible orthognathic surgery at skeletal maturity. The abnormal attachment of the muscles of the soft palate in a cleft palate alters the tension on the pharyngeal drainage of the eustachian canal, increasing the incidence of ear infections. Myringotomy and grommet tube placement is performed in the majority of infants at the time of either the lip repair or the palate repair to prevent the development of hearing abnormalities.

Isolated Cleft Palate

The infant with isolated cleft palate is examined carefully to ascertain if there are manifestations of the Pierre Robin sequence (micrognathia, glossoptosis, and airway obstruction). The etiopathogenesis of the cleft palate in the Pierre Robin sequence is thought to be obstruction of the palatal shelves as they swing from a vertical to horizontal orientation during palate fusion. The micrognathia and associated glossoptosis causes this obstruction, resulting in the characteristic wide "horseshoe" cleft palate associated with this sequence. If the Pierre Robin sequence is present, appropriate measures are instituted, the mainstay of which is prone positioning. In severe cases, treatment may include around-the-clock prone positioning, nasopharyngeal airway protection, gavage feedings, and apnea monitoring. Very few of these patients will require temporary endotracheal intubation or tongue–lip adhesion. In extreme cases, tracheostomy is required to manage the airway if the mandible is not lengthened surgically by early distraction osteogenesis. In Pierre Robin patients, palatoplasty may be delayed for several months, compared to other cleft palate closures, to ensure adequacy of the airway.

Submucous Cleft Palate

The submucous cleft palate is traditionally defined by a triad of deformities: a bifid uvula, a notched posterior hard palate, and muscular diastasis of the velum. Submucous clefts vary considerably, however, and muscular diastasis can occur in the absence of a bifid uvula. The majority of patients with submucous cleft palate are asymptomatic, although approximately 15% will develop velopharyngeal insufficiency (VPI). VPI correlates with short palatal length, limited mobility, and easy fatigability of the palate. Because the majority of patients with submucous cleft palate remain asymptomatic, a nonoperative approach is recommended until speech can be adequately evaluated.

PRESURGICAL ORTHOPEDICS

The cross-specialty collaboration between plastic surgery and dentistry has produced some of the most exciting advances in cleft care. It has also generated some of the most animated discussions about the perceived advantages and disadvantages of presurgical orthopedics in the literature and at national conferences. Because this field continues to be controversial, it is important to relate advances in presurgical orthopedics from a historical perspective.

Historical Perspective of Combined Presurgical and Surgical Treatments

Surgeons have long recognized the challenge of the bilateral cleft deformity. The main obstacles to the repair are the protruding premaxilla and the deficient columella. During the 16th, 17th, and 18th centuries, the surgical treatment involved excision of the premaxilla followed by a surgical union of the prolabium to the lateral lip segments. At a later age, prosthetic replacement of the anterior dentition was recommended to improve facial appearance. In the 19th century, surgeons finally accepted that excision of the premaxilla removed the upper incisors and deprived the lip of bony support, causing midface deficiency, maxillary constriction, malocclusions, and an apparent mandibular prognathism. The focus became preservation and retraction of the premaxilla to achieve optimal lip repair. Two treatment philosophies evolved: surgical correction alone and surgical correction following presurgical orthopedics.

Surgical Correction

Surgical options for premaxillary retraction included fracture of the vomer, resection of part of the vomer or nasal septum, partial resection of the anterior portion of the premaxilla, and a full-thickness vertical incision of the septum, which allowed the proximal and distal segments to slide over each other. Although these techniques achieved the primary goal of retracting the premaxilla, they were associated with significant complications. Both long-term clinical observations and animal studies demonstrated that resection of the nasal septum produced severe growth arrest of adjacent bones. The technique had other limitations, including lingual inclination of upper incisors caused by a lingually displaced premaxilla, nasal airway obstruction, and flat facies.

Another surgical approach that attempted to achieve premaxillary retraction and lateral segment approximation was lip adhesion, which is still used at some centers. Johanson and Ohlsson (1961) described the use of lip adhesion before primary bone grafting. Millard (4) reported the use of lip adhesion in the upper third of the cleft lip segments in preparation for the rotation-advancement technique of final lip closure. Randall (1965), using short, broad, triangular flaps, claimed that closure of the soft tissues molded the underlying bony structures, reduced tension in the lip, and repositioned the alar base. Randall undermined the lateral lip if necessary when there was a large cleft gap.

The disadvantages of lip adhesion include the risks of an additional surgical procedure, scarring of the involved tissue, loss of the local mucosal flaps used in some techniques for nasal lining repair, and potential dehiscence of the surgical site. In addition, the tension of the surgically adhered lip over the alveolar segments is an uncontrolled force that does not always align the segments in an ideal position, frequently causing collapse of the dental arches. Lip adhesion should be limited to those cases in which the maxillary segments are expanded without collapse. If the segments are medially collapsed, lip adhesion is of no use and a technique that provides alveolar expansion is preferable.

Presurgical Infant Orthopedics

The concept of presurgical treatment originated in the 16th century, when excision of the protruded premaxilla in bilateral clefts was the recommended treatment. Dissatisfied with the long-term results of this treatment modality, surgeons and dentists explored new avenues to achieve more optimal results. Franco (1561) described a head cap for extraoral therapy. Hoffmann (1686) used a head cap with facial extensions over the cheeks and lips to narrow the cleft by pressing over the premaxilla. Louis (1768), Chaussier (1776), and Desault (1790) used bandages over the prolabium to simulate muscle retraction, compressing the premaxillary region. In 1844, Hullihen, an American dentist, used facial adhesive strapping to "prepare" the cleft before surgery. He believed that closing the alveolar cleft prior to surgery during the first months of life was crucial in order to properly perform lip closure. Other early contributors to this field include Von Bardeleben (1868), who used a compression bandage with a bonnet; Thiesch (1875), who used rubber bands; and Von Esmarch and Kowalzig (1892), who employed an elastic band attached to a head cap. Brophy (1927) adapted an intraoral approach, passing wires through the alveolar bone proximal to the cleft on both sides. By slow tightening of the wires, he achieved approximation of the segments.

The concept of modern presurgical infant orthopedics (PSIO) started with the work of McNeil, who, disappointed with the maxillary collapse created by the available techniques, used an oral prosthesis similar to an obturator to approximate the cleft alveolar segments. In his technique, a maxillary impression was taken of the newborn and an acrylic appliance was made from a plaster model that was cut and modified with the cleft gap slightly closed. By repeating this step and frequently modifying the appliance, McNeil was able to close not only the alveolar gap, but also the hard palatal cleft by influencing bone growth direction. He believed that alveolar and palatal surgery could be avoided completely, implying that a soft tissue and even a bony continuity could be achieved. He also stated that the technique improved speech function, feeding, and deglutition, and could eliminate the need for orthodontic treatment. McNeil's exaggerated claims damaged the credibility of the technique, and controversy has surrounded the subject ever since. Moved by the intrigue, W.R. Burston (1958) evaluated McNeil's work and became one of the most loyal proponents of the technique. At the same time, Schuchardt used the method, especially in preparation for primary bone grafting.

Many variations in presurgical orthopedic techniques have evolved during the last 40 years. The appliances can be described as active or passive, although there is no uniform consensus or universal agreement on their classification. Huebener and Liu classified the appliances as (a) presurgical versus postsurgical, (b) active versus passive, and (c) extraoral versus intraoral.

Generally, active appliances use a hard acrylic plate and controlled forces, sometimes from extraoral traction (bonnet with straps), to move the maxillary alveolar segments into approximation. One of the best-known active appliances is the pin-retained variety used by Latham (1980), which is designed to exert a forward force to the lesser posterior segment of the unilateral cleft maxilla. It consists of a two-piece maxillary splint that overlies the palatal shelves and is retained by short medial pins. An expansion screw connecting the two pieces can be moved to adjust the widths of the lateral palatal segments. An orthodontic elastic chain is used to retract the premaxilla. By adjustment of these independent controls, the premaxilla is brought back into its proper position in the arch before the primary repair. The Latham device requires a surgical procedure to introduce the device and to remove it.

Passive appliances generally consist of an alveolar molding plate made of a hard outer shell and a soft acrylic lining. By gradual alteration of the tissue surface of the acrylic plate, the alveolar segments are gently molded into the desired shape and position by direction of alveolar growth. This method was initially described by Gnoinski and developed by Rosenstein (1963), Rosenstein and Jacobson (1967), and Monroe (1968). The devices allowed continued growth by a passive molding action without permitting medial movement of the buccal segments. Once the segments were in proper position, early lip repair and bone grafting could be performed. This passive molding approach has evolved into the more recent technique of NAM, which addresses the alveolar, labial, and nasal abnormalities as discussed later in the chapter.

The Controversy

One of the most outspoken opponents of PSIO is Pruzansky. In 1964, he published a dissenting opinion challenging McNeil's presurgical orthopedic technique. He believed that spontaneous retropositioning of the premaxilla following lip repair obviates the need for intervention with orthopedic devices. It is generally agreed that PSIO does not enhance growth of the maxilla, the orthodontic benefits are limited, and non-surgical closure of palatal bone and soft tissue is impossible. Proponents of PSIO report that the aesthetic result of the cleft lip and nasal repair is improved and the number of surgeries are minimized. Opponents are concerned about the added cost and the risk of iatrogenic malocclusion and midface retrusion. Despite this ongoing controversy, presurgical orthopedics continues to be widely used, and it has been cited by Brogan and McComb as the superlative example of cooperation within the cleft rehabilitation team. Hotz et al. reported that, in 1984, 22 of the 32 cleft lip and palate rehabilitation centers in Zurich indicated that they used presurgical orthopedics treatment. In 1990, Asher-McDade and Shaw indicated that 40 of 45 British cleft palate teams reported the use of presurgical orthopedics. In a recent unpublished survey of cleft teams in the United States, Huebener and Marsh (1993) showed that appliance use has increased over the past 5 years.

The inability to resolve the controversy surrounding PSIO through clinical trials or reviews of the literature stems from a variety of problems. The variation in the treatment modality and in the timing and use of bone graft, as well as the absence of normative data are some of the difficulties encountered when comparing results from different centers.

The Effect of Presurgical Infant Orthopedics on Maxillary Growth

One of the most controversial issues surrounding PSIO is about its effect on maxillary growth. The dilemma becomes more complicated if the surgeon performs gingivoperiosteoplasty (closure of the alveolar cleft) at the time of the primary lip repair. Ross (1987) showed in a major multicenter study that there is no difference in facial growth between cleft patients treated with or without PSIO. On the other hand, Robertson (1983), in a 10-year follow-up study by a single surgeon, demonstrated that better facial growth was achieved in patients treated with PSIO than in control subjects. In another long-term single-surgeon study, Lee et al. (2004) showed that maxillary growth was not inhibited in patients ages 9 to 13 years who had previously undergone presurgical orthopedics and primary gingivoperiosteoplasty. In contrast, Berkovitch (2004) has been openly critical of the Latham and Millard technique of presurgical orthopedics, gingivoperiosteoplasty (GPP), and presurgical orthopedic, periostoplasty, lip adhesion (POPLA). He reports a higher incidence of anterior and buccal crossbite at 3, 6, 9, and 12 years of age after POPLA when compared to no presurgical orthopedics with no GPP. Millard (1999) reviewed this same clinical database and also reported a higher incidence of anterior crossbite in the POPLA group, but a lower incidence of buccal crossbite. He noted that the two groups had different orthodontic treatment protocols by different orthodontists, and that this could have a confounding effect on the results. These two reports focused on dental relationships as the outcome measure instead of facial skeleton landmarks, which are a more accurate representation of facial growth or impaired growth. It is important to distinguish between dental malocclusion and maxillary hypoplasia. Both can result in anterior crossbite, but dental malocclusion can be treated by orthodontics, whereas marked midface hypoplasia requires or-

thognathic surgery. This distinction emphasizes the need for a standard outcome measure for PSIO, and the difficulty in interpreting previous studies.

It is logical that restoring the normal anatomy of the maxillary segments presurgically allows lip repair under less tension. Ross and MacNamera stated that one possible benefit of PSIO is that the lip surgery should be easier, enabling a more precise repair with less tension. If the aesthetic outcome is improved, this is a powerful incentive to adopt presurgical infant orthopedic procedures.

Presurgical Nasoalveolar Molding

Presurgical nasal and alveolar molding includes as its objectives the active molding and repositioning of the nasal cartilages and alveolar processes, and lengthening of the deficient columella. A description of the protocol for treatment of the patient with bilateral cleft deformity was introduced by Grayson et al. (1).

This modification of the traditional approach to presurgical molding plate therapy takes advantage of the plasticity of cartilage in the newborn infant during the first 6 weeks after birth. Matsuo, Hirose, and Tonomo postulated that the high degree of plasticity and lack of elasticity in neonatal cartilage is caused by high levels of hyaluronic acid, a component of the proteoglycan intercellular matrix. As the estrogen level increases, the level of hyaluronic acid increases and the elasticity of the cartilage decreases. With the neonatal levels of maternal estrogen highest immediately after birth, the period of plasticity is slowly lost during the first months of postnatal life. It is during this first 2 to 3 months after birth when active soft tissue and cartilage-molding plate therapy is most successful.

After the successful application of molding therapy to deformed auricular cartilage, Nakajima and Yoshimura, and Matsuo and Hirose applied the same method to the unilateral cleft lip nasal structures. A combined technique for nasal and alveolar molding has been refined, critically analyzed, and documented by the Cleft Palate Team of the Institute of Reconstructive Plastic Surgery at New York University Medical Center. This technique has been demonstrated to have a positive influence on the outcome of the primary nasal, labial, and alveolar repair, and has been adopted by an increasing number of cleft teams, including the Craniofacial Center at Children's Hospital in Seattle.

Correcting the Unilateral Cleft Lip and Nasal Deformity with Nasoalveolar Molding

In the unilateral cleft, the ipsilateral lower lateral cartilage is depressed and concave, and separated from the contralateral cartilage. This results in depression and displacement of the nasal dome and is associated with overhang of the ipsilateral nostril apex. The columella and nasal septum are inclined over the cleft with the base deviated toward the noncleft side. In addition, the orbicularis oris muscle in the lateral lip element contracts into a bulge with some fibers running along the cleft margin toward the nasal tip.

Shortly after birth, an impression of the intraoral cleft defect is made using an elastomeric material in an acrylic tray. A conventional molding plate is constructed on the maxillary study model from clear orthodontic resin. The molding plate is applied to the palate and alveolar processes, and secured through the use of surgical adhesive tapes applied externally to the cheeks and to an extension from the oral plate that exits the horizontal labial fissure. The molding plate is modified at weekly intervals to gradually approximate the alveolar segments. This is achieved through the selective removal of acrylic from the region into which one desires the alveolar bone to grow ("negative sculpting"). At the same time, soft denture liner is added to line the appliance in the region from which one desires the bone to be moved. The ultimate goal of this sequential addition and selective removal of material from the inner walls of the molding plate is to align the alveolar segments and achieve closure of the alveolar gap. The effectiveness of the molding plate is enhanced by adequately supporting the appliance against the palatal tissues, and by taping the left and right lip segments together between clinical visits.

The goal of presurgical NAM in the patient with unilateral cleft deformity is to align and approximate the alveolar segments, and correct the malposition of the nasal cartilages and the alar base on the affected side, as well as to idealize the position of the philtrum and columella. These changes benefit the patient and surgeon by decreasing tension on the incision line and subsequent scar, controlling alveolar contact, facilitating creation of a natural curvature to the alar rim, and decreasing the amount of surgical dissection required. Alveolar approximation does occur to a variable degree after lip adhesion or after approximation of the orbicularis muscle with surgical repair of an unmolded cleft lip, but these changes are uncontrolled and often result in collapse of the lesser alveolar segment and variable cleft closure. With NAM, alignment and approximation of the alveolar segments is controlled to create a natural arch form.

NAM also permits the surgeon to offer the patient a limited-dissection GPP at the same time as the cleft lip repair if the alveolar edges are vertically aligned and in close contact (2). The gingivoperiosteal flaps are raised within the alveolar cleft, without any dissection on the anterior face of the alveolus. The two sets of flaps create a periosteum-lined "tunnel" between the exposed bone surfaces of the alveolar cleft. This promotes tissue-guided regeneration as bone forms across the alveolar gap. This limited dissection GPP following NAM differs markedly from the previously reported GPP techniques of Skoog, which required extensive subperiosteal dissection to achieve closure of the unmolded cleft.

The nasal changes of NAM are achieved by the use of a nasal stent rising from the labial vestibular flange of the acrylic intraoral molding plate. The medio-lateral position of the nasal stent is adjusted as it lifts the nasal tip. The shape of the nostrils and alar rims is carefully molded to resemble the normal configuration of these structures through modifications gradually made to the nasal stents.

Correcting the Bilateral Cleft Lip and Nasal Deformity with Nasoalveolar Molding

In the bilateral cleft, the alar cartilages have failed to migrate up into the nasal tip and cause growth of the columella. The prolabium lacks muscle tissue and is attached on the end of the short columella. The alar cartilages are positioned along the alar margins and are stretched over the cleft as flaring alae. In the complete bilateral cleft, the premaxilla is suspended from the tip of the nasal septum and the lateral alveolar segments remain behind.

The objective of presurgical nasal and alveolar molding in the patient with bilateral deformity is to lengthen the columella, elongate the prolabium, reposition the nasal cartilages toward the tip, and align the alveolar segments, including the premaxilla. This is accomplished through the use of nasal stents that are based on the border of a conventional oral molding plate, adhesive surgical tape, and elastic bands (Fig. 23.2). The first stage of treatment involves repositioning of the everted premaxilla into the space between the lateral alveolar segments using progressive modifications of an acrylic intraoral plate in conjunction with elastic bands that are adhered to the cheeks. In the second stage, as the alveolar segments gradually approximate one another, the nasal stents are built from the anterior rim of the oral plate and enter the nasal apertures. This provides support and gives shape to the dome and alar cartilages

in the immediate neonatal period. The nasal stents advance the lateral alar cartilages into the nasal tip and provide stretch to the columellar skin. In the bilateral cleft deformity, the columella at birth is often from 0 to 2 mm in length; following NAM it is expanded to 4 to 7 mm. The normal columellar length for children at this age is 3.2 mm. Overcorrection of the columellar length is intended to account for some postsurgical relapse. Attached to the two nasal stents, is a horizontal prolabial band that stabilizes the columellar base at the nasolabial angle, serving as a fulcrum for the distracting forces of the nasal stents upwards on the columella envelope, and of the labial tapes downward on the prolabium. This controlled elongation of the linear distance from the top of the columella to the bottom of the prolabium provides sufficient tissue for the surgeon to create both nasal projection (columella) as well as central lip length (prolabium), a feat that is frustratingly difficult in an unmolded nose.

Evaluation of Nasoalveolar Molding

Previous studies on presurgical infant orthopedics, including the Latham device, cannot be extrapolated to the technique of NAM. Previous studies focused on dental relations, such as crossbites, as the outcome measure of facial growth, instead of maxillary dimensions, which are a more direct measure. NAM also has implications on nasal morphology, soft-tissue relationships, and the ability to perform a limited dissection gingivoperiosteoplasty. These were not considerations in previous studies. To address this lack of objective data on the outcome of NAM patients, the Cleft Team at NYU evaluated their cases with the following findings:

1. The presurgical alignment and correction of deformity in the nasal cartilages minimize the extent of primary nasal surgery required and therefore minimize the extent of scar tissue formation, leading to more consistent postoperative results. An average of 4 years after surgery, superimposition analysis of molded and unmolded unilateral cleft noses demonstrated increased symmetry in the group undergoing NAM as compared with the control group who had alveolar molding without nasal molding.

2. Presurgical closure of the alveolar gap enables the surgeon to perform a GPP at the time of primary lip repair. Santiago et al. have reported that GPP eliminates the need for secondary alveolar bone grafts during the period of the mixed dentition in more than 60% of the cases studied.

3. The quality of the generated bone in the alveolar cleft of NAM + GPP cases is equal to the quality of unmolded clefts that underwent secondary bone grafting. Of the 40% of NAM + GPP clefts that required secondary bone grafting, the outcome of the secondary bone graft was superior to unmolded clefts, presumably because of the intact nasal floor and the bone bridge that had been generated as a result the GPP.

4. The distance from posterior to anterior nasal spine as a measure of maxillary projection an average of 11 years after the primary surgery was not significantly different between molded patients who had a GPP at the time of cleft lip repair and unmolded patients who did not. Although it will be a few more years before this cohort can be examined at skeletal maturity, after this initial study, the alveolar cleft of the control group was closed by secondary bone grafting. Thus both groups will have intact alveolar arches on future analysis.

5. There is a cost benefit to NAM with GPP. The cost savings in not needing to perform secondary alveolar bone grafting in 60% of infants with a GPP outweighs the orthodontic fees for presurgical NAM. This study did not

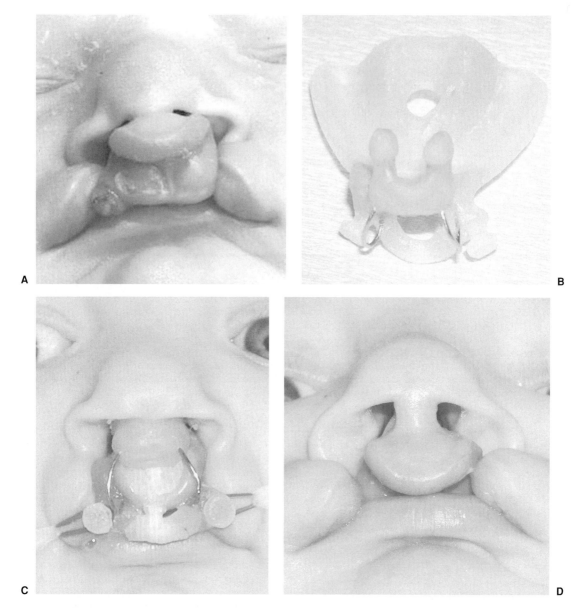

FIGURE 23.2. Nasoalveolar molding (NAM) of the bilateral cleft deformity. **A:** Bilateral complete cleft lip and palate in a newborn. **B:** Nasoalveolar molding plate with nasal extensions. The projecting buttons are used to secure the plate to the patient's cheeks with tape and elastics. The nasal extensions are not added to the molding plate until the alveolar cleft is less than 5 mm wide so as to avoid overstretching the nostril. **C:** Molding plate and nasal extensions in place. **D:** Presurgical result of the same patient after a course of NAM. The alveolar segments and premaxilla are aligned, the columella is lengthened, the alar bases are in a more medial position, the alar rims are curved, and the prolabium is of sufficient size to reconstruct the central lip with minimal tension.

include the possible additional cost benefit of decreased secondary nasal revisions in molded noses.

PRIMARY UNILATERAL CLEFT LIP REPAIR

Numerous methods have been described for repair of the cleft lip deformity. Early techniques involved a straight-line closure (Fig. 23.3), and these procedures still find applicability in the repair of microform (forme fruste) clefts. Repairs involving a combined upper and lower lip flap were advocated by Skoog and Trauner and Trauner. Modern repairs have in common the

use of a lateral lip flap to fill a medial deficit, a concept that can be accredited to Mirault. The LeMesurier repair involves a lateral, quadrilateral flap, whereas the Tennison repair employs a lateral triangular flap (Fig. 23.3) (3). Both procedures introduce tissue in the lower part of the lip.

In 1955, Millard described the concept of advancing a lateral flap into the upper portion of the lip combined with downward rotation of the medial segment. The technique preserves both the Cupid's bow and the philtral dimple, and it has the additional advantage of placing the tension of closure under the alar base, thereby reducing flare and promoting better molding of the underlying alveolar processes (4).

At our two institutions we employ a modification of the technique initially described by Mohler, which, in turn, is based

STRAIGHT LINE

Rose-Thompson

LOWER LIP Z-PLASTIES

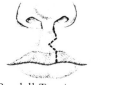

Randall-Tennison   LeMesurier

UPPER LIP Z-PLASTIES

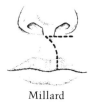

Millard

UPPER AND LOWER LIP Z-PLASTIES

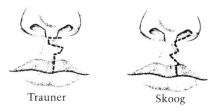

Trauner   Skoog

FIGURE 23.3. Variations of surgical repair of the unilateral cleft lip deformity.

on the technique of Millard (5). Compared to the traditional Millard technique, this technique minimizes the alar base skin incisions and places the back-cut used to rotate the medial lip element at the base of the columella instead of the upper lip. With these modifications, the upper lip scar parallels the contralateral philtrum instead of curving across the philtral groove.

There is no agreement on the ideal timing and the technique of repair among established and experienced cleft surgeons. This underscores the fact that more than one treatment plan is acceptable, and that comparable outcomes can be achieved with different philosophies. Successful approaches have in common a surgeon who is knowledgeable about the variation in abnormal anatomy among clefts, is comfortable with the details and limitations of their technique, and is able to combine these two qualities to achieve the optimum surgical result.

The remainder of this section focuses on the modified Mohler technique used by the authors.

Timing and Treatment Planning

Whenever possible, all complete unilateral cleft lips undergo preoperative NAM at our institutions. Presurgical orthodontic treatment is initiated in the first or second week following birth, with the maximum response occurring during the first 6 weeks. The primary lip repair is scheduled when the patient is approximately 12 weeks of age, at which time closure of the anterior nasal floor and a primary tip rhinoplasty are also performed. If the alveolar segments are appropriately aligned and <2 mm apart, the family is offered a GPP at the time of the surgery. Bone grafts are *not* employed with early closure of the alveolus. If collapse is present or the gap is too wide, the GPP is deferred.

Correction of the nasal deformity in unilateral clefts is coupled with the rotation-advancement repair. Septal repositioning and nasal osteotomies are deferred until late adolescence unless the deformity is severe, in which case they are performed concomitantly with secondary bone grafting of the alveolar cleft (if a GPP was not done) at the time of mixed dentition. We believe that it is important to minimize the number of secondary surgeries to the nose during the growth phase to minimize scarring and to optimize the final result of a formal open rhinoplasty in adolescence.

Anesthesia

General anesthesia is used for all stages of lip repair. A straight, cuffed endotracheal tube is taped to the chin by the surgeon to avoid distortion of the lower lip and alteration of landmarks. The eyes are protected with Tegaderm patches. After markings, 0.5% lidocaine with 1:200,000 epinephrine is injected in the planned dissection planes of the lip, in the supraperiosteal plane of the cleft side maxilla, and between the skin and cartilage of the planned nasal dissection. Accurate injection with a minimal volume of fluid maximizes hemostasis and facilitates dissection.

Unilateral Complete Cleft Lip Operative Technique

The markings for the modified Mohler rotation-advancement repair are applied as shown in Figure 23.4. The depth of the Cupid's bow on the medial lip segment is marked as point 1, with point 2 being the white roll at the height of the Cupid's bow on the non-cleft side, and point 3 being equidistant on the cleft side. Ideally, the distance between each point should be approximately 2.5 mm, for a final Cupid's bow width of 5 mm; however, this can be adjusted based on the patient's anatomy. Point 4 is selected by a number of considerations, the least important of which is the traditional technique of matching the distance from the commissure to Cupid's bow on the non-cleft side. Instead, it is selected by matching the vermilion and white roll thickness, or bulk of the lateral lip segment with that of the medial site at the Cupid's bow peak. This point should coincide as closely as possible with the point on the white roll that intersects the arc of a line drawn from the alar base whose length equals the vertical lip height of the non-cleft side (the height from point 4 to point 5 equals that from point 6 to point 2). The vertical incision of the lateral lip segment that will be approximated to the medial segment to reconstruct the philtral ridge originates from point 4, crossing perpendicular to the white roll, then curves sharply toward point 7 at the nasal sill. The triangle formed by points 4, 5, and 7 is isosceles, with the height from point 4 to point 7 equaling that from point 4 to point 5. It is important that the base of this isosceles triangle

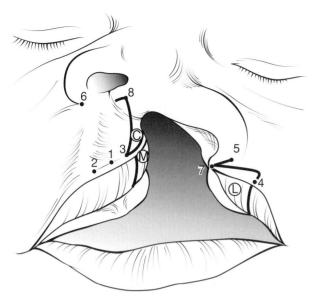

FIGURE 23.4. Markings for unilateral complete primary cleft lip repair. *M*, medial mucosal flap; *L*, lateral mucosal flap; *C*, central cutaneous flap. See text for details.

does not violate the nasal sill. Consequently, the line from point 5 to point 7 tends to slope slightly inferior. Point 4 can be chosen on most cleft lips using these two guidelines. In some cases, however, the lateral lip element is vertically deficient, resulting in a point 4 that is too laterally displaced (too close to the commissure) to achieve a minimal tension repair. In these cases, the curvature of the lateral vertical incision from point 4 to point 7 can be increased to lengthen the lateral lip segment, or the horizontal incision under the cleft side alar base from point 5 to point 7 needs to borrow skin from the nasal sill. If the dry red lip thickness at point 4 is more than 1 mm less than that under the non-cleft Cupid's bow, a triangular mucosal flap of dry vermilion from the medial lip segment can be interdigitated into a corresponding cut at the dry–wet lip junction on the lateral lip segment.

For the medial lip segment incisions, point 8 is chosen as the location of the back-cut of the C flap. Unlike the traditional Millard repair, this point is located approximately 1 mm up on the columella and three-fifths along the width of the columella, toward the non-cleft side. This allows the back-cut scar to be hidden at the base of the columella, instead of on the upper lip. It also creates a vertical scar that mirrors the non-cleft philtral ridge and does not violate the philtral groove. The incision from point 3 to point 8 is the vertical philtral incision of the medial lip segment and defines the non-cleft border of the C flap. Unlike the traditional Millard repair, this incision has only a slight medial curvature in order to create a vertical philtrum. The cleft border of the C flap parallels the junction of the medial lip skin and the oral mucosa. It is important not to include any mucosa in the C flap, as it will be rotated into the base of the columella to fill the skin deficiency after downward rotation of the medial lip segment. The cleft border of the C flap terminates at the anterior aspect of the septum, behind the footplates of the lower lateral cartilages.

Points 3 and 4 on the white roll are tattooed with needle and ink to facilitate alignment at the end of the repair. The lip is then infiltrated with lidocaine and epinephrine as described above (see Anesthesia). After the skin incisions are complete, the red lip portions of the medial and lateral segments are everted to equal fullness, and a no. 11 blade is used to transect the red lip from point 3 and 4 respectively, and the superior

labial arteries are cauterized. The anterior border of the L flap is marked by the incision from points 4 to 7. This continues as a back-cut of the lateral nasal wall behind the lateral crus of the cleft lower lateral cartilage. The posterior border of the L flap is at the level of the palatal shelf inside the nose, such that when the L flap is elevated, it is a posteriorly based mucosal flap pedicled off the lateral nasal wall, posterior to the lateral crus of the lower lateral cartilage. The base of the L flap is left thick by dissecting in the subperiosteal plane on the piriform aperture. With elevation of the L and M flaps in a submucosal plane, the underlying orbicularis muscle can be judiciously separated from the overlying skin. With dissection of the muscle of the medial lip segment, care must be taken not to violate the midline of the philtrum to avoid distorting the natural groove. The red lip mucosa and white roll are not separated from the underlying muscle in order to permit normal animation of this area. The nasal and perioral components of the orbicularis oris muscle are separate at the exposed muscle edge of the lateral lip segments. The nasal component will be used to control the position of the alar base, and the perioral component will be rotated inferiorly to join the medial lip muscle in constructing the transverse orbicularis oris muscle sling.

The medial lip segment is lengthened and rotated inferiorly by sequentially releasing the skin with a back-cut at the base of the columella described above, then the muscle with a separation of the nasal and perioral components of the orbicularis oris, and, finally, the mucosa at the frenum. Care is taken not to fully release the frenum if possible to avoid creating a long lip deformity. At the end of the medial lip segment release and rotation, points 1, 2, and 3, the landmarks of the Cupid's bow, should be aligned horizontally with minimal tension.

Angled Converse nasal tip scissors are used to dissect between the footplates of the lower lateral cartilages by accessing them underneath the C flap (Fig. 23.5). A vertical incision is made through the nasal mucosa in the area of the membranous septum between the anterior edge of the cartilaginous septum and the posterior edge of the ascending limb of the lower lateral cartilage within the cleft-side nostril. This releases the cleft-side lower lateral cartilage footplate, allowing differential elevation of this cartilage and associated nasal tip relative to the non-cleft side. Scissor dissection then continues between the ascending limbs of the lower lateral cartilages, over the nasal tip, and along the alar component of the cleft-side lower lateral cartilage. The skin is carefully separated from the lower lateral cartilage over the alar rim to allow the skin envelope to redrape when the cartilage is repositioned. This dissection pocket between the cartilage and overlying skin is extended up to the upper lateral cartilage of the non-cleft side. This continuous dissection plane between the non-cleft upper lateral and cleft lower lateral cartilages will later be used to place subcutaneous Tajima suspension sutures to adjust the alar rim contour.

The final dissection involves releasing the abnormal attachments of the cleft alar base to allow tension-free approximation across the cleft. An upper gingivobuccal sulcus incision is performed on the cleft side and continued as a supraperiosteal dissection over the face of the maxilla. Through this incision, the abnormal fibrous attachments of the cleft side accessory nasal cartilages to the lateral piriform aperture are released. Along with the small back-cut in the nasal lining behind the cleft lower lateral cartilage, this will allow tension-free mobilization of the lateral lip segment and alar base in even the widest unilateral clefts. All areas are checked carefully for hemostasis before the closure begins.

Closure begins with the nasal floor. The L flap is rotated, trimmed, and sutured into the defect created in the lateral nasal lining when the cleft alar base is advanced into the appropriate position (Fig. 23.6). With the alar base advanced, the inferior edge of the L flap and lateral nasal lining is sutured to an opposing septal mucosal flap to close the nasal floor from the nasal

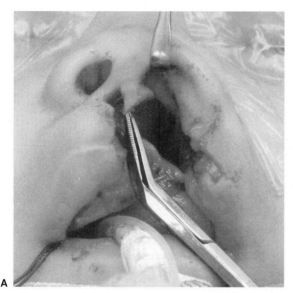
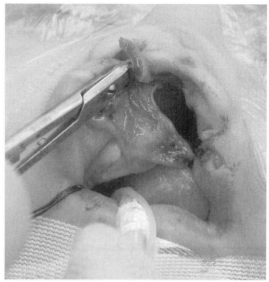

FIGURE 23.5. Primary tip rhinoplasty for unilateral cleft deformity. A: Converse nasal tip scissors are used to access the interdomal space by dissecting underneath the C flap between the footplates of the lower lateral cartilages. Note how the back-cut at the base of the columella is opening to allow elevation of the cleft alar rim. The C flap will later be inset into this defect. B: The scissors are then angled to dissect down to the alar rim on the cleft nostril. See text for details.

sill back to the incisive foramen. At the end of this closure, the posterior displacement of the cleft alar base should be corrected. Closure of the nasal floor to the incisive foramen at the time of primary lip repair will avoid any oronasal or nasolabial communication after the remaining nasal floor reconstruction during the later cleft palate repair. If this detail is omitted from the lip repair, the child will be forced to deal with an anterior nasolabial fistula until closure can be performed at the time of secondary alveolar bone grafting.

Lip construction is achieved by everting the red lip on either side of the cleft to even fullness and then advancing and closing the lateral lip segment mucosa to the medial lip segment mucosa. The M flap can be rotated into the defect from the releasing back-cut at the frenum if necessary, or it can be used to augment the labial sulcus. After the lip mucosa is closed, the white roll should be aligned across the cleft, and the red lip should have equal fullness. If the lateral red lip is thin, the lateral mucosal flap had not been adequately advanced toward the midline. The perioral components of the medial and lateral lip segments are approximated across the cleft using buried horizontal mattress sutures of 5-0 Vicryl to create a philtral ridge and construct the oral sphincter. The vertical incision of the lip is closed with sparse, nonstrangulating, 6-0 interrupted nylon sutures, with care taken to ensure that the tattooed marks of the white roll on either side of the cleft are aligned.

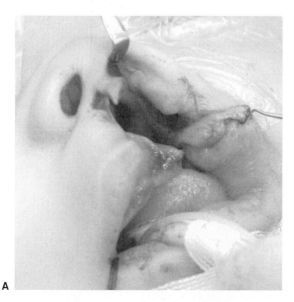
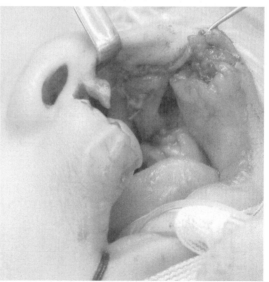

FIGURE 23.6. Nasal lining release and inset of L flap. A: The constricted lateral nasal lining is released with an incision behind the lateral crus, and the mucosal L flap is elevated from the lateral lip element. B: The L flap is pedicled off the lateral nasal wall and inset into the lining defect to support the new position of the alar base.

At this point of the repair, the lip anatomy has been corrected, leaving the nasal deformity. Either 4-0 polydioxanone suture (PDS) or clear nylon is used to secure the dermomuscular pennant under the cleft alar base to the muscle and periosteum of the anterior nasal spine. Two or three sutures are used to place the cleft alar base in the desired medial position. A retractor is used to slightly overcorrect the cleft alar rim and underlying lower lateral cartilage in an advanced and superior position. This slides the released cleft lower lateral cartilage footplate toward the nasal dome in relation to the non-cleft side. A series of 4-0 PDS transfixation sutures are used to secure this new relationship of the ascending limbs of the lower lateral cartilages to the anterior septum. This elevation of the cleft side alar rim and lengthening of the columella leaves a defect from the back-cut at the base of the columella. The C flap is trimmed to fit and rotate into this defect. The rotation point of the C flap creates a natural flare to the base of the columella of the cleft nostril.

The final sculpting of the nostril shape is achieved with 4-0 PDS subcutaneous Tajima suspension suture. The needle enters the nasal surface of the cleft lower lateral cartilage at the point of desired elevation, enters into the previously described nasal tip dissection pocket, exits into the non-cleft nostril at the level of the upper lateral cartilage, and then returns on its path, such that tightening of the suture will elevate the cleft alar rim. Lateral alar cinch sutures of 4-0 PDS can also be used to contour the lateral alar rim and nasal lining in the new position, by exiting and entering the same percutaneous hole in the alar groove. The number of suspension and cinch sutures required will depend on the degree of the deformity. We perform a GPP if the alveolar segments are in appropriate alignment following nasoalveolar molding.

With this approach, the lip and nasal deformities can be addressed in a single surgery (Fig. 23.7).

Unilateral Incomplete Cleft Lip Operative Technique

The unilateral incomplete cleft lip deformity is treated with the same surgical technique and dissection that was described for the complete cleft lip, but with a few modifications. Failure to address all the lip and nasal abnormalities in the incomplete

cleft lip with the same detail paid to the wide complete cleft will result in a suboptimal result.

Compared to the complete cleft lip repair, the incomplete cleft repair does not involve intranasal incisions. If possible, the nasal sill is not violated by the vertical incision. If the nasal base is wide compared to the non-cleft side, a small wedge can be removed from the nasal sill to create symmetry. If any nasal sill is resected, it is vital that the excision be minimal, because overresection with scarring will result in the recalcitrant micronostril deformity.

The L flap and M flap are not required for the incomplete cleft lip repair because the nasal floor is intact. To correct the alar base malposition, the abnormal attachments of the nasal cartilages to the piriform aperture must be released as in the complete cleft technique, but, also, the nasal floor lining must be dissected free from the piriform rim. The thin nasal floor is firmly attached to the edge of the piriform opening, and can easily be perforated if care is not taken. Failure to release the nasal lining from the underlying bone will make it impossible to mobilize the alar base into the desired advanced and medial position.

The nasal deformity is addressed with the same dissection as the complete cleft; however, the vertical nasal lining incision behind the ascending limb of the cleft lower lateral cartilage is not available for improved access to the nasal tip. Angled nasal tip scissors are used to access the nasal tip between the footplates of the lower lateral cartilages; if necessary, the nasal tip can be approached laterally from the supraperiosteal maxillary dissection plane.

Microform Cleft Operative Technique

The critical factor when evaluating the microform cleft is the vertical height of the lip. If the vertical height of the affected side approximates that of the normal side, imperfections in the vermilion along the skin furrow can be eliminated with an elliptical excision and a straight-line repair. Triangular flaps of the white roll and vermilion can be used to balance the closure.

When the vertical difference exceeds 1 to 2 mm, the modified Mohler rotation-advancement repair described above (see Unilateral Complete Cleft Lip Operative Technique) is used. The additional scar underneath the sill and columella is preferable

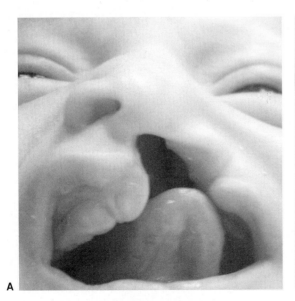
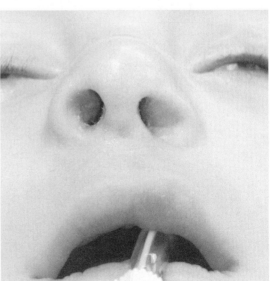

FIGURE 23.7. Mohler unilateral cleft lip repair. **A:** Preoperative complete cleft lip and nasal deformity. **B:** Postoperative result 9 months later.

to a loss of definition in the involved philtral column, which invariably results with straight-line closure when the elliptical excision is extended to provide the desired lengthening.

The correction of a very mild nasal deformity is deferred in the microform cleft requiring a straight-line repair, as the repair does not necessitate a perialar incision. If the deformity remains minimal, treatment is postponed until late adolescence, when a definitive rhinoplasty is performed. With a moderate nasal deformity and with mild deformities requiring a rotation-advancement lip repair, correction of the nasal deformity is carried out with the lip repair.

Lip Adhesion

Lip adhesion is still used by some centers for wide clefts and those with lateral maxillary collapse that does not respond to presurgical maxillary orthopedics, but lip adhesion is not used by us. Supporters of lip adhesion believe that it improves maxillary arch alignment and enables a more predictable correction of the cleft nasal deformity in select patients. The improved nasal results are thought to be secondary to improved alar base arch support, which reduces the strain and relapse tendency for the mobilized lower lateral cartilage.

The adhesion is classified as a straight line muscle repair and begins with the complete marking of a rotation-advancement cheiloplasty. An L flap is elevated from the lateral segment beginning approximately 3 mm medial to the Cupid's bow peak. This flap length provides adequate tissue for nasal release. The flap is turned 90 degrees into the nasal release along the lateral floor of the nose, which follows the piriform rim and the lateral portion of the nasal bones. A contiguous, maxillary sulcus incision is made through this nasal mucosal incision, and the lateral lip and cheek muscle mass is elevated in continuity from the maxilla and piriform aperture. The L flap is sutured into the nasal defect, and the lateral lip element is advanced medially for closure.

An M flap is also raised 3 mm from the Cupid's bow peak to maintain symmetry of repair. The mucosal flap is based on the maxillary alveolus and is turned into the alveolar cleft to augment closure. All dissection is maintained outside the margins for primary lip repair. No medial muscle dissection is done at this stage.

Closure is achieved with sutures placed in the undissected orbicularis layer along the pared margin and is reinforced with a chromic catgut mucosal closure between the M flap and the lateral lip mucosa. Skin is generally closed with interrupted 5-0 chromic catgut, with sutures placed outside the markings for definitive cheiloplasty. The adhesion effectively closes the nasal sill and upper two-thirds of the lip. The forces from the overlying muscle closure have an immediate effect on the position of the alveolar segments.

Postoperative Care

The infants are kept in soft arm restraints for 2 weeks after lip repair. An infraorbital nerve block with bupivacaine can be used to minimize the early need for analgesics. Care must be taken not to overuse morphine in these patients.

Some surgeons prefer feedings with a catheter-tip syringe fitted with a small, red, rubber catheter for the first 10 days postoperatively to minimize strain on the muscle and skin sutures and to avoid trauma to the repaired velum. Many others do not impose restrictions and allow return to the preoperative routine immediately. Diet is advanced to full-strength formula or breast milk on the day of surgery to pacify the infant.

Suture line care consists of regular cleansing with half-strength hydrogen peroxide followed with a light coating of polymyxin B–bacitracin ointment. Sutures are removed on the fifth to seventh postoperative day. Postsuture removal taping and silicone scar gel can be used if desired. Parents are told to expect firmness in the lip scar and temporary shortening across the repair that generally becomes maximum 4 to 6 weeks after surgery. Scars typically soften between 3 and 6 months postoperatively.

PRIMARY BILATERAL CLEFT LIP REPAIR

Bilateral cleft lip repair is recognized by surgeons as more difficult than a unilateral cleft lip repair. As previously described in this chapter (pages 203–204), the anatomy of the bilateral cleft lip deformity creates numerous challenges. Although the lip repair is made more difficult by the deficiency of skin and muscle overlying the premaxilla, it is the associated bilateral nasal deformity that was previously recalcitrant to correction. The treatment of the complete bilateral cleft and associated nasal deformity remains in transition. Only recently, because of NAM, have the results of one-stage primary bilateral cleft lip and nose repair begun to approach those of unilateral cleft lip and nose repair. Previous multistage techniques often produced a lip and nose that were still quite abnormal, with a confluence of scars at the lip–columella junction, a broad nasal tip, an unstable premaxilla, and often large nasolabial fistulas. Results fell short of ideal because the condition was viewed as a purely cutaneous deformity. Over the past decade, techniques have recognized the importance of addressing the contribution of the nasal tip cartilages to the cleft deformity. This shift from a skin-based to a cartilage-based paradigm has produced a number of techniques with improved outcomes.

Construction of the Central Lip Vermilion

There are two general methods for constructing the central lip vermilion. One involves using the mucosa visible on the inferior aspect of the prolabial skin to form the central vermilion, such as used in the Manchester repair. The original Manchester repair did not create an orbicularis oris sling across the upper lip, but instead sutured the muscle to the edges of the premaxilla. As there was no muscle under the prolabium or within the buccal mucosa, this approach did not provide sufficient bulk to serve as the central lip vermilion, and resulted in an abnormal appearance with animation of the central upper lip. A number of techniques have been described to address this limitation, including bringing strips of muscle across this area from the lateral lip, and de-epithelializing the buccal mucosa or subcutaneous tissue from the lateral sides of the prolabium and folding them behind the inferior prolabial mucosa. An advantage of using the prolabial or buccal mucosa to create the central vermilion is that very little bulk of the lateral segment of the vermilion is required, thereby decreasing the tension required for closure across the cleft. The disadvantages of this technique are that (a) there are two parallel scars across the vermilion, (b) the central red lip does not have sufficient bulk, resulting in a whistle deformity, and (c) the central buccal mucosa does not possess the same minor salivary gland distribution as the lateral vermilion tissues, often resulting in a dry, chapped, central vermilion segment.

A second approach is to use the vermilion tissue from the lateral lip segments to create the central vermilion as a variation of the technique described by Millard. The muscle of the lateral lip elements rotates down with the full-thickness vermilion flaps and can create a satisfactory central vermilion construction with a single vertical scar under the depth of the Cupid's

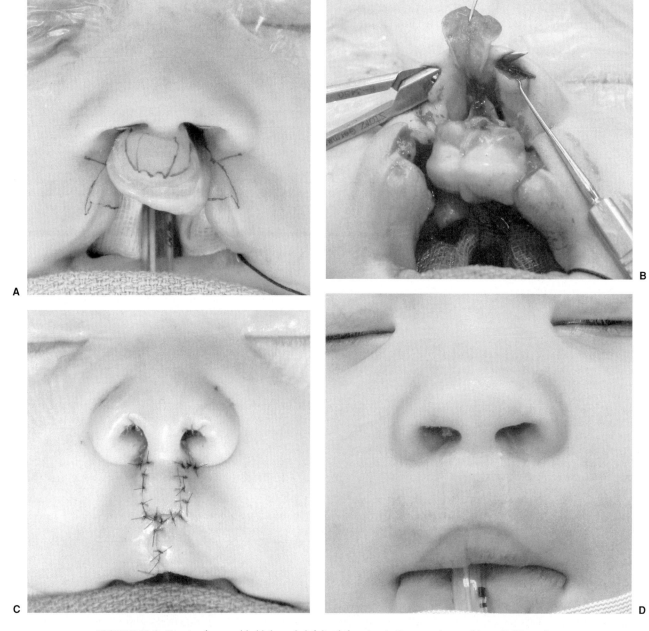

FIGURE 23.8. Repair of nonmolded bilateral cleft lip deformity. **A:** Preoperative markings. **B:** Dissection of nasal cartilages through bilateral alar rim incisions. Elevation of the prolabial flap also allows retrograde central access to the interdomal space. **C:** Immediate postoperative result. The columella length has been achieved by redistributing the nasal tip skin envelope. **D:** Nine months after the operation. There is good symmetry with minimal labial scars. The width of the prolabium and interdomal space have slightly increased at the expense of the columella height. Presurgery NAM may have minimized these postoperative changes.

bow. We prefer to include the white roll with the lateral lip segments that are used to create the central tubercle (Fig. 23.8). By placing two hemicircular incisions at the inferior aspect of the prolabial skin, the combination of the scar on top of the natural white roll and vermilion from the lateral elements produces a satisfactory Cupid's bow.

Skin Paradigm of Bilateral Cleft Lip and Nose Repair

Until relatively recently, methods of bilateral cleft lip repair focused on the skin imbalance evident in the primary defor-

mity. The columella is usually short or absent, whereas the prolabium hanging directly from the nasal tip skin is generally too broad and is vertically deficient. A natural approach is to take the excess in prolabial width and use it, usually in two stages, to create both a columella and a central white lip. We refer to this approach as the skin paradigm of bilateral cleft repair.

One early approach was to bring the lateral lip elements together in the midline to close the lip and to use the prolabium to elongate the columella. This approach has been abandoned, because it produces an unnatural looking lip with a midline scar in place of a Cupid's bow and an upper lip that is tight horizontally. In most of the techniques described in this section, the wide prolabium is split vertically in some fashion to provide skin for both the area of the white lip between the philtral columns, as well as to form a neocolumella.

The next evolution of techniques involved a staged approach to the lip and the nasal deformity. At the initial operation, the lip is approximated to the wide prolabial tissue. This is followed by a second stage in which the extra width of the prolabial tissue is advanced up into the columella. The lip reconstruction is addressed as either a one-stage or two-stage bilateral triangular or rotation-advancement closure, using the techniques described for unilateral deformities. This approach can result in a lip that is too long; it also produces scars that cross Langer lines and that frequently meet in the midline either under the columella (rotation-advancement approach) or above the Cupid's bow (triangular flap techniques). The muscle is either repaired underneath the prolabium to create an intact orbicularis sling across the cleft, or is attached to the sides of the prolabium. Advocates of not repairing the muscle across the cleft state that if the premaxilla is not retracted before lip repair, muscle repair is often difficult and requires much lateral undermining. Similarly, if the prolabium is hypoplastic, suturing of the muscle to its sides will result in stretching of the prolabium, which facilitates later use for the columella. Other surgeons believe strongly that the muscle should be repaired behind the prolabium. If the muscle is not repaired, the resulting lip is frequently too thin in the anteroposterior dimension. Similarly, the pull on the sides of the prolabium can cause it to get very wide in the postoperative period. In the currently employed one-stage cartilage paradigm repairs, which are described later in the chapter (page 215, Cartilage Paradigm of Bilateral Cleft Lip and Nose Repair) the muscle is always repaired under the prolabium, because widening of the interphiltral distance is undesirable.

After the first-stage procedure, the patient has a prolabium that is too wide and an absent columella. The second-stage procedure, when this extra prolabial width is used to create a columella, can be performed several months after the initial lip repair. The more common approach, however, is to wait until age 4 to 5 years. The second-stage columella reconstruction is usually approached using two different methods. In the first technique, forked flaps from the lip are advanced into the columella (6). In the second method, a midline V-to-Y flap advances the prolabium excess into the columella. The forked flap approach produces a new vertical scar in the midline of the columella. Midline V-to-Y from the prolabium into the columella avoids the new vertical scar on the columella but produces a new vertical scar in the central upper lip. In both instances a confluence of scars at the lip-columella junction is produced, usually under considerable tension. If the lip scars have widened, forked flaps permit revision of the lip scars. The vertical scar in the middle of the columella will be seldom seen in short individuals. In a tall male, a central V-to-Y flap has some advantages. The columella is more visible and will not have a scar, and if the individual grows a moustache, the lip scars will be camouflaged. The prolabium, however, has poor terminal hair growth compared to the lateral lip.

A banked forked flap repair, in which the forked flaps are "banked" under the alar bases at the time of the primary lip repair, previously enjoyed widespread popularity. This "banking" allows a one-stage lip repair that is usually quite satisfactory. The lateral "forks" from either side of the prolabium are inserted into incisions at the alar labial junction. The forks are "unbanked" at a second stage and advanced up to form a columella. This second stage is similar to the procedure described by Cronin (6). Just as in the secondary forked flap approach previously discussed, a new vertical scar in the columella is produced along with a confluence of secondary scars under tension at the lip-columella junction.

Criticisms of the Skin Paradigm

Although the skin paradigm has been the most common approach to the bilateral repair in the last 100 years, it produces a number of unsatisfactory effects on nasal form. Techniques based on this approach concentrate on redistributing the available skin of the prolabium to correct the deformity, while ignoring the basic underlying anatomic derangement of the nasal tip lower lateral cartilages.

With all of the techniques described above, advancement of the prolabial skin into the columella has the potential of worsening the underlying cartilaginous tip deformity. The neocolumella produced by advancement of the prolabial skin does not contain cartilage to provide support of the nasal tip. The footplates of the medial crura have been advanced into the nasal tip, while the domes of the lower lateral cartilages, which represent the true nasal tip, are thrust laterally. Later growth of these divergent tip cartilages results in a bulbous nasal tip with an abnormal skin envelope, which is difficult to correct in tertiary procedures. The lack of cartilaginous structure in the neocolumella can result in a lip–columella junction that pulls inferiorly, blunting the angle, or conversely may contract up toward the caudal septum, producing a retracted columella. This latter result is compounded by the absence of the anterior nasal spine described earlier.

In addition to the requisite parallel vertical scars at the philtral columns on either side of the prolabium, approaches based on the skin paradigm produce an additional visible vertical scar. The central V-to-Y technique leaves a new vertical scar in the midline of the lip, whereas the forked flap approach produces a new midline scar in the columella. With both of these approaches, a confluence of secondary scars across a tight lip–columella junction is produced.

Dissatisfaction with the long-term results of these earlier skin paradigm techniques prompted surgeons to consider the underlying cartilage displacement to be as important as the skin deformity, creating a shift over the past 10 years to the cartilage paradigm.

Cartilage Paradigm of Bilateral Cleft Lip and Nose Repair

A number of techniques have been developed that place primary emphasis on the nasal tip cartilage deformity and assign the skin deformity secondary importance. Common factors to these techniques are that (a) the absent columella skin is recruited from the nasal tip skin instead of the prolabium, (b) the lower lateral cartilage domes are repositioned with the hope that subsequent cartilage growth will create columellar skin and nasal projection, and (c) columella skin can be produced by presurgical columella elongation.

McComb Method

McComb described a two-stage approach to correction of the complete bilateral cleft that focuses on the nasal deformity (7). A V-to-Y "gullwing" incision is performed on the skin of the nasal tip at the time of the first procedure. This allows direct visualization of the nasal tip cartilages with elevation of the nasal tip skin. The laterally displaced domes of the lower lateral cartilages are mobilized and sutured together in the midline to a more normal relationship, displacing the intervening fibrofatty tissue into the nasal tip. Closure of this gullwing incision in a V-to-Y manner recruits the width of the nasal tip skin into the production of a columella. A lip adhesion is done at the time of the first nasal procedure. Lip repair is performed at a second stage.

Mulliken Method

Mulliken initially described an approach that uses a vertical incision in the midline of the nasal tip along with bilateral incisions at the nostril apices to allow dissection of the nasal tip cartilages. As with the McComb technique, this allows the surgeon to mobilize the domes and suture them together in the midline. The vertical incision in the nasal tip was proposed rather than McComb's V-to-Y incision to maintain better blood supply to the prolabium, allowing one-stage lip and nose repair. No primary columella elongation was performed at the time of the initial repair save that produced by nostril apex incisions extended out onto the nasal tip.

Mulliken has since modified his initial technique (8). The vertical tip incision is omitted, and all cartilage dissection is performed through bilateral alar rim incisions. Through these limited incisions, the domes of the nasal cartilages can be visualized and approximated at the midline to encourage future anterior growth of the nasal tip. Mulliken also describes skin redundancy in the soft triangles and lateral columella that becomes apparent after positioning of the nasal cartilages, and should be trimmed.

Prolabial Unwinding Flap

Cutting (1993) described the prolabial unwinding flap. In this approach, the wide prolabium is "unwound" to produce columella skin and lip skin without any scar in the nasal tip columella or prolabium. This approach is possible as a result of the circumferential prolabial artery. Nasal tip cartilages are dissected retrograde through transfixion incisions that extend in front of the membranous septum but completely behind the prolabium. This technique is a hybrid of the two paradigms. The problem with this approach was that it is an asymmetric design, is a difficult technique, and still pushes the footplates of the medial crura up into the columella.

Trott Method

In this approach, a one-stage open rhinoplasty is performed where the prolabial flap is carried on the end of the columellar skin (9). This allows the best possible exposure to the displaced dome cartilages for mobilization and suturing in the midline. Furthermore, it does not produce any scars in the nasal tip or at the lip–columella junction. The blood supply to the prolabium may be quite precarious. It should be noted that the columella is not elongated in any way by this approach. This method and that of Mulliken share a common feature. Both rely on the growth of the medial crura, which have been placed into a correct anatomic relationship, to produce columellar skin secondarily over time.

Presurgical Columella Elongation

Although the techniques focused on correcting the nasal cartilage deformity lead to more favorable nasal tip growth, they are limited in creating sufficient skin for creation of a columella without a nasal tip incision. As described earlier in the chapter (pages 203–204, Complete Bilateral Cleft Lip), the vertical distance from the nasal tip to the inferior prolabium is decreased in the bilateral cleft lip deformity, and this limited skin is needed to create both nasal projection and central lip height. In severe deformities, this leads to a satisfactory lip reconstruction at the cost of a flattened nose.

Presurgical orthopedics is enjoying a revival, largely as a result of the ability to create adequate skin for both an optimum lip and nasal repair. Techniques such as NAM retract the premaxilla, elongate the prolabium, and create the skin for a neocolumella (1). The nasal lining is stretched and the depressed nasal domes are elevated anteriorly and carried toward the midline. This allows one-stage repair of the alveolus on both sides (gingivoperiosteoplasty), lip repair using a narrow central prolabial flap, and nasal repair with retrograde

dissection and suturing of the domes in the midline. Initially, it had been hoped that no nasal surgery would be necessary using this method; however, the fibrofatty deposit between the displaced dome cartilages cannot be corrected with presurgical columella elongation alone. After presurgical nasal molding, retrograde dissection of the skin and fibrofat from between the separated nasal domes is necessary along with suturing of the dome cartilages in the midline. No scars from the nasal tip to the Cupid's bow are produced. Presurgical molding requires a dedicated molding and surgical team and parents who are prepared to spend the time to achieve the desired result, but when possible, it is our method of choice.

PRIMARY CLEFT PALATE REPAIR

Although cleft lip and cleft palate surgeries are linked by a shared patient population, and both require a complete understanding of the abnormal anatomy by the surgeon, they are surprisingly different. A cleft lip repair is an artistic, flexible technique tailored to the unique three-dimensional anatomy of each child, whereas a cleft palate repair is a precise technical exercise whose success is based on performing the dissection reliably and atraumatically. Following a cleft lip repair, the parents appreciate the hours of work of the surgeon because of the visible incisions and facial difference, whereas following a cleft palate repair, the key portions of the operation, namely the nasal closure and the intravelar veloplasty, are hidden in the mouth by the transposed oral flaps. The success of the cleft lip repair can be predicted at the end of the operation; results of the cleft palate repair take years to assess, and cannot be evaluated definitively until commencement of speech and completion of facial growth. Despite the lack of surgical glamour associated with a palatoplasty, the patient with a cleft palate requires multidisciplinary evaluation and treatment, a precise, technically sound operation, and standardized postoperative care to achieve the desired results while minimizing the potentially severe complications.

Timing of Surgery

The optimum timing of cleft palate repair balances the benefit of normal velopharyngeal function to optimize speech development against the potential disadvantage of impaired facial growth secondary to early surgical trauma. Graber's description in the late 1940s of restricted maxillary growth following early palate closure was accompanied by a recommendation to delay surgery until 4 to 6 years of age. Because of the deleterious implications of this recommendation on speech development, the conventional timing for cleft palate repair was arbitrarily set at 18 to 24 months as a compromise between speech and facial growth. The current consensus, based on an increased understanding of speech development, is that cleft palate repair should be completed before 18 months of age; however, there is no general agreement regarding how early the surgery can be performed. Since Graber's earlier work, there have been a number of studies supporting the theory that impaired maxillary growth in cleft patients is independent of cleft palate repair, and can result from the lip repair alone or is more a result of intrinsic restriction rather than early surgical trauma.

Results from previous retrospective studies examining the effect of timing of cleft palate repair on speech development are inconsistent and are compromised by small study numbers and potentially confounding variables. Kirschner recently retrospectively reviewed Randall's and LaRossa's cases at Children's Hospital of Philadelphia, using two relatively homogenous cohorts undergoing soft palate repair either before or after 7 months of age, and found no significant benefit of early closure over later repair with respect to speech outcome. These authors emphasized the one thing that the surgical community agrees on: that long-term well-designed prospective studies are required before the optimum timing of cleft palate repair can be decided.

There are currently two common approaches to the timing of cleft palate repair in North America: (a) two-stage repair, with the soft palate repair and veloplasty performed at the time of lip adhesion or primary lip repair, and the hard palate repaired before 18 months, or delayed further with the use of an obturator, and (b) single-stage repair around the age of 11 to 12 months. Our two centers practice the latter approach, delaying the surgery until the time when the child starts to demonstrate the introduction of plosives (b, d, and g) in their speech. It is at this time that they require an intact velopharyngeal sphincter to continue with normal speech mechanics. In children with airway issues, such as that associated with micrognathia of Pierre Robin sequence, the surgery can be delayed until age 14 to 18 months to allow further mandible growth and to decrease the chance of postoperative airway compromise.

Cleft Palate Repair Operative Technique

At our two centers we perform a single-stage, two-flap palatoplasty with intravelar veloplasty as a modification of the technique described by Veau, Wardill, and Kilner (the "Oxford" palatoplasty). This technique is described below.

The patient is placed in the supine position, with a shoulder roll to extend the neck. A number of mouth retractors have been designed for the operation, but all retract the lips and tongue, open the jaws, and keep the endotracheal tube out of the operative site. Care must be taken not to hyperextend the neck, not to strangulate the tongue, and not to bruise the lips. The mouth and nasal cavities are cleaned with normal saline and a small throat pack is placed. The hard and soft palates and the nasal septum are infiltrated with lidocaine and epinephrine, avoiding injection directly around the greater palatine vascular pedicle. With pressure, the mucoperiosteum can be hydrodissected from the hard palate with the injection to facilitate elevation of the flaps.

The bilateral posteriorly based mucoperiosteal flaps are incised laterally at the junction between the hard palate mucosa and the attached gingiva, and then elevated from the hard palate. With a curved elevator, through this lateral incision, the nasal mucosa can be elevated from the lateral nasal wall and posterior nasal spine in continuity with the oral flaps. We find it easier to perform this dissection before separating the oral and nasal flaps along the length of the cleft. The medial aspects of the bilateral mucoperiosteal flaps are then released and the incision continued along the visible line between the oral and nasal mucosa to the tip of the uvula. Care must be taken not to leave the nasal flaps deficient. The oral flaps can always be mobilized to the midline, whereas the mobility of the nasal flaps is limited if they are cut too short. The anterior tips of the mucoperiosteal flaps can then be elevated to expose the greater palatine pedicle, which is carefully preserved and dissected circumferentially.

Two structures tether the mucoperiosteal flaps and limit their mobilization across the cleft at the level of the posterior nasal spine. The first is the greater palatine pedicle, and the second is the abnormal attachment of the levator veli palatini and tensor palatini muscles to the posterior hard palate. A number of techniques have been described for lengthening of the pedicle, including osteotomies of the foramen. Sharp release of the periosteal sheath of the pedicle allows the pedicle to be stretched without compromising perfusion of the flaps. With the pedicle on stretch, a beaver blade is placed behind the pedicle at the edge of the hard palate. The periosteal sheath is lightly stroked until the underlying perivascular fat starts to herniate, at which point the incision follows the length of the pedicle along the long axis of the flap. Scissors are placed behind the pedicle, with one blade resting on the posterior hard palate shelf. Gradual opening of the scissors will create a palpable pop as the remaining periosteal sheath is released by the stretch. Sufficient pedicle length is created to allow tension-free closure of wide clefts. The pedicle dissection must be performed before release of the muscle from the posterior hard palate. If the pedicle is compromised during the dissection, the muscle attachments are required to perfuse the mucoperiosteal flaps.

The nasal lining is then separated from the muscles of the soft palate using sharp fine scissors. There is no reliable dissection plane within the first 2 or 3 mm of the cleft edge, and we prefer to leave this edge of the nasal lining flap thick to help with suturing. Immediately beyond the cleft edge, however, there is a defined, gray, smooth dissection plane under the muscles. Care must be taken not to leave muscle fibers on this undersurface of the nasal mucosa of the soft palate. The dissection continues back to the skull base so that the nasal flaps can be approximated across the cleft with minimal tension.

The final stage of the dissection is the intravelar veloplasty, which is essential for normal speech development. As described by Sommerlad, the normal velum consists of the levator muscle in the middle 40% and the tensor aponeurosis in the anterior 33%. In the cleft palate anomaly, the two muscles are closely related, with the tensor aponeurosis attaching to the posterior border of the hard palate and the levator inserting at the margins of the cleft in the anterior half of the velum. The abnormal attachment of the tensor can be directly visualized at the posterior shelf of the hard palate as obliquely oriented fibers. The fibers are sharply released from the edge of the hard palate, and the tensor tendon is divided medial to the hamulus. This maintains the attachment of the lateral component of the tensor to the hamulus, maintaining muscle tension for normal eustachian function. The medial release of the tensor tendon, however, allows mobilization of the levator muscle, so that it can be retrotransposed across the cleft. The levator is dissected sharply from the palatoglossus on its oral surface to increase its mobility. This leaves a thick, well-perfused oral mucosa flap that can be advanced medially across the cleft, independent of the posterior-medial rotation of the levator sling. The fibrous component of the tensor that was released from the posterior edge of the hard palate travels with the levator to provide more substantial tissue for anterior suture placement when the levator muscle sling is approximated across the cleft. This intravelar veloplasty not only serves to create an intact circumferential levator-pharyngeal sphincter for nasopharyngeal closure and speech, it also serves to lengthen the soft palate.

Sommerlad's intervelar veloplasty, which was developed independently of the technique of Cutting described above, shares much in common with Cutting's technique but has a number of features that distinguish it: (a) mucoperiosteal palatal flap elevation is not performed, (b) the velar muscles are exposed by raising oral mucosa in a plane underneath the mucous glands, (c) the nasal closure is completed before muscle dissection and repositioning in order to place the dissection plane on stretch, and (d) the operation is performed under a dissecting microscope with a knife, rather than loupe magnification with scissors. Readers are encouraged to read Sommerlad's paper for a detailed description of the velar anatomy (10).

The palate is repaired sequentially; the nasal closure from anterior to posterior, followed by the oral closure from posterior to anterior. In a bilateral cleft of the secondary palate, bilateral mucosal flaps are elevated from the caudal edge of the vomer with a midline incision and sutured to the opposing lateral nasal flaps using buried interrupted 5-0 Vicryl sutures. The posterior extent of the vomerine flaps is at the posterior nasal spine. At this point, the nasal closure continues with direct approximation of the nasal lining of the soft palate across the cleft back to the uvula. With a unilateral cleft, only one vomerine flap is required. If there is an associated cleft of the primary palate, the nasal lining is repaired as far anterior as possible. Ideally, the nasal floor should have been repaired by the earlier cleft lip repair back to the incisive foramen, such that oronasal separation can be completed at the time of the palate repair. This saves the child the inconvenience of an anterior oronasal fistula during the years after the palate repair, but also makes a secondary alveolar bone graft easier and potentially more successful as nasal closure has already been achieved.

Various techniques have been described for uvuloplasty, including bilateral Y incisions and truncating the tip of the uvula to create a broad raw surface. None are ideal. With wide cleft repairs under increased tension, the uvula tends to widen at the base and decrease in projection. All techniques have in common accurate eversion of the mucosal lining of the uvula and repair of the muscle bundle at the base of the uvula to decrease postoperative widening and prevent fistula formation.

After nasal closure, the mobilized levator sling is transposed across the cleft. The tension of the muscle repair is based on surgeon experience. A repair that is too tight can lead to a decreased nasopharyngeal aperture and potential postoperative airway compromise. A repair that is too loose will compromise function of the levator sling during speech. We repair the muscle sling with approximately three buried horizontal mattress sutures of 3-0 Vicryl.

Oral closure is achieved using 4-0 chromic vertical mattress sutures. Two 3-0 chromic sutures are used to grasp the underlying nasal lining closure as part of the mattress suture. These are left as delayed ties to close the dead space between the oral and nasal lining. Delayed ties of 3-0 chromic are also used to secure the anterior tips of the mucoperiosteal flaps directly to the alveolus. In a bilateral cleft, the flaps are also secured to the posterior aspect of the premaxilla, where a very limited mucoperiosteal dissection is performed to create an edge to receive a suture. The original description of the two-flap palatoplasty included a "pushback" to lengthen the palate, which left the anterior hard palate exposed. This pushback technique has been discontinued following evidence of impaired facial growth, and is unnecessary for lengthening if a proper levator muscle transposition is performed.

Meticulous hemostasis is essential during the cleft palate repair. If there is any sign of oozing from the flaps or lateral defects, the bleeding is stopped prior to waking the patient. Some surgeons suture absorbable hemostatic material in the lateral defects, but recognize that this does not replace surgical hemostasis. Any blood that has collected in the oropharynx is suctioned. The patient is placed in soft arm restraints, and the endotracheal tube is not removed until spontaneous breathing and purposeful movement is established. We recommend postoperative oxygen saturation monitoring and close observation in the recovery room for 1 to 2 hours prior to discharge to the ward. ICU level care may be indicated in syndromic or other complex patients.

Other Operative Techniques

Although the principles of palatoplasty are consistent across techniques, there are variations for mucosal closure. Along with the two-flap modified Veau-Wardill technique described above (see Cleft Palate Repair Operative Technique), variations of the von Langenbeck two-flap technique are also common. With the von Langenbeck closure, the anterior tips of the bilateral mucoperiosteal flaps are left attached to the anterior hard palate and are mobilized as bipedicled flaps that transpose to the midline. The Furlow double opposing Z-palatoplasty can be used for secondary palate lengthening to treat velopharyngeal insufficiency, but is also commonly employed for primary cleft palate closure, especially for isolated clefts of the secondary palate. With this technique the levator muscles are transposed as opposing limbs of a Z-plasty in the soft palate (Fig. 23.9). Lengthening of the palate is achieved by the differential transposition of the Z-plasty. The short limb of the Z is placed on the midline, and the long axis across the cleft. When the flaps are transposed, the lengthening of the palate is achieved at the expense of increased tension in closure of the lateral mucosa.

Complications Following Cleft Palate Repair

Complications of cleft palate repair include bleeding, respiratory obstruction, infection, dehiscence, and oronasal fistula formation. Significant postoperative bleeding is rare, but if it occurs, it requires re-intubation and exploration for hemostasis. Respiratory obstruction is also rare in the absence of excessive bleeding, but it may be life-threatening. The airway is monitored carefully in the recovery room and only after adequate assessment should the baby be transferred to the floor. We recommend oxygen saturation monitors to be employed on the floor or the patient can be monitored in an ICU setting if

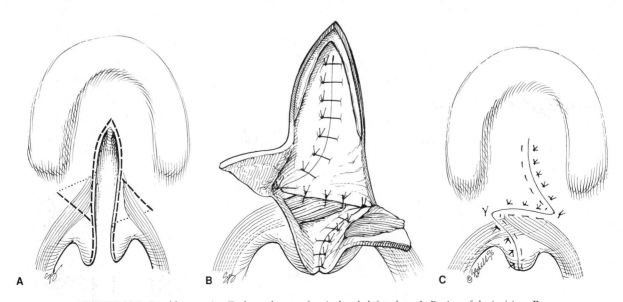

FIGURE 23.9. Double opposing Z-plasty closure of an isolated cleft palate. **A:** Design of the incisions **B:** Muscle included in the posteriorly based flap. **C:** Final result with recreation of the levator sling.

the airway is tenuous. Monitors alone are not a fail-safe prophylaxis. They are only as good as the response of personnel to the alarm. Pain control should be handled by experienced staff, as overmedication with narcotics can easily lead to respiratory arrest in these patients. Infants with Pierre Robin sequence or other congenital anomalies affecting the airway are at highest risk for airway problems.

Palatal fistulas may present as asymptomatic holes or may cause such symptoms as speech problems, nasal regurgitation of fluids, or difficulty with oral hygiene. The most common locations are at the region of the incisive foramen, at the posterior nasal spine, and the uvula. Fistula rate has previously been reported at 10% to 15%, but in experienced hands is now 5% or less. Meticulous surgical technique to create intact, well-perfused flaps that are carefully approximated across the cleft with minimal tension is the best prophylaxis against fistula formation. The use of biomaterials, such as acellular cadaveric human dermis, has been described as a reinforcing layer on top of the nasal closure for wide clefts. With a well executed technique this should rarely, if ever, be indicated. Oronasal fistulas are treated early with local mucosal flaps if they are symptomatic, or are left unrepaired until the time of another surgery, such as alveolar bone grafting, if they are asymptomatic.

Orthodontic and Orthognathic Treatment Following Cleft Palate Repair

Studies on unrepaired cleft palates in developing countries suggest that the surgical intervention of cleft palate repair impairs future maxillary growth. Some individuals with cleft palate may also have an intrinsic limited growth potential. Decreased maxillary width and the resulting lingual crossbite are common and are managed by orthodontic maxillary expansion with a fixed appliance. Once expansion is completed, the optimum time for bone grafting is chosen according to the stage of canine development. If the graft is performed too early, it can result in bone resorption as a consequence of a lack of mechanical stimulation from a tooth. If the graft is performed too late and the erupting canine root does not have sufficient bone support, the tooth may be lost.

Maxillary retrusion or midface hypoplasia resulting in an Angle class III occlusal relationship with anterior crossbite can be managed in childhood with a distraction device such as a Delaire mask to aid horizontal growth, but eventually requires orthognathic advancement. A plan of treatment is formulated on the basis of clinical examination, photographs, cephalometric studies, and dental models. If surgery is indicated, presurgical orthodontics is required to align dental arches and to eliminate crowding and dental compensations. LeFort I maxillary advancement is performed at the time of epiphyseal closure at skeletal maturity, approximately age 16 years for a girl and 18 years for a boy. Large advances greater than 1 cm can be difficult as a result of restriction from palatal scarring related to palate repair or previous pharyngeal flaps, and are prone to relapse. These cases can either be treated with an accompanying bilateral sagittal split-mandibular osteotomy setback to minimize the maxillary advancement required, or can be treated with LeFort I maxillary distraction osteogenesis.

Polley and Figueroa have studied and popularized LeFort I maxillary distraction osteogenesis using an external cranial halo-based device. Once the permanent teeth have descended below the osteotomy site, the LeFort I osteotomy is performed as with traditional surgery, and the maxillary dentition is attached to the halo-based distraction device via an occlusal splint or other orthodontic attachment. The segment can then be advanced at a rate of 1 mm a day into the desired position of overcorrection. This is followed by a period of wearing the device without advancement during which ossification occurs within the osteotomy and consolidates the new maxillary po-

sition. The original consolidation period of 8 weeks has been decreased to 2 to 3 weeks by the use of a removable, elastic-traction, traditional, orthodontic face mask that is attached to the oral splint after removal of the halo. Polley and Figueroa's studies demonstrated stability of large maxillary advancements with distraction osteogenesis and that there is minimal detrimental effect on speech.

OPERATIVE TREATMENT OF VELOPHARYNGEAL INSUFFICIENCY

Speech and Language Development

All children born with a cleft palate require examination by a speech pathologist at regular intervals to allow timely intervention if a significant delay develops in receptive or expressive language. The diagnosis and work-up of language difficulties requires the multidisciplinary involvement of the speech pathologist, audiologist, otolaryngologist, psychologist, and pediatrician, as the delay is not always secondary to mechanical problems of the velopharynx. Other potential contributing factors include hearing difficulties, abnormal speech habits, psychosocial delay, and tongue restriction. VPI is the inability to achieve closure of the velopharyngeal port during sustained speech. The most common cause of VPI is a cleft of the secondary palate; however, other less-common causes include submucous cleft palate, neuromuscular abnormalities, adenoidectomy, and congenital VPI of unknown etiology. Once other causes of language delay have been ruled out, a formal VPI work-up is performed to diagnose the underlying dynamics of the velopharynx, and to recommend appropriate treatment.

Velopharyngeal Incompetence

Intelligible speech production requires reliable and voluntary function of the velopharyngeal valve that controls communication between the oral and nasal cavities. The valve is closed by contraction of the pharyngeal muscles to advance the lateral and posterior pharyngeal walls, as well as the levator sling that pulls the soft palate (velum) posteriorly. If this palatopharyngeal sling is incompetent, abnormal coupling of the nasal and oral cavities occurs, which results in hypernasality, nasal emission, imprecise consonant production, decreased vocal intensity (loudness), and short phrases. These are the typical signs of velopharyngeal incompetence, which may be caused by either a structural defect or a physiologic dysfunction.

Tissue deficiency, pharyngomegaly, and neurogenic paresis of the velopharynx can all cause VPI; however, not all patients who exhibit glottal stops, pharyngeal fricatives, or nasal emission have VPI. Learned articulatory compensations such as glottal stops and pharyngeal fricatives may be confused with velopharyngeal dysfunction. Phoneme-specific nasal emission is often confused with VPI, even though no resonance disorder exists. Other aspects of phonatory, articulatory, and prosodic breakdowns may be unrelated to the competency of the velopharyngeal valve. If opening of the velopharyngeal valve, instead of closing, is the problem, abnormal uncoupling of the nasal and oral cavities results in hyponasality. This can be found in individuals with hypertrophic adenoid tissue and must be recognized before considering surgical intervention. Nonsurgical treatments of VPI include speech therapy, prosthetic management with speech bulb or palatal lift appliances, and posterior pharyngeal injections or implants. This section focuses on the surgical treatment of VPI.

Preoperative Velopharyngeal Insufficiency Evaluation

The goal of surgical intervention of patients with VPI is to provide a mechanism for functional speech. The design of the surgical procedure is based on the velopharyngeal anatomy and the function, which is determined by a series of clinical and radiographic tests. Clinical examination includes a formal recording of the child's speech before, during, and after therapeutic intervention. Typical speech samples include isolated phonemes, words, phrases, and nonnasal reading passages with the nares occluded and unoccluded to detect acoustic differences associated with cul-de-sac resonance. Dynamic study of the pharynx by multiview videofluoroscopy and nasopharyngoscopy is usually indicated. This test provides information regarding the posterior and superior movement of the velum as well as the degree of medial excursion of the lateral pharyngeal walls during speech. In patients who have been referred from another center, intraoral examination and nasopharyngoscopy will determine if an intravelar veloplasty was performed at the time of cleft palate repair, and if the levator sling is functioning appropriately. With these tests, the VPI team can determine if the problem is insufficient length and/or excursion of the velum, or poor excursion of the pharynx, which will determine whether correction requires a secondary palate lengthening procedure such as a Furlow palatoplasty, or if pharyngeal surgery is indicated.

After pharyngeal flap surgery, patients are followed closely by both the surgeon and the speech pathologist. Clinical evaluations and tape recordings are obtained at least every 3 months for the first year and then annually for 3 to 5 years. Periodic acoustical analyses with the sound spectrograph are used to monitor speech characteristics postoperatively, and should validate more subjective, perceptual ratings in judging the success of surgery.

Pharyngeal Surgery for Velopharyngeal Insufficiency

The nonvelar surgical management of VPI usually consists of pharyngeal flap or sphincter pharyngoplasty. At NYU, we prefer a superiorly based pharyngeal flap, whereas at Children's Hospital, a sphincter pharyngoplasty is employed. Both are useful techniques with advantages and disadvantages.

Pharyngeal Flaps

Pharyngeal flaps may be superiorly or inferiorly based. Most studies in the literature have not found a difference on speech outcome between the two dissections. The mucosal flaps are raised from the posterior pharyngeal wall and attached to the soft palate so as to create a midline obstruction of the oral and nasal cavities between two lateral openings (ports). The amount of lateral pharyngeal wall motion will determine how wide the flap needs to be to achieve velopharyngeal competence. If the flap is too narrow, hypernasality will persist from inability of the lateral pharyngeal walls to close the ports on either side of the flap. If the flap is too wide, passive occlusion of the lateral port can occur, and the patient will develop mouth breathing, hyponasality, and possibly obstructive sleep apnea. Hogan (1973) popularized the concept of lateral port control based on his appreciation of the previous work by Warren et al. in the 1960s. These pressure-flow studies demonstrated that oropharyngeal air pressure decreases markedly when the port cross-section exceeds 10 mm², whereas nasal escape of air is audible above 20 mm². Sphrintzen et al. introduced the concept of "tailor-made" flaps based on preoperative evaluation of lateral pharyngeal excursion (11).

The technique of pharyngeal flap surgery involves longitudinal incisions through the mucosa and muscle down to the prevertebral fascia on each side of the posterior pharyngeal wall. Dissection is continued along the prevertebral fascia. A superiorly based flap is transversely incised inferiorly and raised to a level above the palatal plane, which usually corresponds to 1 to 2 cm above the tubercle of the atlas. An inferiorly based flap is incised just below the adenoid pad. The flap is usually inset with turn-back flaps on the nasal side of the uvula, with or without opening the midline palate repair. The turn-back flaps from the nasal mucosa are used to line the raw surface of the pharyngeal flap to minimize postoperative contraction. The pharyngeal donor defect of the flap is closed primarily. In patients with velocardiofacial syndrome, the internal carotid arteries can have an anomalous course that approaches the midline. The pharynx is observed and palpated carefully for any abnormal pulsations in the region of the proposed flap. Some authors have advocated preoperative computerized tomography (CT) or magnetic resonance imaging (MRI) angiograms in these select patients.

Complications following pharyngeal flap surgery are considerable compared to those of primary cleft lip and palate repairs. The Hospital for Sick Children in Toronto published retrospective data from a 7-year period in 1992 and reported an 8.2% risk of bleeding, a 9.1% risk of airway obstruction, and a 4.1% risk of sleep apnea. Five percent of their cohort required eventual surgical revision of the flap. With changes instituted by this group based on their review, including closer observation and monitoring, increased education, and decreased number of surgeons performing the procedure, the total rate of complications decreased from 11% to 3.2%. Bleeding decreased to 1.4%, airway obstruction to 3.2%, and hospital stay decreased from 5.8 to 3.8 days. These two valuable reports emphasize the potential complications associated with pharyngeal surgery, and the benefit of constant vigilance and quality improvement at all centers.

As expected, sleep apnea or upper airway obstruction is a potential complication of an operation whose purpose is to decrease the velopharyngeal airway. Although studies report up to a 35% incidence of abnormal polysomnograms following pharyngeal flap surgery, the vast majority of these patients resolve within 5 months. Lesavoy (1996) concluded that "the surgeon may sometimes need to accept some transient upper airway obstruction to achieve correction of velopharyngeal insufficiency."

Sphincter Pharyngoplasty

The sphincter pharyngoplasties performed today are modifications of either the Hynes or the Orticochea techniques. In both techniques, the sphincter is constructed from bilateral superiorly based flaps raised from the posterior tonsillar pillars including mucosa and the palatopharyngeus muscle. In the Hynes pharyngoplasty, the flaps are transposed to the midline and inset into a defect created by a transverse incision at the level of the flap base. In the Jackson modification of the Orticochea technique, the flaps are sutured together with a small, superiorly based, posterior pharyngeal flap (12). Subsequent authors and studies have emphasized that the level of the sphincter is the most important predictor of success in both of these techniques. The pharyngeal constriction must be high, at the level of palatopharyngeal closure. The tightness of the pharyngoplasty can be controlled by the degree of overlap of the tonsillar flaps.

The procedure achieves both static and dynamic reduction in the velopharyngeal port with no disruption of the velum. It is ideal when there is poor medial excursion of the lateral pharyngeal walls and a short anteroposterior component of velar competency. It has the advantage of allowing revision if necessary by re-elevating the flaps and adjusting the tightness of the sphincter.

In both sphincteroplasties and pharyngeal flaps, the adenoid pad can limit the superior dissection and placement of the obstruction. For these patients, the otolaryngologist on the cleft team should be consulted to determine if an adenoidectomy is in the best interest of the child.

Pharyngeal Flap Compared to Sphincter Pharyngoplasty

Studies comparing the two pharyngeal surgeries have not documented a significant difference in speech outcome. Both techniques have advantages and disadvantages and potential complications, and require an experienced surgeon for success. An ongoing international prospective trial under the direction of Shaw in Manchester, UK comparing these two surgeries hopefully will improve our understanding of their relative values.

TREATMENT OF THE ALVEOLAR CLEFT

The preconference symposium of the 2004 American Cleft Palate–Craniofacial Association (ACPA) annual meeting focused on treatment of the alveolar cleft. Three approaches were presented and debated: (a) early alveolar bone grafting in the first year of life with autogenous rib cortical graft as a separate operation; (b) presurgical NAM with primary GPP at the time of primary lip repair; and (c) secondary alveolar bone grafting as a separate operation during mixed dentition with autogenous iliac crest cancellous graft. No conclusions regarding the superiority of one technique over another could be drawn at the end of the symposium. Each approach has been studied by its proponents to provide data justifying its use. Secondary bone grafting at the time of mixed dentition remains by far the most common technique for treatment of the alveolar cleft, and as such remains the standard by which other techniques are compared (13). The ideal treatment for the alveolar cleft would be a minimal surgical intervention performed without an additional anesthetic, with no donor-site morbidity, and no detrimental effect on facial growth or dental eruption. To date, NAM with primary GPP is the closest to this goal, but as described earlier in this chapter (page 206, Presurgical Nasoalveolar Molding), it requires presurgical orthopedics by a trained team, is associated with a 60% chance of avoiding secondary bone grafting, and requires further evaluation to confirm that it has no detrimental effect on maxillary growth. As prospective standardized multicenter data is gathered on the effect of these different surgical approaches on facial growth, bone quality, tooth survival, and patient satisfaction, we will have an increased understanding of their relative advantages and limitations.

Advances in tissue engineering and bone substitutes will generate an increasing number of materials that can be used for "off-the-shelf" replacement of missing alveolar bone. Although exciting, these materials still require a surgical procedure for introduction into the cleft. As with all new techniques, they should undergo the same stringency of evaluation prior to widespread use, including an emphasis on cost-effectiveness and potential side effects.

SECONDARY CLEFT LIP AND NOSE SURGERY

Increased understanding of the primary cleft abnormal anatomy with an associated improvement in the technique of primary repair has reduced the severity of residual deformities and the need for secondary corrections. Perfection in a single surgery, however, remains elusive. The goals of early cleft lip and nose reconstruction are that the cleft be undetectable by peers at conversational distance by school age to minimize psychosocial stigmata, and that an optimal final surgical result using up-to-date techniques be complete by skeletal maturity. This is rarely achieved by one surgery in wide, complete clefts, resulting in the need for secondary cleft lip and nose surgeries. These secondary interventions should be kept to a minimum while striving to achieve these two goals.

Each surgery is approached with the following guidelines in mind:

- Identify the primary repair that has been performed to appreciate how it will affect the planned revisions.
- Recognize the optimum age to achieve the surgical goals. If the child is too young, small, temporizing procedures are performed to minimize the deformity and scarring until the definitive procedure can be performed.
- Find the normal landmarks and return them to their normal positions.
- Do not remove any tissue until certain that it will not be useful.
- Treat each case individually—there is no routine secondary procedure.
- Use the basic plastic surgery principle of transferring tissue from areas of excess to areas in need.
- Replace lost tissue with similar tissue when prior surgery, growth, or the lack of growth is responsible for the deficiency.

Indications for Surgery

The indication for a secondary surgical procedure is a correctable deformity given the age of the patient, which if not repaired, will remain or will result in psychosocial or functional problems. The surgeon must recognize that there are four perspectives of anatomic abnormalities to be considered: those of the surgeon, those of the patient, those of the parent, and those of peers or other members of society. Which perspective is predominant affects both the indication for surgery and the chance of a successful outcome.

When addressing a patient with a secondary deformity, it is first necessary to recognize the cause of the deformity. Steffensen (1953) outlined reasonable requirements for lip repair: (a) accurate skin, muscle, and mucous membrane union; (b) proper rotation of the deflected medial and lateral orbicularis oris muscle into a horizontal position; (c) a symmetric nostril floor and nostril tip; (d) an even vermilion border with reproduction of the Cupid's bow; (e) slight eversion or pouting of the central upper lip; and (f) a minimal scar. Failure to meet one or more of these requirements may indicate the need for secondary repair.

Timing of Secondary Repair

As mentioned above, the goals of secondary repair of cleft lip and nasal deformities are that the cleft be undetectable by a peer at conversational distance by school age, and that an optimal final surgical result is complete by skeletal maturity. To achieve this, we perform presurgical nasoalveolar molding in early infancy, followed by a primary lip repair with repositioning of the nasal cartilages when the patient is approximately 3 months old, and defer any revisions until just prior to school age. At that time, any indicated lip revisions are completed to facilitate the child's interaction with peers in a school environment. In the case of an obvious residual nasal deformity, such as that following repair of an unmolded wide bilateral cleft, a minor nasal tip rhinoplasty through limited intranasal incisions can be offered. The optimal time to complete the nasal reconstruction, however, is in adolescence, when a formal open rhinoplasty with cartilage grafting, septoplasty, and/or osteotomies can be done. If orthognathic surgery is anticipated, the rhinoplasty is best deferred until after this is complete, as the appearance of the nose will change following repositioning of the bone that supports the nasal base.

Unilateral Cleft Lip

Deformities of the unilateral lip repair are mainly asymmetries and disproportions. One of the most readily visible deformities is an asymmetry between the vertical heights of the peaks of the Cupid's bow. If the Cupid's bow is not level, the cause should be identified and a surgical solution created. Vertical shortening of the cleft lip scar is not uncommon in the first few months following surgery, but should settle within a year postoperatively.

Deep to the cutaneous cleft lip repair is the orbicularis muscle. Proper reconstruction of the oral sphincter is key to preventing secondary contraction after repair. Discontinuity of the orbicularis oris is seen less often following unilateral repairs than following bilateral repairs. When discontinuity is present, a subcutaneous groove or trough appears and the scar contracture, which is normally seen only in the first few months after a repair, persists. The groove is more readily apparent on lip animation, with bulging of the lateral muscle segments caused by unbalanced contraction.

Secondary deformities of the unilateral cleft lip are diagnosed on physical examination. They include the deficient tubercle, vermilion deficiency and irregularities, the short upper lip, long upper lip, tight upper lip, and unfavorable scars.

Deficient Tubercle

A deficient or poorly pronounced tubercle following unilateral lip repair may be ameliorated by using a V-Y advancement of the labial mucosa. In rare cases, a dermal graft may be used to provide an autogenous lip augmentation. A fine mosquito clamp is used to create a tunnel along the horizontal length of the tubercle and within the substance of the orbicularis oris muscle. This procedure can yield a natural-appearing lip, especially during lip animation, but has the associated risk of asymmetry and fibrosis.

Vermilion Deficiency and Irregularities

The most common irregularity is a notch or whistle deformity. Notching is usually caused by inadequate approximation of the orbicularis marginalis muscle within the red lip. Deficiency of the free edge of the lip can often be treated by reopening of the inferior incision, symmetric eversion of the medial and lateral lip elements, and accurate layered approximation of the orbicularis marginalis and mucosa. If the primary repair had resulted in deficiency of tissue, local rearrangement of tissue is required: V-Y advancement, Z-plasty, or bilateral opposing advancement flaps of the labial mucosa. Z-plasty is especially useful when notching of the vermilion border is combined with scar contracture. The frenulum should always be examined if there is a red lip asymmetry, to ensure that a tight frenulum is not contributing to the problem. If the lip is excessively thick on the cleft side, a transverse ellipse can be excised at the wet–dry junction. Loss of the Cupid's bow after repair of a unilateral cleft can be corrected using the unilateral Gillies operation. This technique involves a triangular skin excision above the

mucocutaneous line (to preserve this landmark). The excision is then closed horizontally.

Short Upper Lip

Short lip following unilateral repair refers to a diminished distance from the Cupid's bow to the base of the columella. The most common cause of the short lip is failure to adequately lengthen the lip at the primary repair. A short lip is more common when straight-line and rotation-advancement methods were used for the primary repair if the techniques were not executed properly. It can be a difficult deformity to repair. Careful evaluation is warranted, as recreation of the defect and complete revision is often necessary. As mentioned, shortening of the lip scar is not uncommon in the first few months after surgery, and it may be severe. Asymmetry generally exists during this time and is maximal 6 to 8 weeks after surgery. Softening and relaxation of the scar returns the lip to its immediate postoperative position when a proper muscular repair exists. However, if the lip is short on the operating table, it will always remain short. Techniques available for lip lengthening include (a) rotation-advancement flaps, (b) Z-plasties, (c) V-Y or forked flaps, (d) muscle advancements, and (e) Abbe flaps.

If a straight-line repair was performed primarily, it will not interfere with a subsequent rotation-advancement revision, which will advance the alar base medially and lengthen the columella on the cleft side. The ideal indication for rotation-advancement following a straight-line repair includes (a) the philtral scar on the cleft side is short; (b) the Cupid's bow is pulled up toward the nostril; (c) the nostril floor is wide; and (d) the ala is displaced laterally and downwards.

A short upper lip following a Millard-type rotation repair usually requires revision with recreation of the defect and repeat rotation-advancement. Simple rerotation and advancement of skin only, without complete takedown of the muscular repair, should be reserved for minimal deficiencies. Additional lengthening may be obtained by adding a Z-plasty placed close to the sill of the nostril so that it is not readily apparent.

Long Upper Lip

The long lip is more commonly found in bilateral than unilateral clefts. Compared to the rotation-advancement techniques, the quadrangular (LeMesurier) or triangular (Tennison) repair have been blamed for vertically long lips on the side of the cleft. The excess can be easily corrected by excising the exact amount of excess height from the horizontal components of the quadrangular repair.

It is unusual to find a rotation-advancement that has been rotated too much. A long lip deformity following a Millard-type repair may be corrected by total take-down of the repair with partial derotation of the medial segment. It may be necessary to shorten the vertical height of the lateral element to match the new rotation edge by a horizontal excision under the alar base.

Tight Upper Lip

In a unilateral cleft lip repaired using a triangular method, a common secondary deformity is a tight upper lip. It is a horizontal tightness of the upper lip across the upper alveolus. This tightness is best corrected using a Z-plasty. Many early straight-line designs not only destroy the Cupid's bow but also result in a horizontal tightness. In time, this tightness might improve as the displaced maxillary segments approximate. The tight upper lip tends to restrain anteroposterior facial growth and gives the relative appearance of a pouting lower lip. Severe tightness requires an Abbe lip switch flap for correction. This is more commonly used for treating bilateral cleft lip secondary deformities and is described in that section (see Bilateral Cleft Lip below).

Unfavorable Scars

Unfavorable scars alone may require revision. Scars causing concern are generally either hypertrophic or widened, or are in an unacceptable position. Patients with multiple previous procedures may have a network of visible scars on the upper portion of the lip under the columella. If the scars are not hypertrophic and the lip–nose relationship is favorable, there is very little that can be done to improve the appearance. Hypertrophic scars most commonly appear about 1 month after the operation. They are red, raised, and firm. We make an effort to maintain tape on our lip repairs for up to 3 months to prevent these scars. Silicone scar management products can also be used. Wide scars may result from any of the previously discussed techniques, and are often associated with inaccurate approximation of the underlying orbicularis muscle. Revision is the usual solution. A pink scar may persist over time, and may be treated with a laser (see Chapter 56).

Upper lip hair will not grow in cleft lip scars. A patchy moustache formation can either be treated with scar revision, or with individual hair transplants.

Bilateral Cleft Lip

Bilateral cleft lip repair more typically leads to secondary deformity than does unilateral cleft lip repair. The secondary deformities listed above (see Unilateral Cleft Lip) can also occur following bilateral cleft lip repair and some may treated in a similar fashion. In the repair of the bilateral cleft lip, the goal is to achieve a narrow philtrum with a Cupid's bow, an adequate vermilion tubercle, and sufficient horizontal laxity to permit natural animation. Paradoxically, it is often easier to achieve lip symmetry with a bilateral repair than with a unilateral one. Horizontal (distance from philtrum to commissure) asymmetry is usually less obvious than vertical asymmetries. The contribution of the bony components of the cleft to the secondary deformity needs to be considered. It may be necessary to set back a projecting premaxilla before lip or nasal revision can be adequately addressed.

The most frequent secondary deformity of the bilateral cleft lip is paucity of the central lip. The thin central vermilion (whistle deformity) is more commonly seen after a Manchester-type repair, where the central lip has been corrected with abnormal prolabial mucosa that is deficient in bulk and often dry or flaking. The single-stage Millard-type bilateral repair, in which the red lip component of the lateral segments creates the central vermilion, usually leads to better symmetry and a fuller vermilion tubercle.

If a whistle deformity is present following a Manchester-type repair, the best treatment is often to recreate the defect and reconstruct the central lip from the lateral lip elements. If there is insufficient lateral lip bulk, a portion of the old prolabial mucosa may be maintained under the Cupid's bow. Attenuation of the inferior contour of the vermilion free border can also be improved with bilateral mucosal advancements, dermal grafting, or a V-Y advancement.

Once good symmetry is achieved in the bilateral cleft, the result may be compromised by a wide philtrum. We plan our philtrum to be 5 mm wide at the time of primary repair, understanding that this will stretch to a variable degree with time. The narrower the philtrum at the time of primary repair, the more vermilion is available for reconstruction of the central tubercle from the lateral lip elements. If there is excess philtral width in a secondary deformity, this redundant tissue may be used to lengthen the invariably short columella, and should not be excised until the decision has been made not to use it. When narrowing a wide philtrum by direct excision, the redundant dermis can be preserved to provide bulk underneath the new philtral margins.

A tight upper lip that cannot be corrected sufficiently with local flaps requires a donation of tissue from the lower lip via an Abbe flap. The Abbe flap improves the balance between the upper and lower lips by bringing comparatively excessive tissue from the pouting lower lip to the tight upper lip that is deficient of tissue. The scar on the upper lip is excised, creating a central defect. A full-thickness flap is designed centrally on the lower lip to reconstruct the aesthetic subunit of the upper lip philtrum. The donor defect on the lower lip should not violate the mental crease. The flap is rotated on a mucosal bridge containing an intact labial artery and vein that are found at the level of the vermilion border on the lingual (inner) side of the lip. The pedicle is divided after 10 to 14 days, and the flap is inset. The white roll of the flap segment must line up perfectly with that of the lateral lip elements. Up to one-third of the lower lip can be harvested while still achieving primary closure of the donor defect. If the muscle sphincter of the upper lip is in continuity, the Abbe flap can be designed as a skin/mucosal flap to wrap around the native orbicularis muscle.

Deficiency of the central labial sulcus is, unfortunately, a common secondary deformity following a bilateral repair. It results when the labial sulcus height has not been set at the time of the primary repair by suturing the turn-down mucosal flap from the prolabium to the periosteum of the premaxilla. The upper labial sulcus must be of sufficient length to provide a free upper lip for normal animation and speech. If deficiency of the labial sulcus is caused by an adhesion, the adhesion can be split horizontally with the resulting defect closed using Z-plasty flaps from the lateral lip mucosa. If there is insufficient tissue from the lateral lips to reconstruct the central sulcus, a mucosal graft can be used. It is placed inside-out over a stent, which is then inserted into the defect between the premaxilla and lip. This last technique, however, is prone to recurrence of the contracture.

Premaxillary Setback

The complete bilateral deformity is characterized by protrusion of the premaxilla and collapse of the lateral alveolar segments. Following repair of the orbicularis oris at the time of the primary repair, the segments are typically naturally molded by the muscle tension. In some cases, persistent premaxillary protrusion may occur. With the help of the team orthodontist, the decision is made whether a premaxillary setback is required as an orthognathic procedure. Premaxillary setback should only be performed by an experienced surgeon, as the vascular supply of the premaxilla is precarious and loss of the entire premaxilla and central teeth can occur. In some cases, the lip repair has formed a constricting band superior to the premaxilla forcing the premaxilla inferiorly. Not only does the premaxilla continue to project, but its severe inferior malposition may result in the incisor teeth biting into the lower gingivobuccal sulcus. In this circumstance, resection of a short section of vomer stem with repositioning of the premaxilla, mucosal repair, and alveolar bone grafting may be required. Premaxillary setback and repositioning should only be performed with the guidance of an orthodontist to plan for future dental rehabilitation and facial contour aesthetics.

Secondary Cleft Lip Nasal Repair

The literature is replete with numerous approaches to secondary repair of the cleft lip nasal deformity (Fig. 23.10). Many older techniques are still useful in certain circumstances, but should be used within the current paradigm of a systematic

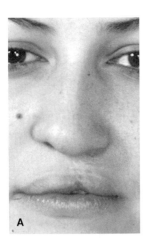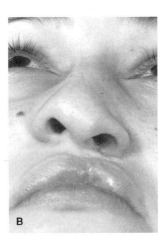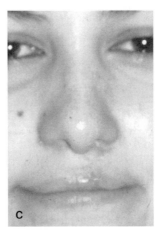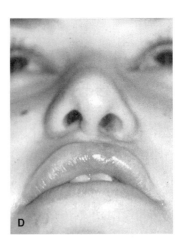

FIGURE 23.10. Secondary rhinoplasty. **A** and **B:** Frontal and worm's-eye view of a nasal deformity secondary to unilateral cleft lip. The nasal tip is wide and underprojected because of divergence of the nasal domes and a shortened left columella. The left alar rim is depressed and flattened secondary to a deformed lower lateral cartilage. The left alar base is laterally and posteriorly displaced. The bony pyramid of the nasal dorsum is asymmetric. The patient also had a deviated septum and collapsed internal nasal valve. **C** and **D:** Frontal and worm's-eye view of the same patient after an open Dibbell tip rhinoplasty, submucous resection of the cartilaginous septum, a spreader strut graft, and monobloc nasal osteotomy.

anatomic evaluation of the deformity followed by an equally systematic treatment plan. Just as techniques first used in the treatment of cleft patients formed the basis of the aesthetic rhinoplasty, many of the techniques that have recently evolved in aesthetic plastic surgery have been adopted by cleft surgeons. Each component of the deformity must be addressed in an orderly manner: skeletal base, nasal dorsal bone and cartilage, nasal tip cartilage, and, finally, the skin envelope (14).

Skeletal Base

Like all facial structures, the nose is supported by the underlying skeleton. The cleft deformity is not restricted to the skin and cartilage. In the unilateral deformity, the piriform rim under the ipsilateral alar base is deficient of bone and is retrusive. During the primary cleft lip surgery, the abnormal attachment of the nasal accessory cartilages to the piriform rim is released in order for the alar base to be moved anteriorly, medially, and superiorly into the desired position. Because of the lack of skeletal support, the alar base on the cleft side can, in some cases, become retropositioned with growth, even following an appropriate primary correction. If the patient is undergoing secondary alveolar bone grafting at the time of mixed dentition, this is the best time to augment the deficient piriform rim with autogenous cancellous onlay bone graft. The bone graft will elevate and support the alar base to achieve symmetry, and provide a stable base for the remainder of the nasal reconstruction in the teenage years.

In the bilateral cleft deformity, the anterior nasal spine is absent, and the footplates of the lower lateral cartilages rest on the muscle repair over the premaxilla. Prior to the definitive secondary rhinoplasty, the position of the premaxilla must be assessed. If the patient has not yet undergone orthodontic treatment, the premaxilla can be retrusive or protrusive. Both deformities will affect the appearance of the nose and lip, and should be corrected before a rhinoplasty is undertaken. In the unfortunate event that the premaxilla is absent, either because of inappropriate resection or iatrogenic loss, prosthetic replacement is needed to provide a base support for the nose and lip.

A number of cleft patients will require orthognathic surgery following orthodontics because of midface retrusion. Ideally, the definitive rhinoplasty should be delayed until after the maxillary advancement has been completed. The LeFort segment contains the anterior nasal spine, which will affect the columella–labial angle and nasal tip projection.

Nasal Dorsal Bone and Cartilage

The unilateral cleft lip nasal deformity often includes a deviated bony and cartilaginous nasal septum with or without deviation of the nasal bones. All of the techniques described in the cosmetic rhinoplasty literature can be employed. If the nasal bony pyramid is symmetric, it can be mobilized as a "monobloc" and centralized, as described by Vilray Blair (1930). If the pyramid is asymmetric, independent movements of the nasal bones will be required. We used a 3-mm osteotome percutaneously to control the nasal osteotomies.

The deviated nasal septum can be treated with a septoplasty, using sutures and scoring to straighten the nasal passage, or, alternatively, with a submucosal resection if cartilage graft is required for the nasal tip, leaving a 1-cm dorsal and ventral L strut for support. In both cases, the base of the septum is mobilized and centralized using a permanent suture through the periosteum of the nasal spine. If the septal cartilage is too weak to support the new position, onlay strut grafts are used to reinforce the nasal tip projection.

As with any rhinoplasty, the preoperative evaluation includes an intranasal examination. If the patient has collapse of the internal nasal valve with nasal obstruction on inspiration, spreader grafts between the upper lateral cartilage and septum are needed. It is important to inform the patient preoperatively that this will widen the nasal dorsum, which is often opposite to what the patient wants esthetically.

The bilateral cleft lip nasal deformity frequently has a broad nasal dorsum. This can be treated with bilateral nasal osteotomies and in-fracturing to narrow the nasal pyramid and increase dorsal projection. This maneuver will narrow the nasal passage, and needs to be balanced with the functional goals of the surgery.

Nasal Tip Cartilages

The medial and lateral feet of the lower lateral cartilages in the secondary deformity are often displaced posteriorly on the cleft side, with the lateral foot displaced laterally. This causes collapse of the nasal tripod, alar rim hooding, and lateralization of the genu of the nasal dome. Older techniques transposed subsections of the displaced cartilages, and are rarely indicated. The current consensus is to reposition the entire lower lateral cartilage structure using an open tip rhinoplasty. Unlike a non-cleft rhinoplasty, simple repositioning with nasal tip sutures is typically insufficient to correct the cleft deformity. After the native cartilage framework is reconstructed, autogenous cartilage grafting is required to strengthen the new position and to augment the nasal tip projection.

In the unilateral deformity, a "springboard" graft is often required to maintain alar rim curvature. The graft is harvested from the septum, and is anchored in a subcutaneous pocket at the alar base. The graft is then bent under mild tension over the lower lateral cartilage and secured to the nasal dome. The lateral crus is then secured to the undersurface of the graft. The springboard effect of the graft will create and maintain the desired alar rim curvature when the skin is redraped. Other useful techniques are modifications of the Dibbell (1982) bipedicle chondrocutaneous flap (15). A bipedicled flap of nasal floor skin is elevated in continuity with a chondrocutaneous flap of medial crus with incisions below the crus and above it in the membranous septum. The depressed medial crus is advanced up into the tip, and the alar base is carried medially by the bipedicle nasal floor flap. This is performed in conjunction with an open approach, using a Tajima (1977) "inverted U" nostril apex incision to address the soft triangle (16). Tajima suspension sutures anchored to the upper lateral cartilages are useful to elevate the alar rim in both these techniques.

In the bilateral cleft lip nasal deformity the displaced lower lateral cartilages are addressed in a fashion similar to that described above. Compared to the unilateral deformity, however, the nasal tip projection and support is more deficient. Columella cartilage strut grafts or septal extension grafts as described by Byrd (1997) are required to provide support to the nasal tip construct. After medialization of the genu of the lower lateral cartilages to the midline to create a nasal dome, multiple onlay tip or Sheen grafts are usually required to achieve the desired shape and projection.

Skin Envelope

A principal argument for an aggressive primary rhinoplasty in infancy is the frustration associated with attempts to correct the deformed, deficient, and scarred skin envelope of a secondary or tertiary rhinoplasty. All cleft surgeons have experienced the satisfaction of constructing a formidable cartilage framework, only to see it compromised under compression when the skin is redraped. The delicate anatomy of the natural soft triangle and nasal dome cannot be created with current secondary techniques, but should remain our goal.

In the unilateral deformity, the deformed skin envelope often overhangs the nostril apex. The Tajima "inverted U" nostril apex incision can help to address this problem. The skin flap left attached to the inferior edge of the lower lateral cartilage turns over to form the inner lining of a constructed soft triangle. A similar turn-over flap approach can be used secondarily if the underlying cartilage is already in the correct position.

In the bilateral cleft lip nasal deformity, the skin envelope is deficient vertically, from the nasal tip to the base of the columella. When closing the open rhinoplasty, the relatively lax lateral tip skin is advanced toward the nasal tip when the rim incisions are closed, in order to create sufficient skin for the nasal tip and columella closure. In severe deformities, however, the skin envelope is too tight to drape over the cartilage construct with tension-free closure at the columella incision. As described in previous sections, techniques that borrow skin from the lip, such as a V-Y advance, result in considerable scarring at the lip–columella junction. Conversely, techniques that borrow from the horizontal laxity of the nasal tip skin, such

as the McComb and Brauer alar lift incisions, result in additional scars on the nasal tip. Both approaches therefore have limitations, but no ideal alternative currently exists.

Nostril Stenosis

Nostril stenosis is the most difficult late complication associated with cleft lip repair. It is considerably easier to narrow a nostril than to enlarge it. In general, any circumferential nasal lining incision is associated with a high incidence of nostril stenosis. With a rotation-advancement repair, placement of the L flap in the nasal vestibule helps to provide adequate nasal lining and can reduce the incidence of stenosis. Once formed, nostril stenosis is a challenge to release. Intranasal Z-plasties or composite grafts are frequently used. Long-term postoperative use of nasal stents is required to minimize the chance of recurrence, but, unfortunately, is limited by patient compliance.

CONCLUSION

Many plastic surgeons were drawn to their surgical specialty after seeing their first cleft lip repair. Cleft care stands out as a rare opportunity in plastic surgery to have a huge impact on an infant's future psychosocial well-being, and to follow these children over the formative years of their lives. The surgeon is reminded of the success, as well as of the failure, of the surgeon's primary operations for years to come. Modern cleft surgical techniques, preoperative orthodontics, and specialized multidisciplinary team care enable us to achieve consistently favorable primary surgical results. Repair of secondary nasal deformities, however, remains a challenge, and is still best treated by preventative surgery at the time of the primary repair. Recent "inductive" techniques, such as nasoalveolar molding and distraction osteogenesis, have improved cleft care over the past decade, and as comparable advances in plastic surgery occur in the future, a child born with a cleft can look forward to fewer operations with better aesthetic and functional results.

References

1. Grayson B, Cutting C, Wood R. Preoperative columella lengthening in bilateral cleft lip and palate. *Plast Reconstr Surg.* 1993;92:1422.
2. Wood R, Grayson B, Cutting C. Gingivoperiosteoplasty and growth of the midface. *Plast Surg Forum.* 1993;16:229.
3. Brauer RO, Cronin TD. The Tennison lip repair revisited. *Plast Reconstr Surg.* 1983;71:633.
4. Millard DR. Refinements in rotation-advancement cleft lip technique. *Plast Reconstr Surg.* 1964;33:26.
5. Mohler LR. Unilateral cleft lip repair. *Plast Reconstr Surg.* 1987;80:511.
6. Cronin T, Upton J. Lengthening of the short columella associated with bilateral cleft lip. *Ann Plast Surg.* 1978;1:75.
7. McComb H. Primary repair of the bilateral cleft lip nose: a 15-year review and a new treatment plan. *Plast Reconstr Surg.* 1990;86:882.
8. Mulliken JB. Primary repair of bilateral cleft lip and nasal deformity. *Plast Reconstr Surg.* 2001;108:181.
9. Trott JA, Mohan N. A preliminary report on one stage open tip rhinoplasty at the time of lip repair in bilateral cleft lip and palate: the Alor Setar experience. *Br J Plast Surg.* 1993;46:215.
10. Sommerlad BC. A technique for cleft palate repair. *Plast Reconstr Surg.* 2003;112:1542.
11. Shprintzen RJ, Lewin ML, Croft ML, et al. A comprehensive study of pharyngeal flap surgery: tailor-made flaps. *Cleft Palate J.* 1979;16:46.
12. Jackson IT, Silverton JS. The sphincter pharyngoplasty as a secondary procedure in cleft palates. *Plast Reconstr Surg.* 1977;59:518.
13. Abyholm EE, Bergland O, Semb G. Secondary bone grafting of alveolar clefts. *Scand Reconstr Surg.* 1981;15:127.
14. Cutting CB. Secondary cleft lip nasal reconstruction: state of the art. *Cleft Palate Craniofac J.* 37:538.
15. Dibbell D. Cleft lip nasal reconstruction: correcting the classic unilateral defect. *Plast Reconstr Surg.* 1982;69:264.
16. Tajima S, Maruyama M. Reverse-U incision for secondary repair of cleft lip nose. *Plast Reconstr Surg.* 1977;60:256.

CHAPTER 24 ■ NONSYNDROMIC CRANIOSYNOSTOSIS AND DEFORMATIONAL PLAGIOCEPHALY

JOSEPH H. SHIN AND JOHN A. PERSING

Craniosynostosis is the pathologic condition that results from premature fusion of one or more sutures in the cranial vault; it is associated with a deformity of the vault and cranial base. Most cases of nonsyndromic craniosynostoses demonstrate a sporadic pattern of occurrence. When a suture fuses prematurely, the skull and the growing brain beneath the suture are restricted, leading to expansion into regions of the skull with less restriction. This "compensatory" growth of the skull occurs largely in planes parallel to the affected suture, resulting in consistent, recognizable cranial deformities. The incidence of nonsyndromic craniosynostosis is seen more commonly with a reported frequency of between 0.4 and 1/per 1,000 live births (syndromic craniosynostosis is discussed in Chapter 25).

The development of craniofacial surgery has been profound in the previous 30 years. Technologic advances and greater safety in the care of these patients is the result of craniofacial teams incorporating the expertise of all necessary specialties: genetics, neurosurgery, plastic surgery, pediatric anesthesiology, ophthalmology, otolaryngology, orthodontics, speech therapy, physical therapy, and psychology.

HISTORY AND PATHOGENESIS

Virchow, in 1851, noted that premature fusion along the suture lines resulted in compensatory growth along a plane parallel to the fused suture and a decrease in the growth of the skull in relation to the perpendicular axis (Fig. 24.1). This hypothesis of skull maldevelopment remained unchanged for nearly 100 years until Van der Klaauw, in 1946, and Moss, in 1959, proposed that the cranial base was the source of abnormal physical stress leading to dural abnormalities that yielded premature sutural fusion, that is, the "functional matrix theory." Subsequent animal studies (1) have, however, elucidated that the cranial vault abnormalities typical of synostosis can be produced with experimental fusion of developing cranial vault sutures. Moreover, cranial base deformities are secondarily induced by restrictions in growth of cranial vault sutures. Mooney et al. corroborated the importance of suture fusion in the development of cranial vault and cranial base changes in a rabbit model (2). Moreover, cranial base, and even deformities of the facial skeleton, may develop secondary to the cranial vault suture restrictions. Further supportive evidence for the primacy of cranial vault suture pathology in most cases of nonsyndromic craniosynostosis comes from the clinical observation by Marsh and Vannier that following cranioplasty in patients with individual suture craniosynostosis in which surgery altered only the cranial vault structure, previously developed cranial base abnormalities were ameliorated (3). More recently

Opperman, Ogle, Longaker, and others have demonstrated developmental and biologic abnormalities in prematurely fusing sutures (4,5).

Surgical treatment of craniosynostosis began with Lane (1892) and Lannelongue (1890). Both performed strip craniectomies for fused cranial vault sutures in young infants. To the present day, modifications of this approach continue to be used to treat patients with cranial deformities. Tessier's recommendations include the use of wide exposure, the intracranial approach to correcting some forms of facial deformity, the liberal and exclusive use of autogenous bone grafting, and reliance on rigid bony fixation. Subsequent developments include three-dimensional radiographic visualization and precise computer-guided modeling. Improved pediatric anesthesia, critical care, and monitoring contribute to overall safety and effectiveness while decreasing morbidity and mortality. Rigid fixation and the development of resorbable plates and screws and bone substitutes have also greatly improved the efficacy of the surgery. The development of the techniques of distraction osteogenesis applied to both the cranial vault and the facial skeleton also have radically altered and expanded surgical options for correction of these deformities.

CRANIAL ANATOMY AND THE DEVELOPMENT OF ANOMALIES

The cranial vault is composed of a series of bone plates, the junctions of which constitute the cranial sutures (Fig. 24.1). The major cranial sutures are the metopic, sagittal, coronal, and lambdoid. A partial list of other minor sutures includes the temporosquamosal, the frontonasal, and the frontosphenoidal. In some cases, brain growth is retarded by prolonged restriction of the cranial vault secondary to fusion of the overlying sutures. In most cases, fusion of a solitary suture does not result in gross neurologic impairment by currently available measuring techniques, although more subtle learning disabilities may be more frequent (6) (see Increased Intracranial Pressure below). When multiple sutures are involved, the possibility of compression of underlying brain increases significantly (7). Some cases of craniosynostosis are not detectable at birth because the manifestations may be mild. When craniosynostosis is suspected, the infant should be evaluated by a craniofacial team.

The most common types of craniosynostosis are (a) metopic synostosis producing a trigonocephaly deformity, (b) sagittal synostosis producing a scaphocephaly deformity, (c) unilateral coronal synostosis resulting in a plagiocephaly deformity, and (d) bilateral coronal synostosis resulting in a brachycephaly deformity. Lambdoid synostosis is a distinctly

the inherent risks and benefits associated with a careful review of the outcomes both as a group and individually.

CLINICAL OBSERVATIONS AND MANAGEMENT

Isolated Craniosynostosis

Metopic Synostosis

The metopic suture is the first cranial suture to fuse, occurring at approximately 7 to 8 months of age. Premature closure of the metopic suture results in a well-recognized "keel"-shaped deformity known as trigonocephaly (Fig. 24.2). Metopic synostosis is relatively uncommon and accounts for less than 10% of isolated suture, nonsyndromic craniosynostoses. Brain development is not usually impaired, although Renier has noted elevated ICP in approximately 4% of patients, and trigonocephaly may be associated with underdevelopment of the frontal lobes as a primary brain anomaly (7). Such problems of development may be a result of primary brain maldevelopment. Hypotelorism is evident and often accompanied by upward slanting of both the lateral canthi and the lateral portions of the eyebrows, as well as flattening of the supraorbital ridges.

When the metopic suture is prematurely fused, bone growth is apparently reduced along all margins of the frontal bones adjacent to the stenotic suture. There is a compensatory increase in bone deposition at the abutting sagittal suture, resulting in enlarged parietal bones. The triangular shape is a result of the flattening of the frontal bones, anterior displacement of the coronal sutures, and flaring of the parietal bones. This shape is exaggerated by the lack of lateral projection of the supraorbital rims and narrowing of the temporal regions (Fig. 24.3).

There is wide variation in the degree of deformity, and an individualized and properly timed correction is ideal. The basic operative management in all but the mildest deformities includes overcorrection of the bilateral dimension.

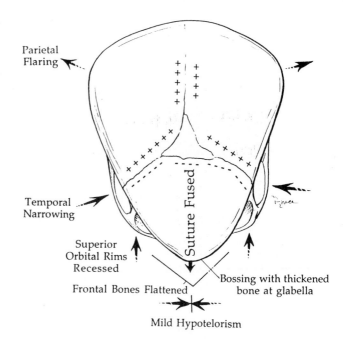

FIGURE 24.3. Skull shape abnormalities seen with metopic synostosis.—, Regions of reduced bone deposition; +++, regions of compensatory increased bone deposition. (From Shaffrey ME, Persing JA, et al. Surgical treatment of metopic synostosis. In: Pershing JA, Jane JA, eds. *Neurosurgical Clinics of North America*, Philadelphia: WB Saunders; 1991:622, with permission.)

Operative Procedure. Early correction (younger than 1 year of age) is performed with the patient in the supine position (Fig. 24.4). A bifrontal craniotomy is performed, and the frontal and parietal bones are removed as a single bone graft (Fig. 24.5). Remodeling of the bifrontoparietal bone graft is performed using a shaping burr and radial osteotomies (Fig. 24.6). Care is taken to avoid the detachment of the orbital rims at the frontozygomatic suture. Our current technique advances the orbital rims by the bowstring technique. This appears to reduce the potential to compromise the supraorbital rim blood supply and allows angulation of the orbital rim pivoting on the frontozygomatic suture. We believe this is important for supporting the orbital rim and frontal bone, preventing a superior flattening of the supraorbital/frontal region that may yield a less-than-satisfactory outcome. We maintain the temporalis muscle attachment to the underlying bone and squamous bone overlay, attempting to prevent the "temporal hollowing" that may be seen following techniques that detach fully, then reattach the temporalis muscle with suture. The anterior temporal bone and muscle are outfractured as a composite unit. The frontal bone graft is secured to the supraorbital rims either with wire or suture fixation. As a general rule, bone grafting is required when the defect is greater than the size of a quarter. Otherwise the small defects ossify spontaneously in children younger than 1 year of age.

In children between the ages of 1 and 3 years, the bony remodeling techniques are altered to allow reshaping of the more mature cranial vault. The bone in this age group is more brittle, making bending less effective. The major difference in technique in this age group involves selective weakening of the bone by the placement of endocranial channels or "kerfs" in the bone. These patients (those older than 1 year of age) usually require bone grafting, as the defects tend to be larger.

In children older than 3 years of age, surgical correction requires further modifications. Cranial vault and brain growth are approximately 85% complete by 3 years. At this point there is greater emphasis on direct reshaping and fixation of formed

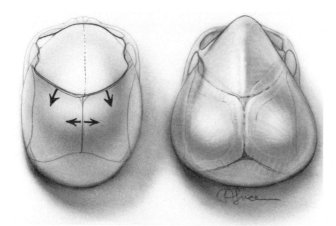

FIGURE 24.2. Metopic suture synostosis. **Left:** Schematic predicting the directions of abnormalities *(arrows)* in the skull. **Right:** Fusion of the metopic suture results in reduced growth in the frontal bone medially, producing bifrontal narrowing; asymmetric compensatory expansion at the coronal suture associated with symmetric expansion at the sagittal suture results in the characteristic trigone-shaped skull. (From Persing JA, Jane JA, Edgerton MT. Surgical treatment of craniosynostosis. In: Persing JA, Edgerton MT, Jane JA, eds. *Scientific Foundations and Surgical Treatment of Craniosynostosis*. Baltimore: Williams & Wilkins; 1989:124, with permission.)

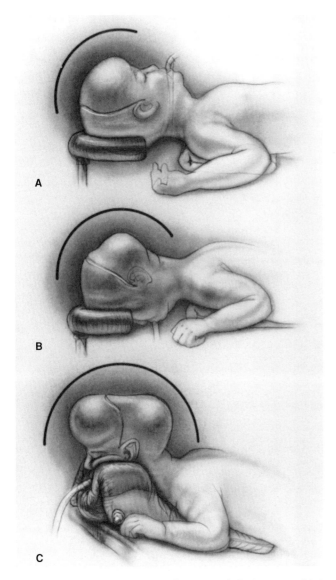

FIGURE 24.4. Operative positions for surgery. **A:** Supine on a padded horseshoe head rest. **B:** Prone on a horseshoe head rest allowing access to the posterior half of the skull. **C:** Modified prone position with chin support in a padded "bean bag" to allow simultaneous access to the anterior and posterior skull. (From Persing JA, Jane JA, Edgerton MT. Surgical treatment of craniosynostosis. In: Persing JA, Edgerton MT, Jane JA, eds. *Scientific Foundations and Surgical Treatment of Craniosynostosis.* Baltimore: Williams & Wilkins; 1989:134, with permission.)

bone segments in their "normal" adult positions. These basic principles of bone remodeling and cranial fixation apply to the treatment of all forms of nonsyndromic craniosynostosis.

Sagittal Synostosis

Sagittal synostosis, the most common form of craniosynostosis, is associated with a skull deformity known as scaphocephaly. This skull shape is the result of premature fusion of the sagittal suture, and characterized by a skull with increased anteroposterior length and decreased width, yielding a "boatlike" shape. Sagittal synostosis is typically sporadic, with only a 2% genetic or familial predisposition. The male-to-female incidence ratio is 4:1.

Following sagittal suture fusion, the coronal and lambdoid sutures, which are adjacent to the restricted parietal bone plate, compensate by enhanced bone deposition at the edge of these

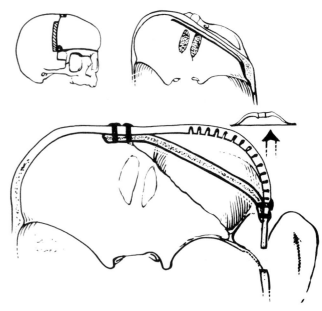

FIGURE 24.5. Figure depicts osteotomy performed and schematic of the principle of the bowstring canthal advancement technique (horizontal view). (From Knoll B, Shin JH, Persing JA. Bowstring canthal advancement: a new technique to correct the flattened supraorbital rim in unilateral coronal synostosis. *J Craniofac Surg.* 2005. In press; with permission.)

sutures (in the frontal and occipital bones, respectively). The metopic suture compensates with symmetric bone expansion along its sutural borders. The compensatory growth process produces the characteristic frontal and occipital prominence seen in sagittal synostosis. Because the squamosal sutures are distant to the fused suture, they do not participate significantly in the compensatory growth process and, as such, there is no prominent projection of the temporal (squamous) regions bilaterally. The entire sagittal suture might not be involved so that deformity may be predominantly anterior, predominantly posterior, or both.

Operative Procedure. Treatment of sagittal synostosis varies according to the age of the patient. The younger patients, especially those younger than 1 year of age, present with cranial

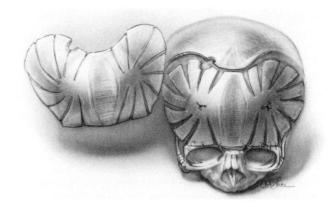

FIGURE 24.6. Operative technique in metopic synostosis. The bifrontal bone graft is remodeled using radially oriented osteotomies in the frontal bone and controlled fractures using the mallet and Tessier rib bender. (From Persing JA, Jane JA, Edgerton MT. Surgical treatment of craniosynostosis. In: Persing JA, Edgerton MT, Jane JA, eds. *Scientific Foundations and Surgical Treatment of Craniosynostosis.* Baltimore: Williams & Wilkins; 1989:167, with permission.)

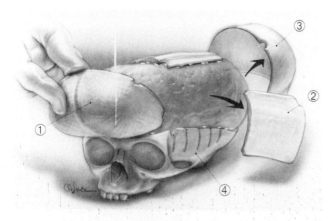

FIGURE 24.7. Operative technique in sagittal synostosis. Bifrontal *(1)*, separate parietal *(2)*, and biparietal occipital craniotomies *(3)*, are performed in serial order. Laterally oriented barrel staves are placed in the temporal bone region *(4)*. (From Persing JA, Jane JA, Edgerton MT. Surgical treatment of craniosynostosis. In: Persing JA, Edgerton MT, Jane JA, eds. *Scientific Foundations and Surgical Treatment of Craniosynostosis.* Baltimore: Williams & Wilkins; 1989:188, with permission.)

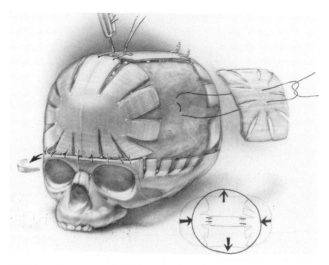

FIGURE 24.8. Operative technique in sagittal synostosis. Reduction in anteroposterior skull length is achieved frontally by removing a segment of midline bone. Triangular wedges of frontal bone are removed just cephalad to the supraorbital margins to allow for posterior inclination of the forehead. The frontal bone laterally is remodeled to create a neocoronal suture. As the wires are cinched down frontally, bulging occurs in the parietal region, for which the parietal bone is reshaped to add increased contour laterally. (From Persing JA, Jane JA, Edgerton MT. Surgical treatment of craniosynostosis. In: Persing JA, Edgerton MT, Jane JA, eds. *Scientific Foundations and Surgical Treatment of Craniosynostosis.* Baltimore: Williams & Wilkins; 1989:190, with permission.)

vault bones that are malleable and easily reshaped. Reshaping is more difficult in older patients because of the increased "brittleness" of the bones. The primary operative goals are to release the stenosis and reshape the cranial vault by increasing the parietal and temporal width and decreasing its anteroposterior dimension.

If access to both the anterior and posterior deformities is necessary, the patient is placed in the modified prone position (Fig. 24.4). Supraperiosteal dissection is performed extending from the glabella anteriorly to the posterior lip of the foramen magnum posteriorly. After appropriate burr hole placement, craniotomies are performed to separate the bifrontal and biparietal-occipital fragments (Fig. 24.7). The narrowing of the low temporal and parietal regions is addressed by placement and outfracturing of parallel vertical "barrel stave" osteotomies. The cone-shaped occiput is remodeled after radial osteotomies and bending of the bone to provide a more gradual convex curvature. The bifrontal fragment is similarly reshaped after placement of radial osteotomies. Shortening of the anteroposterior (AP) length of the skull is accomplished by resecting a portion of the frontal and parietal bones at the midline. The remaining parietal bone fragments are remodeled with the goal of increasing the lateral convexity, particularly in the parietal regions.

Once the bone fragments are remodeled satisfactorily, they are secured with wire or suture fixation in the midline (Fig. 24.8). The frontal segment is secured anteriorly to the superior orbital rims, and posteriorly to the parietal bone segment overlying the sagittal sinus. The occipital segment is attached to the basal occiput posteriorly and to the parietal bone anteriorly. The remodeled parietal bone segments are attached to the underlying dura but are not fixed to adjacent bone so as to encourage further widening of the skull postoperatively.

In older children, the techniques of bone remodeling require several modifications. Kerfs, or channels, placed on the internal surface of the bone oriented perpendicular to the long axis of the bone segment, allow for selective weakening of the bone and easier reshaping and molding.

Unilateral Coronal Synostosis

Premature fusion of one of the coronal sutures results in plagiocephaly (a Greek term meaning oblique skull) (Fig. 24.9).

This is an uncommon disorder, occurring in 1 in 10,000 live births.

In unilateral coronal synostosis, fusion at the coronal suture results in a single frontoparietal bone plate ipsilateral to the fused suture, with an apparent reduced growth potential. This impairment prevents the ventral expansion of the anterior cranial fossa, resulting in a shortened anterior cranial fossa ipsilateral to the fused suture. Growth superiorly results in

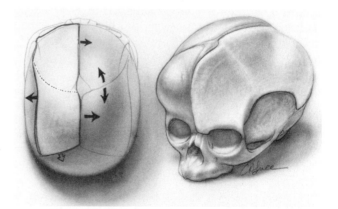

FIGURE 24.9. Left: Predicted skull deformities associated with unilateral coronal synostosis. **Right:** Fusion of the left coronal suture results in flattening of the left frontoparietal region and bulging of the ipsilateral squamous portion of the temporal bone related to asymmetric bone deposition along the squamosal suture. Similar asymmetric expansion at the perimeter metopic and sagittal sutures results in parietal bulging contralateral to the fused suture. The right coronal suture in line with the fused suture demonstrates significant, *symmetric* bony expansion. (From Persing JA, Jane JA, Edgerton MT. Surgical treatment of craniosynostosis. In: Persing JA, Edgerton MT, Jane JA, eds. *Scientific Foundations and Surgical Treatment of Craniosynostosis.* Baltimore: Williams & Wilkins; 1989:125, with permission.)

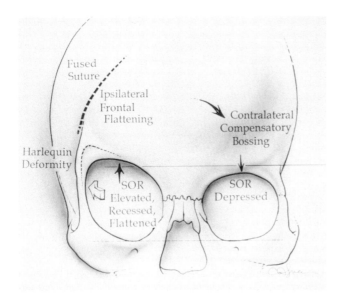

FIGURE 24.10. Unilateral coronal synostosis. Demonstration of the harlequin deformity, the changes in the superior orbital rim, and the frontal bones, both ipsilateral and contralateral to the fused suture. SOR, superior orbital rim.

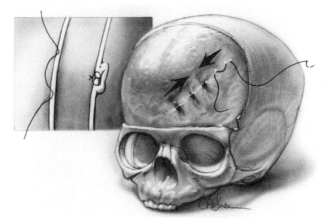

FIGURE 24.11. Dural plication. In areas where there is an increase in prominence of the brain and dura, a needle is passed between the two leaves of dura and plicated so as to reduce the prominence of the dura locally. Because the stitch is placed above the arachnoid, the potential for injury to underlying brain and vasculature is minimized. Plication can also be performed by localized application of the bipolar cautery. (From Persing JA, Jane JA, Edgerton MT. Surgical treatment of craniosynostosis. In: Persing JA, Edgerton MT, Jane JA, eds. *Scientific Foundations and Surgical Treatment of Craniosynostosis.* Baltimore: Williams & Wilkins; 1989:160, with permission.)

elongation of the forehead, whereas inferiorly directed growth produces deformity of the middle cranial fossa with ventral bowing of the greater wing of the sphenoid. The deformity of the sphenoid results in effacement of the temporal fossa, which, combined with shortening of the lateral wall of the orbit, produces proptosis of the globe. The "harlequin" orbit seen on AP radiographs is pathognomonic for unilateral coronal synostosis and is secondary to the lack of descent of the greater wing of the sphenoid during development. Compensatory overgrowth of bone occurs asymmetrically at all perimeter sutures that border the now fused single frontoparietal bone plate that incorporates the coronal suture. This accounts for the bulge in the ipsilateral squamous portion of the temporal bone, contralateral frontal and parietal bones, and, to a much lesser degree, contralaterally in the occipital bone. The fused coronal suture may demonstrate prominent ridging, and the ipsilateral frontal and parietal bones are flattened.

Clinical facial features include widening of the ipsilateral palpebral fissure, superior and posterior displacement of the ipsilateral orbital rim and eyebrow, and deviation of the nasal root toward the flattened side of the frontal bone (Fig. 24.10). The chin point deviates to the contralateral side, and the malar eminence is frequently anterior on the same side as the flattened side forehead (and fused coronal suture) when compared to the contralateral malar eminence.

Operative Procedure. The patient is placed supine and a bifrontal craniotomy is performed. The greater wing of the sphenoid, which is thickened and displaced superiorly, is rongeured to the level of the lateral supraorbital fissure. A supraorbital rim osteotomy is performed bilaterally, and the orbital rims are contoured to symmetry, then advanced. Where the prominence of the brain and dura is increased, dural plication can be performed gently with the bipolar cautery or with suture. In unilateral coronal synostosis, the dura is plicated in the frontal bone region contralateral to the fused coronal suture to achieve frontal region projection symmetry (Fig. 24.11). An advancement of the supraorbital rim is performed unilaterally. The affected side must be overcorrected or reversion to the preoperation asymmetry is assured. The frontal bone is remodeled using radially oriented osteotomies, and selective fractures are

performed to achieve the desired form. The frontal bone plate is attached to the orbital rims superiorly and laterally, but not posteriorly so as to allow further growth of skull at the "neo"-coronal suture.

Bilateral Coronal Synostosis

Bilateral coronal synostosis is characterized by a tower-shaped, but short, head, or turribrachycephaly (Fig. 24.12). The skull is shortened anteroposteriorly, widened mediolaterally, and elongated vertically. The anterior cranial base is shortened, and the orbital rims are retrusive. The superior frontal and squamous temporal bones are protuberant, and the occiput usually is flattened. There may be ridging of the coronal suture and

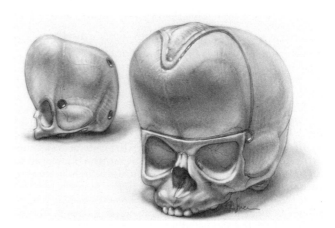

FIGURE 24.12. Bilateral coronal synostosis. The skull in bilateral coronal synostosis demonstrates flattening occipitally and bulging frontally with an anteriorly displaced vertex. Burr holes are placed as indicated (*left*). A bifrontal bone graft is elevated (*right*). (From Persing JA, Jane JA, Edgerton MT. Surgical treatment of craniosynostosis. In: Persing JA, Edgerton MT, Jane JA, eds. *Scientific Foundations and Surgical Treatment of Craniosynostosis.* Baltimore: Williams & Wilkins; 1989:180, with permission.)

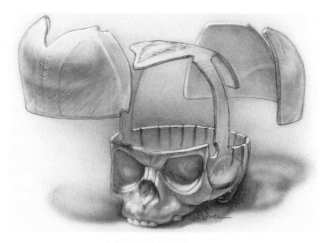

FIGURE 24.13. Bilateral coronal synostosis. A biparietal-occipital bone graft is developed posteriorly with a bony bridge between the two hemicrania located below the level of the torcula. The remaining occipital bone undergoes barrel stave osteotomy. (From Persing JA, Jane JA, Edgerton MT. Surgical treatment of craniosynostosis. In: Persing JA, Edgerton MT, Jane JA, eds. *Scientific Foundations and Surgical Treatment of Craniosynostosis.* Baltimore: Williams & Wilkins; 1989:181, with permission.)

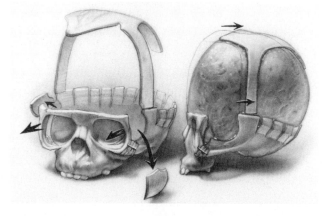

FIGURE 24.14. The orbital rims are advanced by orbital osteotomy. The squamous portion of the temporal bone is elevated and remodeled (*left*). The vertex of the skull is shifted posteriorly by severing the parietal bones and relocating them posteriorly (*right*). This reduces the prominence of the frontal "bossing." (From Persing JA, Jane JA, Edgerton MT. Surgical treatment of craniosynostosis. In: Persing JA, Edgerton MT, Jane JA, eds. *Scientific Foundations and Surgical Treatment of Craniosynostosis.* Baltimore: Williams & Wilkins; 1989:182, with permission.)

flattening of the caudal portion of the frontal bones and supraorbital ridges. Radiographically, bilateral harlequin abnormalities may be present.

Operative Procedure. The patient is placed either supine or, in a majority of cases, in a modified prone position. If the primary focus of involvement is the frontal bar/orbital rim with only mild involvement of the occipital region, then the supine position is preferred. If there is absolute elevation of the height of the skull associated with shortening in an anteroposterior direction then, through the modified prone position, the height of the skull can be shortened and the anteroposterior dimension can be elongated. A biparietal-occipital bone graft is elevated and reshaped by a combination of radial osteotomies and controlled fractures of the bone segments (Fig. 24.13). Barrel stave osteotomies are placed in the occipital region, which are "outfractured" to increase the bony "capacity" of the intracranial compartment. The thickened and elevated superior portion of the greater wing of the sphenoid is removed by rongeur to the level of the supraorbital fissure. Osteotomies can be done in both orbits to increase orbital rim projection bilaterally (as described earlier; Fig. 24.5, Unilateral Coronal Synostosis). The remaining parietal bone struts are severed and shifted posteriorly approximately 1 to 2 cm (Fig. 24.14). The height of the skull is reduced while ICP is monitored. Throughout the procedure, the ICP can be monitored in order to maintain an adequate cerebral perfusion pressure of approximately 60 mm Hg. The reshaped bone segments are replaced and a postoperative skull molding cap is used to guide skull shape for 2 to 3 months.

Lambdoid Synostosis

True lambdoid synostosis is extremely uncommon, and represents the least-common form of craniosynostosis. It is characterized by bony fusion of the lambdoid suture, flattening of the ipsilateral occiput, posterior/inferior displacement of the ear ipsilateral to the fused suture, and distortion of the posterior cranial base. It is to be distinguished from deformational plagiocephaly, which is common and characterized by a "parallelogram" skull deformity (Fig. 24.15) (12). In both deformational plagiocephaly and unilateral lambdoid synosto-sis skull deformities the occiput is asymmetrically flattened. In patients with lambdoid synostosis, the ear is positioned posteriorly and inferiorly on the side of suture fusion and occipital flattening. In patients with deformational skull deformity (plagiocephaly), the ear is positioned anteriorly (compared to the opposite side ear) on the side of occipital flattening (Table 24.1).

Radiographically, lambdoid synostosis is characterized by bony bridging of the lambdoid suture and deviation of the foramen magnum toward the side of the fused suture (9,13). In deformational plagiocephaly, the cranial base midline is unaltered and there is no bony bridging of the lambdoid suture. Premature infants tend to have positional deformities more often simply because they are less mobile because of gestational age. The distinction between deformational plagiocephaly and lambdoid synostosis is important because deformational plagiocephaly ordinarily will improve without surgery, whereas lambdoid synostosis skull deformity will not improve without surgery. The occipital flattening deformity

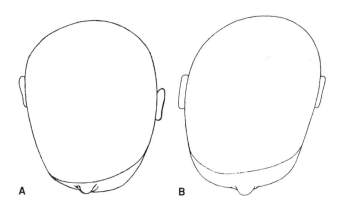

FIGURE 24.15. Illustration of differences between left synostotic (**A**) and left deformational (**B**) frontal plagiocephaly. Note opposite configuration of left malar eminence and opposite position of ears. (From Hansen M, Mulliken JE. Frontal plagiocephaly: diagnosis and treatment. *Clin Plast Surg.* 1995;21(4):547, with permission.)

TABLE 24.1

ANATOMIC FEATURES THAT DIFFERENTIATE CORONAL SYNOSTOSIS FROM DEFORMATIONAL PLAGIOCEPHALY

Anatomic Feature	Coronal Synostosis	Deformational
Major deformity	Forehead	Occiput
Ipsilateral brow	Up	Normal
Ipsilateral ear	Normal	Anterior
Nasal root	Ipsilateral	Midline
Nasal tip	Contralateral	Midline
Ipsilateral palpebral fissure	Wide	Normal

From Hansen M, Mulliken JE. Frontal plagiocephaly: diagnosis and treatment. *Clin Plast Surg.* 1994;21(4):547, with permission.

(i.e., deformational plagiocephaly), when unilateral, is usually seen on the right side, which is most likely related to consistent decubitus positioning in infancy. The decision to recommend surgical repair for unilateral lambdoid synostosis depends on the severity of the deformity. The treatment varies depending on whether the condition is unilateral or bilateral, but the operative exposure and craniotomy lines are similar.

Operative Procedure. The patient is placed in the prone position and the occipital bone is fully visualized to the level of the foramen magnum. A bilateral parieto-occipital bone segment is elevated (Fig. 24.16). Barrel stave osteotomies are performed bilaterally in the flattened basal occipital bone to increase the convex projection of the occipital bone locally. In patients with moderate unilateral lambdoid synostosis defor-

mity, the barrel staves are placed primarily ipsilateral to the fused suture in the occipital bone. In more severe cases, bilateral barrel staves are performed, "infracturing" the normally convex, and "outfracturing" the flattened, portion of occipital bone. The biparietal-occipital bone graft is cut radially and remodeled to achieve a normally rounded, symmetric posterior skull (Fig. 24.17). Cranial bone struts, secured by resorbable plates maintain the normal occipital convexity and symmetry postoperatively. The dura is plicated in areas of excess projection before bone remodeling. The bone graft is replaced and secured to the dura without attaching it to surrounding bone. If the parieto-occipital abnormality is accompanied by significant frontal abnormality (a rare clinical presentation), a bifrontal craniotomy is also performed. The frontal bone is remodeled by radial osteotomies and controlled fractures as

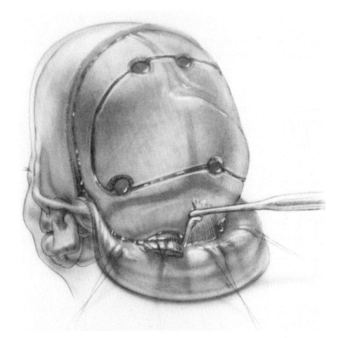

FIGURE 24.16. Lambdoid synostosis For the occipital abnormality a biparietal-occipital craniotomy is performed. (From Persing JA, Jane JA, Edgerton MT. Surgical treatment of craniosynostosis. In: Persing JA, Edgerton MT, Jane JA, eds. *Scientific Foundations and Surgical Treatment of Craniosynostosis.* Baltimore: Williams & Wilkins; 1989:200, with permission.)

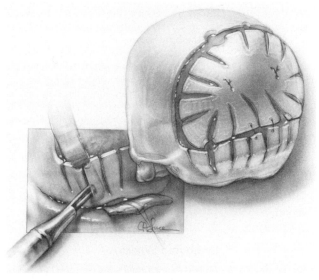

FIGURE 24.17. Barrel staves are performed in the occipital bone to increase projection ipsilateral to the fused suture. A retractor is used to protect the transverse and sagittal sinuses during the osteotomies *(insert).* (From Persing JA, Jane JA, Edgerton MT. Surgical treatment of craniosynostosis. In: Persing JA, Edgerton MT, Jane JA, eds. *Scientific Foundations and Surgical Treatment of Craniosynostosis.* Baltimore: Williams & Wilkins; 1989:201, with permission.)

described earlier for the parietal segments. The frontal bone is secured to the surrounding bone with nonabsorbable suture material.

COMPLICATIONS

Complications in general are relatively infrequent and may be divided into those that are acute and those that are late. Acute complications include blood loss, air embolus, dural tear with CSF leak, and infection and respiratory complications. Blood loss occurs nearly continuously intraoperatively and accounts for most complications. Consequently, vigilant attention to accurate blood replacement is paramount to avoid coagulopathy secondary to dilution of clotting agents. Blood loss may also be rapid and hemodynamically significant with a tear of the venous sinus or major cortical vein. Abnormal transosseous veins in some syndromes, such as the Carpenter syndrome, in the region of the torcula may be torn during the bone dissection and require immediate control. Generally, however, in the presence of sutural fusion, the dural connection to the underlying sinus is often attenuated and the risk of a tear of the sinus is generally reduced. Air embolus has been documented in children undergoing cranioplasty and may occur in any operative position, including supine. It is appropriate to consider the placement of precordial Doppler monitors as well as end-tidal CO_2 monitors to ascertain entrainment of air into the venous system, and central venous lines for blood volume assessment (and resuscitation) and air embolus evacuation. Ongoing blood loss may continue for 12 to 24 hours following cranioplasty and intensive care unit monitoring is essential. Dural tears may lead to CSF leak with or without infection. Immediate repair is indicated in most cases. Postoperative CSF leak may be controlled with a lumbar drain, but if persistent may require surgical closure. Loss of continuity of the osteogenic dura may result in a thinning of the overlying bone, resulting in a cranial defect. Of acute complications, infection represents an uncommon but potentially life-threatening problem. Generally, infection is associated with a CSF leak and persistent communication of the intracranial cavity to the nasal cavity or frontal sinus. Because the frontal sinus develops quite late in childhood, the latter is seen as a consequence of surgery in the older child or adolescent. Whitaker et al. reported an approximate 7% infection rate for patients undergoing craniofacial surgery (13).

Acute airway problems may be related to inadvertent transection of the nasotracheal tube during frontofacial advancement. This may require immediate change to an oral endotracheal tube or possibly tracheostomy. In a retrospective analysis of 542 patients undergoing 579 craniofacial procedures at the Hospital for Sick Children, Crysdale et al. reported that 18% of patients required tracheostomy for management of the airway (14). Those patients who were intubated for longer than 24 hours experienced considerably more complications. Currently, the use of small-caliber fiberoptic flexible bronchoscopy greatly facilitates nasotracheal intubation in those patients previously considered incapable of endotracheal intubation.

Late complications generally are associated with the sequelae of abnormal bone healing and impaired bone growth. Children older than 1 year of age have a decreased ability to fill cranial defects compared to younger patients. In a series of 592 patients following cranioplasty, Prevot et al. reported that 5% of patients had inadequate ossification (15). Generally, defects greater than 2 cm in children older than age 1 year should be filled with split calvarial bone grafts in order to prevent postoperative cranial defects. Significant bone loss requiring bone grafting may occur in the setting of infection and subsequent resorption.

From its inception, the use of miniplate and microplate rigid fixation has greatly improved the outcome of craniofacial surgery. However, Persing et al. have reported significant transcranial plate migration in the growing child (16). Although no harmful effects have been reported, the potential for risk and difficulty posed for reoperative surgery have been noted. We currently use resorbable plating as well as suture fixation in the young child when it is feasible.

With complete and adequate cranioplasty, relapse and recrudescence to the original defect of the cranial vault is uncommon, assuming normal brain growth and development. However, in the region of the orbits and midface, if operated on at a very young age, bone contour may relapse significantly. The degree of relapse depends on the severity of the phenotype as well as the continued effect of cranial base restriction. The constricting force of the soft-tissue envelope and resorption of bone grafts may contribute to further relapse. The advent of distraction osteogenesis is of particular interest in the prevention of relapse as soft-tissue expansion is combined with new bone development. Orthodontic occlusal management is also important in ensuring stability of the final result in the older patient.

Overall the morbidity and mortality from the treatment of craniofacial syndromes is quite low. Mortality has been variously reported to range between 1.5% and 2%. In 1979, Whitaker et al. reported the experience of six craniofacial centers and reported on 13 deaths representing a 1.6% mortality (13). It is likely that ongoing advances in monitoring and anesthetic techniques, as well as refinements in surgical techniques, will continue to yield similar or better results.

In spite of the significant problems that these children and their families face, the future continues to be bright, with the technical advances providing a multiplicity of diagnostic and treatment alternatives that will impact our ability to provide care to these patients.

CONCLUSION

Nonsyndromic craniosynostoses are relatively common, and gross brain damage as a consequence of restriction of skull growth appears to occur infrequently. More subtle abnormalities in learning are now appreciated as being more likely. Skull deformities are significant, however, and surgical correction to reshape skulls to normal contours is indicated. The complication rate is usually low with an experienced team and a state-of-the-art facility.

References

1. Persing JA, Babler WJ, Jane JA, et al. Experimental unilateral coronal synostosis in rabbits. *Plast Reconstr Surg.* 1986;77:369–376.
2. Mooney MP, Losken HW, Tschakaloff A, et al. Congenital bilateral coronal suture synostosis in a rabbit and craniofacial growth comparisons with experimental models. *Cleft Palate Craniofac J.* 1993;30:121–128.
3. Marsh JL, Vannier MW. Cranial base changes following surgical treatment of craniosynostosis. *Cleft Palate J.* 1986;23(suppl. 1):9.
4. Opperman LA, Ogle RC, et al. Tissue interactions with dura mater inhibit osseous obliteration of developing cranial sutures. *Dev Dyn.* 1993;198:312.
5. Longaker MT, Duncan BW, et al. An in-utero model of craniosynostosis. *J Craniofac Surg.* 1992;3:70.
6. Magee SN, Westerveld M, et al. Long-term neuropsychological effects of sagittal craniosynostosis on child development. *J Craniofac Surg.* 2002;13:1.
7. Renier D. Intracranial pressure in craniosynostosis: pre- and postoperative recordings—correlation with functional results. In: Persing JA, Edgerton MT, Jane JA, eds. *Scientific Foundations and Surgical Treatment of Craniosynostosis.* Baltimore: Williams & Wilkins; 1989: 263.
8. Gault DT, et al. Intracranial pressure and intracranial volume in children with craniosynostosis. *Plast Reconstr Surg.* 1992;90:377.

9. Posnick J C, et al. Metopic and sagittal synostosis: intracranial volume measurements prior to and after cranio-orbital reshaping in childhood. *Plast Reconstr Surg.* 1992;89:299.

10. Kapp-Simon KA, et al. Longitudinal assessment of mental development in infants with nonsyndromic craniosynostosis with and without cranial release and reconstruction. *Plast Reconstr Surg.* 1993;92:831.

11. Camfield PR, Camfield CS. Neurologic aspects of craniosynostosis. In: Cohen MM, ed. *Craniosynostosis: Diagnosis, Evaluation, and Management.* New York: Raven; 1986: 215.

12. Turk, McCarthy, Thorne, et al. The "back to sleep campaign" and deformational plagiocephaly: is there cause for concern? *J Craniofac Surg.* 1996;7(1):12.

13. Whitaker LA, Munro IR, Salyer KE. Combined report on problems and complications in 793 craniofacial operations. *Plast Reconstr Surg.* 1979;64: 198.

14. Crysdale WS, Kohli-Dang N, Mullind GC, et al. Airway management in craniofacial surgery: experience in 542 patients. *J Otolaryngol.* 1987;16:207–215.

15. Prevot M, Renier D, Marchac D. Lack of ossification after cranioplasty for craniosynostosis: a review of relevant factors in 592 consecutive patients. *J Craniomaxillofac Surg.* 1976;4:131.

16. Persing JA, Posnick J, Magee S, et al. Cranial plate and screw fixation in infancy: an assessment of risk. *J Craniofac Surg.* 1996;7: 267–270.

CHAPTER 25 ■ CRANIOSYNOSTOSIS SYNDROMES

SCOTT P. BARTLETT

Craniosynostosis can involve any of the sutures in the skull: metopic, sagittal, lambdoidal, or coronal (Chapter 24, Nonsyndromic Craniosynostosis and Deformational Plagiocephaly). In simple craniosynostosis, one suture is prematurely fused. In multiple-suture synostosis, two or more sutures are prematurely fused. Craniosynostosis can occur as an isolated event resulting in *nonsyndromic* craniosynostosis, or it can occur in conjunction with other anomalies in well-defined patterns that make up clinically recognized syndromes. Most cases of isolated nonsyndromic craniosynostosis occur sporadically with a reported frequency of 0.6 in 1000 live births. **Syndromic craniosynostosis is most often genetic in nature, and patterns of autosomal dominant, autosomal recessive, and X-linked inheritance have been observed.** More than 90 reported syndromes are associated with craniosynostosis, with most involving associated anomalies of the limbs, ears, and cardiovascular system.

The Apert, Crouzon, Pfeiffer, Saethre-Chotzen, and Carpenter syndromes represent the more commonly identified craniosynostosis syndromes seen by plastic surgeons. **These familial craniosynostosis syndromes share many common features, including midface hypoplasia, cranial base growth abnormalities, abnormal facies, and limb abnormalities.** In fact, the craniofacial features are clinically similar among the various syndromes so that the digital anomalies of the hands may be the differentiating feature between the various syndromes. Although it is clear that synostosis of the cranial sutures is significantly involved in the development of the abnormal craniofacial features in these syndromic children, there probably exists a mesenchymal defect in the cranial base that also contributes to the craniofacial deformity.

The exact etiology of the craniosynostosis in these syndromic children remains unclear. Advances in molecular genetics provide insights into a possible link between mutations identified in fibroblast growth factor receptor (FGFR) genes and several autosomal dominant skeletal disorders. Fibroblast growth factors participate in the regulation of cell proliferation, differentiation, and migration, and play a role in controlling normal bone morphogenesis via complex cell-signaling pathways. The transduction of a fibroblast growth factor signal to the cytoplasm is mediated by a group of transmembrane tyrosine kinase receptors known as the fibroblast growth factor receptors. **Mutations in three of the four known *FGFR* genes located on chromosomes 8, 10q, and 4p have been identified in the Pfeiffer, Apert, Crouzon, and Jackson-Weiss syndromes.** Achondroplasia, a skeletal disorder that causes the most common form of short-limb dwarfism, also is linked to a mutation in the FGFR complex. The Pfeiffer syndrome is linked to a mutation in both the *FGFR1* and *FGFR2* genes, whereas the Crouzon and the Apert syndromes are linked with mutations in the *FGFR2* complex.

CROUZON SYNDROME (ACROCEPHALOSYNDACTYLY TYPE II)

The Crouzon syndrome is characterized by premature fusion of calvarial sutures, midface hypoplasia, shallow orbits, and ocular proptosis (Fig. 25.1). The clinical features were first described by Crouzon, a French neurologist, in 1912. The pattern of inheritance is autosomal dominant. The reported frequency is 1 in 25,000 live births. The variability in expression of the dominant features that make up Crouzon syndrome is widely recognized.

Premature fusion of both coronal sutures, resulting in a brachycephalic head, is the most common calvarial deformity, but scaphocephaly and trigonocephaly, as well as the cloverleaf skull deformity, have been observed. The craniosynostosis is often complete by 2 to 3 years of age, but occasionally the sutures are fused at birth. The cranial base sutures are frequently involved, resulting in maxillary or midface hypoplasia. The maxillary hypoplasia is evidenced by a reduced dental arch width and a constricted high palatal arch. Normal mandibular growth leads to a class III malocclusion. The midface hypoplasia is reflected in the shallow orbits with exorbitism, which is a consistent finding and can result in exposure conjunctivitis or keratitis. Exorbitism can be so severe that herniation of the globe through the eyelids may occur, requiring immediate reduction. Acuity problems, strabismus, and hypertelorism have all been reported. A conductive hearing deficit is not uncommon. There are no commonly reported anomalies of the digits in this population of patients.

APERT SYNDROME (ACROCEPHALOSYNDACTYLY TYPE I)

Apert, in 1906, described a syndrome characterized by craniosynostosis, exorbitism, midface hypoplasia, and symmetric syndactyly of both hands and feet (Fig. 25.2). The incidence is reported to be 1 in 160,000 live births. Most cases are sporadic, although several cases with autosomal dominant transmission have been reported. The cranial vault deformity in these patients is variable but most often presents as a short anteroposterior dimension with craniosynostosis involving the coronal sutures resulting in a turribrachycephalic skull. The typical craniofacial appearance includes a flat, elongated forehead with bitemporal widening and occipital flattening. The midface hypoplasia is accompanied by orbital proptosis, downslanting palpebral fissures, and hypertelorism. The nose is downturned at the tip, the bridge is depressed, and the septum deviated.

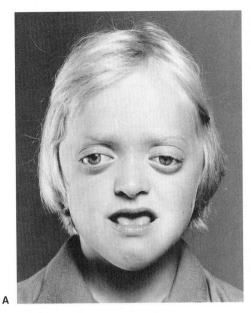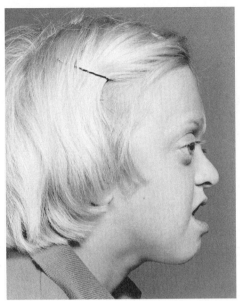

FIGURE 25.1. Crouzon syndrome in a young male. Note the midface hypoplasia, shallow orbits, and ocular proptosis. **A:** Frontal view. **B:** Profile view.

The maxillary hypoplasia results in a class III malocclusion. The hand syndactyly, which is pathognomic for the condition, most often involves fusion of the second, third, and fourth fingers, resulting in mid-digital hand mass, but the first and fifth fingers may also be joined to the mid-digital mass (Fig. 25.3). When the thumb is free, it is broad and deviates radially. In the feet, the syndactyly also usually involves the second, third, and fourth toes. These hand anomalies are so severe and functionally debilitating that referral to a hand surgeon with special expertise in this area is essential.

An extensive review of central nervous system (CNS) problems in patients with Apert syndrome shows an increased incidence of delayed mental development, but many of these patients develop normal intelligence.

PFEIFFER SYNDROME (ACROCEPHALOSYNDACTYLY TYPE V)

This syndrome was described by Pfeiffer in 1964 and consists of craniosynostosis, broad thumbs, broad great toes, and, occasionally, a partial syndactyly involving the second and third

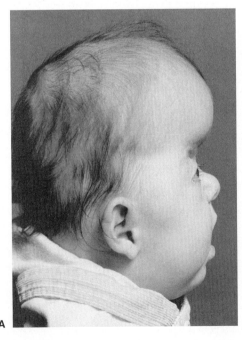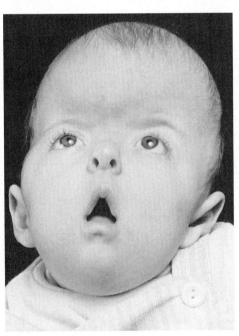

FIGURE 25.2. Apert syndrome in an infant. Note the midface hypoplasia, elongated forehead with temporal widening, and beaked nose.

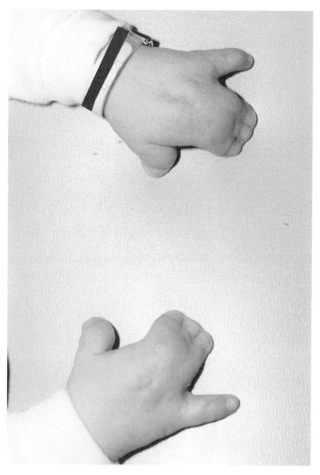

with resulting midface deficiency leads to shallow orbits and exorbitism. Hypertelorism and downslanting palpebral fissures are also common. The nose is often downturned with a low nasal bridge. Intelligence is reported to be normal in the more common form of Pfeiffer syndrome. **The broad thumbs and great toes are the hallmark of the syndrome,** but the findings are frequently subtle. The partial syndactyly of the hands usually involves digits 2 and 3. A partial syndactyly of toes 2, 3, and 4 has also been noted.

SAETHRE-CHOTZEN SYNDROME (ACROCEPHALOSYNDACTYLY TYPE III)

This syndrome was first described by Saethre in 1931 and by Chotzen in 1932. The predominant features include a brachycephalic skull, a low-set frontal hairline, and facial asymmetry with ptosis of the eyelids (Fig. 25.6). The mode of inheritance is autosomal dominant with wide variability in expression.

The craniofacial features, which involve a brachycephalic skull, are secondary to a bicoronal synostosis. The low-set hairline is also a constant feature of this syndrome. The facial asymmetry is often accompanied by deviation of the nasal septum and maxillary hypoplasia with a narrow palate. Intelligence is usually normal. A partial syndactyly involving the second and third digits is often observed, and short stature is also a frequent finding.

CARPENTER SYNDROME

This is a rare genetic disorder characterized by a craniosynostosis of various sutures, leading to an asymmetric head, partial syndactyly of the digits, and preaxial polysyndactyly of the feet. The syndrome was first described by Carpenter in 1901, but not recognized as a significant clinical syndrome until 1966, when it was reported by Temtamy. The mode of transmission is autosomal recessive.

The craniofacial features are variable and are significantly influenced by the shape of the skull. Because the craniosynostosis can involve the lambdoid, sagittal, and coronal sutures, the head shape may vary from brachycephalic

FIGURE 25.3. Syndactyly of second, third, and fourth fingers in infant with Apert syndrome.

digits (Figs. 25.4 and 25.5). Symptoms vary, ranging from very mild to severe. The mode of inheritance is autosomal dominant.

The craniofacial features are similar to those of Apert syndrome. The skull is turribrachycephalic secondary to the coronal and occasional sagittal synostosis. Maxillary hypoplasia

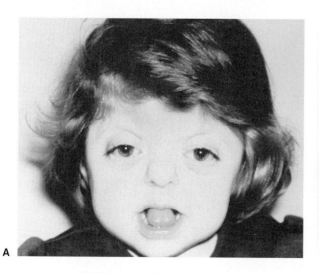

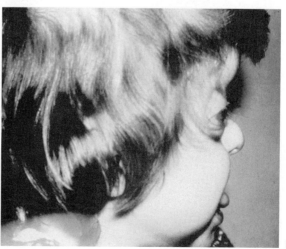

A   B

FIGURE 25.4. Pfeiffer syndrome in an infant female. Note the midface hypoplasia, hypertelorism, and turribrachycephalic skull. Chromosome analysis of this patient revealed a splice mutation in exon B of *FGFR2*. (Reproduced with permission from Schnell U, Hehr A, Feldman G J, et al. Mutations in *FGFR1* and *FGFR2* cause familial and sporadic Pfeiffer syndrome. *Hum Mol Genet.* 1995;3:323.)

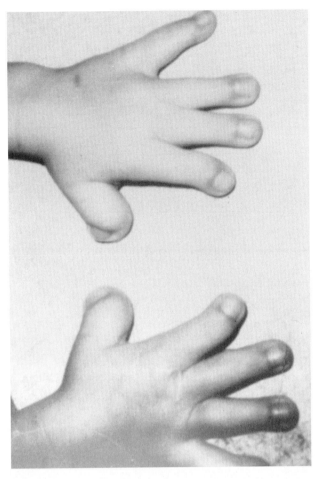

FIGURE 25.5. Broad thumbs in a child with Pfeiffer syndrome. Digital findings in the Pfeiffer syndrome are frequently less obvious than in this case.

to turricephalic. Low-set ears and lateral displacement of the inner canthi are also prominent features. Mental deficiency has been reported, and congenital heart defects have been reported in as many as 33% of cases. The soft-tissue syndactyly of the hands usually involves the third and fourth digits.

FUNCTIONAL ASPECTS

To fully appreciate the surgical treatment of children with these craniosynostosis syndromes, it is necessary to understand the craniofacial growth process and how it relates to certain functional aspects of development. Normal craniofacial growth is directed by two general processes: displacement and bone remodeling. **During the first year of life the brain triples in size and continues to grow rapidly until about 6 or 7 years of age.** The growth of the brain causes displacement of the overlying frontal, parietal, and occipital bones in the presence of open functioning sutures, and this stimulates bone growth and remodeling in the skull and cranial fossa. The growth and maturation of the face follows a craniocaudad gradient, progressing from late childhood to adolescence, with maturation of the upper face followed by maturation of the midface and finally the mandible. The functional aspects of development, which are directly or indirectly influenced by abnormal craniofacial growth, are examined individually below.

Intracranial Pressure

The size of the brain triples during the first year of life and continues to grow rapidly until about age 6 or 7 years. In the patient with craniosynostosis there can be restricted growth of the cranial vault, resulting in a disparity between brain size and intracranial volume, which leads to increased intracranial pressure.

Increased intracranial pressure (ICP) can be recognized clinically by the finding of papilledema on funduscopic

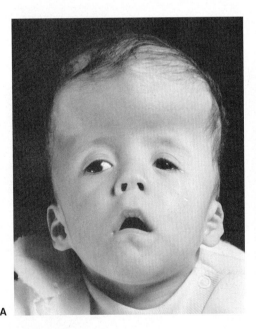
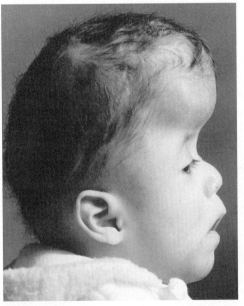

FIGURE 25.6. Saethre-Chotzen syndrome in an infant. Note the brachycephalic skull, low-set frontal hairline, and ptosis of eyelids. Chromosome analysis of this infant and his mother with the Saethre-Chotzen syndrome demonstrated a balanced translocation at the 7p2 region. (Reproduced with permission from Reid CS, McMorrow LE, McDonald DM, et al. Saethre-Chotzen syndrome with family translocation at chromosome 7p22. *Am J Med Genet.* 1993;47:637.)

TABLE 25.1

SYNDROMIC CRANIOSYNOSTOSIS TREATMENT OPTIONS

Procedure	Timing (age)	Comments
Craniectomy, fronto-orbital advancement	4–12 mo	Repeat procedure may be indicated in childhood or adolescence for continued growth restriction or abnormal growth of the skull.
LeFort III osteotomy and advancement—conventional or by distraction osteogenesis	4–8 y	If performed in this age group, a secondary LeFort III may be required in teenage years.
LeFort III osteotomy and advancement—conventional or by distraction osteogenesis	9–12 y	Delaying to this age in less-severe cases may obviate the need for a second major midface advancement.
LeFort I ± mandibular osteotomy	14–18 y	Required to establish neutral dental occlusion after facial growth has ceased.
Monobloc frontofacial advancement—conventional or by distraction	4–12 y	Simultaneously improves forehead, orbital, and midface aesthetics. Suitable for a patient whose deformity allows simultaneous advancement.
Contouring via reduction, onlay bone grafts, bone substitutes, or alloplasts	15–19 y	Performed as the final procedure to enhance aesthetics after all growth has ceased.

examination and, in later stages, "thumb printing" or the beaten-cooper appearance on plain radiographs. **Unfortunately, there does not yet exist a reliable indicator of increased ICP on computerized tomographic scan.** In a study that evaluated ICP by an epidural sensor in 358 children with various types of craniosynostosis, it was found that children with multiple suture synostosis had higher rates of increased ICP (26% to 54%), and in the syndromic population increased ICP was noted in 66% of the patients with Crouzon syndrome and in 43% of those with Apert syndrome. Although it has been documented by three-dimensional computerized to-mography (CT) studies that increases in intracranial and ventricular volume occur following cranial vault reshaping, and that ICP pressure decreases, we cannot yet accurately determine by means of CT scan alone which group of patients with craniosynostosis will develop increased ICP.

Visual Changes

Craniosynostosis can result in abnormal growth of the skull and, in the syndromic population of patients, this is often

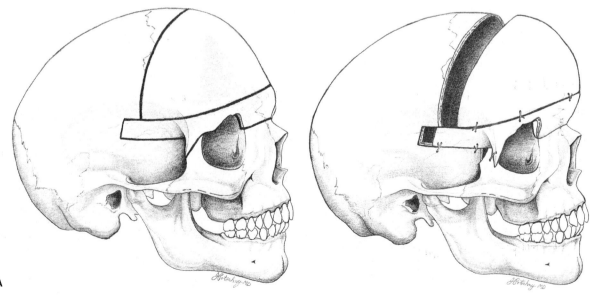

A   B

FIGURE 25.7. Fronto-orbital advancement. **A:** Lines of osteotomy for forehead and supraorbital bar advancement. **B:** Fronto-orbital advancement in a tongue-in-groove manner and fixation with wires.

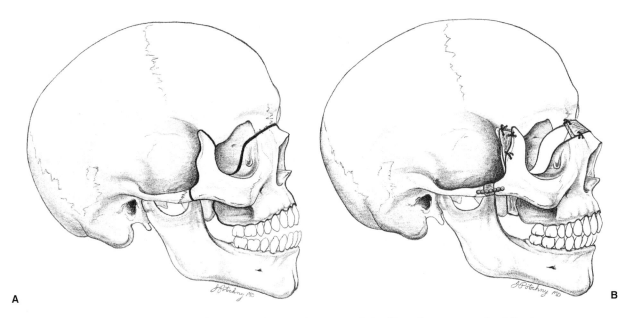

FIGURE 25.8. Le Fort III advancement. **A:** Lines of osteotomy. **B:** Midface advancement and stabilization with bone grafts and miniplates.

accompanied by midface hypoplasia. Underdeveloped shallow orbits or abnormally shaped orbits can cause the eyes and periorbital structures to be displaced from their normal position; this is termed *exorbitism*. Exorbitism can result in corneal exposure and the development of keratitis, pain, infection, corneal scarring, and, at worst, ulceration and blindness. Occasionally, the degree of exorbitism is so great that immediate surgical intervention is required to protect the globe.

Ocular motility problems frequently arise secondary to the abnormal size and shape of the orbits. Strabismus with exotropia is a common finding. Abnormal development and position of ocular muscles have also been frequently reported in children with Crouzon or Apert syndrome.

Increased ICP leading to papilledema and optic atrophy can result in blindness. Whether the optic atrophy is secondary to increased ICP or is secondary to damage to the nerve from compression or a compromised vascular supply is not entirely clear.

Hydrocephalus

Although the incidence of hydrocephalus and craniosynostosis is rare, it appears that among children with craniosynostosis syndromes, the incidence of hydrocephalus is significantly higher, with reports ranging from 4% to 10%. There is clearly a higher incidence of hydrocephalus among children with Apert syndrome. The etiology of hydrocephalus remains unclear, but it has been postulated that it is caused by increased venous pressure in the sagittal sinus secondary to obstruction of the venous outflow caused by the craniosynostosis. Both communicating and noncommunicating forms of hydrocephalus have been identified, but the communicating form is more common.

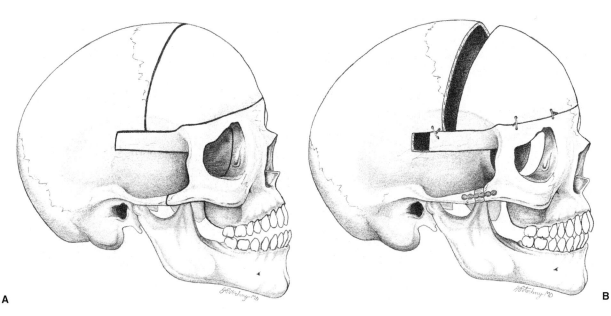

FIGURE 25.9. Monobloc advancement. **A:** Lines of osteotomy for monobloc osteotomy. **B:** Advancement of midface, orbits, and frontal bone and stabilization with bone grafts and miniplates.

Hydrocephalus can present without either marked head enlargement (which may be difficult to detect in the patient with syndromic craniosynostosis) or signs of increased ICP. Preoperative CT scanning or ultrasonography help define the population at risk. At the earliest sign of progressive ventricular enlargement, a shunting procedure should be performed to prevent cerebral injury.

SURGICAL MANAGEMENT

The surgical treatment of patients with craniosynostosis syndromes dates from the late 19th century, when the first techniques were aimed at correcting only the functional aspects of the deformity. The earliest techniques, linear craniectomy and fragmentation of the cranial vault, still are useful in some of the more severe deformities to provide temporary brain and eye protection until a more definitive craniofacial procedure can be undertaken. Simple craniectomy or morcellization performed in infancy, unfortunately, is accompanied by a high rate of re-

ossification and will give only modest results when mobilization of the orbits and midface is not performed concurrently. Additionally, the reossified bone is of poor quality, making definitive correction more difficult. In 1967, Tessier first published his results following correction of the recessed forehead and supraorbital regions using an intracranial approach that allowed accurate osteotomy, mobilization, and repositioning. The current surgical treatment approach for children with syndromic craniosynostosis and accompanying midface deficiency involves an initial fronto-orbital and cranial vault remodeling, a midface advancement procedure with or without distraction (Le Fort III or monobloc), and secondary orthognathic surgery to correct any dentofacial deformities (Le Fort I, mandibular osteotomies).

Surgical intervention for the correction of craniofacial deformities in patients with syndromic craniosynostosis can be divided into those procedures that are performed early in life (4 to 12 months) for suture release, cranial vault decompression, and upper orbital reshaping/advancement, and those that are performed at a later age (4 to 12 years) for midface

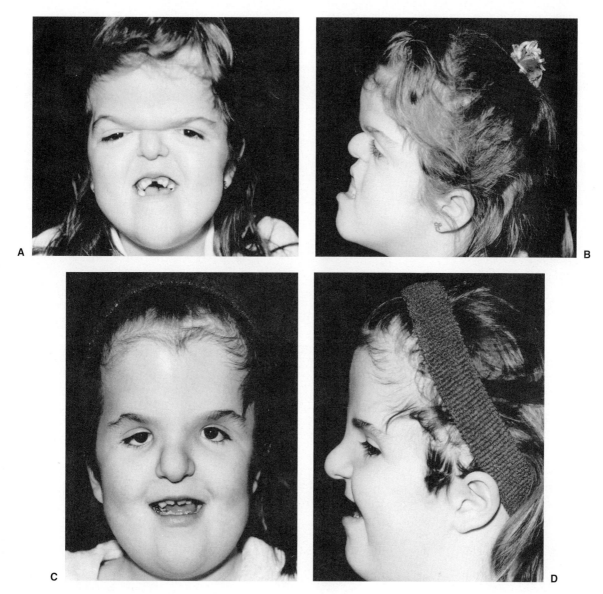

FIGURE 25.10. Midface advancement at age 10 years using a Le Fort III procedure in a child with Apert syndrome. **A:** Preoperative frontal view. **B:** Preoperative profile view. **C:** Eight months postoperative view. **D:** Postoperative profile view.

deformities and jaw surgery (14 to 18 years). The exact timing and sequence for each of the aforementioned surgical procedures is dependent on both the functional and the psychological needs of the patient (Table 25.1). The area of largest controversy centers around the timing of midface osteotomies. Two approaches are currently practiced: (a) waiting until all midface and lower face growth is complete before doing a definitive osteotomy and advancement, or (b) performing a midface advancement in childhood with the realization that a second advancement will be necessary when mandibular growth is complete. Because midface advancement is usually performed using distraction techniques, the complications of blood loss and infection have been reduced, making the procedure more common in childhood.

Fronto-Orbital Advancement

The surgical goals of a fronto-orbital advancement are threefold: (a) to release the synostosed suture and decompress the cranial vault, (b) to reshape the cranial vault and advance the frontal bone, and (c) to advance the retruded supraorbital bar, providing improved globe protection and an improved aesthetic appearance. The procedure is performed through a coronal incision. With the assistance of a neurosurgical team, a frontal craniotomy is performed to release the synostosed suture and elevate the frontal bone. In certain instances, the child may have previously undergone a prior frontal craniotomy by the neurosurgical staff to release the coronal suture when elevated ICP was suspected. Reossification usually has occurred by 1 year of age. Once the frontal bone is removed, the brain is gently retracted, exposing the underlying retruded supraorbital bar, which is advanced in a tongue-in-groove manner and secured with resorbable plates or sutures (Fig. 25.7). Cranial vault remodeling is dependent on the preoperative head shape. For severe turricephaly, a total cranial vault reshaping is performed; this procedure allows for a significant reduction in the vertical height of the skull. For the child with mild turricephaly, only the anterior two-thirds of the vault is remodeled. The supraorbital bar and forehead are advanced into an overcorrected position to allow room for further brain growth.

Following this initial fronto-orbital advancement and cranial vault remodeling procedure, the child is seen on a 6- to 12-month basis by the craniofacial team. Continued growth of the cranial vault and midface are monitored closely by means of three-dimensional CT scans, as well as clinical observation. **Although fronto-orbital advancement provides excellent**

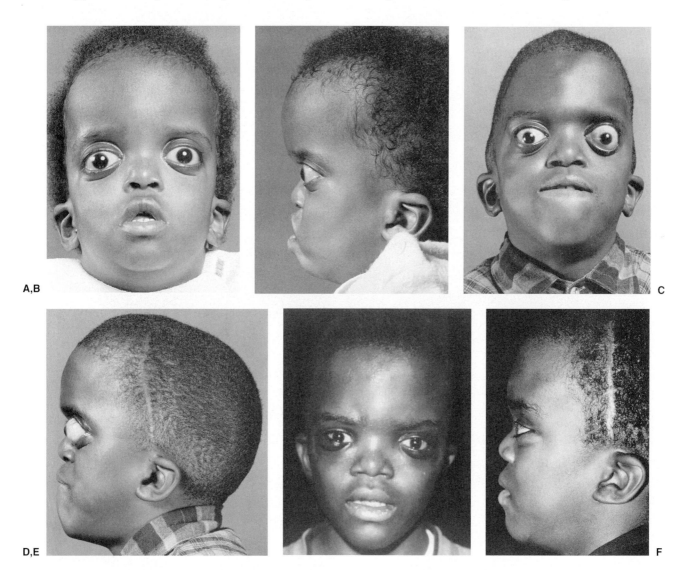

FIGURE 25.11. Child with Pfeiffer syndrome. **A, B:** Before fronto-orbital advancement. **C, D:** After fronto-orbital advancement. **E, F:** After Le Fort III osteotomy.

decompression of the craniosynostosis and moderate improvement in the shape of the cranial vault in the early postoperative period, continued growth restriction in both the cranial vault and the midface region often produces poor long-term aesthetic results in these syndromic patients. If signs of increased ICP, severe exorbitism, or an abnormally shaped cranial vault develop, a second and, occasionally, a third fronto-orbital advancement and cranial vault remodeling procedure are indicated.

Surgical Correction of the Midface Deformity

The first attempt to correct the midface deformity in a syndromic craniosynostosis patient was made by Sir Harold Gillies, who performed a Le Fort III procedure. The procedure, initially abandoned by Gillies, was later popularized by Tessier (Fig. 25.8). The Le Fort III can be performed alone or, if all permanent teeth have erupted, in conjunction with a Le Fort I advancement. The monobloc frontofacial advancement procedure, which involves the advancement of the Le Fort III fragment in coordination with the frontal bar, was developed by Ortiz-Monasterio (Fig. 25.9). The monobloc procedure, while offering the advantage of simultaneously correcting the supraorbital and midface deformity, is associated with greater blood loss and a higher infection rate, which is most likely a result of the direct communication between the cranial and nasal cavities. This increased risk makes the monobloc procedure in the neonatal period contraindicated. Currently, the Le Fort III via a subcranial approach is probably the procedure of choice for correcting the midface deformity, although good results with the monobloc, especially via distraction (see Distraction Osteogenesis of the Midface, below), have been reported (Figs. 25.10 and 25.11). **The exact timing of midface correction**

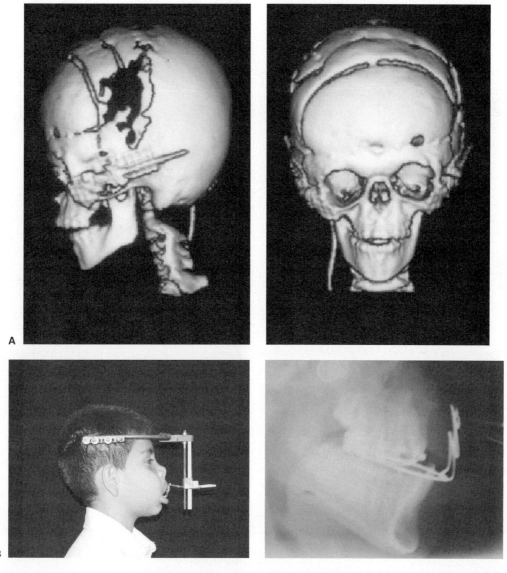

FIGURE 25.12. A: Three-dimensional CT scan depicting a buried LeFort III distractor following monobloc advancement. The distal foot plate is affixed via mesh and screws to the mobile facial segment while the proximal foot plate is affixed to stable temporal bone. The flexible cable through which one activates the device to cause separation of the bone segments exits through the skin posteriorly. **B:** An external halo-type distractor. The frame is affixed to the temporal bone with external screws. The vertical bar links the device to the mobile Le Fort segment via a dental appliance. Activation of the fixture will pull the segment forward as new bone forms.

remains a controversy among craniofacial surgeons. Some craniofacial centers advocate early surgical correction between the ages of 4 and 7 years; others prefer to wait until skeletal maturity is reached at around puberty, unless airway obstruction or severe exorbitism dictates immediate early surgery. The advocates of delayed surgical correction cite evidence of a high incidence of recurrent class III malocclusion in patients who undergo surgery earlier (4 to 9 years), often requiring a secondary Le Fort III procedure in the teenage years. Advocates of early correction of the midface deformity believe the overall aesthetic improvement will have a significant positive psychological effect and improve self-esteem in these children, and they accept a secondary Le Fort III or monobloc osteotomy as a standard step in the treatment of these patients.

Distraction Osteogenesis of the Midface

In recent years, an alternative to the one-stage Le Fort III or monobloc procedure was developed. Because the overlying soft tissue envelope may physically limit the amount of advancement possible and contribute to bony relapse, advancement via gradual distraction osteogenesis, initially used in the appendicular skeleton and mandible has been employed. The procedure involves a standard LeFort III or monobloc osteotomy, *without* acute advancement, with semiburied placement of an external or semiburied distractor (Fig. 25.12). This device that allows for slow stretching/adaptation of the soft tissue and advancement of the face while new bone forms in the osteotomy gaps. At days 5 to 7 postoperatively, after early callus has occurred at the osteotomy site, the device is activated, allowing for advancement of 1 mm per day until the desired forward movement is achieved. This is followed by a period of several months during which the new bone formed in the osteotomy gaps is allowed to consolidate (calcification of the osteoid). Distractor removal is then performed.

Advantages of distraction include (a) less blood loss and shorter operative time at the initial procedure; (b) greater advancement (up to 20 mm or more) as compared to standard advancement techniques (6–10 mm maximum); (c) absence of need for bone grafts as new bone forms at the osteotomy sites (hence the term *distraction osteogenesis*); (d) less risk of infection with the monobloc procedures; and (e) less relapse. Disadvantages include the (a) prolonged time needed for distraction

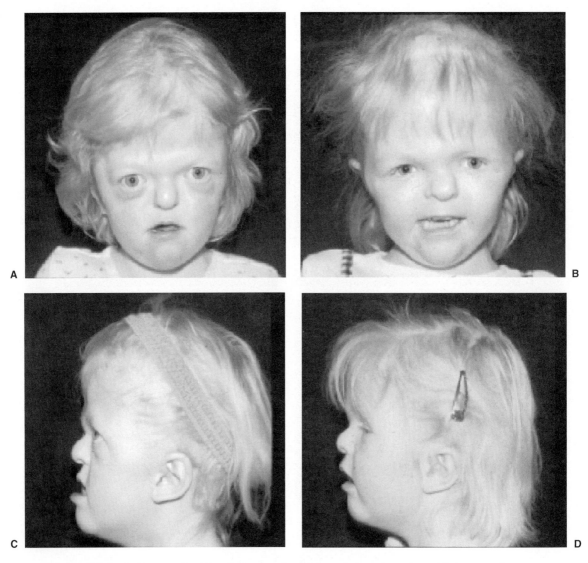

FIGURE 25.13. Preoperative (**A**) and postoperative (**B**) frontal view of a patient with Apert syndrome following monobloc fronto-facial advancement utilizing distraction osteogenesis. Preoperative (**C**) and postoperative (**D**) lateral view. Note dramatic improvement in midface projection and exorbitism.

and consolidation; (b) need for a second procedure to remove the buried devices; and (c) need for wearing an external device for a prolonged period.

Overall, distraction osteogenesis has improved the results obtainable for midface advancement while minimizing the complications. Figure 25.13 is an example of a patient so treated by osteodistraction.

Orthognathic Surgery

The abnormal patterns of facial growth in children with craniosynostosis syndromes often result in significant dentofacial deformities. The class III malocclusion, secondary to midface retrusion, is the most commonly seen deformity and often develops despite appropriate midface surgical treatment. The team approach to the management of these jaw abnormalities usually involves an orthodontist, a dentist, and a craniofacial surgeon. Following the completion of growth of both the maxilla and the mandible and any needed presurgical orthodontic therapy, surgical correction involving at least a Le Fort I osteotomy with a sliding genioplasty may be indicated. These surgical procedures are usually performed between the ages of 14 and 18 years, when the facial skeleton is mature.

Final Facial Contouring

At the completion of facial growth and all major osteotomies, contour irregularities of the facial skeleton may still remain. Final contouring procedures are often performed at this time. They include smoothing down irregularities, adding bone grafts or bone substitutes to different areas (e.g., calcium carbonate cements), and resuspending soft tissues such as the midface or canthus.

CONCLUSION

In the past, children with craniosynostosis syndromes were stigmatized as being mentally challenged because of their craniofacial features when, in fact, they were often of normal intelligence. The advent of craniofacial surgery techniques, although far from perfect, offer these children a chance of obtaining a more normal facial appearance and the opportunity to grow, develop, and integrate socially with their peers. The application of newer operative techniques to craniofacial surgery, including endoscopic surgery and osteodistraction, is expected to offer improved results with fewer complications. Distractive osteogenesis has yielded promising results in the cranium and midface.

The real future of children with craniosynostosis syndromes, however, lies in the hands of the molecular geneticists. The advances in this field have allowed for the identification of the gene and associated mutation for several craniosynostosis syndromes. Ultimately, the ability to genetically screen for these DNA mutations will allow for appropriate family counseling and perhaps, in the future, gene therapy for the correction of the mutation.

Suggested Readings

Bachmayer DI, Ross RB, Munro IR. Maxillary growth following Le Fort III advancement surgery in Crouzon, Apert, and Pfeiffer syndromes. *Am J Orthod Dentofacial Orthop.* 1986;90:420.

Cohen MM Jr, ed. *Craniosynostosis: Diagnosis, Evaluation, and Management.* New York: Raven Press; 1986.

Cohen SR, Boydston W, Burstein FD. Monobloc distraction osteogenesis during infancy: report of a case and presentation of a new device. *Plast Reconstr Surg.* 1998;101:1919.

Fearon JA. The LeFort III osteotomy: to distract or not to distract. *Plast Reconstr Surg.* 2001;107:1091–1106.

Fearon JA, Whitaker LA. Complications with facial advancement: a comparison between the Le Fort III and monobloc advancements. *Plast Reconstr Surg.* 1993;91:990.

Gosain AK, Santoro TD, Havlik RJ, et al. Midface distraction following LeFort III and monobloc osteotomies: problems and solutions. *Plast Reconstr Surg.* 2002;109:1797–1808.

McCarthy JG, LaTrenta GS, Breitbart AS, et al. The Le Fort III advancement osteotomy in the child under 7 years of age. *Plast Reconstr Surg.* 1990;86:633.

Molina F, Ortiz-Monasterio F. Mandibular elongation and remodeling by distraction: a farewell to major osteotomies. *Plast Reconstr Surg.* 1995;96(4):825.

Ortiz-Monasterio F, Fuente delCampo A, Carillo A. Advancements of the orbits and the mid-face in one piece, combined with frontal repositioning for the correction of Crouzon's deformities. *Plast Reconstr Surg.* 1968;61:507.

Polley JW, Figueroa AA. Management of severe maxillary deficiency in childhood and adolescence through distraction osteogenesis with an external adjustable, rigid distraction device. *J Craniofac Surg.* 1997;8:181–187.

Tessier, P. The definitive plastic surgical treatment of the severe facial deformities of craniofacial dysotosis: Crouzon's and Apert's disease. *Plast Reconstr Surg.* 1971;48:419.

Whitaker LA, Bartlett SP, Shut L, et al. Craniosynostosis: an analysis of the timing, treatment, and complications in 164 consecutive patients. *Plast Reconstr Surg.* 1985;80:195.

Whitaker LA, Munro IR, Salyer KE, et al. Combined report of problems and complications in 793 craniofacial operations. *Plast Reconstr Surg.* 1979;64:198.

CHAPTER 26 ■ CRANIOFACIAL MICROSOMIA

JOSEPH G. McCARTHY

Craniofacial microsomia, a variable hypoplasia of the skeleton as well as of the overlying soft tissue, is the second most common congenital syndrome of the head and neck region, with an incidence as high as 1 in 3,500 live births.

The deformity has been known by a variety of terms. In continental Europe, the term *dysostosis otomandibularis* has been used. Gorlin and Pindborg preferred *hemifacial microsomia*, but this term implies that the syndrome is unilateral and that the deformity is confined to the face. I prefer the term *unilateral craniofacial* microsomia or, when there is bilateral involvement, *bilateral craniofacial microsomia*.

Craniofacial microsomia can be confused with Treacher Collins syndrome (see Chapter 29), but the latter shows a well-defined pattern of inheritance and, unlike bilateral craniofacial microsomia, the pathology is symmetrical. Treacher Collins syndrome has other distinguishing features (absence of the medial lower eyelashes and antegonial notching of the mandible), findings that are absent in craniofacial microsomia. Likewise, craniofacial microsomia should be distinguished from micrognathia of the developmental or posttraumatic type. In the latter, the underdevelopment is restricted to the mandible and there is no evidence of facial paralysis, ear anomalies, or soft-tissue hypoplasia of the cheeks.

ETIOLOGY

The hypoplasia can be variably manifest in any of the structures derived from the first and second brachial arches (Table 26.1), accounting for the wide spectrum of deformity observed in this syndrome.

There is no evidence of genetic transmission of the syndrome. In a series of 102 affected patients, only four had a sibling or parent with evidence of craniofacial microsomia; indeed, only a few pedigrees of the syndrome have ever been reported. Despite the possibility of an occasional autosomal dominant transmission, only a 2% to 3% recurrence rate was found in a study of first-degree relatives.

Several theories have been proposed in an attempt to understand the mechanisms involved in the etiopathogenesis of craniofacial microsomia. Stark and Saunders invoked the concept of mesodermal deficiency, currently in vogue as the cause of cleft lip and palate.

The most commonly accepted is a teratogen theory of a vascular insult, with hemorrhage and hematoma formation in the developing first and second branchial arches and subsequent maldevelopment of the latter. The stapedial artery is a temporary embryonic collateral of the hyoid artery, which forms connections with the pharyngeal artery, only to be replaced by the external carotid artery. Defects of this temporary vessel may result in hemorrhage, accounting for injury to the developing first and second branchial arches.

Laboratory phenocopies of craniofacial microsomia have been created following the administration of triazine to the developing mouse and thalidomide to the monkey. Histologic studies demonstrated hematoma formation with varying amounts of hemorrhage before formation of the stapedial artery. The spectrum of the pathology varied depending on the volume of hemorrhage, ranging from involvement of only the external ear and auditory ossicles to a larger defect involving the zygomatic complex and the entire mandible on the affected side of the mouse model. Moreover, the laboratory finding was supported by the clinical documentation in Germany of approximately 1,000 severe cases and an additional 2,000 less severe cases of craniofacial microsomia following the widespread use of thalidomide as a tranquilizer in pregnant women.

Tessier, in a classification system of orbitofacial clefts, invoked a clefting mechanism as he described three types of clefts involving the orbitozygomatic complex in patients with craniofacial microsomia.

EPIDEMIOLOGY

The incidence of the syndrome is not accurately known in the United States but has been reported to be as low as 1 in 3,500 live births. One study suggested an incidence of 1 in 5,642 live births and another author cited an incidence of 1 in 4,000 live births. If all infants with preauricular skin tags and so-called isolated microtia are included, the incidence of maldevelopment of the first and second arches is obviously higher.

Similarly, the sex ratio is not accurately known; in a series of 102 patients, 63 were males and 39 were females. Another series reported an almost equal sex ratio (59 males and 62 females).

The incidence of bilateral involvement is said to be 10% to 15%. The true incidence is probably higher when one considers the presence of preauricular skin tags and subtle radiographic abnormalities of the mandible on the contralateral of "unaffected" side.

CLINICAL FINDINGS

There is a wide variety of pathologic expression of craniofacial microsomia in the following anatomic regions: jaws, other skeletal components, muscles of mastication, ears, nervous system, and soft tissue (Fig. 26.1).

Jaws

The most obvious deformity is the mandible, especially the ascending ramus, which can be absent or reduced in the vertical dimension. The size of the condyle usually reflects the degree of

TABLE 26.1

STRUCTURES DERIVED FROM THE FIRST AND SECOND BRANCHIAL ARCHES AND THE OTIC CAPSULE

First branchial arch		
	Maxillary process	Maxilla
		Palatine bone
		Zygoma
	Mandibular process	Trigeminal nerve
		Anterior part of auricle
		Mandible
		Head of malleus
		Body of incus
		Tympanic bone
		Sphenomandibular ligament
First branchial groove		External auditory meatus
		Tympanic membrane
First pharyngeal pouch		Eustachian tube
		Middle car cavity
Second branchial arch		Facial nerve
		Posterior part of auricle
		Manubrium of malleus, long process of incus, stapedial superstructure, tympanic surface
		Stapedial artery, styloid process, stylohyoid ligament
		Lesser cornu of hyoid
Otic capsule		Vestibular surface of stapes, internal acoustic meatus
		Inner ear

Modified from Pearson, A. A., and Jacobson, A. D. The development of the ear. In: Manual of the Am. Academy of Ophthmology & Otolaryngology, Portland: University of Oregon Printing Dept., 1967 and from Converse, J. M. *Reconstructive Plastic Surgery.* Philadelphia: Saunders, 1977.

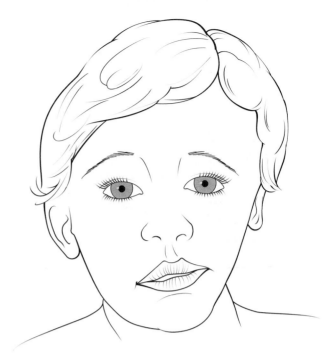

FIGURE 26.1. Patient with left-sided craniofacial microsomia demonstrating the characteristic occlusal cant upward on the affected side with associated cheek hypoplasia and ear anomaly.

hypoplasia of the ramus. Involvement of the temporomandibular joint (TMJ) can range from mild hypoplasia to only a pseudoarticulation at the cranial base. In addition to being short, the ramus is usually displaced toward the midline. Because of the hypoplastic ramus, the mandibular plane angle is increased and the body of the affected mandible can show an increased horizontal dimension.

The chin is deviated toward the affected side and there is a corresponding cant of the mandibular occlusal plane, which is paralleled in the corresponding planes of the floors of the maxillary sinuses and the pyriform apertures. Similarly, the maxillary and mandibular dentoalveolar complexes are also reduced in the vertical dimension on the affected side. In addition to crowding, there is often delayed eruption of the deciduous and permanent teeth; the molars can also be absent.

Pruzansky proposed a classification of the mandibular deficiency, which was later modified by Mulliken and Kaban (Fig. 26.2):

Type I. Mild hypoplasia of the ramus, and the body of the mandible is minimally or slightly affected;

Type II. The condyle and ramus are small; the head of the condyle is flattened; the glenoid fossa is absent; the condyle is hinged on a flat, often convex, infratemporal surface; the coronoid may be absent.

Type III. The ramus is reduced to a thin lamina of bone or is completely absent. There is no evidence of a temporomandibular joint.

The above classification was subsequently modified by subdividing the type II mandible according to the pathology of the temporomandibular joint region. In type IIA, although the ramus and condyle are abnormal in size and shape, the glenoid fossa–condyle relationship is maintained because the glenoid fossa has a position in the temporal bone similar to that of the contralateral side. Temporomandibular joint function is almost normal. In contrast, in Type IIB, the condyle is hypoplastic and malformed and displaced toward the midline relative to the contralateral side. Patients open with restricted hingelike functioning of the mandible on the ipsilateral side.

Other Skeletal Components

The maxilla is reduced in the vertical dimension and, depending on the degree of hypoplasia of the mandible, there is a corresponding cant of the occlusal surface of the maxillary dentition. The maxillary molars are consequently slow to erupt.

The zygomatic complex can be reduced in all of its dimensions; the zygomatic arch can be decreased in length or even absent. These findings, combined with soft-tissue deficiency of the cheek, result in a reduction or shortening in the distance between the oral commissure and tragus (often rudimentary) on the affected side.

The temporal bone can also be involved, although the petrous portion is usually spared. The mastoid process can be hypoplastic and there can be partial or complete lack of pneumatization of the mastoid air cells. The styloid process can be shortened or absent. The orbit is often reduced in all dimensions, and occasional patients have microphthalmos. The frontal bone can be flattened, giving the illusion of a plagiocephaly without radiographic evidence of synostosis of the ipsilateral coronal structure.

Malformations of the cervical vertebrae are not uncommon and include the presence of hemivertebrae, fused vertebrae, and even a basilar impression syndrome. Goldenhar described a variant of craniofacial microsomia characterized by epibulbar

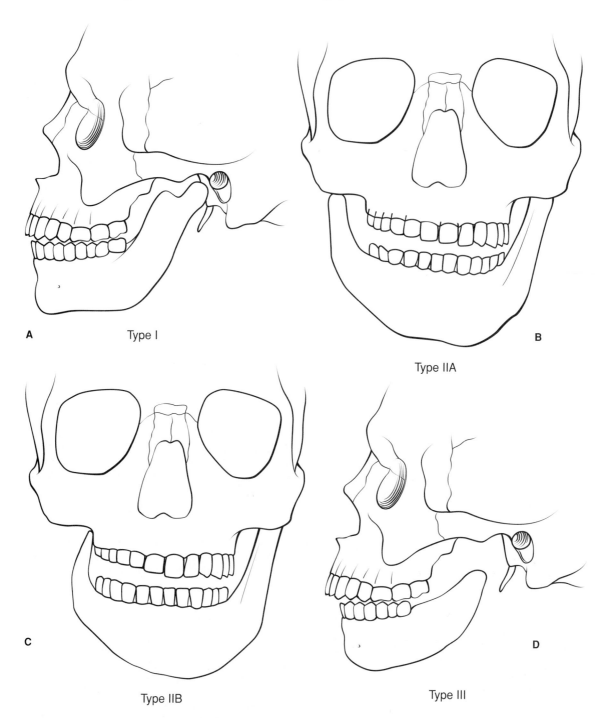

FIGURE 26.2. Pruzansky's proposed (1969) classification of the mandibular deformity seen in craniofacial microsomia as modified by Mulliken and Kaban (1987). **A:** Type I: The condyle and ramus are reduced in size but the overall morphology is maintained. **B:** Type IIA: The ramus and condyle demonstrate abnormal morphology but the glenoid fossa has maintained a position in the temporal bone similar to that of the contralateral side. **C:** Type IIB: The ramus/condyle is hypoplastic, malformed, and displaced outside the plane of that of the contralateral side. **D:** Type III: The ramus is essentially absent without any evidence of temporomandibular joint.

dermoids/lipodermoids, associated vertebral (usually cervical), and occasional rib anomalies.

Muscles of Mastication

The syndrome is not restricted to the skeleton; the associated muscles of mastication are hypoplastic. The deficiency is not always proportional to the skeletal deficiency. A three-dimensional computed tomography (CT) scan study compared the volume of the mandibular deformity to that of the adjacent muscles of mastication and noted that there was not always a 1:1 relationship in the degree of pathologic involvement.

Muscle function is impaired, as is especially evident with lateral pterygoid muscle function on the affected side. The lateral pterygoid muscle is responsible for movement of the mandible and chin point to the contralateral side. Consequently, in patients with unilateral craniofacial microsomia who attempt a protrusive chin movement, the chin deviates to the affected side during opening and during forceful protrusion. The hypoplastic lateral pterygoid muscle on the affected side is overpowered by its unaffected counterpart. Moreover, mouth opening is also adversely affected by the hypoplastic ramus and malpositioned temporomandibular joint.

Ears

Involvement of the auricle occurs in most patients. Meurmann proposed a classification of the external ear deformities: Grade I, distinctly smaller malformed auricle but all components are present; Grade II, only a vertical remnant of cartilage and skin with complete atresia of the external auditory canal; Grade III, almost complete absence of the auricle except for a small remnant, usually a soft tissue lobule. There is not a direct correlation between the auricular deformity, as classified using Meurmann's proposal, and the hearing function as measured by audiometry and temporal bone tomography.

Nervous System

Cerebral abnormalities, although rare, can occur and include hypoplasia of the cerebrum and corpus callosum, as well as hydrocephalus of the communicating and obstructive types. The brainstem can be involved secondarily because of anomalies of the cervical vertebrae, resulting in disturbances such as impression of the brainstem.

The most common cranial anomaly is a facial palsy of varying degrees, attributed to the following (alone or in combination): absence of the intracranial portion of the facial nerve and nucleus in the brainstem, aberrant pathway of the nerve in the temporal bone, or angenesis of the facial muscles. Absence of facial nerve function in the distribution of the marginal mandibular branch is seen in approximately 25% of patients, with weakness of other components, such as the buccal and zygomatic branches, occurring in a smaller percentage.

Soft Tissue

On the affected side, preauricular skin tags are common, and the skin and subcutaneous tissue of the cheek region show varying degrees of hypoplasia. As shown in Figure 26.1, the muscles of mastication are also involved, and hypoplasia or aplasia of the parotid gland has been documented. The soft-tissue deficiency is multidimensional and may result in a marked reduction in the distance between the oral commissure and the rudimentary ear on the affected side.

Lateral facial clefts (macrostomia) are common associated findings and also contribute to the overall cheek hypoplasia.

Overt clefts of the soft palate are said to occur in 25% of patients, and the soft palate may deviate to the affected side on voluntary function.

CLASSIFICATION

Several classifications have been described based on the clinical findings of the patient with unilateral craniofacial microsomia. Harvold, Vargervik, and Chierici proposed the following classification:

I (A). The classic type characterized by unilateral facial underdevelopment without microphthalmos or ocular der-

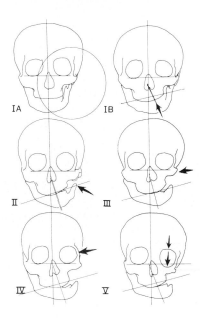

FIGURE 26.3. Classification of unilateral craniofacial microsomia proposed by Munro and Lauritzen in 1985. The circle in Figure 26.1A designates the usual site of skeletal involvement. The midsagittal, midincisor, occlusal, and orbital planes are designated. See text for details of each type. (From McCarthy JG, Grayson BH, Coccaro PJ, et al. Craniofacial microsomia. In: McCarthy JG, ed. *Plastic Surgery.* Philadelphia: WB Saunders; 1990, with permission.)

moids but with or without abnormalities of the vertebrae, heart, or kidneys.

I (B). Similar to type I (A) except for the presence of microphthalmos.

I (C). Bilateral asymmetric type in which one side is more severely involved.

I (D). Complex type that does not fit the above but does not display limb deficiency, frontonasal phenotype, or ocular dermoids.

II. Limb-deficiency type—unilateral or bilateral with or without ocular abnormalities.

III. Frontonasal type. Relative unilateral underdevelopment of the face in the presence of hypertelorism with or without ocular dermoids and vertebral, cardiac, or renal abnormalities.

IV. (A) Unilateral or (B) bilateral. Goldenhar type with facial underdevelopment in association with other dermoids, with or without upper lid coloboma.

Munro and Lauritzen proposed a clinical classification system (Fig. 26.3) that was designed as an aid in planning surgical correction:

Type IA: The craniofacial skeleton is only mildly hypoplastic and the occlusal plane is horizontal.

Type IB: The skeleton is as in IA, but the occlusal plane is canted.

Type II: The condyle and part of the affected ramus are absent.

Type III: In addition to the findings in type II, the zygomatic arch and glenoid fossa are absent.

Type IV: This is an uncommon type with hypoplasia of the zygoma and medial and posterior displacement of the lateral orbital wall.

Type V: The most extreme type has inferior displacement of the orbit with a decrease in orbital volume.

Vento et al. proposed the nosologic OMENS classification system in an effort to standardize reporting between treatment centers. The acronym OMENS designates each of the five major areas of involvement in craniofacial microsomia: O = orbital, M = mandibular, E = ear, N = facial nerve, and S = soft tissue. The orbital gradations were based on size and position, the mandible was scored as noted above, the ear anomaly was categorized essentially according to the previously described Meurmann classification, the facial nerve according to which branches were involved, and the soft tissue according to the degree of subcutaneous and muscular deficiency.

PREOPERATIVE ASSESSMENT

A complete clinical evaluation is mandatory, because other organ systems, such as the kidneys and heart, can be involved. Medical photographs are obtained, including frontal, lateral, oblique, submental vertex, and occlusal views. Cephalograms (posteroanterior, lateral, and basilar) and a panoramic roentgenogram (panorex) are likewise obtained. The optimal way to define the various skeletal deformities is with a three-dimensional CT scan (Fig. 26.4), which can be reformatted to give a dentascan and document the location of tooth follicles in the younger patient in whom cephalograms and panorex cannot be obtained.

TREATMENT

It must be recognized that there is no prescribed treatment program for the child with craniofacial microsomia. The pathology, as emphasized before, is variable, and other factors, such as growth and development and prior therapy, must be considered before recommending an individualized treatment program.

Surgical correction of the unilateral deformity is challenging. Consequently, all treatment plans must be customized according to the needs and age of the individual patient.

Younger than Two Years of Age

Excision of the preauricular skin tags and cartilage remnants is often satisfying to the parents, because it removes some of the stigmata of the syndrome. Likewise, macrostomia can also be corrected by a commissuroplasty on the affected side or on both sides in bilateral craniofacial microsomia. In the occasional patient with involvement of the fronto-orbital region, characterized by severe retrusion of the supraorbital bar and frontal bone, a fronto-orbital advancement–cranial vault remodeling can be performed as a combined craniofacial surgical procedure.

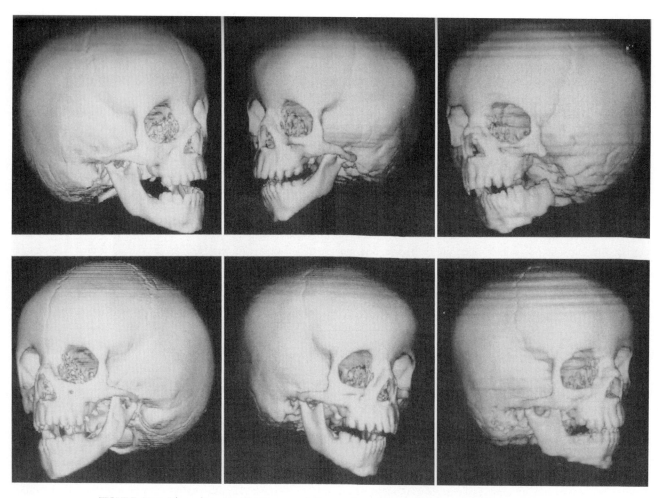

FIGURE 26.4. Three-dimensional CT scans of three unilateral craniofacial microsomia cases demonstrating increasing severity from left to right. The affected side of each case is on the top panel, with the corresponding normal contralateral side on the lower panel. The three cases correspond to the modified Pruzansky classification of mandibular deformity: class 1 *(left)*, class II *(center)*, class III *(right)*. (Reproduced from Mathes S. J. *Plastic Surgery*. Philadelphia: WB Saunders; 2005, with permission.)

Mandibular distraction (Chapter 12) is indicated in the newborn or infant with sleep apnea (with or without a tracheostomy). It can correct not only the sleep apnea but also the associated alimentary or feeding problems (e.g., swallowing, reflux).

Two to Six Years of Age

In the child with mild deformity, such as Pruzansky type I mandible and a horizontal occlusal plane (Munro and Lauritzen type IA), no surgical treatment is recommended at this age.

In the child with severe reduction in the vertical height of the mandibular ramus (Pruzansky types I and II) and obvious aesthetic deformity, the technique of distraction osteogenesis (Fig.

26.5) can be considered after the child has attained at least 2 years of age. Sufficient clinical experience with mandibular distraction has accumulated to demonstrate that this technique not only lengthens the affected ramus, but also augments the associated soft tissue and muscles of mastication. The latter finding and the gradual nature of the distraction process lowers relapse rates. Studies also demonstrate that the distracted ramus/condyle assumes a more anatomic size, shape, and position.

In the patient with a Pruzansky type III deformity without evidence of a ramus, condyle, and glenoid fossa (or zygomatic arch), a preliminary costochondral rib graft reconstruction should be performed at approximately age 4 years. In this technique, the glenoid fossa, zygomatic arch, and ascending ramus are reconstructed in a singular surgical procedure (Fig. 26.6). If there is a persistent

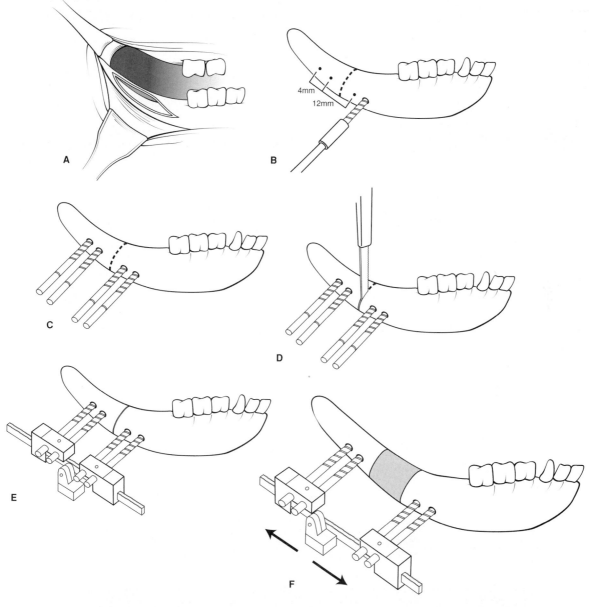

FIGURE 26.5. The technique of mandibular distraction. **A:** An intraoral incision is made along the oblique line of the mandibular remnant. **B:** Sites of the pinholes and proposed osteotomy *(interrupted line).* **C:** The pins are inserted. **D:** The osteotomy is performed. **E** and **F:** Commencement of distraction with the appliance in position. The *arrows* designate the movement of the mandibular segments with formation of bony regenerate (shaded) in the resulting gap. (Reproduced from Mathes S. J. *Plastic Surgery.* Philadelphia: WB Saunders; 2005, with permission.)

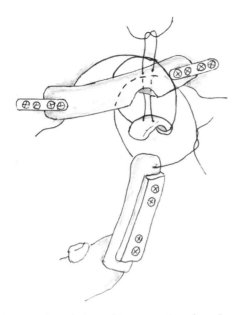

FIGURE 26.6. The technique of reconstruction of an absent ramus. Zyomatic arch and the temposomandibular joint with rib grafts. Note the cartilage graft simulating the disc and the cartilaginous portion of the rib graft simulating the condile. (Modified from Munro IR, Lauritzen C. G. Classification and treatment of hemifacial microsomia. In: Caronni EP, ed. *Craniofacial Surgery*. Boston: Little, Brown; 1985:391–400, with permission.)

mandibular deficiency, distraction, as a secondary procedure, could be considered.

In the child with bilateral craniofacial microsomia (Pruzansky types I and II mandibular deformity) with associated sleep apnea (with or without tracheostomy), bilateral mandibular distraction can be performed after sleep studies have established the diagnosis and the latter has been confirmed by endoscopy. In these children, the treatment can result in removal of the tracheostomy. If there is no evidence of the mandibular rami, bilateral costochondral rib graft reconstruction is the treatment of choice.

Six to Fifteen Years of Age

This is the period of orthodontic treatment, including possible functional appliance therapy to promote eruption and growth of the dentoalveolus on the affected side. Distraction can be considered in the patient with chronic low-grade sleep apnea, and in the patient with severe deformity who has never received treatment. Ear reconstruction is often undertaken during this period. Insertion of a microvascular free flap to augment the facial soft tissue and improve facial contour on the affected side frequently results in considerable aesthetic improvement.

Older than Fifteen Years of Age

Surgery is often indicated in the period of skeletal maturity because of residual deficiency resulting from inadequate growth

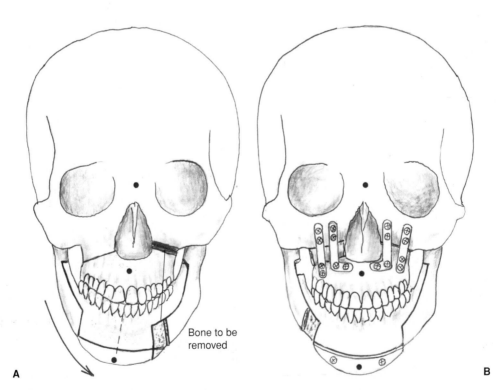

FIGURE 26.7. The combined Le Fort I osteotomy, bilateral sagittal split of the mandible, and genioplasty in a patient with right-sided hemifacial microsomia. **A:** *(left)* Lines of osteotomy. The ostectomy and site of vertical impaction are illustrated on the left maxilla. The *solid circles* designate the midpoints of the chin, maxilla, and orbital region. The *arrow* shows the direction of the jaw movements. **B:** *(right)* Following movement of the maxillary, mandibular, and chin segments and the establishment of rigid skeletal fixation. Note the interposition bone graft in the right maxilla. The *solid circles* line up along the craniofacial midsagittal plane. (Modified from Obwegeser H. L. Correction of the skeletal anomalies of stomandibular dysostosis. *J Maxillofac Surg.*1974;2:73, with permission.)

and development on the affected side, severe malocclusion, or failure of the patient to seek treatment previously.

At this point in time, when craniofacial growth and development are almost complete, the following procedures could be considered: (a) limited autogenous bone grafting of deficient portions of the craniofacial skeleton; (b) bilateral mandibular advancement in patients with mild to moderate mandibular micrognathia; (c) combined Le Fort I osteotomy, bilateral mandibular osteotomy, and genioplasty (Fig. 26.7); and (d) microvascular free flap to augment the soft tissue of the face on the affected side.

Suggested Readings

Gorlin RJ, Pindborg JJ. *Syndromes of the Head and Neck.* New York: McGraw-Hill, 1964.

Gosian AK, McCarthy JG, Pinto R.S. Cervico-cerebral anomalies and basilar impression in Goldenhar syndrome. *Plast Reconstr Surg.* 1994;93:489.

Grayson B, Boral S, Eisig S, et al. Unilateral craniofacial microsomia. Part I–mandibular analysis. *Am J Orthod.* 1983;84:225.

Longaker MT, Siebert JW. Microvascular free flap correction of hemifacial atrophy. *Plast Reconstr Surg.* 1995;96:800.

McCarthy JG, Fuleihan NS. Commissuroplasty in lateral facial clefts. In: Stark RB, ed. *Plastic Surgery of the Head and Neck.* Boston: Little, Brown; 1986.

McCarthy JG, Schreiber JS, Karp NS, et al. Lengthening of the human mandible by gradual distraction. *Plastic Reconstr Surg.* 1992;89:1.

Meurmann Y. Congenital microtia and meatal atresia. *Arch Otolaryngol.* 1957;66:443.

Molina F, Ortiz-Monasterio F. Mandibular elongation and remodeling by distraction: a farewell to major osteotomies. *Plast Reconstr Surg.* 1995;96:825.

Mulliken JB, Kaban LB. Analysis and treatment of hemifacial microsomia in childhood. *Clin Plast Surg.* 1987;14:91.

Munro IR, Lauritzen CG. Classification and treatment of hemifacial microsomia. In: Caronni EP, ed. *Craniofacial Surgery.* Boston: Little, Brown; 1985:391–400.

Obwegeser HL. Correction of the skeletal anomalies of otomandibular dysostosis. *J Maxillofac Surg.* 1974;2:73.

Vento AR, La Brie RA, Mulliken JB. The O.M.E.N.S. classification of hemifacial microsomia. *Cleft Palate Craniofac J.* 1991;28:68.

CHAPTER 27 ■ ORTHOGNATHIC SURGERY

STEPHEN B. BAKER

Orthognathic surgery is the term used to describe surgical movement of the tooth-bearing segments of the maxilla and mandible. Candidates for orthognathic surgery have a dentofacial deformity that cannot be ideally treated with orthodontic therapy alone. These patients have malocclusions caused by skeletal discrepancies secondary to congenital anomalies or trauma. Approximately 2.5% of the American population has occlusal discrepancies severe enough to warrant surgical correction (1). Regardless of the etiology, the patient examination and treatment planning principles remain the same. **The goal of orthognathic surgery is to establish ideal dental occlusion and to optimize facial aesthetics.**

BASIC DENTAL TERMINOLOGY

The following terms are used frequently to describe dental anatomy and concepts:

Apertognathia: An occlusion characterized by a vertical separation of the maxillary and mandibular anterior teeth, frequently described as anterior open bite.

Articulator: A mechanical device that represents the temporomandibular joints and jaws to which the maxillary and mandibular casts may be attached for treatment planning.

Buccal: Pertaining to or adjacent to the cheek.

Cast: A plaster replica of the teeth and surrounding tissues.

Centric occlusion: The relation of opposing occlusal surfaces that provides the maximum planned contact or intercuspation.

Centric relation: The relationship of the mandible to the maxilla when the condyles are in their most posterosuperior unstrained positions in the glenoid fossa

Cephalometric radiograph: A lateral radiograph of the head taken with precise reproducible relationships between X-ray source, subject, and film.

Class I occlusion: The mesiobuccal cusp of the first permanent maxillary molar occludes in the buccal groove of the permanent mandibular first molar.

Class II malocclusion: The mesiobuccal cusp of the first permanent maxillary molar occludes mesial to the buccal groove of the permanent mandibular first molar.

Class III malocclusion: The mesiobuccal cusp of the first permanent maxillary molar occludes distal to the buccal groove of the permanent mandibular first molar.

Distal: Away from the median sagittal plane of the face and following the curvature of the arch.

Labial: Pertaining to the lip, especially in reference to the surface of a tooth.

Lingual: Pertaining to the tongue, especially in reference to the surface of a tooth.

Mesial: Situated toward the midline of the dental arch.

Palatal: Pertaining to the palate, especially in reference to the surface of a tooth.

Proclination: Anterior angulation of the anterior teeth.

Prognathic: A forward position of the mandible in relation to the cranial base.

Retroclination: Posterior angulation of the anterior teeth.

Retrognathic: The condition of a mandible that is posteriorly positioned in relation to the cranial base.

ESTABLISHING THE DIAGNOSIS

History

It is important to obtain a thorough medical and dental history from every patient. Systemic diseases such as juvenile rheumatoid arthritis, diabetes, and scleroderma can affect treatment planning. With jaw asymmetries, a history of hyperplasia or hypoplasia secondary to a syndrome, traumatic accident, or neoplasm affects treatment considerations. Each patient should be questioned regarding symptoms of temporomandibular joint (TMJ) disease or myofascial pain syndrome. Motivation and realistic expectations are important for an optimal outcome. It is important for the patient to have a clear understanding of the procedure, the recovery, and the anticipated result. Orthognathic surgery is a major undertaking and the patient must be appropriately motivated to undergo necessary preoperative and postoperative orthodontic treatment and rehabilitation.

Physical Examination

The patient must demonstrate evidence of good oral hygiene and periodontal health prior to orthodontic treatment and surgery. The occlusal classification is determined, and the degrees of incisor overlap and overjet are quantified. Often, the clinician can get a sense of the degree of dental decompensation on physical examination, but radiographic analysis is necessary to quantify the degree of compensation (see below). The surgeon should assess the transverse dimension of the maxilla. If a crossbite is present, models should be obtained to assess if it is a relative crossbite or a true crossbite (see Cephalometric Analysis and Dental Models below). A true crossbite is a result of maxillary constriction and requires either orthopedic (orthodontic appliance) or surgical expansion for correction. If the mandibular third molars are present, they must be extracted 6 months prior to sagittal split osteotomy. Any missing teeth or periapical pathology should be noted, as should be any sign or symptom of TMJ dysfunction.

The facial evaluation begins with assessment of the vertical facial thirds: trichion to glabella, glabella to subnasale, and subnasale to menton. Each of these facial thirds should be about equal. If the lower two-third of the face is short, it can be increased by inferiorly positioning the maxilla, which will result in increasing the distance from the glabella to pogonion. In contrast, a long lower face may benefit from a maxillary impaction, which would have the opposite effect. **The most important factor in assessing the vertical height of the maxilla is the degree** of incisor showing while the patient's lips are in repose. A man should show at least 2 to 3 mm, whereas as much as 4 to 5 mm is considered attractive in a woman. If the patient shows the correct degree of incisor in repose, but shows excessive gingiva in full smile, the maxilla should not be impacted. It is more important to show the correct degree of incisor in repose than it is to be concerned about showing excessive gingiva in full smile. The surgeon certainly would not want to bury the incisors in repose just to reduce the degree of gingiva in a full smile. If lip incompetence or mentalis strain is present, it is usually an indicator of vertical maxillary excess.

The intercanthal distance should be about the same as the distance between the medial and lateral canthus of each eye. The inferior orbital rims, malar eminence, and piriform areas are evaluated for the degree of projection. If these regions appear deficient, maxillary advancement is indicated; if they are excessively prominent, posterior repositioning may be necessary. The alar base width should also be assessed prior to surgery since orthognathic surgery may alter the width. Asymmetries of the maxilla and mandible are documented on physical examination, and the degree of deviation from the facial midline is noted. The soft-tissue envelope of the upper face is evaluated for descent of the malar fat pads, the severity of the nasolabial creases, and folds. These changes are associated with aging; however, skeletal movements of the maxilla will affect these areas. **It is important for the surgeon to realize that skeletal expansion (anterior or inferior repositioning of the jaws) will improve the creases and folds, whereas skeletal contraction (posterior or superior movements of the jaws) will accentuate these problems (2).** The surgeon must avoid the creation of a prematurely aged patient. However, the surgeon can frequently take advantage of skeletal expansion to reduce some of these soft-tissue creases, giving the patient a youthful appearance and reducing the signs of aging (See Developing a Treatment Plan). In evaluating the chin, the clinician assesses the labiomental angle. **An acute angle may indicate a short or prominent chin, and effacement of the crease typically excessive vertical length or insufficient anterior projection.**

The profile evaluation focuses on the projection of the forehead, the malar region, the upper and lower jaws, the nose, the chin, and the neck. An experienced clinician can usually determine whether the deformity is caused by the maxilla, the mandible, or both just by looking at the patient. This assessment is made clinically and verified radiographically. If the jaws appear to be aligned but the chin projection is either pronounced or deficient, a geniplasty may suffice. The proper position of the nose relates to the upper lip, which is supported by the maxillary incisors, and the chin. Because both of these structures may be altered by orthognathic surgery, it is important to predict how the dimensions of the nose will fit into the new facial proportions. A rhinoplasty may be necessary to maintain proper facial proportions. The soft tissues of the neck are also assessed. The patient with submental laxity will not benefit aesthetically from posterior positioning of the mandible. Mandibular advancement, however, will improve the laxity and improve the cervicomental angle. In a patient with prominent submental fat in whom mandibular advancement is contraindicated, suction-assisted lipectomy is helpful in removing the adipose deposits. Redundant skin requires direct excision.

The maxillary and mandibular dental midlines are assessed to determine if they are congruent with each other and the facial midline. Deviations are noted and quantified. The presence and degree of dental compensation is also recorded. The term *dental compensation* is used to describe the tendency of teeth to tilt in a direction that minimizes the dental malocclusion. For example, in a patient with an overbite (class II malocclusion), retroclination of the upper incisors and proclination of the lower incisors minimize the malocclusion. The opposite occurs in a patient who has dental compensation for an underbite

(class III malocclusion). **Thus, dental compensation, often the result of orthodontic treatment, will mask the true degree of skeletal discrepancy.** Precise analysis of the dental compensation is done on the lateral cephalometric radiograph.

If the patient desires surgical correction of the deformity, presurgical orthodontics will upright or decompensate the occlusion, thereby reversing the compensation that has occurred. This has the effect of exaggerating the malocclusion, but allows the surgeon to maximize skeletal movements. If the patient is ambivalent or not interested in surgery, mild cases of malocclusion may be treated by further dental compensation. Compensation will camouflage the deformity and restore proper overjet and overlap. The importance of a commitment to surgery prior to orthodontics lies in the fact that the dental movements for decompensation and compensation are in opposite directions, so this decision needs to be made prior to orthodontic therapy (3).

Cephalometric Analysis and Dental Models

A lateral cephalometric radiograph is performed under reproducible conditions so that serial images can be compared. This film is usually taken at the orthodontist's office using a cephalostat, an apparatus specifically designed for this purpose, and head frame to maintain consistent head position. It is important to be certain the surgeon can visualize both bony and soft-tissue features on the image so as to facilitate tracing all the landmarks. A piece of transparent acetate tracing paper is secured with tape over the radiograph and the following landmarks are traced: sella turcica, inferior orbital rim, nasion, frontal bone, nasal bones, maxilla, maxillary first molar and central incisor, external auditory meatus, the condylar head and mandible, and the mandibular first molar and incisor. The soft tissue of the forehead, nose, lips, and chin are also traced. Once the normal structures are traced, several planes and angles are determined (Fig. 27.1).

The maxillary plane is a line drawn between the anterior nasal spine (ANS) and posterior nasal spine (PNS). The occlusal plane is drawn between the occlusal surfaces of the teeth. The mandibular plane is drawn between menton and gonion, and the Frankfort horizontal plane is delineated between the superior portion of the external auditory meatus (porion) and the inferior orbital rim (orbitale). Analysis of these planes aids in establishing an accurate diagnosis. A steep mandibular plane is usually associated with a class II malocclusion, anterior open bite, and a short mandible. A shallow mandibular plane is associated with a deep bite, class III malocclusion, and a long mandible.

The sella-nasion-subspinale (SNA) and sella-nasion-supramentale (SNB) are the two most important angles in determining the positions of the maxilla and mandible relative to each other, as well as to the cranial base. These angles are determined by drawing lines from sella to nasion to A point or B point, respectively. By forming an angle with the sella and nasion this position is related to the cranial base. A point provides information about the anteroposterior position of the maxilla. If the SNA angle is excessive, the maxilla exhibits an abnormal anterior position relative to the cranium. If SNA is less than normal, the maxilla is posteriorly positioned relative to the cranial base. B point is used to relate the mandibular position to the cranial base. The importance of the cranial base as a reference is that it allows the clinician to determine if one or both jaws contribute to the deformity. For example, a patient's class III malocclusion (underbite) could develop from several different etiologies: a retrognathic maxilla and normal mandible, a normal maxilla and a prognathic mandible, a retrognathic mandible and a more severely retrognathic maxilla, or a prognathic maxilla and a more severely prognathic

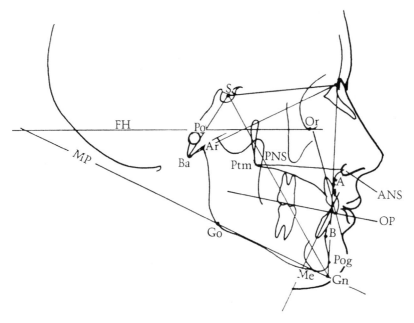

FIGURE 27.1. Standard lateral cephalometric tracing with landmarks. S, sella—the center of the pituitary fossa; N, nasion—the most anterior point of the nasofrontal suture in the midsagittal plane; Ar, articulare—the intersection of basisphenoid and the posterior border of the condyle; A, subspinale—the deepest point of the anterior border of the maxilla between the anterior nasal spine and prosthion, usually around the level of the apex of the maxillary central incisor; Pog, pogonion—the most anterior point of the contour of the chin; B, supramentale—the deepest point between infradentale and pogonion at the level of apices of the mandibular incisors; ANS, anterior nasal spine—the most anterior point of the nasal floor; Me, menton—the lowest point of the contour of the mandibular symphysis; GN, gnathion—the midpoint between Pog and ME created by bisecting the facial line (N-Pog) and the mandibular plane (Go-Me); PNS, posterior nasal spine—the most posterior point on the contour of the hard palate; MP, mandibular plane—a plane constructed from menton (Me) and gonion (Go); NF, nasal floor—a plane constructed from PNS to ANS; Go, gonion—located by bisecting the posterior ramal plane and the mandibular plane angles: It is the midpoint of the curvature connecting the ramus and the mandibular body. (From Wolfe AA, Berkowitz S. *Plastic Surgery of the Facial Skeleton.* Boston: Little, Brown and Co., 1989:57, with permission.)

mandible. All of these conditions yield a class III malocclusion, yet each requires a different treatment approach. The surgeon can delineate the true etiology of the deformity by the fact that the maxilla and mandible can be independently related to a stable reference, the cranial base.

Plaster dental casts are also obtained during the treatment planning process. Casts allow the surgeon to evaluate the occlusion by articulating the casts. Analysis of the potential postoperative occlusion gives the clinician an idea of how intensive the presurgical orthodontic treatment plan will be. Casts also allow the clinician to distinguish between absolute and relative transverse maxillary deficiency. Absolute transverse maxillary deficiency presents as a posterior crossbite with the jaws in a class I relationship. A relative maxillary transverse deficiency is commonly seen in a patient with a class III malocclusion. A posterior crossbite is observed in this type of patient, leading the surgeon to suspect inadequate maxillary width. However, as the maxilla is advanced or the mandible retruded, the crossbite is eliminated. Articulation of the casts into a class I occlusion allows the surgeon to easily distinguish between relative and absolute maxillary constriction.

DEVELOPING A TREATMENT PLAN

Once the data are obtained, the surgeon can determine which abnormalities the patient exhibits and the extent to which

these features deviate from the norm. The treatment plan is the application of these data to provide the best aesthetic result while establishing a class I occlusion. The goal is not to "treat the numbers" in an attempt to "normalize" every patient. **The appearance of the soft-tissue envelope surrounding the facial skeleton is the most crucial factor in determining the aesthetic success of orthognathic procedures, and the jaws should be positioned so they provide optimal soft-tissue support.**

Historically, skeletal movements that expanded the soft tissue of the face were less stable, so posterior and superior movements were preferred. Although these movements were more stable, they resulted in contraction of the facial skeleton with the associated soft-tissue features of premature aging. Since the introduction of rigid fixation, osteotomies that result in skeletal expansion have been achieved with a great degree of predictability. An attempt is made to develop a treatment plan that will expand or maintain the preoperative volume of the face (2). If a superior or posterior (contraction) movement of one of the jaws is planned, an attempt should be made to neutralize the skeletal contraction with an advancement or inferior movement of the other jaw or the chin. It is important to avoid a net contraction of the facial skeleton as this may result in a prematurely aged appearance.

As skeletal expansion is increased, soft-tissue laxity is reduced and facial creases are softened. These effects increase the definition of the face, creating a more attractive appearance. **It has been shown that skeletal expansion is aesthetically pleasing even if facial disproportion is necessary to achieve the** expansion (4). Women with successful careers as fashion models often exhibit slight degrees of facial disproportion and are considered beautiful. The aesthetic benefits the patient receives by expanding the facial envelope frequently justify the small degree of disproportion necessary to achieve them. Even in young adolescent patients who do not show signs of aging, one must not ignore these principles. A successful surgeon will incorporate these principles into the treatment plan of every patient so that as the patient ages, the signs of aging will be minimized and a youthful appearance will be maintained as long as possible (Fig. 27.2).

An example demonstrating these principles is an adult woman who presents for surgery with a slightly prognathic mandible, submental laxity, jowl descent, and deep nasolabial creases. If a treatment plan was developed based solely on cephalometric values, a mandibular setback would be the appropriate procedure. This procedure would do nothing for the upper face and would accentuate the submental laxity and jowl descent. In contrast, if one were to accept the slight prognathism and advance the maxilla to a class I relationship, the nasolabial crease and jowl descent would be improved, and the submental laxity would not be made worse. Thus, moving the normal maxilla into a class I occlusion with a prognathic mandible establishes a normal occlusion and achieves excellent aesthetics despite being slightly disproportionate. The surgeon treats patients not radiographs.

A class I occlusion can be achieved with the jaws in a variety of different positions. The goal in treatment planning is to use the data from the patient's examination to predict the location of the jaws that will optimize the soft-tissue features of the face. By reducing the emphasis on normal values and increasing the awareness of the soft tissue effects of skeletal movements, it is realized that skeletal disproportion often leads to a more favorable result.

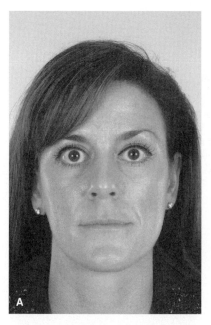

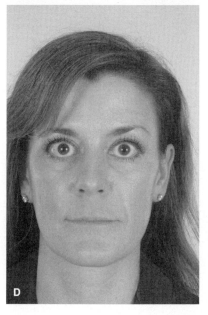

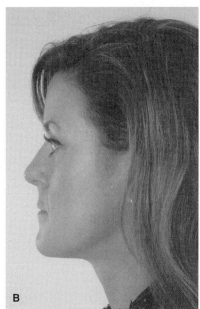

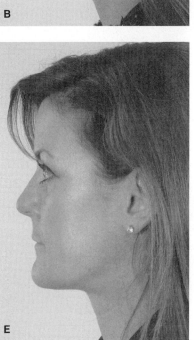

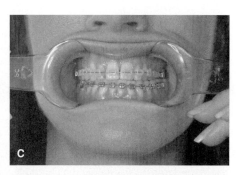

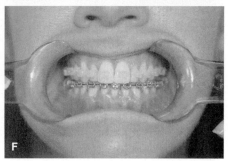

FIGURE 27.2. This patient exhibited a left unilateral crossbite, a prominent chin, and malar deficiency (she is missing a central incisor). She did not desire two-jaw surgery and her malocclusion was treated with bilateral sagittal split osteotomy. Her midface deficiency was corrected with prosthetic malar and piriform augmentation. A: Frontal exam preoperation. B: Profile preoperation. C: Occlusion preoperation. D: Frontal postoperation. Note attenuated nasalabial creases from malar implants. E: Profile postoperation. Noted improved malar projection achieved and alloplastic augmentation. F: Postoperation occlusion.

BASIC APPROACHES TO COMMONLY ENCOUNTERED PROBLEMS

It is important to discuss the basic treatment principles in commonly encountered dentofacial deformities. The surgeon must recognize there are multiple solutions to a single problem; this is where the proper application of the previously discussed principles is crucial to achieving the best aesthetic result.

Skeletal Class II Occlusion

A skeletal class II malocclusion is almost always caused by mandibular retrognathia and is almost always best treated by mandibular advancement (Fig. 27.3). The mandible is small, and forward positioning is an expansile movement that enhances facial form. If the maxilla is also slightly deficient or in a normal position, one may consider a bimaxillary advancement to further enhance facial soft-tissue definition. If the malocclusion is minimal and there is little pre-existing dental compensation, one may choose to have the orthodontist intentionally compensate the dentition to correct the occlusion and avoid surgery. In contrast, if the malocclusion appears minimal but there is dental compensation, the skeletal discrepancy will be more significant after the orthodontist decompensates the dentition, and the patient may be a good surgical candidate.

Skeletal Class III Malocclusion

A prominent lower jaw may be treated by advancing the maxilla, by posteriorly positioning the mandible, or by combining these procedures. It is important to consider the contributions of the mandible and the chin separately as each may require different treatments to achieve aesthetic goals. If some poste-

rior positioning of the mandible is necessary, one may advance the maxilla to counteract the skeletal contraction produced from the mandible. Additionally, the patient may benefit from a genioplasty that can counteract any skeletal contraction that occurs from a mandibular setback. As in the class II patient, a minor malocclusion with minimal dental compensation may be corrected with orthodontic treatment alone. In contrast, a minor malocclusion with dental compensation may become a significant malocclusion after dental decompensation.

Maxillary Constriction

Patients can exhibit a maxilla that is narrow in the transverse dimension. Maxillary constriction may occur as an isolated finding or as one of multiple abnormalities. Up to about 15 years of age, the orthodontist can expand the maxilla nonsurgically with a palatal expansion device. If orthopedic expansion cannot be done, a surgically assisted rapid palatal expansion can be performed (5). If the maxilla requires movement in other dimensions, a two-piece Le Fort I osteotomy can be performed to place the maxilla in its new position while simultaneously achieving transverse expansion (Fig. 27.4).

Apertognathia

An anterior open bite is caused by a premature contact of the posterior molars. The recommended treatment is a posterior impaction of the maxilla. By reducing the vertical height of the posterior maxilla, the mandible can come into occlusion with the remaining mandibular teeth. Posterior maxillary impaction does not necessarily result in incisor impaction; the posterior maxilla is simply rotated upward using the incisal tip as the axis of rotation. Therefore, incisor show should not be affected. If a change in incisor show is also desired, the posterior impaction

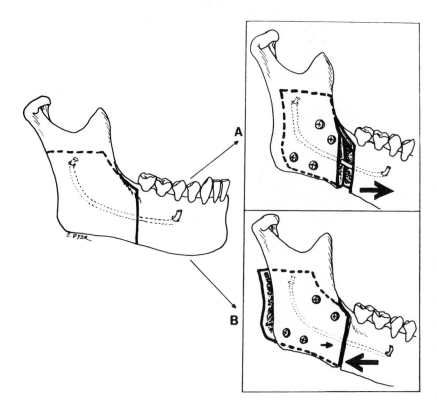

FIGURE 27.3. The sagittal splitting procedure is the most versatile ramus osteotomy, as it can be used for both mandibular advancement (**A**) and mandibular setback (**B**). The procedure is performed through an intraoral approach and requires special instrumentation to be performed with ease. Three or four screws are placed percutaneously to effect rigid fixation. It is vital that the mandibular condyles be properly seated at the end of any mandibular osteotomy. If they are not, when intermaxillary fixation is removed they go back into the glenoid fossae with a resultant anterior open bite.

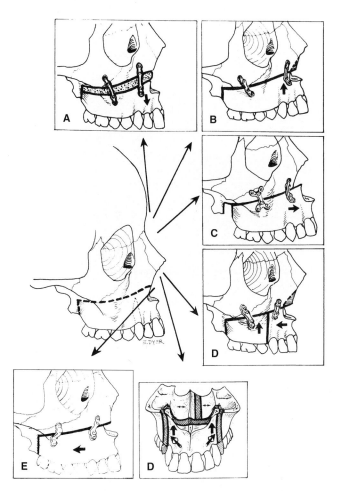

FIGURE 27.4. The Le Fort I osteotomy sections the maxilla transversely at a level between the roots of the teeth (note that the root of the cuspid may extend as high as the piriform rim) and the infraorbital foramen. After the lower portion of the maxilla is mobilized, movement in a number of directions is possible. **A:** Lengthening of the maxilla with an interpositional bone graft (note the use of miniplates for fixation). **B:** Shortening of the maxilla after resection of bone above the osteotomy line. **C:** Advancement of the maxilla. **D:** Segmentalization of the maxilla after downfracture and extraction of teeth. **E:** Setback of maxilla.

is done and then the whole maxilla can be inferiorly positioned or impacted to its new position (Fig. 27.5).

Vertical Maxillary Excess

Vertical maxillary excess is typically associated with lip incompetence, mentalis strain, and an excessive degree of gingival show (long face syndrome). The treatment approach is to impact the maxilla to achieve the proper incisor show with the lips in repose. Impaction results in skeletal contraction, so the surgeon must consider anterior repositioning of the jaws to neutralize the associated adverse soft-tissue effects. As the maxilla is impacted, the mandible rotates counterclockwise to maintain occlusion. This rotation results in anterior positioning of the chin and is called mandibular autorotation (Fig. 27.6). The opposite occurs if the maxilla is moved in an inferior direction. In this case, the chin point rotates in a clockwise direction, which results in posterior positioning of the chin point. It is important to note these effects on the cephalometric tracing during treatment planning because a genioplasty may be required to re-establish proper chin position.

Short Lower Face

A short lower face is marked by insufficient incisor show and/or a short distance between subnasale and pogonion. Treatment is aimed at establishing a proper lip–incisor relationship. The facial skeleton should be expanded to the degree that provides optimal soft-tissue aesthetics. As the maxilla is inferiorly positioned, clockwise mandibular rotation will occur, leading to posterior positioning of the chin. The surgeon needs to assess the new chin position on the cephalometric tracing to determine if an advancement genioplasty is now necessary to counter the effects of mandibular clockwise rotation.

PREPARING FOR SURGERY

Preoperation Cephalometric Tracing

Cephalometric tracings give the surgeon an idea of how skeletal movements will affect one another as well as the soft-tissue profile. They also allow the surgeon to determine the distances the bones will be moved. Different tracing methods are used for isolated maxillary, isolated mandibular, or two-jaw surgeries. All cephalometric tracing begins by securing a clear piece of acetate tracing paper over the cephalometric radiograph. The anatomy and aforementioned cephalometric points are then marked on the tracing paper (Fig. 27.5A).

Mandibular Surgery

When isolated mandibular surgery is indicated, a second piece of acetate is used to trace only the mandible and the soft tissue of the chin and lower lip. This second tracing of only the mandible is then placed into the desired occlusion against the maxilla from the first tracing. The differences in distance between the B point and the first molar cusps, when comparing the new and original positions of the mandible, denote the distance that the mandible will be anteriorly or posteriorly positioned. The new soft-tissue profile is estimated from the tracing.

Maxillary Surgery

In isolated maxillary surgery, a second piece of acetate with only the maxilla, first molar, upper incisors, and lip is placed into the desired position. The incisal edges of the incisors should be placed at least 3 to 4 mm below the lower margin of the upper lip. The anterior positioning of the maxilla is determined by placing the maxillary teeth against the mandibular teeth in a class I occlusion (Fig. 27.5B).

An anterior open bite will dictate posterior maxillary impaction until the mandibular teeth contact the maxillary teeth in normal occlusion. The appropriate degree of posterior maxillary impaction is verified by using a tracing of the mandible and rotating it counterclockwise with the condyle remaining in the original position (Fig. 27.5C). The proper position of the maxilla is determined by establishing a class I occlusion with the incisal edges 3 to 4 mm below the upper lip. The movement required in each portion of the maxilla can be determined by measuring the distance between landmarks of the new maxillary position and the original position. Useful landmarks for the maxilla are the incisal edge, the mesial cusp of the first molar, ANS, and PNS. The anteroposterior position of the maxilla is determined by soft-tissue aesthetics and the occlusion. If soft-tissue aesthetics require moving the maxilla into a position that precludes a class I occlusion, a mandibular osteotomy is also necessary.

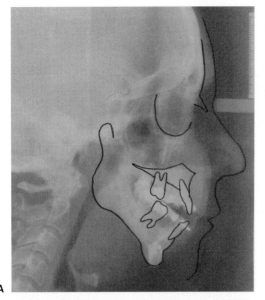

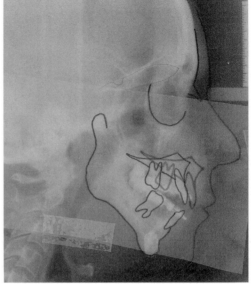

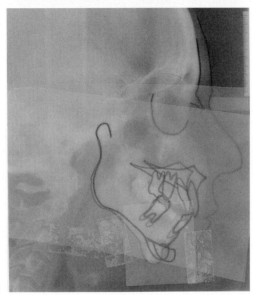

FIGURE 27.5. **A:** This patient exhibits an anterior open bite, but has good incisal show on repose. The normal landmarks on the cephalogram are recorded. **B:** The maxilla is then traced and is put into ideal position. Because incisal show is good, the anterior maxilla is not lowered and the occlusion is achieved with a posterior impaction. **C:** The mandible is then rotated into its new position using another piece of acetate that includes the mandible. The condyle is the center of rotation when moving the mandible. Because the mandible cannot be advanced without creating a malocclusion, the chin is moved forward to advance pogonion.

Two-Jaw Surgery

In two-jaw surgery, the maxilla is positioned on the cephalometric radiograph as above, and then the new position of the mandible is placed using separate pieces of acetate overlying the original cephalometric tracing. By measuring the difference between the new landmarks and the original landmarks, the surgeon determines the distance to move the maxilla and/or mandible in each dimension (6). Computer imaging may be useful at this point. **The patient should be told the computer-generated image is not a guaranteed result, only a guide to the surgeon's goals.** It is useful to make sure the patient and the surgeon are in agreement about the goals prior to surgery. The next step is to simulate these movements on plaster casts of the jaws.

Model Surgery

Model surgery begins by obtaining accurate casts of the patient's occlusion. If the surgeon does not have a dental laboratory, the orthodontist will obtain the casts. **The success of the**

technical portion of orthognathic procedures correlates directly with the accuracy of the model surgery and splint fabrication.

Isolated Mandibular Surgery

It should be noted that if isolated mandibular surgery is being performed, the casts can be hand articulated into the desired occlusion. The Galetti articulator is a useful tool that allows securing of the casts with a screw mount. A universal joint allows the casts to be set to the desired relationship. Surgical splints can then be made from the articulator. If the maximum intercuspal position is the desired postoperative occlusion, a splint is unnecessary. The surgeon can osteotomize the mandible and secure it into its new position using the maximum intercuspal position as the guide to the new position. The surgeon should always verify the desired postoperative occlusion with the orthodontist prior to surgery.

Isolated Maxillary and Two-Jaw Surgery

A face bow is a device that is used to accurately relate the maxillary model to the cranium on an articulator. If a maxillary

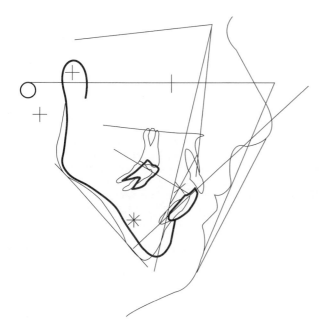

FIGURE 27.6. A counterclockwise mandibular rotation will produce an increase in the anterior position of the chin. Clockwise rotation will posteriorly position the chin. The final anticipated projection of the chin needs to be cephalometrically assessed to determine if it will require surgery to move it into a more aesthetic position.

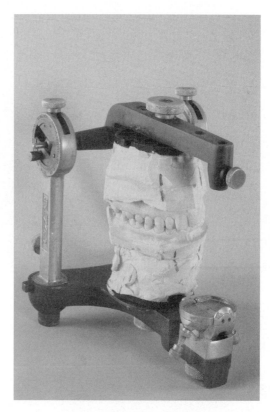

FIGURE 27.7. A semiadjustable articulator with mounted casts enables assessment of occlusal cants, malocclusion, and skeletal relationships.

osteotomy is being performed, one set of models should be mounted on an articulator using the face bow (Fig. 27.7). Two other sets of models are used in treatment planning. Next, an Erickson model block is used to measure the current position of the maxillary central incisors, cuspids, and the mesiobuccal cusp of the 1st molar (7). The face bow-mounted maxillary cast is placed on the model block. The maxillary model is then measured to the tenth of a millimeter vertically, anteroposteriorly, and end-on (Fig. 27.8). By having numerical records in three dimensions, the surgeon can reproduce the maxillary cast's exact location, as well as determine a new location. Reference lines are circumferentially inscribed every 5 mm around the maxillary cast mounting. The distances the maxilla will move in an anteroposterior, lateral, and vertical direction have been determined from the previous cephalometric exam. These numbers are added or subtracted from the current values measured on the model block to determine the new three-dimensional position of the maxillary cast. The occlusal portion of the maxillary cast is removed from its base using a saw. As much plaster is removed from the cast as is necessary to accommodate the new position of the maxilla. Soft wax is inserted in the gap between the base of the cast and the occlusal portion. The wax allows slight manipulations of the occlusal portion of the cast while providing some stability. The tooth cusps are measured in three dimensions until they match the desired postoperative position of the maxilla. Once the model block verifies the maxilla is in its new position, the cast is secured with sticky wax or plaster to the mounting ring (Fig. 27.9). Now it can be placed on the articulator. At this point, the surgeon has a mounting of the postoperative maxilla related to the preoperative position of the mandible. An acrylic splint is made at this point. This splint is called the intermediate splint and is used in the operating room to index the new position of the maxilla to the preoperative position of the mandible. A second mounting with the casts in the occlusion desired by the orthodontist is used to make a final splint that represents the new position of the mandible to the repositioned maxilla. This is fabricated in a manner similar to the splint for isolated mandibular surgery

(Fig. 27.10). If the occlusion is good, intercuspal position can be used to position the mandible without a splint.

OVERVIEW OF TREATMENT PRIOR TO SURGERY

The patient has multiple visits at the surgeon's office and has undergone a thorough discussion of the surgical options. Having heard all options available to treat the problem, the patient has agreed with the surgeon on the proposed plan. Good oral health has been achieved. Any TMJ problems have been addressed and appropriate clearance has been obtained. The patient has had preoperative orthodontic therapy to level, align, and decompensate the occlusion. Based on the physical and radiographic examinations, a treatment plan has been developed that will achieve a class I occlusion and optimize the facial soft-tissue aesthetics. Cephalometric tracings have been used to determine the distances the jaws will have to move to achieve the desired result, and model surgery has been performed to develop surgical splints that will position the jaws intraoperatively into the position determined by the cephalometric tracing. If a sagittal split osteotomy is planned, the mandibular third molars require removal 6 months prior to surgery to reduce the chance of an unfavorable split. Similarly, if a segmental osteotomy is planned, the orthodontist will have diverged the root apices on either side of the proposed osteotomy to minimize the chance of tooth root damage. The surgeon should verify that the splints fit and that stable surgical lugs have been applied to the arch wire. Soldered lugs work the best. If the lugs break intraoperatively, the proper application of the splint can be compromised,

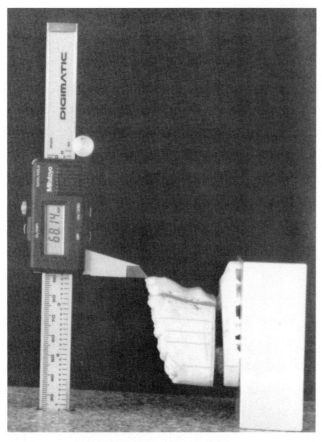

FIGURE 27.8. The preoperative maxillary position is recorded in the three dimensions shown with the Erickson model block. The landmarks are the incisal edge, the canine cusp, and the mesiobuccal first molar cusp. The movements in an anteroposterior, transverse, and vertical direction were determined by the physical and radiographic examinations. These measurements are added to or subtracted from the preoperative measurements.

making an ideal result much more difficult. In two-jaw surgery, autodonation of packed red blood cells is useful.

SURGICAL PROCEDURES

Pertinent Anatomy

The important structures in the mandible that may be injured in the mandibular osteotomy are the mental nerve, the inferior

alveolar nerve, and the teeth apices. The third branch of the trigeminal nerve enters the mandibular foramen to become the inferior alveolar nerve. It runs below the tooth roots and exits at the level of the first and second premolars through the mental foramen to become the mental nerve. The region where it is most medial to the outer cortex is located near the external oblique ridge. This is where the vertical portion of the bilateral sagittal split osteotomy is made because it affords the largest margin of error.

The maxilla is associated with the descending palatine artery, the infraorbital nerve, the tooth roots, and the internal maxillary artery. The internal maxillary artery runs about 25 mm above the pterygomaxillary junction, and the descending palatal artery descends in the posteromedial maxillary sinus. The infraorbital nerve exits the infraorbital foramen below the infraorbital rim along the midpupillary line. The maxillary tooth roots extend within the maxilla in a superior direction. The canine has the longest root and is usually visible through the maxillary cortical bone.

General Principles

Several principles have broad application to jaw surgery. Blood loss can be substantial in maxillofacial surgery. Standard techniques of head elevation, hypotensive anesthesia, blood donation, and administration of erythropoietin are useful adjuncts to reduce blood loss. Before the incisions are made, an antimicrobial rinse is helpful to minimize the intraoral bacterial count. A topical steroid is applied to the lips to reduce pain and swelling associated with prolonged retraction. Intravenous steroids may also be useful to reduce postoperative edema.

The occlusion desired may not be the same as maximum intercuspal position. The splint is useful in maintaining the occlusion in the desired location when it does not correspond to maximal intercuspal position. It is easy for the orthodontist to close a posterior open bite, but very difficult to close an anterior open bite with orthodontic treatment. At the end of the case it is important to have the anterior teeth and the canines in a class I relationship without an open bite.

Guiding elastics are useful postoperatively to control the bite. Class II elastics are placed in a vector to correct a class II relationship (maxillary lug is anterior to mandibular lug). Class III elastics are applied to correct a class III discrepancy. With rigid fixation, the elastics will not correct malpositioned jaws. They serve only to help the patient adapt to his new occlusion. Minor malocclusions can be corrected with postoperative orthodontic treatment.

Certain skeletal movements are inherently more stable than others. Stable movements include mandibular advancement and superior positioning of the maxilla. Movements with intermediate stability include maxillary impaction combined with mandibular advancement, maxillary advancement combined

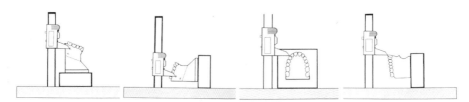

FIGURE 27.9. The cast is divided with enough plaster removed to allow the desired manipulation. The maxilla is moved into its new position and secured with sticky wax. This cast is then reattached to the articulator and the intermediate splint is made. The final splint can be made on a Galetti articulator as shown in Figure 27.10.

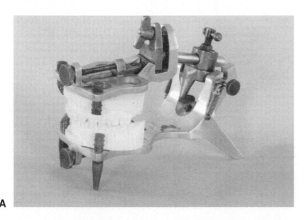
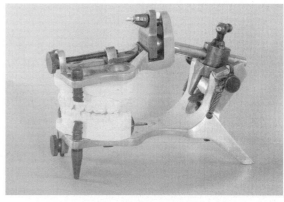

A   B

FIGURE 27.10. **A:** The Galetti articulator enables articulation of models for mandibular surgery. **A:** This photograph demonstrates the preoperative occlusion. **B:** This photograph shows the desired occlusion by the orthodontist. The anterior occlusion has no open bite and the midlines are congruent. The posterior open bite is easily closed with postoperative orthodontics; in this case, a splint was used to preserve the posterior open bite intra- and postoperatively. The splint minimizes the risk of the posterior bite closing, which would compromise the anterior occlusion.

with mandibular setback, and correction of mandibular asymmetry. **The unstable movements include posterior positioning of the mandible and inferior positioning of the maxilla. The least-stable movement is transverse expansion of the maxilla.** Long-term relapse with rigid fixation has not been demonstrated to be clearly superior to nonrigid fixation in single-jaw surgery. However, in two-jaw surgery, rigid fixation results in less relapse (8). The judgment of the surgeon will dictate the extent to which the facial skeleton can be expanded without resulting in unacceptable relapse.

Le Fort I Osteotomy

The first step in any facial osteotomy is satisfactorily securing the nasal endotracheal tube; my preference is a nasal RAE endotracheal tube. The vertical position of the maxilla is recorded by measuring the distance between the medial canthus and the orthodontic arch wire. These vertical measurements are absolutely critical. The maxillary vestibule is injected with epinephrine prior to patient preparation. An incision is made with needle-tip electrocautery 5 mm above the mucogingival junction from first molar to first molar. A periosteal elevator is then used to expose the maxilla around the piriform rim and infraorbital nerve. Obwegeser toe-in retractors are held by the assistant at the head of the operating table. As the dissection extends laterally, it is important to remain subperiosteal to avoid exposure of the buccal fat pad. A Woodson elevator is used to initiate reflection of the nasal mucosa, and a periosteal elevator is used to complete the dissection of the nasal floor and lateral nasal wall. A double-balled osteotome is used to release the septum from the maxilla and a uniballed osteotome is used to release the lateral nasal wall. The surgeon can insert a finger on the posterior palate to help feel when the cut is complete. A periosteal elevator is used to protect the nasal mucosa and then a reciprocating saw is used to make a transverse osteotomy from the piriform aperture laterally until the cut descends just posterior to the last maxillary molar and drops through the maxillary tuberosity. The cut should be made at least 5 mm above the apices of the teeth. This distance is determined from the Panorex radiograph. If cuts are complete, the maxilla is downfractured with manual pressure. An alternative is to use the Rowe disimpaction forceps. These fit into the piriform aperture and on the palate to provide increased

leverage for the downfracture. Pressure should be applied in a slow, steady, controlled fashion, not in a series of quick movements. If the maxilla is not mobilized with relative ease, the cuts are likely not complete and should be reevaluated. Once the downfracture is complete, a bone hook can be used by the assistant to hold the maxilla down while any remaining bony interferences are removed. The descending palatine arteries will be seen near the posteromedial maxillary sinus. These can be clipped prophylactically without compromising the blood supply to the maxilla. The splint is then used to place the maxilla in its proper position. Intermaxillary fixation is then applied with 26-gauge wires around the surgical lugs. The amount the maxilla will be impacted or elongated was determined in the treatment plan. This distance is added or subtracted from the medial canthal–incisor distance to determine the new vertical position of the maxilla. Four 2-mm plates, usually L-shaped, can be used to secure the maxilla. The mandibulomaxillary fixation (MMF) is released and occlusion verified prior to closure. If the alar base is wide, an alar cinch can be performed to normalize the width. Lip shortening may also result from closure. A V-Y closure at the central incisor can help alleviate this effect.

In patients who require increased cheek projection, a high Le Fort I osteotomy can be performed. This differs in that the transverse osteotomy is made as high as the infraorbital nerve will allow. If further cheek projection is necessary, bone grafts can be added. In the case of inferior or anterior positioning, gaps between the segments greater than 3 mm should be grafted with either autogenous bone, cadaveric bone, or block hydroxyapatite. Finally, if simultaneous expansion of the maxilla is necessary, the maxilla can be split into two or more pieces to allow simultaneous expansion.

Surgically Assisted Rapid Palatal Expansion

Correction of transverse maxillary constriction can be corrected in adolescence with nonsurgical orthodontic appliances. As the sutures begin to close during late adolescence, relapse increases. A multipiece Le Fort osteotomy can be performed to provide simultaneous maxillary expansion, but the degree of relapse is high. In the young adult, the preferred procedure is the surgically assisted rapid palatal expansion (SARPE). The orthodontist places a palatal expander prior to the procedure.

A Le Fort I osteotomy is performed to completely mobilize the maxilla from the upper face. A small osteotome is used to make a thin cut between the roots of the central incisors. The midline split is completed to the posterior nasal spine. Separation is verified by activating the device. The maxilla is widened until the gingiva blanches and is then relaxed several turns to avoid ischemia (5). The SARPE offers the best stability for maxillary expansion in the young adult and older patient (9,10). Transverse deficiencies of the mandible can be corrected with a similar technique, that of distraction osteogenesis.

Bilateral Sagittal Split Osteotomy

The endotracheal tube placement and epinephrine injection are similar to the Le Fort osteotomy. The cut is made with electrocautery about 1 cm from the lateral aspect of the molars and extends from midramus to the region of the second molar. If insufficient tissue is left on the dental side of the incision, closure is more difficult. A periosteal elevator is used to expose the lateral mandible and the anterior coronoid process in a subperiosteal plane. As the coronoid process is exposed, placement of a notched coronoid retractor may facilitate the dissection. A curved Kocher with a chain can be clamped to the coronoid process and the chain secured to the drapes. To optimize blood supply, subperiosteal dissection is limited to those areas required to complete the osteotomy. A J-stripper is used to release the inferior border of the mandible from the attachments of the pterygomasseteric sling. The external oblique ridge and inferior border of the mandible should be exposed. The medial aspect of the ramus is also dissected subperiosteally. The mandibular nerve should be identified. A Seldin elevator is inserted medial to the ramus and above the nerve. The superior edge of the elevator is rotated medially, exposing the medial ramus and protecting the nerve. A Lindemann side-cutting burr is used to make a cut on the medial ramus that is parallel to the occlusal plane and extends about two-thirds of the distance to the posterior ramus. The cut extends from medial to lateral until the burr is in the cancellous portion of the ramus, which is about half the width of the ramus. Mandibular body retractors are then placed and a fissure burr or a reciprocating saw is used to make a cut from the midramus down along the external oblique ridge, gently curving to the inferior border of the mandible. The cuts are verified with an osteotome, and then large osteotomes are inserted and rotated to gently separate the segments. The tooth-bearing segment is referred to as the distal segment, and the condylar portion as the proximal segment. The inferior alveolar nerve should be identified and found in the distal segment. If part of the nerve is located within the proximal segment, it should gently be released with a small curette. After both osteotomies are complete, the distal segment is placed into occlusion and secured by tightening 26-gauge wire loops around the surgical lugs. If a surgical splint is necessary to establish the required occlusion, it is placed between the teeth prior to intermaxillary wiring. The proximal segment is then gently rotated to ensure it is seated within the glenoid fossa. When the condyle is comfortably seated within the fossa, it is rotated to align the inferior borders of the two segments and secured into position with a clamp. Three lag screws are placed at the superior border of the overlapping segments on each side of the mandible. To ensure that the transbuccal trocar will be in the proper place, a hemostat is placed at the proposed screw location and pointed out toward the cheek. A small stab incision is made in the skin, and the trocar is placed through the tissue bluntly until the tip enters the oral incision. The trocar is then exchanged for a drill guide, and the 2.0-mm and 1.5-mm drills are used in the lag sequence to make three holes through the overlapping portion of the proximal and distal segments. The screw lengths are measured and the screws inserted. The

intermaxillary fixation is released, and the mandible is gently opened and closed. The teeth should meet in a class I occlusion. If a malocclusion is noted, the most likely etiology is that one or both condyles are not seated properly during application of fixation. The screws should be removed and replaced until the correct occlusion is established. The wounds are irrigated and closed with interrupted 4-0 chromic sutures.

Intraoral Vertical Ramus Osteotomy

A second technique for correcting mandibular prognathism or asymmetry is the intraoral vertical ramus osteotomy (IVRO). The incision is the same as described above. A subperiosteal dissection is performed from the lateral ramus and a LeVasseur-Merrill retractor is used to hold this tissue laterally. An oscillating saw is then used to make a vertical cut from the sigmoid notch to the inferior border of the mandible. The cut must be made posterior to the mandibular foramen on the medial side. The antilingula is a useful landmark. It is an elevation on the lateral mandible that indicates the approximate location of the mandibular foramen. After both sides are complete, the distal segment is moved into occlusion, making sure that the proximal segments remain lateral to the distal segments posteriorly. Because rigid fixation is difficult to apply, a single wire or no fixation is used, and the patient remains in intermaxillary fixation for 6 weeks. This osteotomy can be done from an extraoral approach but this incision results in a scar on the neck.

Two-Jaw Surgery

Moving the maxilla and the mandible in one procedure requires osteotomizing both jaws and precisely securing them into the position determined by the treatment plan. If proper treatment planning, model surgery, and splint fabrication are performed, each jaw should be able to be placed into its desired position with precision. The mandibular bony cuts are made first but terminated prior to osteotomy completion. The maxillary osteotomy is made, and the maxilla is placed into its new position using the intermediate splint. The splint is used to wire the teeth into intermaxillary fixation. The intermediate splint indexes the new position of the maxilla to the preoperative (uncorrected) position of the mandible. With the condyles gently seated, the maxillomandibular complex is rotated so that the maxillary incisal edge is at the correct vertical height. The maxilla is plated into position, the intermaxillary fixation is released, and the intermediate splint is removed. Now the mandibular osteotomies are completed and the distal segment of the mandible is placed into the desired occlusion using the final splint. If the teeth are in good occlusion without the splint, the final splint may not be necessary to establish the desired occlusal relationship. Wire loops secure the occlusal relationship and the rigid fixation is completed as previously described.

COMPLICATIONS

Improper positioning of the jaws is noted by poor occlusion or an obvious unaesthetic result. If the complication results from improper condyle position during fixation or improper indexing of the splint, fixation must be removed and reapplied. It is wise to verify splint fit prior to surgery. Meticulous treatment planning prior to surgery minimizes splint-related problems.

Measures to reduce the chance of a bad split should always be employed. Removal of mandibular third molars 6 months prior to the osteotomy allows time for the sockets to heal, which decreases the chance of a bad split. If the segments do not appear to be easily separating, the surgeon should verify that the osteotomies are complete. One does not want to use excessive force that could increase the chance of an uncontrolled mandibular split. If a bad split occurs, the segments can be plated to reestablish normal anatomy, and the proximal and distal segments can then be secured into the desired position with rigid fixation.

Bleeding may occur from any area but most commonly occurs from the descending palatine artery in the maxilla. This can be stopped with packing or by placing a hemoclip on the artery. Bone wax is useful for bleeding bony edges.

Nerve damage is rare but can occur. The nerves associated with these procedures are the infraorbital, the inferior alveolar, and the mental nerves. If a transection is witnessed, coaptation with 7-0 suture is recommended if possible. The patient should be informed that there is approximately a 70% chance of some paresthesia immediately after surgery but permanent changes are seen only in 25% of patients.

Nonunion or malunion is rare after surgery. If a malunion occurs, the jaw may need to be osteotomized again to move it into the proper position. A nonunion requires secondary bone grafting to establish osseous continuity.

References

1. Morris AL, et al. *Handicapping Orthodontic Conditions*. Washington, DC: National Academy of Sciences, 1975.
2. Rosen HM. Facial skeletal expansion: treatment strategies and rationale. *Plast Reconstr Surg*. 1992;89:798.
3. Tompach PC, Wheeler JJ, Fridrich KL, et al. Orthodontic considerations in orthognathic surgery. *Int J Adult Orthod Orthognath Surg*. 1995;10:97.
4. Rosen HM. Aesthetics in facial skeletal surgery. *Perspect Plast Surg*. 1993;6:1.
5. Betts NJ, Vandarsdall RL, Barber HD, et al. Diagnosis and treatment of transverse maxillary deficiency. *Int J Adult Orthod Orthognath Surg*. 1995;10:75.
6. Proffit WR, Sarver DM. Treatment planning: optimizing benefit to the patient. In: Proffit WR, White RP, Sarver DM, eds. *Contemporary Treatment of Dentofacial Deformity*. St. Louis: Mosby; 2003:213–223.
7. Erickson K. *An Instructional Manual for the Model Platform and Model Block*. Great Lakes Tonawanda, NY: Orthodontics, Ltd, 1990.
8. Proffit WR, Turvey TA, Phillips C, et al. Orthognathic surgery: a hierarchy of stability. *Int J Adult Orthod Orthognath Surg*. 1996;11:191–204.
9. Stromberg C, Holm J. Surgically assisted rapid maxillary expansion in adults: a retrospective long-term follow-up study. *J Craniomaxillofac Surg*. 1995;23:222.
10. Silverstein K, Quinn PD. Surgically assisted rapid palatal expansion for management of transverse maxillary deficiency. *J Oral Maxillofac Surg*. 1997;55:725.

CHAPTER 28 ■ CRANIOFACIAL CLEFTS AND HYPERTELORBITISM

JAMES P. BRADLEY AND HENRY KAWAMOTO, JR.

Congenital craniofacial clefts are anatomic distortions of the face and cranium with deficiencies or excesses of tissue in a linear pattern. They are among the most disfiguring of all facial anomalies. Craniofacial clefts exist in a multitude of locations and varying degrees of severity. Although they appear bizarre and unexplainable, most craniofacial clefts occur along predictable embryologic lines. They are expressed either unilaterally or bilaterally. In addition, one cleft type may manifest on one side of the face, while a different cleft type is present on the other side.

TESSIER CLASSIFICATION

Classification systems have been developed to describe rare craniofacial clefts. The Tessier classification is the most complete and has withstood the test of time. This descriptive classification links clinical observations with underlying skeletal deformities seen with preoperative three-dimensional computed tomography (CT) scan imaging and confirmed during surgery. Newer neuroembryologic theories that allow for mapping of developmental zones of the face have confirmed the value of the Tessier classification to embryologists and geneticists, not just surgeons.

In the Tessier classification, clefts are numbered from 0 to 14, depending on the relationship to the orbit (Fig. 28.1). The orbits divide the face into upper and lower hemispheres and separate the cranial clefts from the facial clefts. At times, facial clefts extend through the orbit to become cranial clefts. The clefts are numbered so that the facial component of the cleft and the cranial component always add up to 14: 0 and 14, 1 and 13, 2 and 12, 3 and 11, 4 and 10, 5 and 9, and 6 and 8. Tessier cleft number 7 is the lateral-most craniofacial cleft. The soft-tissue and skeletal components of a cleft are seldom affected to the same extent. The skeletal landmarks tend to be more constant and reliable than the soft-tissue landmarks. The order of description below consists of facial clefts from medial to lateral followed by cranial clefts from lateral to medial.

DEFINING FEATURES OF CRANIOFACIAL CLEFTS

Number 0 Cleft

The number 0 Tessier craniofacial clefts are unique in that they may present with either a deficiency or an excess of tissue.

Deficiency of Midline Structures

A deficiency may manifest as hypoplasia or agenesis in which portions of midline facial structures are absent (Fig. 28.2A).

This developmental arrest may range from the mildest form of hypoplasia of the nasomaxillary region and hypotelorism cyclopia, ethmocephaly, or cebocephaly. The severe form is often fatal. A CT scan of the brain can differentiate patients with poor differentiation of the brain who may die in infancy from those with a better prognosis. **Soft-tissue deficiencies** with this midline facial cleft include the upper lip and nose. Agenesis or hypoplasia may result in a median cleft of the lip and absence of philtral columns. When a wide central cleft exists, it typically extends the full height of the upper lip and up into the nasal floor. With nasal anomalies the columella may be narrowed or totally absent. The nasal tip may be depressed from lack of septal support. The septum is usually vestigal with no caudal attachment to the palate. **Skeletal deficiencies** range from separation between the upper central incisors to absence of the premaxilla and a cleft of the secondary palate. Nasal deficiency may include partial or total absence of nasal bones and the septal cartilage. The bone defect may extend cephalad into the area of the ethmoid sinuses and result in hypotelorism or cyclopia. An encephalocele may fill the defect or void from the frontonasal junction back to the foramen cecum or sphenoid body.

Excess of Midline Tissue

Midline excess is noted as widening or duplications of structures (Fig. 28.2B). **Soft-tissue midline excess** tissue may be manifested as a true median cleft lip with broad philtral columns. A duplication of the labial frenulum may also exist. The nose may be bifid with a broad columella and mid-dorsal furrow. The alar and upper lateral cartilages may be displaced laterally. **Skeletal excess** (Fig. 28.2C) in a widened number 0 facial cleft can be seen as a diastema between the upper central incisors. A duplicate nasal spine may exist. A characteristic keel-shaped maxillary alveolus is seen. Anterior teeth are angled toward the midline creating an anterior open bite. Central midface height is shortened. The cartilaginous and bone nasal septum is thickened or duplicated. The nasal bones and nasal process of the maxilla are broad, flattened, and displaced laterally from the midline. Ethmoidal and sphenoidal sinuses may be enlarged contributing to symmetrical widening of the anterior cranial fossa and hypertelorism. The cribriform plate is low and the breadth of the crista galli is exaggerated. The body of the sphenoid is broadened with displacement of the pterygoid plates away from the midline.

Number 1 Cleft

Soft-Tissue Involvement

The number 1 cleft, similar to the common cleft lip, passes through the Cupid's bow and then through the alar cartilage

268

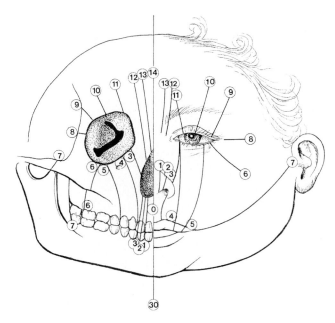

FIGURE 28.1. Tessier classification of craniofacial clefts. The left half (right side of face) depicts the various clefts relative to the skeletal landmarks and the right half (left side of face) outlines the locations based on soft tissue landmarks. Facial clefts = numbers 0 through number 7 and cranial clefts = numbers 8 through number 14. Mandibular midline facial cleft number 30 is also seen.

dome. Notching in the area of the soft triangle of the nose is a distinct feature (Fig. 28.3A). The columella may be short and broad. The nasal tip and nasal septum deviate away from the cleft. Soft-tissue furrows or wrinkles may be present on the nasal dorsum if the cleft extends in a cephalic direction. The cleft is evident medially to a malpositioned medial canthus and telecanthus may result. With a cranial extension as a number 13 cleft, vertical orbital dystopia may be present.

Skeletal Involvement

A keel-shaped maxilla with the anterior incisors facing toward the cleft creates an anterior open bite (Fig. 28.3B). An alveolar cleft is rare but would pass between the central and lateral incisors. This paramedian cleft separates the nasal floor at the pyriform aperture just lateral to the nasal spine. The cleft may extend posteriorly as a complete cleft of the hard and soft palate. Extension of the cleft in a cephalad direction is through the junction of the nasal bone and the frontal process of the maxilla. The nasal bones are displaced and flattened. Ethmoidal expansion leads to hypertelorism. Also, there is asymmetry of the greater and lesser sphenoid wings, the pterygoid plates, and anterior cranial fossa.

Number 2 Cleft

Soft-Tissue Involvement

This cleft may also begin in the region of the common cleft lip (Fig. 28.4A). However, the nasal deformity is in the middle third of the alar rim and distinguishes the number 2 cleft from other clefts. In the number 2 cleft, the ala is hypoplastic, whereas in the number 1 cleft, the ala is merely notched at the dome. The lateral aspect of the nose is flattened and the dorsum is broad. The eyelid is not involved; the cleft passes medially to the palpebral fissure. Although the medial canthus is displaced, the lacrimal duct is usually not involved. If the cleft continues

in a cephalad direction as a cranial number 12 cleft, distortion of the medial brow is noted.

Skeletal Involvement

The number 2 cleft begins between the lateral incisor and the canine (Fig. 28.4B). It extends into the pyriform aperture, lateral to the septum and medial to the maxillary sinus. A hard and soft palate cleft may occur. The nasal septum may be deviated away from the cleft. The cleft distorts the nasal bones as it passes between the nasal bones and the frontal process of the maxilla. Ethmoidal sinus involvement may result in orbital hypertelorism. Asymmetry of the greater and lesser sphenoid wings and anterior cranial base is present.

Number 3 Cleft

The number 3 cleft or the oronasal-ocular cleft is the most common of the Tessier craniofacial clefts.

Soft-Tissue Involvement

The number 3 cleft begins similar to a number 1 and number 2 clefts, passing through the philtral column and floor of the nose (Fig. 28.5A). Deficiency of tissue between the alar base and lower eyelid results in displacement of the alar base and a shortened nose on the affected side. The cleft passes between the medial canthus and the inferior lacrimal punctum. The lacrimal system, particularly the lower canaliculus, is disrupted. Blockage of the nasolacrimal duct and recurrent infections of the lacrimal sac are common. The inferior punctum is displaced downward and drainage can occur directly onto the cheek instead of into the nasal cavity.

The medial canthus is inferiorly displaced and may be hypoplastic. Colobomas of the lower eyelid are medial to the inferior punctum. In mild forms, colobomas may be the only obvious evidence of this cleft, but it is important to check a CT scan for bony involvement and to maintain an index of suspicion for disruption of the lacrimal system. Involvement of the globe is rare, but microphthalmia can occur. Typically, the eye is malpositioned inferiorly and laterally. Injury to the normal eye, including corneal erosions, ocular perforation, and loss of vision in affected eye, may result from desiccation unless the globe is protected.

Skeletal Involvement

Osseous characteristics of this facial cleft include involvement of the orbit and direct communication of the oral, nasal, and orbital cavities (Fig. 28.5B). The cleft begins between the lateral incisor and the canine. In contrast to the number 1 and number 2 facial clefts, the anterior maxillary arch is flat in the number 3 cleft. The number 3 cleft disrupts the frontal process of the maxilla and then terminates in the lacrimal groove. In the severest form the cleft is bilateral and the skeletal disruption is significant (Fig. 28.5C, D). With bilateral cases the contralateral facial cleft may be a number 4 or 5 cleft. There may be narrowing of the ethmoid and sphenoid sinuses. Both the orbital floor and anterior cranial base are displaced inferiorly.

Number 4 Cleft

The number 4 cleft occurs lateral to the nose and other median facial structures.

Soft-Tissue Involvement

As opposed to numbers 1, 2, and 3 facial clefts, the number 4 cleft begins lateral to Cupid's bow and the philtral column and

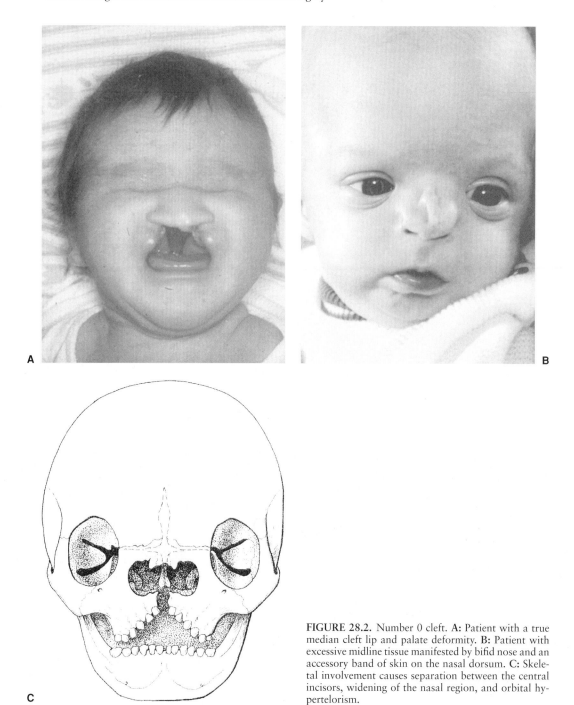

FIGURE 28.2. Number 0 cleft. **A:** Patient with a true median cleft lip and palate deformity. **B:** Patient with excessive midline tissue manifested by bifid nose and an accessory band of skin on the nasal dorsum. **C:** Skeletal involvement causes separation between the central incisors, widening of the nasal region, and orbital hypertelorism.

medial to the oral commissure (Fig. 28.6A). The orbicularis oris muscle is located in the lateral lip element with no muscle centrally. The cleft passes lateral to the nasal ala. Although the ala is not involved and the nose is intact, it is displaced superiorly. Bilateral involvement pulls the nose upward. The cleft extends through the cheek and into the lower eyelid lateral to the inferior punctum. The lower eyelid and lashes may extend directly into the lateral aspect of the cleft. The medial canthus and nasolacrimal system are normal. The globe is typically normal but microphthalmia and anophthalmos may be seen.

Skeletal Involvement

Skeletal involvement (Fig. 28.6B) is usually less extensive than in the number 3 cleft. The alveolar cleft begins between the

lateral incisor and the canine. The cleft extends lateral to the pyriform aperture to involve the maxillary sinus. The medial wall of the maxillary sinus, is intact. A confluence exists between the oral cavity, maxillary sinus, and orbital cavity but not the nasal cavity. The cleft then passes medial to the infraorbital foramen. This landmark defines the boundary between the medial number 4 facial cleft and lateral number 5 facial cleft. The number 4 cleft terminates at the medial aspect of the inferior orbital rim. With an absent medial orbital floor and rim, the globe may prolapse inferiorly. In bilateral cases the medial midface and premaxilla are protrusive. The sphenoid body is asymmetric and pterygoid plates are displaced but the anterior cranial base is unaffected. Bilateral number 4 clefts are not unusual (Fig. 28.6C).

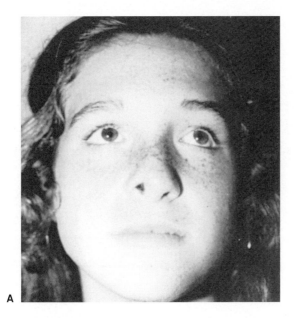
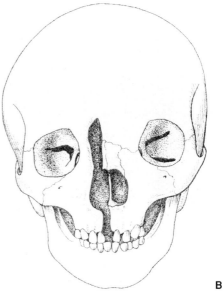

FIGURE 28.3. Number 1 cleft. A: Patient with notched right alar dome and orbital hypertelorism. B: Skeletal involvement is through the piriform aperture just lateral to the nasal spine and septum. The orbit is displaced laterally.

Number 5 Cleft

This facial cleft is extremely rare.

Soft-Tissue Involvement

The number 5 facial cleft begins just medial to the oral commissure and courses along the cheek lateral to the nasal ala (Fig. 28.7A). The cleft terminates in the lateral half of the lower eyelid. Although the globe is typically normal, microphthalmia may occur.

Skeletal Involvement

The alveolar cleft begins lateral to the canine in the region of the premolars (Fig. 28.7B). In contrast to the number 4 cleft, the number 5 cleft courses lateral to the infraorbital foramen and terminates in the lateral aspect of the orbital rim and floor. The cleft is separated from the inferior orbital fissure. The maxillary

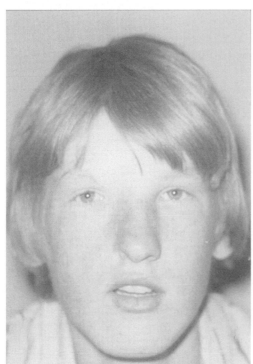
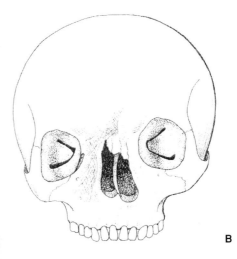

FIGURE 28.4. Number 2 cleft. A: Patient with hypoplasia of the middle third of the right nostril rim causing the appearance of alar base retraction. The lateral nose is flattened. The medial border of the eyebrow is also distorted as evidence of a number 12 cranial cleft. There is also telorbitism and displacement of the right medial canthus. B: Skeletal involvement shows deformity of the piriform aperture and nasal bone.

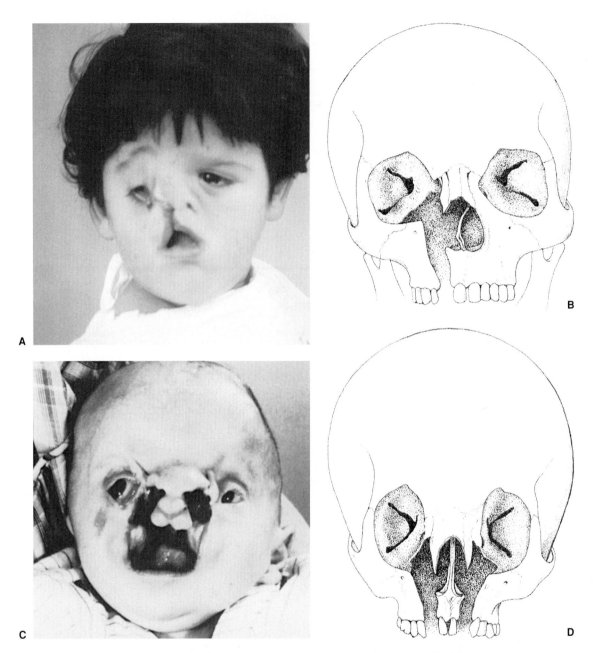

FIGURE 28.5. Number 3 cleft. **A:** (Unilateral) Patient with complete form has a right cleft lip and palate and severe shortening of tissues between the right alar base and medial canthus. The right nasal ala is displaced superiorly, the medial canthus is displaced inferiorly, and the nasolacrimal system is disrupted. **B:** (Unilateral) Skeletal involvement is between the lateral incisor and the canine extending up through the lacrimal groove. The cleft creates communication among the orbital, maxillary sinus, nasal, and oral cavities. **C:** (Bilateral) Patient with bilateral cleft lip and palate and retraction of alar bases extending above the level of the medial canthi. **D:** (Bilateral) Skeletal defects are extensive, with only the nasal septum dividing the cavities of the midface.

sinus may be hypoplastic. Prolapse of orbital contents through the lateral orbital floor defect into the maxillary sinus causes vertical orbital dystopia. The lateral orbital wall may be thickened and the greater sphenoid wing abnormal. The cranial base is normal.

Number 6 Cleft

This zygomaticomaxillary cleft represents an incomplete form of Treacher Collins syndrome. Similar and often more severe

cleft facial features are seen in Nager syndrome. Nager syndrome patients also may have radial club deformities of the upper extremities.

Soft-Tissue Involvement

The cleft is often identified as a vertical furrow, as a result of hypoplastic soft tissue, from the oral commissure to the lateral lower eyelid (Fig. 28.8A). This line of hypoplasia runs through the zygomatic eminence along an imaginary line from the angle of the mandible to the lateral palpebral fissure. The lateral palpebral fissure is pulled downward. The lateral canthus is

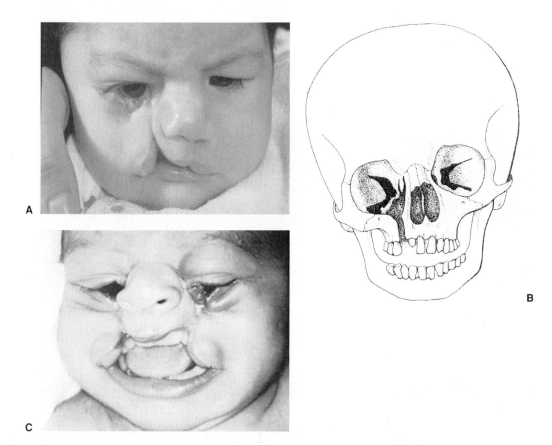

FIGURE 28.6. Number 4 cleft. **A:** (Unilateral) Patient with right cheek cleft. The cleft lip begins lateral to Cupid's bow and terminates in the lower eyelid medial to the punctum. **B:** (Unilateral) Skeletal involvement begins between the lateral incisor and canine and extends through the maxilla between the infraorbital foramen and the piriform aperture. The orbit, maxillary sinus, and oral cavities communicate. **C:** (Bilateral) Patient with bilateral involvement has a cleft of the upper lip lateral to Cupid's bow and malar extension to the lower eyelids with colobomas present. Notching is also seen in the upper lids as evidence of a number 10 cranial cleft.

displaced inferiorly. This may create an appearance of a severe lower lid ectropion and an antimongoloid slant. Colobomas appear in the lateral lower eyelid and mark the cephalic end of the cleft.

Skeletal Involvement

The number 6 facial cleft is along the zygomatic–maxillary suture separating the maxilla and zygoma (Fig. 28.8B). There is no alveolar cleft, but a short posterior maxilla may result in an occlusal tilt. Choanal atresia is common. The cleft enters the orbit at the lateral third of the orbital rim and floor. It connects to the inferior orbital fissure. The zygoma is hypoplastic with an intact zygomatic arch. There is narrowing of the anterior cranial fossa. The sphenoid is normal.

Number 7 Cleft

This temporozygomatic facial cleft is a common craniofacial cleft. It is often seen with craniofacial microsomia (oculo-auriculo-vertebral spectrum). The number 7 cleft is also seen in Treacher Collins syndrome.

Soft-Tissue Involvement

The cleft begins at the oral commissure and varies from a mild broadening of the oral commissure with a preauricular skin tag to a complete fissure extending toward a microtic ear

(Fig. 28.9A). Typically the cleft does not extend beyond the anterior border of the masseter. However, the ipsilateral tongue, soft palate, and muscles of mastication (cranial nerve V) may be underdeveloped. The parotid gland and parotid duct may be absent. Facial nerve weakness (cranial nerve VII) may be present. External ear deformities range from preauricular skin tags to complete absence. Preauricular hair is usually absent in patients with craniofacial microsomia. Patients with Treacher Collins syndrome often have preauricular hair from the temporal region pointing to the oral commissure. The ipsilateral soft palate and tongue are often hypoplastic.

Skeletal Involvement

There is a wide range of osseous anomalies in a number 7 cleft (Fig. 28.9B). The skeletal cleft passes through the pterygomaxillary junction. Tessier believed that the cleft is centered in the region of the zygomaticotemporal suture. The posterior maxilla and mandibular ramus are hypoplastic in the vertical dimension, creating an occlusal plane that is canted cephalad on the affected side. The coronoid process and condyle are also often hypoplastic and asymmetric, which contributes to a posterior open bite on the affected side. The zygomatic body is severely malformed, hypoplastic, and displaced. In the most severe form, the zygomatic arch is disrupted and is represented by a small stump. The malpositioned lateral canthus is caused by a hypoplastic zygoma that results in the inferiorly displaced superolateral angle of the orbit. Occasionally, severely deforming number 7 clefts can cause true orbital dystopia.

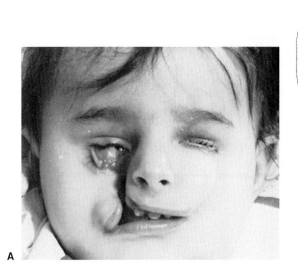

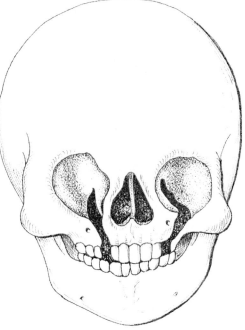

FIGURE 28.7. Number 4 cleft *(right)* and number 5 cleft *(left)*. **A:** This patient demonstrates that the number 4 cleft begins lateral to Cupid's bow and extends up to the medial third of the lower eyelid, whereas the number 5 cleft begins just medial to the oral commissure and extends up the lateral cheek to the middle of the eyelid. **B:** Skeletal involvement in the number 4 cleft begins between the lateral incisor and canine and passes medial to the infraorbital foramen. In the number 5 cleft, the cleft begins at the premolars and extends lateral to the infraorbital foramen.

The abnormal anterior zygomatic arch continues posteriorly as a normal zygomatic process of the temporal bone. The cranial base is asymmetric and tilts causing an abnormally positioned glenoid fossa. The anatomy of the sphenoid is abnormal and there can be a rudimentary medial and lateral pterygoid plate.

Number 8 Cleft

This frontozygomatic cleft divides the facial clefts from the cranial clefts. The number 8 cleft rarely occurs alone but is usually associated with other craniofacial clefts. It appears to be the

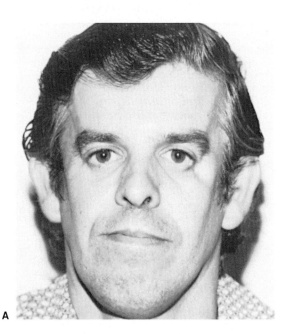

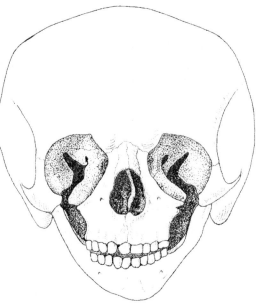

FIGURE 28.8. Number 6 cleft. **A:** Patient with an incomplete form of Treacher Collins syndrome shows bilateral linear malar hypoplasia. **B:** Skeletal involvement occurs in the region of the zygomatic-maxillary suture. The zygoma is hypoplastic.

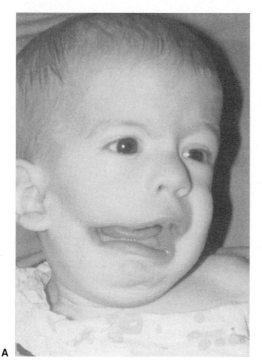

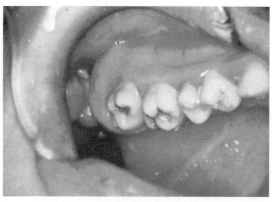

FIGURE 28.9. Number 7 cleft. A: Patient with a complete fissure of the oral commissure that extends toward the external ear, resulting in macrosomia. B: Cleft of posterior maxillary alveolus (↑) between second and third molar.

cranial extension of the number 6 cleft. The bilateral occurrence of the combination of numbers 6, 7, and 8 craniofacial clefts is unique. Tessier believed that this pattern of clefts best describes the Treacher Collins syndrome. Infants with craniofacial microsomia and unilateral involvement typically have more soft-tissue involvement, whereas those with Treacher Collins syndrome tend to have more severe bony abnormalities.

Soft-Tissue Involvement

The number 8 cleft extends from the lateral canthus to the temporal region (Fig. 28.10A). A dermatocele may occupy the coloboma of the lateral commissure. Occasionally, abnormal hair manifestations can be seen along a line between the tempo-ral area and the lateral canthus. The soft-tissue malformation presents as a true lateral commissure coloboma (dermatocele) with absence of the lateral canthus. Abnormalities of the globe, in the form of epibulbar dermoids, are also often present, especially in Goldenhar syndrome.

Skeletal Involvement

The bony component of the cleft occurs at the frontozygomatic suture (Fig. 28.10B). Tessier noted a notch in this region in patients with Goldenhar syndrome (combination numbers 6, 7, and 8 clefts). In the complete form of Treacher Collins syndrome (combination numbers 6, 7, and 8 clefts) (Fig. 28.11), the zygoma may be hypoplastic or absent and the lateral orbital

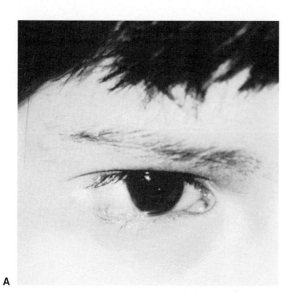

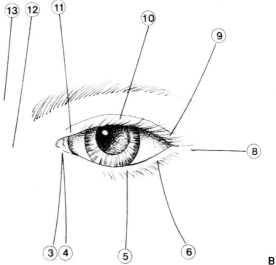

FIGURE 28.10. Number 8 cleft. A: The lateral commissure of the palpebral fissure in this patient's left eye is obliterated by a dermatocele. B: This illustration depicts the number 8 cleft as the boundary or "equator" between the facial clefts (3, 4, 5, 6) and cranial clefts (9, 10, 11) that involve the eyelids and orbit.

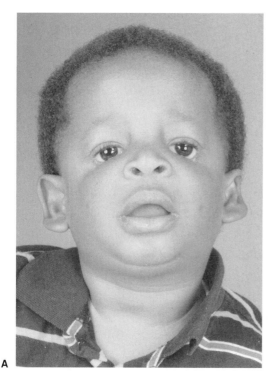

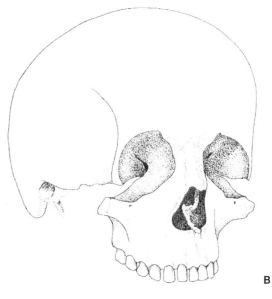

FIGURE 28.11. Combination numbers 6, 7, and 8 clefts. **A:** Patient with Treacher Collins syndrome demonstrates malar hypoplasia, antimongoloid slant to palpebral fissure, and a retruded chin. **B:** Skeletal involvement in the complete form includes absence of the zygoma, lateral orbital wall (greater wing of sphenoid provides remaining portion of the lateral wall), and lateral orbital floor.

wall missing. Thus, the lateral palpebral fissure's only support is the greater wing of the sphenoid and downward slanting occurs. With this defect there is soft-tissue continuity of the orbit and temporal fossa.

Number 9 Cleft

This upper lateral orbit cleft is the rarest of the craniofacial clefts. The number 9 cleft begins the march from lateral to medial of the cranial clefts.

Soft-Tissue Involvement

Abnormalities of the lateral third of the upper eyelid and eyebrow are the hallmarks of the number 9 cleft (Fig. 28.12). The lateral canthus is also distorted. In the severe form, microphthalmia is present. The superolateral bony deficiency of the orbits allows for a lateral displacement of the globes. The cleft then extends cephalad into the temporoparietal hair-bearing scalp. The temporal hairline is anteriorly displaced and a temporal hair projection is often seen in the number 9 cleft. Furthermore, a cranial nerve VII palsy in the forehead and upper eyelid is common.

Skeletal Involvement

The bony defect of the number 9 cranial cleft extends through the superolateral aspect of the orbit. Distortion of the upper part of the greater wing of the sphenoid, the squamosal portion of the temporal bone and surrounding parietal bones may be present. This hypoplasia of the greater wing of the sphenoid results in a posterolateral rotation of the lateral orbital wall. The pterygoid plates may be hypoplastic. There may be a reduction in the anteroposterior dimension of the anterior cranial fossa.

Number 10 Cleft

Soft-Tissue Involvement

The number 10 cleft begins at the middle third of the upper eyelid and eyebrow. The lateral eyebrow may angulate temporally

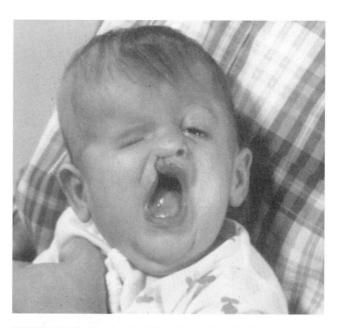

FIGURE 28.12. Number 9 cleft. Patient with left side, rare number 9 cleft through the superolateral orbital roof. The right cleft lip and microphthalmia are additional findings.

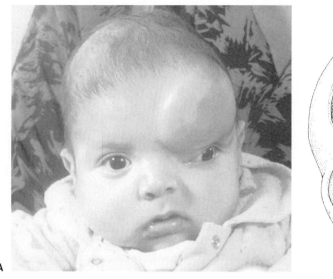

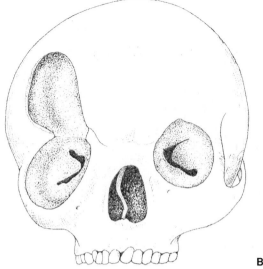

FIGURE 28.13. Number 10 cleft. **A:** Patient with fronto-orbital encephalocele seen in the middle of the left forehead. This fills the void left by the cleft defect in the center of the left superior orbital rim. **B:** Skeletal defect and asymmetric hypertelorism is demonstrated on the right.

(Fig. 28.13A). The palpebral fissure may be elongated with an amblyopic eye displaced inferolaterally. The entire upper eyelid may be absent in severe forms (ablepharia). Colobomas and other ocular anomalies may be present. Frontal hair projection may connect the temporoparietal region to the lateral brow.

Skeletal Involvement

The bony component of the number 10 cranial cleft occurs in the middle of the supraorbital rim just lateral to the superior orbital foramen (Fig. 28.13B). Often an encephalocele occupies the defect through the frontal bone and a prominent bulge is observed in the forehead. The orbit may be deformed with a lateroinferior rotation. Orbital hypertelorism may result in severe cases. The anterior cranial base may also be distorted.

Number 11 Cleft

Soft-Tissue Involvement

The medial third of the upper eyelid may show involvement with a coloboma (Fig. 28.14). The upper eyebrow may have a disruption that extends up to the frontal hairline. A tonguelike projection at the medial third of the frontal hairline may also be identified.

Skeletal Involvement

The number 11 cleft may be seen as a cleft in the medial third of the supraorbital rim if it passes lateral to the ethmoid bone. If the cleft passes through the ethmoid air cells to produce extensive pneumatization, orbital hypertelorism is seen clinically. The cranial base and sphenoid architecture, including the pterygoid processes, are symmetric and normal.

Number 12 Cleft

Soft-Tissue Involvement

The soft tissue cleft lies medial to the medial canthus, and colobomas extend to the root of the eyebrow (Fig. 28.15A).

There is a lateral displacement of the medial canthus with an aplasia of the medial end of the eyebrow. There are no eyelid clefts. The forehead skin is normal with a short, downward projection of the paramedian frontal hairline.

Skeletal Involvement

The number 12 cleft passes through the flattened, frontal process of the maxilla (Fig. 28.15B). It then travels superiorly, increasing the transverse dimension of the ethmoid air cells, producing orbital hypertelorism and telecanthus. The frontal and sphenoid sinuses are also pneumatized and enlarged. The remainder of the sphenoid and frontal bones are normal. The frontonasal angle is obtuse. Because the cleft is located lateral to the olfactory groove, the cribriform plate is normal in width. Encephaloceles have not been observed with this cleft. The anterior and middle cranial fossae are widened on the cleft side, but are otherwise normal.

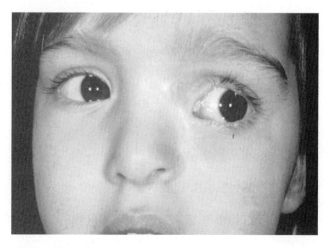

FIGURE 28.14. Number 11 cleft. Patient with small coloboma in medial third of left upper eyelid extending through the medial third of the eyebrow.

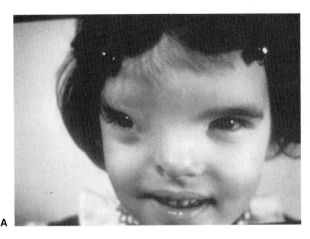

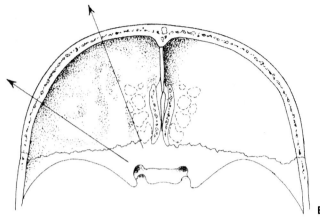

FIGURE 28.15. Number 12 cleft. **A:** Patient with right cleft has orbital hypertelorism and a disturbance of the left medial eyebrow. **B:** Axial view of floor of the anterior cranial fossa with lines demonstrating the axis of the orbit. As the ethmoid air cells widen medially, the orbit is displaced laterally and hypertelorism results.

Number 13 Cleft

Soft-Tissue Involvement

There is typically a paramedian frontal encephalocele, which is located between the nasal bone and the frontal process of the maxilla (Fig. 28.16). The soft-tissue cleft is medial to intact eyelids and eyebrows. The medial end of the eyebrow, however, can be displaced inferiorly. A V-shaped frontal hair projection can also be seen.

Skeletal Involvement

Changes in the cribriform plate are the hallmark of a number 13 cleft. The paramedian bony cleft traverses the frontal bone before coursing along the olfactory groove. There is widening of the olfactory groove, the cribriform plate, and the ethmoid sinus, which results in hypertelorism. A paramedian frontal encephalocele can cause the cribriform plate to be displaced inferiorly, leading to orbital dystopia. Unilateral and bilateral forms of the number 13 cleft exist, similar to most of the other craniofacial clefts. When the cleft is bilateral, some of the most extreme cases of hypertelorism can be seen.

Number 14 Cleft

Soft-Tissue Involvement

Similar to its facial counterpart, the number 0 cleft, the number 14 cleft may produce an agenesis or an overabundance of tissue (Fig. 28.17A; also Fig. 28.2B). When agenesis occurs, orbital hypotelorism is generally seen. Included in this group of craniofacial malformations are the holoprosencephalic disorders, which include cyclopia, ethmocephaly, and cebocephaly. The cranium is typically microcephalic and there is hypotelorism. Malformations of the forebrain are usually proportional to the degree of facial abnormality.

At the other end of the spectrum, hypertelorism is associated with the number 14 cleft. Lateral displacement of the orbits can be produced by midline masses such as a frontonasal encephalocele or a midline frontal encephalocele. Flattening of the glabella and extreme lateral displacement of the inner canthi are also seen. The periorbita, including the eyelids and eyebrows, may be normal or dysplastic. A long midline projection of the frontal hairline marks the superior extent of the soft-tissue features of this midline cranial cleft.

Skeletal Involvement

The frontal encephalocele herniates through a medial frontal defect (Fig. 28.17B). The caudal aspect of the frontal bone is flattened giving the glabellar region a flattened and indistinct position. No pneumatization of the frontal sinus is evident, however, the sphenoid sinus is extensively pneumatized. The crista galli and the perpendicular plate of the ethmoid are bifid and there is an increased distance between the olfactory

FIGURE 28.16. Number 13 cleft. Patient with a facial left cleft that begins as a number 1 cleft through the right alar dome and extends to the frontal bone to cause right-sided telorbitism.

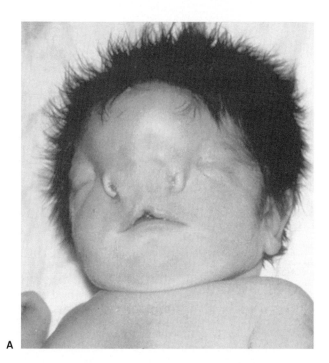
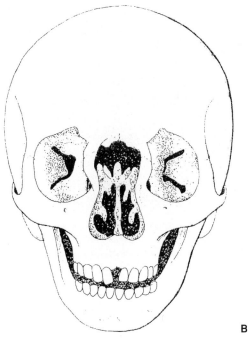

A   **B**

FIGURE 28.17. Number 14 cleft: **A:** Patient with a large frontonasal encephalocele has a true median cleft lip, a wide bifid nose, and orbital hypertelorism. **B:** Skeletal involvement shows displacement of the frontal process of the maxilla, the nasal bones, and medial orbital walls laterally. Often, this large defect is occupied by an encephalocele.

grooves. When the crista galli is severely enlarged, preservation of the olfactory nerve is often not possible during the surgical correction of hypertelorism. The crista galli and ethmoids are widened and caudally displaced. Consequently, the cribriform plate, which is normally located 5 to 10 mm below the level of the orbital roof, can be causally displaced up to 20 mm. The greater and lesser wings of the sphenoid are rotated and result in a relative shortening of the middle cranial fossa. The anterior cranial fossa is upslanting, causing a harlequin eye deformity on plain radiographs.

Hypertelorbitism

With cranial clefts 10 through 14 the distance between the medial canthi may be increased (telecanthus) and the bony interorbital distance may be increased (orbital hypertelorism or hypertelorbitism). The bony interorbital distance is typically measured with a CT scan as the interdacryon (the most medial region of the orbit) distance. Excessive interdacryon distance or hypertelorbitism may be mild (30 to 34 mm), moderate (35 to 39 mm), or severe (>40 mm). In the growing child, excessive distance may be considered anything greater than 25 mm.

Orbital dystopia may be either vertical or horizontal. The midline number 14 cleft may have horizontal or transverse dystopia with the bony orbits displaced laterally (orbital hypertelorism) or medially (hypotelorism), whereas, the lateral number 10 through 13 clefts may have a component of vertical dystopia or asymmetric orbital hypertelorism with the orbits on different horizontal planes.

Correction of hypertelorbitism may be achieved with a facial bipartition or orbital box osteotomy. A facial bipartition involves coronal and gingivobuccal sulcus incisions, a craniotomy for exposure, orbital and midface osteotomies, central wedge ostectomy (between the orbits), rotation of the orbits to an intradacryon distance less than 17 mm and rigid fixa-

tion. Medial canthi bolsters and correction of excessive glabellar soft tissue is necessary. In addition to narrowing the orbital distance, a facial bipartition procedure will also widen a constricted palatal arch. Alternatively, an orbital box osteotomy can be used to narrow orbital distance or correct vertical dystopia, with no effect on the palate or upper dental arch.

Number 30 Cleft

The median cleft of the lower jaw was first described by Couronne. These median clefts of the lower lip and mandible are caudal extensions of the number 14 cranial cleft and number 0 facial cleft.

Soft-Tissue Involvement

Soft-tissue involvement (Fig. 28.18) of this midline cleft may be as mild as a notch in the lower lip. However, often the entire lower lip and chin may be involved. The anterior tongue may be bifid and attached to the split mandible by a dense fibrous band. Ankyloglossia and total absence of the tongue have been reported with midline mandibular clefts.

Skeletal Involvement

Skeletal involvement is typically a cleft between the central incisors extending into the mandibular symphysis. This anomaly is thought to be caused by failure of fusion of the first branchial arch. However, associated neck anomalies are believed to be caused by failure of fusion of other lower branchial arches. For instance, the hyoid bone many times is absent and the thyroid cartilages may fail to completely form. The anterior neck strap muscles are often atrophic and replaced by dense fibrous bands that may restrict chin flexion.

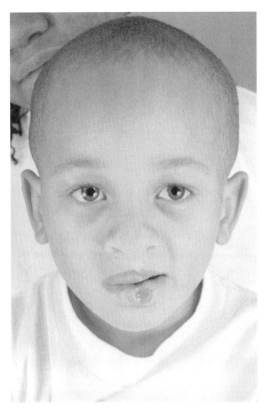

FIGURE 28.18. Number 30 cleft. Patient with a lower lip midline cleft and notching of his mandibular midline alveolar ridge.

TREATMENT OF CRANIOFACIAL CLEFTS

Standardized treatment plans are not possible because of the variety of craniofacial clefts and levels of severity. However, guiding principles are helpful in determining the proper timing and stages for corrective surgery. **If the malformation is severe, or if there are functional problems, like ocular exposure, surgery is performed early. If the malformation is mild, surgery should be delayed. During infancy (3 to 12 months of age), cranial defects and soft-tissue clefts are corrected. Midface reconstruction and bone grafting are performed in older children (6 to 9 years of age). Orthognathic procedures are delayed until skeletal maturity (14 years of age or older).**

Surgical techniques used for correction of craniofacial clefts depend on the anatomic regions involved. The original descriptions for correction of soft-tissue craniofacial clefts involved the use of Z-plasty flaps. Presently, flaps are designed to respect aesthetic units by leaving scars along aesthetic lines. For the nose (as in cleft numbers 0 thru 3), the cleft is excised, nasal cartilages are repaired with the use of cartilage grafts or composite grafts, and local rotation flaps are used for alar retraction. Secondary nasal reconstruction may be performed with cantilevered cranial bone grafts. For the upper lip (as in cleft numbers 0 thru 5), correction of cleft defects involves aligning the vermilion and restoring the muscular continuity, as in common cleft lip repair. If the cleft is lateral to the philtral column,

the intervening tissue is excised. For the oral commissure (as in cleft number 7), the lateral element is closed in a straight line. The medial aspect is closed with a Z-plasty so that the vertical limb is along the nasolabial fold. For the lower lip (as in cleft number 30), V-excision and layered closure is performed.

For the mandibular reconstruction (as in cleft combinations 6, 7, and 8 in both craniofacial microsomia and Treacher Collins syndrome), costochondral grafts may be used for severe deformities and distraction osteogenesis may be used for moderate deformities in mid-childhood (6 to 8 years of age). Mild maxillary deformities should be corrected as an adult with a Le Fort I osteotomy with or without a concomitant mandibular procedure.

Surgical correction of the periorbital region is necessary in many craniofacial clefts. For the eye, urgent intervention is necessary if the eye is exposed and at risk for corneal ulceration. However, early reconstructive procedures for globe protection must be balanced to allow enough eye opening to prevent deprivation amblyopia. For the eyelid, "lid-switch" transposition flaps are used for skin/muscle deficiencies. Accurate repositioning of the medial canthus may be performed with transnasal wiring. Lateral canthopexies are sometimes needed to achieve symmetry. Palatal grafts may be used for lower lid conjunctival lining. Correction of number 8 (lateral eye) clefts are performed with Z-plasty flaps. For the lacrimal apparatus, disruption of the canalicular system may be corrected with silastic stents or formal dacryocystorhinostomy. For the orbit, bone grafts are used to correct dystopia or restore continuity. As mentioned above, orbital dystopia is corrected with a facial bipartition, orbital box osteotomy, or subcranial Le Fort III.

Conclusion

Craniofacial clefts are highly variable and range from a mild, barely noticeable form fruste (microform), to disfiguring, complete defects of the skeletal and soft tissue. Tessier's description of craniofacial clefts based on bony and soft tissue landmarks provides a classification that has been validated by the neurometric theory of neuroembryology.

Suggested Readings

Carstens M, Development of the facial midline. *J Craniofac Surg.* 2002;13:129–187.

Converse JM, Horowitz LS, Coccaro PJ, et al. The corrective treatment of the skeleton asymmetry in hemifacial microsomia. *Plast Reconstr Surg.* 1973;52: 221.

Converse JM, Ransohoff J, Mathews ES, et al Ocular hypertelorism and pseudohypertelorism. Advances in surgical treatment. *Plast Reconstr Surg.* 1970;45:1.

David DJ, Moore MH, Cooter RD. Tessier clefts revisited with a third dimension. *Cleft Palate J.* 1989;26:163.

Gorlin RJ, Jue KL, Jacobsen U, et al. Oculoauriculovertebral syndrome. *Pediatr J.* 1963;63:991.

Kawamoto HK Jr. The kaleidoscopic world of rare craniofacial clefts: order out of chaos (Tessier classification). *Clin Plast Surg.* 1976;3:529.

Kawamoto HK Jr. Rare craniofacial clefts. In: McCarthy JG, ed. *Plastic Surgery.* Philadelphia: WB Saunders; 1990:2922–2973.

Longaker MT, Lipshutz GS, Kawamoto HK Jr. Reconstruction of Tessier no. 4 clefts revisited. *Plast Reconstr Surg.* 1997;99:1501.

Obwegeser HL. Correction of skeletal anomalies of otomandibular dysostosis. *J Maxillofac Surg.* 1974;2:73.

Tessier P. Anatomical classification of facial, cranio-facial and latero-facial clefts. *J Maxillofac Surg.* 1976;4:69.

CHAPTER 29 ■ MISCELLANEOUS CRANIOFACIAL CONDITIONS
Fibrous dysplasia, moebius syndrome, romberg's syndrome, treacher collins syndrome, dermoid cyst, neurofibromatosis

ROBERT J. HAVLIK

This chapter includes a diverse spectrum of disorders that do not "fit" together with other conditions in plastic surgery, or for that matter, with other conditions in medicine. As such, they represent the "outliers." With the exception of neurofibromatosis, they are distinctly uncommon.

FIBROUS DYSPLASIA

Fibrous dysplasia is a benign disorder of bone that affects both the axial and the craniomaxillofacial skeleton. Fibrous dysplasia is not "classically" a congenital disorder, as it is not usually evident at birth, but becomes clinically evident during late childhood or adolescence. It occurs sporadically, and genetic transmission has not been documented. Fibrous dysplasia has been traditionally divided into three main categories: monostotic (or monocystic) fibrous dysplasia, polyostotic fibrous dysplasia, and the McCune-Albright syndrome. The majority of patients (~70% to 80%) present with a single area of bony involvement (monostotic or monocystic fibrous dysplasia), whereas the balance of patients present with multiple sites of bone involvement (polyostotic fibrous dysplasia). Of the patients with polyostotic fibrous dysplasia (20% to 30%), approximately 3% present with a triad of polyostotic fibrous dysplasia, precocious puberty, and skin pigmentation known as the McCune-Albright syndrome. This skin pigmentation presents as "café-au-lait" spots present with a highly irregular border, described as being similar to the coastline of Maine. In addition to this classic triad, McCune-Albright syndrome is also associated with several different endocrine disorders, all caused by autonomous hormonal overproduction, such as pituitary adenomas secreting growth hormone, hyperthyroid goiters, and adrenal hyperplasia.

The craniomaxillofacial structures are involved in approximately 25% of cases with monostotic fibrous dysplasia and up to 50% of cases with polyostotic involvement. The most common presentation in the craniofacial skeleton is that of a painless, enlarging mass of bone. The maxilla is the bone most often involved, followed in frequency by the frontal bone, but all bones of the craniomaxillofacial skeleton may show involvement. The clinical manifestations of fibrous dysplasia include expansive growth leading to aesthetic and functional compromise. Maxillary lesions can lead to dental malocclusions, tilting of the occlusal plane, or significant facial deformity and asymmetry. In lesions with orbital involvement, visual disturbance, ocular proptosis, and orbital dystopia can occur. In lesions with sphenoid involvement, blindness may occur as a result of impingement on the optic nerve.

The difficulty in the diagnosis of fibrous dysplasia varies with the extent of presentation of the disease. The polyostotic and McCune-Albright forms of fibrous dysplasia are relatively easily diagnosed based upon clinical and radiologic investigation, whereas establishing the diagnosis of the monostotic form is more difficult because of the number of other important lesions that are included in the differential diagnosis. In the axial skeleton, the lesions frequently appear as well-circumscribed radiolucent lesions with a thin sclerotic periphery. In contrast, the lesions of the craniofacial skeleton are more poorly defined and more radiopaque. Bone biopsy in many areas of the axial skeleton in fibrous dysplasia is generally avoided, especially where the risk of pathologic fracture is high. However, in the mandible, where monostotic involvement is most frequent in the craniomaxillofacial skeleton and therefore there is the greatest difficulty differentiating this from other solitary bony lesions, bone biopsy has not been reported to cause a pathologic fracture in fibrous dysplasia. Malignant degeneration of fibrous dysplasia has been reported to occur in 0.5% of cases with monostotic involvement, and in up to 4% of cases with McCune-Albright syndrome. Notably, the most frequent site for sarcomatous degeneration is the craniofacial skeleton.

Pathogenesis

The basis of this disorder is centered on a structural and functional change in the cellular transduction mechanism involving G-proteins. The G-protein is a membrane-bound intracellular signaling mechanism that carries the message of extracellular hormone into the cell. The G-proteins themselves have an intrinsic activity that causes hydrolysis of guanosine triphosphate (GTP) to guanosine diphosphate (GDP). In fibrous dysplasia, the G-protein has a decreased ability to hydrolyze GTP, resulting in the G-protein remaining in an activated state, leading to continued stimulation of cyclic adenosine monophosphate (cAMP) and multiple other effects. Significantly, many of the adrenal, pituitary, thyroid, and gonadal cells of patients with McCune-Albright syndrome show the same mutations, thereby leading to increased "ON" activity, and constitutively increased hormone production.

The somatic mutation theory implies that fibrous dysplasia arises from the development of cellular mosaicism. It has been postulated that the timing at which this mutation occurs may determine the clinical extent of the disease. In other words, a mutation that occurs late in embryologic development will lead to a decreased number of cells with the mutation and to the development of monostotic bone involvement. In contrast, a mutation that occurs in early embryologic development would lead to a larger number of afflicted cells and multicentric involvement (polyostotic fibrous dysplasia). If the mutation occurs early enough in development, it may lead to the involvement of additional tissues (endocrine disorders, McCune-Albright syndrome, etc.). As noted above, there are no documented cases of genetic transmission of fibrous dysplasia, and it may be that a germline mutation, or a mutation that occurs early enough in embryologic development, is a lethal mutation.

Treatment

Treatment of fibrous dysplasia in the craniofacial skeleton is determined by the functional or aesthetic problems created by the disease process. The mere existence of fibrous dysplasia does not mandate treatment. In bones of the axial skeleton, the expansile process, coupled with cortical resorption, can lead to decreased structural strength and pathologic fracture. This is seldom the case in the craniomaxillofacial skeleton, and indications for treatment are more frequently related to aesthetic imbalance, facial disfigurement, distortion of the functional occlusion, orbital dystopia, ocular proptosis, and impingement on neural foramina. Impingement on the optic nerve has led to visual disturbance and blindness.

Older publications suggest that fibrous dysplasia will "burn out" in the postpubertal adolescent state. Unfortunately, there is no data to support this contention.

Surgical treatment is designed to counter the effects of mass expansion and the consequent deformity that occurs in the facial skeleton. **In most cases, surgery of the craniofacial skeleton consists of either a contour reduction of the afflicted area, or resection and replacement of the afflicted bone.** Contour reduction is a more limited operation; however, it is accompanied by a higher likelihood of recurrence. Resection and replacement overrides cure. A decision is made regarding the rate of tumor growth, or the "aggressiveness" of this benign process. Resection is followed by reconstruction with either alloplastic materials or bone autograft.

In the cranial vault, the frontal bone is the most frequently involved bone, followed by the sphenoid bone. The case illustrated in Figure 29.1 used both resection and contour reduction techniques for treating areas of hyperostotic fibrous dysplasia in the right fronto-orbital region and the right parietal region. The resection and cranial bone autograft reconstruction was performed in the right orbit and frontal bone, where the potential problems with recurrent tumor and repeat resection would be more problematic. The parietal bone was completely removed, and contour reduction was performed down to the level of cortical plate. When fibrous dysplasia involves the skull base, the surgeon must assess the risk of continued expansion versus the risk of resection and the potential outcomes of the planned treatment.

Fibrous dysplasia of the orbit raises several special considerations. First, the mass effect of bone growth can lead to dystopia and visual disturbances. The potential problems of recurrence in this area, particularly with the potentially more difficult surgery in the recurrent field from scarring, swing the balance toward resection of the afflicted bone and replacement.

Second, specific to the orbit is the concern that growth of fibrous dysplasia can lead to optic nerve compression, subsequently leading to visual change and blindness. Visual loss has been cited as the most common neurologic complication of fibrous dysplasia involving the skull.

Although optic nerve decompression in patients with fibrous dysplasia of the sphenoid surrounding the optic canal and with documented visual changes is widely accepted, "prophylactic" decompression of the optic nerve is generally not recommended. Furthermore, decompression after visual decrement or visual loss may not restore the visual deficit (1). The risks involved with surgical decompression of the nerve include a lack of improvement in vision, which occurs in 5% to 33% of cases, and blindness resulting from the surgery (1,2).

Fibrous dysplasia involving the maxilla leads to overgrowth, aesthetic irregularities, tilting of the occlusal plane, and other occlusal irregularities. Successful surgical treatment relies on two key outcomes: an acceptable aesthetic result and an acceptable and functional occlusal result. If the dentition is to be maintained, surgical correction can be obtained by either contour reduction or resection of the maxilla in the plane above the Le Fort I level, coupled with reconstruction of the orbital floor and free tissue transfer for obliteration of the defect. The alternative treatment is formal maxillectomy and reconstruction with free tissue transfer. Treatment planning involves maintaining the existing dentition or a suitable alternative—either reconstructive or prosthodontic.

Fibrous dysplasia of the mandible presents as a mass lesion with cortical expansion. Because the presentation with mandibular disease is frequently monostotic, bone biopsy may be indicated to establish or confirm the diagnosis. As noted previously, biopsy of the mandible can be safely accomplished in fibrous dysplasia without a significant risk of fracture. Depending on the severity of the involvement, either contour reduction or resection can be performed. In lesions involving the ramus in which the temporomandibular joint (TMJ) is spared, every effort should be made to plan the resection and reconstruction using the existing joint. In larger lesions, resection of the tumor with free fibula reconstruction is a reasonable approach (see Chapter 41).

Until recently, surgical treatment was the only option for the treatment of fibrous dysplasia. Recently, several small series have been published using medical therapy with pamidronate, an aminobisphosphonate. This treatment has resulted in an increase in bone mineral density and radiologic signs of healing with the thickening of cortical bone in some cases. In many cases, there has also been a significant decrease in pain with pamidronate therapy. **Radiation therapy is contraindicated because of an increased propensity for malignant transformation.**

MOEBIUS SYNDROME

Moebius syndrome is a rare disorder characterized by paralysis of the cranial nerves. Classically, Moebius syndrome is defined by paralysis of the sixth and seventh cranial nerves resulting in a masklike facies, incapable of animation, and an inability to laterally deviate the eyes (abducens palsy) (3). Facial expression forms a fundamental and important component of human communication and socialization, and the inability to show a facial response to verbal and nonverbal communication is a devastating deficiency (see Chapter 40). In the United Kingdom, there were approximately 90 cases of Moebius syndrome in a population of 50 million people, yielding a prevalence of 1 in 550,000 (4). By extrapolation, approximately 500 cases would be expected in the United States. In some publications, Moebius syndrome is defined more broadly, including

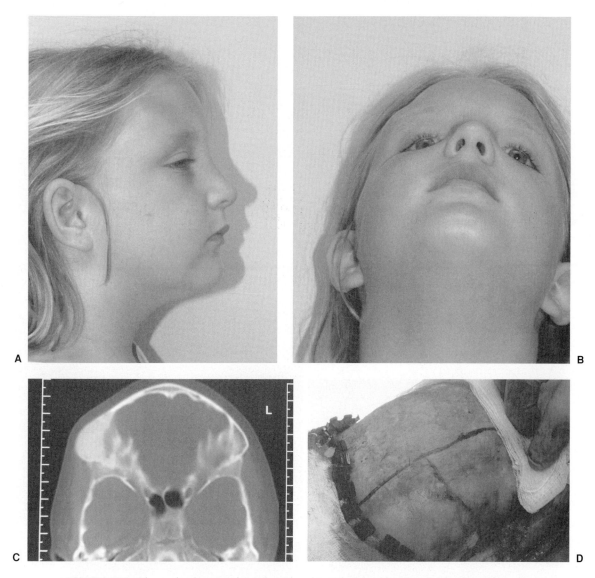

FIGURE 29.1. Fibrous dysplasia involving the right orbit, right frontal bone, and right parietal bone. **A:** Pre-operative lateral view. **B:** Preoperative "worm's eye" view. **C:** Preoperative axial computed tomography (CT) image. **D:** Intraoperative view showing increased density of fibrous dysplasia involving right frontal and right parietal bones. **E:** Planned split-graft donor site using metallic template fabricated in F (*illustration by Min Li, MD*). **F:** Intraoperative view following completed resection of tumor and reconstruction of orbital roof and supraorbital bar using split cranial bone grafts from left parietal bone and contour reduction of right parietal bone. **G:** Completed reconstruction using contour reduction of right parietal bone. **H:** Three-year postoperative "bird's-eye" three-dimensional CT scan showing symmetry of reconstruction and no evidence of recurrence. **I:** Three-year postoperative frontal view. **J:** Three-year postoperative "worm's-eye" view.

patients with additional facial nerve palsies. Involvement of nearly all of the facial nerves has been documented, but the third, ninth, tenth, and twelfth nerves are most commonly involved (3). In addition to the characteristic facies associated with the sixth and seventh nerve palsies, ptosis, nystagmus, or strabismus may be present, and epicanthal folds are frequent (Fig. 29.2). The nose typically has a high, broad bridge, and this increased breadth extends to the nasal tip. The mouth opening is typically small. In addition, there can be hypoplasia of the tongue, either unilaterally or bilaterally. There frequently is poor palatal mobility, poor suck, inefficient swallowing, and drooling. The mandible tends to be hypoplastic. These factors can contribute to difficulty feeding during the first year of life, frequently leading to poor growth. A coarse voice and speech impairment can be present, although hearing is usually normal. As the child grows, the ability to open the mouth and feed

tends to improve. The facial paralysis and masklike facies tend to bias early estimates of psychomotor activity. Only 10% to 15% of children are mentally retarded (3).

Etiology and Pathogenesis

The etiology of this disorder has not been elucidated. It occurs sporadically and, in cases of "classic Moebius syndrome" involving only sixth and seventh cranial nerves, genetic transmission is rare. For Moebius syndrome, four separate and distinct, although not mutually exclusive, pathogenetic mechanisms have been advanced: (a) aplasia/hypoplasia of the cranial nerve nuclei; (b) destruction of the cranial nerve nuclei; (c) peripheral nerve abnormalities; and (d) primary myopathy.

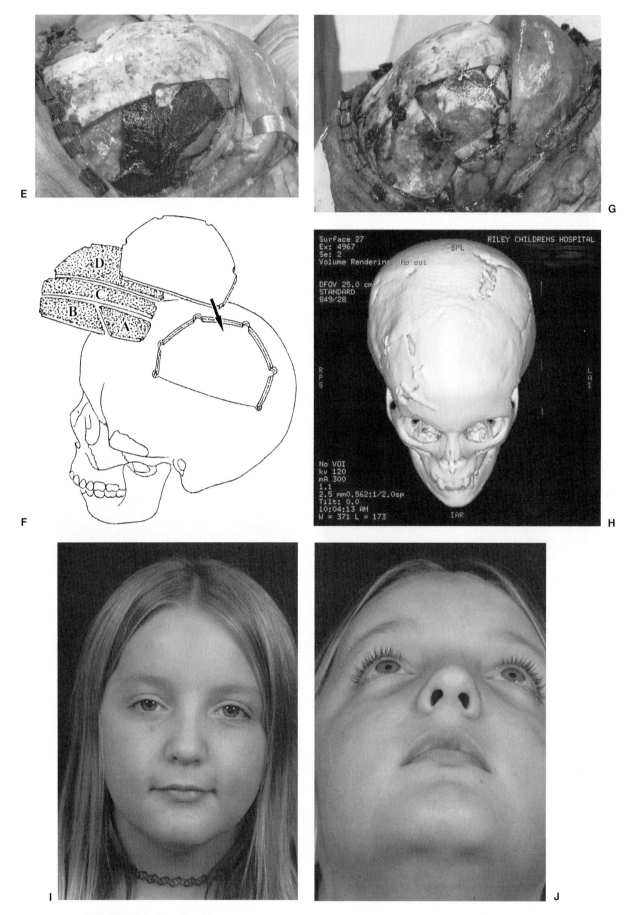

FIGURE 29.1. *(Continued).*

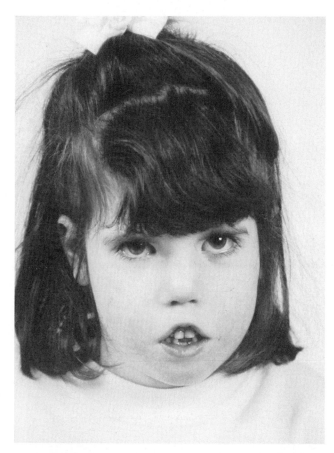

FIGURE 29.2. Moebius syndrome with typical mask-like facies and downslanted oral commissures. *(Photo courtesy of Ron Zuker, MD.)*

Operative findings and postmortem examinations have supported each of these four mechanisms (3,5).

Treatment

Treatment has progressed more rapidly than our understanding of this rare disorder, and focuses on one of the most socially devastating problems of this disorder—the inability to show a facial response. Facial reanimation surgery is effective in restoring function in many different etiologies of facial nerve deficits, and this treatment has been extended to Moebius syndrome. **Zuker et al. have reported excellent results with microvascular free tissue transfer of the gracilis muscle to the face, and this procedure represents the state of the art (5).** Although they initially used the hypoglossal or accessory nerve, they have refined their technique to use the branch of the trigeminal nerve to the masseter muscle as the motor nerve of choice (see Chapter 40). This motor nerve has the advantage of being largely spared in Moebius syndrome, and the function can reliably be assessed preoperatively. The nerve is located in proximity to the transfer, in the region of the sigmoid notch of the mandible. Furthermore, the innate function of this motor nerve is relatively synergistic with the desired posttransplant function of facial animation. The surgery is accomplished in two separate stages, one stage for each side of the face. Zuker et al. report a series of 10 patients who had an average movement of their oral commissures following bilateral microvascular transfers of 1.37 cm, allowing for meaningful and deliberate facial animation (5). In addition, the children showed improvement with

drooling and an improved ability to drink. The surgery also has a definite benefit on speech.

ROMBERG DISEASE (PROGRESSIVE HEMIFACIAL ATROPHY)

Progressive hemifacial atrophy (PHA) is widely known by the eponym of Romberg disease. In an era of molecular and genetic analysis, PHA remains as perhaps the most enigmatic of the craniofacial disorders. The etiology of this disorder remains unknown.

Clinical Findings

PHA may involve any or all of the facial tissues, typically involving skin and subcutaneous tissue, but also potentially muscle, cartilage, and bone. Pensler et al. (6) have reviewed the clinical course in 41 patients and report that the initial presentation involved the distribution of V_1 (first division of trigeminal nerve) in 35% of cases, the distribution of V_2 in 45% of cases, and the distribution of V_3 in the remaining 20% of cases. Either side of the face is equally likely to be involved, and involvement is unilateral in 95% of cases. The initial presentation typically involves the skin and may be quite subtle, sometimes including pigment changes in which there may be either a brownish or bluish discoloration, or even hypopigmentation. Alternatively, the disorder may first present as a limited area of atrophy of the subcutaneous fat. A striking archetypal presentation often includes a nearly vertical linear depression of the forehead extending into the eyebrow and frontal hairline, known as the *coup de sabre*, or "cut of the saber" (Fig. 29.3). This "clinical sign" was thought to be pathognomonic for Romberg disease, but can also been noted in linear scleroderma, a subtype of localized scleroderma, leading to a potential overlap of these diagnoses.

PHA is not a congenital disorder, with the typical onset being in the first or second decade of life. The hallmark of the disorder is a slowly progressive course, with an "active phase" of disease characterized by involution, or "wasting away" of the skin, subcutaneous tissue, and muscle. This "active phase" lasts from 2 to 10 years. The subcutaneous tissue is the most severely involved, followed by substantial involvement of the skin and muscle. The facial musculature undergoes thinning, but usually maintains sufficient power to animate the face. The muscle involvement commonly includes atrophy of the tongue and palatal tissues. Patients with an early age of onset (during facial growth), are much more likely to have significant skeletal involvement. Pensler et al. (6) report that 65% of their patients had osseous involvement, and **they found a strong correlation between the age at onset and the degree of bone hypoplasia.** However, in their review, they noted no correlation between the other findings of severity of soft-tissue atrophy, the duration of the disease, the initial site of skin changes, and the eventual location or magnitude of the skeletal involvement.

In cases where the disease occurs during the first decade of life, there can be profound skeletal hypoplasia of the afflicted side of the face. This stands in distinct contrast to those cases that present initially in the second decade of life. In these cases, there is typically limited impact on the facial skeleton, with the gross morphologic changes being confined to skin and subcutaneous tissue. The patient in Figure 29.3 had disease onset at 10 years of age. There is clinical involvement of the skin, eyebrow, and periocular tissues. There is clearly hypoplasia or atrophy of the right nasal sidewall and cartilaginous atrophy of the nasal ala. Her dental development and occlusal relations show no signs of involvement. In view of this strong correlation

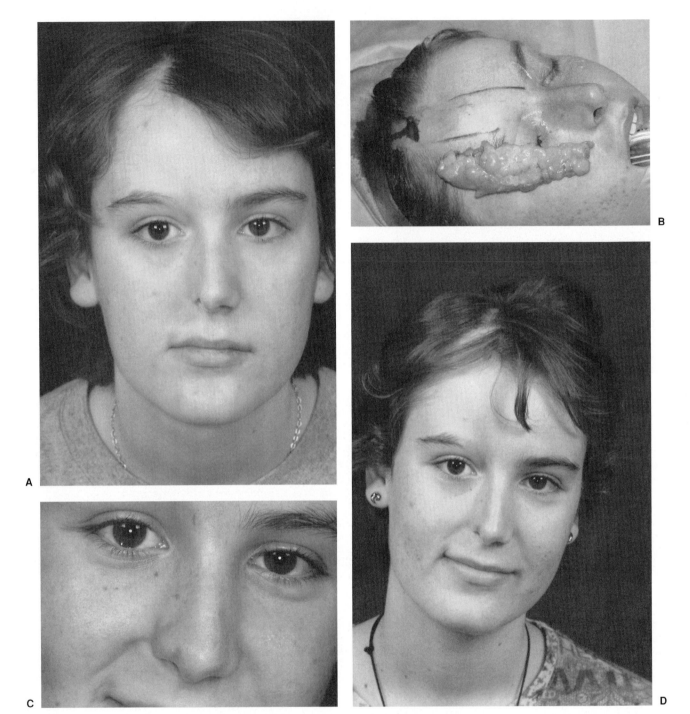

FIGURE 29.3. Progressive hemifacial atrophy in a 14-year-old adolescent with onset at age 10 years. **A:** Frontal view illustrates large area of alopecia of scalp, mild soft-tissue depression, loss of medial eyebrow, and vertical deficiency of right alar rim consistent with a mild *coup de sabre*-type deformity. The nose not only shows vertical deficiency, but also thinning and collapse. Radiographic evaluation revealed no evidence of skeletal irregularity. **B:** Intraoperative view showing dermal fat graft in position for grafting soft-tissue deficiency of forehead. An ear cartilage conchal bowl composite graft was used to reconstruct the alar deficiency. **C:** Initial postoperative result of ala reconstruction. Unfortunately, she developed a late *Pseudomonas* infection, and although she has a significantly improved patency of her internal and external nasal valves, the vertical correction has diminished as seen below. **D:** Postoperative result. The dermal fat graft initially led to significant overcorrection of the deficiency, but now yields a favorable result.

of the severity of this disorder with the age of onset, it is unclear whether the facial skeleton actually undergoes atrophy. More likely the bone fails to develop fully in the field of overlying atrophy of skin and subcutaneous tissue. The skeletal "atrophy" in PHA is more accurately termed *hypoplasia*.

In early onset cases, the skeletal involvement often involves the mandible and midface, with concomitant implications for the occlusal relationships and facial appearance. There can be hypoplasia of the mandible, including significant vertical undergrowth of the ramus and a deficiency in posterior facial height. The mandible may also show significant sagittal undergrowth. The maxilla may also manifest both vertical and sagittal undergrowth in the sagittal plane. Because the involvement is unilateral, profound tilting of the occlusal plane develops. When PHA involves the V_1 distribution of the nerve, the periocular tissues are typically involved as well. In these cases, enophthalmos is a frequent finding. Pensler et al., based on radiographic orbital measurements, suggest that the enophthalmos is not caused by a skeletal change in the orbital volume, but that it is related to atrophy of the periorbital soft tissues (6).

PHA can be associated with many other findings, including areas of skin and subcutaneous atrophy elsewhere on the body distinct from the face. The disorder is associated with nervous system dysfunction, including Horner syndrome, trigeminal neuralgia, and unilateral mydriasis. Central nervous system involvement has been reported in smaller series by several authors, ranging from magnetic resonance imaging (MRI) changes to seizure disorders. However, the relative paucity and inconsistency of data at this point preclude any definitive correlation between these reports.

Etiology

The etiology of PHA is unknown. PHA does not show any genetic predilection, is found in all races, and there is no evidence of a hereditary basis. It does occur more frequently in females in most series. Patients will frequently remember an "initiating event" in PHA, and the onset of the disorder is often linked to an episode of trauma or infection. However, it is unclear whether this is simply an event that calls attention to a subtle area of initial clinical involvement, or whether there are true pathogenetic associations. Traditionally, three theories have been advocated for the etiology of Romberg disease: the infection hypothesis, the trigeminal-peripheral neuritis hypothesis, and the sympathetic hypothesis. The infectious hypothesis was historically linked to an irritation of nerves. In the current era of a new understanding of infectious agents (viruses, prions, mad cow disease, chronic wasting disease of deer, etc.), the infectious hypothesis may be remain a tenable etiology until a definitive understanding of this disorder is truly established. The trigeminal-peripheral neuritis hypothesis suggests a neuritis involving the trigeminal nerve, and is supported by episodes of pain in the involved areas prior to the onset of tissue involution. The sympathetic hypothesis is based on an association of Horner syndrome, pilomotor reflex changes, unilateral mydriasis, vasomotor disorders, unilateral migraine, and perspiration disorders. Based on current evidence, no definitive etiology has been established.

The insightful work of Pensler et al. has provided some enhanced understanding. First, in their clinical review, as previously noted, they found no evidence of sensory, sympathetic, parasympathetic, or sudomotor dysfunction. Muscles of mastication and facial expression were found to be fully functional. Biopsies revealed epidermal atrophy and a variable perivascular mononuclear cell infiltrate, with morphologic characteristics of lymphocytes and monocytes, that were grouped around dermal neurovascular bundles. Many of the venules were noted to have striking degenerative alteration in the lining epithelium with reduplication of the basal lamina. Significantly, they also noted that elastic fibers were present and morphologically intact (in contrast to linear scleroderma). They interpret these findings as lymphocytic neurovasculitis, and they advance this theory as a pathogenetic mechanism.

Understanding the pathogenesis of this disease is complicated further by the apparent overlap between the disorder of linear scleroderma and PHA. It is very likely that many of the cases that have historically been termed Romberg disease may include cases of linear scleroderma, as differentiating the two clinically is difficult, if not impossible. Linear scleroderma may also show monocytic infiltrates. The only finding that has been reported as useful to differentiate these two disorders is the absence of elastic fibers in the scleroderma group, and their preservation in the PHA group (4).

Treatment

Many surgeons will defer treatment until the disease "burns out," or reaches a stable plateau phase. For milder asymmetry and atrophy of the skin and subcutaneous tissue, injection of collagen and hyaluronic acid derivatives or fat injection may provide some short-term benefit.

For small areas of asymmetry, dermal grafts, fat grafts, or dermal-fascial-fat grafts are considered. These can be tailored to smaller defects and provide an acceptable improvement with a limited operative approach and limited operative time and risk (Fig. 29.3). However, because of the variability in graft survival, overcorrection is necessary. In addition, there is typically a postoperative period that is characterized by induration. **Overall, the experience in the literature with nonvascularized transfer of fat tissue, particularly with larger transfers, has been inconsistent.**

Microvascular free tissue transfer is the gold standard in reconstruction of patients with Romberg disease. Upton et al. (7) reported microvascular transfer of scapular and parascapular flaps in 30 patients, five of whom were patients with Romberg disease. They used long fat-fascial extensions with these transfers to fill isolated areas. They noted no postoperative atrophy in the 30 flaps, but they did note that in patients who gained weight, the flap volume increased. In addition, there were isolated areas, such as the upper lip, that tended to be undercorrected. They also noted no evidence that free tissue transfer altered the natural history of the disease process in PHA.

In children with the early onset of the disorder, there is often distortion of the orbit and the zygomaticomaxillary complex, leading to vertical orbital dystopia. Depending on the severity, this can be corrected either through corrective osteotomies and vertical repositioning of the orbit, or through bone grafting of the orbital floor. Involvement of the V_2 and V_3 distributions of the trigeminal nerve can lead to severe maxillary and mandibular asymmetries, with distortion of both the facial midline and occlusal plane. **Bimaxillary surgery is necessary to correct of the occlusal plane.**

TREACHER COLLINS SYNDROME

Treacher Collins syndrome, or mandibulofacial dysostosis, is a craniofacial disorder that has an incidence of between 1 in 25,000 births and 1 in 50,000 births and is characterized by a range of clinical presentations. The full clinical presentation is characterized by hypoplasia/aplasia of the body and arch of the zygoma, a significantly increased facial convexity, mandibular hypoplasia, a retrusive chin with increased vertical height, and external and middle-ear anomalies. **A key distinguishing feature of this entity is that it is bilateral and symmetrical.** The periorbital soft tissues show an antimongoloid slant of the palpebral fissures. The lower eyelid is hypoplastic with a coloboma located at the junction of the medial two-thirds and lateral third of the lower lid. The deficiency involves both the skin of the eyelid, and the cartilage of the tarsal plate eyelid also lacks eyelashes typically over the medial third. These findings, along with the hypoplastic zygoma, lead to a striking clinical appearance (Fig. 29.4). The nose is broadened in the midnasal dorsum, and can have a slightly elongated appearance. The midface is

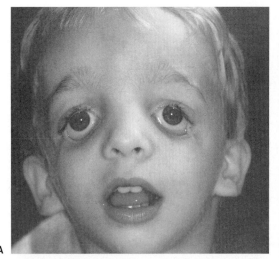

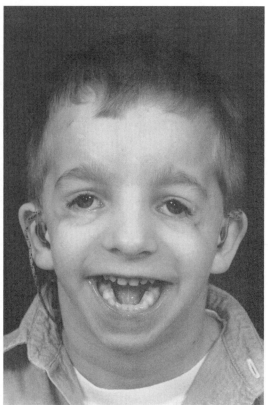

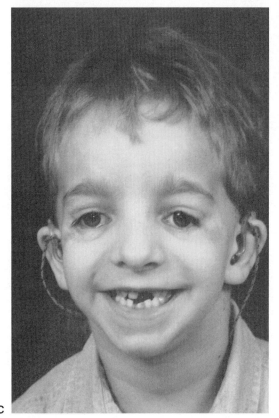

FIGURE 29.4. Treacher Collins syndrome. **A:** Characteristic facies with orbital findings, including vertically deficient lower lid, lower eyelid coloboma, downslanting palpebral fissures (antimongoloid slant), and hypoplastic malar eminences. **B:** Five-year-old male with result of lid-switch procedure with conjunctival grafting and canthopexy performed at age 3 years. **C:** Approximately 1-year result after dermal fat grafting shows improved contour in the malar eminence in 7-year-old.

hypoplastic, particularly at the level of the zygomatic body and arch, but also in the maxillae. The mandible is characteristically hypoplastic, with a chin that has the unusual combination of increased vertical height and deficiency in sagittal projection. An anterior open bite is often present. This combination exacerbates the overall clinical appearance of a facial profile that is much too convex. Cephalometric analysis has revealed that this facial convexity is attributable to the mandibular hypoplasia and position, as the relationship between this midface and the anterior cranial base is essentially within the normal range (SNA angle). In addition, the occlusal plane tends to be quite steep, with a clockwise rotation of the mandibular plane (hypoplastic posteriorly with decreased posterior facial height). There are characteristically significant deformities of both the external and middle ear present, with a low-lying hairline with

tongue-shaped caudal extensions of hair-bearing scalp in the preauricular areas.

Pathogenesis

Treacher Collins is an autosomal dominant disorder, with a markedly variable penetrance. While up to 60% of cases are thought to arise de novo, the variability in penetrance occurs at both the interfamilial and the intrafamilial level. All known cases of Treacher Collins result from mutations in the *TCOF 1* gene. The *TCOF 1* gene has been mapped to the 5q31.3–5q33.3 gene locus. Identification of family specific mutations and tracing these specific mutations through family pedigrees shows that the actual number of cases arising de novo may be less, and the familial transmission rate may actually be higher, as family members previously thought to be unaffected in fact may show the genetic mutation.

Treatment

Patients with Treacher Collins syndrome often require a life-saving tracheostomy at birth. The cranial vault may show a mild deficiency in bitemporal diameter, but this is never of the magnitude to merit surgical intervention. The orbital changes, however, are striking and pathognomonic for this disorder. The orbital changes are consistent with the hypoplasia of the zygoma that characterizes the disorder. Treatment goals include correction of both the lower eyelid deficiency and the zygomatic deficiency.

No perfect procedure exists for the lower eyelids. The cutaneous deficiency can then be addressed through a lid-switch operation. The lid-switch operation, with a laterally based banner flap consisting of skin and orbicularis oculi muscle, has the advantage of providing vascularized tissue with an excellent skin color match (Fig. 29.4). The lid switch also has a salutary benefit of vertical repositioning of the lateral canthus contributing to the correction of the antimongoloid slant of the palpebral fissure. This flap, however, may become edematous and remain "prominent" for an indefinite period of time. It is of critical importance that the cutaneous reconstructions be coupled with adequate conjunctival release with a widely offset incision and appropriate conjunctival reconstruction.

Several different techniques have been described for reconstruction of the hypoplastic zygoma, including split-thickness and full-thickness cranial bone grafts, vascularized calvarial grafts based on a temporalis muscle pedicle, and rib grafts. The cranial bone grafts are typically cut as one-piece T-shaped grafts that serve to reconstruct both the body of the zygoma, the zygomatic arch, and the inferior orbital rim. Technical problems include the paucity of soft tissue in the malar eminence that is available for coverage of the skeletal reconstruction, a soft-tissue problem exacerbated by the net volume expansion required with the reconstruction. Bone grafts in this area of craniofacial skeleton eventually undergo resorption. This may be partially a result of the overlying soft-tissue "matrix" in this disorder, and partially attributable to the inherent tendency of bone grafts to undergo resorption with revascularization. The deficiency of soft-tissue coverage may also influence the problems with graft revascularization.

A component of the controversy regarding reconstruction of the zygoma includes consideration of the timing of reconstruction of the zygoma and the age of the patient. Posnick et al. (8) have reported favorable results with reconstruction of the zygoma using full-thickness bicortical grafts for reconstruction of the zygoma at an age of 5 to 7 years. An alternative in the younger child about to start school is the use of dermal fat grafts to help correct the soft-tissue deficiency and effectively camouflage the skeletal deficiency (Fig. 29.4). Siebert has employed bilateral soft-tissue free flaps to camouflage the skeletal deficiency with results that rival or exceed any skeletal reconstruction (9).

The nasal deformity in Treacher Collins includes a broad midnasal dorsal hump, further accentuated by the retrusive chin. The nasal dorsum is correctable through conventional rhinoplasty approaches and procedures, with the usual caveats regarding avoiding airway obstruction.

Approximately one-third of Treacher Collins patients have a cleft of the palate. Strict attention is directed to ventilatory status before considering repair of the cleft palate, to avoid ventilatory obstruction. In many cases, this requires correction of the hypoplastic mandible or tracheostomy prior to attempts at closure of the palatal cleft.

Ears

The ears are characteristically involved in Treacher Collins syndrome, and this includes the auricle, the external auditory canal, and the middle ear. Both left and right sides are afflicted, and the deficiencies tend to be symmetrical. Middle-ear malformations are common, and include aplasia, hypoplasia, and/or ankylosis of the ossicles. Most patients (96%) have a moderate or greater degree of hearing loss. This is critical to recognize and treat appropriately as adequate hearing is essential for speech development and speech production. External hearing assistance through hearing aids is often necessary (see Chapter 30).

The external ear deformities pose unique problems. First, the low hairline and "tongue" of hair-bearing scalp that descends in the preauricular area often precludes reconstruction with native mastoid skin and requires the alternative use of a temporoparietal fascial flap with skin graft. Second, the external auricle reconstruction must be coordinated with the mandibular reconstruction and the reconstruction of the zygoma. If there is inadequate non–hair-bearing mastoid skin for ear reconstruction, as is often the case, incisions in proximity to the ear must be carefully planned to preserve the superficial temporal artery. If there is favorable mastoid skin for reconstruction, no incisions should be planned prior to placement of the cartilage framework, as these violate the blood supply and can contribute to skin breakdown above the tension of a cartilage framework reconstruction. **Because the mandibular reconstruction must take into consideration obstructive airway concerns and the timing of palatal closure, careful planning and coordination of each step in the child's reconstruction is necessary.**

Mandible

The mandibular deformity in Treacher Collins syndrome is extremely variable and can include the entire spectrum of mandibular hypoplasia. There is typically an exaggerated antegonial notch, clockwise rotation to an anterior open bite deformity, and the appearance of excess facial convexity. There is a decreased posterior facial height and an increased height of the lower anterior face, partly as a result of the increased vertical height of the chin. The mandibular body is also foreshortened in sagittal dimension. The Kaban-Mulliken modification of the Pruzansky classification of the mandibular deformity in hemifacial microsomia is directly applicable and widely used to characterize the deficiency in Treacher Collins syndrome (Fig. 29.5) (10).

In general, patients with types I and IIA deformities have normal TMJ function that should be preserved. Mandibular deficiency in most of these patients can be corrected during adolescence using conventional orthognathic procedures including sagittal split osteotomy of the mandibular ramus and Le Fort I osteotomy of the midface to correct the angle of the occlusal plane and to close any anterior open bite. In addition, an osseous genioplasty designed to decrease the vertical height of the chin and improve the sagittal projection of the chin is routinely added.

In patients with type IIA mandibles with a significant loss of posterior facial height, and in patients with type IIB mandibles, reconstruction can often best be obtained using the technique of mandibular distraction osteogenesis. The technique uses a mandibular osteotomy, followed by application of an external framework, and slow lengthening of the bone segments. It has the advantages of predictably lengthening bone with a minimal degree of relapse, unlike conventional bone grafting techniques.

In type III mandibles, there is only a cortical shell of a mandible behind the dentition. This anatomy often precludes distraction osteogenesis. These children often require a tracheostomy in the perinatal period for mandibular hypoplasia. These children require reconstruction of the mandibular

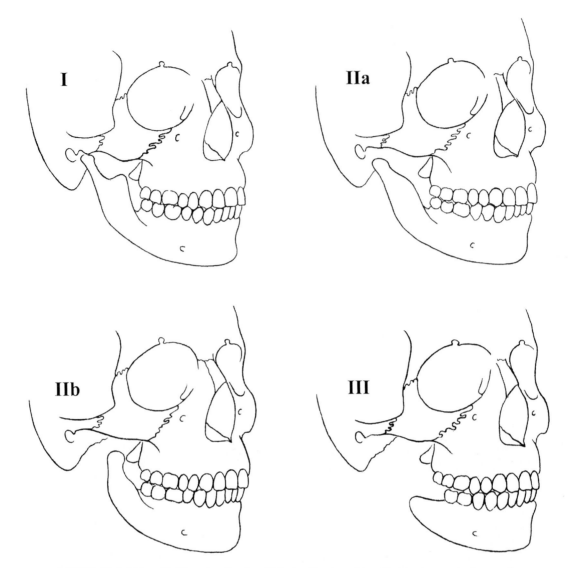

FIGURE 29.5. Kaban-Mulliken classification. This classification of hemifacial microsomia that can be extended to classify and discuss the mandible of Treacher Collins patients. Hypoplasia of the mandible is broken into four groups: Type I—normal architecture but smaller dimensional size of mandible and TMJ; type IIA—moderate hypoplasia of mandible with hypoplasia of ramus and condyle but some TMJ development adequately positioned for symmetrical opening of the joint; type IIB—moderate to severe hypoplasia of ramus, condyle, and TMJ joint that is malpositioned inferiorly, medially, and anteriorly and is "operationally equivalent" to a type III child; type III—total absence of mandibular ramus behind dentition making it unsuitable for bone distraction. *(Illustration by Min Li, MD.)*

ramus using a costochondral graft designed and positioned to abut against the skull base, because there is hypoplasia of the glenoid fossa. The costochondral rib grafts are harvested and positioned through Risdon (neck) incisions. Incisions in the preauricular are frequently necessary to assist in reconstruction of the zygomatic arch and glenoid fossa. This creates a posterior "stop" for the costochondral graft and facilitates mandible function. This surgery can be performed at 6 to 10 years of age, as the costochondral grafts are of adequate caliber to perform the surgery at that age. Significantly, these steps should be postponed until after ear reconstruction is completed, for the reasons of skin tension and vascularity previously noted. Ultimately, these children will require secondary double-jaw surgery to correct the malpositioned midface, correct the occlusal plane angle, and correct the facial height discrepancies discussed above. A Le Fort I osteotomy and a sagittal split osteotomy of the rib graft can be used, but obvious care must be taken in the rib graft osteotomy.

CONGENITAL DERMOID TUMORS

Congenital dermoid inclusion cysts of the face are common entities most commonly located in the upper lateral orbit and the upper lateral orbital rim, although they also can be found in the forehead and nasal areas (11). These lesions are benign, and embryologically these cysts represent displacement or retention of dermal and epidermal cells into embryonic lines of development. These benign tumors are more common in females than males (11). Surgical removal is the only effective treatment, and complete resection is necessary for successful management.

Clinical Findings

Congenital dermoid inclusion cysts can be subdivided into two groups, those involving the orbital/periorbital area (including

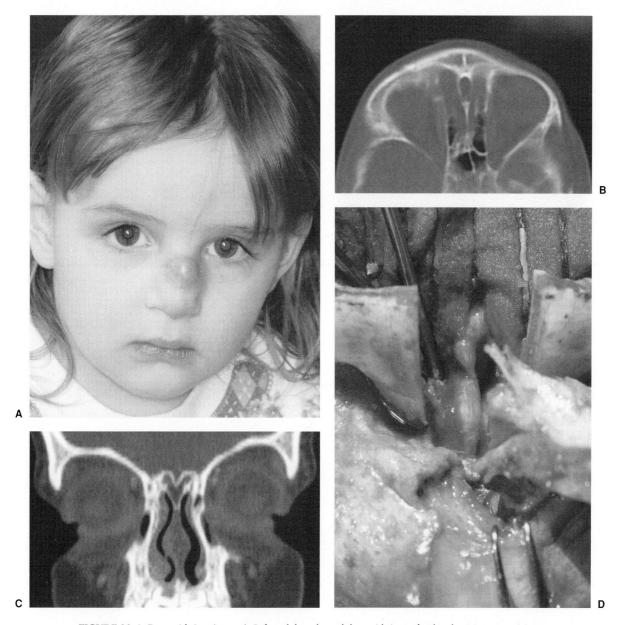

FIGURE 29.6. Dermoid sinus/cysts. **A:** Infected dorsal nasal dermoid sinus after local attempt at excision; this lesion extended intracranially. **B:** Patent foramen cecum in anterior skull base that transmitted dermoid sinus intracranially. **C:** Bifid crista galli on coronal CT scan. **D:** Intraoperative photograph of intracranial extension of nasal dermoid sinus cyst after "keystone" portion of supraorbital bar was removed.

the midline lower forehead) and those involving the nasal area. The lesions typically present at birth as firm, but not hard, nodular lesions involving the upper lateral orbital rim or the central forehead above the nose that slowly increase in size. They range in size from a few millimeters to a few centimeters, but most are between 1 and 2 cm in diameter. In lesions in the orbital and lower forehead areas, the presence of an external ostium or punctum is uncommon, whereas in the nasal dermoid lesions the presence of a punctum occurs frequently. In a recent large series of patients, 80% of the lesions in this series were located in either the upper lateral orbit or the upper lateral orbital rim (11); 10% of the lesions involved the upper medial orbit. The nasal lesions account for approximately 5% to 10% of all dermoid lesions, and have a distinct clinical presentation and a distinct etiology. Nasal dermoid cyst/sinuses are typically located in the midline and they can have multiple presentations, including nasal pits, hair growth within a punctum,

intermittent drainage of sebaceous material, chronic draining sinus tracts, abscess, and soft-tissue infections, including cellulitis. They can also present as recurrent lesions after failed incision and drainage procedures (Fig. 29.6A).

Etiology and Pathogenesis

The etiology of orbital and periorbital congenital dermoid inclusion cysts is thought to be related to migrating tissue being "trapped" below the surface along lines of embryologic fusion as embryologic development progresses. Dermoid inclusion cysts are distinguished from simple epidermoid inclusion cysts by the presence of dermis and skin adnexa in the wall of the lesion. Because the cysts have skin adnexa present, the cysts or sinuses can contain cellular debris, sebum, and hair. The lesions subsequently enlarge over time.

The etiology of nasal dermoid inclusion cysts and sinuses is distinct from that of orbital or periorbital dermoids. Although three separate theories have been advocated to account for these nasal dermoid sinus/cysts, the one that has been most often acknowledged is the "nasocranial deep trilaminar" theory. During normal embryogenesis the nasal and frontal bones develop by intramembranous ossification, but remain separated by a small fontanelle called the fonticulus nasofrontalis. A prenasal space between the nasal bones and cartilaginous nasal capsule extends from the skull base to the nasal tip. Dura extends through the fonticulus nasofrontalis, into the prenasal space, and comes into contact with skin. Normally, the dura and skin separate as the nasal process of the frontal bone grows. The dura recedes and the fonticulus nasofrontalis and foramen cecum fuse, forming the cribriform plates. **Nasal dermoid cysts and sinuses are formed when the dura remains fused to the overlying skin, instead of separating.** As the dura recedes intracranially, it pulls ectodermal tissue with it, most frequently along the tract through the foramen cecum. A sinus tract is formed when the misplaced dermal and epidermal lined tract maintains a connection with the skin, whereas a cyst is formed when ectoderm is trapped without egress to the skin, trapping the sloughed contents below the surface.

Treatment

Complete surgical removal of these benign lesions is the only successful therapeutic strategy. For the 90% of these lesions that are located in the orbital or forehead areas, no preoperative diagnostic evaluation is warranted. The lesions can be approached through a supratarsal fold upper-eyelid incision. Dissection is carried through the orbicularis muscle and directly down onto the cyst wall. The dissection then meticulously proceeds on the cyst wall around the lesion. The lesions are frequently below the periosteum, so incision of this slightly tougher layer must occur as part of the complete excision of the cyst.

For the 10% of these lesions that are true nasal dermoids, the critical issue in management is to establish whether or not there is intracranial extension of the cyst/sinus. The midline location is a harbinger of the potentially more complicated problem. If the lesion extends intracranially, a formal craniotomy is often necessary. Preoperative imaging with fine-cut computed tomography (CT) scan through the anterior cranial base is essential and can differentiate whether there is a patent foramen cecum and a bifid crista galli present, two signs of intracranial extension (Fig. 29.6B and C). Although the presence of a bifid crista galli and an open cecum does not confirm intracranial extension, it is agreed that a normal size and appearance of the crista galli and foramen cecum rules out intracranial extension. If the CT findings are positive, an MRI may provide additional insight. If the MRI is positive with an obvious intracranial extension, then surgical planning should include neurosurgical involvement and a formal craniotomy. If a coronal incision and formal craniotomy are required, then the majority of the dissection and retrieval should be accomplished from the coronal approach. This can be facilitated by outfracture of the "keystone" portion of the supraorbital bar (12) (Fig. 29.6D). If the MRI findings are equivocal or absent but the CT findings are positive, a frequent clinical scenario, then planning should still include the possible need for a craniotomy and neurosurgical consultation and evaluation. In this case, the nasal lesion can be approached by an incision around the lesion and dissection cephalad, or through an open rhinoplasty approach with a small incision around the base of the nasal punctum. The dissection proceeds cephalad, meticulously dissecting the stalk of the lesion dorsal to the cartilage but deep to the nasal bones. If the stalk can be completely removed, there

is no need for the craniotomy. Otherwise, the craniotomy is required to ensure complete removal (Fig. 29.6D). Recurrence rates have been reported to be as high as 12%, and incomplete removal can be associated with complications such as infection and osteomyelitis.

NEUROFIBROMATOSIS

Neurofibromatosis is common, with an estimated 100,000 cases in the United States alone. The disorder can involve both the central and peripheral nervous systems. **The clinical hallmark of the disorder is the development of multiple cutaneous and subcutaneous nodular tumors.** The disease has protean manifestations, a variable age of onset, a variable presentation, variability in clinical findings, and a variable but progressive course. Over the past 20 years, our understanding of neurofibromatosis has advanced significantly. Critical to this advance was a National Institutes of Health Consensus Statement in 1987 that established the diagnostic criteria for "peripheral neurofibromatosis," now known as neurofibromatosis-1, and "central neurofibromatosis," now known as neurofibromatosis-2 (Table 29.1). Although refinements of these criteria have been proposed, the establishment of the criteria in 1987 effectively focused thought about neurofibromatosis throughout the world. **Surgical resection remains the mainstay of treatment for enlarging or symptomatic tumors.**

TABLE 29.1

CLINICAL DIAGNOSTIC CRITERIA FOR NEUROFIBROMATOSIS

1987 National Institutes of Health Consensus Conference

Neurofibromatosis-1

Diagnostic criteria are met in an individual if two or more of the following are found:

- Café-au-lait spots (six or more larger than 5 mm in greatest dimension in prepubertal individuals and larger than 15 mm in postpubertal individuals)
- Two or more neurofibromas of any type or one plexiform neurofibroma
- Freckling in the axillary or inguinal region
- Optic glioma
- Two or more Lisch nodules (hamartomas of the iris)
- A distinctive osseous lesion such as sphenoid wing dysplasia or thinning of long bone cortex with or without pseudoarthrosis
- A first-degree relative (parent, sibling, or offspring) with neurofibromatosis-1 by the above criteria

Neurofibromatosis-2

Diagnostic criteria are met in an individual who has:

- Bilateral eighth nerve masses seen with appropriate imaging techniques
- A first-degree relative with neurofibromatosis-2 and either:
   1. Unilateral eighth nerve mass, or
   2. Two or more of the following
      - Neurofibroma
      - Meningioma
      - Glioma
      - Schwannoma
      - Juvenile posterior subcapsular lenticular opacity

Clinical Presentation

Plastic surgeons and craniofacial surgeons are primarily concerned with the manifestations of neurofibromatosis-1 (NF-1). The clinical presentation of is most commonly heralded by the appearance of café-au-lait spots. These lesions are cutaneous hyperpigmented areas, typically 20 to 30 mm in diameter, with greater than six lesions found in 90% to 99% of all cases (11). These lesions can be difficult to differentiate from congenital nevi, but this can be accomplished by a punch biopsy. Most children present with café-au-lait spots as the earliest and as the only manifestation of NF-1, but more than 80% will develop additional signs of the disorder. Axillary freckling generally appears before age 5 years and is seen in approximately 80% of all cases of NF-1 (13,14). Lisch nodules are pigmented, dome-shaped nodules seen on the surface of the iris that are best seen by ocular exam with slit-lamp microscopy. They usually have an onset by 10 years of age and are present in nearly all NF-1 cases by 20 years of age. The NF-1 gene is a tumor-suppressor gene that regulates cell proliferation, and intracranial tumors are frequent occurrences in these NF-1 patients. Optic pathway gliomas are the most common central nervous system tumors, occurring in ap-

proximately 15% of cases, and are histologically identified as low-grade pilocytic astrocytomas (13,14). NF-1 patients also have an increased incidence of brainstem gliomas, as well as an apparent increase in the occurrence of benign and malignant astrocytomas, ependymomas, meningiomas, medulloblastomas, and malignant schwannomas. Skeletal abnormalities associated with NF-1 include sphenoid wing aplasia, macrocephaly, scoliosis, and thinning of long bone cortex, causing anterior tibial bowing. The sphenoid wing aplasia is present in 5% to 7% of NF-1 cases and is characterized by unilateral agenesis of the greater wing of the sphenoid (Fig. 29.7A and B). This agenesis creates a large communication between the middle temporal fossa and the orbit, and can lead to ocular proptosis, pulsatile exophthalmos, and exposure problems for the eye. It can also be associated with neurofibromas within the cone of periocular tissues.

Neurofibromas, the hallmark of the NF-1 disease, are nerve sheath tumors that arise anywhere along a nerve sheath from the dorsal root ganglion to the terminal nerve branches (13,14). They are composed of Schwann cells, fibroblasts, mast cells, and perineural cells. Neurofibromas occur in five main types: localized cutaneous neurofibromas, diffuse cutaneous neurofibromas, localized intraneural neurofibromas, massive soft-tissue neurofibroma, and plexiform neurofibromas.

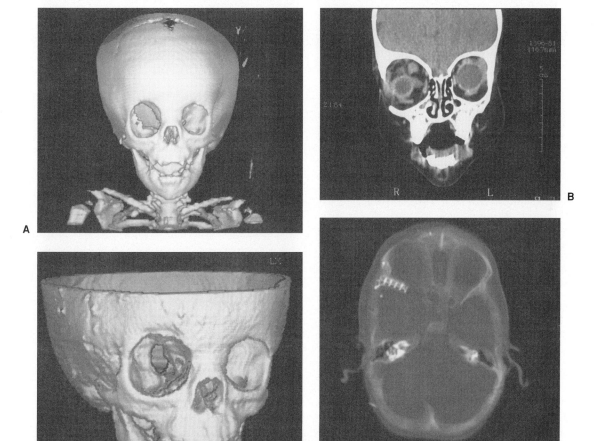

FIGURE 29.7. Neurofibromatosis. **A:** Three-dimensional CT scan demonstrating large defect in sphenoid wing. **B:** Coronal CT scan of orbit revealing expanded orbit, vertical dystopia, and intraorbital neurofibromas. **C:** Postoperative three-dimensional CT scan showing decrease in size of aperture between orbit and middle fossa. This aperture allows passage of the ophthalmic nerve and contents of the superior orbital fissure. **D:** Postoperative CT scan showing titanium and bone graft composite reconstruction of posterior sphenoid wing. **E:** Massive plexiform neurofibromatosis of right face showing significant overgrowth with extensive distortion evident on frontal view. **F:** Postoperative result following staged resection and suspension of soft tissue from zygomatic arch using sutures and fascia lata suspension. The recurrent laxity is evident.

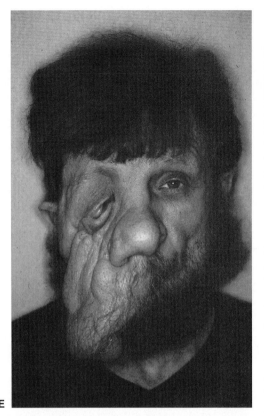
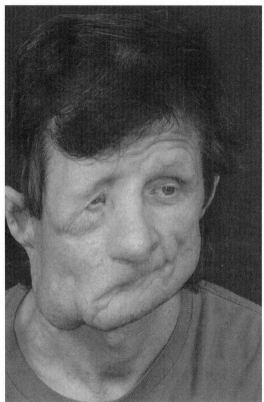

E   F

FIGURE 29.7. *(Continued)*

Plexiform neurofibromas are virtually unique to NF-1 and are composed of nerve sheath cells that proliferate along the length of a nerve. Plexiform neurofibromas are frequently associated with hypertrophy of the soft tissue and hyperpigmentation or hypertrichosis of the overlying skin. Their growth can cause destruction or compression of local tissue, causing significant morbidity. Plexiform lesions occur in 16% to 40% of patients with NF-1, and are found on the trunk in 43% to 44%, the extremities in 15% to 38%, and the head and neck in 18% to 42% of patients (15). Craniofacial plexiform neurofibromas most frequently involve the second and third divisions of the fifth cranial nerve and each occur in approximately 5% of patients with NF-1. In contrast to the other types of neurofibromas, these plexiform neurofibromas are believed to be congenital in origin, and usually become clinically evident by 2 years of age. Their growth is unpredictable, but occurs frequently during early infancy and times of hormonal change such as preadolescence/adolescence and pregnancy. Craniofacial neurofibromas cause significant facial disfigurement.

Malignant degeneration of peripheral nerve sheath tumors is more frequent than may be appreciated by conventional wisdom, occurring in up to 13% of patients with NF-1 (16). Malignant peripheral nerve sheath tumors, which were formerly known as neurosarcomas or malignant schwannomas, arise from Schwann cells. More than 50% of patients with malignant nerve sheath tumors have NF-1. Only the plexiform neurofibromas have a high propensity for malignant degeneration. Medium and large nerves, such as those involving the thigh, the buttock, the brachial plexus, and the paraspinal nerves, are most frequently involved. **Pain is the most reliable indicator of malignant degeneration.** Prompt medical attention is warranted and surgical biopsy is indicated. Once diagnosed, management consists of an aggressive attempt at total surgical resection. Metastases are common. Malignant soft-tissue neo-

plasms occur approximately 34 times more frequently than in a control group, and accounted for 9.4% of the deaths of patients with NF-1 (11). Despite treatment, the 5-year survival rate of malignant peripheral nerve sheath tumors is estimated to be between 16% and 52%.

Etiology and Pathogenesis

Plastic surgeons and craniofacial surgeons are primarily concerned with the manifestations of NF-1, which is more than 10 times more common than neurofibromatosis-2 (NF-2). The gene for NF-1 has been localized to band 11.2 of the long arm of chromosome 17, clearly distinct from that for NF-2, which has been localized to the middle of the long arm of human chromosome 22. NF-1 is transmitted as an autosomal dominant disorder with variable penetrance and expressivity. Families must be counseled that there is a 50% chance of an affected individual having an affected child.

Treatment

The craniofacial problems associated with NF-1 typically are of two types: the orbitopalpebral neurofibromas associated with sphenoid wing dysplasia (cranio-orbital neurofibromatosis) and the plexiform neurofibromas involving the soft tissue of the face, largely in the distribution of the trigeminal nerve. These two types may exist together in the same patient, but most frequently occur separately. Several core issues must be addressed in treatment planning. First, the surgery is treating the deformity only. The underlying process of neurofibromatosis remains, and the recurrence of the neurofibromas is common. Second, both the timing of surgery and the extent of surgery must be carefully considered. Third, neurofibromas of the face and cranio-orbital region tend to bleed significantly during surgery, the bleeding is difficult to control with electrocautery, and blood loss can be substantial. Jackson reported the option of packing the facial wound open with compression, and returning in 48 hours to complete the operation (17). Appropriate patient monitoring and intravenous access must be a component of preoperative planning, and consideration should be given to hypotensive anesthesia (17,18). Fourth, the resected tumor is prone to recurrence. The soft tissue of the face in neurofibromatosis, including the skin, ligaments, tendons, and subcutaneous tissues, appears to have a decreased tensile strength, and there is a strong tendency toward stretch and "relaxation," with recurrence of the original deformity. Finally, the surgical management of this disorder must balance aesthetic outcome with the preservation of function. While these considerations are acknowledged, surgery is the most powerful tool for helping these patients, and these patients are often extremely grateful and appreciative of surgical intervention, even though the aesthetic result may be less than the surgical team had desired. Surgical approaches vary from limited surgery at intervals to massive "one-stage" surgical resections of the involved tissues. It is likely that the optimal approach lies somewhere between these two ends of the spectrum, and should be decided by the surgeon based on the degree of the deformity and in consultation with the patient and family.

Management of Cranio-Orbital Disorders

The orbital-palpebral neurofibromas associated with sphenoid wing dysplasia form a discrete subtype of neurofibromatosis, frequently described as cranio-orbital neurofibromatosis (17–19). The principal findings in this disorder are pulsatile exophthalmos, an enlarged bony orbit, orbital neurofibroma, dysplasia or aplasia of the sphenoid wing with the presence of a herniation of the temporal lobe into the orbit, and a bulging temporal fossa. In addition to the exophthalmos, there is also frequently vertical dystopia of the globe. Overall, cranio-orbital-temporal neurofibromatosis has been found to exist in from 1% to 10% of patients with NF-1. Although several etiologies have been advocated for the sphenoid dysplasia, including a direct effect of the orbital neurofibroma on the bone versus a congenital mesodermal maldevelopment with defective ossification of the sphenoid bone, the etiology of the sphenoid defect has not been clearly demonstrated.

The management of the orbital structures is one of the most complex issues in neurofibromatosis. In most cases, when vision exists in the afflicted eye, although potentially compromised, the eye is preserved. In patients with functional vision, Jackson approaches mild cases with little change in orbital volume through the upper eyelid, whereas in cases with significant bony enlargement, he recommends use of a coronal flap, and a C-shaped osteotomy through the lateral orbital wall, zygoma, and horizontally through the maxilla below the inferior orbital nerve. The neurofibroma is resected through either approach, although he notes that it may be inadvisable to remove the tumor completely in the plexiform variety where there is significant involvement of the neuromuscular structures, as this may cause a disturbance of eye movement and resultant diplopia. The sphenoid wing is reconstructed with a bone graft, using either split-rib grafts or cranial bone graft. The greatly stretched levator aponeurosis is repaired directly to the tarsal plate, but Jackson cautions against excess shortening of the levator aponeurosis and also against excess skin resection. In patients with a loss of vision, an orbital exenteration is performed. The temporal lobe is reduced into the middle cranial fossa, and the entire defect in the sphenoid wing is reconstructed using a bone graft. The eyelid skin is invaginated into the orbit and used as skin cover. Once healing is complete, the orbital defect is fitted with prosthesis.

An alternative way to approach these ocular problems is through the use of a coronal incision and a frontal craniotomy. The incision placement can be selected to allow for a forehead lift and direct excision of skin in those cases with involvement of the forehead and eyebrow and resultant ptosis of the eyebrow. The supraorbital bar and orbital roof are removed, allowing both direct exposure of the entire orbit and the opportunity to reposition the supraorbital bar in cases of dystopia or orbital volume change. The coronal approach allows for excellent visualization and separation of the dura from the periorbital structures. It also allows favorable visualization as dissection proceeds medially and the ophthalmic nerve and vessels are approached. The cranial bone graft is cut precisely and placed to allow for separation of the middle cranial fossa from the orbital contents, minimizing the area of defect that must remain to allow passage of the ophthalmic nerve and contents that usually pass through the superior orbital fissure (Fig. 29.7B and C). Many surgeons have commented about the tendency for these grafts to absorb over time, and the use of a "composite" graft of cranial bone and titanium mesh is often useful to tolerate the pulsations of the brain and provide osseous healing and stability (Fig. 29.7D).

As difficult as the skeletal reconstruction may be, the soft-tissue structures are problematic as they appear to have a decreased tensile strength, tending to stretch and "relax" and recreate the original deformity. The management of the medial and lateral canthal structures is performed using standard techniques, but it should be noted that these tissues are subject to relaxation and, therefore, relapse (18). Similarly, this same problem can occur with the ptosis correction, which frequently must be repeated. One must avoid the temptation to overcorrection of the ptosis, as a foreshortened eyelid with ocular exposure is a disastrous complication. It is much better to repeat the surgery and repair the levator aponeurosis again. As is true of many aspects of management of neurofibromatosis, improvement can be significant, but correction is both difficult to achieve and harder to maintain.

Management of Plexiform Neurofibromas of the Face

Plexiform neurofibromas involving the face typically involve either the temporal fossa, or originate from one or more divisions of the trigeminal nerve. Grabb et al. have said that neurofibromas "are woven into the normal fabric of the face and usually defy all but partial treatment." The plexiform neurofibromas that originate from one or more divisions of the trigeminal nerve cause significant distortion of the facial soft tissue and skeletal framework. The characteristic overgrowth of the soft tissue leads to distortion of the eyebrow, thickening of the eyelids, ptosis, visual obstruction, dysconjugate gaze, glaucoma, ectropion, and can lead to visual loss. Epiphora is frequently present. The cheek is usually grossly involved and ptotic. There can be hypertrophy of the nose and distortion of the nasal soft and cartilaginous tissue (Fig. 29.7E and F). There can be significant dental involvement and distortion of the maxillary and mandibular occlusal plane. Plexiform infiltration of the mandibular division of the trigeminal nerve can lead to compromise of buccal, oropharyngeal, and retropharyngeal tissue causing speech apraxia and oropharyngeal dysfunction. These patients can have such profound disfigurement that they suffer from profound psychosocial problems related to the facial deformity, and they can be desperate for any improvement in appearance.

Surgical management of neurofibromatosis of the temporal fossa needs to include a careful assessment of risks and expected outcomes. These are benign tumors that seldom cause major problems in this location. Certainly, the simple presence of a neurofibroma in this location, as elsewhere, does not warrant surgery. Many times there is a simple, subtle enlargement of the soft tissue of the temporal fossa. If pain and considerable enlargement supervene, then surgery can be considered. Occasionally, these lesions will cause deformity of the mandible and maxilla by a mass effect. The temporalis muscle can be densely infiltrated by the neurofibromas. The caveat of blood loss during these procedures in NF-1 patients must be acknowledged and planned for in these corrective skeletal procedures. Following resection, the most obvious problem is frequently a soft-tissue deficiency. Reconstruction can be performed using microvascular free tissue transfer, dermal-fascial-fat grafts, or onlay of the skull using bone substitutes. The exact method for reconstruction depends on the severity of the soft-tissue deficit, with free tissue transfer typically being reserved for larger deficiencies.

Soft-tissue plexiform neurofibromas of the forehead can be approached through a coronal or "hairline" frontal incision. These approaches allow excellent exposure, and can be used to lift the redundant skin vertically as needed, thereby allowing correction of eyebrow ptosis. Separate incisions may be necessary to address orbital changes.

Surgery to correct the hypertrophy of the cheek, nose, and lips should follow skeletal correction, if this is planned. Similar to the principles for reconstruction of congenital defects, the skeletal framework correction should be performed first. In general, this consists of reduction of osseous structures with leveling of the occlusal plane through modifications of standard orthognathic approaches and techniques. The correction of the soft tissue of the cheek, nose, and lip can then be undertaken. The redundancy of the cheek skin can be approached through a facelift incision/approach or a Weber-Ferguson approach. If the facelift incision is used, every attempt should be made to preserve the function of the facial nerve. Although many of the facial muscles may have limited function as a result of involvement by a neurofibroma, the nerve should be preserved wherever possible. Direct full-thickness excision of redundant tissue is necessary. The skin incisions usually heal very favorably and do not tend to be either prominent or noticeable after surgery. The tendency toward relapse should be counteracted by using permanent sutures to anchor the tissue to the bony skeleton at the zygomatic arch and wherever possible. In severe cases of redundancy, it may be worthwhile considering the use of tensor fascia lata slings to suspend the soft-tissue structures and minimize the tendency toward relapse of the position of the soft tissue. In cases with significant redundancy of the soft tissue, facial animation may not occur to any appreciable extent, and static suspension of the soft tissues is appropriate and yields a significant clinical improvement. The redundancy of the tissue of the lip and nose should be addressed through direct excision. Both vertical and horizontal excisions may be necessary to obtain the desired position of these structures, and considerable improvement can reliably be obtained.

Surgery for plexiform neurofibromas of the face must consider the initial deformity, the blood loss, the aesthetics of the expected result, and the likely durability of that result, given the laxity of the soft tissues and the tendency toward recurrence of the deformity. Surgery can provide tremendous improvement both aesthetically and functionally. Although we can seldom provide complete correction, amelioration is a desirable and significant goal.

References

1. Chen Y-R, Breidahl AMS, Chang C-N. Optic nerve decompression in fibrous dysplasia: indications, efficacy, and safety. *Plastic Reconstr Surg.* 1997; 99(1):22.
2. Sassin JF, Rosenberg RN. Neurologic complications of fibrous dysplasia of the skull. *Arch Neurol.* 1968;18:363.
3. Gorlin RJ, Cohen MM, Levin LS. Syndromes of the head and neck. 3rd ed. Oxford, England: Oxford University Press; 1990:642.
4. Harrison DH. Facial reanimation in children with Mobius syndrome after segmental gracilis muscle transplantation (discussion). *Plastic Reconstr Surg.* 2000;106:9.
5. Zuker RM, Goldberg CS, Manktelow RT. Facial animation in children with Mobius syndrome after segmental gracilis muscle transplant. *Plastic Reconstr Surg.* 2000;106:1.
6. Pensler JM, Murphy GF, Mulliken JB. Clinical and ultrastructural studies of Romberg's hemifacial atrophy. *Plastic Reconstr Surg.* 1990;85:6669.
7. Upton J, Albin RE, Mulliken JB, et al. The use of scapular and parascapular flaps for cheek reconstruction. *Plastic Reconstr Surg.* 1992;90:959.
8. Posnick JC, Goldstein JA, Waitzman A. Surgical correction of the Treacher Collins malar deficiency: quantitative CT scan analysis of long term results. *Plastic Reconstr Surg.* 1993;92:12.
9. Siebert JW. Unpublished findings.
10. Kaban LB, Moses MH, Mulliken JB. Surgical corrections of hemifacial microsomia in the growing child. *Plastic Reconstr Surg.* 1980;82:9.
11. Barlett SP, Lin KY, Grossman R, et al. The surgical management of orbitofacial dermoids in the pediatric patient. *Plastic Reconstr Surg.* 1993;91: 1208.
12. van Aalst JA, Luerssen TG, Whitehead WE, et al. "Keystone" approach for intracranial nasofrontal dermoid sinuses. *Plastic Reconstr Surg.* 2005;116:13.
13. Friedman JM. Neurofibromatosis 1: clinical manifestations and diagnostic criteria. *J Child Neurol.* 2002;17:548.
14. Young H, Hyman S, North K. Neurofibromatosis 1: clinical review and exceptions to the rules. *J Child Neurol.* 2002;17:613.
15. Rosser T, Packer RJ. Neurofibromas in children with neurofibromatosis 1. *J Child Neurol.* 2002;17:585.
16. Rasmussen S, Yang Q, Friedman J. Mortality in neurofibromatosis 1: an analysis using U.S. death certificates. *Am J Med Genet.* 2001;68:1110.
17. Jackson IT. Neurofibromatosis of the skull base. *Clin Plast Surg.* 1995; 22(3):513.
18. Poole MD. Experiences in the surgical treatment of cranio-orbital neurofibromatosis. *Br J Plast Surg.* 1989;72:155.
19. Jackson IT, Laws ER, Martin RD. The surgical management of neurofibromatosis. *Plastic Reconstr Surg.* 1983;71:751.

CHAPTER 30 ■ OTOPLASTY AND EAR RECONSTRUCTION

CHARLES H. THORNE

PROMINENT EARS

The term *prominent ears*, for the purposes of this chapter, refers to ears that, regardless of size, "stick out" enough to appear abnormal. When referring to the front surface of the ear, the terms *front*, *lateral surface*, and *anterior surface* are used interchangeably. Similarly, when referring to the back of the auricle, the terms *back*, *medial surface*, and *posterior surface* are used synonymously.

The normal external ear is separated by less than 2 cm from, and forms an angle of less than 25 degrees with, the side of the head. Beyond these approximate normal limits, the ear appears prominent when viewed from either the front or the back.

Anatomic Causes of Prominent Ears

To correct prominent ears, the anatomic abnormality must be determined (Fig. 30.1). The three most common causes of prominent ears may be present alone or in combination:

1. *Underdeveloped antihelical fold.* As a result of inadequate folding of the antihelix, the scapha and helical rim protrude. This anatomic abnormality causes prominence of the upper third and, in many cases, the middle third of the ear.
2. *Prominent concha.* The concha may be excessively deep, the concha/mastoid angle may be excessive, or there may be a combination of these two factors. This anatomic abnormality causes prominence of the middle third of the auricle.
3. *Protruding earlobe.* The protruding earlobe causes prominence of the lower third of the ear.

Although most prominent ears are otherwise normal in shape, some prominent ears have additional deformities. The conditions enumerated below are examples of abnormally shaped ears that may also be prominent. The term *macrotia* refers to excessively large ears that, in addition to being large, may be "prominent." *Constricted ears* (Fig. 30.2) are abnormally small but tend to appear "prominent" because the circumference of the helical rim is inadequate, causing the auricle to cup forward. The *Stahl's ear deformity* (Fig. 30.3) consists of a third crus, in addition to the crura of the triangular fossa, which traverses the scapha. This may give the ear a "Mr. Spock" pointed appearance in addition to being prominent. *Cryptotia* (Fig. 30.4) describes the auricle in which the upper pole of the helix is buried beneath the temporal skin. *Question mark ears* earn their name because deficiency of the supralobular region gives the ear the shape of a question mark.

Goals of Otoplasty

The goal of otoplasty is to set back the ears in such a way that the contours appear soft and natural, the setback is harmonious and there is no evidence of surgical intervention. When examined from the various angles, the corrected auricle should have the following characteristics:

1. *Front view.* When viewed from the front the helical rim should be visible, not set back so far that it is hidden behind the antihelical fold.
2. *Rear view.* When viewed from behind, the helical rim should be straight, not bent like a "C" or a "hockey stick." If the helical rim is straight, the setback will be harmonious; that is, the upper, middle, and lower thirds of the ear will be setback in correct proportion to each other. If, for example, the middle third is set back too much relative to the upper and lower thirds, the helical rim will form a "C" when viewed from behind, creating the so-called telephone deformity. Similarly, if the earlobe is insufficiently set back, the rear view will reveal a hockey stick appearance to the helical rim contour.
3. *Lateral view.* The contours should be soft and natural, not sharp and "human-made."

Timing of Otoplasty

There is no absolute rule about when otoplasty should be performed. In young children with extremely prominent ears, a reasonable age is approximately 4 years. In cases of macrotia associated with prominence, the author has performed the procedure as early as age 2 years, thinking that any restriction of growth is an advantage. Regardless of the exact age, the procedure requires general anesthesia. In other cases, usually more minor, the parents may choose to wait until the child can participate in the decision. This may allow the procedure to be performed under local anesthesia, although it is a rare child that can tolerate local anesthesia before age 10 years, and many not until they are adults.

Operative Procedure

Numerous methods have been described for correcting the anatomic abnormalities described above. **The techniques that have stood the test of time are the simplest, most reliable, and least likely to cause complications or an "operated" look.** The techniques described below are used alone or in combination depending on the anatomic deformity and the choice of the surgeon.

297

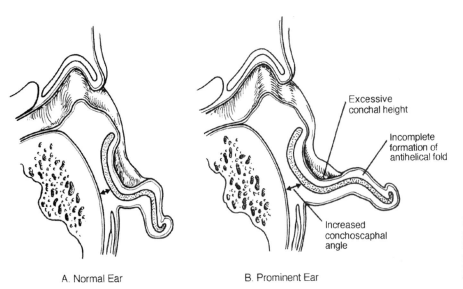

FIGURE 30.1. Comparison of normal and prominent ear anatomy. **A:** Normal ear. **B:** Components of the prominent ear. (Reproduced with permission of Charles H. Thorne, MD. Copyright Charles H. Thorne, MD.)

Antihelical Fold Manipulation

- *Suturing of cartilage.* Mattress sutures are placed from the scapha and/or triangular fossa to the concha, as described by Mustarde, and are tied with sufficient tension to increase the definition of the antihelical fold, thereby setting back the helical rim and scapha (Fig. 30.5).

- *Stenstrom technique of anterior abrasion.* The anterior surface of the antihelical fold cartilage is abraded, causing the cartilage to bend away from the abraded side (principle of Gibson) toward the side of intact perichondrium (Fig. 30.6).
- *Full-thickness incisions.* A single full-thickness incision along the desired curvature of the antihelix permits folding with slight force, creating an antihelical fold (Luckett procedure). Because the fold is sharp and unnatural

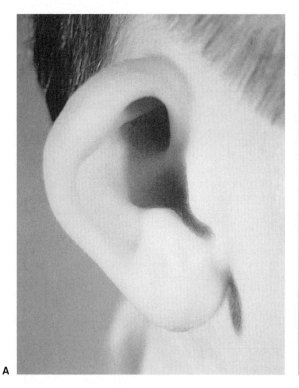
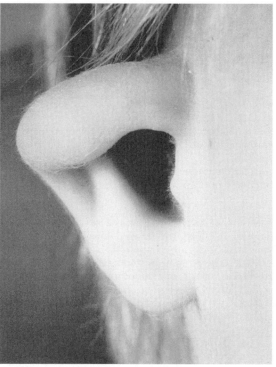

FIGURE 30.2. Constricted ear. **A:** Mildly constricted ear. Otoplasty requires increasing the circumference of the helical rim by advancing the crus of the helix into the helical rim (see Fig. 30.7). **B:** Severely constricted ear. This degree of constriction can only be repaired by discarding some of the cartilage and performing an ear reconstruction as in microtia. (Courtesy of David Furnas, MD.)

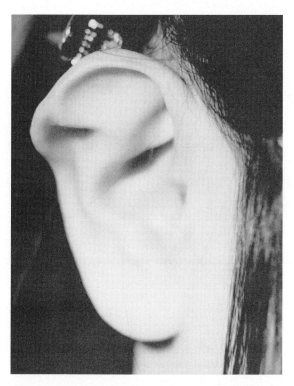

FIGURE 30.3. Stahl's ear. Note the third crus that traverses the scapha. (Courtesy of David Furnas, MD.)

appearing, this single-incision technique was modified. In the Converse/Wood-Smith technique, a pair of incisions is made, parallel to the desired antihelical fold, and tubing sutures are placed to create a more defined fold.

Conchal Alteration

- *Suturing.* The angle between the concha and the mastoid skull can be decreased by placing sutures between the concha and the mastoid fascia as described by Furnas (Fig. 30.5).
- *Conchal excision.* From either an anterior or posterior approach, a full-thickness crescent of cartilage is removed from the posterior wall of the concha (taking care not to violate or deform the antihelical fold), thereby reducing the conchal height. The conchal defect is meticulously closed with sutures to avoid a visible ridge within the concha. The excision is designed so that the eventual closure will lie at the junction of the floor and posterior wall of the concha where it is least conspicuous and causes the least distortion of the normal auricular contours (Fig. 30.5).
- *A combination of Furnas suture and Conchal excision techniques* (Fig. 30.5).

Correction of Earlobe Prominence

Earlobe prominence is not corrected by the above maneuvers. In fact, these maneuvers may increase the prominence of the earlobe, making earlobe repositioning the most difficult and neglected part of the procedure. An auricle that has been repositioned in its upper two thirds but still has a prominent lobule will appear just as abnormal and disharmonious as the original deformity. It has been said that suturing the tail of the helical cartilage to the concha will correct earlobe prominence. Unfortunately the tail of the helix does not extend into the lobule and setting it back does not reliably set back the earlobe. Other authors have described techniques involving skin excision and sutures between the fibrofatty tissue of the lobule and the tissues of the neck. The best technique in the author's experience is the technique described by Gosain, or a variation

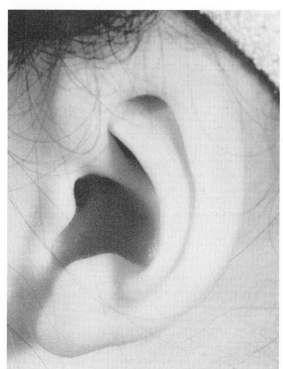

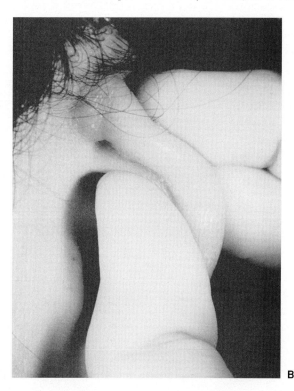

A   **B**

FIGURE 30.4. Cryptotia. **A:** Patient in whom a relatively normal helical rim is buried in the temporal soft tissues. The upper portion of the auricle can be exposed by outward traction on the ear. **B:** Outward traction (in a different patient) causes the upper portion of the ear to emerge from its hiding place. (Courtesy of David Furnas, MD.)

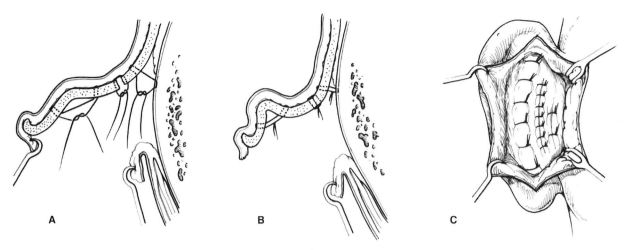

FIGURE 30.5. Otoplasty technique. The combination of a Mustarde scapha-conchal suture, conchal resection with primary closure, and a Furnas conchal-mastoid suture. Note that the conchal closure is at the junction of the floor and posterior wall of the concha. **A:** Sutures placed. **B:** Sutures tightened to create the desired contour. **C:** Same sutures as seen through the retroauricular incision. (Reproduced with permission of Charles H. Thorne, MD. Copyright Charles H. Thorne, MD.)

thereof, in which skin is excised on the medial surface of the earlobe. When this defect is closed with sutures, a bite of the undersurface of the concha is taken, which pulls the earlobe toward the head.

Alteration of the Position of the Upper Auricular Pole

Depending on the degree of prominence preoperatively of the upper third of the ear, the antihelical fold creation may be inadequate to correct the position of the helical rim, near the root

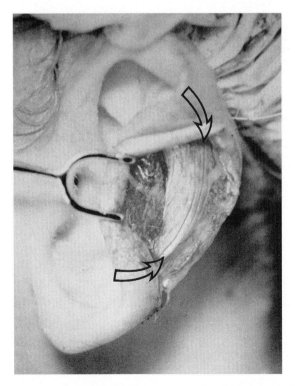

FIGURE 30.6. Stenstrom technique. The antihelical fold is scored. The cartilage bends away from the scoring, moving the helical rim closer to the head and increasing the prominence of the antihelix.

of the helix. An additional mattress suture between the helical rim and the temporal fascia may be required.

Choice of Otoplasty Technique

The final operative plan for an otoplasty is a combination of surgical maneuvers based in part on the anatomic diagnosis of the deformity, and in part on the surgeon's personal preferences. The author's preferred technique involves Mustarde sutures to recreate the antihelix and setback the upper and middle thirds of the ear. **The abrasion techniques are unreliable, uncontrollable, and unnecessary and may result in sharp edges or an overdone appearance.** In the conchal region, the author frequently uses both a conchal resection and Furnas conchal mastoid sutures as shown in Figure 30.5. The combination allows the resection to be small (1–2 mm), minimizing iatrogenic deformity. When conchal excision is used alone, a deformity of the posterior wall of the concha may result. When Furnas sutures are used alone the correction may be inadequate, the patient may have pain, the external auditory canal can be narrowed, and the depth of the retroauricular sulcus is decreased. As mentioned above, earlobe repositioning is the most difficult part of the procedure. The Webster technique of repositioning the helical tail has not been effective in the author's hands for correction of earlobe prominence. **Rather, the Webster technique appears to reposition the ear just above the earlobe, exaggerating the earlobe prominence.**

Other Deformities

Macrotia. To reduce the size of the ears, the incision is made on the lateral surface of the ear, just inside the helical rim. The scapha is reduced and a segment of helical rim is excised and closed primarily to avoid redundancy.

Constricted ear. In mild cases, the crus of the helix is advanced out of the concha and into the helical rim and standard otoplasty techniques are used in addition (Fig. 30.7). In severe cases, the cartilage is discarded and a complete auricular reconstruction performed as in microtia.

Stahl ear. Various techniques have been described to excise the extra crus. None is perfect.

Cryptotia. The superior aspect of the auricular cartilage is pulled out from under the scalp (Fig. 30.4), an incision is made

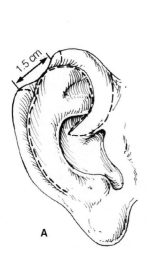
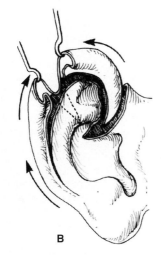
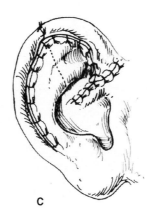

A   **B**   **C**

FIGURE 30.7. Antia-Buch helical advancement. **A:** An incision is designed inside the helical rim and around the crus of the helix. **B:** The incision is made through the skin and the cartilage, but not through the posterior skin. The helical rim is advanced to allow closure and a dog-ear of skin (*dotted line*) is removed on the back of the ear. **C:** Closure showing the crus of the helix advanced into the helical rim. (Reproduced with permission of Charles H. Thorne, MD. Copyright Charles H. Thorne, MD.)

around the now-visible helical rim, and the medial surface of the freed cartilage is resurfaced with a graft or flap. In some cases, the buried cartilage is quite normal, and in other cases, it is markedly abnormal.

Question mark ear. The deficiency is variable and is usually treated with a cartilage graft and a V-Y advancement flap from the retroauricular skin. Often there is excess in the upper third of the ear requiring reduction. In severe cases, the entire ear is reconstructed as in microtia.

Postoperative Care

A bulky, noncompressive dressing is placed for a few days. Excessive pressure from the dressing will cause pain, increase swelling, and may lead to abrasion or even necrosis of auricular skin. When the dressing is removed, the patient wears a loose headband at night for 6 weeks. Again, the headband should only be tight enough that it does not fall off. The purpose is to prevent the corrected ear from being pulled forward when the patient rolls over in bed. A tight headband can erode the lateral surface of the ear, creating an open wound.

Nonoperative Technique in Infants

During the early weeks of infancy, the auricular cartilage has unusual plasticity, attributed to circulating maternal estrogens. During this privileged period, prominent ears and related deformities can be corrected permanently by molding the ears into the correct shape with tape and soft dental compound. The splints and tape are replaced regularly and the skin is checked compulsively for erosion. The process is continued for several months or until there is no further improvement in auricular contour. This ability to mold cartilage is currently being exploited in presurgical molding of the cleft nasal deformity (Chapter 23). It is not clear how long cartilage retains this "moldability" and therefore it is not clear when infants are too old to have this technique attempted.

Complications

Hematoma. Hematomas are one of the few early complications of otoplasty. Excessive pain or bleeding necessitates immediate removal of the dressing to rule out and, if necessary, evacuate a hematoma.

Infection. Cellulitis is rare after otoplasty but is treated aggressively with intravenous antibiotics in an attempt to avoid chondritis. The latter may require debridement and leave the ear permanently disfigured.

Suture complications. By far the most common complication of otoplasty in the author's experience is related to suture extrusion in the retroauricular sulcus. Such sutures are easily removed but may be associated with unattractive and/or painful granulomas. The use of absorbable sutures might eliminate this complication but the author has not had the courage to abandon permanent sutures. Monofilament sutures are more likely to protrude but are less likely to create granulomas. Braided sutures are the opposite: Less likely to protrude but more likely to be associated with granulomas.

Overcorrection/unnatural contours. The most common significant complication of otoplasty is overcorrection. Attention to the principles outlined above will minimize overcorrection and the creation of unnatural contours.

My personal thoughts about otoplasty are as follows:

1. *Incisions*. The incision is best placed in the retroauricular sulcus, not up on the back of the ear. The latter is more convenient for the surgeon and more expeditious, but may leave a scar that is visible when the patient is viewed from behind. Specific indications (macrotia, constricted ear, or ears with inadequate helical rim) call for an incision on the front (lateral surface) of the ear, where it is ideally made just inside the helical rim.
2. *Skin excision*. **Skin excision is unnecessary, does not contribute to the correction, and may lead to hypertrophic or undesirable scars.** The only exception is the earlobe where it may be necessary. When performing the latter, care is taken to remove only enough skin, adjacent to the retrolobular sulcus, to allow repositioning and to leave a full, free earlobe for ear piercing and an aesthetically normal earlobe.
3. *Techniques*. The simplest techniques are best. Techniques that involve abrasion or full-thickness incisions and/or tubing to create the antihelical fold are unnecessary and should be avoided.
4. *Choice of sutures*. The author has returned to monofilament permanent sutures because of occasional granulomas associated with braided sutures such as Mersilene. A long-lasting monofilament suture such as polydioxanone suture (PDS) may be the best choice, but the author has no experience with this suture and therefore cannot credibly recommend it.

5. *Degree of correction.* Overcorrection of the ears is the most common problem. Contours should be soft, round, and natural rather than sharp and surgical in appearance.

PARTIAL ACQUIRED DEFECTS

Most auricular deformities are acquired, partial defects for which there is a good solution. The more superior on the ear the defect is located, the more choices there are for reconstruction. Reconstruction of the lobule is the most difficult and is aesthetically the most important.

Although some defects can be closed by soft tissue alone, cartilage is frequently needed for support. For smaller defects, a conchal cartilage graft may suffice. **However, for larger defects the rules of Firmin are extremely helpful: Defects that consist of 25% or more of the helical rim *or* involve more than two planes (i.e., involve antihelix as well as helix and scapha) will require rib cartilage for support. Conchal cartilage will not provide sufficient support in these cases.**

Specific Regional Defects

External Auditory Canal

Stenosis is best treated by a full-thickness graft applied over an acrylic mold, provided a reasonable recipient vascular bed can be prepared. Occasionally, multiple Z-plasties are used to relieve webbing of the orifice, or a local flap is used to line the canal and break up the contracture. An acrylic stent is then used for several months to counteract the inexorable tendency toward contracture.

Helical Rim

Acquired losses of the helical rim vary from small defects to major portions of the helix. The former, which usually result from tumor excisions or minor traumatic injuries, are best closed by advancing the helix in both directions, as described by Antia and Buch (Fig. 30.7). The success of this excellent technique depends first on freeing the entire helix from the scapha via an incision in the helical sulcus that extends through the cartilage but not through the posterior skin. The posterior auricular skin is undermined, dissecting just superficial to the perichondrium until the entire helix is hanging as a chondrocutaneous flap on the posterior skin. Extra length can be gained by a V-Y advancement of the crus helix, as described in the correction of the constricted ear, and defects up to 2 cm can often be closed with moderate tension. The surgeon can "cheat" by removing some of the scaphal cartilage, which will take tension off the reapproximated helical rim. Although originally described for upper-third auricular defects, this technique is also effective for middle-third defects, as well as for defects at the junction of the middle and lower thirds.

If the helical rim alone is missing, as may occur in burn injuries, a thin tube of retroauricular skin can be applied to the residual scapha with acceptable results (Fig 30.8). This is one example where cartilage may not be necessary. The disadvantage of this technique is that it requires three stages to "waltz" the tube into place: (a) formation of the tube in the sulcus, (b) transfer and insetting of one end of the tube, and (c) transfer and insetting of the other end of the tube.

Upper-third Defects

Techniques available for upper-third defects in increasing order of size and complexity are as follows (Fig. 30.9):

1. Local skin flaps (Fig. 30.9A, B)
2. Helical advancement (Fig. 30.9C, D).
3. Contralateral conchal cartilage graft covered with a retroauricular flap (Fig. 30.9E, F).
4. Chondrocutaneous composite flap. (Fig. 30.9G, H).
5. Rib cartilage graft covered with retroauricular skin or temporoparietal flap/skin graft (see Fig. 30.11).

Middle-third Defects

Techniques available for middle-third defects are as follows:

1. Primary closure with excision of accessory triangles (Fig. 30.10).

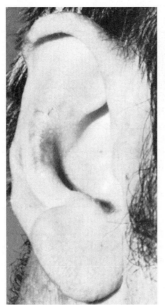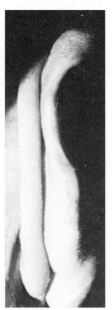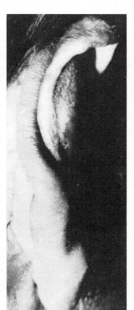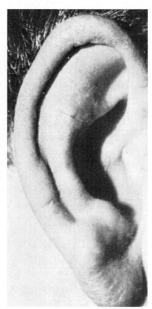

A,B   C,D

FIGURE 30.8. Helical reconstruction with a thin caliber tube flap. **A:** Burn deformity of the helix. **B:** Construction of the tube flap in the retroauricular sulcus. **C:** Transfer of one end of the tube. **D:** Final result. (Courtesy of Burt Brent, MD.)

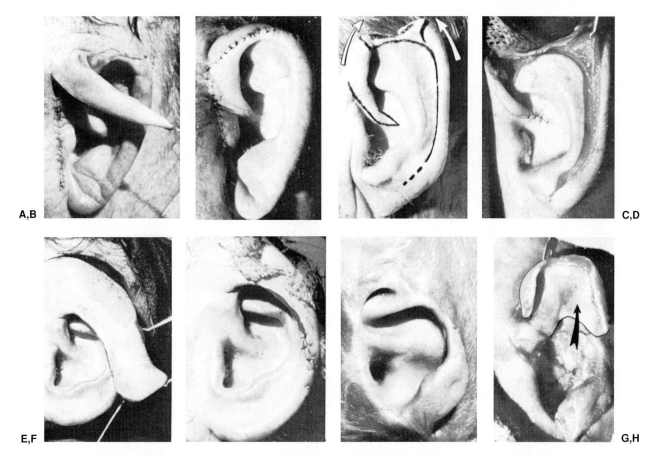

FIGURE 30.9. Four techniques for repairing upper-third auricular defects. **A** and **B**: Preauricular flap. The flap is transposed to repair a minor rim defect. **C** and **D**: Antia-Buch helical advancement. **E** and **F**: The combination of a retroauricular flap and conchal cartilage graft. **G** and **H**: Chondrocutaneous conchal flap to reconstruct the helical rim. Of the upper-third techniques, the only one not shown is a rib cartilage graft, which is shown in Figure 30.11. (Courtesy of Burt Brent, MD.)

2. Helical advancement.
3. Conchal cartilage graft and retroauricular flap.
4. Rib cartilage graft and retroauricular flap and/or temporoparietal flap (Fig. 30.11).

Cartilage grafts can be inserted via the Converse tunnel procedure in which the skin is not detached at the junction of the residual ear and the retroauricular skin. The problem is that precise placement of the graft with exact coaptation to remaining cartilage is difficult using this approach, and a detached retroauricular flap (Fig. 30.11) is often necessary. Middle-third auricular tumors are excised and closed by either a wedge resection with accessory triangles (Fig. 30.10) or a helical advancement, as previously described.

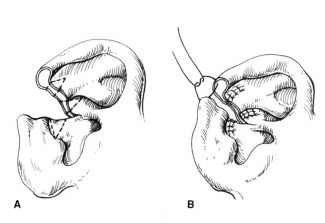

FIGURE 30.10. Wedge resection and primary closure with excision of accessory triangles. **A**: Wedge excision performed and accessory triangles designed. **B**: Closure of the defect. The accessory triangles help prevent the auricle from cupping forward. (Reproduced with permission of Charles H. Thorne, MD. Copyright Charles H. Thorne, MD.)

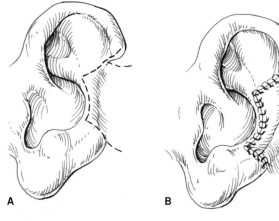

FIGURE 30.11. Reconstruction of a partial defect using rib cartilage framework and retroauricular flap. The technique is a workhorse for partial defects. **A**: The incision is designed. **B**: The cartilage has been placed and the flap closed over it. (Reproduced with permission of Charles H. Thorne, MD. Copyright Charles H. Thorne, MD.)

Lower-third Auricular Defects

Various techniques have been described to reconstruct earlobe defects using soft-tissue flaps. These techniques are not as effective as those that employ cartilaginous support. Like the alar rim, the normal earlobe does not contain cartilage. A reconstructed earlobe, however, maintains its shape better if cartilage is included, analogous to the nonanatomic alar rim grafts to the nose. The author prefers to use thin, flat cartilage obtained from the nasal septum. The cartilage is placed beneath the cheek/retroauricular skin in the first stage. In the second stage, an incision is made around the cartilage graft and the flap is advanced beneath the earlobe as in a facelift (Fig. 30.12).

MICROTIA

Microtia literally means small ear. The simplicity of the term belies the vast complexity of this entity, both in terms of the variable clinical presentation and the difficulty of surgical reconstruction.

History

Gillies is credited with the first use of rib cartilage for construction of an auricular framework in 1920. The importance of his contribution was temporarily obfuscated by several reports using allogeneic cartilage. The allogeneic cartilage, whether from a living donor such as the patient's parent or preserved cadaver cartilage, always underwent gradual resorption.

The modern era of auricular reconstruction began with Tanzer who reintroduced the technique of autogenous costal cartilage grafts as a method of auricular reconstruction.

Tanzer's results inspired Brent who modified, improved, and standardized a four-stage technique of auricular reconstruction. Nagata developed a more complex technique that condensed microtia repair to two stages. The Nagata technique, requires more cartilage and the construction of a higher profile, more detailed framework than the Brent technique. Firmin analyzed those characteristics of a "Brent ear" that fall short of a normal ear and reported a large series using her modification of the Nagata technique.

Although the technique of autogenous auricular reconstruction was evolving, silastic was also used, instead of rib cartilage, as the auricular framework. This material, as well as other artificial materials, led to a high incidence of extrusion. More recently, the use of porous polyethylene frameworks has been explored and has become the standard treatment offered by some surgeons. The largest series was reported by Reinisch. Early attempts were associated with a 42% incidence of framework extrusion leading to modifications of the original technique and coverage of the framework using a temporoparietal fascial flap. According to Reinisch, this drastically reduced the complication rate and is the technique of choice in his opinion.

Finally, an auricular prosthesis is another option. The introduction of titanium osseointegrated fixtures by Branemark has made prosthetic reconstruction of the auricle a more stable and user-friendly alternative. The role of prosthetic reconstruction in microtia will also be discussed below.

Anatomy and Surgical Challenge

The ear is composed of a delicate and complex-shaped cartilage framework covered on its visible surface with thin, tightly adherent, hairless skin. A reconstructed auricular framework

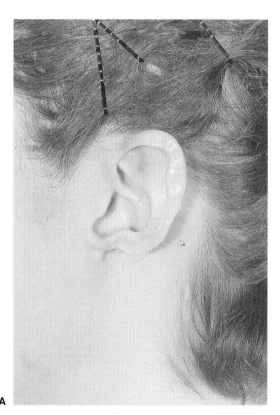
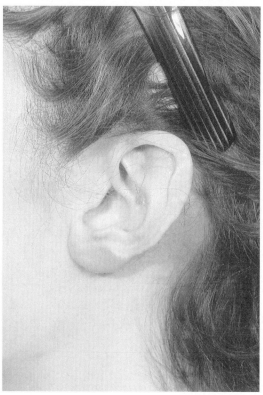

FIGURE 30.12. Earlobe reconstruction using nasal septal cartilage. **A:** Original defect secondary to discoid lupus erythematosus. **B:** Final result after two-stage reconstruction using thin cartilage from the nasal septum. (Courtesy of Charles H. Thorne, MD.)

must be more rigid than the cartilage framework of a normal ear. When the auricular framework is placed beneath the skin in the temporal region, a combination of the tight skin envelope and the progressive scar contracture will gradually obliterate the fine details if the framework is built to mimic the delicate framework of the normal ear. **As such, any reconstructed ear that maintains its projection and definition in the long-term will be more bulky and will lack the flexibility of the normal ear.**

Consequently, even the best result using current techniques for auricular reconstruction is imperfect. The deficiencies of current techniques make it even more important that the reconstructed auricle be the correct size, be located in the proper position such that one earlobe is not higher than the other, and be properly angulated relative to the other facial structures.

Embryology

The middle and external ears are derived from the first (mandibular) and second (hyoid) branchial arches. Most patients with microtia have atresia (absence) of the external auditory canal and tympanic membrane with variable deformities of the middle ear ossicles. Rarely a patient will present with microtia and a patent, stenotic canal. Least common but most difficult to repair are patients with an auricular vestige that is markedly abnormal in position. Because the meatus can only be moved a limited distance, the surgeon must consider complete excision of the canal.

The inner ear is derived from totally separate embryologic tissues from the middle/external ear and is, therefore, almost always normal in patients with microtia. In other words, the hearing loss in microtia/atresia patients is conductive in nature.

Incidence/Genetics

The incidence of microtia varies widely among ethnic groups. Textbooks cling to the figure of 1 in every 6,000 births. The incidence is higher in patients of Asian ethnicity. In addition, microtia is almost twice as common among males as females and almost twice as common on the right side compared to the left. Bilateral microtia occurs in somewhere between 10% and 20% of patients with microtia.

Most cases of microtia occur in an isolated fashion. Only rarely does microtia appear to run in families. One exception is Treacher Collins syndrome, which frequently presents with bilateral microtia and is inherited in an autosomal dominant fashion.

Microtia in Hemifacial Microsomia

Older publications suggest that isolated microtia and hemifacial microsomia are distinct entities. In fact, microtia is part of the spectrum of hemifacial microsomia deformities, all of which owe their origin to maldevelopment in the first and second branchial arches. At one end of the spectrum is the patient with microtia who appears to have an otherwise symmetrical face. At the other end of the spectrum is a patient who manifests underdevelopment of all tissues on one side of the face including microtia, aural atresia, underdevelopment of the mandible, underdevelopment of the soft tissues of the cheek, and underdevelopment of the facial nerve. Microtia and hemifacial microsomia should *not* be considered as separate entities (Chapter 26).

Canaloplasty and Middle Ear Reconstruction

Patients with unilateral microtia/atresia usually have normal hearing in the contralateral ear. This should be verified by an otologist as early as possible after birth. The main goal then becomes protection of the better hearing ear throughout development. It is important that otitis media in the ear with normal hearing be treated completely and that a hearing test be repeated after completion of treatment. Residual middle ear fluid in the only normal ear may result in hearing impairment and consequently interference with speech development.

Patients with unilateral microtia do well from an otologic point of view. These patients have some difficulty localizing sounds but, in many cases, require no amplification device and no special treatment in the classroom. There is, however, a movement in the otologic community to be more aggressive with bone conduction aids that result in binaural hearing.

Patients with bilateral microtia/atresia are in an entirely different situation. These patients are functionally deaf with complete conductive hearing loss bilaterally. These patients are fitted with a bone-conduction hearing aid as early as possible in life and benefit from a bone-anchored hearing aid retained with a titanium abutment when they get older.

Approximately one-half of the patients with microtia/aural atresia have middle ear anatomy that can be reconstructed surgically. In bilateral cases, this is extremely important and may eliminate the need for a hearing aid or at least decrease total dependence on such a device.

The issue in the unilateral case is not as clear because, as stated above, these patients function reasonably well. **Most otologists around the world do not recommend canaloplasty in patients with unilateral microtia.** The surgical results are prone to stenosis of the external auditory canal meatus as well as scar contracture of the reconstructed tympanic membrane. The hearing in the reconstructed ear tends to worsen with time. This nonsurgical recommendation, however, is not universal and good results have been reported by Jahrsdorfer in unilateral cases. The timing of the auricular reconstruction relative to the canaloplasty is important. **The auricular reconstruction is best performed before the canaloplasty.** Auricular reconstruction is possible after canal surgery but the result is compromised by the scarring in the region.

Classification

The microtia deformity itself is enormously variable. At one end of the spectrum is an auricle that is slightly small but otherwise normal in appearance. At the other end of the spectrum is the patient with complete anotia. Various classifications have been proposed to deal with this vast variability in clinical presentation. The Nagata classification is useful because it correlates with the surgical approach.

- *Lobule type.* These patients have an ear remnant and malpositioned lobule but have no concha, acoustic meatus, or tragus.
- *Concha type.* These patients present with an ear remnant, malpositioned earlobe, concha (with or without acoustic meatus), tragus, and antitragus with an incisura intertragica.
- *Small concha type.* These patients present with an ear remnant, malpositioned lobule, and a small indentation instead of a concha.
- *Anotia.* These patients present with no, or only a minute, ear remnant.
- *Atypical microtia.* These patients present with deformities that do not fit into any of the above categories.

Surgical Reconstruction

The following are the three options for reconstruction of microtia:

1. Autogenous reconstruction.
2. Composite autogenous/alloplastic reconstruction using an alloplastic ear framework.
3. Prosthetic reconstruction.

Autogenous Reconstruction

The two main techniques described for autogenous reconstruction of the auricle using a rib cartilage framework are the Brent technique and the Nagata technique.

The Brent technique involves four stages:

1. Creation and placement of a rib cartilage auricular framework (Figs. 30.13 and 30.14).
2. Rotation of the malpositioned ear lobule into the correct position (Fig. 30.15).
3. Elevation of the reconstructed auricle and creation of a retroauricular sulcus (Fig. 30.16).
4. Deepening of the concha and creation of the tragus (Fig. 30.17).

The Nagata technique is performed in two stages:

1. Creation of an auricular framework including the tragus and rotation of the lobule into the correct position (in other words, combining stages 1, 2, and 4 from the Brent technique) (Figs. 30.18 and 30.19).
2. Elevation of the reconstructed ear and creation of the retroauricular sulcus (Fig. 30.20).

Technical Details of the Two Techniques. The patient is examined standing and the location of the earlobe on the normal side is transferred to the affected side. This is the single most important marking because symmetrical earlobes is one of the primary goals of the procedure. The normal ear is traced on clear x-ray film and sterilized. Using this tracing, additional templates are made. A template of the desired framework is made, approximately 3 to 4 mm shorter and narrower than the eventual ear. If the Nagata technique is performed, additional templates are constructed of the antihelix/triangular fossa piece and the tragus/antitragus piece.

The exact location and orientation of the desired auricle are drawn on the patient. Decisions are made about the location of the incisions. In the Brent technique, an incision is designed that can be used again at the time of lobule rotation and at the time of tragus construction. If the Nagata technique is used, the incision is designed as shown in Figure 30.19, to allow rotation of the lobule. The incision is made and the cartilage remnant is removed, carefully preserving the skin and avoiding buttonholes if possible. The pocket is dissected beyond the outline of the eventual auricle. In the Nagata technique, a pedicle is maintained to the dissected flap to improve blood supply.

Attention is turned to the chest. Although a transverse incision will heal more favorably than an oblique incision, the latter provides better exposure. The rectus abdominis muscle is divided. In the Brent technique, two pieces of cartilages are harvested. In the Nagata technique, five pieces are required. In addition to the synchondrosis of two cartilages and a free rib for the helical rim, the Nagata technique requires removal of a piece for the antihelix/triangular fossa, a piece for the tragus/antitragus, and a piece to be banked in the chest for the second stage. This piece is wedged into the sulcus at the second stage to provide projection of the auricle. Nagata harvests the cartilages in a subperichondrial plane, leaving the perichondrium in the chest when the cartilages are removed. The author tends to take the cartilages with the perichondrium and has not noticed a significant difference in the chest wall deformity. If a pneumothorax is created, a catheter is placed into the pleural cavity. After the incision is closed the catheter is withdrawn while the anesthesiologist applies positive pressure ventilation. An additional catheter is left in the wound for the administration of Marcaine postoperatively.

Details are applied to the base using gouges. In the Nagata technique, the antihelix/triangular fossa piece is attached. The helical rim is attached in a similar fashion in both techniques. The difference is that Nagata recommends waiting until

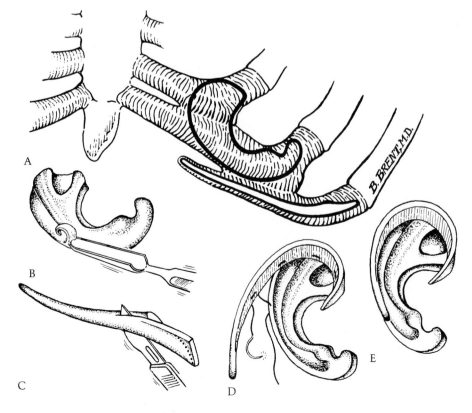

FIGURE 30.13. Fabrication of ear framework from rib cartilage. Brent technique, stage 1. **A:** The base block is obtained from the synchondrosis of two rib cartilages. The helical rim is obtained from a "floating" rib cartilage. **B:** Carving the details into the base using a gouge. **C:** Thinning of the rib cartilage to produce the helical rim. **D:** Attaching the rim to the base block using nylon sutures. **E:** Completed framework.

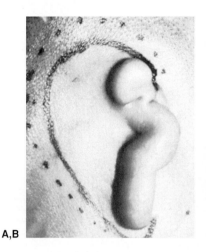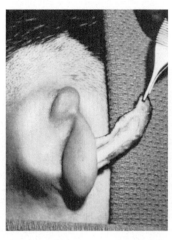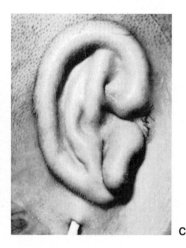

A,B   C

FIGURE 30.14. Insertion of the ear framework. Brent technique, stage 1. **A:** Preoperative markings indicating the desired location of the framework (*solid line*) and the extent of the dissection necessary (*dotted line*). **B:** Insertion of cartilage framework. **C:** Appearance after the first stage. A suction catheter is using to suck the skin into the interstices of the framework. (Courtesy of Burt Brent, MD.)

the child is 10 years old, which yields cartilages that are long enough to reconstruct the crus of the helix. Finally, the tragus/antitragus piece is attached in the Nagata technique. Nagata uses wire sutures. The author has used nylon sutures, rather than wire, for both the Brent and Nagata techniques, with adequate fixation and a low incidence of suture extrusion.

The framework is inserted into the pocket along with two suction drains. Once the closure has been accomplished and the dressing has been applied, the drains are attached to Vacutainer tubes. The tubes are changed every half hour for 2 hours, then every hour for 2 hours and then every 4 hours overnight. The dressing is removed on the second postoperative day and the patient is discharged.

Complications. Complications of the Brent technique are rare in experienced hands. Complications of the Nagata technique, at least in the author's hands, are relatively common. The most common complication is exposure of the cartilage framework. Management requires experience, but these wounds usually heal without surgical intervention unless they are large. Exposed areas of more than 1 cm in greatest dimension require urgent coverage with a temporoparietal flap and skin graft. In fact, if there is the slightest question about whether an exposed area will heal, then flap coverage is indicated. **One never re-**

grets performing flap coverage of an exposed area of cartilage framework, but one may certainly regret *not* performing such a procedure.

Elevation of framework. In the third stage of the Brent technique and the second stage of the Nagata technique, the previously placed framework is elevated and the retroauricular sulcus is resurfaced. Nagata adds a piece of rib cartilage covered with a temporoparietal flap. The cartilage is banked under the skin at the time of the first stage and is wedged into the sulcus to provide projection to the reconstructed auricle in the second stage. The fascial flap covers the graft and provides a bed for skin grafting. (Fig. 30.20) In both techniques the scalp is advanced into the depth of the sulcus and the medial surface of the elevated framework is resurfaced with a skin graft.

Both Nagata and Brent recommend a split thickness graft for this stage. The grafts contract significantly, however, in some cases obliterating the reconstructed sulcus. For this reason the author prefers a full thickness graft from the groin. The disadvantage is a visible scar but the full thickness graft resists contracture and is more likely to result in maintenance of the reconstructed sulcus.

Composite Autogenous/Alloplastic Reconstruction

In these patients, an auricular framework composed of porous polyethylene (Medpor) is used instead of costal cartilage. Reinisch originally reported a 42% incidence of implant exposure. He modified the technique, adding temporoparietal flap coverage of the framework, and reports a vastly decreased complication rate.

Prosthetic Reconstruction

Prior to the introduction of implant retention of prostheses, prosthetic reconstruction depended on adhesive retention and was impractical. Branemark osseointegrated titanium implants have made prosthetic reconstruction somewhat more practical but this technique remains, in the author's opinion, a second choice to autogenous reconstruction (see Chapter 34).

Children are poor candidates for prostheses, often refusing to wear them regardless of the retention mechanism. Children also tire of the maintenance required of the abutments and the surrounding soft tissue. If adequate hygiene is not maintained, the skin/abutment interface becomes inflamed and use of the prosthesis must be discontinued awaiting resolution of the inflammation. Additionally, the daily removal and replacement of the prosthesis serves as a constant reminder of the deformity. In contrast, children with an autogenous reconstruction

FIGURE 30.15. Rotation of lobule. Brent technique, stage 2. The earlobe is rotated from its vertical malposition into the correct position at the caudal aspect of the framework. **A:** Design of lobe rotation is made such that the same incision can be used in stage 4, tragus construction. **B:** After rotation of the lobule. (Reproduced with permission of Charles H. Thorne, MD. Copyright Charles H. Thorne, MD.)

A   B   *after Brent*

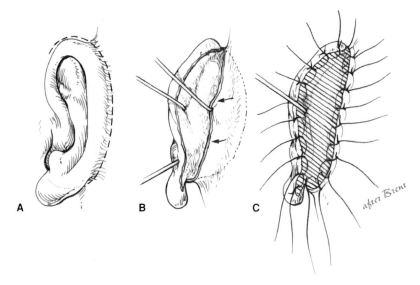

FIGURE 30.16. Elevation of framework and skin graft to sulcus. Brent technique, stage 3. **A:** Incision is designed behind the ear. **B:** The retroauricular scalp is advanced into the sulcus so that the eventual graft will not be visible. **C:** Full-thickness graft to the exposed medial surface of the auricle. (Reproduced with permission of Charles H. Thorne, MD. Copyright Charles H. Thorne, MD.)

incorporate the new ear into their sense of self. Finally, prostheses lack the warmth and texture of autogenous reconstructions and, despite the superior details, are not more "lifelike."

It is important to note that prostheses require replacement every several years for the life of the patient and, therefore, prosthetic reconstruction is more expensive in the long-term than autogenous reconstruction.

To this author's thinking, the only absolute indication for prosthetic reconstruction in a child with microtia is failed autogenous reconstruction with inadequate soft tissue for either a second autogenous reconstruction or a Medpor reconstruction. In such a patient, a prosthesis may represent the only salvage procedure available.

Relative indications for the use of prosthetic reconstruction include a very low hairline where a temporoparietal flap would be required to allow autogenous reconstruction or extreme hypoplasia of the tissues with a concavity where the auricle will eventually be located.

Personal Thoughts on Surgical Reconstruction

The author has extensive experience with both the Brent and the Nagata techniques of auricular reconstruction and it is on the basis of that experience that the following comparative statements are made.

The Nagata procedure was designed to address the perceived weaknesses of the Tanzer/Brent technique, particularly the region of the concha, crus of the helix, tragus, and incisura intertragica. As such, the best possible Nagata-type result may have superior details to the best possible Brent-type result. The problem is that the "best possible results" do not occur most of the time.

The Nagata procedure, at least in the hands of this author, is definitely associated with a higher complication rate. The framework is much higher profile, much more complex in its details, and contains many more sutures. As such, the chance of cutaneous necrosis with framework exposure is significantly greater using the Nagata technique. On the other hand, these areas of exposure are generally small and heal without further surgical intervention and do not necessarily compromise the result.

The individual surgeon must decide, factoring in his/her experience, whether the possibility of a superior result is worth the increased risk of the Nagata procedure. In his own practice, this author currently uses the Nagata/Firmin technique in most patients. In patients with extremely tight skin, or the presence

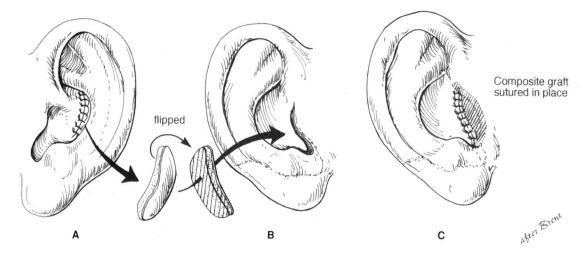

FIGURE 30.17. Construction of tragus. Brent technique, stage 4. **A:** The conchal graft is taken from the posterior conchal wall of the contralateral ear. **B:** An L-shaped incision is made and the graft is inserted with the skin surface down. **C:** The graft healed nicely. (Reproduced with permission of Charles H. Thorne, MD. Copyright Charles H. Thorne, MD.)

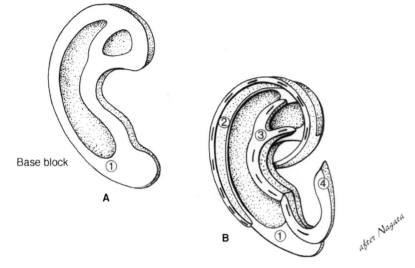

Base block

A

B

Reconstructed ear
using 3-D cartilage framework

after Nagata

FIGURE 30.18. Fabrication of ear framework from rib cartilage. Nagata technique, stage 1. **A:** In a manner similar to Brent, the base and its details are carved from the synchondrosis of two adjacent ribs. **B:** The four pieces of cartilage that make up the cartilage framework are seen and numbered. The base and helical rim are present as they are for the Brent technique. There is an additional antihelix-triangular fossa piece and an additional tragus-antitragus piece that are unique to the Nagata procedure. (Reproduced with permission of Charles H. Thorne, MD. Copyright Charles H. Thorne, MD.)

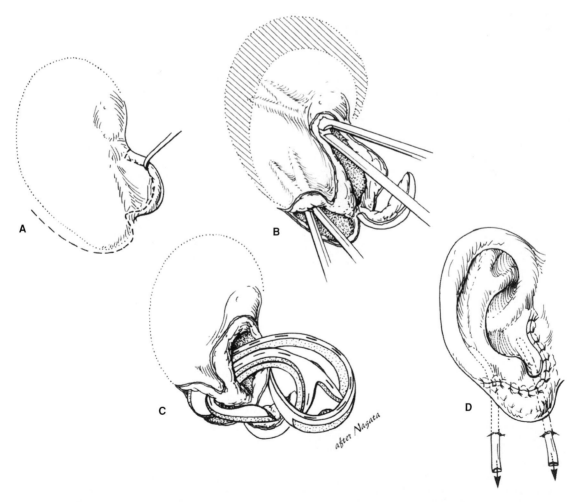

after Nagata

FIGURE 30.19. Insertion of the cartilage framework. Nagata technique, stage 1. **A:** The incision is designed, robbing most of the skin on the medial surface of the lobule that will be necessary to line the concha. **B:** The pocket is dissected, leaving an intact "pedicle" at the caudal end of the flap. **C:** The framework is inserted. **D:** Appearance of the framework after stage 1. Suction drains are in place to coapt the skin to the underlying cartilage. (Reproduced with permission of Charles H. Thorne, MD. Copyright Charles H. Thorne, MD.)

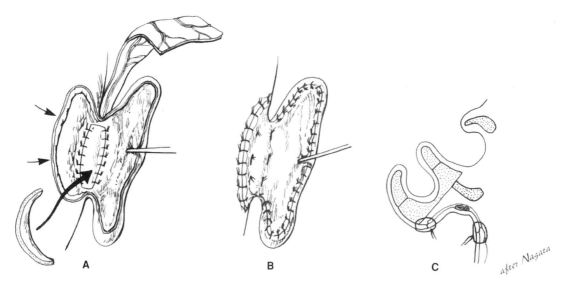

FIGURE 30.20. Elevation of framework. Nagata technique, stage 2. **A:** The auricle is elevated, the scalp is advanced into the sulcus (*arrows*), the cartilage graft is wedged into the sulcus, and the graft is covered with a temporoparietal flap and skin graft. **B:** The skin graft is in place. Nagata described the use of split-thickness skin but this author has noted tremendous shrinkage of the thin grafts and recommends full-thickness graft. **C:** Cross-section showing the cartilage graft in place providing projection as well as the temporoparietal flap covering the temporoparietal flap. (Reproduced with permission of Charles H. Thorne, MD. Copyright Charles H. Thorne, MD.)

of other scars, the Brent technique is used because of its safety and reliability.

The other issue involves the chest donor site. The Nagata technique requires harvesting twice as much cartilage as the Brent technique. While Nagata harvests all cartilage subperichondrially, no detailed study has been performed comparing the chest wall deformity created by the Nagata technique at age 10 years with the deformity created by the Brent technique at age 6 years. Although the donor site is an issue not to be ignored, it tends not to be an issue regardless of which technique is used. Patients simply do not complain about the chest unless they are extremely thin.

Proponents of the composite alloplastic/autogenous reconstruction using Medpor cite the lack of chest donor-site scars/deformity as an advantage. Although that is true, these same reports fail to mention the scars/deformity that replace the chest deformity. For example, the composite technique robs the contralateral normal ear of *all* the skin behind it, resulting in obliteration of the sulcus or a skin graft donor-site scar if the retroauricular defect is replaced with partial-thickness skin. Additionally, this technique requires a scalp scar to harvest the temporoparietal flap. These scars are frequently hypertrophic and/or associated with thin strips of alopecia, which may be more troublesome to the patient than a chest wall scar.

Severe Facial Asymmetry

Placing the reconstructed ear in the best location is straight forward if the face is symmetrical or near symmetrical. In cases of significant asymmetry, however, compromises must be made. The surgeon cannot rely on measurements from landmarks such as the lateral canthus or oral commissure, because the entire side of the face is so much smaller than the other side. If such measurements were used, the ear would be placed far too posteriorly, and would appear strikingly abnormal. Of equal importance, however, the ear must not be place too low or too anterior. The author attempts to place the ear in the correct

craniocaudal position so that the earlobes are at the same level and then determines the anteroposterior positioning based on the relationship to the sideburn. No ear will look normal unless there is a sideburn in front of it.

Acquired Deformity versus Microtia

Total auricular reconstruction of the acquired deformity differs from congenital microtia. There is always less skin available. In microtia, removal of the cartilaginous remnant provides some supple, unscarred skin to supplement the retroauricular skin. In the acquired situation, there may be no residual ear skin and the presence of scarring from the traumatic or surgical removal of the ear restricts the skin pocket. In many cases, a temporoparietal flap with skin graft is required in addition to the native skin. The flap provides an unlimited amount of vascularized tissue, but the combination of the flap and the skin graft never has the definition or color match of the native skin. In addition, the presence of an external auditory meatus limits the access incisions, the extent of the skin pocket and the risk of infection. The canal is colonized with bacteria, frequently *Pseudomonas* species, which adds additional problems not encountered in microtia cases.

SPECIAL SITUATIONS

Acute Auricular Trauma and Cauliflower Ear

A hematoma may result from trauma and frequently occurs in wrestlers. Unless evacuated, the blood tends to become cartilaginous, resulting in the so-called cauliflower ear. Once fully developed, the cauliflower ear is extremely difficult to correct. Hematomas may require repeated aspirations or an incision to fully evacuate. Suturing gauze bolsters to the auricle to

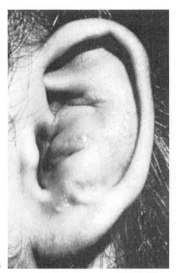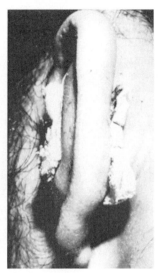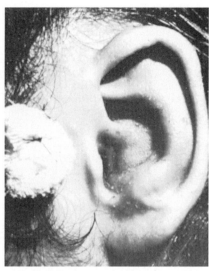

A,B   C

FIGURE 30.21. Management of an acute othematoma. **A:** Recurrent conchal hematoma. **B:** Through-and-through bolster sutures, after evacuation of the hematoma. **C:** Appearance of ear after the compression dressing has been removed at 10 days. (Courtesy of Burt Brent, MD.)

compress the skin against the cartilage usually prevents reoccurrence (Fig. 30.21).

Amputated Ear

Most attempts to replace an amputated ear will fail, resulting in additional incisions/scars and "burning bridges" that may be useful for secondary reconstruction. The patient, however, will not easily accept the decision to discard the amputated part without an attempt at replacement. There is no easy answer.

Replantation of amputated ears has been reported and some excellent results have been obtained. The vessels are small, however, and failure is common. Any attempt at replantation must consider that success is unlikely and may result in scars that limit later reconstructive attempts. Incisions for exposure of recipient vessels are kept to a minimum.

Reattaching large pieces of auricular tissue as composite grafts is doomed to failure. The good news is that such an attempt does not disrupt the surrounding tissues, does no harm, and makes the patient feel that "something" is being done.

Removing the skin from the cartilage and burying it beneath retroauricular skin is a poor choice. The thin, delicate cartilage will not maintain its shape sufficiently against the forces of scar contracture. An alternative is to cover the de-skinned cartilage with a temporoparietal flap. The esthetic result will be poor for the reasons mentioned above and this useful tissue will not be available for secondary reconstruction.

Several successful cases have been reported in which the posteromedial skin was removed from the amputated part, the cartilage was "fenestrated," retroauricular skin was excised, and the part was placed on the healthy bed. The anterolateral auricular skin is vascularized through the cartilage fenestrations by direct contact with this healthy, vascularized bed.

In the opinion of the author, the ideal scenario for an amputated ear is an attempt at microvascular replantation through the available wound, without additional incisions. If unsuccessful, secondary reconstruction with rib cartilage grafts is performed, with or without a temporoparietal flap. If replantation is not an available option, the part should be replaced as a composite graft (knowing it will fail), or the part should be discarded.

Acute Auricular Burns

Acute burns may result in chondritis. Characterized by tenderness, erythema, warmth, and induration, chondritis usually occurs several weeks after the initial injury. Once chondritis is diagnosed, aggressive steps are taken to eradicate the infection and prevent subsequent deformity. Drainage and placement of an irrigation system is an appropriate first step. If this therapy fails, the involved cartilage must be debrided. When the latter becomes necessary, incisions are planned judiciously to minimize the effect on secondary reconstruction.

Skin Cancer/Malignant Melanoma

Cutaneous malignancies of the helical rim can be excised and closed with helical advancement as described above (Fig 30.7). Lesions in the concha or over the antihelix can usually be excised and skin grafted. If the cartilage is involved, it can be excised and the graft placed directly on the posterior skin. Malignant melanomas should be excised with the same margins as melanomas of the equivalent depth in other parts of the body. Melanoma in situ does not require a full-thickness excision. These lesions are excised with a 5-mm margin, preserving the perichondrium, and skin grafted. Invasive melanomas of the helical rim require wedge resection to achieve adequate margins, eliminating helical advancement as an alternative for closure. These defects may be large and require secondary reconstruction as in Figure 30.11.

Earring Complications

While ingenious techniques have been described to reconstruct traumatic clefts in the lobe caused by earrings, the most reliable method is to excise and close the defect in one stage and re-pierce the ears 6 weeks later, or whenever the induration subsides.

Another complication of earrings is keloid formation. Small keloids can be excised and closed primarily and may not recur.

If the patient is truly prone to keloids, then excision, triamcinolone injection, and pressure earrings are warranted. If the keloid recurs, excision with immediate irradiation offers the best chance of avoiding recurrence.

Finally, piercing through the cartilage in the upper portion of the ear can result in severe infections. While not common, chondritis can lead to severe, permanent disfigurement of the auricle. Infections therefore are treated aggressively. If cartilage requires debridement, it is performed early to limit the deformity and incisions are planned carefully to minimize these deformities.

Suggested Readings

Al-Qattan MM, Hashem FK. An alternative approach for correction of Stahl's ear. *Ann Plast Surg*. 2004;52(1):105.

Antia NH, Buch MS. Chondrocutaneous advancement flap for the marginal defect of the ear. *Plast Reconstr Surg*. 1967;39:472.

Brent BD. Technical advances in ear reconstruction with autogenous rib cartilage grafts—Personal experience with 1,200 cases. *Plast Reconstr Surg*. 1999;104:319.

Davis J. Reconstruction of the upper third of the ear with a chondrocutaneous composite flap based on the crus helix. In: Tanzer RC, Edgerton MT, eds.

Symposium on Reconstruction of the Auricle. St. Louis: Mosby; 1974: 247: 51.

Demir Y. Correction of constricted ear deformity with combined V-Y advancement of crus helices and perichondrioplasty technique. *Plast Reconstr Surg*. 2005;116(7):2044.

Firmin R. Ear reconstruction in cases of typical microtia. Personal experience based on 352 microtic ear corrections. *Scand J Plast Surg*. 1998; 32:35.

Gault DT, Grippaudo FR, Tyler M. Ear reduction. *Br J Plast Surg*. 1995; 48:30.

Gosain AK, Recinos RF. A novel approach to correction of the prominent lobule during otoplasty. *Plast Reconstr Surg*. 2003;112(2):575.

Harris PA, Ladhani K, Das-Gupta R, et al. Reconstruction of acquired sub-total ear defects with autologous costal cartilage. *Br J Plast Surg*. 1999;52(4):268.

Janis JE, Rohrich RJ, Gutowski KA. Otoplasty. *Plast Reconstr Surg*. 2005;115(4):60e.

Matsuo K, Hayashi R, Kiyono M, et al. Nonsurgical correction of congenital auricular deformities. *Clin Plast Surg*. 990;17(2):383.

Nagata S. A new method of total reconstruction of the auricle for microtia. *Plast Reconstr Surg*. 1993;92:187.

Noguchi M, Matsuo K, Imai Y, et al. Simple surgical correction of Stahl's ear. *Br J Plast Surg*. 1994;47(8):570.

Thorne CH, Brecht LE, Bradley JP, et al. Auricular reconstruction: Indications for autogenous and prosthetic techniques. *Plast Reconstr Surg*. 2001;107(5):1241.

Vogelin E, Grobbelaar AO, Chana JS, et al. Surgical correction of the cauliflower ear. *Br J Plast Surg*. 1998;51(5):359.

CHAPTER 31 ■ SOFT TISSUE AND SKELETAL INJURIES OF THE FACE

LARRY HOLLIER, JR. AND PATRICK KELLEY

The treatment of the facial trauma patient continues to evolve with progress in imaging, bone fixation technology, and the application of microsurgical reconstructive techniques and distraction osteogenesis. Many of the principles of access and fixation remain constant, but the application of these principles has been greatly facilitated with improvements in instrumentation and osteosynthesis technology. Facial trauma continues to be treated by a variety of specialists, including plastic surgeons, otolaryngologists, and oral surgeons. Plastic surgeons, however, are uniquely trained to handle the full range of issues present in the trauma patient.

INITIAL MANAGEMENT

Facial injuries themselves are rarely life-threatening, but are indicators of the energy of injury. Initial care of all trauma patients should focus on the algorithmic protocol of ATLS (Advanced Trauma Life Support). Facial injuries should alert the examiner to the possibility of airway compromise, cervical spine injuries, or central nervous system injuries.

Airway

Airway compromise is the result of either direct laryngeal injury, foreign bodies (including aspirated teeth and bone fragments), or excessive bleeding from an upper airway source. **Treatment of the compromised airway is complicated by the likelihood that 10% of facial trauma patients have cervical spine injuries.** Often upright positioning with cervical spine protection will improve airway function compromised by excessive bleeding or foreign bodies. Foreign bodies can be mechanically removed by the finger-sweep technique. Airway compromise can also occur when the floor of mouth and tongue lose support from a comminuted mandible fracture and can be alleviated by simple anterior traction on the mandibular symphysis.

The trauma team should have a low threshold for definitive airway protection via endotracheal intubation. The use of blind nasal intubation should be carried out with caution. Nasal intubations can exacerbate nasal and nasopharyngeal bleeding. Additionally, the tube may be inadvertently placed ultracranially in the obtunded patient with a skull-base fracture. Endoscopic nasal or oral intubation improves safety by avoiding the cervical spine manipulation; it further provides immediate confirmation of tracheal intubation.

Emergent tracheotomy is considered in the unusual circumstance of laryngeal fracture or inability to secure an upper airway route to intubation. Tracheotomy performed in the controlled environment of the operating room is far superior to either emergent tracheotomy or cricothyrotomy. There should be a low threshold for a controlled, temporary tracheotomy

in the patient with significant soft-tissue trauma to the floor of mouth and tongue, especially the base of tongue. These injuries are more commonly penetrating in nature and initially misleading in that there may be minimal signs of distress. The swelling in the first 24 to 48 hours, however, may be significant enough to compromise the airway, forcing tracheotomy under less-than-favorable circumstances.

Hemorrhage

The dense vascularity of the head and neck can cause significant blood loss from soft-tissue injuries. Fortunately, most of these injuries allow sufficient access for direct pressure to control hemorrhage. The control of bleeding vessels should be accurate and directed. A number of critical structures can become collateral victims by clamping sources of bleeding with poor exposure and visualization. Bleeding that cannot be controlled with direct pressure requires packing. Packing in the nasal cavity is usually effective and only rarely requires augmentation with a transnasal balloon catheter in the nasopharynx. Nasopharyngeal balloon catheters only serve to impede blood from entering the oropharynx where it can more easily enter the lungs. Massive hemorrhage should be approached with emergent intubation followed by packing and direct pressure. The source of bleeding is most commonly a branch of the external carotid system, which is most appropriately controlled with angiographic embolization. The radiologist usually requires the assistance of the surgeon to remove the packing so that the source of bleeding can be more readily identified. Type-specific blood should be readily available. Surgical ligation of the external carotid artery will not control bleeding from its injured branches because of the robust collateralization present and should not be attempted (Fig. 31.1).

Central Nervous System

Neurologic injury is commonly associated with severe facial trauma. In a series of 1,068 patients with facial fractures, 79.4% were associated with some form of traumatic brain injury (1). Patients with facial trauma rarely die from facial injuries, but can die from associated injuries of the central nervous system. As part of a complete trauma evaluation most patients with facial trauma undergo computed tomography (CT) scanning to rule out head injury. The most widely accepted method for expressing the degree of neurological injury is the Glasgow Coma Score (GCS). This evaluates the motor, verbal, and eye-opening responses of the patient on initial evaluation, rating the patient from a lowest score of 3 to a highest score of 15 (Table 31.1).

As a general rule, concomitant head injury is not a contraindication to facial fracture repair assuming the neurologic

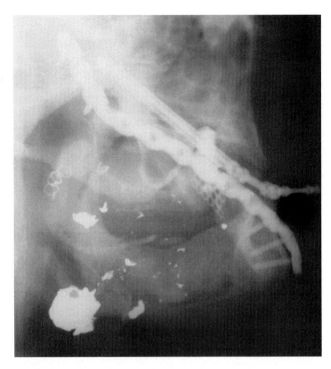

FIGURE 31.1. Hemorrhage treated by embolization. Patient with gunshot wound to mandible requiring embolization of lingual artery (note coil) to prevent exsanguination. Segmental defect is treated with a distraction device.

injury is stable and not in the process of evolution. In the event of acute brain injury, surgical repair of facial fractures generally is delayed to avoid the fluid overload associated with surgery and, most importantly, to avoid undetected decline of neurologic function during the period of general anesthesia when clinical neurologic examination cannot be performed. Once the central nervous system injury and concomitant swelling have stabilized, facial fracture repair can generally be undertaken safely.

Ten percent of patients with facial trauma suffer some form of cervical spine injury. Suspicion for injury and vigilant care of the cervical spine are key elements in the care of

TABLE 31.1

GLASGOW COMA SCALE

Eye opening	Spontaneous	4
	To voice	3
	To pain	2
	None	1
Verbal response	Oriented	5
	Confused	4
	Inappropriate	3
	Incomprehensible	2
	None	1
Motor response	Obeys commands	6
	Localizes	5
	Withdraws (pain)	4
	Flexion	3
	Extension (pain)	2
	None	1
Glasgow Coma Score (Total)		3–16

facial trauma patients. Cervical spine precautions are mandatory until the spine is cleared both clinically and radiographically. For the obtunded patient, the cervical spine is best evaluated with a CT scan, although a negative exam does not rule out unstable ligamentous injury. These patients require additional examination when the sensorium is clear, and possibly flexion/extension radiographs or magnetic resonance imaging (MRI) to definitively evaluate the cervical spine.

FACIAL TRAUMA EVALUATION

History

Use of the AMPLE acronym (allergies, medications, past history, last meal, events surrounding the accident) facilitates a complete trauma history.

Head and Neck Examination

A thorough head and neck examination serves as the starting point and is performed in a logical and consistent manner to avoid missing something. The examiner should not be distracted by the more impressive injuries because of the likelihood of overlooking less obvious but potentially significant problems. In the acutely injured patient with facial trauma, the physical exam is greatly impaired by facial swelling. Asymmetries that are secondary to fractures are usually concealed. Additionally, it may be difficult to elicit tenderness because of simultaneous distracting injuries.

The examiner carefully assesses the face for neurologic deficits, including the trigeminal and facial nerves. Sensory disturbances in the forehead, cheek, and lower lip should be well documented as should any deficits in facial nerve function. Undocumented preoperative nerve injuries may be attributed postoperatively to surgical intervention. Lacerations, contusions, and abrasions of the skin may focus the exam by indicating which nerves are at risk.

A complete ocular examination includes the evaluation of ocular history, acuity, light and red light perception, ocular motility, pupillary exam, and examination of the conjunctiva and eyelids. Each eye requires assessment individually to prevent confusion to the patient and examiner. Much of the long-term morbidity of facial trauma is associated with ocular and orbital injury. Although there should be a low threshold to involve the ophthalmologist, the physician treating facial trauma should be well versed in the ocular examination.

Examination of the oral cavity is essential, especially in the obtunded patient who may have loose teeth, bone fragments, or foreign bodies. Identification and removal of prosthetics (e.g., dentures) is essential. The occlusion and intercuspation is carefully evaluated, as both mandibular and maxillary fractures can result in malocclusion. Patients are capable of sensing the slightest change in their occlusion. Even in patients with unusual bites, careful analysis of the wear facets may enable the surgeon to determine if an underlying malocclusion is present.

Proper record keeping of facial injuries includes rough sketch drawings in the medical chart and photographs to document injuries. These photographs may prove invaluable in the treatment of secondary deformities and can also be beneficial in medicolegal disputes. As such, photographic consents should routinely be obtained as part of the treatment consent upon entrance to the emergency department.

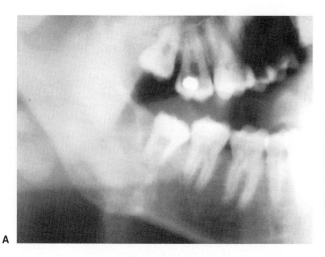
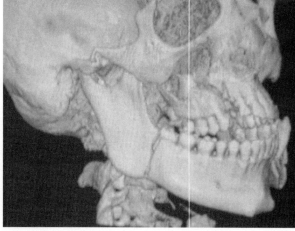

FIGURE 31.2. Fracture missed by Panorex. **A:** The mandible appears normal on panoramic radiograph. **B:** CT scan of same patient revealing complete fracture. Although panoramic radiographs provide valuable information about the mandible and dentition, distortion in the image can conceal fractures.

Imaging

Most patients presenting to the emergency department with a history of facial trauma will undergo a facial trauma series consisting of plain radiographs (anteroposterior [AP], lateral, Caldwell, and Water views). This is a useful screening tool for the emergency room physician when the index of suspicion is fairly low; however, **plain radiographs do not give the degree of information regarding the fracture in terms of severity and displacement that is required for the surgeon.**

In most patients with significant facial impact, CT scanning should be performed. With modern helical CT scanners, it takes a few additional minutes to scan the face. In a busy emergency room, this approach saves both time and expense. Facial CT scans are not only extremely sensitive and specific in their evaluation of the facial skeleton, the cost is comparable to that of a full series of plain radiographs. Additionally, a complete radiographic facial trauma series requires cervical spine clearance for completion. This is unnecessary with modern helical CT scanners.

The CT scan should be performed with axial cuts no greater than 3 mm apart, from the top of the cranium through the bottom of the mandible. Although older models of CT scanners could only perform coronal imaging by hyperextending the neck (requiring cervical spine clearance), most scanners are now capable of rotating their plane of imaging so as to eliminate the need to manipulate the patient's head position and mobilize the neck. This capability is a tremendous asset in the sense that the scan can be performed immediately at the time of the head and abdominal CT scans, which are usually performed quickly and prior to the time of cervical spine clearance. When coronal cuts cannot be taken, most scanner software now provides for digital reconstructions of the coronal plane from the axial images. Additionally, in cases of complex facial trauma, it may be helpful to have a three-dimensional reconstruction of the facial skeleton formatted so as to provide for a better overall orientation.

As a general rule, the CT scan is acceptable for the diagnosis of essentially all facial fractures. The one area where this exam may not be entirely sufficient is the mandible. Although the CT is essentially 100% sensitive and specific for the fractures, it does not give detailed information about dental structures. This is most critical in the region of the mandibular angle with respect to the condition of the third molars. Information re-

garding root damage and tooth position relative to the fracture is critical in the planning and treatment of angle fractures. When using CT scanning for mandible fractures, complications can be related to this factor. As such, a panoramic radiograph is helpful in the evaluation of mandibular fractures. Certain imaging equipment allows the patient to be supine, whereas the more common equipment requires upright positioning and cervical spine clearance. These radiographs place an entire image of the mandible, condyle to condyle, on a single film. They provide excellent detail of the condyles and dentition. Care must be taken when interpreting fractures based solely on a panoramic radiograph of the mandible, especially the symphysis and parasymphysis, as distortion of these regions can be misleading. A supplemental posteroanterior (PA) film of the mandible complements the panoramic image by providing additional detail of the region. Lateral radiographs and CT scans can provide additional information about the regions posterior to the parasymphysis (Fig. 31.2).

TREATMENT OF SOFT-TISSUE INJURIES

Preparation and Anesthesia

Facial injuries frequently involve contaminated wounds. The most important initial responsibility of the surgeon is to convert the contaminated wound to a clean one and then perform wound closure. Wounds should be closed as soon as possible. Although facial wounds can usually tolerate up to a 24-hour delay in repair, the longer the wound is open, the greater chance of infectious complications. Cleansing of wounds is best performed with a mild surgical soap with the light use of a scrub brush. More extensive wounds or those with a great deal of contamination should be irrigated with a pulsed lavage system. All foreign debris must be removed from the wound prior to closure. Adequate cleansing usually requires total anesthesia of the region of concern and a cooperative patient. These are the primary factors that dictate the method of anesthesia necessary.

Although general anesthesia may be necessary for some wounds, many facial wounds can be repaired under a regional nerve block. If regional blockade is impractical, a field block may be necessary to avoid direct infiltration of excessive amounts of local anesthetic, distorting anatomic landmarks that may be useful in restoring the tissues to their anatomic positions.

Only 1 to 2 mL of anesthetic at the site of the nerve trunk is needed to provide complete anesthesia for the respective region. Often multiple regions require blockade. We recommend 1% lidocaine with 1:100,000 epinephrine solution mixed at a 9:1 ratio with 8.4% sodium bicarbonate solution (e.g., 9 mL lidocaine with epinephrine and 1 mL of bicarbonate solution). The bicarbonate solution neutralizes the pH of the lidocaine, which has two important benefits. First, it minimizes the pain of the injection. Second, the lidocaine more effectively crosses the neural membrane to affect its sodium ion channel in the neutral state and, therefore, has a quicker onset of action. Topical cocaine (4%) is an excellent choice for anesthesia in the nasal cavity as it also stimulates vasoconstriction of the nasal mucosa providing for a painless and bloodless field.

Traumatic Wounds

Traumatic wounds can be variously described as lacerations, punctures, contusions, abrasions, and crush injuries. **The wound configuration, whether linear or stellate, is much less important to the final result than the degree of crush, contusion, and vascular compromise of the tissues.** The importance of wound cleansing prior to closure cannot be overemphasized. Removal of all foreign bodies is essential as they are the source of a prolonged inflammatory response and possibly infection. Abrasions with residual foreign bodies will form a traumatic tattoo when not properly debrided. When tissue laxity allows removal of crushed tissue margins, a judicious sharp debridement of the wound margins is undertaken. Clearly devitalized tissue is excised. Freshening the wound margins contributes to rapid healing and improves the final result.

Perhaps the most important step in repair of skin lacerations is excellent approximation of the deep dermal layer. By placing the tension of the closure deep to the skin the resulting scar is improved. A good choice of the suture material for this deep layer is poliglecaprone 25 (Monocryl, Ethicon, Somerville, NJ). Because of the monofilament nature of this suture, it may have a lower likelihood of suture contamination and extrusion. It also maintains tensile strength for a sufficient period of time to allow for uncomplicated wound healing.

The choice of suture for the skin depends a great deal on the patient. Assuming a good deep dermal layer has been placed, the skin suture serves only to more accurately approximate and evert the skin edges. In children, it is beneficial to avoid a permanent suture to obviate the need for suture removal. An excellent choice in this case is 5-0 or 6-0 fast-absorbing gut suture. This suture type dissolves so rapidly that suture marks are not left on the face. It provides very little tensile strength, however, requiring the use of adhesive strips. If a skin adhesive is chosen in the pediatric population, one must take great care not to place any within the wound itself, as placing any within the wound may cause a profound inflammatory response, resulting in breakdown of the closure.

A subcuticular skin suture is also an option in the face. If this is to remain in place, Monocryl is again a good suture material choice. Should one desire to remove the suture, polypropylene tends to be the best choice as it slides out of the skin easily. Skin edges under a greater degree of tension are usually best closed using interrupted nylon or Prolene. In heavily contaminated wounds the use of interrupted sutures or running sutures in short segments can be used. This allows for removal of focal areas of suture in the case of infection, avoiding a complete wound dehiscence. As a general rule, sutures in the face can be removed by 5 to 7 days when they are load bearing. When

a layer of reliable deep dermal sutures are in place, superficial skin sutures can be removed as soon as 3 days to avoid suture marks.

Injuries to Special Facial Regions

Eyelids

The most important aspect of evaluating trauma to the eyelids is ensuring that injury to the globe has not occurred. A thorough ocular examination is an essential element. It is important to remember that the Bell phenomenon results in an upward and lateral rotation of the globe. As such, one may find penetrating injuries to the globe in locations that do not intuitively correspond to the eyelid injury.

Often a general anesthetic is required to provide sufficient anesthesia to explore eyelid injuries and allow for adequate exploration of the globe. General anesthesia is particularly recommended in the pediatric population where additional damage can be caused by working with sharp needles and instruments around the orbit in an uncooperative child. Direct injuries to the globe warrant urgent ophthalmologic consultation.

Perhaps the most critical step in suturing the eyelid is to place an everting stitch along the lid margin. This not only facilitates proper anatomic alignment, but also prevents notching of the lid margin. The suture in the lid margin can be left long and taped down to the cheek to prevent the suture ends from irritating the eye. In general, all layers of the eyelid (inner, middle, and outer lamellas) should be repaired. Although the conjunctiva will heal well without sutures, injuries associated with significant deformity should be sutured with plain gut suture, paying careful attention to bury the knots so as to avoid irritation of the globe. The middle lamella, including the tarsus, should be sutured with a resorbable suture. Following this, the skin of the eyelid should be sutured. Sutures should be removed within 5 days. Depending on the magnitude of the injury, it may be helpful to place a Frost suture to support the lid position during the healing, especially in injuries to the lower lids.

Ears

Ear lacerations can usually be sutured in one layer, addressing the skin only. It is typically unnecessary to place a separate layer of sutures within the cartilage. The firm adherence of the skin to the underlying cartilage framework of the ear ensures that skin approximation accurately aligns the cartilage.

The two most prominent concerns in ear injuries are hematoma and chondritis. Collections of blood in proximity to the cartilage can result in cartilage resorption or a reactive chondrogenesis, which ultimately leads to the cauliflower ear deformity. Hematomas must be evacuated as quickly as possible to avert this adverse sequela. Hematoma can be easily drained through incisions in the overlying skin, making an effort to conceal incisions if possible. Because of the robust perfusion to the auricular skin, a bolster is often required to prevent re-accumulation of the hematoma. Alternatively, a small suction drain or Penrose-type drain may be used. A compression dressing should be employed regardless of the type of drainage technique employed. Following treatment of significant lacerations, one should line the convolutions of the ear with antibiotic-impregnated gauze and place a light head wrap, providing gentle compression of the ear.

One should warn the patient regarding significant pain following these injuries. As a general rule, ear trauma is not terribly painful. The development of pain in the posttreatment period usually signifies the development of a hematoma or infection. Therefore, the delayed onset of pain warrants immediate inspection of the ear. Chondritis is a serious complication of these injuries. As cartilage has such poor blood supply, it is difficult to treat these infections with oral antibiotics. These patients typically require admission for intravenous antibiotics and possibly debridement. It is rare to develop a significant chondritis without concomitant pain.

Nose

Soft-tissue injuries of the nose are somewhat different from auricular trauma. When lacerations involve the underlying cartilaginous support system of the nose, all layers should be repaired after appropriate anatomic reduction. Simple re-approximation of the overlying skin does not necessarily align the underlying cartilage. As such, any lacerations or transections of the upper or lower lateral cartilages should be separately addressed. Because of the difficulty in achieving adequate anesthesia and control of bleeding with the use of local anesthetic alone, general anesthesia is warranted to maximize patient comfort and control.

Lips

The most important consideration in repairing soft-tissue injuries involving the lips involves accurate re-approximation of the injured structures, especially the vermilion. A discrepancy in alignment of the vermilion border as little as 1 mm is noticeable at conversational distance. As such, prior to infiltration of any local anesthetic, the location of the vermilion border on either side of a laceration should be tattooed using a needle with methylene blue. The vermillion should be accurately re-approximated using a 6-0 nylon or similar suture.

Great care must be taken to separately reapproximate the underlying orbicularis oris muscle. Failure to do so will result in bunching of the muscle on either side of the laceration with attempted animation, and typically results in a shortened scar with an exaggerated notching of the lip. Mucosal lacerations are repaired using a resorbable suture such as chromic or Vicryl (Ethicon, Somerville, NJ).

A careful examination is performed to rule out underlying damage to the dentition. Any loose or damaged teeth are documented. Particularly unstable teeth may benefit from a bridle wire securing them to adjacent stable teeth. Panoramic radiographs or periapical images may help to better delineate underlying dental trauma.

Facial Nerve

Soft-tissue injuries to the face involving the facial nerve are particularly devastating. In examining the patient with facial soft-tissue injury, particularly penetrating wounds, facial motion is examined carefully. One should specifically test elevation of brow, forced closure of the eyes, voluntary smile, and eversion of the lower lip. Eversion of the lower lip is not very well tested by asking a patient to purse the lips; rather, it is best seen in attempted full-denture smile. Deficits in the presence of a penetrating injury likely represent transection of a facial nerve branch. As a general rule, all such injuries should be explored operatively. The exception may be suspected injuries to the buccal branches medial to the lateral cantus of the eye. As a consequence of the extensive arborization of the nerve at this level, most such injuries will undergo spontaneous reinnervation over a 3- to 6-month period. Injuries lateral to this and any deficit in brow elevation, eye closure, or lower lip depression should be explored.

Timing is of importance in these situations. The ability to identify the distal transected nerve end is facilitated by stimulating with a facial nerve stimulator and detecting the facial motion. **After approximately 48 to 72 hours, the distal nerve end can no longer be stimulated, greatly complicating accurate** identification because of the small size of the nerve and the inflammatory response in the surrounding tissues. These injuries should be repaired using microscopic magnification and 9-0 or 10-0 nylon epineural sutures. The time to recovery for a repaired nerve can be approximated by measuring the distance between the site of injury and the target muscle. Nerve regeneration typically occurs at a rate of 1 mm per day after a 1-month lag (Chapter 9).

Parotid Gland/Duct Injuries

The most significant concern in parotid injuries is the possibility of facial nerve injury. The facial nerve separates the parotid into a superficial and deep lobe, and lacerations in this region frequently injure both the parotid gland and facial nerve. A parotid gland injury does not require intervention unless the underlying parotid duct is involved. Involvement of the Stensen duct will result in a parotid fistula unless corrected. These injuries may be difficult to identify and may only be seen following repair of a skin lacerations with subsequent accumulation of saliva. Duct injuries should be repaired over a stent to allow healing. It may be easiest to repair the duct through the open wound in the cheek. Identification and access to the distal segment of the Stensen duct can also be facilitated by cannulating the papilla opposite the maxillary second molar with a blunt parotid or lacrimal probe. The ends of the duct should be freshened and repaired over a stent. We often employ a 5-French pediatric feeding tube brought through the papilla and secured intraorally to prevent accidental displacement during the healing period.

FACIAL FRACTURES

Orbital Fractures

Orbital Examination

In any patient presenting with facial trauma involving the orbit, a thorough examination of the globe and associated structures is mandatory. Unrecognized trauma to any of the orbital contents can be disastrous. There is a great deal of information that can be ascertained from examination in the emergency department. A focused history and examination begins by determining if the patient has had any previous history of iatrogenic globe penetration, such as cataract surgery or radial keratotomy. This substantially increases the risk for globe rupture following trauma. A careful assessment is also made of the contralateral, uninjured eye.

A visual examination is performed on every patient. This can be combined with a visual fields exam by having the patient close one eye with the examiner closing the corresponding eye. That is, if the patient is asked to close his left eye, the examiner, facing the patient, should close her right eye. The exam should be performed using a light source at 90 degrees to the visual axis of the examiner and examinee. This is a good assessment for both gross vision and visual fields. Visual field assessment is important, as any damage to the optic nerve may manifest first as a limitation in the visual field rather than a significant change in gross acuity.

Additionally, one should test for color desaturation. Perhaps the first indication of optic nerve compression is red color desaturation. The easiest way to test this in the emergency department is to dim the lights and hold a pen light up to the finger. The light through the skin appears red. The patient should be asked with alternate eyes closed whether there is any difference in the intensity of the red color between the two eyes.

Direct and consensual pupillary responses are elicited to determine the function of the second and third cranial nerves. Anisocoria may be an indication of second or third nerve damage, or direct trauma to the iris. A relative afferent pupillary defect (APD) is indicative of optic nerve injury that can be elicited by a swinging flash light test. Range of motion testing of each eye will determine the function of the third, fourth, and sixth cranial nerves. Restrictions in the range of motion of the globe should be confirmed with a forced duction test to determine if the restriction is caused by mechanical entrapment or by injury to the nerves or muscles. These emergency department maneuvers, although potentially quite informative, are no substitute for a thorough dilated exam by an ophthalmologist. Ophthalmologic consultation should be considered in every case of orbital trauma.

Indications for Surgery: Orbital Floor

Indications for repair of orbital fractures are an area of great controversy. There are, however, several well-established indications. The most significant is evidence of mechanical entrapment of an extraocular muscle causing diplopia. This may be demonstrated on forced duction testing or on imaging studies. A second is evidence of enophthalmos. **With the initial swelling present secondary to the trauma, any enophthalmos that is manifest indicates a significant deformity as it would be expected to worsen with the resolution of swelling.** Deferring surgery will complicate the eventual repair that is required.

Defect size is the most controversial parameter in determining the indication for surgery. Various authors have used different guidelines (2). Many believe that any defect greater than 1 cm^2 benefits from surgical repair because of the likelihood of subsequent enophthalmos. Other authors have tried to quantitate, via CT imaging, the actual increase in orbital volume compared to the uninjured side. This volume is then used to assess the risk for postinjury enophthalmos. Currently, there are no firm data confirming the usefulness of this approach.

There is some benefit, regardless of the indications for surgery, in delaying surgery until there is a modest improvement in swelling. As a successful outcome in these injuries is dependent on reestablishing the proper anteroposterior projection of the globe, it is helpful to have most swelling largely resolved. Because the surgical exploration of the floor evokes some degree of swelling, the cumulative effect can make it difficult to gauge the degree of correction necessary. However, whether the surgery is performed early or late (early, 1 to 3 days; late, 7 to 10 days), the operated eye is overcorrected so that it projects a little farther than the uninjured eye immediately following surgery.

Incisions/Technique

The most common complication from incisions used to access the orbital floor is lower eyelid retraction. This may result in ectropion or entropion. The subciliary approach, so often used for blepharoplasty, clearly has the highest risk of associated retraction when one examines the literature. The transconjunctival approach has consequently gained popularity. One may approach this dissection in either the preseptal or postseptal plane. Avoiding dissection of the skin and orbicularis diminishes the risk of postoperative retraction. Although some authors believe that a lateral canthotomy is unnecessary, there is no question that detaching the lateral canthus improves exposure. If a lateral canthotomy is performed, a canthopexy must be performed at the conclusion of the case in order to reestablish the appropriate position of the lateral canthal ligament.

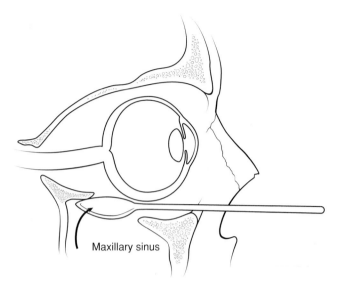

FIGURE 31.3. Identification of posterior ledge in orbital floor fractures. Technique of safely identifying the posterior limit of an orbital floor defect. The elevator is placed into maxillary sinus and used to identify the posterior ledge by sweeping upward and forward.

The subtarsal incision can also be employed, especially in older patients with prominent lower lid rhytides within which the incision can be concealed. This incision is the most direct access to the orbital floor and avoids dissection of the lower lid proper. Consequently, it is very unlikely to cause lower lid retraction.

Dissection of the lower lid should be directed toward exposing the periosteum of the infraorbital rim and incising it on the outer margin of the rim. This affords a greater degree of control and ensures that the proper plane is obtained prior to entering the orbit. A periosteal elevator is then used to dissect posteriorly. The infraorbital nerve is encountered within the orbital floor, usually about halfway back. The nerve is protected and kept down with the bone. The orbit is conically shaped with a superior-medial slant toward the orbital apex. The goal of the dissection is to identify the portion of the floor that is still intact and contiguous with the orbital apex. Whatever material is used to reconstruct the floor must be suspended on this posterior ledge to ensure accurate anatomic reconstruction. At times, the posterior ledge can be difficult to identify in the subperiosteal plane. In these cases, it can be safely identified by placing the elevator straight posteriorly into the maxillary sinus and gently walking the elevator superiorly (Fig. 31.3). The posterior floor is then encountered. The anterior ledge of the intact posterior floor can be safely identified by working the elevator anteriorly until the defect is encountered. Once the margins of the defect are defined, reconstruction can proceed.

Floor Implants

In the past, there was a general consensus among maxillofacial surgeons that bone was the best implant for reconstruction of the floor. Classically, this was harvested from the outer table of the skull. Although this is clearly a reliable option, it does entail a longer operative time, potential donor-site morbidity, and some degree of resorption of the graft postoperatively.

Alloplastics enjoy several advantages over bone grafts, including immediate availability and no risk of resorption. The disadvantage is obviously the potential risk of implant infection and extrusion, which is a rare complication. Among the implants available are titanium mesh, high-density porous polyethylene, and resorbable materials. Very large orbital defects, particularly those involving the medial wall, are best reconstructed using titanium mesh because of the support provided and the ease of contouring. Resorbable implants may be useful in smaller defects, particularly in children, where there is some reluctance to use permanent implants because of growth concerns. Silastic, although used commonly in the past, is best avoided as a floor implant because of a relatively higher risk of late extrusion and infection.

Complications

The most common complications following surgery for orbital fractures are lower-eyelid retraction and enophthalmos. As was previously discussed, lower-eyelid retraction can be minimized by appropriate choice of incision. This should be an uncommon complication if the subciliary incision is avoided. It may also be helpful postoperatively to place a Frost suture maintaining the lower eyelid in an elevated position for 24 hours following the procedure. If retraction is noted in the early postoperative period, the patient should begin aggressive lower-eyelid massage and forced eye-closure exercises. This resolves the problem in the vast major of cases. Early operative intervention for lid retractions should be avoided unless the patient is experiencing problems with corneal exposure as indicated by constant irritation of the eye. In the absence of this, operative intervention for lid retraction should only be considered after failure of conservative measures for 4 to 6 months. Regardless of the initial incision, patients with postoperative lid retraction should be approached through the transconjunctival approach. The typical cause is scarring of the middle lamella. This should be released and a spacer such as hard palate mucosa placed.

Enophthalmos is particularly resistant to secondary correction and is most frequently caused by inaccurate reconstruction of the orbital floor and excessive orbital volume. As a result of the superior incline of floor, placement of the floor implant must be directed superiorly to anatomically reconstruct the defect. Dissecting straight back rather than cephalically results in the implant being placed within the maxillary sinus (Fig. 31.4). This maintains the expansion in the orbital volume and results in subsequent enophthalmos. One must also remember that appropriate reconstruction of the orbital floor results in the operated eye being slightly proptotic in the early postoperative period when compared to the uninjured side. Failure to achieve this at the time of surgery is an almost certain guaran-

tee of enophthalmos when the swelling resolves. Although fat atrophy may also increase orbital volume somewhat postoperatively, the contribution of this mechanism to enophthalmos is likely not significant. The most direct approach for correction of this problem is accurate and anatomic reconstruction of the orbital floor. Secondary reconstruction is much more difficult. However, established postoperative enophthalmos never improves and, if bothersome to the patient, will require reoperation.

Persistent diplopia may also be seen following repair of orbital fractures. This is most troublesome if it is in the primary field of gaze or in downgaze, as walking may become problematic. In avoiding this complication, it is very important to perform a forced duction test at the termination of the operation to ensure that implant placement has not resulted in a mechanical interference with globe movement. In the event that the patient complains of new-onset diplopia in the immediate postoperative period, a CT scan should be performed to evaluate this possibility. If no mechanical impedance is appreciated, the patient should be followed conservatively with ophthalmologic consultation to assist with care. Although this problem is usually a result of low-grade neurapraxia, muscle contusion, or swelling, which resolves spontaneously within several months, rebalancing of the extraocular muscles may ultimately be required.

Orbitozygomatic Fractures

Diagnoses/Examination

The physical examination in orbitozygomatic fractures is important, but often misleading. Swelling from the injury frequently conceals the malar recession and any evidence of enophthalmos. Anesthesia in the distribution of the infraorbital nerve is common and should be documented on initial examination. Additionally, severely displaced fractures may cause trismus secondary to impingement of the coronoid process on the mandible by the displaced posterior aspect of the zygomatic arch. The orbital aspect of these injuries necessitates careful ophthalmologic examination and is perhaps the most important aspect of the preoperative work-up.

The decision to operatively reduce an orbitozygomatic fracture is largely dependent on the CT scan data, as swelling often precludes accurate determination of the degree of deformity. When evaluating the CT scan, it is most useful to look at the lateral orbital wall on the axial cuts, which represents the articulation of the zygoma with the greater wing of the sphenoid. This broad articulation will manifest any displacement present and determine the degree of deformity. One must also assess four other articulations for displacement, including the infraorbital rim, the zygomaticomaxillary buttress, the zygomaticofrontal suture, and the zygomatic arch.

Nondisplaced fractures may be safely managed with a nonchew diet and close clinical follow-up. A nonchew diet will prevent the activation of the masseter from displacing the fracture segment. Displacement of the fracture is a definitive indication for operative reduction and fixation, as the results of early operative repair far exceed those of delayed repair. Repositioning of a displaced fracture in a delayed setting requires osteotomy of all buttresses and extensive craniofacial exposure. It is best to reduce and fixate fractures anatomically in the acute setting.

Operative Techniques

The operative treatment of orbitozygomatic fractures depends largely on the degree of displacement and comminution. The majority of patients can be accurately reduced and fixated

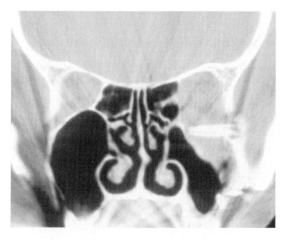

FIGURE 31.4. Incorrectly placed orbital floor prosthesis. Orbital floor implant misplaced directly posteriorly into the maxillary sinus. Note the flat lie of the implant, which should incline superiorly.

using incisions in the upper gingivobuccal sulcus, lower eyelid (transconjunctival), and the lateral extent of the supratarsal fold of the upper eyelid. The coronal incision is necessary only when the zygomatic arch must be exposed and reduced as a guide to appropriate alignment of the zygoma. This is typically only necessary when there is so much comminution of the infraorbital rim and zygomaticomaxillary buttress that these cannot be used as an accurate guide to reduction. In practice, only three of the four buttresses require reduction as long as the zygoma is a single, large, fracture segment.

As a general rule, the intraoral incision is typically performed first. In lower-energy fractures, it is occasionally possible to elevate the displaced zygoma using an instrument placed behind the zygomatic arch. If the fracture reduces with this maneuver, a plate may be placed across the zygomaticomaxillary buttress and the operation terminated. Even if this does not allow anatomic reduction of the fracture, it is still beneficial in that it moves the zygoma to a more anatomic location, facilitating the lower-eyelid dissection of the orbital rim. As with orbital fractures, the subciliary incision is typically best avoided. Generally, either the transconjunctival or subtarsal incision is best. If a coronal incision has not been used, the zygomaticofrontal suture requires exposure through the lateral extent of the supratarsal fold. Although eyebrow incisions have been used in the past, these may leave prominent scars and provide less-direct access to the suture.

Once all of the articulations of the zygoma have been visualized, they should be aligned and the fracture stabilized. It is very useful to first align the zygomaticofrontal suture using either a wire or a 1.0-mm plate. This sets the vertical height of the zygoma while still allowing rotation and further alignment at the level of the rim and the zygomaticomaxillary buttress. Once this suture is stabilized, the surgeon should anatomically reduce the other two buttresses. Reduction may be facilitated by using a Carol-Gerard screw placed through the lower-eyelid incision into the body of the zygoma (Fig. 31.5). It acts like a joystick and allows easy control of the fracture fragment in three dimensions.

A 1.5-mm plate is typically placed along the superior aspect of the infraorbital rim rather than anteriorly to avoid either visibility or palpability by the patient postoperatively. The buttress that provides the most stability to the reduced fracture is the zygomaticomaxillary. A 2.0- or 1.5-mm L-plate is most commonly used at this buttress. In the most severe fractures, when the arch has to be exposed to align the zygoma, this is

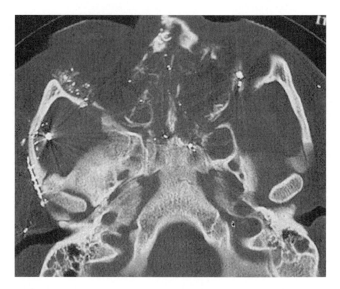

FIGURE 31.6. Incorrect reduction of the zygomatic arch. CT scan of a zygomatic arch that was inappropriately reconstructed as an arch. The normal arch lies in an almost straight anteroposterior direction, as can be seen on the normal side.

best plated first with a 2.0-mm plate to reestablish the width and projection of the zygoma.

It is not necessary to provide three or four points of fixation for every zygoma fracture. Although this number of plates is commonly used, it is usually a result of the sequence of steps used in aligning the fracture. Although three or four plates may be necessary in high-energy injuries, many fractures can be adequately fixated using a single 2.0-mm L-plate along the zygomaticomaxillary buttress.

When the zygomatic arch is significantly displaced and comminuted it requires full exposure and reconstruction. There is a tendency for surgeons to view the arch as an arch when in reality it is much more of a straight anteroposterior structure. If reconstructed as an arch it will result in excessive facial width and prominence to the region relative to the contralateral side. In addition, the malar eminence will not be projected as far forward as it should. This is an especially important factor when there is significant destruction to the malar and arch complexes bilaterally and the surgeon must reestablish facial width in proportion to facial height without the benefit of an internal reference (Fig. 31.6).

Arch Fractures

Isolated fractures of the zygomatic arch are treated differently from true orbitozygomatic injuries. Isolated arch fractures frequently do not require operative reduction. Operative treatment of these fractures is indicated for severe depression of the arch causing either a cosmetically significant contour depression or impingement on the coronoid process and trismus.

The fracture may be approached intraorally through an upper buccal sulcus incision or an incision in the temporal scalp. The intraoral approach, although more difficult, avoids an external scar. The scalp incision, commonly referred to as the Gillies approach, allows more direct access to the fracture site. The incision is placed vertically within the temporal hairline and dissection is carried directly through the temporoparietal fascia and deep temporal fascia. The elevator is then placed in plane between the deep temporal fascia and the temporalis muscle and advanced to a position deep to the arch. Any resistance to sliding the arch inferiorly usually indicates that the plane of dissection is too superficial. Outward pressure

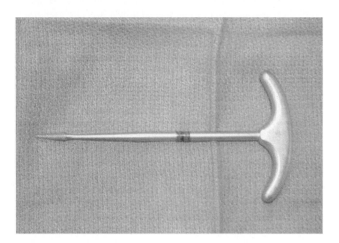

FIGURE 31.5. Carol-Gerard screw. This instrument can be used to gain control of the zygoma in orbitozygomatic fractures. It can be placed either through an intraoral incision or percutaneously.

on the arch forces the fracture into an anatomically reduced position.

Occasionally, arch fractures essentially snap back into position and are stable. In the majority of cases, however, the fracture is unstable in the reduced position. In such situations, it is helpful to splint the reduced arch using permanent sutures placed transcutaneously and encircling the arch. The suture is tied over a metal eye shield to provide constant upward and outward traction. Typically two sutures are required to hold the arch in position. Excessive tension on the sutures may lead to skin necrosis at the margins of the eye shield.

Complications

The most common complication following repair of orbitozygomatic fractures is enophthalmos. This results from malreduction of the fracture. As in orbital floor injuries, displaced orbitozygomatic fractures almost always expand orbital volume, as the zygoma constitutes a large portion of the orbital floor and lateral wall. Both the increased orbital volume and the malar recession must be addressed in the treatment of the malreduced fracture. To address this, the zygoma is best osteotomized, repositioned in its appropriate anatomic location, and secured with plates. Occasionally, the malar recession is not significant and treatment can be directed at correction of the orbital volume alone. As in an orbital floor fracture, additional alloplast may be placed in the floor or along the wall of the orbit to diminish volume and correct the enophthalmos. Maxillary sinusitis and persistent numbness in the infraorbital nerve distribution may complicate orbitozygomatic fractures less frequently.

Nasal Fractures

Diagnosis/Examination

The diagnosis of a nasal fracture is clinical. Patients presenting with a history of acute trauma with evidence of a deviated nose have an underlying nasal fracture. Radiographs, although frequently obtained, are superfluous.

When examining a patient with a suspected nasal fracture, an intranasal inspection is mandatory to identify a septal hematoma. Untreated septal hematomas may lead to resorption of the cartilaginous septum and result in a saddle nasal deformity. Septal hematomas should be expeditiously evacuated. Reaccumulation can be prevented with the use of either septal quilting sutures or intranasal splints.

Treatment

Treatment of nasal fractures can be divided into early and late phases. If one sees a patient with nasal fracture immediately following the injury, it is beneficial to perform a closed reduction. This may be done in the emergency department using local anesthesia and an intranasal vasoconstrictor. Although closed reduction can be performed any time in the first 2 to 3 weeks, the swelling may be so severe as to camouflage the magnitude of the deformity and complicate accurate reduction. Swelling usually improves significantly 10 to 14 days after injury facilitating closed reduction.

The late phase is defined as a period where sufficient bony union has taken place such that osteotomy is required to anatomically reduce the fracture fragments. Correction in the late phase should be viewed as a complete rhinoplasty. The contribution of the septum to the deviation should be appreciated and addressed. Simply performing osteotomies is unlikely to correct the deformity in the face of septal involve-

ment, particularly in high dorsal deviations. Extensive septal mobilization, resection, and scoring may be necessary. Airway compromise should also be a focus of the subsequent rhinoplasty.

Maxillary Fractures

Diagnosis

Fractures of the maxilla have been classically described as Le Fort I, II, and III patterns. These patterns, by definition, are fractures that detach the maxilla from the skull base. The maxilla is mobile and may result in malocclusion. Although it is not uncommon in facial trauma that the anterior wall of the maxillary sinus, and even the zygomaticomaxillary and nasomaxillary buttresses, are fractured, injury to these structures alone does not constitute a true Le Fort injury. The fracture must extend through the pterygoid plates to create a complete Le Fort fracture (Fig. 31.7).

The Le Fort I injury classically passes through the maxilla transversely, somewhere between the tooth roots and the infraorbital rims, with preservation of the integrity of the infraorbital rims. The Le Fort II fracture extends through the infraorbital rim and nose and is sometimes referred to as a pyramidal fracture. The Le Fort III fracture involves the zygomatic arch, lateral orbital wall, and the nasofrontal region. Le Fort fractures rarely exist in pure form. More commonly, patients will present with a combination of injuries such as a Le Fort I on one side and a Le Fort III on the contralateral side.

Preoperative evaluation should be focused on the occlusal relationship. Any sign of malocclusion should be evaluated carefully. Correction of the occlusion to the preinjury state will guide the appropriate anatomic reduction.

Operative Technique

Le Fort I injuries can be adequately exposed through an upper gingivobuccal sulcus incision and maxillary degloving. Le Fort II injuries often require a lower lid incision. As in orbital fractures, a transconjunctival incision is preferred over a subciliary incision. In older patients, a subtarsal incision can be concealed in a lower-lid crease. Le Fort III injuries may be approached through a combination of buccal sulcus and lower-lid incisions in low to moderate impact injuries. More severe injuries require a coronal approach for exposure of the nasofrontal and medial orbital regions and the zygomatic arch. Following mobilization of all of these fractures, the patient should be placed in maxillomandibular fixation and the zygomaticomaxillary and nasomaxillary buttresses stabilized with plates.

Nasoorbitoethmoid Fractures

Diagnosis and Examination

Fractures of the nasoorbitoethmoid (NOE) region involve the medial orbit, nasal bones, septum, and nasofrontal junction. On examination, patients with nasoorbitoethmoid injuries may exhibit substantial loss of dorsal nasal support. Additionally, telecanthus may be present secondary to lateral displacement of the bone fragments bearing the medial canthal tendon. These patients demonstrate an increased distance between the medial canthi and rounding of the medial canthal angle.

The CT scan is the most helpful radiologic tool in determining the location of the injury and the degree of comminution—the two factors critical to determining the appropriate treatment. Analysis of the axial cuts should focus on the lacrimal

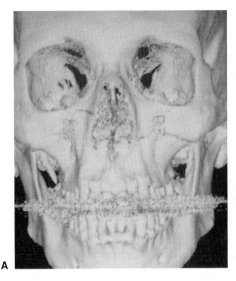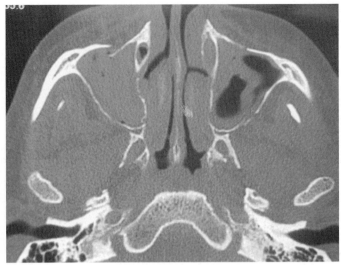

A   B

FIGURE 31.7. Incomplete Le Fort I fracture. **A:** Three-dimensional CT demonstrating a midface fracture that appears to be present at the Le Fort I level. **B:** Axial CT scan of the same fracture revealing intact pterygoid plates. This fracture was completely stable on examination under anesthesia and thus does not require stabilization.

fossa and the start of the nasolacrimal duct. This region identifies the level of insertion of the medial canthal tendon. A great deal of comminution at this level may require transnasal fixation of the bone fragments bearing the medial canthal ligaments. Bilaterally mobile medial canthal tendons represent a significant challenge to reconstruction as there is no normal frame of reference with which to judge preoperative location of the medial canthi.

On occasion, it is difficult to definitively make the diagnosis of nasoorbitoethmoid injury. Definitive diagnosis can be made by examination under anesthesia by placing a hemostat in the nose to the level of the medial canthus. With a finger palpating externally over the medial canthus and outward pressure on the internally positioned hemostat, one can determine the degree of mobility, and consequently the need for operative stabilization.

Operative Technique

The majority of nasoorbitoethmoid injuries should be exposed through both coronal and lower-eyelid incisions. As the fracture is dissected, one must take great care not to strip the insertion of the medial canthal tendon off of the fracture fragments. Markowitz et al. (3) have devised a classification scheme based on the relation of the insertion of the medial canthal tendon to the fracture. Type 1 fractures involve a very large bone fragment to which the medial canthal tendon is inserted. These injuries may be treated essentially by fixation of the bone fragment to adjacent surrounding bone. Type 2 fractures involve more extensive comminution; however, the medial canthal tendon is still attached to a bone fragment that can be stabilized directly. When the fragment is too small for fixation, transnasal wiring can be used to position the fragment and medial canthal tendon appropriately. Additional bone grafting may be required. Type 3 injuries involve avulsion of the medial canthal tendon from its skeletal insertion. In addition to appropriate reduction of bone fragments and bone grafting, these patients require transnasal fixation of the medial canthal tendon.

When transnasal medial canthoplasty is necessary, it must be performed so that the direction of pull on the canthal tendon is posterior and superior. A common mistake is to reattach the canthal tendon too anteriorly, resulting in persistent telecanthus. The procedure is performed by drilling from the contralateral side through the nasal bones with the exit point planned at approximately the level of the superior aspect of the lacrimal fossa. This is an appropriate vector for pull on the tendon. The medial canthal tendon is grasped either from the underside of the coronal incision, or looped from an anterior incision medial to the medial canthal angle. The wire or permanent suture is then placed through the drill hole using a wire-passing drill bit toward the contralateral side. The suture or wire can be affixed to a screw placed on contralateral side.

Many of these injuries involve substantial loss of nasal support that cannot be restored by direct plating. In these situations onlay bone grafting of the nasal dorsum will reestablish the appropriate projection and width of the nasal radix. Multiple techniques have been described to stabilize bone grafts in this region including miniplates, lag screws, and K-wires.

A soft-tissue bolster over the medial canthal valley is also often necessary to restore the normal contour to this region. The medial canthal valley is a unique region of the face where the skin is intimately adherent to the underlying skeleton. The soft-tissue bolster prevents the subcutaneous accumulation of blood and fluid that interferes with the healing of the skin directly to the underlying bone. These bolsters are usually left in place for 7 to 10 days. The skin underlying the bolster should be watched carefully for necrosis and the bolster should be tied in such a way to allow for adjustment of tension postoperatively.

The most common complication following nasoorbitoethmoid fractures is telecanthus. This is a very difficult problem to correct secondarily. Once it is established, the area must be approached in a similar fashion, the scar contractures completely released, bone grafts placed to reestablish contour, and transnasal canthoplasties performed. The results of secondary repairs are always disappointing when compared to accurate acute repair.

Frontal Sinus

Diagnosis and Examination

Patients with frontal sinus fractures may present with obvious contour deformities of the forehead, but often the swelling

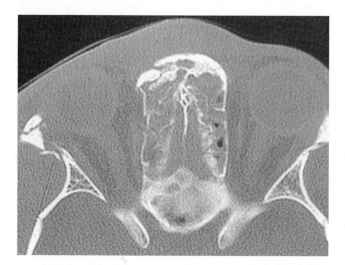

FIGURE 31.8. Axial CT scan of the frontoethmoidal region revealing complete obliteration of the nasofrontal duct by bone fragments. The frontal sinus requires obliteration in the case of a nonfunctioning duct to avoid development of a mucocele.

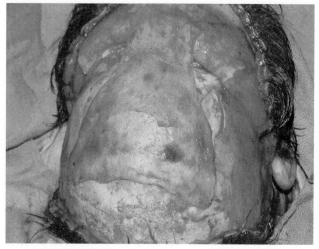

FIGURE 31.9. Pericranial flap. This tissue is often used to interrupt the communication between the ethmoid sinuses and nose with an obliterated frontal sinus.

associated with the injury blunts the degree of deformity. Injury to the frontal sinus is commonly associated with injury to the central nervous system, and early evaluation should focus on this possibility. Axial cuts of the CT scan are useful in determining the degree of injury and involvement of anterior table, posterior table, and the nasofrontal duct. These three structures are used in the classification of frontal sinus fractures as well as subsequent treatment.

Isolated anterior table fractures may be treated simply by reduction and plate fixation via a coronal incision or through existing cuts in the forehead. The function of the nasofrontal duct should be kept in mind at all times. In many cases, involvement of the nasofrontal duct is obvious from the CT scan (Fig. 31.8). This is particularly true for fractures located inferior and medially in the sinus, where the meatus typically originates. During operative exploration, direct instillation of dye (fluorescein) into the region of the nasofrontal duct within the sinus cavity can be used to test the function of the duct. The presence of dye on pledgets placed intranasally indicates a functional duct system. Any compromise of this drainage requires frontal sinus obliteration.

The first step in frontal sinus obliteration is removing the anterior table entirely. The limits of the sinus may not be obvious based on direct examination, particularly in small fractures. Placing one arm of a bayonet forceps into the sinus until the limits of the sinus are reached can help delineate the margins so that the sites of the antrostomy can be determined. Additionally, the operating room lights may be turned down and a light source placed within the sinus, defining the margins of the sinus. Finally, a 1:1 posteroanterior radiograph of the skull may be used to obtain a template of the shape and location of the sinus. This may be cut out from the radiograph, sterilized, and used as a guide for antrostomy.

Once the anterior table is removed, all mucosa must be removed from the sinus. Because of small mucosal invaginations into the bone, termed the *vascular crypts of Breschet*, a burr should be used to ensure complete mucosal obliteration. Once this has been accomplished, the nasofrontal drainage system must be plugged to prevent ingrowth of the mucosa from the ethmoid sinus and nose below. This may be accomplished with a graft of muscle, bone, fat, or a pericranial or galeal flap. At this point, many surgeons fill the sinus cavity with graft material, most frequently fat. This has been challenged by some on the basis of the concept of osteoneogenesis. Mickel and

Rohrich (4) demonstrated spontaneous obliteration by bone in cat frontal sinuses that were surgically burred out and not filled with graft material. This technique has been used by the authors for years without evidence of any increase in complication rates over those published in the literature. From a conceptual standpoint, one must question the superiority of filling a bone cavity with nonvascularized material over simply not filling it at all. In reality, the pericranial or galeal flap used to obliterate the nasal communication may in itself completely fill smaller sinus cavities (Fig. 31.9).

Fractures of the posterior table of the frontal sinus place the patient at risk for acute meningitis and late intracerebral mucocele formation. Fractured fragments of the posterior table may develop trapdoor-type phenomena leaving small bits of mucosa within the cranial cavity. These areas of trapped mucosa are at risk for mucocele formation. Evaluation of the axial cuts through the frontal sinus will reveal displacement of the posterior table within the cranial cavity. Any significant posterior displacement or the presence of a cerebrospinal leak is considered an indication to cranialize the sinus. Cranialization involves performing a frontal craniotomy and removing the entire forehead as a bone flap. The posterior table is then removed and the mucosa of the anterior table burred out. As in obliteration, the nasal communication is eliminated using a pericranial or galeal flap. The bone flap is then plated back into position and the brain is allowed to expand into the space previously occupied by the sinus.

Complications

The most significant complications related to frontal sinus fractures are infectious in nature. In cases in which the frontal sinus has been preserved, one must give consideration to serial CT scans in the postoperative period to assess adequate drainage of the sinus. Failure of the sinus to clear radiographically may indicate impaired drainage that may lead to infection. Evacuation of a poorly draining sinus should be achieved with aggressive medical therapy, including topical and systemic decongestants and mucolytics, or via an endoscopic or open surgical drainage procedure. Mucocele formation may be a late complication of these fractures (Fig. 31.10). Unfortunately, most mucoceles and infections present very late following these injuries. It is not uncommon for this to occur years following the injury or surgery. Such delayed presentation makes accurate data regarding the success of the various treatment options difficult to obtain.

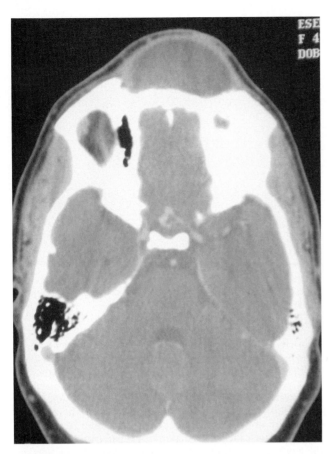

FIGURE 31.10. Frontal sinus mucocele. Axial CT scan of a mucocele several years following a frontal sinus obliteration with bone cement.

Mandible Fractures

Diagnosis and Examination

Mandible fractures typically result in some degree of malocclusion. As patients are capable of detecting even the slightest degree of change in their occlusion, a complaint of malocclusion is a reliable indication of a mandible fracture. Care must be taken in the evaluation of mandible fractures to determine the effect on the occlusion that the fracture has caused. Because the goal of treatment is to restore the mandibular arch to its preinjury occlusal state, as much information as possible must be obtained from the patient history, including orthodontic treatment and any history of dental extraction. The wear facets of the dentition are perhaps the most valuable indicators as to the

patient's preinjury occlusion. Stable mandible fractures with no evidence of malocclusion can occasionally be treated with a nonchew diet for a period of 4 to 6 weeks, depending on the age, state of dentition, and compliance of the patient. For the most part, this is the exception and not the rule, as patients suffering mandible fractures tend to be young, male patients notorious for their noncompliant demeanor.

Because of the constant motion of the lower jaw in normal daily function, mandible fractures tend to be painful until stabilized. Some of the immediate discomfort is relieved by temporary immobilization of the fracture with a wire joining the teeth adjacent to the fracture site. This must be done carefully to avoid dislodging the teeth, which may be destabilized by the fracture. Careful documentation of mental nerve function is performed. Mental nerve neurapraxia often indicates involvement of the body of the mandible between the mental foramen and the mandibular foramen. Because of the likelihood of further neurapraxia related to surgical correction, it is wise to discuss the condition of the nerve and its clinical course prior to undertaking the operative repair.

As with all facial fractures, radiographic evaluation is mandatory. An excellent single test for mandibular fractures is the panoramic radiograph. This requires that the patient be able to sit upright with a mobile neck, so cervical spine clearance is obligatory. The panoramic radiograph places the entire mandible on one film. It provides an excellent evaluation of the condyles and dental anatomy. Because of the nature of the technique in which it is taken, there can be significant distortion in the region of the symphysis, which may conceal fractures in this region (Fig. 31.2). The symphysial region is best evaluated with a plain, posteroanterior radiograph of the mandible.

The CT scan, which is frequently obtained in the emergency center to evaluate facial trauma, is very sensitive and specific in detecting mandibular fractures. On the other hand, it provides a very little information about the dental anatomy, especially in the region of the mandibular angle. The relationship of fractures in the region of the mandibular angle to the surrounding teeth, particularly the third molars, is critical to successful treatment and is best evaluated with a panoramic radiograph. We routinely obtain a Panorex radiograph as an adjunct to the CT scan when the CT scan has already been obtained in the emergency department and indicates a mandible fracture.

Fixation

Choice of fixation must be predicated on the specifics of each fracture. One must choose between rigid fixation (loading bearing) and what one might term functionally stable fixation (load sharing) (5). When internal fixation was first applied to the mandible, it was generally felt that absolutely rigid stabilization was required. Since then it has become appreciated that not all fractures require this, and may indeed do just as well with less-rigid stabilization (Table 31.2).

TABLE 31.2

STABILITY OF FIXATION FOR MANDIBLE FRACTURES (5)

Rigid fixation	Functionally stable fixation (nonrigid)
Reconstruction bone plate (± arch bar)	One 4-hole 2.4-mm compression plate without arch bar
Two bone plates (miniplates, compression plates, or combinations of these) (± arch bar)	One 2.0-mm miniplate + arch bar
Two lag screws (± arch bar)	One lag screw + arch bar
One bone plate plus one or more lag screws (± arch bar)	One 2.0-mm miniplate without arch bar for angle fracture
One 4-hole 2.4-mm compression plate + arch bar	
One 6-hole 2.4-mm compression plate (± arch bar)	

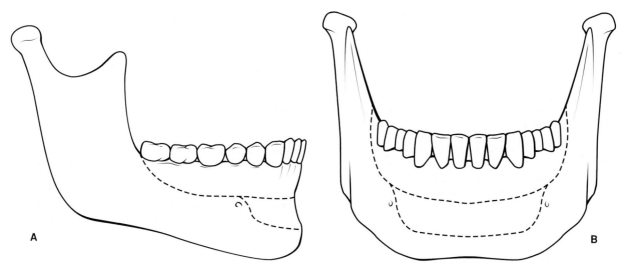

FIGURE 31.11. Champy's lines of osteosynthesis.

Rigid fixation typically implies plates that accommodate screws that are 2.4 or 2.7 mm in diameter. Functionally stable fixation most often uses plates accommodating screws 2.0 mm in diameter or smaller. The decision as to the type of fixation should be determined largely by the fracture pattern and its intrinsic stability. Patients with severely displaced fractures or with multiple mandible fractures have lost more of the intrinsic stability of the mandibular arch and may require fixation that is more rigid and bears more of the functional mandibular load. Additionally, patients at high risk for poor healing, such as those with atrophic mandibles or established infection, usually benefit from absolutely rigid fixation. Uncomplicated, isolated mandible fractures heal uneventfully using smaller plates and screws placed along the lines of osteosynthesis as delineated by Champy (Fig. 31.11).

Operative Technique

Symphysis/Parasymphysis Fractures. As with most mandible fractures, the operative procedure should begin by reestablishing the patient's occlusion using maxillomandibular fixation. In severely displaced fractures, it may be beneficial to expose the fracture first to achieve some degree of initial reduction. If the arch bars are applied initially without some degree of reduction, the arch bar itself will essentially lock the arch into a malreduced position and consequently a malocclusion.

Displaced symphysis fractures typically require internal fixation. Maxillomandibular fixation does not usually achieve sufficient immobilization and stabilization of symphysial fractures because of the lack of intercuspation of the anterior dentition in most patients. These fractures may be adequately stabilized with either large or small plates. Placement of a single, large plate (≥ 2.4 mm) along the inferior border using bicortical screws is sufficient. It should be noted, however, that contouring a 2.4-mm plate to the acute curvature of the symphysial or parasymphysial region can be difficult and time-consuming. Equally rigid fixation can be achieved by placing a 2.0-mm plate with bicortical screws at the inferior border and a 2.0-mm tension band with monocortical screws just below the root apices. A well-placed arch bar can take the place of the tension band and be left in place until bone union. We prefer the use of a tension band as we use it to assist with reduction prior to placing the inferior border plate. After the patient is placed into maxillomandibular fixation, two small holes are drilled into the inferior border on each side of the fracture to accommodate a reduction clamp. With the bone aligned and

the patient in occlusion, the monocortical tension band plate is applied. With this in position, the bone reduction clamp may be removed without impacting the reduction, and the inferior border plate placed onto a relatively stable platform. Most of these fractures may be treated via an intraoral incision. External incisions are typically reserved for only the most severe fractures in this region (multiple fractures and comminuted fractures).

Body Fractures. Mandibular body fractures are treated with either maxillomandibular fixation alone (for 4 to 6 weeks) or internal fixation. Most practitioners prefer to perform an open reduction and internal fixation in these cases. As with symphysial and parasymphysial fractures, a single 2.4-mm inferior border plate or two 2.0-mm plates may be used. Care must be taken to avoid the mental nerve with the screws when treating these injuries. As with symphysial fractures, all but the most severe fractures are treated using an intraoral incision.

Angle Fractures. Mandibular angle fractures are associated with the highest risk for infection and postoperative complications. The presence of a partially erupted or impacted third molar is the cause of the majority of complications. Partially erupted or impacted third molars predispose the angle region to fractures by weakening the bone in the region. The fracture site is frequently described as open secondary to its direct communication with the third molar socket. Although the decision to remove or retain the third molar is controversial, it may be generally believed that any significantly damaged or diseased third molar should be removed, as should any third molar that prevents reduction.

Mandibular angle fractures have been treated with a variety of fixation techniques. Ellis et al. (6) advocate using a single miniplate along the external oblique ridge of the mandible along the lines of Champy. When comparing this to all other forms of fixation, the authors found their complication rate to be the lowest. Additionally, the fracture may be plated along the buccal cortex using a single 2.4-mm plate or two 2.0-mm miniplates. Intraoral exposure and plating is preferred in the majority of patients with simple angle fractures. A small incision in the cheek is required for placement of the screws. However, in complicated or comminuted fractures consideration should be given to an external incision. The external incision provides much greater exposure and control over the fracture.

Subcondylar Fractures. No area of the mandible is as controversial as this region in terms of appropriate treatment. The literature is confusing with regard to terminology in the condylar/subcondylar regions. Injury may occur at the level of the condylar head, the condylar neck, or the region below the sigmoid notch, the subcondylar region. Condylar head injuries are intra-articular and for the most part are not amenable to internal fixation techniques. They are at very high risk for ankylosis. Condylar neck fractures are defined as those that occur between the head and the sigmoid notch.

Historically, most of these injuries have been treated using maxillomandibular fixation for a period of 2 to 6 weeks. Although this results in excellent functional occlusion in many patients, it rarely reduces the fracture into anatomic alignment. Rather, the patient essentially develops a functional occlusal adaptation to the malreduction. Patients frequently continue to deviate to the fractured side with maximal opening and lose some of the contour of the mandibular border on the fractured side.

Many authors advocate open reductions and internal fixation. The concern of many surgeons regarding this is the potential risk of damage to the facial nerve. Although most published series have demonstrated a very low risk of permanent injury to the facial nerve, even neurapraxia is a distressing complication. In an effort to avoid this, endoscopic instrumentation has been developed to fixate these fractures largely through an intraoral incision with small trochar sites externally (7,8).

Zide and Kent (9) published a list of absolute and relative indications for open reduction and internal fixation of condylar fractures. This list has been modified by the body of literature over the years. As a general rule, internal fixation is considered in cases where maxillomandibular fixation is contraindicated (e.g., poorly controlled seizure disorder), fractures in which an acceptable occlusion cannot be reestablished, and bilateral fractures in the panfacial injury (to reestablish appropriate facial height).

When maxillomandibular fixation is chosen as the treatment, the period of fixation varies, depending on the age of the patient and the fracture pattern. Patients with uncomplicated clinical healing should usually be maintained in maxillomandibular fixation for 2 to 3 weeks, followed by an additional 2 to 3 weeks of nonchew diet. As a general rule, the primary determinant of the period of treatment is the occlusion. Patients with no significant occlusal change may not even require maxillomandibular fixation. Additionally, high condylar fractures may have a greater risk of ankylosis and should be immobilized for shorter periods of time. **The same can be said of children in whom maxillomandibular fixation is limited to 2 weeks. Many surgeons advocate the use of elastics rather than wire to guide the occlusion in the postoperative period.** This approach should only be attempted in the highly reliable patient. Using elastics provides control of the patient's occlusion while still allowing constant mobilization of the mandible, avoiding the problems inherent in maxillomandibular fixation.

Complications

The most common complications after mandibular fracture repair is malocclusion, usually secondary to maladaptation of the plate used for fixation. Inappropriately contouring the plate (especially a large plate such as the 2- to 4-mm system) results in the mandible shifting to adapt to the plate. This shift promotes malreduction and, consequently, malocclusion. It is less commonly seen when miniplates are used, as the plates tend to adapt to the bone instead of the reverse. This phenomenon is less likely to occur with locking plates. These are plates designed with threads within the screw hole. As the screw head approaches the plate, it locks into the plate. As such, the screw does not continue to tighten until the head is pulled up to the plate even if the plate is maladapted and is sitting above the plane of the bone. The screw stops when it reaches to the plate.

Once fixation has been applied to a mandibular fracture, maxillomandibular fixation is released and the patient's occlusion carefully assessed. Malocclusion at this point mandates removal of the fixation and recontouring of the plate. One never relies on postoperative maxillomandibular fixation or elastics to correct a malocclusion secondary to a malreduction.

Infection is also a common complication of mandibular fractures, most often as a consequence of mobility at the fracture site or because of loose hardware. During the exploration of an infected fracture that had been previously repaired, the operative site is thoroughly irrigated and the stability of the fixation assessed. In patients in whom the fixation has not failed and continues to provide stabilization of the fracture, the plates and screws are left in place, the wound cultured, and closed over drains. Culture-specific antibiotic therapy is instituted after an appropriate operative culture in obtained. If, on the other hand, the fixation is loose, it is removed and a more rigid fixation applied to ensure stable fixation of the fracture site.

SECONDARY DEFORMITIES IN FACIAL TRAUMA

Enophthalmos

Enophthalmos is defined as posterior displacement of the globe within the orbit. Clinically, it is noticeable when the displacement is 2 mm or greater. Inferior displacement is termed *hypoglobus*. Often there is some element of both enophthalmos and hypoglobus in the presence of malreduced or unreduced orbital injuries.

Failure to reestablish the correct orbital volume is the most common mistake in the repair of these fractures, resulting in late enophthalmos. This occurs if the orbital implant is not appropriately angled superiorly toward the anterior edge of the remaining intact orbital floor but is placed straight back into the maxillary sinus. Some suggest that correct placement of the implant or bone graft should be confirmed with an endoscope placed into the maxillary antrum.

Delayed enophthalmos is evaluated with a maxillofacial CT scan with 1.0-mm cuts through the orbits. Sagittal and coronal reconstructions are useful adjuncts to the orbital analysis and comparison to the normal contralateral side is extremely helpful. Thorough examination of the eye is performed by the ophthalmologist to assess abnormalities in vision or extraocular movement. The most common finding in patients with enophthalmos is diplopia, more often in peripheral than central gaze. Diplopia is most frequently related to disorders of the nerves or muscles controlling ocular motility, but may be related to malposition of the globe. The central nervous system can accommodate a significant degree of ocular displacement before diplopia becomes evident.

Correction of enophthalmos should be directed toward correction of the orbital volume. In the case of fractures of the orbital floor or medial wall, placement of bone grafts or an alloplastic implant in the deficient areas will correct the displacement. We often use titanium mesh, which can be easily molded and contoured, to reconstruct larger and more complex defects. Porous polyethylene is useful in the reconstruction of isolated floor fractures. The orbit is typically approached through a transconjunctival incision in much the same way that it is approached in primary repair. If the problem with globe positioning is strictly one of posterior displacement (enophthalmos) with no vertical component, and there is no well-defined defect to reconstruct, the implant is typically placed posterolaterally in the orbital cone. This achieves forward displacement of the globe without changing the vertical dimension. It is also

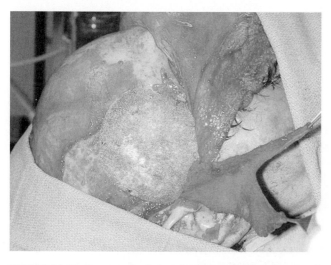

FIGURE 31.12. Porous polyethylene implant used to treat temporal hollowing. The implant is placed in the subperiosteal plane and larger than the anticipated defect.

important to perform a thorough subperiosteal dissection of the orbital cone to prevent the globe from being tethered posteriorly by scar. A slight degree of overcorrection is warranted in these cases to compensate for swelling that occurs during the dissection.

Enophthalmos secondary to malunion of an orbitozygomatic fracture requires careful evaluation. When the malar eminence is displaced in the presence of enophthalmos, corrective osteotomies of the entire zygomatic complex are performed at the level of the zygomaticomaxillary buttress, infraorbital rim, arch, zygomaticofrontal buttress, and sphenoid articulation within the orbit. This is accomplished through the coronal, lower lid, and buccal sulcus incision. Bone grafting is often required to compensate for the inevitable loss of bone that occurs from the original injury.

Malocclusion

Malocclusion is a very difficult problem to correct secondarily once bone union has occurred. It is far easier to avoid it in the first place. Although malocclusion can be related to malunion of maxillary, palatal, or mandible fractures, it is most commonly associated with poorly treated mandible fractures.

It cannot be emphasized enough that the occlusion seen following plating of the fractures must be meticulously evaluated. Any discrepancy seen in intercuspation and alignment of wear facets must be corrected. Removal and replacement of hardware is a minor inconvenience when compared to the inconvenience to both the surgeon and patient of a postoperative malocclusion. To fully assess the corrected occlusion it is vital to release the patient from maxillomandibular fixation at the conclusion of the plating. Maxillomandibular fixation can displace the condyles or bone fragments enough to give the appearance of a good bite. When checking the occlusion at the conclusion of the procedure, the surgeon should use only gentle upward pressure on the symphysis to check the occlusion. Because of the relatively lax configuration of the mandibular articulation with the skull, it requires only a mild degree of force to dislocate the condyles and force the patient into an occlusal state that appears normal, but is not centric. Centric occlusion is seen when the condyles are seated within the articular fossae. The challenge is to ensure that the occlusion at the end of the case is equal to centric occlusion.

When malocclusion is discovered in the immediate postoperative period, Panorex and plain radiographs can often determine if the condition is amenable to operative correction. Minor tooth interferences can be addressed by burring down teeth at the points of contact. Orthodontics is a powerful tool to address less-significant degrees of malocclusion. Orthodontics is often more useful in the malaligned alveolar fracture or segmental fractures of this nature. **The vast majority of postoperative malocclusions, however, should be taken back to the operating room for exploration, removal of hardware, appropriate reduction, and stabilization.** If internal fixation cannot

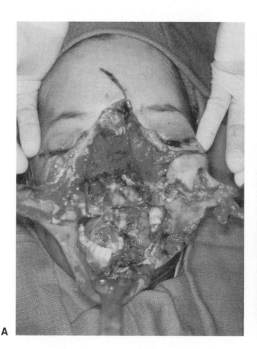

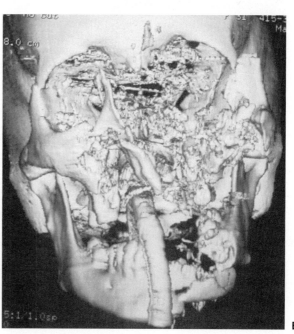

FIGURE 31.13. A and B: Shotgun wounds. Shotguns cause both extensive soft-tissue and skeletal destruction, often resulting in severe comminution of the facial skeleton.

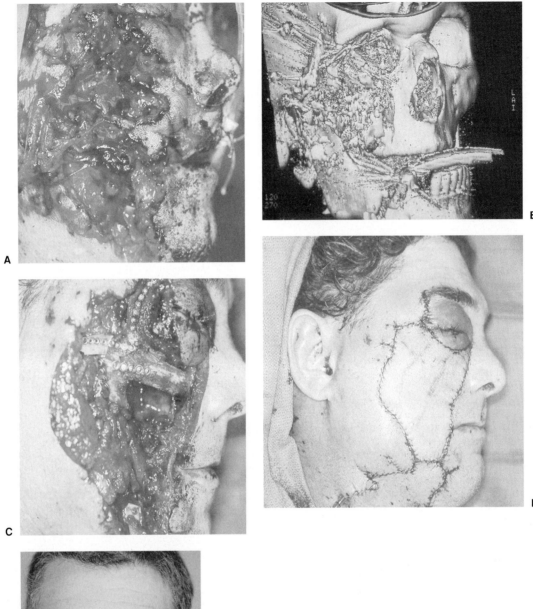

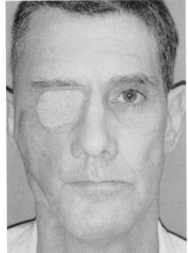

FIGURE 31.14. Complete phases of treatment of facial shotgun wound. A: Initial injury B: Three-dimensional CT scan of initial injury revealing degree of skeletal destruction. C: Reconstruction of the zygomatic complex with extensive primary bone grafts fixed with miniplates. D: Soft-tissue reconstruction with a combination of local flap advancement from cheek and radial forearm free flap for the central region. Stable soft-tissue reconstruction is critical to bone graft survival. E: Two-year follow-up.

be achieved for some reason, then the fail-safe maneuver is 4 to 6 weeks of maxillomandibular fixation.

In the case of malunion, where bone fragments are no longer mobile, osteotomies must be made. This approach requires the fabrication of models and mock surgery. The models are cut to correct the malocclusion, and an occlusal or lingual splint is fabricated to guide the repair. Although reproducing the initial fracture often suffices, in late cases in which there has been some degree of dental compensation, sagittal split and Le Fort I osteotomies may be required.

Temporal Hollowing

Temporal hollowing is caused by injury and subsequent loss of volume within the temporal fat pad. The temporal fat pad lies between the two layers of the deep temporal fascia (the thick layer of fascia immediately superficial to the temporalis muscle) that encompass the fat pad and insert onto the zygomatic arch. In dissection of the temporal region, some surgeons believe it is important to dissect deep to the superficial layer of the deep temporal fascia as one approaches the zygomatic arch in an effort to protect the temporal branch of the facial nerve. This results in some degree of trauma to the fat pad, which may result in devascularization and some loss of volume in this region. Although elevating this fascia does provide protection to the nerve (which runs deep to the temporoparietal fascia), nerve injuries are usually the result of excessive traction, which is not necessarily prevented by this fascial layer. To minimize the risk of devascularization and temporal hollowing, the authors prefer to dissect just on top of the superficial layer of the deep temporal fascia (or temporoparietal fascia) with a moist sponge using a sweeping motion. The dissection should elevate the superficial temporal fascia off of the deep temporal fascia, ensuring that the nerve is raised with the flap, and avoids the fat pad altogether.

Once temporal hollowing has occurred, one effective treatment is placement of a porous polyethylene implant in the subperiosteal plane and secured to the temporal fossa. Because of the deep placement of the implant below the temporalis muscle, the size of the implant is frequently larger than one would anticipate relative to the defect (Fig. 31.12). Porous polyethylene offers several advantages, including availability, permanency, and tissue ingrowth. It can also be stabilized with screws to the temporal region to prevent displacement. For smaller volume defects, autologous fat grafts are also an option.

Telecanthus

Telecanthus is even more difficult to resolve secondarily than it is primarily. The most common findings are tenting of the soft tissues of the medial canthus, lateral displacement of the canthus, and rounding of the medial canthal angle. The goal of revisional surgery is to correct all of the above deformities and ensure that the skeletal contour in the region is correct. Because of the nature of soft tissue in the region, most deformities in bone contour are readily visible. Exposure is obtained most frequently through a coronal and lower lid incisions. The entire soft-tissue envelope is mobilized and scar tissue resected or released. The correct position of the insertion of the medial canthal tendon is at the posterosuperior aspect of the lacrimal fossae. If this area has been distorted, it should be reconstructed to the appropriate contour, using the uninjured side to guide the reconstruction. The same is true for positioning of the medial canthus. The typical error is in reinserting the canthus too

anteriorly. It should always be remembered that it is difficult to overcorrect patients with this deformity.

Redraping the soft tissue of the medial canthal valley is a significant challenge. Transnasal wiring or suturing can be used to set the correct position of the medial canthus, but does little to ensure that the overlying soft tissues adhere down to the bone. It is useful in this regard to employ a soft-tissue bolster to compress the skin to the bone. It is best to use a technique that allows for adjustment of tension on the bolster postoperatively to avoid tissue necrosis. The bolster helps eliminate dead space and evacuate blood so that hematoma formation does not impede soft-tissue adherence.

Gunshot Wounds and Panfacial Fractures

Gunshot wounds can cause any combination of soft-tissue injury and fracture within the craniofacial skeleton. With most gunshot injuries to the face, the entrance wound tends to be inconspicuous relative to the degree of skeletal injury. The exit wounds are more variable and depend to a large degree on the caliber (energy) of the weapon. Shotgun wounds, on the other hand, almost universally impart a great deal of soft-tissue injury along with a significant degree of underlying skeletal injury (Fig. 31.13).

This difference is extremely important with respect to how these injuries are treated. The goal of skeletal reconstruction must first be the restoration of the anteroposterior projection and width of the face. Primary bone grafting has proven a reliable technique in the face of bone loss and severe comminution (10,11). Although the order in which the craniofacial skeleton is addressed is somewhat controversial, the zygomatic arch serves as a useful guide and should be plated early in the sequence. Correct positioning of the arch essentially establishes the proper facial width, framing the face. Failure to accurately reconstruct the arch results in the remainder of the reconstruction being set to the incorrect frame.

When a large soft-tissue component is also present, as occurs with shotgun wounds, soft-tissue reconstruction is an early priority. Stable soft-tissue coverage is vital to restoration of the skeleton, especially when bone grafting is required (12). Additionally, damaged and devitalized tissue can lead to significant scar contractures that ultimately can limit facial form and function. Although debridement of soft tissues in the facial region should be tempered with the goal of preservation of critical structures, all efforts should be made to achieve complete soft-tissue coverage and wound healing within 1 to 2 weeks in an effort to avert scar contractures. At times, this goal can only be achieved with free tissue transfer (Fig. 31.14).

References

1. Martin RC 2nd, Spain DA, Richardson JD. Do facial fractures protect the brain or are they a marker for severe head injury? *Am Surg.* 2002;68(5): 477.
2. Manolidis S, Weeks BH, Kirby M, Scarlett M, et al. Classification and surgical management of orbital fractures: Experience with 111 orbital reconstructions. *J Craniofac Surg.* 2002;13(6):726; discussion 738.
3. Markowitz BL, Manson PN, Sargent L, et al. Management of the medial canthal ligament in nasoethmoidal orbital fractures. *Plast Reconstr Surg.* 1991;87:843.
4. Rohrich RJ, Mickel TJ. Frontal sinus obliteration: In search of the ideal autogenous material. *Plast Reconstr Surg.* 1995;95(3):580.
5. Ellis E. Selection of internal fixation devices for mandibular fractures: How much fixation is enough? *Semin Plast Surg.* 2002;16(3):229.
6. Ellis E. Treatment methods for fractures of the mandibular angle. *Int J Oral Maxillofac Surg.* 1999;28(4):243.
7. Martin M, Lee C. Operative controversies: Thoughts on an intraoral

endoscopic assisted method of condylar fracture repair. *Semin Plast Surg.* 2002;16(3):251.

8. Lee C, Mueller RV, Lee K, et al. Endoscopic subcondylar fracture repair: functional, aesthetic, and radiographic outcomes. *Plast Reconstr Surg.* 1998;102:1434, discussion 1444.

9. Zide MF, Kent JN. Indications for open reduction of mandibular condyle fractures. *J Oral Maxillofac Surg.* 1983;41(2):89.

10. Manson PN, Crawley WA, Yaremchuk MJ, et al. Midface fractures: advantages of immediate extended open reduction and bone grafting. *Plast Reconstr Surg.* 1985;76:1.

11. Gruss JS, Mackinnon SE, Kassel EE, et al. The role of primary bone grafting in complex craniomaxillofacial trauma. *Plast Reconstr Surg.* 1985; 75:17.

12. Gruss JS, Antonyshyn O, Phillips JH. Early definitive bone and soft-tissue reconstruction of major gunshot wounds of the face. *Plast Reconst Surg.* 1991;87:436.

CHAPTER 32 ■ HEAD AND NECK CANCER AND SALIVARY GLAND TUMORS

PIERRE B. SAADEH AND MARK D. DELACURE

The intricate anatomy of the head and neck and its myriad of specific afflictions combine to present powerful treatment challenges with tremendous functional and aesthetic consequences. Several texts comprehensively discuss these topics (1–3). The vast majority of malignant tumors of the head and neck are squamous cell carcinomas, heterogenous in behavior, arising from the mucosal lining of the upper aerodigestive tract. Chapter 16 discusses tumors of the skin and adnexa. Salivary gland tumors are a diverse group of pathologic entities addressed later in this chapter. Successful reconstruction is contingent on communication between members of a multidisciplinary team, familiarity with the anatomy of the region, an appreciation of the terminology used to quantify the severity and prognosis of disease, an understanding of the natural history of the disease process and its treatment goals, a sense of the expected deficit requirements, and a logical approach to reconstruction.

HEAD AND NECK TEAM

The modern standard of care for the treatment of patients with head and neck tumors requires a collaborative effort among the ablative, reconstructive, radiologic, oncologic, radiotherapeutic, dental, speech and swallowing therapy, and psychosocial services.

HEAD AND NECK ANATOMY AND STAGING

A systematic, standardized approach to head and neck anatomy facilitates discussion and treatment. The primary site/subsite approach currently used for head and neck cancer reflects both unique regional tumor behavior and specific treatment-related considerations (functional, reconstructive, etc.). This section of the chapter focuses on sites with the greatest incidence of pathology and on subsites with specific reconstructive challenges. Primary tumor sites include the oral cavity, the nasopharynx, the oropharynx, the hypopharynx, and the larynx (supraglottis, glottis, subglottis). The tumor, node, metastases (TNM) classification developed by the American Joint Committee on Cancer (AJCC) in 2002, is the standard system used to establish stage grouping and to facilitate determination of both prognosis and treatment. Because T stage definitions vary depending on primary site location, these definitions are included with the primary site figures.

Oral Cavity

Table 32.1 defines the primary site locations of the oral cavity. Figure 32.1 demonstrates the anatomy and T staging of the oral cavity.

Nasopharynx

Table 32.2 defines the primary site locations of the nasopharynx. Figure 32.2 demonstrates the anatomy and T staging of the nasopharynx.

Oropharynx

Table 32.3 defines the primary site locations of the oropharynx. Figure 32.3 demonstrates the anatomy and T staging of the oropharynx.

Hypopharynx and Cervical Esophagus

Table 32.4 defines the primary site locations of the hypopharynx and cervical esophagus. Figure 32.4 demonstrates the anatomy and T staging of the hypopharynx.

Larynx

Table 32.5 defines the primary site locations of the larynx. Figure 32.5 demonstrates the anatomy and T staging of the larynx.

Nasal Cavity and Paranasal Sinuses

Table 32.6 defines the primary site locations of the nasal cavity and paranasal sinuses. Figure 32.6 demonstrates the anatomy and T staging of the nasal cavity and paranasal sinuses.

Neck

Table 32.7 defines the primary site locations of the neck. Figure 32.7 demonstrates the anatomy and T staging of the neck. To facilitate and standardize discussion of neck metastases and neck dissection, the neck has been divided into nodal group levels.

STAGING

Figure 32.8 outlines head and neck TNM staging as defined by the American Joint Committee on Cancer. (Figures 32.1 through 32.7 correlate the anatomic site to the respective T stage.)

TABLE 32.1

PRIMARY SITE LOCATIONS OF THE ORAL CAVITY

Lip	Skin–vermilion junction to oral mucosa and including the commissures.
Buccal mucosa	Mucosal lining extending from the pterygomandibular raphe forward. The Stensen (parotid) duct arises next to second maxillary molar.
Alveolar ridge	Gingival mucosa anterior to retromolar trigone.
Retromolar trigone	Mucosa behind the last mandibular molar tooth extending superiorly to the maxillary tuberosity.
Hard palate	Bounded by the superior alveolar ridge and the junction of the soft palate.
Floor of mouth	Bounded by the inferior alveolar ridges and the tongue. Wharton (submandibular) ducts arise in the midline.
Anterior (two-thirds) tongue (oral tongue)	Extends anteriorly from the circumvallate papillae and bounded by the floor of mouth. Motor innervation of the tongue is via the hypoglossal nerve (cranial nerve [CN] XII) whereas sensory innervation is via the lingual nerve (branch of CN V3).

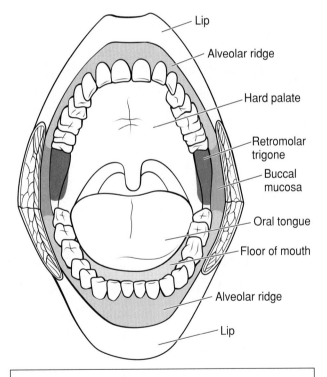

T1   < 2 cm

T2   2–4 cm

T3   > 4 cm

T4   Invades adjacent structures (cortical bone, inferior alveolar nerve, floor of mouth, muscles of tongue, skin); superficial erosion of bone by gingival primary is insufficient for T4 classification

FIGURE 32.1. Anatomy and T staging of oral cavity.

HEAD AND NECK CANCER

Although head and neck cancers are a devastating group of diseases, site- and stage-specific survival reveal that many locally advanced tumors exhibit 50% overall 5-year survivals (Table 32.8). Although a major cause of morbidity and mortality worldwide (500,000 cases in 2001), the incidence of squamous cell carcinoma of the head and neck has been decreasing in the United States, paralleling a decrease in smoking rates (Fig. 32.9). However, it remains the fifth leading cause of cancer incidence and sixth leading cause of cancer death in the United States. Cumulative DNA alterations caused by the synergistic effects of cigarette smoking and alcohol use are thought to underlie a majority of mucosally derived head and neck squamous cell carcinomas. Of note, a link has been identified between oropharyngeal tumors and human papillomavirus (HPV) DNA. As a result of "field cancerization" (7), the entire upper aerodigestive tract mucosa is at risk for both synchronous (5%) and metachronous (5% to 15%) second primary malignancies. The surgical treatment of other oral malignancies (e.g., salivary gland, sarcoma), which account for less than 10% of the malignancies in this region, is generally similar to squamous cell carcinoma and is outlined below.

Oral Cavity

Precancerous lesions of the oral cavity include the leukoplakia, which is common among smokers, and erythroplakia. Dysplastic leukoplakia and erythroplakia require, at minimum, close

TABLE 32.2

PRIMARY SITE LOCATIONS OF THE NASOPHARYNX

Hollow cavity delimited by oropharynx, hard palate, skull base, spine, and nasal cavity.

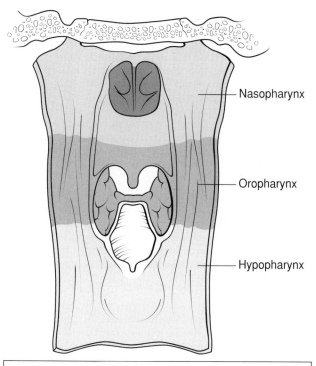

Nasopharynx

Oropharynx

Hypopharynx

T1	Tumor confined to nasopharynx
T2	Tumor extends to soft tissues
T3	Tumor involves bony structures and/or paranasal sinuses
T4	Tumor with intracranial extension and/or involvement of cranial nerves, infratemporal fossa, hypopharynx, orbit, or masticator space

FIGURE 32.2. Anatomy and T staging of nasopharynx.

serial observation. Additionally, treatment options include either chemoprevention (isotretinoin), or ablation with cryotherapy, electrocautery, or surgery.

Because of the accessibility of the oral cavity, and the morbidity of radiation-induced xerostomia, early tumors of this area (T1 and T2) are generally treated surgically. Locally advanced lesions (T3 and T4) are typically treated with combination therapy.

Lip

Squamous cell carcinoma of the lip comprises approximately 30% of oral cavity malignancies and the vast majorities of these occur on the lower lip. The majority of tumors of the upper lip are basal cell carcinomas. Unlike the remaining squamous cell carcinomas discussed in this chapter, sun exposure is thought to play a major role in its pathogenesis. Furthermore, although occult metastatic spread is unusual for most lip tumors, the commissures are associated with a 20% risk. In situ lesions may be treated with shave excision, topical 5-fluorouracil (5-FU), or imiquimod (Aldara, 3M, St. Paul, MN; non-FDA approved as of this writing), whereas later-stage lesions require assessment of possible mandibular and/or mental nerve involvement prior to excision with adequate margins. Because of the difficulty reconstructing the commissure, malignancies of this area may be treated with radiotherapy. Larger lip lesions warrant evaluation of the neck and possible selective neck dissection. Upper lip and commissure malignancies may drain to periparotid nodes, which require evaluation and possible superficial parotidectomy, in selected cases. Lip reconstruction is discussed in Chapter 36.

Anterior (Oral) Tongue

The anterior tongue is the site of malignancy in 25% to 50% of oral cavity cancers, with the midlateral aspect most frequently affected. Because of the lack of anatomic barriers to spread, tongue cancer has a propensity for diffuse, infiltrative involvement, which is often difficult to gauge clinically. Curative resection, therefore, mandates an adequate cuff (generally 1 cm) around the lesion. T1 or T2 lesions are usually amenable to transverse wedge excision. Larger T2 and posteriorly situated lesions are treated with paramedian mandibulotomy, which provides access for both tumor excision and, if indicated, in-continuity neck dissection. Smaller resections are treated with primary closure or skin-grafting, whereas larger defects generally require free tissue transfer (which may be sensate) to maintain tongue mobility and optimize oral function. All patients with tumors thicker than 3 to 5 mm and clinically negative necks should be treated with supraomohyoid neck or postoperative adjuvant radiotherapy dissection because of the relatively high risk of occult metastasis (up to 60%). Lymphoscintigraphy and sentinel node dissection may play a role in further refining the approach to occult neck disease.

Floor of Mouth

Floor of mouth cancer accounts for 30% of oral cavity malignancies and may extend locally into the tongue or the

TABLE 32.3

PRIMARY SITE LOCATIONS OF THE OROPHARYNX

Soft palate	Extends from the hard palate junction to the uvula posteriorly and anterior tonsillar pillars laterally.
Tonsil	Bounded by the tonsillar pillars (faucial arch).
Lateral pharyngeal wall	Extends from posterior tonsillar pillar to posterior pharyngeal wall. The internal carotid artery, internal jugular vein, vagus and sympathetic nerves, and cranial nerves (CN) IX to XII are located in the parapharyngeal space, which is immediately lateral to the lateral pharyngeal wall.
Posterior pharyngeal wall	Bounded by lateral pharyngeal walls and extending from the level of the hard palate superiorly and the hyoid bone inferiorly.
Posterior (one-third) tongue (base of tongue)	From circumvallate papillae to epiglottis (vallecula).

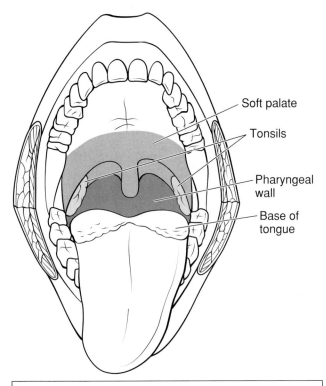

Soft palate

Tonsils

Pharyngeal wall

Base of tongue

T1	< 2 cm
T2	2–4 cm
T3	> 4 cm
T4	Invades adjacent structures (larynx, deep muscles of tongue, pterygoids, hard palate, pterygoid plates, skull base), surrounds carotid artery

FIGURE 32.3. Anatomy and T staging of oropharynx.

agement of the mandible, therefore, is an essential aspect of floor of mouth cancer treatment. Surgical guidelines include 1-cm margins, which results in marginal mandibulotectomy for tumors intimately related to the mandible. Radiologic evidence of cortical invasion mandates segmental mandibulotectomy with bone cuts about 1 cm away from the soft-tissue portion of the malignancy and evaluation of inferior alveolar nerve margins. Preplating the mandible may facilitate reconstruction. Larger tumors that do not require segmental mandibulotectomy may be resected in continuity with planned neck dissection through a transcervical route. This subsite also has a propensity for occult neck metastasis which may be bilateral.

Retromolar Trigone

Tumors of this subsite are generally difficult to treat because of challenging access and because of their locally aggressive nature, which often requires segmental mandibular resection and inferior alveolar nerve sacrifice.

Alveolar Ridge

Malignancies occur in this subsite uncommonly and are treated according to the principles outlined above. Occult metastases are rare. There is an increasing trend towards free bone/soft tissue transfer in the reconstruction of anterior maxillary defects.

Hard Palate

The hard palate is an uncommon subsite for oral cavity malignancy. Up to a third of tumors in this area may be of minor salivary gland origin. Principles of resection are similar to those described above and occult neck metastases are rare. Depending on tumor size and location, resection may be performed perorally, through a transoral midface degloving approach, or through a Weber-Ferguson approach. Reconstruction of the hard palate (to maintain speech, feeding, and the separation of the oral cavity from the nasal cavity), restoration of nasal lining, and, occasionally, reconstruction of the inferior orbital wall may be required. Small defects may be addressed with local flap closure or prosthodontics, but larger defects require free tissue transfer and/or maxillofacial prosthodontics.

Buccal Mucosa

Although also uncommon, buccal mucosal malignancies are locally aggressive and have a propensity to metastasize. Resection of these lesions may result in large, full-thickness soft-tissue deficits with significant cosmetic consequences. Free tissue reconstruction is frequently required.

mandible in the alveolar region. Dentition plays an important role, both as a relative barrier to mandibular invasion by tumor and in the maintenance of alveolar height. Irradiated mandibles lose the characteristic of alveolar invasion and are at greater risk of direct cortical involvement. After cortical breach, tumor infiltrates the cancellous space and may track in a perineural fashion if the alveolar canal is entered. Loss of alveolar height in the edentulous patient places the alveolar canal in proximity to the mucosal surface and affords portal of entry via empty tooth sockets. Oncologically sound man-

TABLE 32.4

PRIMARY SITE LOCATIONS OF THE HYPOPHARYNX AND CERVICAL ESOPHAGUS

Hypopharynx	Arbitrarily divided into three anatomically contiguous regions.
Postcricoid region	Extends from the arytenoids superiorly to the cricoid cartilage inferiorly.
Posterior pharyngeal wall	Anterior to retropharyngeal space and extends from the level of the epiglottis to the level of the cricoid cartilage.
Pyriform sinus	Pyramidal in shape with a base superiorly and an apex inferiorly. Extends from the oropharynx superiorly to the laryngeal ventricles inferiorly. The medial border is the lateral cricoid cartilage while the lateral border is the medial thyroid cartilage. The posterior border is bounded by both the lateral and posterior pharyngeal walls.
Cervical esophagus	Extends from the cricoid level to the sternal notch.

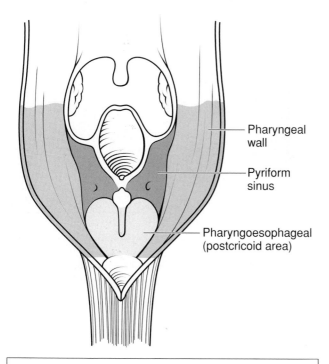

- Pharyngeal wall
- Pyriform sinus
- Pharyngoesophageal (postcricoid area)

T1	< 2 cm and limited to one subsite
T2	2–4 cm without fixation of hemilarynx or invades more than one subsite
T3	> 4 cm or with fixation of hemilarynx
T4	Invades adjacent structures (thyroid/cricoid cartilage, hyoid bone, thyroid gland, esophagus, central compartment soft tissue, prevertebral fascia), encases carotid artery, or involves mediastinal structures

FIGURE 32.4. Anatomy and T staging of hypopharynx and cervical esophagus.

Nasopharynx

Rare in the United States, tumors of the nasopharynx are much more common in China and have an association with Epstein-Barr virus and nitrosamine-containing foods. Although still a factor, cigarette smoking is thought to play a minor etiologic role in squamous cell carcinoma of this subsite. Locally advanced disease with (bilateral) neck involvement is a common presentation. Growth into local structures including the oropharynx, nasal cavity, sphenoid sinus, orbit, spine, or skull base can occur. Skull base extension into the cavernous sinus may present with associated neural involvement (cranial nerves

TABLE 32.5

PRIMARY SITE LOCATIONS OF THE NASOPHARYNX

Consists of the supraglottis, glottis, and subglottis.	
Supraglottis	Includes the epiglottis, arytenoids, aryepiglottic folds, and false cords.
Glottis	Consists of the true vocal cords, the anterior commissure, and the posterior commissure.
Subglottis	Region below the glottis extending to the inferior margin of the cricoid cartilage.

[CNs] III, IV, V_1, and VI [commonest]). The primary treatment for this highly radiosensitive tumor is chemoradiation with surgery reserved for recurrent disease (8).

Oropharynx

Functional outcomes take on greater importance in this subsite as a result of the proximity of the digestive and respiratory tracts to one another. Tumors in this region are characterized by their relatively small size compared to much larger neck metastases (clonal heterogeneity), the propensity of near midline lesions for bilateral neck involvement, and the possibility of retropharyngeal nodal metastasis. Although most tumors are squamous in origin, the higher concentration of lymphatic tissue yields a proportionally higher incidence of lymphomas (mucosal-associated lymphoid tissue [MALT] tumors), which are exquisitely radiosensitive.

Sixty percent of patients present with a mass in the neck, as the primary site is usually asymptomatic or has nonspecific symptomatology. However, CN IX or X involvement may present with referred otalgia and/or ipsilateral soft palate paresis. CN XII invasion can manifest as wasting and ipsilateral deviation of the tongue. In light of functional considerations, early lesions (T1 and T2) that cannot easily be resected are often best treated with radiation therapy. Advances in organ-preservation chemoradiation protocols are increasingly relegating surgery to advanced lesions (T3 and T4) and to salvage for treatment failure or recurrence (9).

The base of the tongue is most frequently affected and, similar to the oral tongue, infiltrative spread is common. While most base-of-tongue tumors are presently treated with chemoradiation and/or brachytherapy, there are multiple approaches to this area. Surgical access, depending on the lesion's location and size, includes transoral excision, lateral pharyngotomy, supra/transhyoid pharyngotomy, lip splitting, and paramedian mandibulotomy. The latter approach implies a larger tumor, which generally mandates advanced reconstruction. Similarly, locally advanced pharyngeal wall tumors require advanced access, laryngopharyngectomy, and reestablishment of digestive continuity. Tumors close to or involving the mandible (ramus: tonsil, pharyngeal arches, lateral pharyngeal wall) require marginal or segmental mandibulectomy, usually with reconstruction, as outlined in the section on oral cavity tumors. Consideration of tracheostomy and/or gastrointestinal feeding tube should be part of the preoperative plan of any extensive resection/reconstruction of the oropharynx. Except for early lesions of the soft palate and posterior pharynx, the propensity for neck metastasis by tumors of the oropharynx mandates treatment of the neck.

Hypopharynx and Cervical Esophagus

Malignancies of the hypopharynx most frequently involve the pyriform sinus with dysphagia and palpable neck disease as frequent presenting complaints. Referred otalgia from tumor invasion of the tympanic branch of the CN IX is also a common symptom. **Locally advanced hypopharyngeal tumors have the highest rate of distant metastases (usually to the lungs).** Tumors of the cervical esophagus are characterized by submucosal infiltration. Traditional surgical treatment of hypopharyngeal cancer commonly involves laryngopharyngectomy because of the proximity of tumor to the larynx and the limited ability to preserve function. There has been a shift in the treatment of hypopharyngeal tumors to concurrent chemoradiation protocols, similar to those used in the treatment of oropharyngeal cancer, which offer the hope of larynx preservation. This remains, however, an area of both controversy and of active

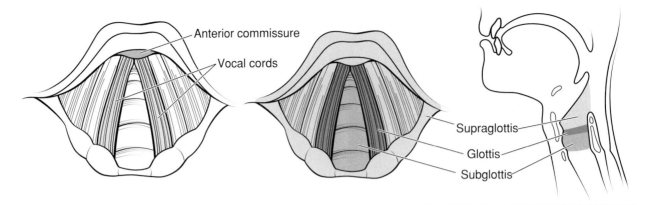

Supraglottis

T1   Limited to one subsite (mobile vocal cords)

T2   Invades mucosa of more than one adjacent subsite (mobile vocal cords)

T3   Limited to larynx with vocal cord fixation and/or invades: postcricoid space, pre-epiglottis, paraglottic space, and/or minor thyroid cartilage erosion

T4   Invades through thyroid cartilage and/or tissues beyond larynx

Glottis

T1   Limited to vocal cord(s) with normal mobility

T2   Extends to supraglottis or subglottis, and/or with impaired vocal cord mobility

T3   Limited to larynx with vocal cord fixation and/or invades paraglottic space, and/or minor thyroid cartilage erosion

T4   Invades through thyroid cartilage and/or tissues beyond larynx

Subglottis

T1   Limited to subglottis

T2   Extends to vocal cords with normal or impaired mobility

T3   Limited to larynx with vocal cord fixation

T4   Invades cricoid or thyroid cartilage and/or invades tissues beyond larynx

FIGURE 32.5. Anatomy and T staging of larynx.

investigation. Surgical treatment is indicated in selected early-stage patients, in patients with extensive, bulky disease, and in chemoradiation failures. Small localized lesions of the pyriform sinus may be treated by partial laryngopharyngectomy (PLP) that typically results in a hemicircumferential defect of the hypopharynx, whereas total laryngopharyngectomy results in complete disruption of gastrointestinal continuity. **Reconstructive options usually favor free tissue reconstruction with fasciocutaneous flaps for resurfacing of hemicircumferential defects and intestinal interposition flaps for complete defects.** Total

TABLE 32.6

NASAL CAVITY AND PARANASAL SINUSES

Nasal cavity	Extends superiorly from the walls of the ethmoid sinus anteriorly and the sphenoid sinus posteriorly down to the hard palate anteriorly and nasopharynx posteriorly. Lateral margins are the medial walls of the maxillary sinus and the nasal cavity is bisected sagittally by the septum.
Four paired sinuses	
Maxillary sinus	Bounded superiorly by the orbital floor, inferiorly by the hard palate, posteriorly by the pterygoid plates and pterygopalatine fossa, and laterally by the pterygoid muscles and mandibular ramus.
Frontal sinus	Above and along the anterior aspect of the ethmoid sinus.
Ethmoid sinus	Between medial orbits, superior to nasal cavity.
Sphenoid sinus	Skull base, posterior to ethmoid sinus.

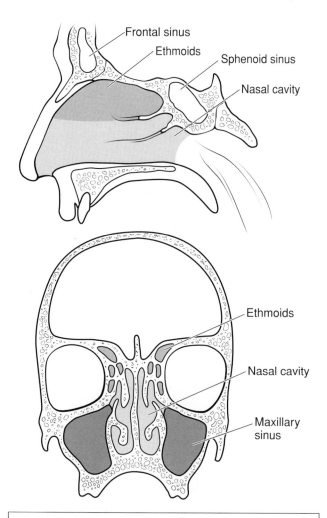

Maxillary sinus

T1 Limited to sinus mucosa without bone invasion

T2 Bone invasion excluding posterior sinus wall and/or pterygoid plates

T3 Invasion of posterior sinus wall, subcutaneous tissues, orbital floor, pterygoid fossa, ethmoid sinuses

T4 Invades orbit, skin of cheek, nasopharynx, pterygoid plates, skull base, dura, brain

Nasal cavity and ethmoid sinuses

T1 Restricted to one subsite, with or without bony invasion

T2 Invades two subsites in a single region or extends to involve an adjacent region within the nasoethmoidal complex, with or without bony invasion

T3 Extends to medial/floor orbit, maxillary sinus, palate, cribiform plate

T4 Invades orbit, skin of cheek, nasopharynx, pterygoid plates, skull base, dura, brain

FIGURE 32.6. Anatomy and T staging of nasal cavity and paranasal sinuses.

esophagectomy is reconstructed with gastric pull up. Pectoralis major flaps are generally reserved for poor free flap candidates, as adjunctive coverage, or for salvage. Complications specific to hypopharyngeal/esophageal reconstruction include fistula, stenosis, and dysphagia, which vary according to the selected reconstructive option. In patients who have undergone la-

ryngectomy, speech may be reestablished through esophageal speech, tracheoesophageal puncture, or with an electrolarynx. Early neck metastases with a propensity for bilaterality warrant an aggressive approach to the neck.

Larynx

Treatment considerations for carcinoma of the larynx center on tumor ablation, local control, and organ/voice preservation. The disease is generally divided into early and late laryngeal cancer.

Early laryngeal cancer (defined as stages I and II) usually involves the glottis and represents 60% of laryngeal cancers. Early glottic tumors generally have a good prognosis with 90% 5-year patient survival for T1 lesions. Because of limited lymphatic drainage, the neck is rarely affected. Historically, single-modality therapy with radiation therapy has been the standard treatment. Treatment options for T1 lesions include transoral laser ablation and other partial laryngectomy procedures. Controversy persists regarding both adequate evaluation and treatment of lesions involving the anterior commissure. Open vertical partial laryngectomy is generally reserved for T2 tumors, radiation failure, or limited local recurrence. Another operative option of increasing interest is supracricoid subtotal laryngectomy.

Early supraglottic cancer is similarly treated with radiation, transoral endoscopic approaches, or open surgery. However, because the rate of neck involvement in the clinically negative neck exceeds 20%, elective treatment of the neck (bilateral for midline or larger lesions) is advocated, usually with the same modality as the primary site treatment. Radiation therapy is most effective in the treatment of smaller volume, superficial lesions without cartilage destruction. Open surgery typically involves horizontal supraglottic laryngectomy and is an effective treatment of both T1, T2, and select T3 tumors. Involvement of the anterior commissure is a similar subject of controversy.

Early subglottic laryngeal carcinoma is very rare, and is amenable to the treatments indicated above. Because of similar outcomes between the various treatment modalities, albeit with some compromise between voice quality and local control rates, the treatment decision must often be made with patient performance status and preferences in mind.

Treatment of patients with advanced laryngeal carcinoma (stages III and IV) has undergone considerable change in the last two decades (10). Although survival has not changed appreciably, newer chemoradiation protocols have dramatically increased laryngeal preservation rates, reserving surgery (usually total laryngectomy) for salvage. Management of the N+ neck depends on the primary modality employed either with surgery performed after radiation or radiation therapy performed depending on clinicopathologic analysis of the surgical specimen.

Free flap reconstruction (commonly radial forearm free flap with palmaris tendon) of the vocal cord deficit in vertical partial laryngectomy defects has increased the predictability of the functional result in conservation laryngectomy (less than total) salvage procedures (11).

Nasal Cavity and Paranasal Sinuses

Similar to the nasopharynx, sinonasal tract squamous cell carcinoma occurs infrequently and has a relatively low association with cigarette smoking. The maxillary sinus is most frequently affected and tumors can grow considerably before becoming symptomatic. Tumors located below the Ohngren line (which extends from the medial canthus to the angle of the jaw) have a better prognosis than tumors located above it. Treatment

TABLE 32.7

SUMMARY OF THE REGIONAL NODAL GROUPS FROM THE MOST RECENT NECK DISSECTION CLASSIFICATION SYSTEM (4)

Level (nodal groups)	Anatomy	Likely primary site
Level I	Submental: nodal tissue superior to the hyoid bone and between the anterior bellies of the digastric muscles (sublevel 1A). Submandibular: nodal tissue between the mandibular border and the digastric muscles, including the submandibular gland (sublevel 1B).	Floor of mouth, anterior oral cavity/alveolar ridge, lower lip Submandibular gland, oral/nasal cavity, midfacial soft tissues
Level II	Nodal tissue along the upper aspect of the internal jugular vein extending from the skull base to the hyoid bone (clinical landmark) or the carotid bifurcation (radiologic landmark). Extends superiorly to the border of the sternohyoid muscle and inferiorly to the lateral border of the sternocleidomastoid muscle. Sublevel IIA represents tissue anterior to the spinal accessory nerve whereas sublevel IIB tissues are located posterior to the spinal accessory nerve.	Oral/nasal cavity, nasopharynx, oropharynx, hypopharynx, larynx, parotid
Level III	Nodal tissue along the middle aspect of the internal jugular vein extending from the lower limit of level II the cricothyroid membrane (clinical landmark) or the omohyoid muscle (radiologic landmark). Anterior and posterior borders are the same as level II.	Oral cavity, nasopharynx, oropharynx, hypopharynx
Level IV	Nodal tissue along the lower aspect of the internal jugular vein extending from the lower limit of level III to the clavicle. Anterior and posterior borders are the same as level III.	Hypopharynx, cervical esophagus, larynx, thyroid
Level V	Nodal tissue along the posterior course of the spinal accessory nerve. Triangle is defined by the lateral border of the sternocleidomastoid muscle, the trapezius muscle, and the clavicle.	Oropharynx, nasopharynx, posterior scalp and neck
Level VI	Nodal tissues delimited by the hyoid bone superiorly, sternal notch inferiorly, and common carotid arteries laterally.	Thyroid, glottic/subglottic larynx, piriform sinus apex, cervical esophagus

of malignancies of this area is generally surgical and consideration must be given to possible involvement of surrounding structures, including the remaining sinuses, the nose, the orbital floor and orbit, and the anterior and middle cranial fossae. The functional and cosmetic deformities resulting from tumor extirpation with uninvolved margins present significant reconstructive challenges, including restoration of hard palate continuity, reconstruction of the orbital floor, dead space elimination, and prevention of cerebral spinal fluid leak. Postoperative radiation is usually indicated.

Management of the Neck

The prognostic and therapeutic implications of nodal neck metastases mandate a standardized approach to both the description of neck anatomy, as outlined previously, and to options of management. The traditional radical neck dissection involves unilateral removal of lymphatic groups I to V and sacrifice of the spinal accessory nerve, internal jugular vein, and sternocleidomastoid muscle. Numerous modifications of this operation have been described in an effort to limit morbidity or to more specifically target occult metastases (Table 32.9 and Fig. 32.7). Neck dissections are classified as comprehensive (radical, modified radical), or selective, based on the nodal levels dissected and nonlymphatic structures preserved.

The proliferation of the various neck dissections is largely based on the observation that cervical metastases in previously untreated patients proceed in a predicable fashion depending on the site of the primary tumor. In the N0 neck, treatment includes surgery or radiotherapy, generally depending on the treatment modality selected for treatment of the primary tumor ("split-modality therapy" describes treating the primary tumor with surgery and the neck with radiation or vice versa). Elective treatment is further dependent on the location of the primary tumor. Occult metastases of oral cavity tumors have been correlated with increasing T stage (T3 or T4) and tumor thickness (>3 mm) and such patients should undergo elective treatment, surgical treatment of which generally involves supraomohyoid neck dissection. Tumors of increasing stage of the oropharynx, hypopharynx, and supraglottic larynx have a high incidence of occult cervical spread and elective treatment of the neck is recommended, surgical treatment of which involves lateral neck dissection. However, because access to the oropharynx often necessitates a mandibulotomy, consideration to an anterolateral neck dissection should be given. Elective surgical treatment of the neck is also indicated in unreliable patients and if the approach of surgical treatment of a primary tumor involves a neck approach (either for extirpation or reconstruction).

Treatment of the N+ neck generally involves comprehensive neck dissection with an effort to spare structures depending on

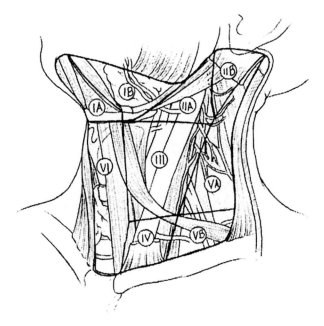

FIGURE 32.7. Anatomy of regional nodal groups.

tumor involvement. Selective neck dissection may be appropriate in many cases because of the rarity of level V involvement (except in nasopharyngeal malignancies) in the absence of multilevel involvement or level IV adenopathy.

As implied above, radiotherapy compares favorably to surgery in the elective treatment of N0 necks with regards to locoregional recurrence. Although there remains some controversy regarding the timing of radiation, radiotherapy is generally indicated in the treatment of N+ necks, particularly in the presence of multiple nodes or extracapsular extension.

Recent and Future Developments

Diagnostic, staging, and surveillance strategies of head and neck cancer are increasingly incorporating positron emission tomography (PET), which exploits the tendency of tumor cells to preferentially take up a radiolabeled glucose analog (fluorodeoxyglucose). PET is particularly useful in detecting recurrence, where traditional anatomically based imaging is limited by postoperative and radiation induced tissue derangements. Additionally, PET has demonstrated usefulness in the localization of occult primary tumors; detecting synchronous, metachronous, or late metastases; and improving the diagnostic accuracy of computed tomography (CT) when used with newer CT-PET fusion technology.

Radiation therapy has evolved. The most significant innovation is three-dimensional conformational radiotherapy (also referred to as intensity-modulated radiation therapy [IRMT]) planning and delivery, sparing radiation-induced damage to normal, uninvolved tissue. Furthermore, standard fractionation schedules have, in many cases, been supplanted by hyperfractionation or accelerated fractionation schedules. Hyperfractionation delivers smaller does of ionizing radiation over an unaltered timeframe, resulting in higher overall radiation doses as a consequence of lowered tissue toxicity. Accelerated fractionation shortens the delivery period of radiation, thereby limiting both duration of therapy and tumor doubling time. These therapies have improved locoregional control by up to 15%. **Mucositis remains a significant side ef-**fect, exacerbated, sometimes severely, by chemoradiation protocols. Other significant developments include paradigm shifts in reradiation schemes (now accepted and increasingly aggressive) (12) and increasing roles for neoadjuvant and combination modality protocols (10). Implant brachytherapy and intraoperative radiotherapy continue to have roles in selected patients.

Although there have not been any dramatic changes in chemotherapeutic agents, the use of these agents in combination with radiation, based on their radiosensitizing characteristics, has dramatically altered the treatment of locally advanced head and neck cancer (13). Chemotherapy can be administered as induction therapy (before other treatments), concurrent with radiation (most common), or as adjuvant therapy (after other treatments). Current clinical trials are evaluating the potential of antiangiogenic agents, such as the antivascular endothelial growth factor agent bevacizumab (Avastin, Genentech, South San Francisco, CA) in the treatment of head and neck cancer.

As in so many other areas of medicine, an improved understanding of the molecular and genetic derangements associated with head and neck cancer will likely play an ever more important role in its diagnosis and management. Disease progression is closely associated with the loss of tumor-suppressor genes p16 (80%) and p53 (50%, more common in smokers), and the elaboration of epidermal growth factor receptor (>90%), which may allow both earlier detection of cancer and the development of novel chemotherapeutic strategies. The discovery of biomarkers will likely aid in the identification of otherwise occult or early-stage tumors and has the potential to improve the prognostic accuracy of staging systems. Additionally, significant research efforts to attenuate or reverse the aforementioned molecular derangements via monoclonal antibodies, tyrosine kinase inhibitors, or even adenovirally mediated p53 gene delivery offer the hope of novel medical therapies for head and neck cancer.

SALIVARY GLAND TUMORS

Neoplasms of the salivary glands are a unique and rare (3% to 6% of all adults) subset of head and neck tumors. Their varied histology and infrequent occurrence, as well as their relationship to critical surrounding structures (facial nerve, mandible), often present a diagnostic and therapeutic challenge.

There are three paired major salivary glands (parotid, submandibular, sublingual; Fig. 32.10) and 600 to 1,000 minor salivary glands distributed primarily throughout the oral cavity (concentrated in the soft palate) and upper aerodigestive tract. Whereas the output of the parotids is primarily serous, that of the submandibular and sublingual is mucous and that of the minor glands mixed. This fact, in addition to the antigravitational anatomic arrangement of the submandibular duct, is responsible for the frequent involvement of that gland in chronic inflammation (sialadenitis) and sialolithiasis (stone) formation, the most common surgical condition of the submandibular gland. In aggregate, the major and minor glands produce 500 to 1,500 mL of saliva daily.

Seventy percent to 85% of all adult salivary gland tumors occur in the parotid gland, 8% to 15% in the submandibular, and 5% to 8% in the minor salivary glands. Sublingual neoplasms are extremely rare (<1%). **In general, the smaller the gland, the higher the probability of malignancy.** More than 66% of parotid, approximately 50% of submandibular, and approximately 25% of minor salivary gland tumors are benign. The most common benign tumor in all locations is the pleomorphic adenoma, or benign mixed tumor. It is also the most common tumor postirradiation. Mucoepidermoid carcinoma

		T			
		1	2	3	4
N	0	Stage I	Stage II	Stage III	Stage IV
	1	Stage III	Stage III	Stage III	Stage IV
	2	Stage IV	Stage IV	Stage IV	Stage IV
	3	Stage IV	Stage IV	Stage IV	Stage IV

Primary Tumor (T)

TX = Primary tumor cannot be assessed

T0 = Noevidence of primary tumor

Tis = Carcinoma in situ

T 1—4 = See respective sites

Metastasis (M)

MX = Distant metastasis cannot be assessed

M0 = No distant metastasis

M1 = Distant metastasis

¥ Table applies to M0 tumors

¥ M1=Stage IV

¥ Tis/N0=Stage 0

Regional lymph nodes (N)

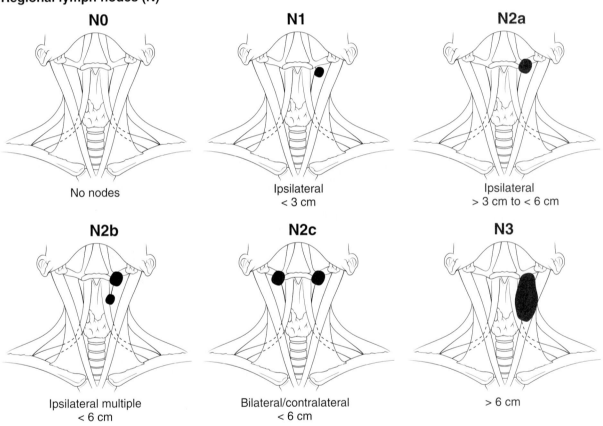

FIGURE 32.8. AJCC staging for head and neck cancer (5).

is the most common malignant tumor of the parotid; adenoid cystic tumor is the most common in the submandibular and minor salivary glands.

Children

Whereas epithelial neoplasms are the most common in adults, nonepithelial neoplasms (vascular malformations) are most frequent in children. Acellular dermal allograft (AlloDerm, Life-Cell Corporation, Branchburg, NJ) has been used in this group (where recurrent disease is not a significant possibility) to ameliorate the typical contour deformity subsequent to parotidec-

tomy. Pleomorphic adenoma is the most common epithelial neoplasm in children, as in adults. The parotid gland is the most frequently involved gland. When vascular malformative lesions are excluded, benign and malignant tumors occur with equal frequency. Females are slightly more likely to develop pediatric salivary gland tumors. Principles of treatment are generally similar to those in adults.

Pathology

Two theories of histogenesis have been postulated to explain the broad variation (more than nine types) in histopathologic

TABLE 32.8

STAGE- AND SITE-SPECIFIC 5-YEAR SURVIVAL RATES (%) BY SURVEILLANCE, EPIDEMIOLOGY, AND END RESULTS (SEER) PROGRAM OF THE NATIONAL CANCER INSTITUTE (1995–1997) (6)

Localized stage[a]	5-year survival rate (%)
Lip	89.6
Oral cavity	72.0
Salivary gland	88.5
Oropharynx	61.0
Nasopharynx	70.5
Hypopharynx	56.0
Larynx	74.3
Other mouth/pharynx	71.4
Regional stage[b]	
Lip	82.7
Oral cavity	43.8
Salivary gland	54.5
Oropharynx	50.6
Nasopharynx	59.3
Hypopharynx	34.6
Larynx	53.2
Other mouth/pharynx	29.3
Distant stage[c]	
Lip	40.0
Oral cavity	35.2
Salivary gland	17.6
Oropharynx	30.2
Nasopharynx	44.8
Hypopharynx	12.9
Larynx	38.3
Other mouth/pharynx	0.0

[a]Localized: neoplasm confined entirely to the organ of origin.
[b]Regional: neoplasm extends beyond the limits of the organ of origin directly into surrounding organs or tissues into regional lymph.
[c]Distant: neoplasm has spread to parts of the body remote from the primary tumor either by direct extension or by discontinuous metastasis.

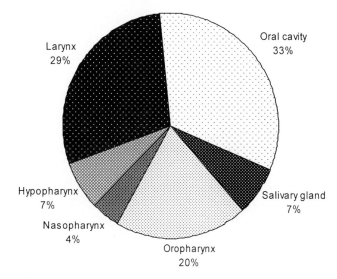

FIGURE 32.9. Distribution of head and neck cancer in the United States (6).

tumor types. In the multicellular theory, mature differentiated cells of the glandular unit give rise to specific tumor histologies, although it requires dedifferentiation for some types. In the second and more popular theory, tumors arise from one of two undifferentiated reserve cells. **The only known predisposition to salivary gland tumors is therapeutic external irradiation (acne, adenoid hypertrophy), with a latency, often, of one to three decades.** Concern regarding the use of cellular phones has not been substantiated.

Unique Tumor Characteristics

Malignant

Adenoid cystic carcinoma is neurophilic with a high incidence of occult perineural spread (outside the immediate operative field) and soft-tissue invasion. This feature mandates the use of postoperative adjuvant radiotherapy in most cases. Hematogenous metastases to liver, lung, and bone are frequent and may occur with a long latency period. Patients may live with significant metastatic tumor burden for an extended period (years).

Survival period statistics may exceed 5 years for this tumor, with survival curves diverging at 10 to 15 years.

Carcinoma ex pleomorphic adenoma (malignant mixed tumor) may arise in isolation, but is more commonly the concomitant of a long-standing pleomorphic adenoma. Malignant transformation is rare, occurring in fewer than 10% of these tumors.

Acinic cell carcinoma is bilateral in 3% of cases, and is the second most common malignant salivary neoplasm in children.

Squamous cell carcinoma is rarely of primary parotid origin and, when it is, is most commonly high-grade mucoepidermoid carcinoma. More commonly, this entity represents metastasis from a frontotemporal scalp cutaneous carcinoma to a peri- or intraparotid lymph node. The mass is noted 1 to 2 years after treatment of the primary (usually large and long-standing) and represents a failure to adequately treat (undertreat) the original lesion, that is, postoperative adjuvant radiotherapy to the primary site *and* regional nodes (levels I, II, and III). Total parotidectomy is often required to remove all intraparotid nodes. Skip metastasis to the upper neck is also observed, but should also include parotidectomy for occult or in-transit disease. These treatment principles also apply to malignant melanomas of the temporal region.

Lymphomas of the salivary glands are characterized by massive enlargement, and the role of surgery is limited to incisional biopsy.

Adenocarcinoma of the parotid gland exhibits a 7:1 female-to-male preponderance.

Benign

Recurrent pleomorphic adenoma may be mono- or multinodular and may occur up to several decades after treatment of the index tumor. **Tumor spill at the first procedure (capsular rupture) is not thought to predispose to this phenomenon.** These recurrent tumors may occur in extraglandular soft tissues and may be aggressive and ultimately fatal (metastatic, locally invasive, skull base). More commonly, this is the result of less-than-adequate surgery (i.e., nodulectomy, less-than-superficial parotidectomy). Treatment is reoperation with significant increase in the risk of permanent damage to the facial nerve with each subsequent procedure. Adjuvant external-beam radiotherapy should be added in most cases of multinodular recurrence.

TABLE 32.9

DESCRIPTION OF TYPES OF NECK DISSECTIONS

Neck dissection type	Nodal levels dissected	Preserved structures
Radical neck dissection	I–V	None
Modified radical neck dissection (type I)	I–V	CN XI
Modified radical neck dissection (type II)	I–V	CN XI, SCM
Modified radical neck dissection (type III)	I–V	SCM, IJV
Supraomohyoid neck dissection	I–III	CN XI, SCM, IJV
Lateral neck dissection	II–IV	CN XI, SCM, IJV
Anterolateral neck dissection	I–IV	CN XI, SCM, IJV
Posterolateral neck dissection	II–V	CN XI, SCM, IJV

CN XI, spinal accessory nerve; IJV, internal jugular vein; and SCM, sternocleidomastoid muscle.

Warthin tumor (benign cystadenoma lymphomatosum) exhibits a 5:1 male-to-female preponderance, typically appearing in the fifth to seventh decade of life. Metachronous bilaterality has been observed in up to 6% of cases.

AIDS-related lymphoepithelioma is related to involvement of intraparotid lymph nodes and may result in ductal obstructive phenomena and multicystic glandular involvement, which may be both deforming and painful. Treatment is external-beam radiotherapy.

Pleomorphic adenoma is the most common deep lobe parotid tumor. Because of their retromandibular position, it is common for deep lobe parotid tumors to achieve a significant size prior to diagnosis, as they are generally nonpalpable. The diagnosis is often made as an incidental finding on diagnostic imaging studies obtained for other complaints. The operative approach is superficial parotidectomy and facial nerve dissection followed by dissection of the nerve branches from the tumor surface. The deep plane tumor is then delivered beneath transposed branches.

Accessory parotid tumors rests of parotid tissue may be present along Stensen's duct and present as an anterior cheek mass. These rare tumors may be positioned so anteriorly that formal superficial parotidectomy may not be required; however, identification of regional branches (zygomatic) should be performed because of proximity to the tumor.

may also be used to justify a conservative policy of observing patients who may present significant operative risks (the very elderly with prohibitive comorbid conditions) for elective surgery. In the case of HIV-related tumors, CT and MRI may demonstrate multicystic (lymphoepithelial) involvement allowing the avoidance of high-risk (to surgical team) elective surgery altogether; radiation therapy is the indicated treatment for this entity. Preoperative knowledge of malignancy via FNAB where it is clinically suspected by palpable regional adenopathy, facial nerve paralysis, or pain, may assist the surgeon in time allocation, as with the addition of neck dissection and total parotidectomy, a 2-hour procedure may balloon into a 6-hour procedure. In cases where lymphoma is suspected (massive glandular involvement, multilevel bilateral adenopathy), flow cytometry on cells obtained via FNAB may allow less than a parotidectomy (lymph node biopsy) to secure the diagnosis with significantly lower morbidity.

Most deep lobe (and parapharyngeal) tumors are disclosed as incidental findings in diagnostic imaging studies obtained in the evaluation of other symptoms such as neck pain, headache, and the like. Rarely is the diagnosis suspected ahead of time because of the difficulty in palpating these tumors due to the

Evaluation of the Patient with a Parotid Mass

The diagnosis of a parotid tumor is a clinical one in most cases. History (usually an asymptomatic swelling in the region) and physical examination will lead to the next course of action (superficial parotidectomy with facial nerve dissection and preservation) in more than 90% of cases. In these, no other test or imaging study is indicated. **Fine-needle aspiration biopsy (FNAB), CT, or magnetic resonance imaging (MRI) will rarely add information that will change this surgical approach.** In the vast majority of cases, these studies are confirmatory of the diagnosis of parotid tumor but neither give histologic information (CT, MRI) nor give the exact location of the tumor to the branches of the facial nerve. Superficial parotidectomy serves as both a diagnostic and definitively therapeutic procedure in the majority of cases.

FNAB should be used selectively to help guide the timing of treatment; for example, those needing to schedule an elective procedure and convalescence around professional or educational demands, in which case knowledge of a benign tumor will allow safe scheduling on the order of months versus a malignant tumor that should be managed within weeks. FNAB

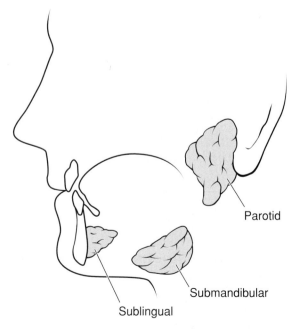

FIGURE 32.10. Location of major salivary glands.

ascending ramus of the mandible. A vague fullness in this region, without discretely palpable superior margin, may represent one of these neoplasms.

In malignant melanomas of the frontotemporal region, lymphoscintigraphy may document first echelon nodes in the parotid region (periparotid or intraparotid). The assessment of such nodes is controversial and is discussed above.

Only approximately 50% of submandibular gland stones are radiopaque. A classical history is of more help in making the diagnosis of chronic sialadenitis/sialolithiasis. This involves multiple episodes of painful gland enlargement, usually around eating. Persistence of symptoms increases, and episodes become more frequent. Severe involvement may require tracheotomy for airway stabilization and/or incision and drainage of consequent neck abscess, with interval gland excision.

Treatment

The minimal operation on the parotid gland is en bloc superficial parotidectomy with facial nerve dissection and preservation. This removes about two-thirds of gland parenchyma and lymph nodes. Lesser approaches are characterized by increased local recurrence. Expansion to total parotidectomy adds the piecemeal removal of tissue deep to the plane of the nerve and gland within the retromandibular and parapharyngeal spaces.

Wide open exposure of the facial nerve (as opposed to keyhole identification through a small aspect of the incision) and prograde dissection of the nerve are techniques that should allow the performance of safe parotidectomy. The operation should begin with elevation of the facial flap over the parotid-masseteric fascia to the anterior border of the gland and inferiorly to the platysma fibers. The tail of the gland is removed from the sternocleidomastoid muscle and steep vertical dissection performed to identify the posterior belly of the digastric muscle. The facial nerve trunk exits the skull base in the plane of the posterior belly about 1.5 cm superior to it. The tragal pointer cartilage is another commonly used landmark, with the nerve exit being about 1 cm inferior and deep to the plane of the pointer tip. Wide open exposure of the interval between these two landmarks affords the most reliable method to identify the trunk exit where possible. Another landmark is the artery to the stylomastoid foramen, which is about 1 mm in diameter and usually lies directly lateral to the nerve and within 1 mm or so of it.

Large tumors directly overlying the area of exit of the nerve may mandate a retrograde approach to the nerve where a major branch is identified at the perimeter of the gland and traced toward the trunk exit from the skull base. A clue to the location of the peripheral nerve branches is that they develop neurovascular territories and are accompanied by small vessels along their course peripherally. The use of nerve stimulators and monitors is optional and may confound a procedure through over stimulation and loss of signal. In general they are rarely used and do not substitute for direct visual identification of the nerve. As such, neuromuscular paralysis is generally used for parotid cases to facilitate those parts of the dissection that take place next to muscle. An intubating dose may be given to allow return of twitches in about 30 to 60 minutes, at which time the nerve trunk is found (and stimulation used if necessary). Once the nerve is identified, the dose can be supplemented to allow completion of the case.

Intraoperative decision making requires experience and judgment and cannot be underemphasized. Where malignancy is suspect because of invasive features, an inability to dissect from facial nerve, or associated adenopathy, the planned procedure may need to be escalated to total parotidectomy (high grade or metastatic cutaneous carcinoma/melanoma) with or without regional lymph node dissection, usually supraomohyoid, clearing levels I, II, and III.

Recurrent malignancies after previous parotidectomy and/or radiotherapy may require mandibulectomy, skin and nerve branch excision, and flap reconstruction, with pectoralis major or radial forearm with antebrachial cutaneous nerves usually serving as conduit interpositional nerve grafts for facial nerve reconstruction. Although interpositional nerve graft healing occurs despite postoperative adjuvant radiotherapy, the time to recovery and extent of recovery are affected by this necessary modality.

Sentinel lymph node biopsy of first-echelon nodes in the parotid region is controversial. In general, superficial parotidectomy should be the procedure to assess such nodes, which may be either intraparotid or periparotid. In only the most expert of hands should intraglandular biopsy be performed without full nerve identification. This should be guided by chromatic (isosulfan blue)-aided identification because of the similarity of appearance of intraglandular nodes and gland parenchyma.

Total excision of the submandibular gland is the treatment for most neoplasms in this location. In cases of direct nerve invasion by adenoid cystic carcinoma, nerve branch excision is added (marginal mandibular), as well as partial mandibulectomy and/or removal of the hypoglossal nerve. Supraomohyoid neck dissection may also be added by extending the submandibular (Risdon-type) incision. Protection of the marginal mandibular branch in submandibular surgery is best done by knowledge of the surgical planes of operation. Direct identification by dissection of the nerve branch (unlike in parotid surgery) is to be discouraged, as damage caused by this effort alone (stretch) will often result in permanent dense neurapraxia and/or paralysis as a consequence of the lack of redundancy in this region.

In general, an incision two fingerbreadths below the inferior border of the mandible and dissection straight down through the platysma muscle at this level (no flap undermining) will allow incision of the gland capsule in its inferior half. Immediate dissection along the capsule with superior dissection taking place along the curvature under the mandible (common error is to dissect above the mandible). Ligation of the facial vessels at the inferior border with transposition of sutures (cut long) above the border is another technique of nerve avoidance and protection. On the deep surface of the gland, the lingual nerve (CN V2) should be visualized, and the distal portion of CN XII visualized and not included in clamped ductal tissue entering beneath the mylohyoid muscle, when delivering the gland. A venous plexus accompanying the glossopharyngeal nerve, just beneath the digastric tendon, must be carefully worked around in order to avoid inadvertent damage to the nerve in the event of hemorrhage (careless clamping).

Reconstructive considerations are usually minimal in salivary gland surgery. In cases of nonrecovery of the marginal mandibular branch, botulinum toxin A (Botox, Chapter 46) injection of the contralateral depressor muscle will equalize (but not normalize) the smile. The majority of patients acclimate to the scaphoid defect resulting from superficial parotidectomy, with only the rare patient seeking amelioration of the defect. Efforts to "fill in" the defect are generally ill-advised in cases involving neoplasms, which have a finite chance of recurrence, the detection of which may be obscured by interposed tissue flaps or implant materials. AlloDerm rolls have been used for this purpose, however, in cases of parotidectomy for pediatric vascular malformations. The doubly modified Blair incision should be the standard surgical approach to parotid surgery, with short scar approaches providing inadequate exposure for many tumors. The cervical component may be extended

TABLE 32.10

HISTOPATHOLOGIC GRADES OF SALIVARY MALIGNANCY

Low grade	High grade
Acinic cell carcinoma	Adenoid cystic carcinoma
Low-grade mucoepidermoid	Squamous cell carcinoma
	Adenocarcinoma
	Carcinoma ex pleomorphic adenoma
	High-grade mucoepidermoid

anteriorly under the mandible to facilitate the addition of supraomohyoid neck dissection in appropriate cases. The incision may be designed to course behind the tragal cartilage in younger patients without a well-defined preauricular skin crease.

Postoperative adjuvant radiation therapy is indicated in the treatment of high-grade malignancies; adenoid cystic carcinomas (tendency to perineural spread beyond surgical field); metastatic adenopathy; close or involved margins of resection; invasion of skin, muscle, or bone; and selected cases of multinodular recurrent pleomorphic adenoma. The addition of therapeutic radiation has improved both local and regional control, as well as improved survival. Adjuvant chemotherapy is of unproven efficacy in the treatment of salivary gland malignancies.

Frey Syndrome

This auriculotemporal nerve syndrome is demonstrated in approximately 80% of patients undergoing parotidectomy by the minor starch iodine test; however, only approximately 20% of patients notice the phenomenon or request treatment for it. When the parotidectomy flap is elevated, sympathetic nerve endings subserving the sweat glands are transected. In the performance of parotidectomy (unlike facelift), auriculotemporal nerve endings are also transected. In the process of healing, nerve ingrowth occurs in a mixed pattern resulting in gustatory sweating. Interposition of an AlloDerm sheet may prevent the development of this phenomenon. Topical scopolamine cream and injected Botox are also used for severe cases.

Results

Benign salivary neoplasms rarely affect survival. Pleomorphic adenoma does have a recurrence rate of 2% to 7% and conversion to carcinoma ex pleomorphic adenoma occurs in approximately 10% of cases.

Univariate analysis has shown histologic high grade (Table 32.10), age greater than 35 to 50 years, site (submandibular, sinus, larynx), clinical stages III and IV (Fig. 32.8), and male gender to have an adverse impact on survival. Multivariate analysis adds histologic grade as one of the two (along with stage) most important features affecting survival. A 90% 10-year survival for stage I, 65% 10-year survival for stage II, and 20% 10-year survival for stage III malignant salivary neoplasms are reported. Overall, high-grade mucoepidermoid and adenocarcinoma fare more poorly than low-grade tumors of the same histology. Squamous and anaplastic carcinomas carry the worst prognosis. Acinic cell and low-grade mucoepidermoid carcinomas fare best. Parotid malignancies do better than those of other subsites. Tumor recurrence rates are 39%, 60%, and 65% for parotid, submandibular, and minor salivary gland malignancies, respectively. Because this may happen years after index treatment, long-term follow-up is essential. Survival for adenoid cystic carcinoma should be measured in decades as survival curves may only begin to diverge from the population around 15 years posttreatment.

References

1. Shah JP, Shah JP. *Head and Neck Surgery and Oncology.* 3rd ed. Edinburgh, UK: Mosby; 2003:732.
2. Shah JP, Patel SG, and the American Cancer Society. *Cancer of the Head and Neck. Atlas of Clinical Oncology.* Hamilton, Ont: BC Decker; 2002:ix, 484.
3. Harrison LB, Sessions RB, Hong WK. *Head and Neck Cancer: A Multidisciplinary Approach.* 2nd ed. Philadelphia: Lippincott Williams & Wilkins; 2004: xvii, 1077.
4. Robbins KT, et al. Neck dissection classification update: revisions proposed by the American Head and Neck Society and the American Academy of Otolaryngology-Head and Neck Surgery. *Arch Otolaryngol Head Neck Surg.* 2002;128(7):751.
5. O'Sullivan B, Shah J. New TNM staging criteria for head and neck tumors. *Semin Surg Oncol.* 2003;21(1):30.
6. Carvalho AL, et al. Trends in incidence and prognosis for head and neck cancer in the United States: a site-specific analysis of the SEER database. *Int J Cancer.* 2005;114(5):806.
7. Slaughter DP, Southwick HW, Smejkal W. Field cancerization in oral stratified squamous epithelium: clinical implications of multicentric origin. *Cancer.* 1953;6(5):963.
8. Lin JC, et al. Phase III study of concurrent chemoradiotherapy versus radiotherapy alone for advanced nasopharyngeal carcinoma: positive effect on overall and progression-free survival. *J Clin Oncol.* 2003;21(4):631.
9. Rudat V, Wannenmacher M. Role of multimodal treatment in oropharynx, larynx, and hypopharynx cancer. *Semin Surg Oncol.* 2001;20(1):66.
10. Forastiere A, et al. Head and neck cancer. *N Engl J Med.* 2001;345(26):1890.
11. Gilbert RW, Neligan PC. Microsurgical laryngotracheal reconstruction. *Clin Plast Surg.* 2005;32(3):293, v.
12. Kasperts N, et al. A review on re-irradiation for recurrent and second primary head and neck cancer. *Oral Oncol.* 2005;41(3):225.
13. Gibson MK, Forastiere AA. Multidisciplinary approaches in the management of advanced head and neck tumors: State of the art. *Curr Opin Oncol.* 2004;16(3):220.
14. Greene FL, American Joint Committee on Cancer, and American Cancer Society. *AJCC Cancer Staging Manual.* 6th ed. New York: Springer-Verlag; 2002:xiv, 421.

CHAPTER 33 ■ SKULL BASE SURGERY

HRAYR K. SHAHINIAN

For decades, the skull base represented a virtual "no-man's land" in terms of surgical treatment. The area is difficult to navigate because of the numerous vital blood vessels and critical cranial nerves that enter and exit the base of the brain (1–3).

Perhaps the most significant recent innovation in the field of skull base surgery has been the introduction of endoscopic minimally invasive techniques for the treatment of complex conditions such as pituitary tumors, microvascular nerve compression syndromes, acoustic neuromas, meningiomas, and a variety of brain and skull base tumors (4,5).

Endoscopic skull base surgery offers dramatic benefits to patients. Using thin, flexible, and precise endoscopic instruments, these minimally invasive approaches eliminate large craniotomies, brain retraction, scarring, and nasal packing. They shorten surgery time, dramatically reduce length of stay in the hospital, and result in faster overall recovery, return to work, and return to normal activities (6,7).

Anatomically, the skull base is divided into three subdivisions: the anterior skull base, the lateral skull base, and the posterior skull base (Fig. 33.1).

ANTERIOR SKULL BASE (ANTERIOR CRANIAL FOSSA)

Midline or paramedian anterior skull base lesions such as olfactory groove or planum sphenoidale meningiomas, esthesioneuroblastomas, and transcranial extensions of orbital or paranasal sinus tumors have traditionally been approached through, "craniofacial," unifrontal, or bifrontal craniotomies with elevation of one or both frontal lobes and requiring retraction of the brain for exposure. The introduction of endoscopic skull base surgery has allowed resection of these tumors through a small (2-cm) incision within the skin crease in the bridge of the nose or within the hair of the eyebrow, depending on the location of the tumor (Figs. 33.2 and 33.3).

Subsequent to the skin and soft-tissue incision, a 1.5-cm craniectomy is performed. If necessary, the frontal sinus is cranialized and the nasofrontal duct obliterated. The dura is incised and cerebrospinal fluid drained. The endoscope is introduced through the keyhole and advanced between the frontal lobe and the floor of the anterior skull base to approach the tumor. A panoramic view of the tumor is displayed on a flat screen monitor. Using a combination of a custom-designed bipolar electrocoagulation system and a micro-Cavitron ultrasonic aspirator, the tumor is gradually resected. This allows complete resection of most anterior skull base tumors through minimally invasive techniques with minimal or no brain retraction. More than 90% of patients undergoing these procedures are discharged from the hospital within 48 hours.

LATERAL SKULL BASE (MIDDLE CRANIAL FOSSA)

Midline lesions confined to the sella and the suprasellar space such as pituitary tumors, craniopharyngiomas, Rathke cysts, and chordomas, can be removed via the transnasal, transsphenoidal, endoscopic approach to the area. A microendoscope, 2.7 mm wide and 20 cm long with an angled tip, is inserted through the right nostril and into the skull base. This technique offers numerous advantages in terms of the surgery and recovery. Because the camera is "placed" at the tip of the endoscope, surgeons have a vivid panoramic view of the brain. The angled endoscopes allow the surgeon to see around corners and make a full assessment. This panoramic view enables the surgeon to remove the entire tumor in most cases. In the traditional, open translabial, transsphenoidal approach, the surgeon had to view the tumor site through a microscope outside the skull at a focal distance that limited visibility. The work was performed through a nasal speculum that restricted both viewing and the ability to maneuver instruments laterally. Because the point of entry for the endoscopic technique is through a nostril, no incision is required. Consequently, no more nasal packing is required and the brain is undisturbed. The time required for the actual surgical procedure, the length of hospital stay, and the overall recovery time are reduced. Patients return home within 24 to 36 hours of surgery and have a rapid overall recovery (Fig. 33.4).

Paramedian tumors (i.e., sphenoid wing schwannomas, neurofibromas of the trigeminal system, or sphenoid wing meningiomas) are approached through a preauricular transzygomatic 1.5-cm craniectomy. The dura is incised and cerebrospinal fluid is drained from the middle cranial fossa. After adequate relaxation of the temporal lobe, an endoscope is inserted, and direct access to the floor of the middle cranial fossa and the entire sphenoid wing is obtained (Fig. 33.5). This technique also provides access to the lateral cavernous sinus and tumors within its lateral triangle. This approach provides access to the foramen ovale and the V3 branch of the trigeminal nerve, and the foramen rotundum and the V2 branch of the trigeminal nerve. It also provides access to the superior orbital fissure and the optic canal. Both the precavernous internal carotid artery segment along the floor of the middle cranial fossa and the postcavernous internal carotid artery segment posterior and medial to the anterior clinoid are accessible.

POSTERIOR SKULL BASE (POSTERIOR CRANIAL FOSSA)

Posterior skull base lesions, such as acoustic neuromas or meningiomas of the cerebellopontine angle, and neurovascular compression syndromes, such as trigeminal neuralgia or hemifacial spasm, can be approached through a dime-size opening

347

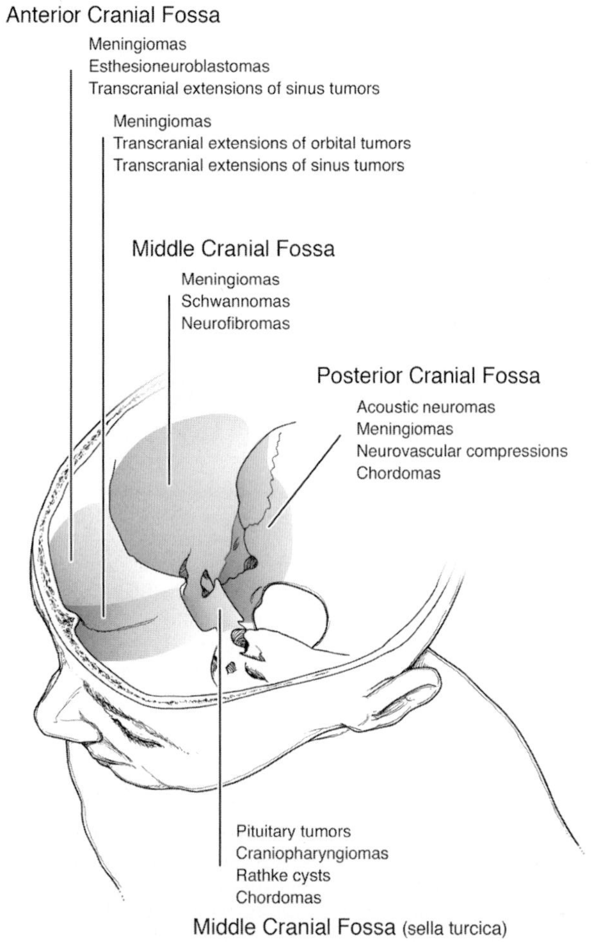

Anterior Cranial Fossa
Meningiomas
Esthesioneuroblastomas
Transcranial extensions of sinus tumors

Meningiomas
Transcranial extensions of orbital tumors
Transcranial extensions of sinus tumors

Middle Cranial Fossa
Meningiomas
Schwannomas
Neurofibromas

Posterior Cranial Fossa
Acoustic neuromas
Meningiomas
Neurovascular compressions
Chordomas

Pituitary tumors
Craniopharyngiomas
Rathke cysts
Chordomas

Middle Cranial Fossa (sella turcica)

FIGURE 33.1. Anatomic subdivisions of the skull base and the most commonly encountered lesions of these regions.

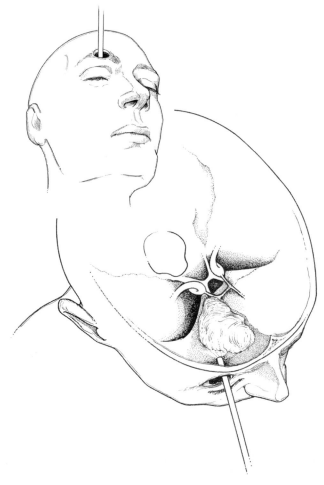

FIGURE 33.3. Endoscopic supraorbital approach to paramedian anterior cranial fossa tumors.

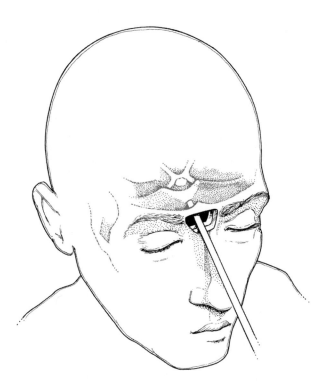

FIGURE 33.2. Endoscopic transfrontal approach to midline anterior cranial fossa tumors.

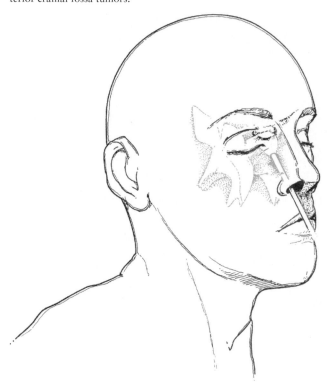

FIGURE 33.4. Endoscopic transnasal transsphenoidal approach to tumors of the sella turcica.

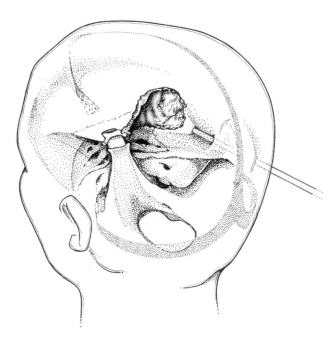

behind the ipsilateral ear. This approach is performed by making a 3-cm retroauricular scalp incision, followed by a 1.5-cm retrosigmoid craniectomy. The dura is incised and cerebrospinal fluid is drained from the posterior fossa. After adequate relaxation of the cerebellum, a 4-mm, zero-degree endoscope is introduced into the posterior fossa and gradually advanced to the ipsilateral cerebellopontine angle (Fig. 33.6). Tumors such as acoustic neuromas and meningiomas are resected using microsurgical techniques and the use of custom-designed microinstruments, a custom-designed bipolar electrocoagulation system, and a micro-Cavitron ultrasonic aspirator. Neurovascular compression syndromes are similarly managed with the use of custom-designed microinstruments that allow the safe dissection of intracranial vessels from cranial nerves and the safe insertion of a Teflon pledget between the vessel and the nerve. This often alleviates the excruciating facial pain in the case of trigeminal neuralgia, and the debilitating facial twitching in the case of hemifacial spasm. More than 95% of these patients spend only one night in the surgical intensive care unit followed by another 24 hours on a regular floor and discharged home within 48 hours.

FIGURE 33.5. Endoscopic transzygomatic approach to sphenoid wing and middle cranial fossa tumors.

CONCLUSION

Advances in fiberoptic technology, customized microinstrumentation, robotic holding devices, xenon lighting, and digital recording equipment have ushered in the era of endoscopic skull base surgery. The principles of minimally invasive approaches, more direct working distances, and the elimination of brain retraction have guided the skull base surgeon in tackling these challenging problems and have enabled the removal of tumors once thought to be "unresectable" (8,9).

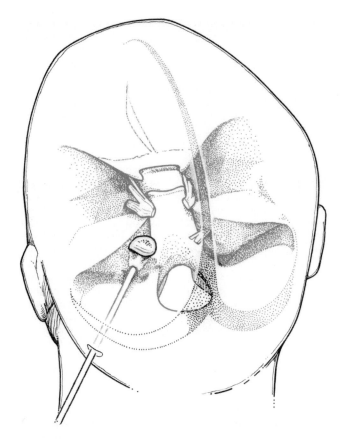

FIGURE 33.6. Endoscopic retrosigmoid approach to cerebellopontine angle tumors.

References

1. Fisch U, Mattox DE, eds. *Microsurgery of the Skull Base*. New York: Thieme Medical Publishers; 1988.
2. Sekhar LN, Janecka IP, eds. *Surgery of Cranial Base Tumors*. New York: Raven Press; 1993.
3. Shahinian HK, Dornier C, Fisch U. Parapharyngeal space tumors: the infratemporal fossa approach. *Skull Base Surg*. 1995;5:5.
4. Jarrahy R, Shahinian HK. Surgical management of pituitary tumors. *Pituitary*. 2000;3:1.
5. Jarrahy R, Cha ST, Berci G, et al. Endoscopic transglabellar approach to the anterior fossa and paranasal sinuses. *J Craniofac Surg*. 2000;11(5):412–417.
6. Jarrahy R, Shahinian HK. Surgical management of pituitary tumors. In: DeGroot LJ, Jameson JL, eds. *Endocrinology*. 4th ed. Philadelphia: WB Saunders; 2000:343–353.
7. Eby J, Cha ST, Shahinian HK. Fully endoscopic vascular decompression of the facial nerve for hemifacial spasm. *Skull Base Surg*. 2001;11(3):189–196.
8. Jarrahy R, Cha ST, Shahinian HK. Retained foreign body in the orbit and cavernous sinus with delayed presentation of superior orbital fissure syndrome. *J Craniofac Surg*. 2001;12(1):82–86.
9. Jarrahy R, Eby J, Shahinian HK. State of the art: a new powered endoscope holding arm for endoscopic surgery of the cranial base. *Minim Invasive Neurosurg*. 2002;45:189–192

CHAPTER 34 ■ CRANIOFACIAL AND MAXILLOFACIAL PROSTHETICS

LAWRENCE E. BRECHT

When surgical reconstruction with autogenous tissue is not possible or provides less than acceptable results, maxillofacial or craniofacial prosthetics offers an alternative method for restoring lost or missing structures. Despite advances in microvascular tissue transfer, the reconstruction of combined hard and soft tissue defects of the nose, orbit, or large facial defects often does not provide the patient with an acceptable aesthetic result. Similarly, autogenous reconstruction for absent or malformed auricular structures may be the treatment of choice in patients with microtia but is often suboptimal for adult patients with posttraumatic and postsurgical deformities where scarring is present. Intraoral defects of the maxilla or mandible following ablative tumor surgery are often best left accessible for examination, yet the patient must be reconstructed in some fashion to restore form and function.

Historically, *maxillofacial prosthetics* was defined as the restoration of hard and soft tissues of the stomatognathic system and surrounding maxillofacial structures that are absent as a result of a congenital anomaly or lost through trauma or ablative surgery. More recently, the term *craniofacial prosthetics* has been employed to describe the restoration of extraoral defects of the head and neck, whereas maxillofacial prosthetics has been used to describe defects more closely associated with intraoral and adjacent structures.

EXTRAORAL CRANIOFACIAL PROSTHESES

Osseointegration

The most significant advance in craniofacial prosthetics over the last several decades has been the application of *osseointegration* to address the problem of retention of extraoral prostheses. The concept of osseointegration was pioneered by Brånemark and describes the phenomenon in which an implant or *fixture* of commercially pure titanium is surgically placed into bone and, following a period of healing, a stable bond capable of supporting a prosthesis forms at the bone/implant interface. The concept of osseointegration was first applied clinically to the edentulous human mandible in 1965 to restore missing teeth (1). In 1979, Tjellström applied the same principles of osseointegration in the mastoid region to retain an auricular prosthesis (2). Since that time, long-term studies in Sweden, Canada, and the United States have demonstrated the successful application of osseointegrated craniofacial fixtures in the retention of prostheses for the ear, orbit, nose, and mid-face, in both irradiated and nonirradiated situations (2,3). Hyperbaric oxygen therapy for irradiated patients has dramatically improved success rates almost to those of nonirradiated patients (4). Studies have demonstrated no major complications such as infection, wound dehiscence, or osteoradionecro-sis associated with craniofacial osseointegrated implants (2). The use of osseointegrated craniofacial fixtures has safely and effectively eliminated the problem of inadequate retention for extraoral prostheses.

Auricular Prostheses

The etiology of defects of the external ear includes congenital anomalies (i.e., microtia associated with hemifacial microsomia), cutaneous malignancies, and trauma (including burns, motor vehicle accidents, animal attacks, human bites, etc.). Autogenous reconstruction of the deformed or missing auricle is one of the most technically challenging plastic surgical procedures (see Chapter 30). The alternative to autogenous reconstruction is an auricular prosthesis made from alloplastic materials, which, despite closely reproducing the form of an intact ear, has suffered until recently from the lack of a suitable mechanism of retention. Since the days of the first auricular prosthesis described by Ambrose Paré more than 400 years ago (5), the attachment of an artificial ear has relied on some form of either mechanical or adhesive retention. These methods have included engaging natural or surgically created anatomic undercuts, providing attachment to eyeglass frames or hearing aids, and using headbands, double-sided adhesive tape, or medical adhesive applied to the prosthesis. Adhesives have been the most widely employed method but are difficult to apply by the patient and often lead to tissue irritation. Adhesives also must be continually reapplied to provide a patient with the sense of confidence that the prosthesis is secure and will not fall off unexpectedly. The solvents in many adhesives also degrade the elastomeric material in the prosthesis, leading to discoloration, loss of flexibility, and a reduced lifespan. **These deficiencies have historically led to poor patient acceptance of conventional adhesive or mechanically retained auricular prostheses and make ear prostheses in children almost completely unacceptable.**

If an auricular prosthesis is chosen, however, osseointegrated implants are the method of choice for securing that prosthesis. Two craniofacial fixtures placed in the temporomastoid region posterior to the external auditory meatus are usually sufficient to support the prosthesis. The surgeon and maxillofacial prosthetist plan the location of the fixtures prior to surgery to maximize the final aesthetic result. Ideally, the site where the implants penetrate the skin and the location where the retentive components are hidden in the prosthesis should both lie deep to the antihelix. A template resembling the final ear is helpful to determine the best location for fixture placement. An incision is made in the overlying skin through which the abutment projects. Percutaneous titanium abutments are connected to the head of the implant fixtures. The abutment allows the implant to eventually be connected to the prosthesis. In situations in which there is adequate bone thickness, the placement of the craniofacial fixtures and the percutaneous abutment connection may be completed in one surgical procedure. After 2 to 3 months of healing, the prosthesis is constructed and placed on the implants. In children and in situations in which the bone is thin or of poor quality, the fixtures are placed and allowed to heal for several months. In a second procedure, the abutments are connected. Additional procedures that enhance the final prosthetic result, including removing remnants of the microtic ear, thinning the skin over the implants, or placing a skin graft, are best performed at a second stage.

The prosthesis is fabricated from heat-cured silicone elastomer that is custom colored to match the surrounding skin. The most life-like appearing prostheses are internally characterized with multiple shades of silicone to modify the basic skin tone shade of silicone (Fig. 34.1). The use of external pigmentation painted on the prosthesis should be kept to a minimum because it tends to discolor and is easily rubbed off with routine use.

Osseointegration allows the ear to be retained mechanically with clips or magnets placed within the prosthesis that attach securely to a bar connecting the implants. Implant-retained ear prostheses are used by patients an average of 12 hours a day,

compared to 2 hours daily for an adhesive prosthesis. Similarly, the majority of patients with implant-retained auricular prostheses also consider the prosthesis an extension of themselves after 18 months of use. The success rate for osseointegrated fixtures placed in the temporomastoid region is approximately 99% in both irradiated and nonirradiated situations.

Autogenous reconstruction remains the first choice for replacing a missing ear because it follows the primary doctrine of reconstructive surgery that the patient's tissue should be used whenever possible. Wilkes (6,7) stated that autogenous reconstruction remains the method of choice (a) in classic microtia, (b) in situations in which the lower one third of the ear remains intact, (c) when the patient preference is for reconstruction, and (d) in patients who are less compliant and are unlikely to maintain a prosthesis. The relative indications for an osseointegrated auricular prosthesis include (a) defects resulting from ablative tumor surgery, (b) failed attempts at autogenous reconstruction, (c) a missing lower one third of the ear, (d) patient preference for a prosthesis, (e) previously irradiated reconstruction site, (f) severely compromised local tissue (i.e., burn patients), (g) patients who have a more involved craniofacial anomaly rather than classic isolated microtia, and (8) patients who may

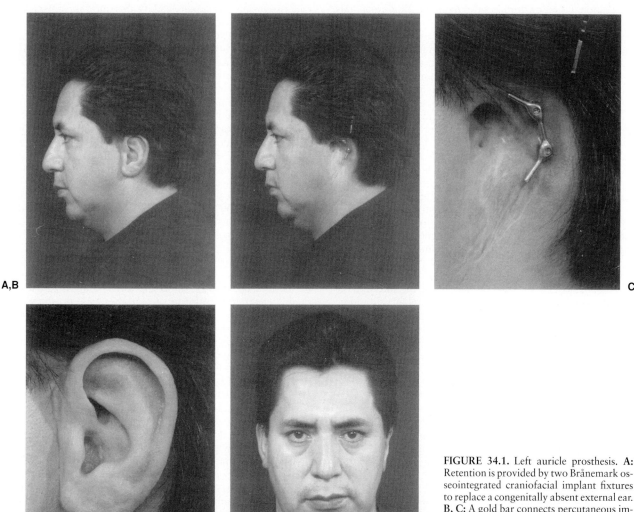

FIGURE 34.1. Left auricle prosthesis. **A:** Retention is provided by two Brånemark osseointegrated craniofacial implant fixtures to replace a congenitally absent external ear. **B, C:** A gold bar connects percutaneous implant abutments to which the ear prosthesis is retained by clips incorporated into the tissue side of the prosthesis. **D, E:** The prosthesis provides an excellent aesthetic result for an adult patient. Note the thin, immobile skin around the abutments.

be a poor operative risk. It should be remembered that children are always better served by autogenous reconstruction if at all possible.

Nasal Prostheses

Acquired defects of the nasal structures are most easily and aesthetically reconstructed with autogenous tissues. Small nasal defects after tumor resection, especially those limited to the soft tissues, are particularly suited to surgical reconstruction. Defects resulting from congenital anomalies should also be reconstructed surgically whenever possible. Prosthetic reconstruction is indicated as the method of choice for nasal rehabilitation only in instances in which bone as well as soft tissue has been resected (i.e., total rhinectomy) or when the defect is so large that reconstruction is not possible. Similarly, traumatic defects after motor vehicle accidents, burns, or gunshot wounds often lead to massive local tissue destruction that precludes the surgical option for reconstruction. Nasal prostheses may also serve as interim restorations after resection and radiation therapy while a patient awaits autogenous reconstruction. Finally, a prosthesis should be considered for the patient who is a poor surgical risk or who prefers a prosthesis rather than the additional surgical procedures required for autogenous reconstruction.

Nasal prostheses have been retained by adhesives, spectacles, through the engagement of tissue undercuts within the defect, and, more recently, with osseointegrated implants. Although less successful in the nasal region than in other bones of the craniofacial region, osseointegration still provides the most reliable method of retaining a nasal prosthesis.

When the need for a prosthesis is anticipated, the surgeon and maxillofacial prosthodontist should work as a team to optimize the functional and aesthetic result. If possible, a presurgical examination and impression of the nasal structures prior to resection should be made to guide the sculpting of the prosthesis. If the entire nose is to be removed, full resection of the nasal bones will improve the form and contour of a prosthesis. The nasal septum should also be sufficiently resected to optimize the defect for a prosthesis. The exposed nasal mucosa should be covered with a skin graft to provide tissue suitable to support a prosthesis whether it is to be retained with adhesives or by implants. Ideally, three implants are placed to retain a nasal prosthesis. The preferable implantation sites include the nasion, both angles at the base of the piriform aperture, and the anterior nasal spine area. Osseointegrated implants should be placed secondarily after the resection. The implants, in turn, should heal for 4 to 6 months before the connection of the percutaneous abutments. The surrounding tissue or skin graft through which the abutments project should be made as thin as possible to prevent any soft tissue movement around the abutment. Thick tissues that move around the abutments lead to tissue irritation and discomfort under the prosthesis.

Implant-supported nasal prostheses are retained mechanically with clips or magnets within the prosthesis that engage a metal bar. The bar serves to connect the implant abutments and distributes loading forces over all the implants. Individual magnets may also be attached directly to the abutments. In situations in which there is a combined intraoral maxillary defect associated with a nasal defect, the retentive bar mechanism for the nasal prosthesis may be modified to provide stability to an intraoral prosthesis as well. Care must be exercised in designing the retentive features of an implant-supported nasal prosthesis or combined intraoral-nasal prosthesis to assure that the implants will not be subjected to excessive loading forces. Overloading of implants placed into the membranous bones of the paranasal region may lead to loss of implant osseointegration.

Because the nose is a projecting midline structure, a prosthesis fabricated from silicone elastomer will reflect light in a fashion different from the surrounding skin. Therefore, even the most aesthetic implant-retained nasal prosthesis will appear dissimilar from the adjacent tissues. This can be minimized by having the patient wear eyeglasses with an appropriate frame design to distract the observer away from the patient's midface and the border between the skin and the prosthesis (Fig. 34.2). Properly thinned, translucent margins on a carefully colored nasal prosthesis also help to make it more lifelike.

Orbital Prostheses

Exenteration, or removal of the entire contents of the orbit including the eye and extraocular muscles, is often indicated to treat malignancy, infection, other aggressive diseases (e.g., fibrous dysplasia, neurofibromatosis, mucormycosis) or after trauma. The bony rim of the orbit, as well as the adjacent soft tissues, may also require resection when a disease process extends outside the anatomic orbit. This includes the nasal structures with medial extension or the frontal sinus with superior extension. Perhaps the most frequent indication for orbital exenteration is the superior extension of maxillary sinus tumors into the orbit. The defect after exenteration with or without a wider resection is best managed by an orbital prosthesis. Only a prosthesis provides an aesthetic alternative to an open eye socket or eye patch.

An orbital prosthesis consists of an *ocular prosthesis* that replaces the missing eye, which is custom fabricated from acrylic or glass, and the soft tissue components made from silicone elastomer, which replace the eyelids and surrounding skin. Historically, the retention of orbital prostheses has relied on skin adhesives, mechanical engagement of tissue undercuts in the defect, attachment to eyeglass frames, or interlocking mechanisms designed into a maxillary obturator. Currently, osseointegrated implants provide the most reliable and predictable method of retention for orbital prostheses while minimizing the soft tissue irritation associated with other forms of retention. In a multicenter clinical trial, osseointegrated craniofacial fixtures demonstrated 100% implant survival in nonirradiated orbits and a 79% survival rate when placed in irradiated orbits (8).

The maxillofacial prosthodontist and the surgeon should evaluate the patient together prior to resection to provide guidance during surgery that will optimize the aesthetics of the orbital prosthesis. Often, removal of the contents of the orbit alone without resection of the surrounding bone yields a shallow, restrictive recipient site for an orbital prosthesis. Intentional widening and deepening of the surgical site provides more space for the retentive framework, ocular component, and bulk of silicone material. Similarly, the flaps used to reconstruct large defects that may include protection for the brain should not be left unnecessarily bulky. When possible, eyebrows should be preserved because they are difficult to reproduce in a prosthesis.

The ideal locations for the placement of osseointegrated implants for retention of an orbital prosthesis include the superolateral rim and the inferolateral rim. The fixtures are placed into the bone along the *inner* aspect of the orbit. This allows the components of the prosthesis to fall inside the boundaries of the orbit without distorting the natural anteroposterior relationship of the eye within the orbit. Without proper positioning of the ocular prosthesis in the orbital prosthesis, the final prosthesis will not be symmetric with the unresected eye. The result will be a hopelessly artificial-appearing prosthesis.

Three implants may be placed in both the superior and inferior orbital rims. These areas provide the greatest thickness and density of bone suitable for implant placement. A minimum of four or five fixtures should be planned to support an

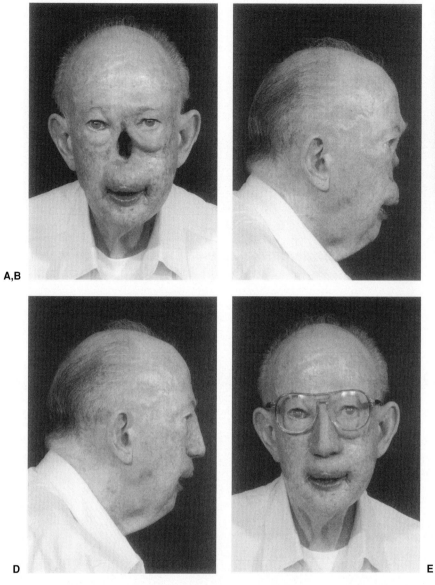

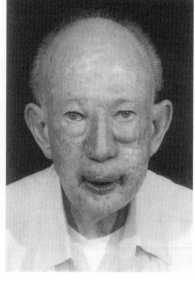

FIGURE 34.2. A, B: An 84-year-old patient with a nasal defect after total rhinectomy to remove multiple basal-squamous cell carcinomas. C, D: Implant-retained nasal prosthesis with one implant in the nasion region. Resection of the bony vault enhances aesthetic control of the contour of the nasal prosthesis and increases stability. E: Eyeglass frames aid in masking the margins of the nasal prosthesis and increase stability.

orbital prosthesis. Ideally, additional fixtures are placed in case some fail to integrate. This is particularly important in patients who have been irradiated prior to surgery. In patients who have received ionizing radiation in the implant area the success rate for fixture osseointegration may be improved by a course of hyperbaric oxygen treatment according to the protocol developed by Granström (9). After a 4- to 6-month healing period, the implants are uncovered during a second procedure in which the percutaneous abutments are connected to the integrated fixtures. The additional implants that will not be used to retain the prosthesis are allowed to remain "sleeping" in the bone for future use, should they be needed. At the second stage, the soft tissues surrounding the implant abutments are thinned as much as possible to prevent tissue movement around the abutments. This may require the placement of a split-thickness skin graft directly on the exposed bone. Failure to aggressively thin the soft tissues in the peri-implant area will lead to tissue irritation, a minor but troubling complication.

Two weeks after abutment connection, the patient may begin to have the implant-supported orbital prosthesis fabricated. An impression of the defect that registers the location of the implant abutments is made and a cast is poured. The ocular component is carefully trimmed and positioned in the defect on the patient to assure a lifelike gaze will be reproduced in

the prosthesis. The position of the ocular must be determined on the patient rather than a cast. Once the ocular position has been verified, the surrounding eyelids and soft tissue details are carefully sculpted in wax and finished with the patient present. The prosthesis is then formed in MDX-4420 heat-cured silicone elastomer that has been custom colored to the patient's skin tone. Multiple small mixes of stronger shades of silicone, such as violet in the medial canthal region or pale blue in the superior palpebrum, are added where appropriate to match the uninvolved orbit (Fig. 34.3).

Eyelashes and eyebrows may also be added to lend a natural appearance. Eyeglasses with a clean, simple frame design are worn to cover margins between the prosthesis and skin that may be easily discerned. However, an implant-supported prosthesis should have thin, clear margins that allow the prosthesis to blend imperceptibly with the adjacent tissues.

An orbital prosthesis may be securely retained by craniofacial implants through a bar and clip arrangement, a bar and magnets, individual magnets on the implants, or individual ball-shaped attachments. The method of retention employed depends on the size of the defect, the quality of the bone at the implant sites, the position, number, and angulation of implants, and the patient's level of manual dexterity.

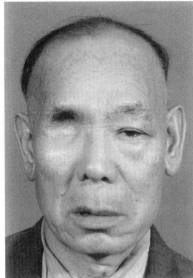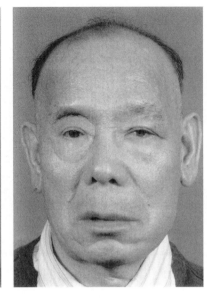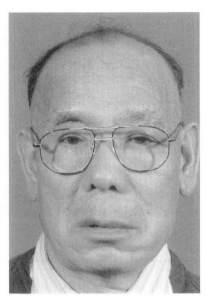

A,B   C

FIGURE 34.3. A: A 72-year-old patient with shallow orbital defect after exenteration. B: Adhesive-retained silicone elastomer prosthesis in place. C: Eyeglass frames mask prosthesis margins, provide stability, and protect the remaining functional eye.

INTRAORAL MAXILLOFACIAL PROSTHESES

Maxillary Defects

Defects of the maxilla resulting from trauma or ablative tumor surgery are most readily managed with an *obturator* prosthesis rather than through surgical reconstruction. The primary goal of obturation of a maxillary defect is to maintain the anatomic separation normally present between the oral and nasal-antral cavities, thus allowing the patient to speak and swallow without fluid or air leakage into the nasal cavity. The use of a removable obturator prosthesis also allows visual inspection of surgical sites to rule out recurrent tumor. Several types of maxillary obturators may be fabricated, depending on the particular postsurgical phase of treatment.

Immediate Surgical Obturator

During the surgical phase of treatment an *immediate surgical obturator prosthesis* or *surgical obturator* is inserted in the operating room immediately after the removal of the tumor and adjacent maxillary structures. The surgical obturator serves as a matrix to hold surgical packing in the defect. It also supports and immobilizes a split-thickness skin graft often used to line the defect (Fig. 34.4). By separating the surgical site from the oral cavity, it also allows the patient to speak and swallow more quickly, thereby reducing the postsurgical hospitalization period.

Preparation for the surgical obturator requires that the patient be evaluated by the prosthodontist as soon as possible after the decision has been made to surgically resect a lesion. At this presurgical appointment, after a thorough clinical and radiographic examination to assess the quality of the patient's dentition, impressions of the dental arches are made and stone casts obtained. Records of the patient's occlusion are also made. The prosthodontist and the surgeon review the planned resection. Tumor-free margins remain the primary goal of resection; however, the surgeon and prosthodontist together should outline the casts and develop a surgical plan that also takes into

consideration the long-term stability and retention for an obturator. Structures such as the zygomatic buttress, pterygoid plates, maxillary tuberosity, infraorbital bony rim, and undercuts created in the residual vertical palatal wall all serve to increase the stability and retention of a maxillary prosthesis. Similarly, a presurgical assessment by the prosthodontist may

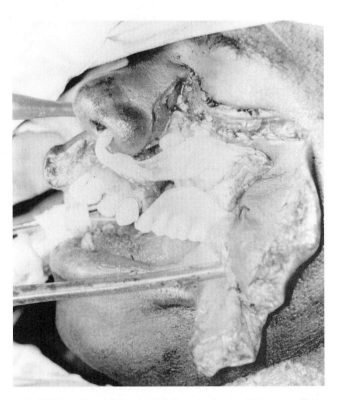

FIGURE 34.4. Immediate surgical obturator inserted into a maxillary defect after resection of ameloblastoma. Wires provide additional retention. The prosthesis supports surgical packing and a buccal split-thickness skin graft lining the mucosal defect.

indicate the need for the removal of the coronoid process of the mandible on the side of the resection. The ipsilateral coronoid process may serve to dislodge an obturator during lateral mandibular excursions after resection of the posterior maxilla.

After the planned resection is outlined on the casts by the surgeon and the prosthodontist, the prosthodontist then performs "model surgery" to alter the cast to accommodate the planned resection. The surgical obturator is fashioned on the modified cast in the dental laboratory. An immediate surgical obturator is fabricated from heat-processed polymethylmethacrylate (PMMA), which provides strength, yet allows it to be easily adjusted with a bur or augmented with a soft denture reline material. Close attention should be focused on the extension of the acrylic around teeth and into undercuts on the modified cast to assure that minimal adjustment in the operating room will be required.

Surgical obturators are often retained through wire fixation to stable bone near the resection site. This may include circumzygomatic wires, more superiorly based craniofacial wiring, circumdental wires (when sound teeth remain), or transalveolar wiring if the residual maxilla is edentulous. A transpalatal screw is also effective in retaining a surgical prosthesis in edentulous situations or when minimal maxillary bone exists. Recessed holes for ligature wires should be predrilled on the prosthesis and polished prior to surgery. Resilient wire clasps may also provide retention when there are sufficient supporting teeth remaining. If the resection involves removing anterior teeth, then replacement teeth are added to the surgical prosthesis to aid in speech production and to improve aesthetics. However, posterior teeth may or may not be added depending on the anticipated stability of the prosthesis. Posterior teeth may interfere with the retention of the prosthesis if the dental occlusion is not properly reproduced in the surgical prosthesis.

Ideally, the maxillofacial prosthodontist should accompany the surgeon in the operating room. After the surgical specimen has been removed and a split-thickness skin graft has been placed by the surgeon, the immediate surgical prosthesis is inserted and checked for proper fit, stability, and the need for possible adjustment. Modifications to reduce the size of the prosthesis should be performed with a Hall drill and a pineapple-shaped bur. This should be done well away from the surgical field. All residual acrylic shavings should be rinsed from the prosthesis and the operator's gloves with a sterile wet sponge prior to returning to the surgical field. Xeroform gauze or sterile foam rubber is then placed superiorly above the prosthesis to fill the defect void and keep the skin graft in close approximation to the underlying wound. The facial contour with the cheek flap in position should be checked and should not be overextended to avoid having the surgeon close the flap under excessive tension. If indicated for additional retention, the immediate surgical prosthesis is secured with 24-gauge stainless steel ligature wires as previously discussed prior to the closure of the flap.

Although its surgical effectiveness has been questioned, the use of a split-thickness skin graft (STSG) to line the lateral portion of the cheek serves to greatly increase the retention of an obturator prosthesis following full healing of the graft and is considered a prosthetic necessity. The usual thickness of the graft to line a maxillary defect is between 0.012 and 0.015 inch. The graft may be perforated depending on the area of coverage required. As the graft heals, there is a differential rate of contracture across the juncture of the STSG with the intact buccal mucosa. This contracture leads to the development of a lateral scar band, which acts as a "purse string" in maximizing the seal of the prosthesis with the surrounding soft tissue. In addition, the keratinized tissue surface from the STSG is better suited to withstand the trauma that is continually applied to the area because an obturator prosthesis moves during mastication, swallowing, and speech.

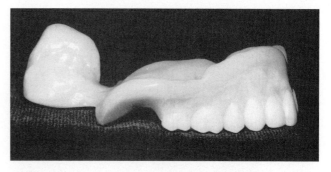

FIGURE 34.5. Definitive maxillary obturator prosthesis for soft palate resection.

The immediate surgical obturator is removed by the maxillofacial prosthodontist 7 to 10 days after surgery in an outpatient setting with mild sedation. The wires are cut and removed. After the prosthesis is removed, the defect is debrided and irrigated. The prosthesis may be modified with soft denture lining material to afford retention without ligature wires, or impressions may be made to fabricate a new obturator to be used during the early healing period.

Definitive Obturator Prosthesis

At 6 to 9 months, after the surgical defect has fully matured and the tissue margins have stabilized, the patient may progress into the fabrication of a *definitive obturator prosthesis* (Fig. 34.5). The progression to the definitive phase of obturator fabrication should be delayed an additional 3 to 6 months for patients who require postsurgical radiation therapy. This prosthesis is fabricated with a durable cast metal base (either gold, titanium, or a chromium-cobalt alloy) that covers the residual palate and has a clasping mechanism on the remaining teeth that provides improved retention. Again, the undercuts within the defect, as well as surrounding soft tissues, are used to provide additional retention and stability for the prosthesis. The defect region is closed with a hollowed acrylic bulb that is polished for comfort and hygiene. The definitive obturator should serve the patient for five years before requiring replacement. A definitive prosthesis should also give support to the facial soft tissues, providing aesthetic benefit, as well as allowing the patient to speak normally and swallow without nasal leakage.

Cleft Palate Prostheses

An obturator is also indicated in certain circumstances for patients with clefts of the palate. During infancy, a presurgical infant orthopedic appliance or *molding plate* is fabricated to guide the alveolar segments together, but it also serves as an obturator to close off the oral and nasal cavities to allow the infant to suckle. This type obturator is therefore often referred to as a *feeding aid appliance* (Chapter 23).

A *speech bulb appliance* may be fabricated for children or adults with primary or secondary velopharyngeal insufficiency or incompetency as a result of unrepaired clefts of the soft palate, central nervous system trauma, tumor surgery, or failed pharyngeal flap surgery (Fig. 34.6). The obturator "bulb" or pharyngeal section is molded by the patient in a thermolabile wax that registers the posterior and lateral pharyngeal wall muscles during movements such as swallowing and speaking to form a well-fitting prosthesis. Nasendoscopy is helpful in objectively assessing the design and fit of a speech bulb appliance.

Adults with unrepaired clefts of the hard and soft palates often are restored with obturator prostheses and elect to remain prosthodontic patients rather than undergo surgical repair of their cleft. A prosthodontic approach to reconstruction of the

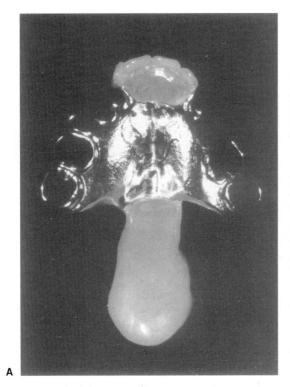
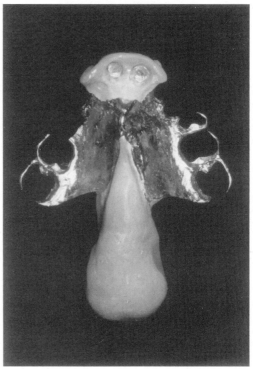

A   B

FIGURE 34.6. Speech bulb obturator prosthesis for an adult with unrepaired cleft palate. **A:** Oral surface, **B:** nasal surface. The cast metal framework is lightweight, and clasps engage undercuts on abutment teeth for retention of the prosthesis. The pink acrylic "bulb" portion is custom molded to the patient's anatomic defect. Prosthetic anterior teeth also replace missing structures.

adult cleft patient with a wide defect offers a predictable non-surgical alternative.

Autogenous Reconstruction and Osseointegration in the Restoration of Maxillary Defects

Patients with maxillary defects that remain free of disease for a period greater than 5 years or whose defect may have been due to trauma may be well served by reconstructive surgical procedures combined with the placement of osseointegrated implants to improve both the functional and aesthetic qualities of a prosthesis. A combined reconstructive and rehabilitative approach should be considered from the time of initial consultation between the prosthodontist and the surgeon prior to resection. Early surgical interventions include the placement of implant fixtures into the remnant of the zygoma on the resected side, as well as into the maxillary tuberosity or edentulous regions of the alveolar process on the unresected side during the ablative surgery. Maxillary defects may also be reconstructed using microvascular free flaps from the iliac crest, fibula, or radial forearm transferred to the defect site (9,10). Osseointegrated fixtures may then be placed during a separate surgical procedure after 4 to 6 months of healing. Direct placement of the fixtures into the grafted bone at the time of reconstructive surgery, although technically feasible, often results in prosthetic compromises due to a lack of precise control of fixture location. The fibula and iliac crest provide the best combination of bone quality, bone quantity, and graft dimensions for implant placement, as well as the potential for soft tissue transfer. In larger defects of the maxilla, the vascularized fibula has a number of characteristics that make it the more suitable alternative. It may be easily osteotomized into the "U" shape of the

maxilla without compromising its periosteal blood supply. It may be harvested with minimal postsurgical morbidity, with or without a soft tissue pedicle.

Although the maxilla may be adequately reconstructed using microvascular tissue transfers taken from the fibula, iliac crest, scapula, or radial forearm, it remains an area of controversy between reconstructive surgeons and restoring prosthodontists as to whether a surgically reconstructed maxillary defect actually provides an improved treatment outcome relative to the prosthetic rehabilitation with an obturator. Yet again, each patient must be thoroughly evaluated prior to surgery by both the surgeon and the prosthodontist before a treatment plan is finalized and implemented.

Functional Restoration of Mandibular Defects

While maxillary resection defects are usually best restored through the use of an obturator prosthesis rather than surgery, mandibular resection defects are best reconstructed using autogenous tissue, with or without any prosthetic dental appliance to restore masticatory function. Mandibulectomy defects may be predictably reconstructed through the placement of a microvascular fibula free flap, iliac crest, or radial forearm graft. The first two of these osseous grafts provide excellent bone quality and quantity to allow the placement of osseointegrated dental implants. These implants then may provide the support for either a fixed dental prosthesis or a removable dental prosthesis that can restore masticatory function as well as improve speech and aesthetics. In addition, microvascular fibula, iliac crest, and radial forearm grafts also allow for soft tissue transfer if indicated.

Mandibular reconstruction with implant placement into the graft may be staged or performed during the same operation after the removal of the tumor. Again, presurgical planning and communication among the surgeon placing the graft, the surgeon placing the implants, and the prosthodontist restoring the dental function will optimize the overall functional and aesthetic results.

References

1. Brånemark PI, Breine U, Adell R, et al. Intraosseous anchorage of dental prostheses. I. Experimental studies. *Scand J Plast Reconstr Surg.* 1969;3:81.
2. Tjellström A, Albrektsson T, Lindström J, et al. The bone-anchored auricular epithesis. *Laryngoscope.* 1981;91:811.
3. Nakayama B, Matsuura H, Ishihara O, et al. Functional reconstruction of a bilateral maxillectomy defect using a fibula osteocutaneous flap with osseointegrated implants. *Plast Recontructr Surg.* 1995;96:1201.
4. Granström G, Bergström K, Tjellström A, et al. A detailed analysis of titanium implants lost in irradiated tissue. *Int J Oral Maxillofac Implants.* 1994;9:653.
5. Conroy BF. The history of facial prostheses. *Clin Plast Surg.* 1979;10:689.
6. Wilkes GH, Wolfaardt JF. Osseointegrated alloplastic versus autogenous ear reconstruction: criteria for treatment selection. *Plast Reconstr Surg.* 1994;93:967.
7. Thorne CH, Brecht LE, Bradley JP, et al. Auricular reconstruction: indications for autogenous and prosthetic techniques. *Plast Reconstr Surg.* 2001;107:1241.
8. Mounsey RA, Boyd JB. Mandibular reconstruction with osseointegrated implants into free vascularized radius. *Plast Recontructr Surg.* 1994;94:457.
9. Granström G. Rehabilitation of irradiated cancer patients with tissue-integrated prostheses: adjunctive use of hyperbaric oxygen to improve osseointegration. *J Facial Stomato Prosthet.* 1996;2:1.
10. Riediger D. Restoration of masticatory function by microsurgically revascularized iliac crest bone grafts using enosseous implants. *Plast Recontructr Surg.* 1988;81:861.

CHAPTER 35 ■ RECONSTRUCTION OF THE SCALP, CALVARIUM, AND FOREHEAD

LOK HUEI YAP AND HOWARD N. LANGSTEIN

There are many causes of scalp and forehead defects, including trauma, burns, resection of benign or malignant lesions, poor wound healing from previous surgery, and congenital abnormalities. As a general rule, reconstruction of scalp and forehead defects is accomplished by the simplest means possible. At the same time, the size and depth of the defect, as well as previous radiation therapy or surgery, dictates the most appropriate technique, which may require a complicated procedure.

ANATOMY

Because the scalp and forehead are anatomically similar, reconstructive principles for defects in these areas are discussed together in this chapter, along with reconstruction of the underlying calvarium. From an anatomic point of view, the scalp and forehead can be considered as a single unit, except that the scalp is usually hair bearing and contains a galeal layer, whereas the forehead has the frontalis muscle. Both the forehead and scalp have five distinct anatomic layers: skin, subcutaneous connective tissue, galea or muscle, loose areolar tissue, and pericranium (Fig. 35.1) (1).

The skin of the scalp is the thickest skin on the body, ranging between 3 and 8 mm. It is connected to the galea aponeurotica via numerous vertical septae that minimize shearing of the skin on the skull. Beneath the skin lies the subcutaneous tissue layer, which contains dense connective and fatty tissue and hair follicles, along with veins, arteries, lymphatics, and sensory nerves of the scalp. **Transection of vessels in the scalp can lead to exsanguination because of vascular density, high blood flow, and tendency for the cut ends of vessels to retract into the fat.**

The galea aponeurotica is part of a broad fibromuscular layer that envelops the forehead and scalp and serves as the central tendinous confluence of the occipitalis muscle posteriorly and the frontalis muscle anteriorly. The occipitalis and frontalis muscles are thin, quadrilateral muscles, each consisting of two bellies joined in the midline by extensions of the galea. The occipitalis muscle arises from the lateral two thirds of the superior nuchal line of the occipital bone and from the mastoid part of the temporal bone. The frontalis muscle has no bony attachments. Medially, its fibers are continuous with those of the procerus muscles. The frontalis muscle fibers join the galea aponeurotica in the upper forehead. The galea aponeurotica, which covers the upper part of the cranium, is continuous with the temporoparietal fascia (superficial temporal fascia). The galea is also contiguous with the subcutaneous musculoaponeurotic system (SMAS) of the face (see Chapter 49).

Beneath the galea lies the loose areolar layer, also known as the subaponeurotic layer, subgaleal fascia, or innominate fascia, which is a relatively avascular plane. This layer enables the layers above it (skin, subcutaneous connective tissue, and galea) to slide as a unit over the cranium. As such, this layer is easily dissected and is often the plane of cleavage in avulsion or "scalping" injuries.

The pericranium is the periosteum of the calvarium and is distinctly separate from the innominate fascia above it. Laterally, at the superior temporal line, the pericranium is continuous with the deep temporal fascia (temporalis muscle fascia). More inferiorly, the deep temporal fascia divides into two layers, deep and superficial, which envelop the superficial temporal fat pad and insert into the superficial and deep aspects of the zygomatic arch, respectively (Fig. 35.2) (2).

Blood Supply

The scalp is supplied by paired arteries that form rich interconnections within the subcutaneous layer (Fig. 35.3). From anterior to posterior, these are the supratrochlear arteries, the supraorbital arteries, the superficial temporal arteries, the posterior auricular arteries, and the occipital arteries. **The superficial temporal and occipital arteries are considered the principal blood supply to the scalp, but the entire scalp will survive in most cases as long as any one of these vessels is preserved, as evidenced by complete scalp survival after replantation of only one artery and vein.**

The blood supply to the anterior scalp and forehead is chiefly from the supratrochlear and supraorbital arteries, which enter the forehead vertically at the level of the supraorbital rim. Above the brow, the vessels become superficial, piercing the frontalis muscle, and ultimately lie in the superficial layer where they anastomose with anterior branches of the superficial temporal arteries and supply blood to the anterior and anterolateral scalp.

The superficial temporal arteries are the largest of the scalp vessels and supply the skin, subcutaneous tissue, and superficial temporal fascia of the lateral scalp with connections to the galea of the central scalp. These arteries are among the terminal branches of the external carotid arteries. The superficial temporal arteries course through the superficial lobes of the parotid glands, becoming superficial and palpable above the zygomatic arch. The superficial temporal arteries lie within the superficial temporal fascia above the zygomatic arch divide into anterior and posterior branches. These branches anastomose liberally with anterior and posterior blood supplies of the scalp. The anterior arterial branch usually crosses the most anterior temporal branch of the facial nerve above the lateral brow, an important anatomic landmark for finding either the nerve or the vessel. The temporalis muscle is supplied separately by the deep temporal vessels. Above the temporal line, vascular connections between the galea and pericranium allow perfusion of portions of the outer cortex of the calvarium based on the superficial temporal arteries (3).

The occipital arteries are the dominant blood supply to the posterior scalp. These arteries run from the external carotid

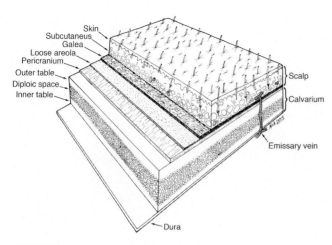

FIGURE 35.1. Layers of the forehead and scalp.

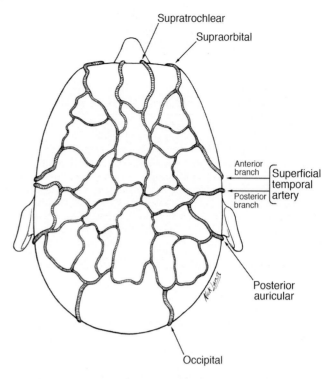

FIGURE 35.3. Blood supply to the scalp and forehead.

arteries along the vertebral muscles and join the scalp through the cranial attachments of the trapezius muscle or in the space between the trapezius and sternocleidomastoid muscles. These arteries are usually found within 2 cm of the midline at the nuchal line and usually divide into medial and lateral branches above this location.

The region of the mastoid is supplied by the posterior auricular arteries, which are smaller than the other regional arteries. They are sufficient for some local flaps in this vicinity but not robust enough to support the entire scalp.

The scalp is drained externally by veins that accompany the named arteries. Venous blood also flows internally through the diploë of the cranium to the dural sinuses via emissary veins. These emissary veins do not have valves, and superficial infections of the scalp, especially in the loose areolar layer, can spread intracranially via these veins (3). The supratrochlear vein and supraorbital vein drain the anterior region of the scalp. The superficial temporal vein descends in front of the auricle and enters the parotid gland. It then joins the maxillary vein to form the retromandibular vein. The anterior division of the retromandibular vein unites with the facial vein to form the common facial vein, which drains into the internal jugular vein. The posterior auricular vein joins the posterior division

of the retromandibular vein to form the external jugular vein. The occipital vein terminates in the suboccipital venous plexus, which lies beneath the floor of the upper part of the posterior triangle.

The scalp lymphatics are located principally in the subdermal and subcutaneous levels. There are no lymph nodes in the scalp region and hence no barriers to lymphatic flow. Lymph from the scalp drains freely toward the parotid, preauricular and postauricular nodes, upper cervical nodes, and occipital nodes. Knowledge of these drainage patterns is important when treating melanoma of the scalp.

Nerve Supply

The muscles of the forehead are innervated by the frontal (otherwise known as temporal) branches of the facial nerve, which cross the midportion of the zygomatic arch. As many as five separate branches course in the loose areolar plane below the SMAS, cross the zygoma, and innervate to join the undersurface of the frontalis muscle via its deep surface (Fig. 35.2). Because of this arrangement, the frontal branches are at risk during dissection below the SMAS and superficial to the zygoma if surgical approach to the zygomatic arch is required.

It is safest to approach the zygoma from within the superficial temporal fat pad by dissecting deep to the superficial leaf of the deep temporal fascia. Once the arch is reached, subperiosteal dissection onto the zygoma effectively avoids the frontal branches.

The temporalis muscles are supplied by motor branches from the third division of the trigeminal nerve.

The sensory nerve supply to the anterior scalp is from the ophthalmic division of the trigeminal nerve. The supratrochlear and supraorbital nerves arise from this branch and leave the skull through the supraorbital foramina or grooves at the middle of the supraorbital rim.

The temporal scalp is supplied by the maxillary division of the trigeminal nerve (zygomaticotemporal nerve) and the

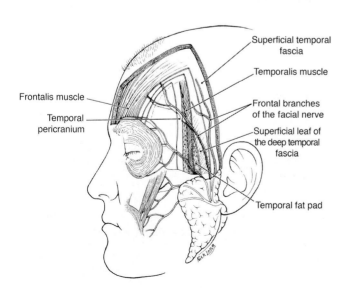

FIGURE 35.2. Anatomic relationships in the temporal region.

preauricular scalp by the mandibular division (auriculotemporal nerves). The postauricular scalp is supplied by dorsal rami of the cervical spinal nerves (greater occipital nerve and third occipital nerve).

SCALP RECONSTRUCTION

Scalp Defects <3 cm

Primary closure is possible for scalp defects up to 3 cm in size. The scalp has a rich vascular supply, which means that some degree of tension is acceptable, but, at the same time, the galea is relatively inelastic and resists closure. Galeal scoring parallel to the axis of the defect can provide some relief of tension and allow wounds of borderline size to be closed (1). Incisions are made 1 to 2 cm apart in the galea and parallel to supplying vessels, although it is practically impossible to completely avoid all subgaleal vessels. One can expect a few millimeters of release for each galeal incision score line, sometimes adding up to 1 cm or more (Fig. 35.4). Undermining of surrounding tissues can also be used to aid closure. **However, in general, neither undermining nor scoring yields a bounty of tissue laxity.**

Small scalp defects or lacerations can and should be closed primarily; larger ones will require scalp flaps, skin grafting, or transfer of distant tissue. Traumatic scalp lacerations are irrigated and the devitalized edges sharply debrided before closure. In situations where primary closure results in excessive tension even after undermining and galeal release, two or more curvilinear incisions can be made in a pinwheel pattern. These small adjacent scalp flaps can facilitate closure, but must be designed so that their donor regions can be closed as well.

The scalp contains tissues that can be used in the closure. The layers of the scalp can be separated from one another, liberating sheets of tissues that can facilitate reconstruction. Pericranial and galeal flaps are useful in some situations. The pericranial flap includes the periosteum of the skull along with the overlying loose areolar innominate fascia (Fig. 35.5). This flap should be based on one of the named scalp vessels or from their general vicinity. Perfusion across the midline, often meager, can be enhanced by including the galea with the flap. This galeal–pericranial flap is a much more robust parcel of tissue that can be separated from the neighboring scalp, placed over bare skull, and covered with a skin graft (1,4). Full-thickness scalp flaps, in

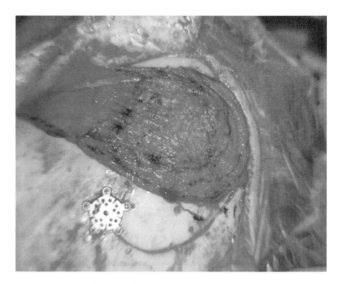

FIGURE 35.5. Closure of a cerebrospinal fluid leak following craniotomy for tumor ablation.

general, provide more reliable coverage of such exposed calvarial defects, but occasionally the pericranial and galeal flaps can be handy adjuncts to reconstruction (Fig. 35.6).

In some instances, healing by secondary intention leads to acceptable outcomes. This principle is used in forehead flap donor closure (see below) and can be employed in the scalp as well, if alopecia is acceptable.

Skin grafts can be used to resurface all locations of the scalp and forehead, provided the periosteum is left intact, but the aesthetic results can be suboptimal because of alopecia or poor color match. One possible exception to this suboptimal outcome is when the aesthetic unit of the full forehead is replaced with a full-thickness graft. Additionally, split-thickness or full-thickness graft resurfacing of non–hair-bearing scalp can sometimes lead to a reasonable appearance. If periosteum is not present, skin grafting can still be performed, provided the calvarial layer is prepared by burring, curettage, or removal of the outer table (Fig. 35.7). Distinct bleeding from the bony surface is required for skin graft take. A pericranial or galeal flap from the remaining scalp placed over the denuded skull, with a skin graft replacing it, improves the chance of "take." A subatmospheric pressure dressing system (vacuum-assisted closure, or VAC), can also be used on exposed calvarial defects to encourage "granulation" and improve the chances of skin graft take. This approach is gaining popularity in preparing many kinds of scalp wounds for grafting, even facilitating closure of some wounds without the need for a graft. Some surgeons advocate performing the skin grafting in a single stage, placing the VAC over the graft, with complete skin graft take reported in a small series (5). If the repaired region of the scalp will receive radiation therapy, a skin graft, split- or full-thickness, might not provide durable coverage and may either break down later or not survive at all. A scalp flap or free tissue transfer may be a better choice. Alternatively, tissue expansion and excision of the previously placed skin graft can be performed at a later date.

Scalp Defects of 3 to 6 cm

Most scalp defects of 3 to 6 cm are amenable to closure with full-thickness scalp rotation-advancement flaps. One should attempt to design such a flap so that the primary and secondary defect can be closed primarily.

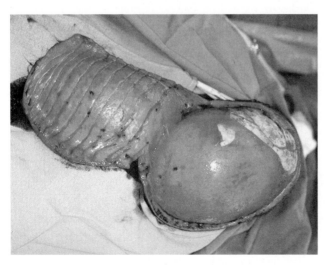

FIGURE 35.4. Scoring of the galea of a scalp flap.

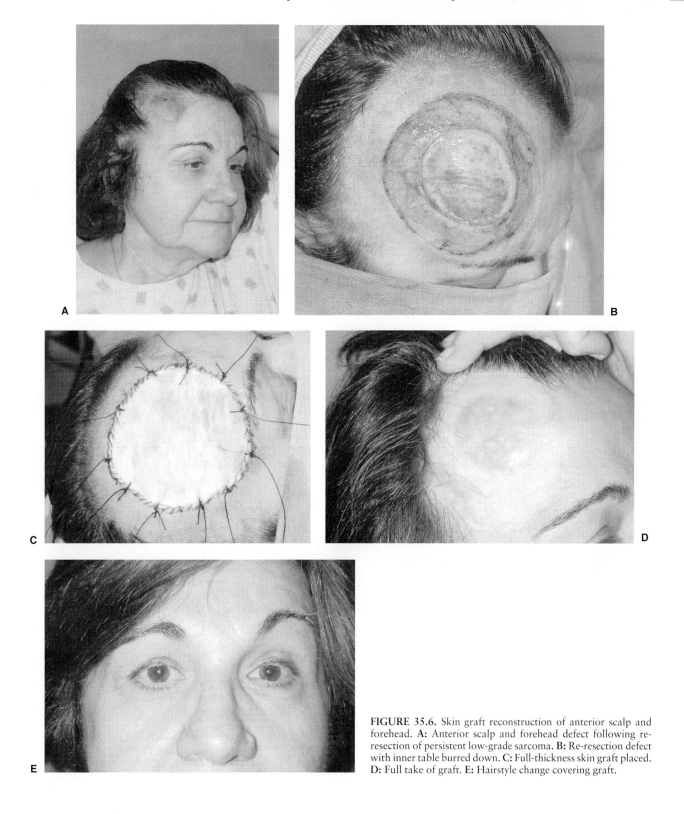

FIGURE 35.6. Skin graft reconstruction of anterior scalp and forehead. **A:** Anterior scalp and forehead defect following re-resection of persistent low-grade sarcoma. **B:** Re-resection defect with inner table burred down. **C:** Full-thickness skin graft placed. **D:** Full take of graft. **E:** Hairstyle change covering graft.

The scalp has rich anastomotic connections between major supplying vessels. Because of these extensive interconnections, a single major vessel, such as the superficial temporal artery, is capable of supplying the entire scalp, and long axial flaps can be harvested for reconstruction. Because scalp flaps almost always need to be rotated and advanced, a long, curvilinear incision (Fig. 35.8) that incorporates at least one named vessel allows for maximal excursion. Scalp flaps should be raised below the galea. One should use as wide-based a flap as possible to fa-

cilitate maximal rotation and advancement. The length of the rotation flap should exceed five times the diameter of the defects to prevent excessive tension. When incising hair-bearing scalp, an attempt is made to bevel the cut parallel to the hair shaft direction to avoid follicular damage and incisional alopecia. Once the flap is cut, rotation and advancement are facilitated by a combination of galeal scorings and back cutting, in that order. Usually, a good deal of the scalp must be undermined in order to close the donor site. The spherical shape of the

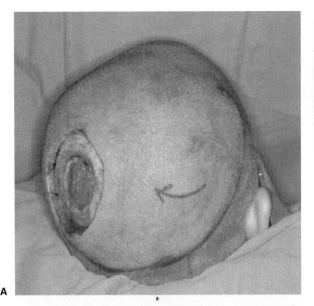

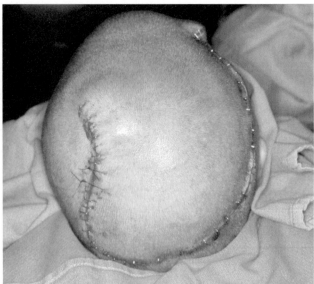

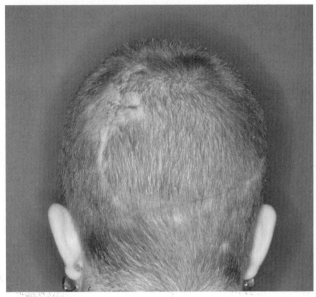

FIGURE 35.7. Scalp flap reconstruction for defect following melanoma resection. **A:** Postresection defect extending down to inner table. **B:** Both primary and secondary defects closed primarily. **C:** Early postoperative result showing complete healing.

scalp as a globe means that the flap must advance more than is generally anticipated, and often a substantial back cut is required to provide the necessary movement of the flap (1,6).

Scalp Defects of 6 to 9 cm

For defects ranging from 6 to 9 cm, one large scalp flap based on a major pedicle can be used, but the secondary defect may require skin grafting. For this reason, it is important to preserve the pericranium in the donor defect. A "bucket-handle" flap, based on both superficial temporal vessels, can be used to resurface anterior scalp defects, and the requisite skin graft can be placed in the vertex, which can be covered by hair. Alternatively, a tissue expander is placed in the donor region. Primary closure of the donor site becomes possible once the flap is advanced and the expander removed (Fig. 35.9). The use of tissue expansion reduces the need for skin grafting. This principle is used to prepare the scalp of conjoined twins for separation. Tissue expansion of hair-bearing scalp was formerly used in the treatment of bald areas but has been largely replaced with modern hair transplantation techniques. In general, one

or more expanders is inserted through remote incision, oriented radially to the defect. It is important to anticipate where the future incisions for the flap advancement will be placed prior to expander insertion. The amount of expansion achieved can be loosely estimated by the difference in distances between the base diameter and the over-the-top distance. **Overexpansion by up to 50%, however, is necessary because the flaps do not yield the theoretical tissue gain.** Appropriate back-cuts are usually required to advance the expanded tissue. The periprosthetic capsule is incised to allow maximal flap movement (see Chapter 10).

The use of multiple (three or four) flaps for scalp reconstruction, popularized by Orticochea, is of historical interest because of tissue expansion (7). This technique involved the elevation of the remaining scalp, with one posterior flap based on the occipital or posterior auricular vessels and two anterior flaps based on the superficial temporal vessels. The posterior flap was based on the side opposite the defect and recruited excess tissue found in the nape of the neck region. These flaps were widely elevated and interdigitated, covering the defect but often leaving an anterior secondary defect that required grafting when the primary defect was posterior.

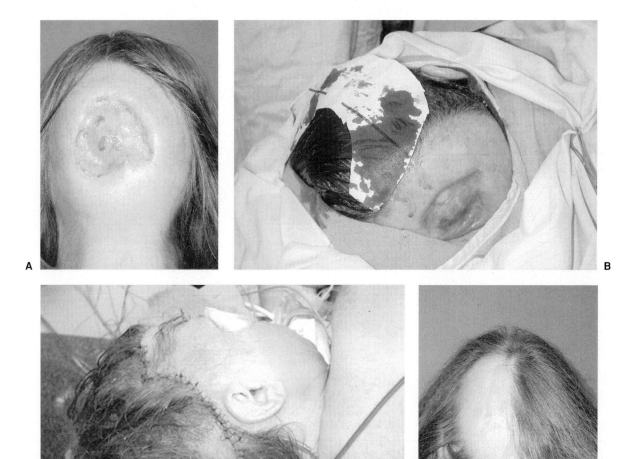

FIGURE 35.8. Tissue expansion and scalp flap reconstruction for unstable skin graft on posterior skull. **A:** Unstable skin graft following dermatofibrosarcoma protuberans excision and radiation therapy. **B:** Placement of large crescent tissue expander at anticipated donor region. **C:** Rotation of expanded scalp allowed coverage of exposed skull. **D:** Postoperative result showing stable wound but persistent alopecia from irradiation.

Conversely, when the defect was anterior, one of the anterior flaps was used to cover the primary defect. The other flaps were pieced together to close secondary and tertiary defects. Skin grafts were used in other locations where the flaps were under tension.

Local flaps or skin grafting may not be possible when prior radiation therapy has been given. Usually reserved for larger defects, free tissue transfers should be considered when such prior therapy makes local flaps unreliable. Alternatively, the scalp flaps can be made more reliable by delaying them, but this involves one or more procedures, which may not be appropriate for every patient.

Scalp Defects >9 cm

Free tissue transfer offers a one-step solution for resurfacing large scalp defects and produces surprisingly good results, especially in patients with preexisting alopecia (1,8). Because the area to be covered usually exceeds the size of any myocuta-neous flap that can be harvested with primary closure of the donor site, muscle-only free flaps along with nonmeshed split-thickness skin grafts are used, and lead to very acceptable outcomes. The superficial temporal vessels are frequently available as recipient vessels, although the vein is occasionally inadequate or absent, in which case interpositional vein grafting to the neck is necessary. Alternatively, the transferred muscle's pedicle can be lengthened by an intramuscular dissection, leaving portions of remaining muscle in the preauricular region to reach the neck without vein grafts. This skin-grafted muscle may be secondarily thinned, but this often is not necessary because of significant spontaneous atrophy.

Traditionally, a latissimus dorsi muscle flap has been used to cover large defects of the scalp because of its consistent vascular pedicle and its large muscle (Fig. 35.10). A rectus abdominis muscle flap, covered with a skin graft, is also useful for this purpose. The serratus anterior muscle free flap has a longer pedicle that can reach the neck vessels without the need for vein grafts, and is a good choice for smaller defects. Fasciocutaneous flaps, such as the anterolateral thigh, can also be used, but if

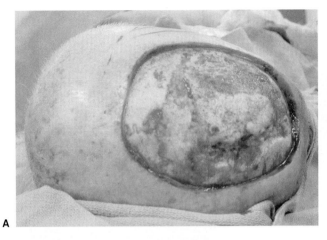

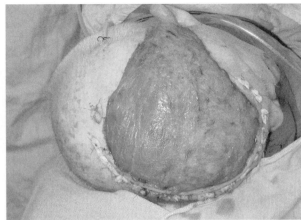

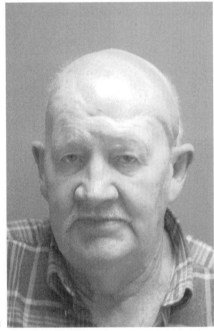

FIGURE 35.9. Free latissimus dorsi flap reconstruction of scalp defect. **A:** Large scalp defect following angiosarcoma resection, radiation therapy, and unsuccessful skin graft placement. **B:** Latissimus dorsi free flap placed on defect with anastomoses to superficial temporal vessels. **C:** Postoperative result with satisfactory contour.

their donor sites are to be closed primarily, these flaps will not cover substantial defects. A large omental flap can be used, covered with a skin graft, but this flap often becomes thin over time and may not be suitable for long-term durable coverage.

The superficial temporal vessels can serve as recipients for free tissue transfer in many cases. These vessels are easily found through a preauricular incision with elevation of the skin flap to the location of the palpable pulse of the artery. The depth of these vessels decreases as the incision advances superiorly, such that they are quite superficial in the temporal region and lie within the parenchyma of the parotid gland more inferiorly. The vein is occasionally located at a distance from the artery or may not be detectable at all. Occasionally, the occipital vessels can be used as recipient vessels.

Free tissue transfer works very well for scalp defects, but may not be appropriate for all clinical situations. Subtotal scalp flaps have been used successfully for defects approaching 50% of the surface area of the scalp in these circumstances. Some lower scalp defects can also be reconstructed with regional pedicled flaps such as the trapezius myocutaneous flap or the latissimus dorsi myocutaneous flap (9). Preliminary delay of these flaps should be considered to enhance vascularity and maximize flap success.

FOREHEAD RECONSTRUCTION

Soft-Tissue Defects

Small defects of the forehead can be closed primarily, but because the forehead is more visible than much of the scalp, incision placement is critical for an aesthetic result. Although there are preferred locations to place incisions in the forehead, there really are no anatomic subunits per se to preserve. Incisions oriented transversely and placed along the eyebrows or anterior hairline lead to the best results. Distortion of the brows and hairline should be avoided when possible, and in some cases, complete replacement of the entire forehead unit with a full-thickness skin graft may yield a better result than gross eyebrow malposition following primary closure.

If primary closure is not possible or desired, local flaps should be used for defects of up to 40% (Fig. 35.10). A rotation-advancement flap can be designed based on the supratrochlear and supraorbital vessels, with the superior incision skirting the anterior hairline. Another approach is to advance the remaining forehead in a V-to-Y fashion to close the defect, basing the flap on or both supraorbital and supratrochlear vessels. An "H" flap can be also used by creating parallel

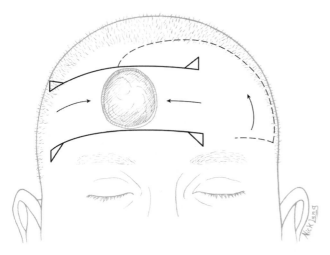

FIGURE 35.10. Reconstructive choices for forehead defects with local flaps. Solid lines, "H" flap advancement; dashed lines, rotation advancement.

transverse incisions from the superior and inferior aspects of the defect and advancing the tissues medially. The Burrow triangles may need to be resected if redundancy is excessive. Sometimes a rotation-advancement flap oriented obliquely and stair-stepped along the hairline is successful. Lateral defects near the eyebrows can be addressed with superficial temporal artery-based hair-bearing flaps. The anterior hairline can be preserved, at least partly, by transfers of hair-bearing scalp flaps, but recognize that any postoperative radiation therapy will cause alopecia and ruin the effect . Near or total forehead defects can also be resurfaced with free radial forearm or groin flaps.

Central defects are harder to close with forehead tissue, and consideration should be given to leaving such a defect to heal secondarily, as one would the donor site of a paramedian forehead flap. Central defects can be closed vertically, but the eyebrows may be positioned too close to each other. Tissue expansion can also be used to recruit enough tissue to replace a poorly healed scar or a temporary skin graft. In some instances, tissue expansion of adjacent forehead provides adequate coverage and is appropriate for removal of large congenital nevi or burn scars in this location.

Sometimes, a forehead defect should be considered as just a specialized scalp defect, and large scalp rotation flaps can be used to rotate large parcels of hair-bearing and non–hair-bearing scalp to resurface the defect. Care must be taken to preserve the hairline when moving the scalp and forehead as one unit. Hairstyle changes can camouflage some hairline aberrations. Lateral forehead defects can sometimes be reconstructed by elevating cheek skin upward along with the sideburn area, recruiting excess facial tissue to fill in temporal deficiencies. An extended paramedian flap that includes immediate subjacent scalp can resurface lateral and temporal defects.

SKULL BASE RECONSTRUCTION

The goals of skull base reconstruction include separation of intracranial contents from the external environment and, for anterior defects, from nasal secretions (see Chapter 42) (10).

The pericranial or pericranial–galeal flap is first harvested during a craniotomy and is placed over the exposed dura or dural repair. All remnants of sinus mucosa are ablated to reduce the incidence of late mucocele. The galeal flap may be better vascularized than the pericranial flap but its use leaves a visi-

ble depression. If additional dead space exists, the temporalis muscle, which can comfortably reach the anterior orbital roof and apex, is used.

Free tissue transfers have revolutionized the repair of skull base defects, especially if the region has been or will be irradiated. Fasciocutaneous flaps, such as the free radial forearm flap, have great utility in and around the orbit, because the long pedicle can often obviate vein grafting. Free muscle flaps with skin grafts on the exposed portions are also useful for delivering bulky soft tissue and well-vascularized tissue to support a dural reconstruction. Muscle is particularly helpful in this regard, because even with a "watertight" closure of the dura, cerebrospinal fluid may leak. In cases where an established cerebrospinal fluid leak is identified, the muscle of the flap may assist in spontaneous closure of the leak over time.

The bone of the skull base rarely needs to be replaced, even in the orbital roof, where "pulsatile" enophthalmos rapidly resolves absence of bony repair.

CALVARIAL RECONSTRUCTION

The two questions that must be answered regarding calvarial reconstruction are (a) should it be done and (b) if it should be done, what material should be used. The goals of reconstructing defects of the calvarium include protection of the underlying contents and restoration of the overlying contour. These can be accomplished with a variety of materials, including nonvascularized autogenous bone grafts (calvarial, split rib, or iliac crest), vascularized autogenous bone grafts, and alloplastic materials (e.g., methylmethacrylate, calcium phosphate cements, and titanium). Many factors influence whether to perform a cranioplasty, such as the size of the defect, cleanliness of the wound, age of the patient, and prognosis.

If calvarial reconstruction is contemplated, autogenous bone is the most reliable material especially when craniofacial growth is anticipated or bone is also advantageous if there is any contamination of the wound. Alloplastic cranioplasty has its place, however, especially if the defects are very large.

Of autogenous materials, iliac crest bone grafts, split-rib grafts, and calvarial bone grafts, can be used. Most commonly, these grafts are used as nonvascularized free grafts, but vascularized grafts are also available. Split-rib grafts can be harvested via an anterolateral incision centered over the seventh rib. Subperiosteal elevation of the bone may allow for bone regrowth of the rib donor site in smaller children. It is advisable to minimize rib harvest to three ribs per side, choosing alternate ribs in order to minimize the contour deformity of the donor site. The ribs are then split longitudinally with an osteotome, curved with a rib bender, tightly packed into the defect, and immobilized by wire, suture, or plate fixation. Bone graft incorporation is generally successful with split-rib grafts, but the final result is a washboard contour, making it less suitable for defects anterior to the hairline.

Calvarial bone grafts allow for better contouring and can be harvested from the same operative field. These grafts are ideally harvested as full-thickness bone and split ex vivo. In situ harvest with a curved osteotome is adequate for small grafts. The skull is thickest in the parietal region, just posterior to the coronal suture, and graft harvest from this region minimizes the risk of violating the inner table or dura.

Vascularized versions of calvarial bone and rib grafts exist and are usually chosen in the setting of an irradiated recipient bed or the presence of infection. A vascularized calvarial bone graft can be transferred based on the superficial temporal vessels, maintaining attachment to the superficial temporal fascia and pericranium (3). For rib grafts to be vascularized, microsurgical anastomoses need to be performed. In this situation, a few slips of serratus anterior muscle are harvested with one or more ribs as a composite free flap in order to deliver bone that can heal more promptly without reliance on vascular ingrowth from a compromised wound bed. Bone chips, paste, or other bone substitutes can be inserted in the small gaps that may remain after reconstruction with either rib or calvarial bone. Rib grafts can also be vascularized by wrapping them with a soft-tissue free flap such as a rectus abdominis flap.

A variety of alloplastic materials have been used for cranioplasties, ranging from metal alloys to biocompatible acrylics and, more recently, "smart" moldable pastes. Metals such as vitallium (cobalt-chromium alloy), titanium, and stainless steel have the advantage of being easy to apply but are prone to infection, are radiopaque, and conduct heat and cold. Polymethylmethacrylate (PMMA), a quick-setting polymer, has been widely used for restoring bony defects because it is easy to apply, is relatively inexpensive, and has a long record of biocompatibility. However, PMMA has a complication rate as high as 23% in the pediatric population and can reach temperatures as high as 100°C (212°F) as it sets up (11). Calcium phosphate cements in conjunction with titanium mesh have also been used for cranioplasty. Fast-setting calcium phosphate cements with favorable handling properties are gaining popularity as cranioplasty material because during curing these materials are less exothermic than similar products, and some of the formulations can harden under wet conditions. The choice of cranioplasty material, however, is ultimately based on the surgeon's preference, material handling characteristics, type and size of the defect, age of the patient, cleanliness of the wound, and reliability of the overlying scalp tissue (see Chapter 7).

References

1. Hoffman JF. Management of scalp defects. *Otolaryngol Clin North Am.* 2001;34(3):571–582.
2. Zide BM, Jelks GW. *Surgical Anatomy of the Orbit.* New York: Raven Press; 1985:13–20.
3. McCarthy JG, Zide BM. The spectrum of calvarial bone grafting: introduction of the vascularized calvarial bone flap. *Plast Reconstr Surg.* 1984;74(1):10–18.
4. Horowitz JH, et al. Galeal-pericranial flaps in head and neck reconstruction. Anatomy and application. *Am J Surg.* 1984;148(4):489–497.
5. Molnar JA, et al. Single-stage approach to skin grafting the exposed skull. *Plast Reconstr Surg.* 2000;105(1):174–177.
6. Worthen EF. Transposition and rotation scalp flaps and rotation forehead flap. In: Strauch B, Vasconez LO, H.-F.E. J., eds. *Grabb's Encyclopedia of Flaps.* Boston: Little Brown and Company; 1990.
7. Orticochea M. New three-flap reconstruction technique. *Br J Plast Surg.* 1971;24(2):184–188.
8. Hussussian CJ, Reece GP, W. U.S.L.M.O.U.S.A. Division of Plastic Surgery. Microsurgical scalp reconstruction in the patient with cancer. *Plast Reconstr Surg.* 2002;109(6):1828–1834.
9. Mustoe TA, Corral CJ, N.U.M.S.U.S.A. Department of Surgery. Soft tissue reconstructive choices for craniofacial reconstruction. *Clin Plast Surg.* 1995;22(3):543–554.
10. Langstein HN, et al. Coverage of skull base defects. *Clin Plast Surg.* 2001;28(2):375–387, x.
11. Taggard DA, et al. Successful use of rib grafts for cranioplasty in children. *Pediatr Neurosurg.* 2001;34(3):149–155.

CHAPTER 36 ■ RECONSTRUCTION OF THE LIPS

SEAN BOUTROS

The lips are the primary aesthetic feature of the lower central face, with functional requirements that include speech, containing oral contents, and kissing. A hallmark of the lips is their mobility, which is critical for natural appearance and function. Reconstruction of lip defects is simple in that reconstruction, in most cases, is feasible, but complex in that a natural-appearing, dynamic reconstruction is often elusive.

ANATOMY

The lip consists of four basic components: the skin and subcutaneous tissue, the muscle, the mucosa, and the vermilion. Each of these structures has unique characteristics that must be considered when planning the reconstruction.

The skin of the lips is typical of facial skin. It is hair bearing with the hair being mostly vellus in women and children, with a downward direction of growth. The skin is of intermediate thickness for facial skin and is rich in sebaceous and sweat glands. The skin thickness and the number of appendages decrease with age. Deep to the skin is a significant amount of subcutaneous fat that makes up the bulk of lip thickness (Fig. 36.1).

The external landmarks of the lips are the philtral columns and the Cupid's bow. The philtral columns are musculocutaneous ridges that diverge slightly in their course from the base of the columella to the vermilion border. The philtral columns merge with the white roll, another ridge formed by the orbicularis muscle. The orbicularis fibers form the philtral dimple in the central lip between the paired philtral columns. There is a low point between the two peaks of the Cupid's bow, which is referred to as the depth of the Cupid's bow (Fig. 36.2).

The primary muscles of the lip are the orbicularis oris muscles. They are paired, mostly horizontally oriented muscles that originate just lateral to the commissure at the modiolus. The modiolus is a crossroads of several other facial muscles, including the levator anguli oris, the risorius, and the depressor anguli oris. The two orbicularis oris muscles join in the midline of the lower lip in a raphe. In the upper lip, it crosses the midline and inserts into the opposite philtral column. The orbicularis also sends fibers to the skin at the base of the ala, nasal sill, and septum, and is the most important muscle for oral competence. It also provides for pouting and eversion of the lip, and some elevation of the lower lip. The buccal branches of the facial nerve innervate the orbicularis muscles.

The second most important, and least understood, lip muscles are the paired mentalis muscles. The mentalis muscles are the main elevators of the lower lip, and this elevation is required for lower-lip positioning and lip competence. These muscles are inaccurately depicted in most anatomy texts, where they are shown as small, striplike muscles. **In fact, they are large trapezoidal/pyramidal-shaped muscles that originate from the mandible just below the attached gingiva and insert horizon-** **tally and inferiorly into the chin pad below the labiomental fold.** The superior extent of the muscles defines the labiomental fold. They travel horizontally and inferiorly from the mandible to the skin of the chin. Contraction of the mentalis muscles elevates the lower lip in order to strongly coapt the upper and lower lip or to push contents out of the gingivobuccal sulcus. The marginal mandibular branch of the facial nerve innervates the mentalis muscles.

The depressors of the lip include the depressor anguli oris (also called the triangularis), the depressor labii inferioris, and, to some degree, the platysma. The marginal mandibular branch of the facial nerve innervates these muscles, with the exception of the platysma that is innervated by cervical branches. The elevators of the upper lip include the levator anguli oris, the zygomaticus major and minor, and the levator labii superioris. They elevate the commissure, the lateral aspect, and the central body of the upper lip respectively. The zygomatic and buccal branches of the facial nerve innervate theses lip elevators.

The inside of the lip is lined by mucosa, which is nonkeratinized epithelium that is rich in minor salivary glands. **The mucosa is distinct from vermilion in its color and appearance.** Vermilion, on the other hand, is the visible portion of the lip inside the white roll. It is duller than mucosa in its appearance. It has a unique light reflection and is nearly impossible to duplicate. The wet–dry line is the junction of the wet vermilion and the dry vermilion. Close observation will show that the vermilion tissue extends for a few millimeters beyond where the lips meet in natural mouth closure. It is in these few millimeters that the vermilion transitions to mucosa.

The sensory innervation of the lip is provided by the mental and infraorbital nerves. The mental nerve is the terminal branch of the inferior alveolar nerve which is, in turn, a branch of the mandibular division of the trigeminal nerve (V3). The mental nerve exits the mandible between the first and second premolars. It divides into several branches, some of which can be seen intraorally. The upper lip receives its sensibility from the inferior orbital nerve, which is a branch of the maxillary division of the trigeminal nerve (V2). It exits the skull through the foramen rotundum, passes through the inferior orbital fissure and travels along the orbital floor before diving into the maxillary sinus and emerging from the bone through the infraorbital foramen. It provides sensation to the upper lip, ala, and nasal sidewall.

These two distinct nerves allow for local anesthesia to be easily and quickly established for lip procedures. Low volumes of solution, placed accurately, will give complete anesthesia. Intraoral injections have the advantage of being less painful, and simpler to achieve complete blockade as they are based on bony landmarks (teeth) and the entire path of the needle parallels the bone. The mental nerve is injected by placement of the needle at the depth of the gingivobuccal sulcus in line with the canine. The needle is advanced for 1 cm and a depot of 1 to

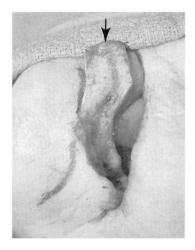

FIGURE 36.1. Cross-section of the lip from the vermilion to the labiomental fold. Note the labial artery (arrow) just below the junction of the wet and dry vermilion and the significant amount of subcutaneous tissue making the bulk of the lip.

2 mL of lidocaine is injected. If sharp pain or paraesthesia is felt, the needle is backed out a few millimeters and the remaining volume deposited. The infraorbital nerve is also injected at the height of the gingivobuccal sulcus in line with the canine. The needle is advanced approximately 2 cm along the bone directed towards the lateral commissure of the eye. Again, a depot of 1 to 2 mL of lidocaine is injected, with care to avoid injection if a sharp pain or paraesthesia is felt.

The vascular supply of the lips is both significant and redundant. The main arterial supply is from the labial arteries, which are branches from the facial artery and form a 360-degree loop, allowing for various flap designs. The arteries lie just deep to the orbicularis muscle and can be found in cross section approximately at the wet–dry line (Fig. 36.1). They provide numerous perforators through the orbicularis muscle to the overlying skin. Although it is advised that flaps in the area contain the labial artery, the blood supply is so rich in this region that many authors have described survival of local flaps based only on a segment of mucosa. The venous drainage of the lips does not follow the arterial supply. A dense venous network coalesces in the area of the major names arteries to form the larger veins.

The lymphatic drainage of the lips is important for oncologic considerations. The upper lip drains primarily to the submandibular nodes with some drainage from the commissure to

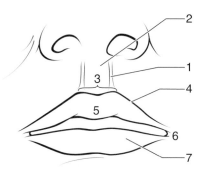

FIGURE 36.2. Topographic anatomy of the lips. *1,* Philtral columns. *2,* Philtral groove or dimple. *3,* Cupid's bow. *4,* White roll upper lip. *5,* Tubercle. *6,* Commissure. *7,* Vermilion. (Redrawn after Zide BM. Deformities of the lips and cheeks. In: McCarthy JE, ed. *Plastic Surgery.* Philadelphia: Saunders; 1990:2009.)

the periparotid nodes. Both of these nodal regions subsequently drain to the ipsilateral jugulodigastric nodes. The drainage is primarily ipsilateral, although there can be some crossover in the midline. The lower lip also drains to the ipsilateral submandibular nodes with the exception of the midline lip, which drains into the submental nodes. These are prone to cross the midline. The submental nodes subsequently drain into the submandibular nodes.

FUNCTION

The lips serve many functions that are accomplished as a result of their unique anatomy, especially the sphincteric muscle anatomy. The muscular content of the lips allow for their tone. Without this muscular support, the tissue would simply lose its support and become ptotic, as seen in patients with facial palsy who inevitably develop lower-lip laxity and lower-incisor show. Similarly if the upper lip was without muscular tone, the normal upper incisor–upper lip relationship would be lost.

The sphincteric function of the lips allows for oral competence in eating and drinking, speech and sound production, forceful blowing, and kissing. The loss of this function with many lip reconstructions is frequently frustrating. Many reconstructions, especially those involving nonlip tissues, may look fine at rest, but appear abnormal in the living, moving patient.

ETIOLOGY

The etiology of most lip defects is tumors or trauma. Lip tumors are either congenital or acquired. Congenital tumors are most often vascular malformations and hemangiomas. Acquired tumors are usually basal cell carcinoma in the upper lip and squamous cell carcinoma in the more sun-exposed lower lip. Melanoma is also quite common on the lip. Other tumors or pathologies are rare. Traumatic defects are different in that they occur in young, health patients.

LIP DEFECTS

When analyzing a lip defect, the most important assessment is the amount of remaining lip vermilion. Vermilion, if present, carries with it muscle that can be used to maintain the sphincteric function of the lip. All methods of vermilion reconstruction by using other tissues are suboptimal. Buccal mucosa and tongue look like buccal mucosa and tongue. They do not take lipstick in the same way, have different light reflection, and have different color. Remaining lip skin is also important, but in general, this tissue can be replaced more easily than vermilion.

When deciding on the operative plan, one must decide whether the lip can be reconstructed with lip tissue, which is preferable, or if the defect will require nonlip tissue. Lip tissue not only replaces "like with like," but most lip reconstruction using lip tissue with orbicularis muscle will eventually have some element of neurotization. This will allow for functional reconstruction that provides a natural appearance both at rest and in conversation. It also allows for the replacement of precious vermilion tissue. Direct lip closure, or closure with sliding lip tissue, is always the first choice.

Flaps such as the Abbe and reverse Abbe flap also satisfy the principle of reconstruction of "lip with lip." These flaps are lip-switch flaps that do not move the commissure. As a result, a normal appearance at the commissure can be expected. The insertion of the muscles at the modiolus is preserved and a more normal dynamic appearance is likely. **They also have the distinct advantage of tightening the donor lip, which helps provide balance with the tightened reconstructed lip.** The Abbe flap's disadvantages are that it is a two-stage procedure and that it has no way to directly preserve innervation of the transferred orbicularis muscle.

Other lip reconstructive flaps such as the Estlander, Gilles, and Karapandzic flaps, slide lip elements around the commissure. The upper lip is recruited to the lower lip as the commissure moves medially and a new commissure is created. These flaps have the advantage of not requiring a secondary flap division and inset. The Karapandzic flap has the advantage of maintaining innervated muscle. These other flaps, however, often require secondary revisions to establish a more normal-appearing commissure. With the exception of the Estlander flap, they do not directly shorten the donor lip and instead move the modiolus and the corresponding muscles from the normal location to the defect.

Some defects are simply too large to allow for reconstruction with lip tissue. In general, if a defect involves more than 40% of the total available upper- and lower-lip area (or greater than 80% of either lip), reconstruction with lip tissue will result in microstomia that is too significant and creation of a new lip must be considered. The Webster-Bernard, McGregor, Nakajima, and free flap reconstructions are examples of reconstructions that create new lip tissue from nonlip tissue (cheek and forearm). Although they are occasionally necessary reconstructions using nonlip tissue result in an unnatural dynamic appearance. In addition, the establishment of lip competence is more difficult.

Vermilion

Because of its importance in lip appearance, the anatomy of the vermilion deserves special attention. The vermilion is a thin layer of nonkeratinized epithelium that is devoid of sebaceous glands and hair follicles. It gets its unique color and spongy nature from the underlying dense capillary network. Beneath this capillary network is the orbicularis muscle. The vermilion is bordered by the white roll, which is a myocutaneous ridge that sits just outside the vermilion border.

The upper-lip vermilion is thickest directly below the high points of the Cupid's bow. Below the depth of the bow, the vermilion often forms a tubercle. This is most obvious in children. The vermilion tapers off toward the commissure where the white roll becomes less prominent.

The lower-lip vermilion is thickest in the midline and is usually more prominent than the vermilion in the upper lip. It tapers slightly until the lateral one-third of the lower lip, where it tapers rapidly.

Alignment of the vermilion is a key element in any lip procedure, from simple lacerations to complex reconstructions with flaps. Stepoffs in the vermilion of 1 mm are noticeable at conversational distance. **Note that it is impossible to accurately identify the vermilion or the white roll after injection of local anesthetic solutions.** The pressure of the anesthetic solutions or vasoconstriction of the epinephrine distorts the distinct vermilion color and obscures the white roll. **Therefore, the vermilion or white roll is marked prior to infiltration of anesthetic solutions.** Consequently, the aforementioned nerve blocks are useful for lip procedures. They have the advantage of complete anesthesia without local deformation of tissues. A useful technique is tattooing of the vermilion border or white roll with a needle dipped in methylene blue. This will provide a reference that can be realigned accurately. Alternatively, a single fine suture can be placed at the white roll or vermilion border prior to infiltration of local anesthesia.

Small, superficial vermilion defects can usually be closed primarily without elevation of flaps. Care must be taken to evert the edges to prevent notching. Lateral, superficial defects more than 2 to 3 mm from the white roll can usually be left to heal by secondary intention. This is less successful centrally where there can be a depression or a notching at the site. Alternatively, V-to-Y advancements from inside the vermilion will result in minimally noticeable scars.

For larger vermilion defects that do not involve the white roll, flaps are indicated. These can include vermilion flaps (lip flaps) or mucosal and tongue flaps (nonlip flaps). Vermilion flaps are best suited for defects that are close to the white roll. They replace vermilion with vermilion and scars in the vermilion itself usually heal well. Techniques include vermilion advancements or vermilion switches from the opposite lip. Vermilion advancements are best suited for central defects. They are robust flaps based on the labial vessel. The external incision is made directly on the vermilion border and the intraoral incision is made well inside the lip (Fig. 36.3). These flaps have a distinct advantage, especially in central defects in that the normal vermilion taper is preserved. This advantage is lost in more lateral defect. For more lateral defects, the distance from the vermilion border to the wet–dry line is measured on both sides of the defect. The taller side is tailored so that the vermilion will not show a significant step off at the wet–dry line.

Vermilion switch flaps are extremely useful. The vermilion is cut exactly as in a vermilion advancement, but is inset in the opposite lip (Fig. 36.4). The reconstruction of the donor lip is with vermilion advancement at the time of flap division. These flaps, like all lip flaps, are divided at 10 days. It is best not to delay division too long, as significant secondary healing will make tailoring and inset time more difficult, especially in the donor lip.

Mucosal advancements are useful for broad defects that are remote from the vermilion border, as these defects will have enough normal appearing vermilion spared. As mucosal flaps contract and retract, they will result in a thinner lip, and this

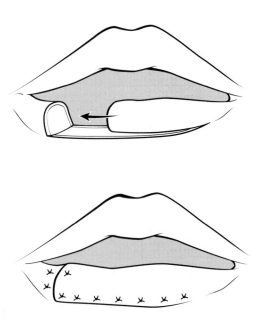

FIGURE 36.3. Vermilion advancement flap. Proper eversion of the sutured edges will prevent notching. The height of the vermilion should be tailored in closure of lateral defects. (Redrawn after Zide BM. Deformities of the lips and cheeks. In: McCarthy JE, ed. *Plastic Surgery.* Philadelphia: Saunders; 1990:2016.)

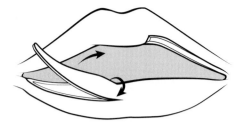

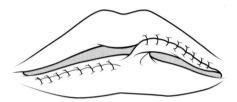

FIGURE 36.4. Vermilion switch flaps can be performed using a portion of the vermilion (as shown here) or the entire vermilion. If the entire vermilion is used, the donor site is closed with vermilion advancement flaps. (Redrawn after Zide BM. Deformities of the lips and cheeks. In: McCarthy JE, ed. *Plastic Surgery.* Philadelphia: Saunders; 1990:2029.)

should be expected. These bipedicled flaps are elevated just below the minor salivary glands and advanced to fill the defect. The donor site is treated with a mucosal graft.

Tongue flaps are another method of reconstruction. The anteriorly based lateral tongue flap is a useful tool as it can provide significant bulk. It, like all other nonvermilion flaps, does not leave a normal-appearing lip and is therefore best reserved for lateral defects. It is elevated from the lateral surface of the tongue, avoiding the papillary tongue. Closure of the donor site is important as the lingual nerve may be exposed in larger flaps.

Upper Lip

Superficial defects of the upper lip must be categorized by their location and size. These defects have the advantage of intact orbicularis and lip bulk. As a result, the reconstruction can often be simplified and still give a good aesthetic result, even with larger defects. Central defects between the philtral columns can be repaired primarily or with a wedge resection if they involve less than half of the central lip segment. The orbicularis muscle must be accurately repaired for normal lip movement. If the superficial defect involves more than half of the central lip, but does not cross or just crosses the philtrum, a full-thickness skin graft from the preauricular area is a reasonable option. This technique has the advantage of hair growth that can often improve the aesthetic appearance. For lateral, superficial defects, wedge resection is usually a good option except for cases where there is greater than half of the lateral lip involved. For these cases, full-thickness grafting will often give an acceptable result.

Full-thickness defects are defects that include significant amounts of the subcutaneous fat and the orbicularis muscle. Treatment is based on their size and location in the upper lip. Defects up to one third will do well with primary closure with local tissue rearrangement and advancement. This local tissue rearrangement will often include perialar crescentic excisions and medial advancement of the nasolabial fold.

For central defects involving up to half of the distance between the philtral columns, primary closure is the best option. This will shift the philtrum in most cases, and will result in a narrow central lip. For defects that include greater than half of the central lip, an Abbe flap will give the best result. The remainder of the central lip, that is, from philtral column to philtral column, should be excised. This excision can, of course extend past the philtral column, knowing that this may result in slight asymmetry.

With elevation and inset of the Abbe flap, certain principles must be followed (Fig. 36.5). The flap is harvested based on the labial artery. As the venous drainage does not follow the

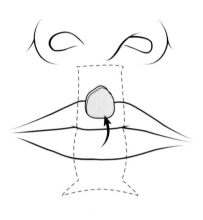

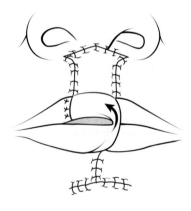

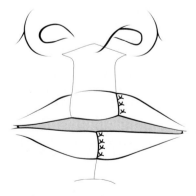

FIGURE 36.5. Abbe flap. **Top:** The Abbe flap is elevated from the central lower lip. For central upper defects, it is elevated to the labiomental fold. For lateral defects, it continues through the central chin pad. **Middle:** It is inset onto the columella, above the columellar base with the extensions to the nasal sill. **Bottom:** The flap is divided and inset at two weeks.

arterial supply, it is best to maintain a several-millimeter cuff of labial mucosa for venous drainage. The Abbe flap should be harvested from the central lower lip. One must remember that the orbicularis muscle is paired. The Abbe flap should include the central raphe so as to leave neurotized orbicularis on both sides of the closure. Whenever possible, the Abbe flap should be in the exact center of the lower lip. Central lip incisions will leave the best donor scar on the lip and chin. The base of the Abbe can be closed with two Burrow triangles on either side so as to leave a small horizontal scar at the labiomental fold. It is rare that the Abbe flap needs to be extended beyond the labiomental fold. This is true because most lateral defects of the upper lip should be treated with concomitant medialization of the cheek and thus the nasolabial fold. This decreases the superior extent of the defect. In cases where the Abbe flap must be extended beyond the labiomental fold, it should be kept directly in the midline. This will avoid disrupting the balance of the paired mentalis muscle and usually leaves an acceptable scar. When the Abbe flap is inset in the upper lip, it should be sutured on the columella, just above the medial footplates. If it is inset below the medial footplates, there will be loss of the normal meniscus that exists between the columella and the upper lip.

The Abbe flap can also be used to replace lateral lip defects larger than a third. This is the preferred technique if the commissure is intact. It is best to combine the Abbe flap with perialar excision and lip advancement. This allows for the tip of the Abbe flap to be inset at the alar base and the cheek tissue to be advanced to fill the lateral portion of the defect. The nasolabial fold is thus advanced medially such that it begins at the alar base, and not at the lateral ala. The remaining lip defect is closed via medial advancement of the lateral lip. This will shift the philtrum slightly and the patient should be forewarned.

For even larger defects, those up to 80% of the upper lip or 40% of the total available lip tissue, the Abbe flap is simply made larger. It is designed with a bilateral Schuchardt advancement because it will allow for medial advancement of the lower lip and closure of the large donor side. This is also combined with bilateral perialar crescentic excision. Overall, this will leave a microstomia, and secondary lip stretching will be necessary. **Remember that a balance in the length of the upper and lower lip is important and the tissue should be near equally shared by the two lips.**

Subtotal (greater than 80%) and total upper lip defects are rare, and reconstruction is basically a salvage operation. Most patients with these defects have lived with deforming tumors for years without seeking care. The exceptions, and most difficult cases, are traumatic lip loss and these patients have higher demands. As mentioned above, procedures employing nonlip tissues rarely appear natural at rest, and even more seldom in the living, moving patient.

Functional reconstruction is not as critical in the upper lip as in the lower lip. A static upper lip can allow for competence if the lower lip is normal. The radial forearm free flap is a useful tool for subtotal or total lip defects. It can provide adequate bulk of tissue and a reasonable color match. It is often folded to provide both intraoral and external tissue. Care should be taken to avoid a lip that is too long, as the new lip will become ptotic with time. The vermilion can be reconstructed with either tattooing or with buccal mucosal grafting. If grafting is used, the forearm flap is de-epithelized in a second stage and buccal mucosa placed. In male patients, good results can be expected with the free occipital flap. It results in a hair-bearing upper lip that allows for camouflage of the nonmobile, poor-color-match lip. The inside of the lip is reconstructed with a thick split-thickness graft. This is advantageous as it will give some stiffness to the lip as the graft contracts.

Lower Lip

Lower-lip defects should be divided into those involving the commissure (or approaching the commissure) and those of the central lip. **The lower lip can tolerate wedge excision for the majority of defects encountered.** This includes most superficial defects, which, unlike the upper lip, are treated in the same fashion as full-thickness defects. The only exception is the rare superficial defect of greater than 50% of the lower lip for which a skin graft is appropriate.

For defects that are not amenable to straight wedge excision, the Schuchardt procedure is the next option (Fig. 36.6). This is a sliding-lip reconstruction that advances the lower lip with an inferior incision along the labiomental fold to the mandibular

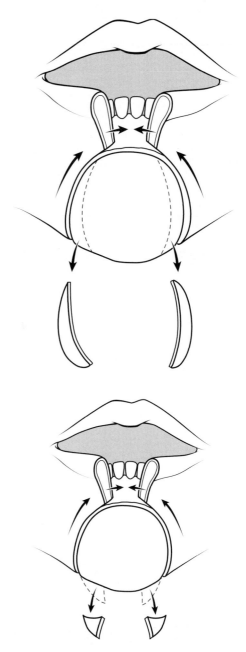

FIGURE 36.6. The Schuchardt procedure rotates and advances the cheek and lip to provide closure. The skin folds are removed as crescents *(top)* or submental triangles *(bottom)*. (Redrawn after Zide BM. Deformities of the lips and cheeks. In: McCarthy JE, ed. *Plastic Surgery*. Philadelphia: Saunders; 1990:2017.)

border. Intraorally, the incisions are on the labial side of the gingivobuccal sulcus. The lip is advanced centrally. It is performed on the side of the lower lip with the greatest amount of tissue as this allows for the greatest advancement. It avoids complex reconstructive procedures and leaves minimal scarring. This technique can be applied to most lower-lip defects as it is easily combined with many of the lip-switching procedures.

Lip-switching procedures are often necessary. The workhorse flap is the reverse Abbe flap, which can be used for either lateral or midline lower-lip defects. These include either the lateral or the central reverse Abbe flaps. The lateral Abbe flap is usually based off the medial labial artery. It differs from the Estlander flap in that it does not move the commissure. The lateral aspect of the flap, and thus the vermilion, is kept medial enough so that it is of sufficient height to match the medial defect of the lower lip. The tip of the Abbe is the perialar crescentic excision in order to allow for primary closure of the upper lip. This is most useful for lateral lower lip defects that cannot be repaired with the Schuchardt alone. It does shift the philtrum towards the Abbe closure.

The central reverse Abbe flap is used for central lower lip defects. This differs from the lateral reverse Abbe flap in that the perialar crescents are not part of the flap, but are discarded in the closure of the upper lip. It also differs in that the vascular pedicle is lateral and not medial. The medial incision for the Abbe flap is at the philtral column and the lateral extent is just at the lateral aspect of the ala. It can be performed as a double central reverse Abbe flap for large lower-lip defects (Fig. 36.7).

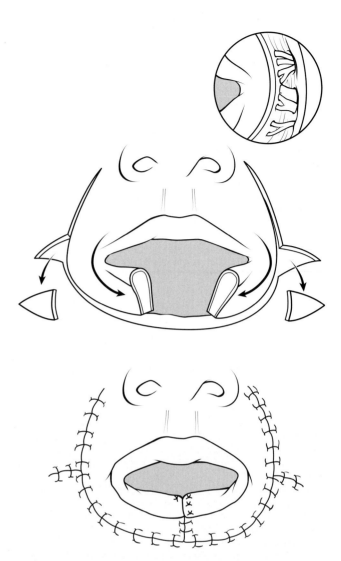

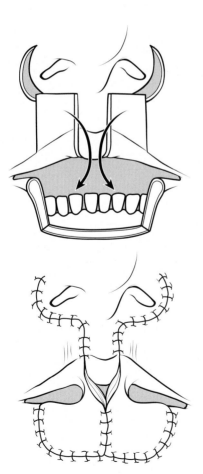

FIGURE 36.7. Double central reverse Abbe flap for closure of large lower-lip defects. This is especially useful as it distributes the total lip tissue without distorting the commissure. (Redrawn after Zide BM. Deformities of the lips and cheeks. In: McCarthy JE, ed. *Plastic Surgery.* Philadelphia: Saunders; 1990:2019.)

FIGURE 36.8. Bilateral Karapandzic flaps for closure of a large lower-lip defect. The Karapandzic techniques preserves the nerves to the orbicularis muscle. (Redrawn after Zide BM. Deformities of the lips and cheeks. In: McCarthy JE, ed. *Plastic Surgery.* Philadelphia: Saunders; 1990:2023.)

With this, bilateral central reverse Abbe flaps are used along with lower lip medial advancement. For these cases, precise measurements are necessary as the goal is to evenly distribute the lip tissue between the upper and lower lip. Again, this can be used for up to 80% defects of the lower lip. The total lip area will be reduced by 40% and secondary stretching will be beneficial.

The sliding lower-lip reconstructive procedures are the Karapandzic and the Estlander flap. The Karapandzic flap is essentially a Gilles flap that maintains the nerve supply to the lower lip and has replaced the Gilles flap (Fig. 36.8). This flap is a rotation-advancement flap along the nasolabial fold that pivots at the commissure and upper lip. The Estlander is a lip-switching flap that involves the commissure and pivots the upper lip to the lower lip (Fig. 36.9). Of these flaps, the Karapandzic is the most useful. Bilateral Karapandzic flaps can be employed for up to 80% defects. The advantage is that the lip is innervated, while the disadvantage is the microstomia, rounding of the commissure, and the misplacement of the modiolus that is inevitably produced.

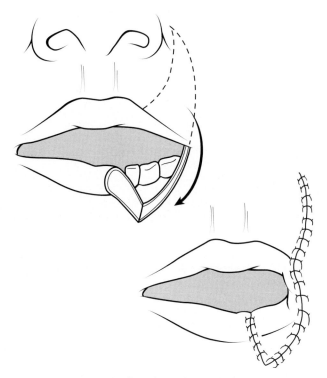

FIGURE 36.9. The Estlander flap rotates the upper lip to the lower lip. It results in a round commissure and loss of the normal taper of the vermilion. (Redrawn after Zide BM. Deformities of the lips and cheeks. In: McCarthy JE, ed. *Plastic Surgery.* Philadelphia: Saunders; 1990:2022.)

For larger defects, nonlip techniques must be employed. The Webster-Bernard operation has stood the test of time (Fig. 36.10). It involves medial advancement of the cheek tissue to create a new lower lip. Excision of tissue at the nasolabial fold allows for this advancement. The vermilion is reconstructed with a bipedicled mucosal sliding flap. The mucosal flap should be brought well outside the lip as it inevitably contracts. It can give good results, although it does result in significant facial scarring. The free radial forearm, as in the upper lip, is a reasonable option. The palmaris tendon can be included with the flap and used to suspend the lower lip. This allows the lower lip to be placed high and provides for oral competence. Hair transplantation to the free radial forearm flap can greatly improve the result. Even if the hair is shaved, it provides texture to the skin that gives a more normal appearance.

Other Reconstructive Tools

Lip reconstructions often require reversionary procedures. Lip-sharing procedures result in some element of microstomia. Because of the superiority of the techniques employing lip tissue, some degree of microstomia is preferable to a reconstruction using nonlip tissues. Established microstomia can be treated with serial stretching. For millennia, the Mursi tribes in present-day Ethiopia have practiced lip stretching by serial placement of larger lip disks (Fig. 36.11). Several techniques have been described for lip expansion and the simplest devices are often the best. Self-retaining spring dental retractors are easy for patients to obtain and can be used at night. These devices are also useful for remodeling the commissure in cases of commissural burns.

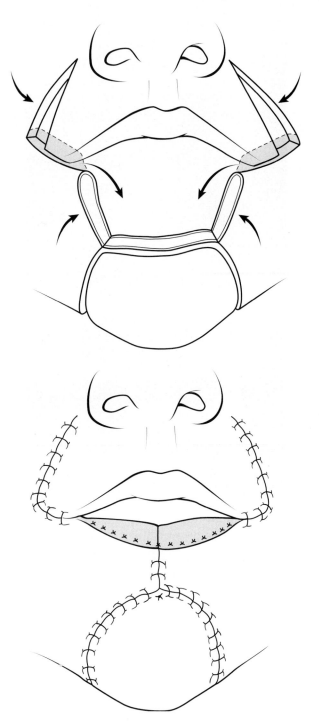

FIGURE 36.10. The Webster-Bernard flap advances the cheek skin medially to replace the lower lip. The vermilion is reconstructed with a mucosal flap. (Redrawn after Zide BM. Deformities of the lips and cheeks. In: McCarthy JE, ed. *Plastic Surgery.* Philadelphia: Saunders; 1990:2020.)

Hair transplants are also very useful. They can camouflage the scars of lip reconstruction and can provide normal texture to the new lip skin even if shaved. They are especially useful in free tissue transfers as they hide nonmobile tissue.

KEY POINTS

1. The mentalis muscles are required for lower lip position and lip competence. They are large trapezoidal/

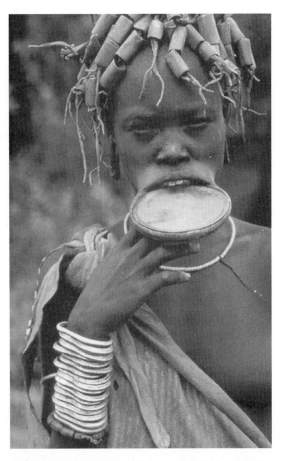

FIGURE 36.11. A Mursi tribeswoman with large lip disk in place. Note how the vermilion tissue is truly expanded.

and inferiorly into the chin pad below the labiomental fold.

2. When analyzing a lip defect, the most important assessment is the amount of remaining vermilion. Lip vermilion carries orbicularis muscle that allows for movement of the lip.
3. The lip vermilion is distinct from mucosa in its color and appearance.
4. The vermilion or white roll is marked prior to infiltration of anesthetic solutions because it is difficult to accurately identify the vermilion or the white roll after injection of local anesthetic solutions.
5. A balance in the length of the upper and lower lip is desirable. With larger reconstructions, total lip tissue should be near equally shared by the two lips.
6. Functional reconstruction of the upper lip is not as critical as in the lower lip.
7. The lower lip can tolerate wedge excision for the majority of defects encountered.
8. Lip-switching procedures have the distinct advantage of simultaneously shortening the normal lip along with reconstructing the opposite lip defect.
9. The Abbe and reverse Abbe flaps have the advantage of not moving the commissure.

Selected Readings

Berkovitz BKB, Moxham BK, Brown, MW, et al. *A Textbook of Head and Neck Anatomy*. London: Wolfe Medical; 1988:154.

Dupin C, Metzinger S, Rizzuto R. Lip reconstruction after ablation for skin malignancies. *Clin Plast Surg*. 2004;31(1):69.

Langstein HN, Robb GL. Lip and perioral reconstruction. *Clin Plast Surg*. 2005;32(3):431, viii.

Sultan MR, Hugo NE. Basic principles of reconstruction of the lip, oral commissure, and cheek. In: Georgiade GS, Riefkhol R, Levin LS, eds. *Plastic, Maxillofacial, and Reconstructive Surgery*. 3rd ed. Baltimore, Md: Williams and Wilkins; 1997.

Zide BM. Deformities of the lips and cheeks. In: McCarthy JE, ed. *Plastic Surgery*. Philadelphia: Saunders; 1990:2009.

pyramidal muscles that originate from the mandible just below the attached gingiva and insert horizontally

CHAPTER 37 ■ RECONSTRUCTION OF THE CHEEKS

BABAK J. MEHRARA

The cheeks represent the largest surface area of the face and frame the central facial units. This anatomic arrangement exposes the skin of the cheek to trauma and to the effects of sun exposure, and, in turn, the frequent need for reconstructive surgery. Reconstruction must be planned carefully and executed meticulously to restore the natural contours, maintain hair patterns, and camouflage scars.

The face can been divided into units based on a number of characteristics, including skin color, skin texture, hair, contour, relaxed skin tension lines, and boundaries between anatomic structures. The cheek, however, is less amenable to "aesthetic unit" analysis. Zide has divided the cheek into three overlapping zones: suborbital, preauricular, and buccomandibular based on reconstructive needs (1). Similarly, Jackson, has divided the cheek into five areas based on reconstructive techniques and anatomic characteristics (lateral, lower, malar, superomedial, and alar base-nasolabial) (2). These classification systems are helpful for planning reconstruction, but principles used for subunit reconstruction in other areas (e.g., resurfacing entire units, discarding remaining tissues of entire units if more than 50% of a unit is missing, using contralateral side to make exact templates) are less applicable to cheek reconstruction.

ANATOMY

The cheek is bounded by the preauricular fold laterally, the zygomatic arch and lower eyelids superiorly, the nasal sidewall and nasolabial fold medially, and the mandibular border inferiorly.

The sensory innervation of the cheek is provided by the maxillary and mandibular divisions of the trigeminal nerve, as well as a small contribution from the anterior cutaneous nerve of the neck and the great auricular nerve, both of which arise from the cervical plexus.

Motor innervation of the superficial facial muscles is provided by the facial nerve and its main branches. The masseter and temporalis muscles are innervated by the trigeminal nerve. The facial nerve is located deep to the parotid masseteric fascia and is protected by the superficial lobe of the parotid gland anterior to the ear.

The arterial supply of the cheek is provided by branches of the external carotid artery including the facial artery, the superficial temporal artery, and the transverse facial artery. Venous drainage follows the arteries and is abundant. The lymphatic drainage of the cheek is provided by lymphatic channels within the parotid nodes and along the facial vessels to the submandibular nodes.

DEFECT ANALYSIS

Analysis of the defect or anticipated defect is a critical part of any reconstructive procedure. Defects may be superficial (simple) and include only the skin and subcutaneous tissues, or may be more complex and include muscle, parotid gland, facial nerve, mucosa, and bone. Ideally, surgical incisions are placed at the cheek margins or within established skin rhytides to camouflage the resulting wound. Care is taken to avoid, if possible, placement of hair-bearing skin into non–hair-bearing areas. Similarly, rotation of non–hair-bearing skin into male beard lines and distortion of sideburns is avoided. Contour deformities and color mismatches are avoided whenever possible by careful planning. Distortion of surrounding structures such as the lower eyelid and upper lip is disfiguring and is an important consideration in planning the surgical approach to reconstruction. According to Zide and colleagues, vertical incisions placed medial to a line drawn from the lateral canthus remain obvious on frontal view and instead should be replaced by incisions along the nasolabial fold or by blepharoplasty incisions (3). Defects involving the full thickness of the cheek can occur from invasion of more superficial cancers, from extensive trauma, or as a result of advanced intraoral cancers. Appropriate reconstruction of all layers, while maintaining reasonable contour, are planned if possible. A successful reconstruction will recreate the missing tissues using the most similar replacement tissues. Thus, as with nasal reconstruction, plans for lining, support, and coverage are developed individually. Secondary revisions for contour may be necessary, particularly for complex reconstructions, and should be described to the patient prior to initiation of therapy.

Facial nerve reconstruction is ideally performed as a planned procedure with the ends of the nerve stimulated and tagged at the time of resection since identification of nerve ends after tumor extirpation is tedious. In addition, nerve transection is performed sharply to avoid cautery damage at the site of neurorrhaphy. Nerve grafts may be harvested from the neck (ansa cervicalis, great auricular nerve) or from distant sites (e.g., sural nerve).

For any given defect, more than one reconstructive option is usually available. **The best option is determined based on the relationship of the defect to the surrounding structures, hair-bearing status, skin laxity, natural wrinkles, previous surgical scars, and relaxed skin tension lines.** Contaminated wounds undergo serial debridement and dressing changes until bacterial content is reduced to an acceptable level before definitive reconstruction is accomplished. A history of previous radiation therapy may prohibit local flap reconstruction.

RECONSTRUCTIVE OPTIONS

Healing by Secondary Intention

The simplest method of closure is healing by secondary intention. Unfortunately, the indications for this technique are limited as large wounds may result in contour irregularities, distortion of surrounding structures, and unstable coverage. This technique may be useful for small (<1 cm), superficial defects located in cosmetically inconspicuous areas (e.g., below the sideburns) in patients with solar-damaged, irregularly pigmented skin.

Primary Closure

Primary closure is the reconstructive method of choice if excessive tension and distortion of surrounding tissues can be avoided. The scars are ideally placed along minimal skin tension lines or within natural skin contours such as the nasolabial or preauricular folds (Fig. 37.1). This technique results in the simplest scar, avoids donor-site deformity, and avoids interpolation of distant tissues into the defect. The size of defect that is suitable for primary closure is variable and depends on the amount of skin laxity present. Wide undermining in an elderly patient with significant skin laxity may allow closure of relatively large defects. Dog-ears created by wound closure should be excised while avoiding excessive lengthening of the scar. The disadvantages of primary closure for larger defects is the long, straight scar. The nonlinear scar from a local flap is preferable in some circumstances.

Skin Grafts

Occasionally, skin grafts are useful for cheek reconstruction. Although skin grafts may be associated with shiny, patchlike, depressed scars, they may be a reasonable option in patients with significant comorbid conditions in whom other proce-

dures may be too risky. Skin grafts have also been advocated by some authors in patients at high risk for local recurrence. In addition, skin grafts may be used to resurface less-critical areas of the cheek (e.g., just below the sideburns) or donor sites of flaps used to resurface more critical areas. Full-thickness skin grafts exhibit less secondary contraction and should be used in situations where contracture would result in distortion of adjacent structures (e.g., lower eyelid). Full-thickness skin grafts have the additional advantage of better color match if harvested from the neck, preauricular/postauricular skin, or upper back. Full-thickness skin grafts are also thicker than split-thickness skin grafts and may be more useful for deeper defects. In general, excisions greater than 5 mm in thickness treated with skin grafts will likely exhibit a permanent contour deformity.

Local Flaps

Advancement Flaps

Advancement flaps are useful for reconstruction of superomedial defects, particularly in elderly patients with significant skin laxity. These flaps may be performed as advancement flaps with excision of Burrow triangles or as V-Y advancement. Ideally, the lesion is excised as a rectangle or square to avoid trapdoor scarring. Advancement flaps are random pattern flaps raised in the subcutaneous plane, and should be of appropriate width to avoid tip necrosis. A base-to-length ratio of 1:1 is considered safe. In addition, advancement flaps should be anchored to the periosteum of zygoma or maxilla with permanent sutures to prevent ectropion.

V-Y advancement flaps are an excellent choice for closure of defects that lie along the medial cheek and alar base,

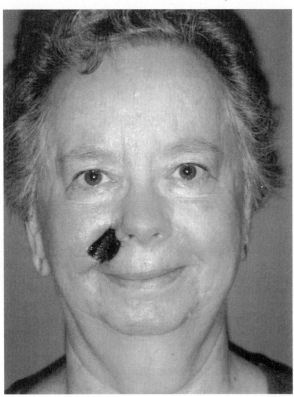

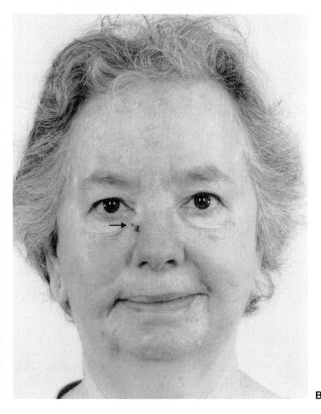

A   B

FIGURE 37.1. Primary closure. Preoperative (A) and postoperative (B) photographs of patient treated with primary closure of Mohs excision for basal cell cancer. Note closure along nasolabial fold with well-concealed scar and minimal distortion. Also note new basal cell cancer excision on nasal sidewall (*arrow*).

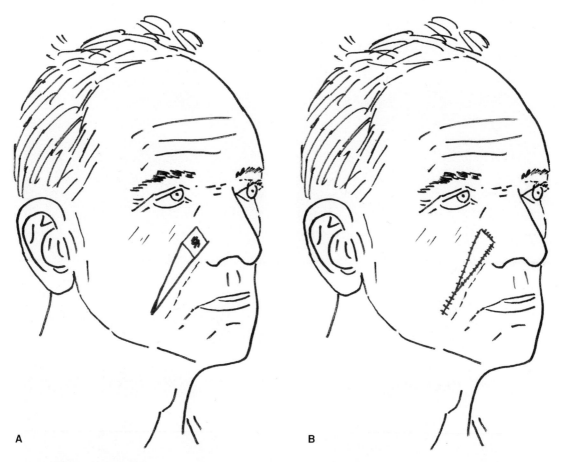

FIGURE 37.2. V-Y advancement flap closure of defect along the medial cheek. **A:** Flap design. **B:** After advancement. Note advancement of nasolabial flap with rectangular excision of the defect.

particularly if primary closure of the defect results in distortion of the lower eyelid or nasal base (Fig. 37.2) (4). The excision is performed as a square or rectangle in the medial cheek or as a wide crescent at the alar base. Skin incisions are preformed to the subcutaneous tissues and the flap is advanced based on a subcutaneous blood supply. The length of the flap should be sufficient to avoid undue tension on the closure.

Zide and colleagues described the deep-plane cervicofacial "hike" repair as an advancement flap that removes dog-ears in a cosmetically acceptable blepharoplasty incision (3). The flap is dissected together with the SMAS (superficial muscu-loaponeurotic system) and is thought to have a better blood supply than subcutaneous flaps. The dissection of the facial nerve is performed with blunt scissors by using vertical spreading, thus enabling advancement of the remaining cheek unit. Resultant dog-ears are excised as an upper or lower blepharoplasty incision. Alternatively, the redundant upper eyelid skin may be used to reconstruct lower-lid defects while the advancement flap is used to reconstruct the cheek defect (Fig. 37.3).

Transposition Flaps

Transposition flaps such as banner flaps, bilobed flaps, and rhomboid flaps are useful for closure of most medium to large defects of the cheek. These flaps are designed to transfer lax skin to repair the defect while the donor site is closed primarily. Although these flaps have some drawbacks (e.g., complex scars, pincushioning, trapdoor scarring, patchlike scarring, and alterations in hair pattern), good results can be obtained in appropriately selected patients and with carefully designed flaps.

Donor scars should be planned carefully to fall as much as possible within relaxed skin tension lines or existing folds. Dog-ears should also be excised without narrowing the base of the flaps.

Banner flaps are the simplest form of transposition flap and transfer skin from the preauricular or nasolabial area to close the defect (Fig. 37.4). Secondary revisions may be necessary to remove remaining dog-ears or to defat pincushioned flaps. Although these repairs usually have excellent contour and reasonable color match, the scars may be conspicuous, particularly with facial animation.

Bilobed flaps are an extension of the banner flap and use a secondary flap to close the defect created by the primary flap (Fig. 37.5). Bilobed flaps are used when the defect created by the primary flap (i.e., the banner flap) is too large to close primarily. The flaps are designed on a 45- to 90-degree axis to the primary defect and the flaps are elevated in the subcutaneous plane. Generally, the primary flap may be drawn somewhat smaller than the defect and is designed, as much as possible, to place the scars along minimal tension lines and within natural skin creases. Flaps designed at 45-degree angles minimize dog-ear formation. The resultant scars are complex and may be quite conspicuous. Pincushioning is a problem with bilobed flaps, particularly relatively small flaps, and may require secondary revisions. **Because of the laxity in the cheek, bilobed flaps have less usefulness on the cheek than on the nose.**

Rhomboid flaps are also a geometric modification of banner flaps and are useful in the treatment of medium to large defects (Fig. 37.6). These flaps are more difficult to design but have a decreased propensity for trapdoor scarring or pincushioning.

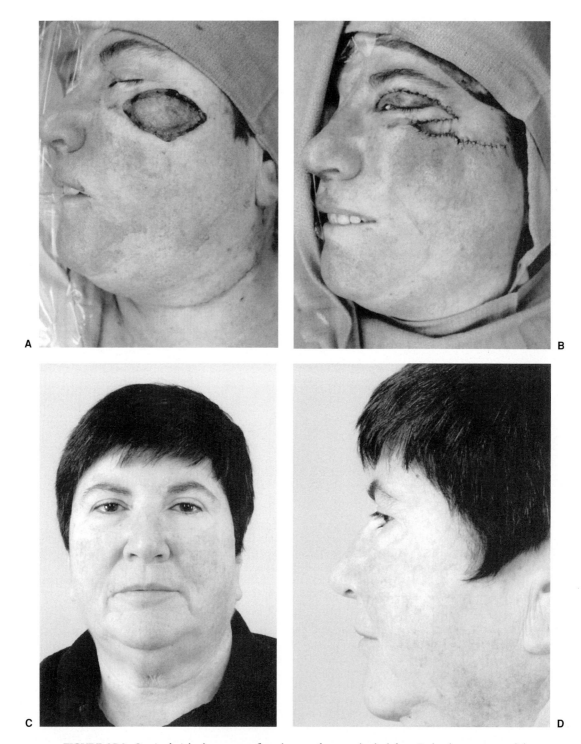

FIGURE 37.3. Cervicofacial advancement flap closure of upper cheek defect. Redundant upper eyelid skin was used to repair lower-eyelid defect while the cheek advancement flap was used to repair the cheek defect. **A:** Defect before operation. **B, C,** and **D:** Postoperative appearance. Note the well-camouflaged scar and lack of lower eyelid distortion.

Rhomboid flaps are useful primarily for lateral, lower cheek, and temporal defects. The excision is performed using a rhombus with 60- and 120-degree angles. The donor flap bisects the 120-degree angle. The flap is drawn to place the donor site incision within normal facial rhytides. This can be determined easily by identifying the area of skin with maximal extensibility. Thus, redundant surrounding skin is transferred to the defect while the donor area is closed primarily. Modifications of the flap may be performed to avoid unnecessary excision of normal

skin, however, more circular excisions resembling banner flaps may be complicated by pincushioning.

Rotation Flaps

Cervicofacial Flaps. Cheek rotation flaps are useful for repair of moderate to large defects of the upper medial region. These flaps use the loose preauricular and neck skin, and are most useful for full-thickness skin and subcutaneous excisions.

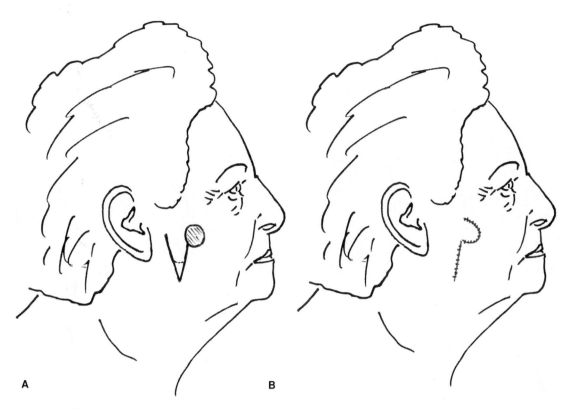

FIGURE 37.4. Banner flap closure of central cheek defect. **A:** Flap design. **B:** After transfer. Note location of final incision corresponds to lines of minimal tension/natural skin creases.

Repair of deeper excisions may result in contour abnormalities.

There are a variety of cheek rotations flaps (Fig. 37.7). In their 1979 description, Juri and Juri popularized the inferomedially based rotation flap. This flap is designed such that the incision starts at the superior aspect of the defect and extends to the outer canthus and along the zygomatic arch (Fig. 37.8). The incision is then brought along the preauricular fold, extended below the ear, and along the retroauricular hairline to the midposterior line of the neck. Wide subcutaneous undermining of the skin flap is then performed, enabling advancement and rotation of the flap into the defect with primary closure of the donor site. **The flap should be anchored to the periosteum of the zygoma and lateral orbital wall with permanent sutures to avoid postoperative ectropion.** Simultaneous lower-lid tightening may be considered, particularly in patients with excessive lower-lid laxity. Skin excess formed at the nasolabial fold is excised carefully so as to avoid narrowing the base of the flap. Occasionally, a full-thickness skin graft is necessary for closure of the donor site to avoid undue tension. This skin graft is best camouflaged below the sideburn. The primary drawback of this procedure is skin necrosis of the distal flap. This complication may be particularly problematic in smokers. In addition, rotation-advancement shifts the normal hair-bearing pattern of the cheek and may result in ectropion or prolonged lower-lid edema. Hematoma may also occur and should be closely monitored as it can lead to large areas of skin necrosis.

Inferolaterally based rotation flaps are designed to transfer the lax skin of the jowls and along the nasolabial fold to reconstruct upper medial defects (Fig. 37.9) (5). The skin incision may be extended across the mandible and back-cut to enable tension-free closure. In addition, extension of the incision to the contralateral neck along an established neck crease may increase the reach of the flap. **These flaps are less likely to un-** dergo necrosis at the distal end than inferomedially based flaps. **The disadvantage is the scar in the central face.** For smaller defects, excision of a Burrow triangle may be necessary to allow rotation-advancement of the flap. These flaps are susceptible to the effects of gravity with resulting ectropion and should therefore be anchored securely to the underlying bone/periosteum. Resections performed close to the lower eyelid may be complicated by lower lid edema, medial ectropion, pin cushioning, and nasolabial fold asymmetry. In addition, scars crossing the mandibular border may be difficult to hide or result in contracture. The use of Z-plasty incisions to cross the mandibular border may obviate this problem.

In an effort to improve the blood supply and reliability of the cheek rotation flap, several authors have described a composite dissection of the skin flap (3,6). This dissection is performed in the deep plane by elevating the skin together with the SMAS. The flap is elevated with vertical spreading below the SMAS and the facial nerve branches are preserved. This modification enables larger flap design and can be used more reliably in smokers and patients with poor skin quality. In addition, the use of composite flaps enables repair of deeper defects without resultant contour abnormalities. Conversely, these flaps may require secondary revision (thinning) if used for the repair of simple excisions.

Cervicopectoral Flaps. Cervicopectoral flaps use the excess skin of the neck and chest to cover lower lateral cheek defects. The upper border of the defects suitable for cervicopectoral flap reconstruction can be estimated by drawing a line connecting the tragus to the lateral commissure. **Reconstruction of defects extending significantly above this line may be complicated by skin necrosis.** The incisions are marked along the posterior aspect of the defect, around the ear lobe and along the retroauricular hairline. The incision is continued in the neck approximately 2 to 3 cm behind the anterior border of the trapezius and across the clavicle at the deltopectoral

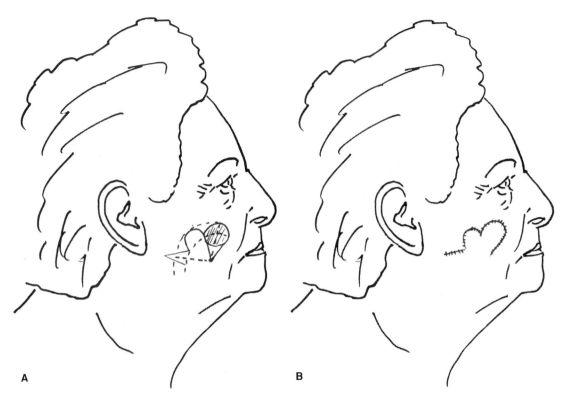

FIGURE 37.5. Bilobed flap closure of central cheek defect. **A:** Flap design. **B:** After transfer. See text for details.

groove. A back-cut may be performed as necessary. Larger defects may require further dissection of the flap by running along the border of the pectoralis muscle and extending across the chest (Fig. 37.10). This flap is based primarily on the internal mammary perforating vessels with variable contribution from perforators emanating from the thoracoacromial artery and vein. Cervicopectoral flaps are raised subcutaneously over the cheek and lower mandible and enter the deep plane below the platysma approximately 3 to 4 cm below the mandibular border. The platysma can be safely transected at this level to improve the reach of the flap. The flap is advanced and rotated into the defect and the donor area of the flap lateral to the pectoralis muscle is closed in a V-to-Y fashion. Skin grafting of the donor site is occasionally necessary to provide tension-free closure. The head is lightly immobilized postoperatively using rolled sheets to avoid violent movements.

Local Composite Flaps

Pectoralis Major Flap. The pectoralis major flap is occasionally useful for repair of lower lateral cheek defects. The pectoralis muscle is supplied by the pectoral branches of the thoracoacromial vessels, which are located along a line drawn from the acromion to the xiphoid process. The vessels emerge from below the clavicle and can be located easily using a Doppler probe. The pectoralis flap is a reliable flap with low total-necrosis rates; however, partial skin necrosis can occur if the flap is not elevated meticulously. The flap tends to be bulky and is primarily used for complex reconstructions involving skin, subcutaneous tissues, parotid, and masseter. Although a folded pectoralis major myocutaneous flap has been described for repair of through-and-through cheek defects to provide both intraoral and extraoral coverage, this option is significantly disfiguring because of excessive bulk and should probably be avoided unless extenuating circumstances are present. The flap may be transferred as a muscle-only flap, or together with an overlying skin paddle. The skin paddle is usually designed as an elliptical excision medial to the nipple areola complex. A width of approximately 6 to 7 cm can usually be closed without undue tension. The superior extent of the skin paddle should ideally preserve the internal mammary perforating vessels to maintain the option for a future deltopectoral flap. Closure of this defect may cause significant distortion of the breast. An alternative is a skin paddle marked below the nipple. This skin paddle has longer reach and a better scar; however, the blood supply may be tenuous. In addition, extensive undermining in a female patient may lead to breast or nipple necrosis. The muscle may be thinned proximally to avoid an unsightly bulge in the lower neck. In addition, near-complete disinsertion of the muscle may prevent postoperative neck contracture and torticollis. Care should be taken when tunneling the flap into the defect to avoid avulsion of the skin paddle, kinking or excessive twisting of the pedicle, or external compression from an inadequate tunnel.

Trapezius Flap. The trapezius flap is similar to the pectoralis major flap in that it is occasionally useful for complex lower lateral cheek defects. **The arterial and venous anatomy of the trapezius (type II Mathes and Nahai vascular pattern) is variable and can be a potential pitfall in dissection.** The dominant pedicle is the transverse cervical artery and vein, which in most instances are branches of the thyrocervical trunk (80%). The distal portions of the muscle receive a variable contribution from the dorsal scapular artery and vein, which course deep to the rhomboid muscles. These vessels are usually branches of the transverse cervical artery and vein, but may arise separately from the subclavian vessels, leading to distal ischemia if divided. Three distinct musculocutaneous flaps based on the trapezius system are available (superior, lateral, and lower). The lower and lateral flaps are more useful for cheek reconstruction because of their arc of rotation. The lower flap is designed with the patient in the lateral decubitus position. The skin flap is marked between the midline and the medial border

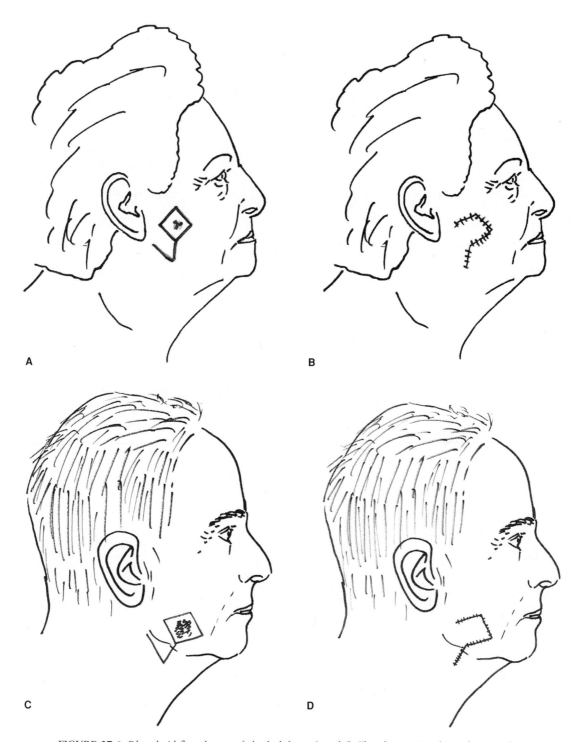

FIGURE 37.6. Rhomboid flap closure of cheek defects. **A** and **C:** Flap design. **B** and **D:** After transfer. Note that flap is drawn along minimal tension lines and within natural skin creases.

of the scapula overlying the inferior aspect of the trapezius muscle. The lower extent of the skin paddle is variable, although the inferior border of the scapula is in general reliable. Skin, subcutaneous tissues, and fibers of the trapezius muscle are incised and the flap is elevated above the plane of the rhomboid muscles. If a large dorsal scapular artery is encountered, the contribution of this vessel to the skin flap perfusion should be assessed using a microvascular clamp. If the dorsal scapular vessels are critical for perfusion of the distal aspect of the flap, these vessels can be mobilized by incising a cuff of rhomboid muscle and ligating their deep branches. Careful dissection can

enable the preservation of the spinal accessory nerve branches to the upper trapezius muscle, thus preserving its function.

Tissue Expansion

When timing of reconstruction is not critical (i.e., excision of a benign lesion), tissue expansion (Chapter 10) may represent an alternative option. In addition, this technique may be useful in secondary revision of existing scars, skin grafts, or excision of skin paddles of previously performed free

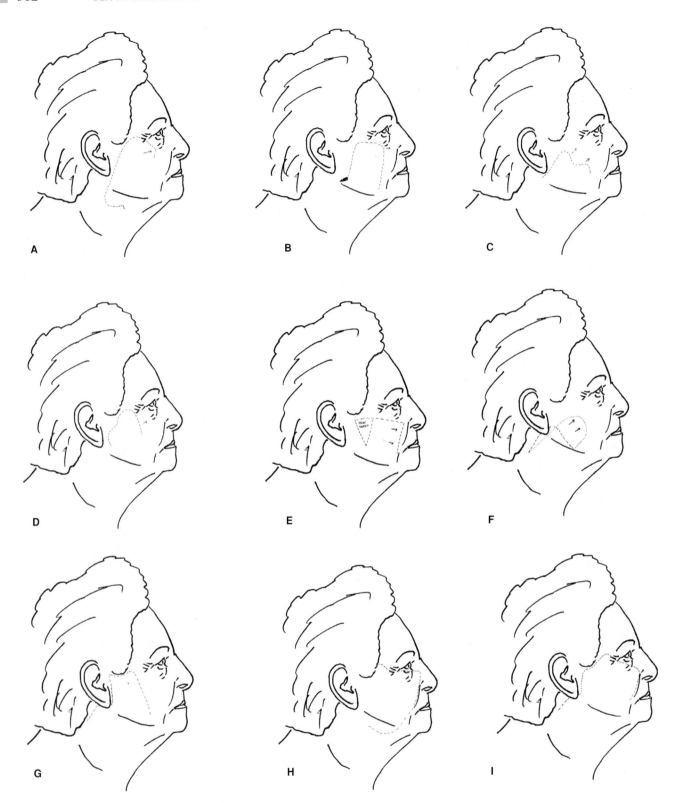

FIGURE 37.7. Various designs for cervicofacial rotation flap closure of cheek defects. **A:** Esser; **(B)** Blascowicz; **(C)** Ferris Smith; **(D)** Mustarde; **(E)** Converse; **(F)** Stark; **(G)** Juri and Juri; **(H)** Zide and Schruder; **(I)** Kroll. (Adapted from Al-Shunnar B, Manson P. Cheek reconstruction with laterally based flaps. *Clin Plast Surg.* 2001;28:283–296, with permission.)

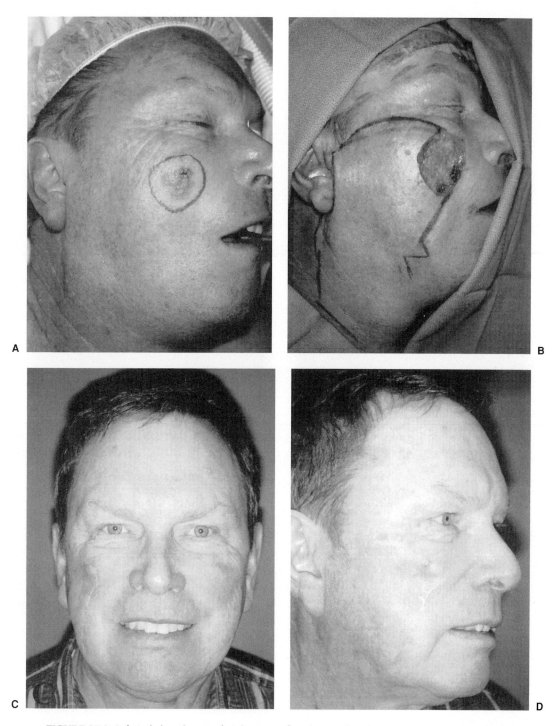

FIGURE 37.8. Inferiorly based cervicofacial rotation flap closure of Mohs resection for basal cell cancer. Note excision of dog-ear along nasolabial fold. **A:** Planned resection. **B:** Defect and flap design. **C** and **D:** Postoperative appearance.

flaps. In these settings, tissue expansion has the advantage of transferring potentially sensate skin that is of similar color, texture, and hair-bearing status while minimizing donor defects.

Although simple in concept, tissue expansion of the cheek is highly technical and can be associated with high rates of complications (7). Despite these difficulties, however, the expanded skin is salvageable in most instances, and successful reconstruction is usually achieved. Careful preoperative planning with regards to patient selection, expander size, and incisions used for

expander and fill-valve placement are critical determinants of success (8).

Wieslander has outlined guidelines for tissue expansion of the head and neck based on his experience with more than 100 patients over a 6-year period (8). These guidelines include the following: the width and length of the expander are at least as large, preferably larger, than the defect; the access incisions are kept small and as far away from the lesion as possible; access incisions are oriented perpendicular to the lesion; expansion of the lesion should be avoided; straight incisions bordering

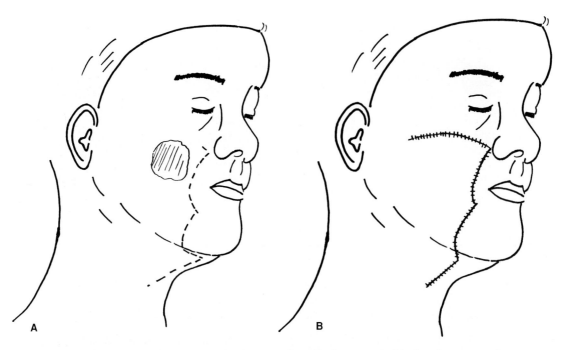

FIGURE 37.9. Laterally based cervicofacial rotation flap. Skin flaps are raised in the subcutaneous plane and rotated/advanced to fill in the defect. **A:** Defect and flap design. **B:** After flap transfer.

the defect are avoided; fill-valves are placed away from (>7 cm) and below or lateral to the expander pocket; expanders are filled intraoperatively to safest maximal amount to avoid seroma/hematoma; postoperative expansion should be delayed for 10 to 14 days; overexpansion by 30% to 50% is recommended; the capsule is incised and capsulectomy is avoided at the time of flap transposition.

Microsurgical Reconstruction

Microsurgical reconstruction is an important option for complex defects involving multiple tissue layers. These techniques are also useful for resurfacing massive skin resections and in patients in whom local flaps may not be available (e.g., previous neck dissection, facial burns) or advisable (contaminated wounds, history of radiation therapy). Resurfacing of extensive intraoral or through-and-through defects and contour deformities are additional potential indications for the use of microsurgical tissue transfer.

Although a number of flap options have been described, the radial forearm, parascapular, rectus abdominus, anterolateral thigh flap, and free fibula flap have been the most useful in our experience. The choice of free flap is dependent on the amount of external skin, intraoral lining, and soft-tissue contour requirements. In addition, the availability and location of the recipient vessels must be carefully determined.

Radial Forearm Flap

The radial forearm flap is a fasciocutaneous flap based on the radial artery. The flap is an excellent source of thin, pliable skin with a long, reliable pedicle. The flap has a dual venous drainage with the cephalic vein and radial vena comitans. Sensate reconstructions may be performed using the lateral antebrachial cutaneous nerve. The forearm flap is an excellent choice for defects requiring a thin coverage of skin (Fig. 37.11). In addition, the flap may be folded upon itself to provide more bulk or to provide coverage of through and through cheek de-

fects (Fig. 37.12). Multiple skin islands may be designed along the length of the flap and the flap may be de-epithelized or thinned to allow soft-tissue contouring. A short segment of the radial bone may be harvested as vascularized bone with the flap. The main drawbacks of this flap include donor-site scarring and color/texture mismatch with local tissues. In addition, the flap may be hair-bearing in some men.

Parascapular Flap

The parascapular flap is also a fasciocutaneous flap based on the circumflex scapular vessels. This flap has more bulk than the radial forearm flap and is useful in reconstruction of composite resections such as radical parotidectomy (Fig. 37.13). The flap may be harvested with a segment of scapular bone (up to 14 cm). In addition, the latissimus dorsi muscle can be harvested on a common pedicle, resulting in a large amount of soft tissues useful in reconstruction of massive defects. In general, this flap has a better color match with facial skin than most other microvascular flaps and is associated with minimal functional deficits, although the donor-site scar tends to widen if large flaps are designed. The flap is not usually useful for through-and-through defects and its pedicle length is shorter and more difficult to dissect than the radial forearm flap. In addition, parascapular and scapular flap dissection requires lateral positioning of the patient, making simultaneous flap harvest and tumor resection difficult.

Rectus Abdominus Flap

The rectus abdominus myocutaneous flap is a workhorse flap for facial reconstruction. The use of this flap for cheek reconstruction is more limited, however. The flap is usually designed with a vertical skin paddle and its primary indications are reconstruction of complex defects including multiple layers. The pedicle vessels are the deep inferior epigastric artery and vein and are highly reliable. Pedicle length may be lengthened through intramuscular dissection and may be as long as 14 to 15 cm. The flap may be bulky, particularly in obese patients, and secondary revisions with liposuction and direct excision

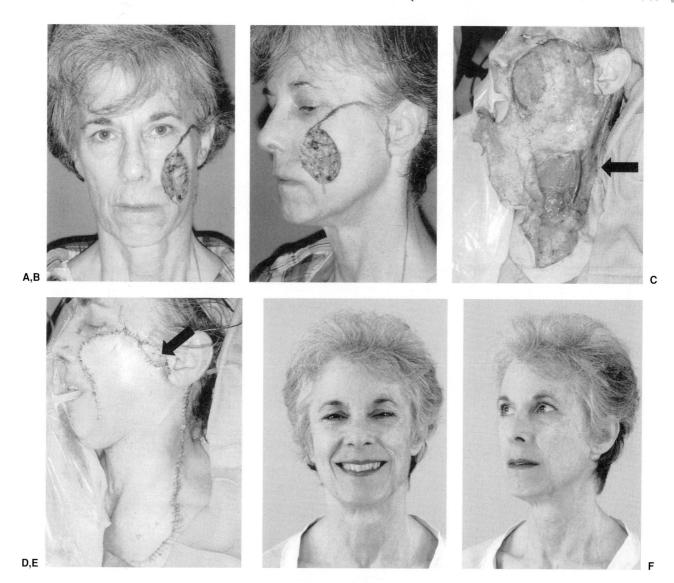

FIGURE 37.10. Cervicopectoral rotation flap. Preoperative (**A, B**), intraoperative (**C, D**), and postoperative (**E, F**) photographs of cervicopectoral rotation flap for large cheek defect resulting from basal cell cancer excision. The flap is elevated in the subcutaneous plane until a point approximately 2 cm below the angle of the mandible at which point the platysma is included with the flap (*dark arrow in C*). A small skin graft was necessary below the hairline to obtain tension-free closure (*arrow in D*). Note good contour and acceptable final scar.

may be required. The flap can be folded upon itself for reconstruction of through-and-through defects of the cheek, but is likely to be too bulky in most patients. The amount of muscle harvested with the flap can be tailored to fit the defect and is particularly useful for obliterating radical resections involving the maxillary sinus and the overlying cheek skin. Recently, perforator flaps (deep inferior epigastric perforator flap) that include only perforating vessels without harvesting rectus muscle have been described for head and neck reconstruction. These flaps have the advantage of being less bulky and may be associated with less donor-site pain and abdominal wall laxity or hernias. The potential drawbacks to the use of the rectus flap for cheek reconstruction include donor-site complications and bulkiness of the flap necessitating secondary revisions.

Anterolateral Thigh Flap

The anterolateral thigh flap is a fasciocutaneous flap based on the perforating vessels of the descending branch of the lateral circumflex femoral artery and vein. The flap may be thin and pliable, depending on the patient's body habitus, and is useful for providing a large amount of skin together with a variable amount of vastus lateralis muscle to fill complex defects (Fig. 37.14). The flap may be thinned somewhat at the time of flap harvest, however, aggressive thining may be associated with partial flap necrosis. Alternatively, secondary revisions with liposuction and direct excision may be required. Thin patients may be good candidates for reconstruction of through-and-through cheek defects based on dissection of multiple perforating branches. Pedicle dissection is more difficult than the radial forearm flap because of anatomic variability; however, large-caliber vessels are available in most instances. Dissection of the pedicle vessels to their origin can result in a lengthy pedicle that enables microvascular anastomosis to the neck vessels while avoiding vein grafting. The advantages of this flap include more favorable donor-site scarring than the radial forearm flap, potential for simultaneous flap harvest and tumor ablation, and the ability to tailor the thickness of the flap by altering the amount of vastus lateralis muscle resection. Knee

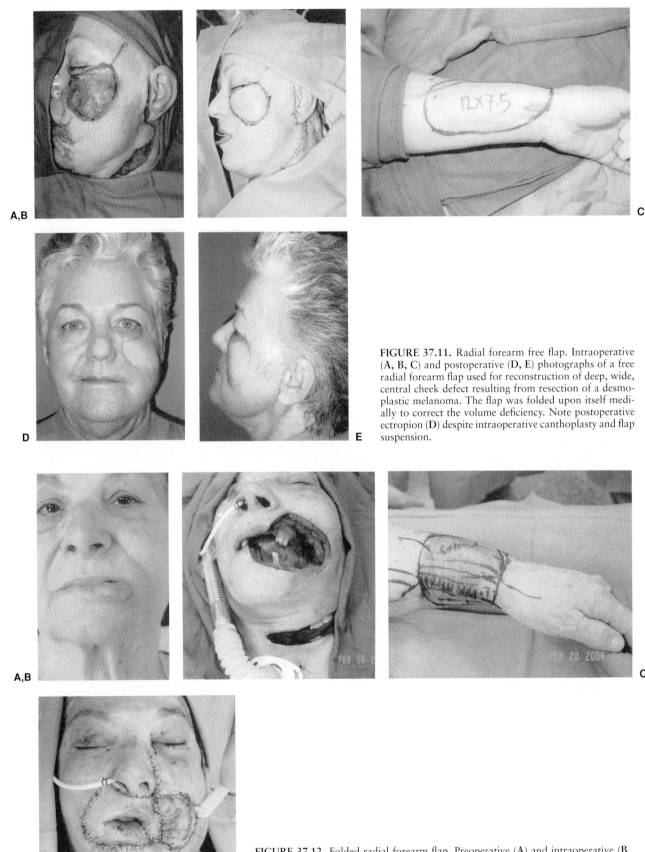

FIGURE 37.11. Radial forearm free flap. Intraoperative (**A, B, C**) and postoperative (**D, E**) photographs of a free radial forearm flap used for reconstruction of deep, wide, central cheek defect resulting from resection of a desmoplastic melanoma. The flap was folded upon itself medially to correct the volume deficiency. Note postoperative ectropion (**D**) despite intraoperative canthoplasty and flap suspension.

FIGURE 37.12. Folded radial forearm flap. Preoperative (**A**) and intraoperative (**B, C, D**) photographs of a folded radial forearm flap for intraoral and external coverage of a complex cheek defect. Note that lip continuity was restored using lip rotation flaps (*right*, Karapandzic; *left*, Estlander) thereby avoiding interposition of the radial forearm flap in the lip defect.

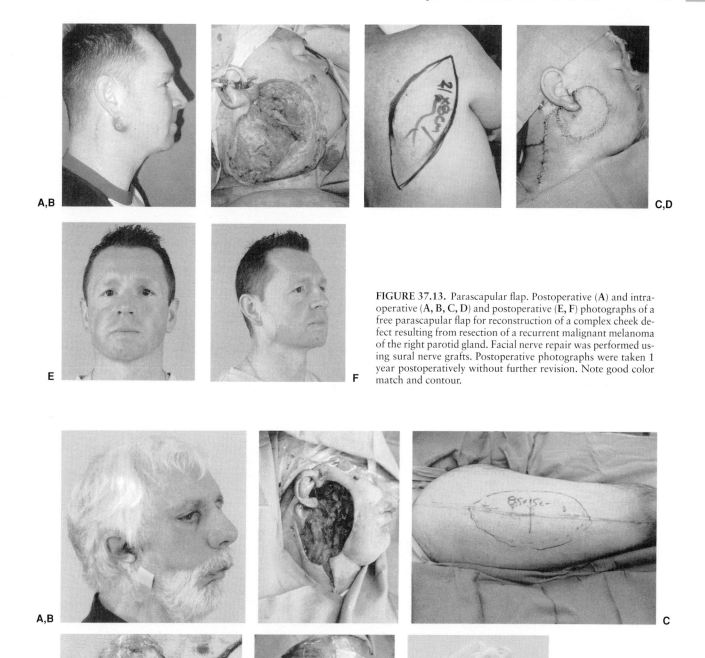

FIGURE 37.13. Parascapular flap. Postoperative (**A**) and intraoperative (**A, B, C, D**) and postoperative (**E, F**) photographs of a free parascapular flap for reconstruction of a complex cheek defect resulting from resection of a recurrent malignant melanoma of the right parotid gland. Facial nerve repair was performed using sural nerve grafts. Postoperative photographs were taken 1 year postoperatively without further revision. Note good color match and contour.

FIGURE 37.14. Anterolateral thigh flap. Preoperative (**A**), intraoperative (**B, C, D, E**), and postoperative (**F**) photographs of a massive cheek and neck defect resulting from resection of osteoradionecrosis and infection of the right mandible. The patient had a previous parotid tumor treated with wide resection, radical neck dissection, and maximal doses of external beam radiation therapy. Note severe atrophy of the surrounding tissues. A thin anterolateral thigh flap together with a small portion of the vastus lateralis muscle (**D**) was used to cover the cheek defect and close the small intraoral defect resulting from resection.

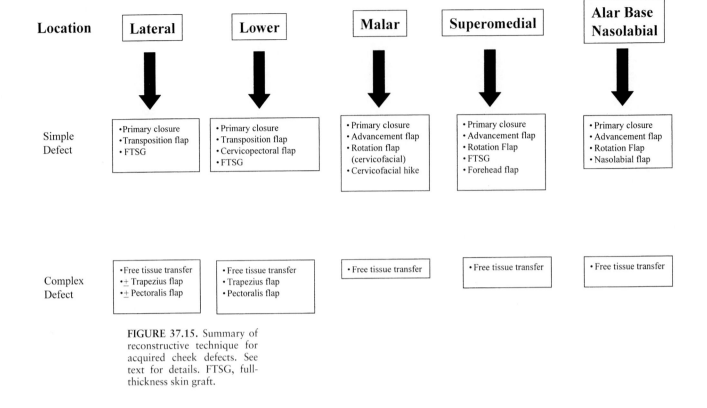

FIGURE 37.15. Summary of reconstructive technique for acquired cheek defects. See text for details. FTSG, full-thickness skin graft.

extension is rarely affected unless there is inadvertent injury to the femoral nerve. Color match to facial skin is poor, however, as is the hair patterns.

Fibula Osteocutaneous Flap

The fibula osteocutaneous flap (Chapter 41) is an excellent source of vascularized bone (up to 30 cm) and a variable amount of skin and soft tissues. Portions of the soleus muscle and flexor hallucis longus muscle can be harvested as vascularized muscle. The flap is based on the peroneal vessels and is useful for reconstruction of segmental mandibular defects that include external skin resections. The flap may be harvested at the time of tumor ablation, and the skin paddle may be folded upon itself to provide both intra- and extra-oral lining. The fibula skin paddle is most reliable in the distal portions of the leg where the perforating vessels tend to follow a septocutaneous pattern. Care must be taken during flap harvest to avoid injury to the neurovascular structures of the lower extremity and to preserve adequate bone proximally and distally to avoid knee and ankle instability, respectively. In addition, the vascular supply of the leg should be carefully evaluated preoperatively, either by physical examination or in combination with radiologic studies, to avoid lower extremity ischemia.

CONCLUSION

Reconstruction of cheek defects requires careful planning and execution. Although the choice of surgical options must be individualized, an overall guide for the practitioner is summarized in Figure 37.15.

References

1. Zide B, Longaker, M. Cheek surface reconstruction: best choices according to zones. *Oper Tech Plast Reconstr Surg.* 1998;5:26.
2. Jackson I. *Local Flaps for Head and Neck Reconstruction.* St. Louis, Quality Medical Publishing, 2002.
3. Longaker M, Glat P, Zide BM, et al. Deep-plane cervicofacial "hike": anatomic basis with dog-ear blepharoplasty. *Plast Reconstr Surg.* 1997;99:16.
4. Chadawarkar R, Cervino A. Subunits of the cheek: an algorithm for the reconstruction of partial-thickness defects. *Br J Plast Surg.* 2003;56:135–139.
5. Al-Shunnar B, Manson P. Cheek reconstruction with laterally based flaps. *Clin Plast Surg.* 2001;28:283.
6. Kroll S, Reece G, Robb G, et al. Deep-plane cervicofacial rotation-advancement flap for reconstruction of large cheek defects. *Plast Reconstr Surg.* 1994;94:88.
7. Antonyshyn O, Gruss J, Zuker R, et al. Tissue expansion in head and neck reconstruction. *Plast Reconstr Surg.* 1988;82:58.
8. Wieslander J. Tissue expansion in the head and neck. *Scand J Plast Reconstr Hand Surg.* 1991;25:47.

CHAPTER 38 ■ NASAL RECONSTRUCTION

FREDERICK J. MENICK

Life is about choices and compromises. For a nasal reconstruction to be successful, the problem must be analyzed, options identified, limitations appreciated, and the best solution chosen to achieve the desired outcome.

THE NOSE

Anatomically, the nose is covered by external skin, supported by a mid layer of bone and cartilage, and lined primarily by mucoperichondrium. If missing, each layer must be replaced. Aesthetically, the nose is a central facial feature of high priority. To appear normal, it must have the proper dimension, position, and symmetry. Its surface can be divided into aesthetic subunits—adjacent topographic areas of characteristic skin quality, border outline, and three-dimensional contour—the subunits of the dorsum, tip, columella, and the paired sidewalls, alae, and soft triangles (Fig. 38.1). Restoration of these "expected" characteristics permits a reconstruction to "appear normal" (1–3). Functionally, the nose must allow unobstructed breathing.

PLANNING

Thoughtful consideration of the patient, the wound, and the available donor materials helps to identify the most appropriate treatment.

The Patient

Most patients want the wound healed and their appearance restored to its preoperative condition. In some cases, however, age, associated illness, or patient desire may dictate a less complicated, quicker repair with minimal surgery or stages. A nasal wound can be allowed to heal by secondary intention. If full thickness, the cover and lining can simply be sutured to one another, accepting a permanent deformity.

If a more complex repair is indicated, the surgeon must be aware that previous surgical treatments for skin cancer, radiation, trauma, or rhinoplasty add scars, may interfere with blood supply, impair healing, or preclude a specific flap option. Operative time, anesthetic requirements, hospitalization needs, the number of stages, and time to completion must be considered.

The Wound

The site, size, depth, and wound condition influence the reconstructive approach. Frequently, the wound is distorted and does not reflect the true tissue loss. It may be enlarged by edema, local anesthesia, gravity, or resting skin tension or diminished by wound contracture due to secondary healing. A preliminary operation may be needed to release an old scar, reposition normal to normal, or open the airway.

In all circumstances, missing tissues must be replaced in the exact amount. If too little is replaced, adjacent landmarks will be distorted, collapsing underlying cartilage grafts. If too much is resupplied, adjacent landmarks will be pushed outward, distorting the external shape or pushing the lining inward, obstructing the airway.

A superficial defect with residual well-vascularized subcutaneous tissue will accept a skin graft. However, exposed cartilage or bone without perichondrium or periosteum will not. The skin of the dorsum and sidewall is thin, smooth, pliable, and mobile. The skin of the columella and alar rim is thin but adherent. The skin of the tip and ala is thick and stiff, pitted with sebaceous glands. Skin grafts, even when taken from a donor site of similar skin quality, will appear shiny and atrophic. Skin grafts are best used within the thin skin of the dorsum or sidewall or the alar rim or columella rather than within the thicker skin of the tip and ala, where they will blend poorly and may appear as a patch. Local flaps because of skin laxity and mobility are most easily used within the dorsum or sidewall.

The nasal bones and cartilage support the nose, impart a nasal shape to the soft tissues both of lining and cover, and brace any repair against the force of the myofibroblast contraction. If missing, support must be replaced. The normal ala is shaped by compact fibrofatty soft tissue and contains no cartilage, but cartilaginous support must be placed along the new nostril margin to maintain shape and projection when an alar rim is reconstructed. In the past, bone and cartilage grafts have been placed secondarily, months after the initial reconstruction. Unfortunately, once the soft tissues have healed in place, they become scarred and can rarely be re-expanded and reshaped by cartilage grafts at a later date. In almost all circumstances, support should be resupplied prior to the completion of wound healing.

Local flaps do not add skin to the nose. They rearrange the residual skin and redistribute it over the entire nasal surface. Under the tension of local skin rearrangement, local flaps may collapse newly positioned cartilage grafts. If cartilage must be replaced, therefore, a regional flap from the cheek or forehead to resurface the nose will be required.

In summary, nasal defects may be classified as small and superficial or large and deep. A small, superficial lesion is one that is less than 1.5 cm in size, with an intact underlying cartilage framework. If a vascularized bed of perichondrium or periosteum is present, a skin graft may be placed or the defect resurfaced with a local nasal flap. If the defect is greater than 1.5 cm, there may not be enough residual skin over the nose to spread over its entire nasal surface without distorting the tip or alar rims. A large, deep defect is one that is greater than 1.5 cm or one requiring the replacement of a cartilage framework or lining. A regional flap from the forehead or cheek will most often be employed for nasal resurfacing.

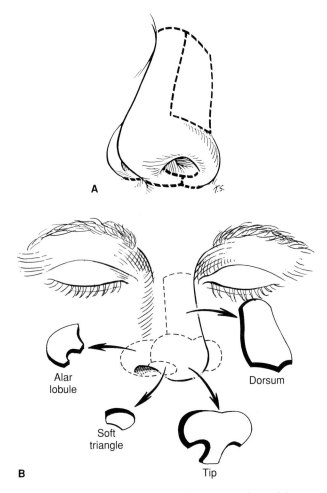

FIGURE 38.1. Aesthetic units and aesthetic junction lines of the nose. A: Lateral wall subunit. B: The nasal lobule and its aesthetic subunits.

Most often, a failure in repair results from a shortage of lining. If the defect is full thickness, lining replacement must be vascular enough to support the early replacement of cartilage grafts, supple enough to conform to their proper shape, and thin enough that it neither stuffs the airway nor distorts the external shape.

Infection or tissue ischemia may preclude immediate reconstruction. Soft tissue foreign bodies, such as injectable or implantable silicone or other allografts, increase the risk of infection, fibrosis, and later extrusion.

The Donor Site

Defects require replacement of variable amounts of cover, support, and lining. Each donor material is chosen by evaluating the quality of the material needed, the available excess (which can be shared from the donor site to recipient site), and its ability to be transferred as a skin graft to a vascular bed or by a pedicle with an adequate arc of rotation.

Covering skin must match the face—only skin from above the clavicle will suffice. Skin grafts lie flat, rarely pincushioning, whereas flaps may trapdoor. The fibroblast contraction under a flap will enhance the repair of a convex surface unit such as the ala but distort the flat sidewall. Skin grafts are best used for superficial defects involving a planar or concave surface. Flaps

are best employed for deeper wounds requiring replacement of soft tissue bulk in convex areas.

GENERAL PRINCIPLES OF REPAIR

1. Establish a goal. The objective may be a healed wound or the reestablishment of normal appearance. Priorities must be set, stages identified, and materials and techniques planned.
2. Visualize the end result. The normal is described in terms of skin quality, outline, and three-dimensional contour. Materials and methods are chosen to achieve this end.
3. Create a plan. Nothing happens by chance. The operative steps and, if necessary, the surgical stages required to transfer tissues for cover, lining, and support are determined.
4. Consider altering the wound in site, size, depth, or position if this will assist the repair. Although all patients have a fear of scars, most nasal wounds heal with minimal scarring. Scars interfere with success only when they distort the expected subunits. If a defect of the convex tip or alar subunit will be covered with a flap and the wound encompasses greater than 50% of that subunit, consider discarding adjacent normal skin within the subunit and resurfacing the entire subunit, rather than just patching the defect. Inevitable trap door contraction (along with cartilage grafts) then contributes to restoration of the expected convexity. If residual tissues are distorted by the old scar, the remaining normal landmarks are returned to their normal position first.
5. Use the ideal or contralateral normal as a guide. Fresh wounds may not represent the true size or shape of the tissues that are actually missing due to the distortion of edema, tension, or gravity. A template of the contralateral normal is made to create a mirror image of the true defect or subunit.
6. Replace the missing tissue exactly to avoid overfilling or underfilling of the defect.
7. Choose ideal donor materials. Covering skin must be thin and conform to the underlying subcutaneous architecture while matching the face in color and texture. Cartilage and bone grafts must be thin but supportive. A nasal framework must extend from the nasal bones superiorly to the alar margin inferiorly and from the tip anteriorly to the maxilla posteriorly. If missing, the support framework must be replaced. Such a reconstruction supports the repair against gravity, shapes the overlying cover and underlying lining, and braces the repair against later scar contraction. Each support graft is carved to create a subsurface framework, which will be reflected through thin, supple covering skin. Lining materials must be vascular enough to support the positioning of early cartilage grafts and supple enough to conform to the shape of the overlying support grafts yet thin enough that they neither stuff the airway nor bulge outward, distorting the external shape.
8. Ensure a stable platform. A composite facial wound that involves nose and adjacent cheek and lip may require a preliminary step. The lip and cheek are repaired before the nose. A shifting lip/cheek platform that has pulled a reconstructed nose inferiorly and laterally under the influence of edema, gravity, and tension will ruin an otherwise beautiful result. Therefore, composite defects are usually reconstructed in stages.

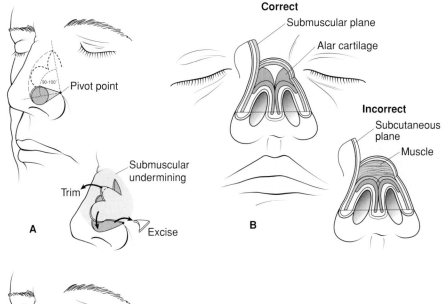

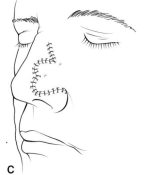

FIGURE 38.2. Bilobed flap. **A:** The skin of the superior two thirds of the nose is mobile and in slight excess, whereas the skin of the tip and ala is adherent and tight. The excess in the superior nose is transferred in one stage to the tip with a bilobed flap. The defect created by the first flap is closed with a second lobe, which can be primarily sutured without distortion. **B:** The flap is elevated in the areolar plane above the perichondrium and includes the fat and nasalis muscles with the skin. **C:** Temporary quilting sutures are useful to close dead space.

SURGICAL TECHNIQUES

Cover: Small, Superficial Defects

Small, superficial defects that lie on planar or concave surfaces and do not border adjacent mobile landmarks that might be distorted by wound contraction can be allowed to heal by secondary intention.

Defects less than 0.5 cm can be closed primarily within the more mobile skin of the dorsum or sidewall.

Full-thickness skin grafts from the forehead, postauricular, or supraclavicular areas are useful within the thin skin zones of the upper two thirds of the nose. Although unpredictable in color and texture, the smooth and atrophic surface of a skin graft tends to blend within these smooth, thin skin zones. Skin grafts are immobilized with a light bolus dressing for 48 hours and must be placed on a well-vascularized bed. The principle of subunit excision is not used when a defect is resurfaced with a skin graft.

Composite chondrocutaneous grafts from the helix, rim, or ear lobe can be used to repair small defects (less than 1.5 cm) along the alar rim and columella. Composite grafts consist of variable amounts of cartilage positioned in a sandwich of an outer and inner layer of skin. Any portion of the graft greater than 5 mm distant from the vascular recipient bed may not survive. So the larger the "skin-only" extension of a composite graft overlapping adjacent vascularized soft tissue, the more likely it is that the composite graft will be successful. Initially, they appear white, but over the next 24 hours, they become blue and congested as vascular flow increases. Over the next 3 to 7 days they become pink as the blood supply is established. Postoperative cooling for the first 36 hours may decrease the

metabolic rate of the skin graft until vascularization occurs and improve "take."

Except as a temporary wound dressing, split-thickness skin grafts are rarely employed. Split-thickness skin grafts provide no bulk, contract significantly, and usually hyperpigment.

Single-lobe transposition flaps (banner) provide an excellent color match. For defects less than 1.5 cm in the lax mobile skin of the upper one third, they are an alternative to skin grafts. Their 90-degree arc of rotation makes them unreliable within the thick, stiff skin of the tip or ala due to dog-ear and vascularity concerns (4).

The geometric bilobe flap is useful for defects up to 1.5 cm in the thick skin zones of the tip and ala (Fig. 38.2) (5). Rules for its design are as follows:

1. Allow no more than 50 degrees of rotation for each lobe.
2. Excise the triangle of dog-ear between the defect and flap pivot point.
3. Undermine widely above the perichondrium on both sides of the incision.
4. Make the diameter of the first lobe equal to the defect. The second lobe may be reduced in width to ease primary closure of the secondary defect.

Dorsal and tip defects can also be resurfaced with a rotation-advancement flap of the residual dorsal skin (6). The dorsal nasal flap (Fig. 38.3) provides good coverage of defects up to 1.5 to 2 cm in size that lie at least .5 cm above the alar rims and no lower than the tip defining points. It has been used with and without a glabella extension.

A superiorly based, single-stage, nasolabial flap can be designed as an extension of a sliding cheek advancement flap (Fig. 38.4). It is useful to resurface defects of the sidewall and ala. A Burow's triangle is excised at the superior pivot point toward

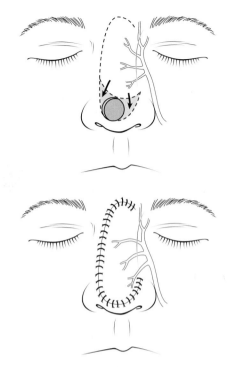

FIGURE 38.3. Dorsal nasal flap. Residual skin and soft tissue of the superior nose is transferred to the dorsum and tip. A Burow's triangle excision in the glabella or nasal root may be needed on closure.

the inner canthus. Periosteal sutures recreate the nasofacial sulcus and minimize tension on the transposed flap. Rather than just redistributing residual nasal skin, this flap adds additional skin from the cheek and avoids the risk of alar rim or tip distortion associated with many of the other local flaps.

Cover: Large, Deep Defects

Two-Stage Nasolabial Flap

A moderate amount of excess skin is available within the nasolabial fold for reconstruction of the ala (7). Although occasionally used as a simple advancement flap to resurface sidewall defects, nasolabial tissue is most commonly transferred in two stages to resurface the ala as a subunit (Fig. 38.5). Its size and

arc of rotation are limited, and it is not useful to recover the tip, dorsum, or a heminasal defect.

When greater than 50% of the ala subunit is missing, residual normal skin is discarded. An exact foil template based on the contralateral normal ala is positioned along the nasolabial crease. The flap is elevated distally with a few millimeters of subcutaneous fat, maintaining a proximal deep superior subcutaneous base, perfused by perforators from the facial and angular arteries. A primary cartilage graft is positioned on residual or repaired alar lining, and the flap is transposed medially to resurface missing alar skin. The donor defect within the nasolabial fold is closed primarily. A few weeks later, the pedicle is divided, the inset is partially re-elevated and excess soft tissue sculpted, and the flap inset is completed. The two-stage nasolabial flap can achieve aesthetic alar subunit reconstruction.

The Forehead Flap

The forehead is acknowledged as the ideal donor for nasal reconstruction due to its superb color and texture match, vascularity, and ability to resurface all or part of the nose. Supplied by a vast arcade of vessels from the supraorbital, supratrochlear, superficial temporal, postauricular, and occipital arteries, the forehead skin has been transposed on numerous pedicles (Fig. 38.6). Most of these designs have only occasional application. Most commonly, a vertical paramedian flap based on a single supratrochlear artery is designed extending from the brow to the hairline. The pivot point can be lowered by incising across the medial brow towards the medial canthus. The flap can be lengthened by including hair-bearing scalp. Hair follicles are later removed by depilation if necessary.

Traditionally the forehead flap is transferred in two stages (8). The forehead is thicker than nasal skin. Initially, the distal flap is thinned by excising frontalis and subcutaneous fat before transposition to the nose. Two weeks later, the pedicle is divided and the proximal aspect debulked while completing the inset.

In smokers or in patients with major defects, the flap is best transposed in three stages. Initially, the flap is transposed without thinning (9). Three weeks after the first operation, the flap is elevated off its bed at a superficial subcutaneous level. The underlying excess bulk of frontalis and subcutaneous fat is excised from the recipient bed. The thin forehead skin is then returned to cover the sculpted recipient site. The pedicle is divided 3 weeks later (6 weeks after the initial transfer). The three-stage method ensures maximal vascularity, precise thinning and soft tissue sculpturing,

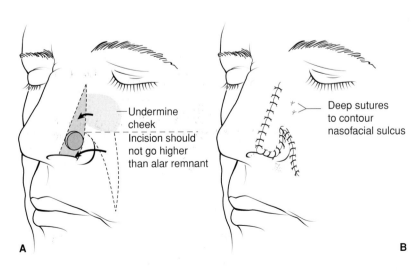

A

B

FIGURE 38.4. The one-stage nasolabial flap. **A:** Defects of the sidewell and ala can be resurfaced by advancement of a cheek flap with a skin extension from cheek excess adjacent to the nasolabial fold. Extra skin may be excised inferior to the defect if does not extend to the rim to hide the scar along the rim. Prime support is placed to brace and suppor the repair. **B:** Deep buried sutures preserve the nasofacial contour.

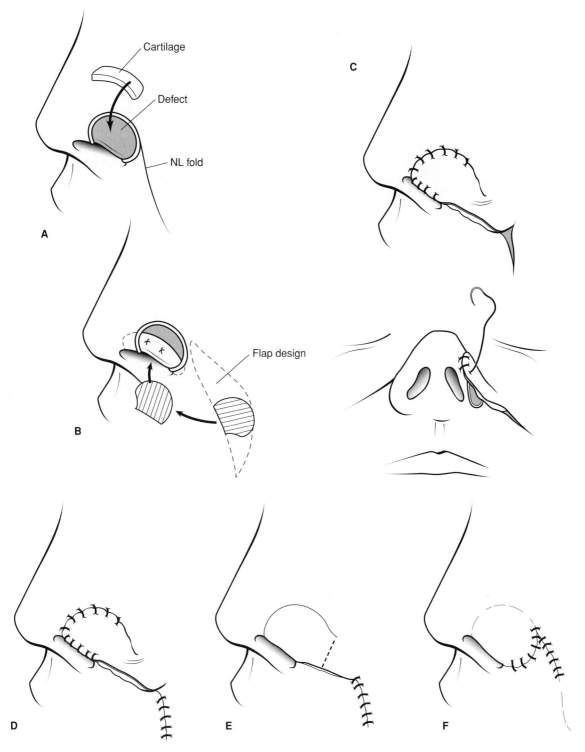

FIGURE 38.5. The two-stage nasolabial (NL) flap. **A:** The ala is best resurfaced with a two-stage flap as a complete alar subunit. Residual normal adjacent skin is discarded with the subunit if the defect is greater than 50% of the subunit. Lining is supported with a primary ear or septal or rib cartilage graft. **B:** Based on an exact pattern of the opposite ala, a template is positioned precisely along the nasolabial fold. Distally the flap is tapered to permit excision of the dog-ear on closure. Proximally, the skin pedicle should be tapered to keep the final scar of closure off the nose while maintaining a wider vascular subcutaneous base during flap elevation. The distal flap is thinned, maintaining 2 to 3 mm of subcutaneous fat. **C, D:** At the first stage the flap is transposed to resurface the entire. The cheek donor site is closed by advancement. **E, F:** Three weeks later the pedicle is transected. The proximal inset is re-elevated, sculpting excess subcutaneous fat and scar into an alar shape, and the skin is trimmed to precisely resurface the lateral alar defect. Excess soft tissue is excised in the medial cheek and the donor closure completed.

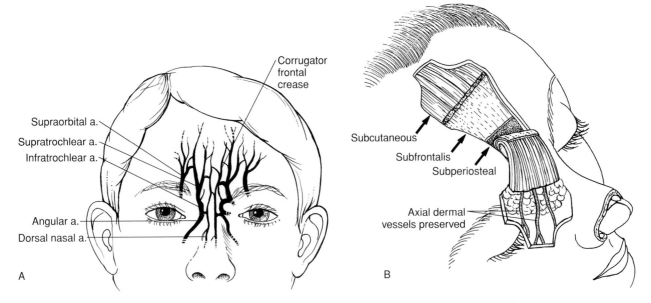

FIGURE 38.6. Forehead flap. **A:** Blood supply is abundant in central forehead. **B:** Paramedian flap design. In the traditional two-stage technique, the frontalis is left on the forehead and skin only is transferred to the defect, as shown here. In the three-stage technique, the full thickness of the forehead is often transferred and thinned at an intermediate stage. A, artery.

and, most important, the useful application of skin grafts or a folded distal extension of the forehead flap for a nasal lining.

The forehead donor defect, although traditionally skin grafted, is best left to heal by secondary intention. Preliminary forehead skin expansion has been recommended to allow primary closure of the forehead defect. However, skin expansion delays the repair, may be associated with secondary late contraction, and has little advantage. It may be useful in secondary nasal reconstruction or in patients with very limited vertical forehead height, less than 3 to 4 cm.

Distant Transfers

Multiple flaps can be taken from the forehead donor site without significant deformity. However, if the forehead is unavailable and the nasal defect too large for repair by a skin graft or local flap, replacement tissue can be brought from distant sites. Arm flaps, cervical flaps, abdominal tube pedicles, and deltopectoral flaps are largely of historical interest. Free flaps, principally the radial forehead flap, have been employed. Unfortunately, distant tissues provide poor color and texture match to adjacent facial skin. The future of free flap nasal reconstruction lies in their use to restore missing lining in the massive, irradiated or cocaine nose, not in its use for nasal cover.

Support

If missing, a supporting framework must be replaced to re-establish support, shape, and resist scar contraction. Each graft is fashioned to mold the overlying skin (and the underlying lining) into the expected nasal shape: a dorsal buttress, a sidewall brace, tip grafts for projection and definition, and an alar batten (even though the ala normally contains no cartilage) (Fig. 38.7). Septal and ear cartilage and rib costicartilage grafts are most commonly used. Traditionally, support grafts have been placed only to support the bridge (cantilever dorsal graft) or alar rim (composite prefabricated rim grafts). Months after the

nasal repair, the shape of soft tissue becomes distorted permanently by scar. Ideally, the support framework should be placed prior to flap division. Supportive grafts are designed to replace the missing nasal bones, upper lateral cartilage, and tip cartilages. Alar reconstructions include cartilage grafts to prevent rim collapse.

In extensive midline defects the septum may be absent. A strong central midline support must be re-established to

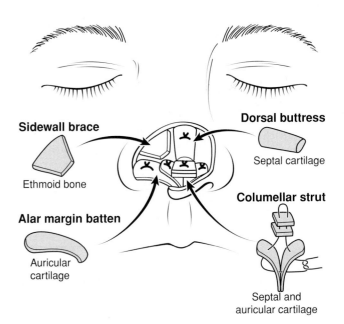

FIGURE 38.7. Primary or delayed grafts of cartilage or bone must be placed before the completion of reconstruction to shape and support the soft tissue against gravity and scar contracture. Support must be present or must be restored to all nasal subunits. (Redrawn after Burget G, Menick F. Nasal support and lining: the marriage of beauty and blood supply. *Plast Reconstr Surg.* 1989;84:189, with permission.)

prevent soft tissue collapse of the tip and dorsum. Several methods are useful, often in combination. When the septal composite lining flap is pivoted anteriorly, both lining and central support are positioned simultaneously. This creates a basic platform on which to rest other grafts. A cantilever dorsal graft of rib or cranial bone can be fixed with wire or a screw to the nasal bones (which are first lowered to avoid excessive radix augmentation). This graft extends from the nasal bones to the tip. A rib cartilage or bone graft in the shape of an "L" can be positioned from the nasal bones to the maxilla, but they tend to create an excessively wide columella.

Lining

Ideally, lining should be thin, supple, and vascular.

Local Hingeover Lining Flaps

If a full-thickness defect is allowed to heal, external skin and scar bordering the defect can be turned over to supply lining, based on the scar along the border of the defect. Such lining flaps are thick and stiff and risk necrosis if greater than 1.5 cm in length. The airway, at the point of the hingeover, is often constricted. Although useful for limited rim defects or in salvage cases, they are not a first choice (10).

Prelaminated Skin Graft and Cartilage for Lining of the Forehead Flap

During a preliminary operation, several weeks before transfer, composite grafts from the ear or septum or separate pieces of skin and cartilage can be placed under the distal end of a forehead flap. These preinstalled lining grafts can create a satisfactory alar margin but may not create an ideal nasal shape after transfer. The technique is most useful for smaller defects in elderly patients in which less complex procedures are indicated due to health concerns.

Intranasal Lining Flaps

Residual nasal lining, although not apparent at first glance, remains within the residual nose and pyriform aperture. The nose is perfused by branches of the anterior ethmoid artery along the dorsum and the angular artery at the alar base and from septal branches of the superior labial artery, which perfuse the right and left septal mucoperichondrial lining leaves (11,12).

In smaller unilateral defects, residual vestibular skin lying above the defect can be incised as a bipedicle flap 6 mm wide, based laterally at the alar base and medially on the septum. This flap is advanced inferiorly to line the alar rim. The defect that remains above is filled by another method (a contralateral septal lining flap or a skin graft).

In larger heminasal defects, a contralateral septal flap (Fig. 38.8) can be hinged and transposed laterally to line the lower vestibule and alar margin. A second mucoperichondrial flap, based dorsally on the anterior ethmoid vessel, is hinged laterally to line the upper vault. (This dorsal flap can be used alone to reconstruct an isolated defect of the sidewall or be combined with the bipedicle vestibular flap).

In some cases an anteriorly based septal mucoperichondrial flap composed of the entire septum can be advanced out of the pyriform aperture based on branches of the right and left superior labial arteries located near the nasal spine (Fig. 38.9). This flap simultaneously supplies dorsal support and bilateral leaves of septal perichondrium, which can be reflected laterally to line the dorsum and vestibules.

Intranasal lining flaps are thin, vascular, and supple and allow the primary placement of cartilage grafts. They are associated, however, with moderate to significant intranasal manipulation and the associated morbidity of bleeding and crusting.

Skin Grafts for Lining

Simultaneous placement of the skin graft on the undersurface of a forehead flap at the time of its transfer has traditionally been unsuccessful. Cartilage grafts are precluded. As the skin graft shrinks, late collapse and distortion follows. However, a full-thickness skin graft of postauricular skin will survive on the deep surface of a forehead flap. Three weeks after transfer, the skin graft becomes integrated into the adjacent normal lining and is no longer dependent on a covering flap. Excess soft tissue can be excised during an intermediate operation, and cartilage grafts are placed. In this manner, a complete cartilage support structure is positioned prior to flap division in a delayed primary fashion, thus preventing significant shrinkage. The simplicity and the avoidance of intranasal manipulation

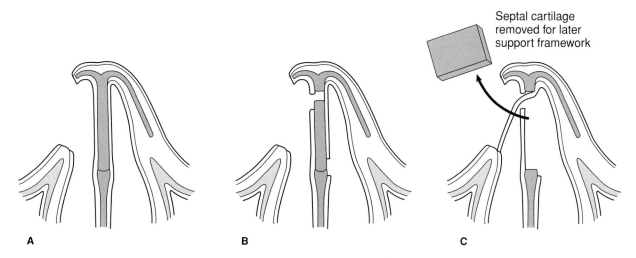

Septal cartilage removed for later support framework

FIGURE 38.8. The contralateral mucoperichondrial flap. Defects of the midvault can be lined with a dorsally based contralateral mucoperichondrial flap perfused by the anterior ethmoid arteries. **A:** Sidewall defect. **B, C:** The flap is passed through a dorsal slit in the ipsilateral septum and will provide lining for the midvault. Septal cartilage is harvested for primary cartilage grafts, which will support and shape the reconstructed midvault. The repaired lining and cartilage flaps are covered with a vascularized flap of cheek or forehead skin.

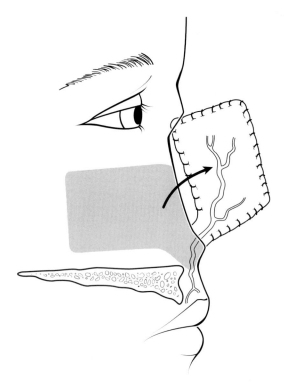

FIGURE 38.9. Septal composite flap. In subtotal nasal loss, the residual septum often remains and can be transposed out of the pyriform aperture based on the right and left septal branches of the superior labial arteries. Fixed superiorly to the residual dorsum, each leaf of the septal mucoperichondrium can be swung laterally to provide lining to the midvault and anterior vestibule.

make this an excellent option for defects less than 1.5 cm along the alar rim.

Folded Forehead Flap for Lining

Although the distal end of a forehead flap can be folded to supply lining, traditionally the technique has precluded the placement of primary support. The resultant alar rim remains thick, shapeless, and unsupported. However, realization that such folded skin becomes revascularized by adjacent lining and is no longer dependent on the covering flap for blood supply permits the elevation of the covering flap, leaving the folded lining in place. Three weeks after transfer, the skin covering aspect of the folded flap is incised along the planned alar rim during an intermediate operation and elevated with 2 to 3 mm of subcutaneous fat. Underlying excess soft tissue is excised from the reconstructed lining, creating thin, supple, and well-vascularized lining. Delayed primary support grafts are placed to support the ala and sidewall as needed. In this way, a complete support framework is positioned prior to pedicle division without intranasal manipulation. Unilateral defects of up to 2.5 cm are readily repaired. This folded technique may become the workhorse for modern nasal repair of full-thickness defects. The technique is simple and can produce excellent results.

References

1. Burget GC, Menick FJ. Subunit principle in nasal reconstruction. *Plastic Reconstr Surg.* 1985;76:239.
2. Menick F. Artistry in facial surgery: aesthetic perceptions and the subunit principle. In: Furnas D, ed. *Clinics in Plastic Surgery*, Vol. 14. Philadelphia: WB Saunders, 1987;723.
3. Millard DR. *Principlization of Plastic Surgery.* Boston: Little Brown, 1986.
4. Elliot RA Jr. Rotation flaps of the nose. *Plast Reconstr Surg.* 1969;44:1a47.
5. McGregor JC, Soutar DS. A critical assessment of the bilobed flap. *Br J Plast Surg.* 1981;34:197.
6. Marchac D, Toth B. The axial frontonasal flap revisited. *Plast Reconstr Surg.* 1985;76:686.
7. Herbert DC. A subcutaneous pedicle cheek flap for reconstruction of ala defects. *Br J Plast Surg.* 1978;31:79.
8. Menick FJ. The aesthetic use of the forehead for nasal reconstruction—The paramedian forehead flaps. In: Tobin G, ed. *Clinics in Plastic Surgery*. Philadelphia, WB Saunders, 1990;607.
9. Menick FJ. Ten-year experience in nasal reconstruction with the three-stage forehead flap. *Plast Reconstr Surg.* 2002;109:1839.
10. Millard DR. Aesthetic reconstructive rhinoplasty. *Clin Plast Surg.* 1981;8:169.
11. Burget GC, Menick FJ. Nasal reconstruction: seeking a fourth dimension: *Plast Reconstr Surg.* 1986;78:145.
12. Burget GC, Menick FJ. Nasal support and lining: the marriage of beauty and blood supply. *Plast Reconstr Surg.* 1989;84:189.

CHAPTER 39 ■ RECONSTRUCTION OF THE EYELIDS, CORRECTION OF PTOSIS, AND CANTHOPLASTY

MARTIN I. NEWMAN AND HENRY M. SPINELLI

EYELID ANATOMY AND PHYSIOLOGY

The eyelids are comprised of an upper and lower lid, a fold of complex, mobile tissue anterior to the globe. Closure of the eyelids affords protection to the globe. Opening of the eyelids is facilitated primarily by elevation of the upper lid and creates the resultant *palpebral fissure*. The lower lid remains essentially stable, but retracts appreciably on downward gaze. When the upper lid is open, it folds upon itself, creating a furrow or *superior sulcus*, superior to the globe and inferior to the supraorbital rim. Disruption of the supporting structures of the upper lid, such as levator dehiscence (see Correction of Eyelid Ptosis Section), may elevate or obliterate this fold. The upper and lower eyelids meet at angles known, respectively, as the medial and lateral *canthi* or *palpebral commissures*. In the normal, youthful, or aesthetically pleasing eye, the lateral canthus is inclined 10 to 15 degrees cephalad to the medial canthal tendon. The *punctum lacrimale* are appreciated at the apex of the *lacrimal papilla* on the margins of both lids with the lower lying more lateral than the upper. Arranged in double or triple rows at the margins of eyelids are the eyelashes or *cilia*. Juxtaposed to the cilia are the openings of the numerous vertically oriented sudoriferous ciliary *glands of Moll* and sebaceous *glands of Zeis* (1–4).

The eyelid may be thought of as a three-layered structure: skin on the outside, a mucosal lining on the inside, and structural elements bridging the space between (Fig. 39.1). The *skin* of the eyelid is extremely thin. In places, the upper lid can measure 1 mm thick, less than 10 cell layers across, and is considered by many to be the thinnest in the body (1,4). The mucosal lining is the *palpebral conjunctiva*. The conjunctiva forms an uninterrupted layer as it arises from the skin at the free edge of one lid and extends over the globe to the free edge of the other. It forms the posterior wall of the lids, folding back upon itself to then form the anterior covering of the globe, the *bulbar conjunctiva*. The apexes of the folds are known as the *superior* and *inferior fornices*. The function of the conjunctiva is to provide a smooth surface facilitating near friction-free movement of the lids over the globe (1,3,4).

Many surgeons consider the elements of the lid between the skin and conjunctiva to form a bilamellar structure. The anterior layer is contiguous with the soft tissues of the face and scalp, and the posterior layer is contiguous with the structures of the orbit. Separating the anterior and posterior lamella is the *tarsofascial layer*. This layer arises from the orbital rim and begins proximally as the *orbital septum*, formed by the confluence of the periosteum of the orbit and the periosteum of the facial bones. As it proceeds distally, the tarsofascial layer continues

as a dividing plane between the anterior and posterior lamella. Distally, the orbital septum fuses with the lid-retracting membrane. In the upper lid, this is the *levator palpebra aponeurosis;* in the lower lid, it is the *capsulopalpebral fascia*. The tarsofascial layer serves as a complete anatomic boundary between the anterior lamella (skin and muscle) and the deeper structures (1–4).

The anterior lamella is composed of skin, subcutaneous tissue, and orbicularis oculi muscle. The *subcutaneous tissue* is sparse and areolar. The *orbicularis oculi* is composed of three concentric oval portions: the innermost *pretarsal portion*, the middle *preseptal portion*, and the outermost *orbital portion*. Together, the pretarsal and preseptal portions form the *palpebral portion,* which contribute to the anterior lamella of the eyelid (1–4).

In the upper lid, the levator palpebra aponeurosis continues distally to fuse with the orbital septum anteriorly and the tarsal plate posteriorly. Deep to the levator palpebra aponeurosis is the Mueller muscle proximally and the tarsal plate distally. On the lower lid, the structures posterior to the tarsofascial layer include the *inferior tarsal muscle* proximally and the tarsal plate distally (1–4).

The *tarsal plates* are the dense cartilaginouslike structures that provide vertical support and rigidity to the eyelids. Composed of dense connective tissue, they measure approximately 2.0 mm in depth and 2.5 cm in length. The *superior tarsus* is larger, semilunar in shape, and 8 to 10 mm in the vertical dimension at the center. The proximal edge of the plate serves as the insertion for the *Mueller muscle*, which is innervated by the sympathetic nervous system. Sympathetic stimulation of this muscle provides an additional 1 to 2 mm of upper lid excursion. The *inferior tarsus* is smaller, elliptical in shape, and has a vertical diameter of 4 to 6 mm. The proximal edge of the inferior plate serves as the insertion for a membrane formed by the confluence of the capsulopalpebral fascia and inferior orbital septum. Here, the capsulopalpebral fascia should be thought of as a structure analogous to the levator palpebral aponeurosis and serves as the lower eyelid retractor. With an origin on both the inferior oblique and rectus muscles, the capsulopalpebral fascia serves to coordinate an unobstructed line of sight on downward gaze.

Along the medial and lateral margins of the palpebral fissure, the tarsal plates become confluent with their respective *palpebral ligaments* or *canthal tendons*. The *lateral canthal tendon* is formed by the confluence of the upper and lower crura, which arise off their respective tarsal plates and create a complex structure known as the *lateral retinaculum*, inserting onto the *Whitnall tubercle*. This key anatomic bony prominence lies 2 mm within the lateral orbit, below the lacrimal fossa. Also contributing to the lateral retinaculum is the lateral horn of the

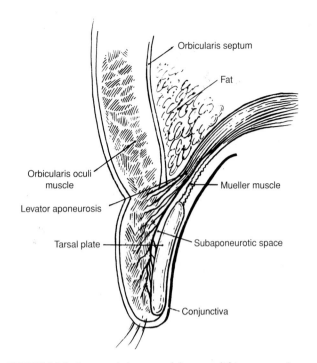

FIGURE 39.1. Structural elements of the upper lid in cross section.

[Labels in figure:] Orbicularis septum; Fat; Mueller muscle; Orbicularis oculi muscle; Levator aponeurosis; Subaponeurotic space; Tarsal plate; Conjunctiva

by the lateral horn of the levator palpebral superioris and the Whitnall ligament. The ducts of the palpebral lobe empty into the upper lateral half of the superior fornix. The ducts of the orbital lobe pass through the palpebral lobe before exiting. In response to stimuli the lacrimal gland elaborates fluid analogous to that of the serous salivary glands. The process of blinking distributes the trilaminar fluid layer across the globe medially where it reaches the puncta and drainage system (1–5).

Tears reaching the medial aspect of the palpebral fissure are drained, or rather pumped, into the nasal cavity by an intricate system of soft tissue consisting of the puncta, canaliculi, lacrimal ducts, muscle fibers of the orbicularis oculi, the lacrimal sac, and, eventually, the nasolacrimal duct. The flow of tear film from the palpebral fissure begins as the fluid passes through the *lacrimal ducts*, also known as the *ductus lacrimalis*, *lacrimal canals*, or *canaliculi* via the *puncta lacrimali* located at the apex of the *papillae lacrimales*, as described above. Both the upper and lower lids contain canaliculi at their medial aspect that dilate along their course into *ampullae* that are enveloped by deep fibers of the orbicularis. The canaliculi come together to a common canaliculus and then empty into the lacrimal sac. The sac sits within the bony *lacrimal fossa* that lies posterior to the insertion of the medial canthal tendon. The lacrimal sac represents the dilated origin of the nasolacrimal duct. Like the lacrimal ducts, the lacrimal sac is enveloped by fibers of the orbicularis muscle, and contraction of the orbicularis, as in blinking, drives the pumping mechanism that both draws the fluid tear film into the lacrimal ducts through the puncta and propels it forward through the canaliculi and lacrimal sac into the nasolacrimal duct where it drains. The *nasolacrimal duct* is approximately 18 mm in length and receives the efflux from the lacrimal canaliculi and lacrimal sac. It directs flow inferiorly into the nasal cavity through the *inferior meatus* of the nose. It runs within a bony canal formed by the maxilla, the lacrimal bone, and the inferior nasal concha. The terminal end of the nasolacrimal duct expands into an imperfect mucosal

levator aponeurosis, the *Whitnall ligament,* which is formed by the fascial condensation of the levator aponeurosis. It helps to direct the forces of the levator palpebral muscle vertically to facilitate lid retraction and serves as a sling providing support to the globe. The *Lockwood ligament* is the lower-lid analog of the Whitnall ligament. Medially, the tarsal plates give rise to the upper and lower crura of the *medial canthal tendon,* which, in turn, gives rise to the medial canthal complex, a tripartite composite structure with posterior, anterior, and superior limbs that insert onto the *medial orbital margin* and nasal bones. The most distal portion of the plates contribute to the free edge of the lids. There, just posterior to the cilia, they are pierced by the ducts of the Meibomian glands. The *Meibomian glands,* also known as the *tarsal glands* or *glandulae tarsales,* are sebaceous. They secrete an oillike substance onto the conjunctiva, which facilitates gliding of the lid over the globe. The glands, which number approximately 10 to 20 on the lower lid and 20 to 40 on the upper lid, may be the site of pathologic inflammatory processes, which may be acute (hordeolum or stye), chronic (noncaseating granulomas, chalazia), or postsurgical (meibomianitis or blepharitis) (1–4).

The vascular system of the eyelid is rich and consists of overlapping contributions from numerous adjacent vessels.

The lacrimal system functions to bathe with and drain the globe of tears (Fig. 39.2). It consists of the lacrimal gland and microscopic accessory glands, which secrete the tears, and the lacrimal ducts or canaliculi, the lacrimal sac, and the nasolacrimal duct, which provides nasal drainage.

Tears form a trilaminar fluid layer composed of a deep mucoprotein layer, a middle aqueous layer, and a superficial lipid layer. Together, these layers act in concert to preserve a moist antimicrobial environment. This layer also serves to bend incoming light before it strikes the cornea and has up to 0.5 diopter of refractile power (1–5).

The *lacrimal gland* proper is composed of two lobes: the main orbital lobe and the smaller palpebral lobe. They are situated in the *lacrimal fossa* of the superolateral orbit and upper lateral eyelid, respectively. They are separated from each other

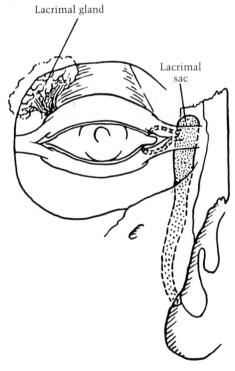

FIGURE 39.2. The lacrimal system is composed of the lacrimal gland, microscopic accessory glands, lacrimal ducts or canaliculi, the lacrimal sac, and the nasolacrimal duct.

[Labels in figure:] Lacrimal gland; Lacrimal sac

valve known as the *plica lacrimalis*, which is formed by a fold of mucous membrane (1–4).

EYELID RECONSTRUCTION

Eyelid defects may result from congenital anomalies, neoplastic processes, ablative surgical procedures, or trauma. Regardless of the etiology, however, the skin, muscle, supporting structures, and conjunctiva must be assessed and, if absent or deficient, reconstructed. The quality and quantity of local, regional, and distal tissues is evaluated, as is the patient's overall health, comorbid conditions, and personal goals.

For congenital defects, it is critical to rule out or identify and treat associated anomalies. If the defect in question follows an ablative surgical procedure, it is necessary to be familiar with the histologic diagnosis and surgical pathology of the underlying neoplastic process. Defects created by the ablation of, for example, a sarcoma may not be amenable to immediate reconstruction, but may better be reconstructed after permanent pathology confirms adequate margins. Any plan for adjuvant treatment, such as radiation therapy, should be considered when planning reconstruction. Finally, lid defects that result from traumatic causes rarely occur in isolation. In these instances, it is important to ensure that all associated injuries have been properly identified and accounted for in the overall treatment plan.

Once the above concerns are addressed, evaluation and treatment of eyelid defects are best approached by dividing the region into zones, each with its own anatomic, functional, and aesthetic considerations (Fig. 39.3) (6). Evaluation of defects with respect to location or zone, and the extent to which each zone is affected (partial or full thickness) may also be predictive of possible postreconstructive complications. With these concepts in mind, and all others factors being equal, defects at risk for postoperative complications should be reconstructed with the most durable techniques available (6).

The following principles serve as guidelines (2,4,7,8).

- All reconstructions should begin with a through evaluation of the defect and function of the lid.
- Components that have been compromised as well as those that remain viable including elements of skin, muscle, tarsus, and conjunctiva should be properly identified and documented.

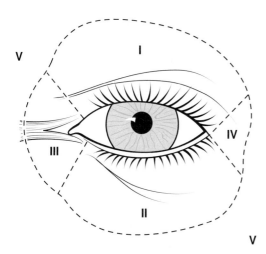

FIGURE 39.3. Periocular zones, each with individual anatomic, functional, and aesthetic considerations. (Adapted from Spinelli HM, Jelks GW. Periocular reconstruction: a systematic approach. *Plast Reconstr Surg.* 1993;91(6):1017–1024, with permission.)

- When feasible, a complete and thorough preoperative ophthalmologic examination, including visual acuity and field testing, as well as a Schirmer test, should be performed and documented. In acute situations, when the luxury of a preoperative evaluation is not possible, ophthalmologic consultation should be considered.
- The eyelids are the focus of much aesthetic attention. Consideration of this detail is important when composing the reconstructive plan. Transverse incisions will help to camouflage scars, and symmetry with contralateral structures should be preserved whenever possible.
- Vertical incisions should be avoided so as to obviate contracture and distortion of eyelid function.
- Debridement of nonviable tissue should proceed, and when doing so, reconstructive goals should be kept in mind.
- When approximating lid margins, alignment of all layers must be achieved. Failure to do so may result in significant functional and/or aesthetic problems.
- Suture material and knots should be placed in an effort to avoid direct contact with the surface of the cornea and globe. Even the finest suture materials can cause extensive irritation and corneal abrasions.
- Ultimately, as in all reconstructive scenarios, the principles of the reconstructive ladder should be appreciated and applied in eyelid reconstruction.

Upper Eyelid Reconstruction: Zone I

Although the structural components of the upper and lower eyelids are analogous, the two differ anatomically and functionally in a few important ways. The upper lid is taller in height, more lax, more mobile, and is the major facilitator of closure.

Zone I defects are considered partial-thickness defects when they involve only skin or skin and muscle (external lamina). Full-thickness defects include loss of the tarsus and conjunctiva as well. It is helpful to divide partial-thickness defects of the upper lid into two categories: those involving less than 50% of the lid length and those involving more than 50% of the lid length. Full-thickness defects of the upper lid are best considered in three categories, defects less than 25% of lid length, defects measuring 25% to 75% of lid length, and defects measuring greater than 75% of upper-lid length.

Partial-thickness defects of the upper lid that measure less than 50% of lid length are, in the author's opinion, best repaired by primary closure with local tissue advancement (Fig. 39.4). The laxity of the upper lid skin facilitates primary closure provided appropriate myocutaneous flaps are raised and advanced appropriately. When possible, scars should be oriented in a transverse direction. In general, vertical scars may result in contracture and related functional and aesthetic problems (6).

Partial-thickness defects of the upper lid that involve more than 50% of the lid length provide a greater challenge (Fig. 39.4). In all likelihood, simple primary closure with local tissue advancement would place too much tension on the underlying tarsus, causing the wound to dehisce, inappropriately scar, or, in extreme cases, buckle the tarsus and disrupt function. For this reason, a tension-free closure is advocated. In our opinion, this is best achieved with a full-thickness skin graft from the contralateral upper lid. A full-thickness graft harvested from the contralateral upper lid provides an excellent match for color and texture and a superior aesthetic result. A composite graft consisting of orbicularis muscle and skin can also be used, however, the added tissue may compromise graft viability. One should note however, that the upper lid is

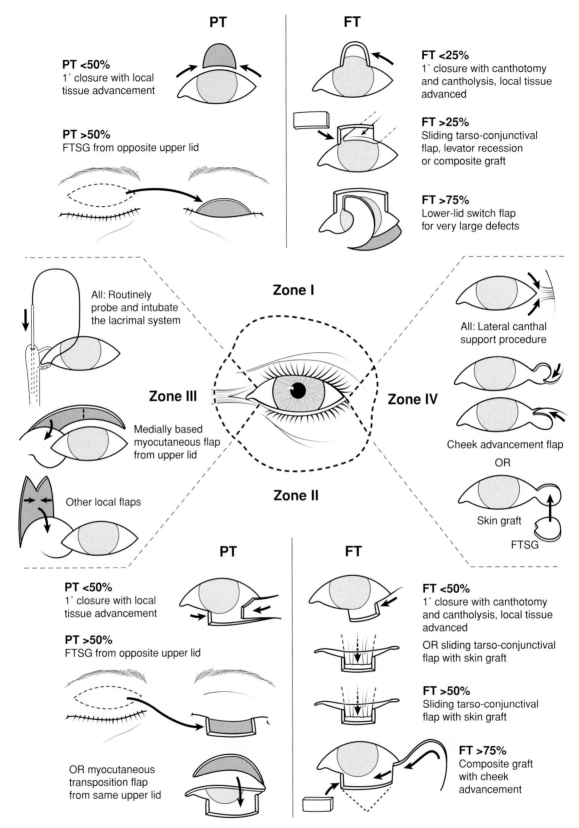

FIGURE 39.4. Reconstructive algorithm based on periocular zones. FT, full-thickness defect; FTSG, full-thickness skin graft; PT, partial-thickness defect. (Adapted from Spinelli HM, Jelks GW. Periocular reconstruction: a systematic approach. *Plast Reconstr Surg.* 1993;91(6):1017–1024, with permission.)

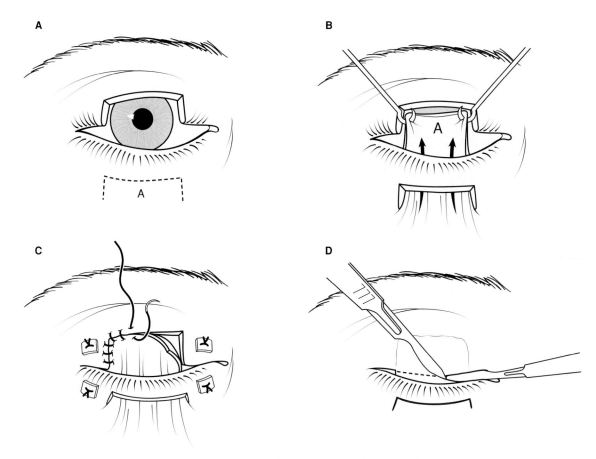

FIGURE 39.5. Modified Cutler-Beard advancement flap.

critical to eyelid function and should a donor-site complication arise, the consequences could be devastating. For this reason, some authors recommend avoiding the upper lid as a donor site unless other options are unavailable, suggesting instead using the postauricular region for the full-thickness skin donor site. Proponents for the use of postauricular skin cite its simplicity of harvest, its large available size providing enough skin to cover a canthal-to-canthal defect, and a cosmetically hidden donor site scar. We prefer contralateral upper lid skin donor sites whenever functional compromise can be avoided (2,8,9).

Full-thickness defects of the upper lid should be divided into three categories, those involving less than 25% of the lid length, those involving 25% to 75% of the lid length, and those measuring greater than 75% of lid length. Full-thickness defects of the upper lid measuring less than 25% of the upper lid length may be reconstructed primarily (Fig. 39.4). The smallest of these defects may be closed applying the principles set forth by Ross and Pham, debriding the wound edges to approximate a pentagon with its apex pointing away from the lid margin. In this manner, dog-ears and notching can be avoided or minimized. Larger defects in this category may also be closed primarily, but might require local myocutaneous flap advancement, canthotomy, and/or cantholysis (2,4,6,9,10).

Full-thickness defects of the upper lid measuring between 25% and 75% are usually not amenable to primary closure (Fig. 39.4). These, we believe, are best reconstructed by either composite grafts or by a sliding tarsoconjunctival flap. Composite grafts, whether they are used to reconstruct upper or lower lid defects, must include a posterior mucosal layer, a structural support layer, and a well-vascularized covering. There are a host of composite grafts described for eyelid reconstruction (2,4,6,8). One of the best choices for a composite graft

reconstruction is to combine a nasal septal cartilage–mucosal graft for the posterior conjunctival-tarsal layer and a transposition myocutaneous flap from an adjacent area for the anterior lamella. Benefits of using the nasal septal mucosal–cartilage for the posterior layer include the pre-existing relationship between the mucosal and cartilaginous layers, and the thinness and pliability of septal cartilage compared to other donor sites. We advocate the use of a pedicled skin–muscle flap for coverage over a composite graft based on its superior blood supply. A full-thickness skin graft may be used as external coverage over a transposition flap of internal lamella structures, providing an excellent functional and cosmetic result. An equally effective option for reconstructing a 25% to 75% full-thickness defect of the upper lid is the Hughes sliding tarsoconjunctival flap from the lower lid. This is accomplished by elevating tarsus and conjunctiva off the remaining lid segment as a proximally based transposition flap and covering it either with a full-thickness skin graft or myocutaneous flap. In general, the skin graft appears and functions more naturally. Another option for repair of full-thickness defects of the upper lid measuring between 25% and 75% is the Cutler-Beard advancement flap. As originally described, reconstruction is carried out by first creating a full-thickness advancement flap from the lower lid, below the tarsal plate, leaving the margin of the lower lid intact (Fig. 39.5). The pedicled flap is then advanced superiorly into the upper lid defect and inset. Division of the pedicle is delayed for 6 to 8 weeks, allowing for maximum ingrowth of local vasculature. The obvious disadvantages to this technique are that (a) the eye must remain closed until division of the pedicle is carried out; (b) the reconstructed portion of the upper lid remains without a supporting structure (e.g., tarsal plate or cartilaginous graft analog); and (c) alteration of lower lid structure and function secondary to full-thickness and long-term scarring. Since its introduction in the 1950s, modifications to the Cutler-Beard advancement flap have been offered, but the need for the eye to remain closed during flap "take," as well as irreversible alteration of lower-lid structure and function, remain major drawbacks to its use.

Full-thickness defects of the upper lid that are greater than 75% of the lid length present a challenge in that donor options are limited (Fig. 39.4). Of the described techniques, our preferred method of reconstruction is a simultaneous lower-lid switch flap with a cheek rotation–advancement as necessary. The lower-lid switch flap was modified for the upper lid by Mustardé (8). This flap uses an intact lower lid to recreate the upper lid by raising the lower-lid tissue as a bilaminar flap based on the marginal artery and rotating it around the medial or lateral palpebral fissure. Closure of the upper-lid defect is achieved by first reducing the size of the defect, up to 25%, by simple advancement of the wound margins, and then by rotating the lower lid to complete the reconstruction. The cheek flap is advanced as length is needed (2,6,8).

On occasion, upper lid defects may extend beyond zone I and involve adjacent periocular tissue. For example, to achieve adequate margins during the excision of a medial upper eyelid neoplasm, ablation of medial canthal tissue (zone III) may be necessary. Large traumatic defects, too, may result in disruption of the upper eyelid in conjunction with nearby adjacent tissue. When faced with these more extensive defects, importation of local tissue should be considered using full-thickness glabella skin or temporoparietal fascia as indicated. The *glabella flap* is based on the supratrochlear blood supply and is discussed below in relation to medial canthal (zone III) defects (6,7). As an interpolation flap, it can be tailored to meet the needs of a wide variety of defects, especially those involving multiple zones. An example of this is the split-finger graft that uses full-thickness glabellar skin to reconstruct a combined defect involving zones I, II, and III (Fig. 39.6). The temporoparietal fascia flap is useful for extensive upper-lid defects that include a lateral perior-

bital component. In these scenarios, the fascia can be harvested through a hemi-coronal incision, tunneled anteriorly, and tailored to meet the needs of the defect. It can be covered with a split-thickness skin graft. A cartilaginous graft can be added to provide support when needed (6,7).

Lower Eyelid Reconstruction: Zone II

As discussed above, the upper and lower lids are analogous in many ways, but each possesses some distinct and specialized anatomic structures and function. For example, the lower lid is shorter in height, less mobile, and contributes only minimally to closure. However, the lower lid is most important in its contribution to passive corneal coverage. Considerations for reconstruction of the lower lid should include lash preservation, appropriate lid position (i.e., avoidance of entropion or ectropion and/or lid retraction), lid tone, marginal notching and irregularities, and overall aesthetic outcome (6).

Similar to defects of the upper lid, we consider defects of the zone II (lower lid) based on the thickness and size of the defect. Partial-thickness defects of the lower lid should be viewed as either those involving less than 50% of the lid length or those involving more than 50% of the lid length. In distinction, full-thickness defects of the lower lid should be further broken down into those less than 50% of lid length, defects measuring 50% to 75% of lid length, and, finally, defects measuring greater than 75% of lid length.

Partial-thickness zone II defects measuring less than 50% of the lid length are best repaired with primary closure, adding local tissue advancement as necessary (Fig. 39.4). As with partial-thickness zone I defects, reconstruction of skin or skin–muscle deficits must provide coverage to the underlying tarsus. Simple primary closure may be adequate when defects are small, but tension-free closures are usually best facilitated by advancement of local, adjacent tissue. Vertical incisions should be avoided if at all possible. This method of reconstruction provides the best color and texture match along with a superior functional and cosmetic result.

Partial-thickness zone II defects that measure greater than 50% cannot be closed primarily without placing, as stated above, undue tension on the tarsus below (Fig. 39.4). For this category of defects, we recommend either a full-thickness skin graft from the contralateral upper lid or a myocutaneous transposition flap from the ipsilateral upper lid.

A full-thickness skin graft from the contralateral lid can provide a fairly large amount of coverage as needed. Full-thickness grafts provide superior coverage, contract less than split-thickness grafts, and offer excellent cosmetic and functional results. If contralateral upper-lid skin is unavailable or undesirable, postauricular skin is an excellent second choice for full-thickness harvest (6,9,10).

Another reconstructive option for repair of partial-thickness zone II defects measuring greater than 50% are local myocutaneous transposition flaps from the ipsilateral upper lid. The two most commonly used examples of these local myocutaneous transposition flaps in lower-lid reconstruction include the unipedicled Fricke flap and the bipedicled Tripier flap. The Fricke flap (Fig. 39.7) is a unipedicled myocutaneous transposition flap composed of the skin and preseptal portion of the orbicularis oculi muscle of the upper lid. The pedicle can be placed either medial or lateral to the palpebral fissure. If a myocutaneous transposition flap is raised on both the medial and lateral pedicle, a bipedicled myocutaneous transposition flap (Tripier) is generated (Fig. 39.8). When constructing either the unipedicled Fricke flap or the bipedicled Tripier flap, inset is performed at initial operation. The unilateral flap will adequately cover defects of the lower lid up to and beyond the midline. For defects requiring a greater length, a bipedicled flap

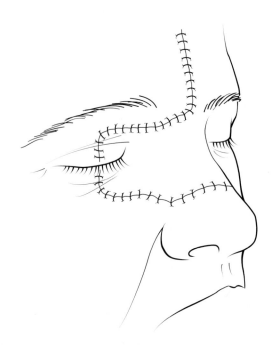

FIGURE 39.6. The split-finger graft is an interpolation flap that can be tailored to meet the needs of a wide variety of defects. (Redrawn after Jackson IT. Eyelid and canthal region reconstruction. In: *Local Flaps in Head & Neck Reconstruction.* St. Louis: Quality Medical Publishing, 2002.)

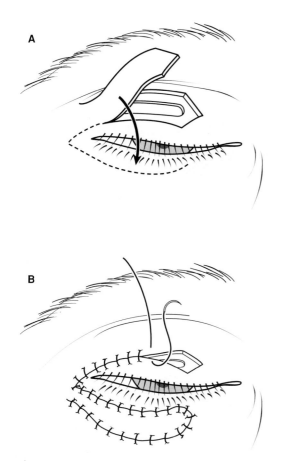

FIGURE 39.7. The unipedicled myocutaneous Fricke transposition flap. (Redrawn after Jackson IT. Eyelid and canthal region reconstruction. In: *Local Flaps in Head and Neck Reconstruction.* St. Louis: Quality Medical Publishing, 2002.)

is usually necessary. Advantages of the Tripier flap include its ease of performance, lack of distal donor sites and facial scars, and maintenance of the visual field. Disadvantages of the Tripier flap include the extremely rare compromise of the upper lid donor site. In general, these myocutaneous transposition flaps are hardy but provide notable bulk that sometimes requires late minor revision procedures for conturing (7).

Full-thickness defects of zone II should be viewed in three distinct categories based on lid length: less than 50%, 50% to 75%, and greater than 75% of lid length. We recommend one of two excellent reconstructive options for repair of full-thickness defects less than 50% of lid length: (a) primary closure with lateral canthotomy, cantholysis, and local tissue advancement (Fig. 39.4), or (b) Hughes tarsoconjunctival flap with skin graft or myocutaneous coverage. Unlike partial-thickness zone II defects, full-thickness defects of up to several millimeters can repaired primarily and dog-ears and notching can be avoided by following the principles set forth by Ross and Pham, debriding the wound edges to approximate a pentagon with its apex pointing away from the lid margin. Some surgeons argue that defects as large as 25% to 33% of the lower lid can be closed in this manner; however, for defects larger than a few millimeters, we find that the addition of lateral canthotomy, cantholysis, and local tissue advancement provides a superior cosmetic and functional result. Of course, this depends on the patient's age and amount of horizontal laxity present (2,4,6,8).

A sliding tarsoconjunctival flap with a skin graft is a versatile technique that can be used to reconstruct zone II defects of less than 50% of lid length, as well as defects that fall into the 50% to 75% category. In this procedure, a superiorly based flap of

the posterior lamella of the upper lid, including the tarsus and the conjunctiva, is advanced to fill the defect of the lower lid. The Mueller muscle can be included in the conjunctival pedicle as it adds increased vascular reliability. The anterior lamella of the lower lid is covered with a full-thickness skin graft or local advancement flap. Donor sites include the contralateral upper lid and postauricular skin. The flap is left on its pedicle for several weeks and later divided. The donor site of the upper lid is not affected as long as 3 to 4 mm of distal tarsus remains intact to ensure upper lid stability. One must recess the upper lid levator by undermining at the second stage division and insetting to avoid upper lid retraction from the advanced upper lid retractors (2,6).

Zone II defects of full-thickness measuring greater than 75% of the lower lid length require a more aggressive approach. In these cases, restoration of the anterior layer can be completed with a cheek flap, and reconstruction of the posterior layer performed by using a composite graft of nasal septal cartilage and lining (2,6,8). This full-thickness cutaneous rotation–advancement flap can be harvested to include the superficial musculoaponeurotic system and provides an excellent color and texture match for zone II defects. Principles to keep in mind when raising a cheek flap include dermal anchorage to the inferior orbit to ensure tension-free closure, superolateral curvature of the incision line to prevent "shortening," and incorporation of a Z-plasty when necessary (2,4,6,8,9,11).

Cervicofacial flaps may be used in place of cheek rotation flaps and, when properly executed, provide excellent coverage of not only of zone II defects but also of defects that extend beyond zone V (12).

Medial Canthal Reconstruction: Zone III

Zone III, the medial canthal region, is the most anatomically and physiologically complex of the periocular zones. The lacrimal papilla, puncta, canaliculi, plica semilunaris, caruncula lacrimalis, and tripartite insertion of the medial canthal tendon are all located within this square centimeter of tissue. Procedures in this zone are associated with a high incidence of complications involving the lacrimal canalicular system and/or medial canthal tendon (6). For this reason, routine lacrimal stenting by silicone tube intubation, as well as measures to insure medial canthal tendon support, are recommended when performing procedures in zone III. Defects of the anterior layers are reconstructed with a medially based, myocutaneous flap from the upper lid based on branches of the infratrochlear vessels. Acceptable alternatives include other local flaps such as the V-Y glabellar flap, and healing by secondary intention (2,6).

Measures to ensure that the medial canthal tendon support remains intact may be simple or complex, depending on the nature of the defect. If the tendon is intact but minor laxity is appreciated, simple plication is recommended. In this procedure, the inferior arm is "tucked" under the canthus. As with all procedures in zone III, care must be taken not to compromise the lacrimal system (10). If the insertion of the tendon is not intact, canthopexy is recommended. In this case, the medial aspects of the upper and lower tarsal plates can be sutured to the nasal periosteum taking care to place the point of fixation below the anterior lacrimal crest. Alternatively, if the tendon is simply avulsed, it can be secured with a wire loop, which is passed and anchored in a transnasal fashion (6).

Lateral Canthal Reconstruction: Zone IV

The critical structure in zone IV, underlying the lateral palpebral fissure, is the lateral canthal tendon. Partial or complete

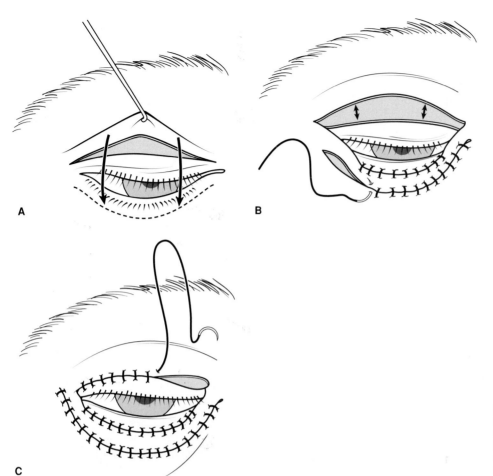

FIGURE 39.8. The bipedicled my-ocutaneous Tripier flap. (Redrawn after Jackson, IT. Eyelid and canthal region reconstruction. In: *LocalFlaps in Head & Neck Reconstruction.* St. Louis: Quality Medical Publishing, 2002.)

ablation or injury to this structure can result in laxity of the lower lid, or, in extreme cases, medial displacement and rounding of the lateral canthus with a shortened horizontal fissure (6,10). For these reasons, we recommend that all reconstructions performed in zone IV include a canthal support procedure or canthopexy. Complete disruptions of the canthus require a canthoplasty. In addition, laxity of the lateral canthus, even when corrected, has a tendency to recur over time. Thus, a slight overcorrection should be the goal (6,10). Options for reconstructing the superficial component of these defects include a cheek advancement flap or full-thickness skin graft.

Simple disruptions of the lateral canthal tendon may be repaired primarily, reattaching the severed portion to the stump as indicated. More significant disruptions, with loss of the lateral aspect, may be reconstructed by anchoring the medial end of the remaining ligament to either the periosteum at the level of the Whitnall ligament or to the bone directly, using small drill holes in the orbital rim (6,10). When the upper portion of the tendon is intact, a lateral canthal sling is used to provide support and tighten an otherwise lax lower lid (6). Finally, when completely obliterated, the lateral canthal ligament can be reconstructed via a lateral tarsal strip procedure. The tarsal plates are sutured to a strip of orbital periosteum raised for this purpose (6,10). Canthopexy and canthoplasty are discussed under Lower Eyelid Reconstruction: Zone II section.

The loss of the superficial components of zone IV defects should be reconstructed with either a local cheek advancement flap or with a full-thickness skin graft. Cheek flaps, as described for zone II defects, may be rotated into defects and provide an excellent color and texture match. Unlike the local advancement cheek flap described above, however, the quan-

tity of tissue required to reconstruct lateral canthal defects is usually minimal. For this reason, flaps may be designed with either superolateral or inferolateral incisions (10). If one elects to reconstruct a zone IV defect with a graft, it should be full-thickness and harvested from a site as close to the recipient bed as possible. Full-thickness grafts provide the necessary texture with less contracture than split-thickness grafts, and postauricular skin provides an excellent color and texture match with minimal donor-site morbidity.

Reconstruction of Periocular Defects: Zone V

Zone V defects are defined as those outside of but contiguous with zones I to IV (6,10). Although Zone V defects do not involve the eyelids or canthi directly, they are relevant to this discussion in that they can affect lid position and function. Normal eyelid form and function results from a fine equilibrium, or balance, between support forces and the counterproductive distraction forces (4,6). Disruption of these forces, by loss or manipulation of the surrounding tissue, can have manifestations within zones I to IV, as discussed in Lower Eyelid Reconstruction: Zone II section. For example, reconstruction of an infraorbital cheek defect following Mohs micrographic surgery without attention to the principles outlined previously can result in ectropion or scleral show (4,6,11). Zone V defects should be reconstructed with attention to the proper functioning and appearance of the lids and canthi in all four of the periocular zones. When necessary, adjuvant procedures, such as lateral canthoplasty and/or canthopexy, should be performed when addressing zone V defects.

Cervicofacial flap reconstruction of the entire cheek illustrates this point. In this example, the patient's lower eyelid (zone II) may lie in a functional anatomic position only until the inferior distraction forces of the flap are applied by way of zone V. Anticipating this, the surgeon should support the lower lid, and the flap, by way of a medial and lateral canthopexy with or without bone fixation, and the flap should be supported independently. In this manner, the lower lid is insulated from the distraction forces of an unsupported flap in zone V.

CORRECTION OF EYELID PTOSIS

Anatomy and Physiology of Eyelid Elevation

The natural state of the upper eyelid is closed. Eyelid elevation in the waking state is mediated primarily by the action of the levator palpebrae superioris muscle with a less-significant contribution made by the Mueller muscle. Together, the levator palpebrae superioris muscle, the levator aponeurosis, and the Mueller muscle form the levator complex responsible for eyelid elevation. In distinction, the action of eye closure and blinking is mediated by the orbicularis oculi muscle (1,3,4).

The *levator palpebrae superioris muscle* originates from the bony orbit, just superior and anterior to the optic foramen. It courses anteriorly, above the superior rectus muscle, following the curve of the globe. As it crosses the Whitnall ligament, the levator muscle fibers dissipate, giving rise to the *levator aponeurosis,* which continues forward, first fusing with the orbital septum and eventually terminating by inserting fibrous connections into the tarsal plate posteriorly and the orbicularis anteriorly (see Eyelid Anatomy and Physiology above) (Fig. 39.1). The fusion of the levator aponeurosis with the orbicularis fibers gives rise to the upper eyelid fold. Disruption at this level—as seen with "levator dehiscence"—results in blunting of the upper eyelid fold, a common characteristic of the senescent eye. The levator palpebrae superioris is innervated by the occulomotor nerve (cranial nerve [CN] III). The *Mueller muscle* arises from the inferior surface of the levator superioris muscle at the level of the Whitnall ligament. From there, it courses anteriorly to insert on the superior margin of the tarsal plate. The Mueller muscle is innervated by sympathetic fibers that arise from the cervical sympathetic ganglion and course through the sympathetic trunk along the internal carotid plexus. In the normal lid, contraction of the levator muscle results in elevation of the upper eyelid. Full excursion of the lid approximates 10 to 15 mm. An additional 1 to 2 mm of elevation is provided by the action of a well-functioning Mueller muscle (1–4).

Classification of Ptosis

The *normal eyelid,* whose position is defined by its margin, should rest one-half way between the pupillary aperture and the corneoscleral junction. *True ptosis* of the eyelid can be defined as a drooping of the eyelid so that its margin falls below the normal anatomic position. True ptosis results from dysfunction of the levator complex (levator palpebrae superioris muscle, levator aponeurosis, and the Mueller muscle) (4) (Table 39.1). An example of true ptosis is levator dehiscence that occurs when the levator aponeurosis separates from the tarsal plate (4). True ptosis is usually compensated for by actions of secondary muscles, for example, contraction of the frontalis muscle. On the other hand, *pseudoptosis* refers to the appearance of an inferiorly displaced lid whose droop is unrelated to the levator complex. A prime example of pseudoptosis is seen in enophthalmos. In this case, retrodisplacement of the globe

TABLE 39.1

GRADES OF PTOSIS AND LEVATOR FUNCTION

Ptosis	Levator Function
Mild: 2–3 mm	Good: 10–15 mm
Moderate: 3–5 mm	Fair: 6–9 mm
Severe: >5 mm	Poor: <5 mm

into the orbit causes the upper lid to drape more inferiorly giving the appearance of ptosis. However, in this case, the eyelid is normal but the globe position is the culprit. Other causes of pseudoptosis include brow ptosis, severe dermatochalasia, hypotropia, and blepharospasm (4).

Prior to surgical intervention, it is imperative to make an accurate diagnosis regarding the etiology of the ptotic lid. Although several classification schemes exist (2), upper eyelid ptosis is conveniently divided as either a syndromic or isolated, intrinsic defect of the levator complex resulting from a specific cause (e.g., mechanical, neurogenic, or other) (4). Syndromic etiologies are associated with neurogenic causes and may include myasthenia gravis (ptosis, orbicularis weakness, exposure keratitis, and intermittent diplopia), Horner syndrome (ptosis, miosis, and anhydrosis), and orbital masses (whether they are contained within the orbit proper or invade the orbit from surrounding structures such as occurs in neurofibromatosis). Syndromic etiologies also may be congenital in nature, and, although rare, include the blepharophimosis syndrome (4).

As opposed to syndromic causes of ptosis, intrinsic dysfunction of the levator complex is usually isolated in nature. Intrinsic dysfunction may also be either congenital or acquired. Congenital ptosis is most often characterized by underdevelopment of the levator palpebrae superioris muscle. In these cases, a detailed patient interview usually reveals a chronic history of ptosis associated with the clinical picture of lagophthalmos and lid lag on downward gaze. Upper-lid deficiency on closure and downward gaze is caused by scar tissue replacing levator muscle fibers. Acquired ptosis is commonly seen in levator dehiscence, where the levator aponeurosis pulls away from the tarsal plate. Levator dehiscence occurs most commonly in the senescent eye, but may also occur after cataract surgery (secondary to surgical trauma or severe edema) or after nonsurgical traumatic injuries. The classical picture of a dehisced levator aponeurosis is ptosis associated with a high or absent lid fold and a superior sulcus deformity (2,4) (Fig. 39.9).

Preoperative Evaluation

As with all patient evaluations, assessment of the patient with eyelid ptosis should focus not only on the chief complaint, but on the patient as a whole. Patients with severe medical or psychiatric conditions should be referred for appropriate consultation.

Gross examination begins with visual acuity testing and attention to topographic landmarks. Symmetry is assessed and documented. The nature of the lid fold (sharp vs. blunted) should be qualified and its position in relation to the lash line quantified. A normal lid fold should rest 7 to 9 mm above the ciliary margin. If the crease is blunted and/or the distance from the margin is greater than the norm, a separation of the levator aponeurosis from the overlying orbicularis should be suspected. If, on the other hand, an excessively deep lid fold (sulcus deformity) exists, separation of the levator from the tarsal plate (levator dehiscence) may be the cause. Test for lagophthalmus by having the patient, with the head held steady, look up then

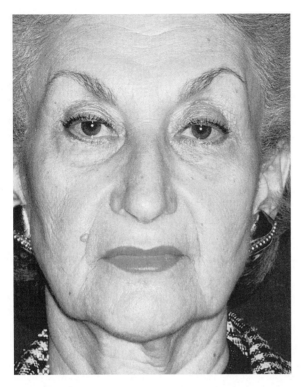

FIGURE 39.9. Levator dehiscence. Demonstrated is the classic picture of a dehisced levator aponeurosis, ptosis associated with a high or absent lid fold, and a superior sulcus deformity. (Reproduced from Spinelli HM. Ptosis and upper eyelid retraction. In: Spinelli HM, ed. *Atlas of Aesthetic Eyelid and Periocular Surgery*. Philadelphia: Elsevier, 2004; 93, with permission.)

down. The presence of lagophthalmos may be associated with congenital ptosis. Bilateral lagophthalmos may be more subtle than unilateral, and harder to detect. The presence and degree of lid lag should be appreciated preoperatively so as to tailor which and to what extent a surgical treatment is applied. Adequate function of the orbicularis oculi muscle is also necessary for globe protection after elevating the upper eyelid. Patients with impaired orbicularis function may be using lid ptosis as a compensatory mechanism to compensate, to protect the globe, and to prevent excessive evaporation of tear film. Elevating the upper eyelid surgically may create symptomatic lagophthalmos. Abnormalities in extraocular muscle function may imply a neurogenic problem, and changes in eyelid location during these versions may indicate aberrant regeneration of CN III. Similarly, other neurologic "cross-wiring" may be associated with ptosis, such as is seen with the Marcus-Gunn jaw-winking phenomenon that results from aberrant connections between CN III and CN V_3. This is demonstrated by changes in upper eyelid position during jaw subluxation. Ptosis procedures may also require modification or be precluded in individuals with poor tear-film coverage. Schirmer testing is helpful for preoperatively identifying these patients. If tear film is marginal, secondary to either underproduction or excessive evaporative loss, eyelid elevation procedures that increase the exposed surface area of the conjunctiva will result in excessive evaporative loss and, in turn, lead to dry eye syndrome. Although the reliability of the Schirmer test has been questioned in the literature, the Schirmer test provides one valuable piece of information that needs to be interpreted in the context of other important tests and findings. Pupils are compared to each other for symmetry and the pupillary reflex is evaluated. Anisocoria, or an abnormal pupillary reflex, should lead the examiner to suspect the

presence of a Horner syndrome or CN III palsy. The position of the upper eyelid should be quantified and documented. Although several methods exist to assess the position of the upper lid (e.g., interpalpebral distance at the midposition), we prefer to use the relationship between the pupillary light reflex and the upper lid margin. In our hands, this has been the most accurate and reproducible method. This distance should be 3.0 to 4.5 mm in the normally functioning lid. On gross examination, the lid margin should rest halfway between the pupillary aperture and the superior margin of the corneoscleral junction (2,4).

The next step in the evaluation of the patient is the quantification and classification of the lid ptosis. The degree of ptosis is divided into mild, moderate, or severe. Ptosis of 2 to 3 mm is mild, 3 to 5 mm is moderate, and greater than 5 mm is severe. Finally, levator function is assessed. Levator function may be influenced by a multitude of factors, including an individual's level of fatigue and serum catecholamine levels. Therefore, the assessment of levator function and the degree of ptosis is repeated at a separate office meeting with the intent to corroborate the initial findings.

To measure levator function, the examiner sits directly across from the examinee (Fig. 39.10). The right eye is measured first, then the left. In measuring the right eye, the examiner places his or her left thumb over the eyebrow to stabilize it (4); otherwise, a patient with severe ptosis and a compensatory elevation of the brow might elevate the brow reflexively during the examination. The examiner holds a clear millimeter ruler in the right hand over the lateral midline of the palpebral fissure and has the subject look up maximally. The ruler is positioned so that this is the zero point. The subject then is asked to look down maximally (Fig. 39.10). The difference between the eyelid apertures from upgaze to downgaze is a measure of levator excursion and function. In normal individuals, levator excursion is usually greater than 12 mm. Levator function is classified as follows: less than 5 mm, poor; 6 to 9 mm, fair; and, 10 to 15 mm, good (2,4).

Selection of the Correct Operation

The degree of ptosis and the extent of levator function determine the operative procedure. When levator excursion is good (10 to 15 mm) and ptosis is mild (2 to 3 mm), most procedures that either plicate, shorten, or otherwise advance the levator muscle will achieve good results. These procedures include levator plication, tarsal conjunctival mullerectomy, and levator advancement. When levator excursion is good, but ptosis is moderate (3 to 5 mm), either levator plication or levator advancement should be considered. When ptosis is severe (>5 mm), however, levator advancement remains the procedure of choice for its superior ability to raise and tailor the upper lid height to the desired level (4).

When levator excursion is moderate (6 to 9 mm) and ptosis is either mild, moderate, or severe, we prefer to perform levator advancement, which affords the versatility and power required. When levator function is poor (<5 mm), as seen in congenital ptosis, regardless of the degree of ptosis, a frontalis sling is required (4).

Regardless of procedure chosen, several principles are applicable:

- Determine the etiology of ptosis prior to planning surgical intervention and rule out pseudoptosis.
- A major goal of all lid procedures is to avoid shortening the upper lid and the creation of symptomatic lagophthalmos.
- Local anesthesia is injected sparingly, so as not to distort lid anatomy. When using epinephrine, the chemical

ASSESSING LEVATOR FUNCTION

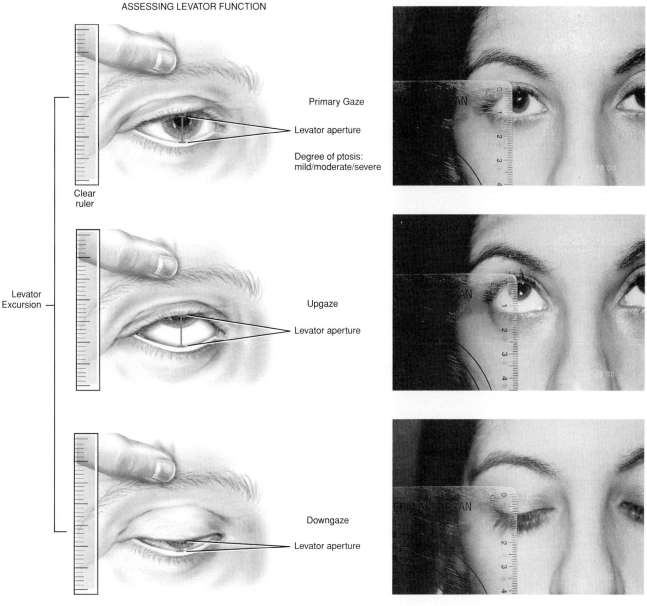

FIGURE 39.10. Assessment of levator function is best confirmed at two separate office visits. (Reproduced from Spinelli HM. Ptosis and upper eyelid retraction. In: Spinelli HM, ed. *Atlas of Aesthetic Eyelid and Periocular Surgery*. Philadelphia: Elsevier, 2004; 96, with permission.)

stimulation of the Mueller muscle will add 1 to 2 mm of elevation to upper lid position.

■ Clear or transparent corneal shields protect the eye and allow for visualization of landmarks intraoperatively.

■ When assessing lid position pre- or intraoperatively, exam lights are lowered to avoid stimulating reflexive squinting.

■ The vertical apex of the corrected upper lid margin should lie directly above the medial margin of the pupil, the nasal pupillary margin.

■ The horizontal margin of the lid should lie approximately halfway between the pupillary aperture and the corneoscleral junction. If orbicularis function is compromised secondary to muscular or neural disorders, the lid should lie closer to the pupillary aperture.

■ The lateral horn of the levator aponeurosis bisects the lacrimal glad and dissections in this region proceed judiciously.

■ Incisions that result in the excision of tissue (e.g., tarsal–conjunctival mullerectomy) should follow the curve of the lid. Failure to do so may result in a tented or pinched appearance.

■ Skin excisions in secondary or tertiary lid procedures are minimized or avoided completely.

Levator Advancement

The levator advancement procedure is the preferred technique for correcting most types of ptosis. It has wide application and may be applied to individuals with mild, moderate, or even severe ptosis. This technique may be used to correct individuals with levator excursion that is fair or better (>6 mm). For these reasons, levator advancement is our procedure of choice for individuals with ptosis secondary to involutional, senescent, traumatic, and certain forms of congenital ptosis. Additionally, it may be performed with or without concomitant blepharoplasty.

As with all lid procedures, levator advancement should begin with tetracaine drops and injection of local anesthetic. When injecting the local anesthetic, care should be taken not to distort the natural anatomy and landmarks. Voluntary muscle function should be preserved whenever possible. A protective corneal shield is inserted. A transparent shield is preferred that allows visualization of the pupillary aperture. The lid is then incised through the orbicularis muscle fibers and the levator aponeurosis is identified. Dissection, using needle-tip electrocautery, continues superiorly past the orbital septum, which is divided at its junction with the aponeurosis. Further cephalad, dissection identifies the preaponeurotic fat. Dissection is next performed inferiorly to just beyond the aponeurotic–tarsal junction. Here, the levator aponeurosis is separated from the tarsal late along its superior margin, and the levator is lifted superiorly. When possible, the Mueller muscle is left behind, lying on the conjunctiva, while elevating the aponeurosis from below. Once the free edge of the levator aponeurosis is mobilized, dissection continues medially and laterally and the horns of the levator aponeurosis are released. Next the aponeurosis is grasped and advanced anteriorly and inferiorly, pulling it like a window shade over the tarsal plate to which it will eventually be resecured. The degree of advancement depends on the degree of ptosis and levator function. In most cases, 1 mm of advancement will provide 1 mm of correction, but as levator function decreases, greater advancements may be necessary to achieve the same results. This is especially true in cases of congenital ptosis where the levator function is, at best, fair. Regardless of the degree of advancement, however, the position of the lid should be evaluated after the first suture is placed intraoperatively in all cooperative patients. This is achieved by advancing the aponeurosis and securing it to the tarsal plate with absorbable suture in temporary fashion. The operating lights are directed off the field to minimize reflexive squinting, and the patient is placed upright and asked to look straight ahead. The cooperative patient is then asked to look up and down in order to assess function and the degree of lagophthalmos. The position of the lid is evaluated with respect to the ideal. The lid should fall halfway between the pupillary aperture and the corneoscleral junction at a vertical line approximating the pupillary nasal margin. Generally, a slight overcorrection by 1.0 to 1.5 mm is necessary to compensate for epinephrine-induced Mueller muscle stimulation. However, one must remember that undercorrection is easier to correct than overcorrection and is usually better tolerated by the patient.

Once the degree of advancement and lid position is determined, the aponeurosis is secured to the superior aspect of the tarsal plate with absorbable sutures. Excess levator tissue is amputated and, if necessary, the skin is secured to the supratarsal levator to recreate the lid fold. The lid incision is then closed with a running intracuticular permanent pullout suture in a medial-to-lateral fashion. If necessary, skin and orbicularis fibers may be excised, thus performing a concomitant blepharoplasty prior to closing the incision. However, it should be noted that, in our experience, resection of skin often is best deferred until a second procedure, after resolution of edema allows for a more accurate evaluation. This is especially true in the previously operated lid. If significant skin excess is left in place, however, a prominent lid fold, distortion of the lash line, or entropion may result.

In summary, the advantages of levator advancement include its broad application and its ability to be performed with or without blepharoplasty. It is technically more demanding, and has a steeper learning curve. However, once mastered, the levator advancement procedure is the most widely useful procedure. It allows adjustments intraoperatively and, most importantly, directly addresses the underlying pathophysiology in most cases (2,4).

Tarsal Conjunctival Mullerectomy

The tarsal–conjunctival mullerectomy (Fasanella-Servat procedure) is indicated for patients with good levator excursion and mild ptosis. In this procedure, a portion of the posterior lamella, including the superior margin of the tarsal plate, the inferior portion of the Mueller muscle, and the associated conjunctiva is removed en block. Anesthesia is provided by instilling topical tetracaine drops and subcutaneous injection of lidocaine with epinephrine, avoiding distortion of the anatomic layers. A minimum of 7 minutes is allowed to elapse for the hemostatic effects of epinephrine to take effect. The lid is everted, presenting the conjunctival surface and underlying cephalic aspect of the tarsal plate and the Mueller muscle. A portion of the posterior lamella, including the superior margin of the tarsal plate extending cephalad, is secured in a pair of identical mosquito clamps, as illustrated in Figure 39.11, leaving a 3- to 4-mm cuff of posterior lamella exposed. It is critical to adjust the placement of the matched clamps so that they parallel the natural curve of the lid. Eccentric clamp placement will result in an unbalanced resection and a "tented" or "pinched" lid. Next, a running, horizontal mattress, monofilament nonabsorbable suture is the brought through the skin on the medial aspect and run laterally under the clamps, exiting through the lateral eyelid skin. Using a scalpel, the tissue above the clamps is amputated and the clamps are removed. The palpebral conjunctiva is smoothed over with the back end of a forceps and the eyelid is reverted to its natural position. The suture tails are tied to each other, and a Steri-Strip is placed as shown. The suture is removed in approximately 1 to 2 weeks—sooner if overcorrection is suspected, and later if undercorrection is supposed. Disadvantages of this procedure include a variable tarsal plate contour, inability to provide graduated tension, a decreased wetting surface, and an increased risk for corneal abrasions in the postoperative period secondary to suture irritation. In contrast to levator advancement, there is little room for flexibility and adjustment intraoperatively with the tarsal conjunctival mullerectomy. Consequently, the individual tailoring aspect of this procedure is somewhat limited (2,4).

Levator Plication

The levator plication, or the levator tuck, is indicated for patients who have mild to moderate ptosis (1 to 5 mm) and good levator function in whom a minimal dissection is desired and required. Plication may be performed with or without other aesthetic or functional procedures such as blepharoplasty or brow lift. Unlike the tarsal conjunctival mullerectomy, the levator plication uses an anterior approach. After anesthetic drops are placed, local anesthesia is administered. A simple curvilinear incision or elliptical upper blepharoplasty incision is made, depending on whether or not skin and orbicularis fibers are to be removed. After identifying the levator aponeurosis, dissection is carried out inferiorly to the tarsal plate and superiorly through the orbital septum exposing the preaponeurotic fat medially and laterally to the margins until the levator aponeurosis is defined. The levator aponeurosis is plicated such that each millimeter of plication results in an equal correction of the ptosis. Some surgeons prefer to correct more so for each millimeter of ptosis, but we have found that a 1:1 ratio is sufficient in patients with fair to good levator function. On the other hand, 2:1 or even 3:1 correction may become necessary when performing this procedure in patients with poor levator function. The patient can be positioned upright and the plication can be adjusted, intraoperatively, accordingly. The first plication suture is placed in a vertical line approximating the nasal pupillary margin, the medial most aspect of the pupillary

TARSAL CONJUNCTIVAL MULLERECTOMY

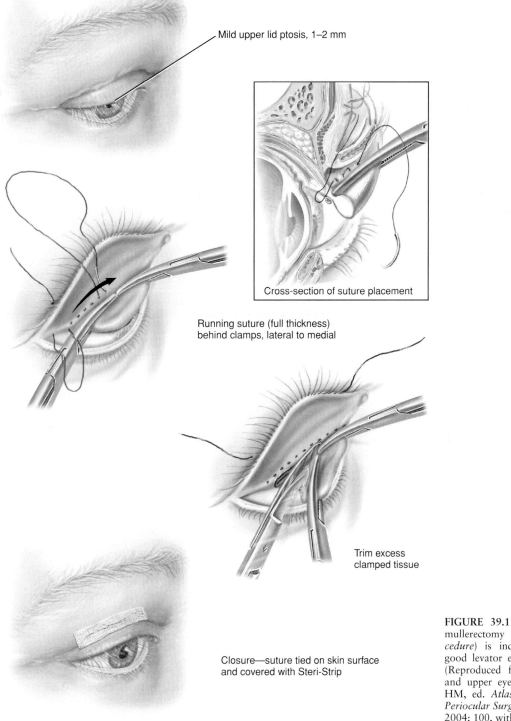

Mild upper lid ptosis, 1–2 mm

Cross-section of suture placement

Running suture (full thickness)
behind clamps, lateral to medial

Trim excess
clamped tissue

Closure—suture tied on skin surface
and covered with Steri-Strip

FIGURE 39.11. The tarsal–conjunctival mullerectomy (*Fasanella-Servat procedure*) is indicated for patients with good levator excursion and mild ptosis. (Reproduced from Spinelli HM. Ptosis and upper eyelid retraction. In: Spinelli HM, ed. *Atlas of Aesthetic Eyelid and Periocular Surgery*. Philadelphia: Elsevier; 2004; 100, with permission.)

aperture. Because the degree of correction required will vary from patient to patient, indeed even from the left to right eyelid, we assess the lid position in the sitting position prior to completing the plication and closure. As in all levator procedures, we err on the side of overcorrection by 1.0 to 1.5 mm in individuals with a competent muscle to compensate for epinephrine-induced Mueller muscle stimulation. After the level of plication is determined, additional plication sutures are placed, medially

and laterally, to complete the tuck. The cuff of levator tissue between our sutures is then assessed. If it is determined that leaving the tissue in place will distort the overlying skin of the lid, it is amputated; otherwise, it is left in place. At this point in the operation, some authors advocate reapproximation of the overlying skin to the levator aponeurosis to recreate the upper lid sulcus. This is especially true in patients in whom the lid height is to be altered. Finally, the skin is closed as in a standard blepharoplasty. The advantages of this procedure are its relative technical ease and the ability to adjust the plication sutures to the correction required. Its disadvantages include its limited application and an inability to be applied to a wide array of ptosis cases (2,4).

Frontalis Sling

When intrinsic levator function is poor (<5 mm) or absent, regardless of the degree of ptosis, upper eyelid elevation must depend upon the action of nearby exogenous muscles linked to the upper lid. Although several procedures have been described for the correction of this form of ptosis, which is often congenital in nature, the generally accepted procedure of choice is the frontalis sling (2,4).

As alluded to above, the frontalis sling essentially tethers the upper eyelid to the frontalis muscle above by way of alloplastic or autologous material tunneled beneath the orbicularis oculi muscle. Elevation of the lid is thereby achieved by elevation of the brow. One prerequisite of this procedure is adequate excursion of the levator complex. The lid must be able to be passively ranged, even if the muscle is completely fibrosed and dysfunctional.

Although numerous materials have been described to create the sling, our preference is to use autologous tissue, such as fascia lata or palmaris longus tendon, which have demonstrated the best overall long-term success. Several configurations of slings have been described. None is perfect and all seek to achieve the same goal. The double-rhomboid design is preferred. It begins by marking seven access points, three above and four below (Fig. 39.12). After anesthesia is administered, four stab incisions, deep to the tarsal plate, are made on the lid approximately 3 mm proximal to the lash line. Three corresponding stab incisions to the periosteum are made approximately 3 mm above the brow line. A strip of fascia or tendon prepared on a back table is then woven under the orbicularis and through the pretarsal area as illustrated. We find that a Wright needle is helpful for this portion of the procedure. Once the slings are in place, we make two assessments. First, we evert the lid to ensure the conjunctiva has not been violated; such a breach can result in a severe postoperative corneal abrasion. Second, we assess the position of the lid as best as possible. Unlike other procedures for ptosis described in this section, adult patients undergoing a frontalis sling procedure are unable to demonstrate lid excursion intraoperatively secondary to a motor block of the frontalis muscle from local anesthesia. In pediatric patients, cooperation is obviated by the level of sedation or general anesthesia. For this reason, landmarks are used to make the assessment. Once the slings are in place, contraction of the frontalis muscle is simulated by action of the surgeon's thumb resting against the patient's forehead. For patients with normal orbiculars function, maximum "excursion" should bring the lid to rest at the level of the corneoscleral junction. If orbicularis function is less than adequate, the lid should rest lower, between the pupillary aperture and the corneoscleral junction. After the final lid position has been appropriately adjusted by way of tightening or loosening the sling, the fascia is knotted and secured with absorbable suture. When possible, the sling is slid under the skin in clothesline fashion to ensure that all knots are buried away from the incision lines. The skin is closed in layers, and a tarsorrhaphy suture is placed. The main advantage of the frontalis sling procedure is that it can simulate, to some degree, levator function in an otherwise unresponsive or underresponsive lid. The major disadvantage of the frontalis sling is that it produces a significant lid lag. Although this is tolerated well, especially in the pediatric population, the lagophthalmos following the frontalis sling procedure can result in significant corneal exposure and

its inherent complications, especially in the immediate or early postoperative period (2,4).

Complications and Management

The most common complication of ptosis surgery is asymmetry. This may be secondary to undercorrection, overcorrection, or differentials in lid crease position and/or contour appearance. Less-common complications include corneal abrasion or keratitis, nerve palsy, entropion, ectropion, wound dehiscence, unfavorable scarring, loss of eyelashes, conjunctival prolapse, infection, and hematoma (2,4).

The most common cause for asymmetry is undercorrection. Undercorrection may be secondary to scarring from previous procedures, insufficient levator advancement, resection or plication, or a technical error. Usually, this is a result of the inexact nature of any of the known methods for assessing levator function intraoperatively. Improvement most often requires a second operative procedure.

Overcorrection occurs less commonly, but results in lagophthalmos (the inability to close the eye completely). Excessive evaporative tear loss may lead to keratitis sicca (dry eye) and corneal irritation. Treatment includes topical lubricants and, if necessary, a temporary tarsorrhaphy. If the condition persists for longer than 3 to 4 weeks, definitive surgical intervention is considered.

Lid crease asymmetry may result from unequal incisions or separation of the skin from the levator aponeurosis. However, reapproximation of the skin to the aponeurosis with absorbable suture through the tarsal plate margin may help reduce this risk.

Less-common complications following ptosis surgery include corneal abrasion or keratitis, which can occur secondary to an intraoperative corneal injury or an exposed suture on the conjunctival surface.

Entropion or ectropion also may be seen when significant imbalances between the anterior and posterior lamella are created during ptosis repair. For example, the presence of an excess of anterior lamella or skin after tarsal–conjunctival mullerectomy can cause the lid to roll inward, creating an entropion. Alternatively, a shortened anterior lamella (skin) following levator advancement with concomitant blepharoplasty, may cause ectropion.

Wound dehiscence may occur after a hematoma or in individuals prone to wound-healing problems (smokers, diabetics, systemic diseases). Scarring is usually favorable following eyelid incisions, but visible scars may occur. Keloid formation following eyelid surgery has been reported. The risk of eyelash loss can be minimized with careful dissection techniques and preservation of the hair follicles. Conjunctival prolapse may be minimized by maximizing atraumatic techniques and using a temporary tarsorrhaphy postoperatively when indicated. Infection is rare, but may occur especially when autologous or prosthetic graft material is used in, for example, frontalis sling procedures. All significant hematomas should be treated expeditiously. Extraocular muscle damage may occur during any orbital procedures as most periocular procedures violate the orbit at its most anterior extent. The internal oblique is the extraocular muscle most commonly injured during blepharoplasty. Finally, the risk of globe perforation, a dreaded complication of any periocular procedure, should be appreciated and avoided (2,4).

CANTHOPLASTY

The ideal lower lid position is 1.5 to 2.0 mm above the inferior corneoscleral junction. The nadir of the curvature should lie halfway between the medial and lateral fissures, and the lateral

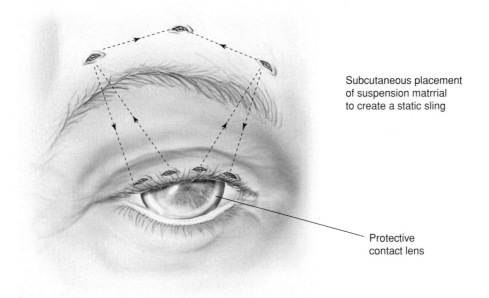

Subcutaneous placement
of suspension matrrial
to create a static sling

Protective
contact lens

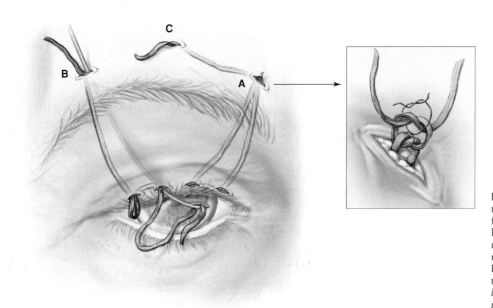

FIGURE 39.12. The frontalis sling tethers the upper eyelid to the frontalis muscle above by way of alloplastic or autologous material tunneled beneath the orbicularis oculi muscle. (Reproduced from Spinelli HM. Ptosis and upper eyelid retraction. In: Spinelli HM, ed. *Atlas of Aesthetic Eyelid and Periocular Surgery.* Philadelphia: Elsevier, 2004; 111, with permission.)

canthus should lie approximately 10 to 15 degrees above a horizontal line that bisects the medial fissure. In the normal state, the intrinsic and extrinsic forces acting on the lower lid maintain a fine balance that holds it approximated to the globe (Fig. 39.13). Imbalances in these forces—as a result of the effects of age, trauma, or previous surgeries—results in malposition of the lower lid. Because the most common cause of lower lip malposition is lid laxity, assessment and treatment of lid laxity are the main issues in canthoplasty. Any patient with scleral show has lid laxity, but early stages of lid laxity may be present even without scleral show (4).

In addition to the assessment of the patient outlined previously in the Selection of the Correct Operation section, evaluation of the lateral canthal region should include an assessment of the lower lid, canthus, and adequacy of the ocular tear film volume, quality, and ability to resist evaporation. A Schirmer test, a "tear film breakup time" examination, a snap-back test, and an evaluation of malar support are all elements of a thor-

ough examination. The *Schirmer test* and the *tear film breakup time* help the surgeon to evaluate the adequacy of tear production and quality, respectively (Fig. 39.14). Marginal tear production or poor quality tears can mitigate against performing some periocular procedures or may force the surgeon to modify the procedure to compensate for a propensity for dry eye (4,5).

The *snap-back test* (Fig. 39.14) should be performed as an evaluation on all patients considered for periocular surgery. Despite some reports to the contrary, we believe the snap-back test is an excellent and reliable clinical measure of intrinsic lid tone. Patients with a weak or moderate snap-back (indicating significant or moderate laxity of the lower lid) are usually candidates for lower-lid tightening procedures, especially when a concomitant procedure that increases distraction forces is entertained (4).

Finally, an evaluation of malar support can be done by simply noting the extent to which the cornea projects beyond the infraorbital rim. The soft-tissue lower-lid support mechanism

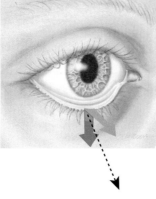

Intrinsic Support Forces (ISF)

Extrinsic Distraction Forces (EDF)

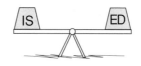

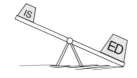

FIGURE 39.13. Intrinsic and extrinsic forces acting on the lower lid maintain a fine balance that holds it approximated to the globe. (Reproduced from Spinelli HM. Anatomy. In: Spinelli HM, ed. *Atlas of Aesthetic Eyelid and Periocular Surgery.* Philadelphia: Elsevier, 2004, with permission.)

(e.g., tarsal plate, orbicularis sling) relies on the underling zygoma as a rigid pillar or weight-bearing structure. The absence of rigid structural support below the lower-lid soft-tissue support structures is clinically seen as a prominent globe or an eyeball that projects beyond the infraorbital rim. A patient on whom the globe does not project beyond the infraorbital rim is said to have a "negative vector" (4).

Surgical options designed to correct lower-lid laxity are numerous and include tarsal tuck canthopexy, the modified lateral tarsal strip procedure, and the common canthoplasty. The choice of procedure(s) depends on the etiology and extent of the problem. To clarify, the term canth*oplasty* implies division of the canthus, in whole or in part. The term canth*opexy* implies that lid support is achieved by plication or redirection without division of the canthus. In performing the *canthopexy,* the lower lid or lateral tendon is not shortened or divided but secured in a new position to a rigid structure like the periorbita. Approximation of the tendon may occur at the Whitnall tubercle or at a point superior and lateral to it. In contrast, *canthoplasty* requires division of either the inferior crus or common crus of the lateral canthal tendon and lateral retinaculum. These are then mobilized and reinserted as a single unit as indicated by the degree of lower-lid laxity. Finally, the *modified lateral tarsal strip procedure* is a canthoplasty. It requires division of the inferior crus of the lateral canthal tendon and reconstruction to provide support by approximating the lateral aspect of the mobilized tarsal plate to the Whitnall tubercle. These procedures are discussed in detail below. The most common error in performing all canthal procedures is insufficient mobilization of the lower eyelid (4).

Surgical Procedures

Tarsal Tuck Canthopexy

The *tarsal tuck* provides support to the lower lid without division of the lateral canthal tendon, the inferior crus, or the tarsal plate. It is not a "lid-shortening" procedure; rather, it is a "lid-

supporting" procedure. It may be performed independently or as an adjunct to a concomitant procedure. Furthermore, it may be performed transcutaneously or through a transconjunctival approach. The indication for the independent tarsal tuck procedure is a patient with mild lower-lid laxity and an intact lateral canthal complex. However, if the laxity is too great, the plicated tissue will tend to buckle, causing the lower lid to lose its apposition with the globe, resulting in an unsatisfactory appearance and poorly functional eyelid. Advantages of the independent tarsal tuck procedure are its simplicity, minimally invasive nature, and ability to concomitantly transpose or resect orbital fat to fill periocular defects. The main disadvantage is that it can only be used when there is minimal lid laxity (4).

Modified Lateral Tarsal Strip Procedure

The tarsal strip procedure has broader application in the treatment of lower-lid laxity. This procedure can serve to restore the natural appearance and function of the lower lid regardless of the manifestation of the lower-lid laxity, whether it be dry eye, ectropion, entropion, or simply scleral show. It may be performed alone or in combination with other procedures, and has proven to be a reliable technique.

This procedure owes some of its evolution to the simple wedge resection in that the lower lid is shortened. Its major discriminating feature is that a new inferior canthal crus is created from the tarsus, which is independently supported.

The lateral tarsal strip procedure begins with a lateral canthotomy and division of the inferior crus of the lateral canthal tendon, proximal to its insertion on the lateral aspect of the tarsal plate (Fig. 39.15). The lower lid is mobilized in the subcutaneous plane, which is accomplished by division of the retinacular elements that secure it to the septum and orbicularis posteriorly. Mobilization of this tissue is the single most important step in achieving satisfactory results. The lateralmost aspect of the lid can be stretched to reach the level of the eyebrow when the mobilization is adequate. Next, the lateral tarsal plate is prepared so that a narrow strip of tarsal plate is created. A minimum of 3 mm of lateral tarsal plate should

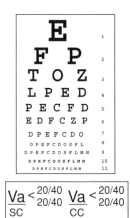

1. Visual acuity via Snellen chart

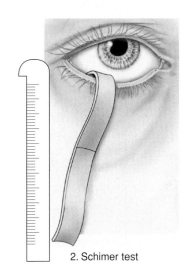

2. Schimer test

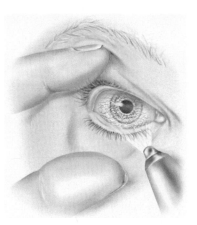

3. Snap-back test

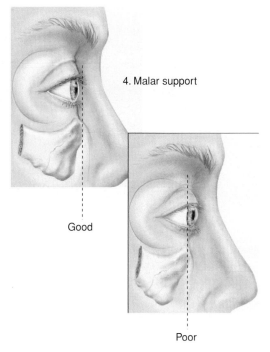

4. Malar support

Good

Poor

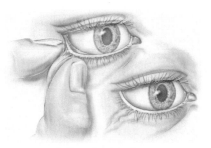

5. Tear film breakup time

FIGURE 39.14. Proper evaluation includes visual acuity, Schirmer test, the snap-back test, and evaluation of malar support and tear film breakup time. (Reproduced from Spinelli HM. Evaluation of the patient. In: Spinelli HM, ed. *Atlas of Aesthetic Eyelid and Periocular Surgery*. Philadelphia: Elsevier, 2004, with permission.)

be exposed. The strip is then de-epithelialized circumferentially of skin from the anterior surface, of lash follicles from the superior margin, and of conjunctiva from the posterior surface. The inferior margin is then separated from the capsulopalpebral fascia below, completely freeing the newly created tarsal strip. This strip will serve as a neocanthal tendon. A double-arm suture is used for fixation. Prior to tying the suture and finalizing the canthoplasty, the position of the lower lid should be assessed in relation to the corneoscleral junction. Here the lid should rest 1.5 to 2.0 mm above the junction. It is helpful at this point to align the gray line of the lower lid with the gray line of the upper lid with a resorbable suture exiting at the lateral commissure (*commissuroplasty*). After determining the appropriate level and tension, the canthal fixation suture is

tied and the overlying elements, including the orbicularis muscle and skin, are trimmed as necessary.

Advantages of the tarsal strip procedure include its wide array of applications and satisfactory long-term results. Disadvantages are few, and for moderate or severe lower-lid laxity manifesting in dry eye, ectropion, entropion, or scleral show, it generally provides satisfactory results. One significant disadvantage to the tarsal strip procedure is that it can create a length discrepancy between the unshortened upper eyelid and the fore-shortened lower lid. This becomes a concern only in the patient with significant redundancy of both the upper and lower lids. In these cases, preoperative planning should be altered accordingly. The length discrepancy can be eliminated by either concomitantly shortening the lateral upper eyelid and creating a

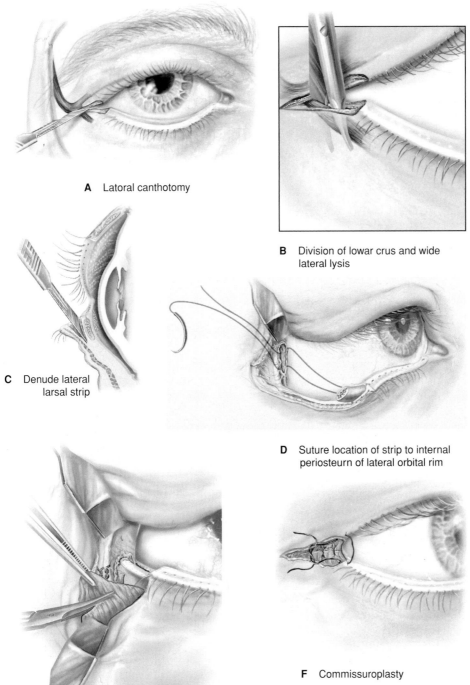

A Lateral canthotomy

B Division of lower crus and wide lateral lysis

C Denude lateral tarsal strip

D Suture location of strip to internal periosteum of lateral orbital rim

F Commissuroplasty

E Trim excess skin and/or orbicularis muscle

FIGURE 39.15. The lateral tarsal strip procedure does not alter the intercanthal distance or disturb the intrinsic–extrinsic balance that supports the lower lid position. (Reproduced from Spinelli HM. Eyelid malpositions. In: Spinelli HM, ed. *Atlas of Aesthetic Eyelid and Periocular Surgery.* Philadelphia: Elsevier, 2004; 39, with permission.)

neocommissure, or by cephalically and laterally tightening the upper and lower eyelids en bloc by performing a common canthoplasty (4,6,10).

Common Canthoplasty and Common Canthopexy

The common canthoplasty is useful alone or in combination with other procedures. It is especially useful when the goal is to correct a shortened intercommissural distance and/or inferior displacement of the entire lateral canthus. It can be applied in both cosmetic and reconstructive scenarios. In addition, consideration should be given to this technique in any patient undergoing a procedure that can compromise the balance of intrinsic and extrinsic forces providing lower-lid support (4).

Access to the lateral canthal tendon can be achieved through an incision of either the upper or lower lid; however, incision of the upper lid is more favorable for achieving the appropriate vector of suspension. Regardless of the access incision, the lateral canthal tendon must be identified and mobilized in its entirety with disinsertion of the common tendon from the

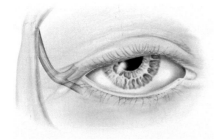

A Eyelid droop due to lateral canthal tendon attenuation

Line of division of lateral retinaculum for common canthoplasty

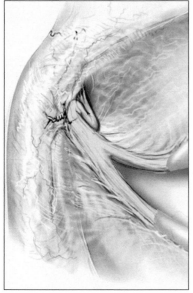

Closeup of common centhopexy

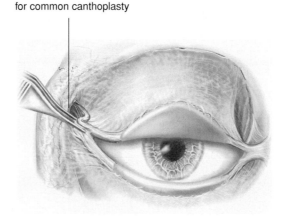

B Common canthal tendon is retracted laterally and superiorly then anchored to periosteum

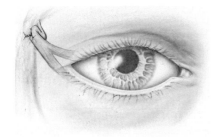

C Effect of completed repair

FIGURE 39.16. The common canthopexy is useful alone or in combination with other procedures. (Reproduced from Spinelli HM. Eyelid malpositions. In: Spinelli HM, ed. *Atlas of Aesthetic Eyelid and Periocular Surgery.* Philadelphia: Elsevier, 2004; 47, with permission.)

Whitnall tubercle. Once the retinacular elements are lysed, the entire lateral canthal complex can be moved cephalically and/or laterally.

Advantages of this procedure, alone or in concert with other procedures, include its ability to correct the attenuation, whether actual or anticipated, of the lateral canthal tendon, restoring the intercanthal distance and elevation of the lateral canthus. Disadvantages are few, and in our opinion, this procedure should be used liberally (4). In contrast to the common canthoplasty, a common cantho*pexy* may be performed and is indicated for those patients with only a minimal amount of lower-lid laxity or simply a slight decrease in intercommissure distance. In this procedure, the lateral canthal tendon is not divided from the lateral retinaculum or from the Whitnall tubercle; instead it is suspended to the periorbita or other nearby rigid structure (Fig. 39.16). In this procedure, mild canthal dystopia, such as is seen with minimal laxity of the lower eyelid or slight decreases in intercommissure distances, can be

corrected. However, because the lateral retinacular elements are not lysed, mobilization is minimal, making this procedure prone to failure unless limited to achieve modest goals.

References

1. Bron AJ, Tripathi RC, Tripathi BJ. *Wolff's Anatomy of the Eye and Orbit.* 8th ed. New York: Chapman & Hall Medical; 1997.
2. Carraway JH. Reconstruction of the eyelids and correction of ptosis of the eyelid. In: Aston SJ, Beasley RW, Thorne CHM, eds. *Grabb & Smith's Plastic Surgery.* 5th ed. New York: Lippincot-Raven; 1997: 529–544.
3. Nesi FA, Lisman RD, Levine MR. *Smith's Ophthalmic Plastic and Reconstructive Surgery.* 2nd ed. New York: Mosby; 1998.
4. Spinelli HM. *Atlas of Aesthetic Eyelid and Periocular Surgery.* Philadelphia: Elsevier; 2004.
5. Spinelli HM, Farris RL. The tear film. In: Byron Smith BC, ed. *Ophthalmic Plastic and Reconstructive Surgery.* St. Louis: Mosby; 1987: 535–545.
6. Spinelli HM, Jelks GW. Periocular reconstruction: a systematic approach. *Plast Reconstr Surg.* 1993;91(6):1017–1024.

7. Jackson IT. *Eyelid and Canthal Region Reconstruction. Local Flaps in Head and Neck Reconstruction.* St. Louis: Quality Medical Publishing; 2002: 273–326.
8. Mustarde JC. Reconstruction of eyelids. *Ann Plast Surg.* 1983;11(2):149–169.
9. Spinelli HM, Suzman MS. Soft-tissue deformities in orbital trauma: evaluation and repair of medial and lateral canthal injury. *J Oper Tech Plast Reconstr Surg.* 2003;8(4):249–258.
10. Spinelli HM, Forman DL. Current treatment of post-traumatic deformities. Residual orbital, adnexal, and soft-tissue abnormalities. *Clin Plast Surg.* 1997;24(3):519–530.
11. Spinelli HM, Sherman JE, Lisman RD, et al. Human bites of the eyelid. *Plast Reconstr Surg.* 1986;78(5):610–614.
12. Kroll SS, Reece GP, Robb G, et al. Deep-plane cervicofacial rotation-advancement flap for reconstruction of large cheek defects. *Plast Reconstr Surg.* 1994;94(1):88–93.

CHAPTER 40 ■ FACIAL PARALYSIS RECONSTRUCTION

RALPH T. MANKTELOW, RONALD M. ZUKER, AND PETER C. NELIGAN

INTRODUCTION

Facial paralysis is a devastating condition. The paralyzed muscles are appropriately called the muscles of facial expression. Lack of facial expression is not an aesthetic issue, but a profound functional disability because the function of the face is to communicate.

Facial paralysis can be congenital or acquired. Reconstruction for facial paralysis is the same, however, regardless of etiology, with one proviso. If the paralysis is recent and reinnervation of the nonfunctional muscles is possible, then certain operations are available. If the paralysis is longstanding, which usually means greater than 1.5 years, then etiology is largely irrelevant to the reconstruction.

ESSENTIAL FUNCTIONS OF THE SEVENTH CRANIAL NERVE

The seventh cranial nerve controls all the superficial facial musculature and thereby controls the appearance of the face, the ability to show expression, and most of the functions about the forehead, eye, cheeks, and mouth.

Unilateral paralysis results in marked asymmetry at rest and with facial animation (Fig. 40.1). Paralysis of the brow results in ptosis of the forehead and eyebrow due to loss of frontalis muscle tone. The older the patient, the more severe is the drooping. Not only an aesthetic problem, frontal paralysis results in obstruction of upward gaze. The depressed position of the forehead gives the impression of unhappiness, anger, or excessive seriousness. Wrinkling of the forehead on the normal side and a smooth forehead on the paralyzed side makes the asymmetry more apparent. Paralysis of the orbicularis oculi muscle causes inability to blink and close the eye. With eyelid closure most of the movement occurs with the upper eyelid. The main function of the lower lid is to maintain the lid margins in contact with the globe and assist in tear drainage. Blinking occurs many times per minute and is an important mechanism for spreading the tear film and preventing the cornea from drying. The ability to close the eyes is also an important mechanism for preventing damage from wind and foreign material. The tone of the eyelids determines the amount of the globe that is visible. In the average adult who is looking straight ahead, the distance between the upper and lower eyelids is 9 to 11 mm at its widest. The upper eyelid usually covers 2 to 3 mm of the superior corneal limbus, and the lower eyelid lies at the level of the inferior corneal limbus. With paralysis, more of the globe is exposed at rest due to the unresisted action of the levator palpebrae and the effect of gravity on the lower lid. Even 1 to 2 mm of scleral show between the cornea and the paralyzed lower lid results in obvious asymmetry.

It is the lack of frequent blinking resulting in corneal desiccation that produces many of the symptoms of discomfort. Drying is accentuated by the lack of tear production that is often present in a high-level facial paralysis. Drying of the eye produces a reflex increase of tear flow that cannot be managed by the canaliculi, resulting in overflow on to the cheek. Thus, we have the paradox of an eye that feels dry having excessive tears. Epiphora can be a significant functional problem, with tears dripping from the cheek onto a work surface, as well as social liability. Patients complain that the eye looks like it is staring. When a person is smiling, the normal eye closes slightly and conveys the expression of pleasure or happiness, whereas the affected eye maintains the widened palpebral aperture (Fig. 40.2).

The orbicularis oris encircles the lips and is necessary for oral competence. Paralysis results in drooling. Orbicularis function is also important for labial sounds such as 'b', 'p' and 'm'. The other muscles around the mouth are retractors, lifting the upper lip, pulling the lower lips down, and retracting the commissure laterally. These muscles are critical for facial expression in the face. Paralysis of the buccinator prevents control of the food bolus, and food tends to pocket in the buccal sulcus. These muscles are critical for facial expression in the lower face.

Although unilateral facial paralysis is more common, bilateral paralysis presents unique problems. Unlike in facial asymmetry at rest, the face is totally immobile and conveys no messages through facial expression. There is symmetric drooping and lack of any expression (Fig. 40.3). Frequently, these patients are treated as if they are emotionally and mentally incompetent. As a result of the paralysis of the orbicularis oris, the lower lip will frequently pout outward, making it difficult to control food and fluids. Labial speech sounds are impossible.

ANATOMY OF THE SEVENTH CRANIAL NERVE

The extratemporal portion of seventh cranial (or facial) nerve begins at the stylomastoid foramen (1). The main trunk of the nerve quickly becomes superficial, making it susceptible to injury. The nerve enters the parotid gland and divides into two trunks, which further divide into five divisions: temporal, zygomatic, buccal, marginal mandibular, and cervical. These divisions are to some extent artificial. There is no distinct separation between zygomatic and buccal branches either in their location or in the muscles that they innervate. As the branches exit from the superior, anterior, and inferior margins of the parotid, there may be 8 to 15 branches making up the five divisions (Fig. 40.4). Distal to the parotid there is significant arborization and interconnection of these branches. Significantly for the surgeon, there is a considerable functional overlap

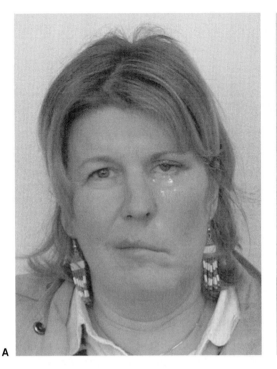

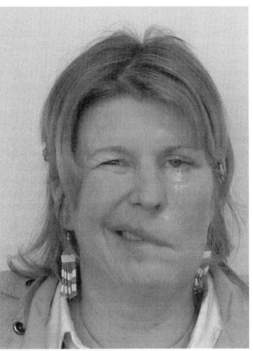

FIGURE 40.1. **A:** Forty-year-old woman with total left facial paralysis seen at rest. **B:** Facial asymmetry is even more apparent on smiling.

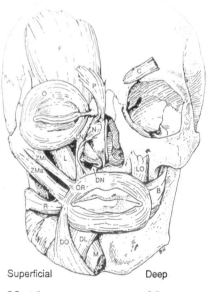

Superficial

F-Frontalis
P-Procerus
O-Orbicularis oculi
OR-Orbicularis oris
N-Nasalis
LN-Levator labii superioris alaeque nasi
L-Levator labii superioris
ZMi-Zygomaticus minor
ZMa-Zygomaticus major
R-Risorius
DO-Depressor anguli oris
DL-Depressor labii inferioris
M-Mentalis
DN-Depressor nasi

Deep

C-Corrugator supercilii
B-Buccinator
LO-Levator anguli oris

FIGURE 40.2. Muscles of facial expression that are controlled by the facial nerve. (Manktelow R. Facial Paralysis. In: Mathes SJ, ed. *Plastic Surgery*, 2nd ed. Philadelphia: Saunders, 2006:887, with permission.)

FIGURE 40.3. With bilateral facial paralysis the face droops and looks the same at rest and with attempted animation.

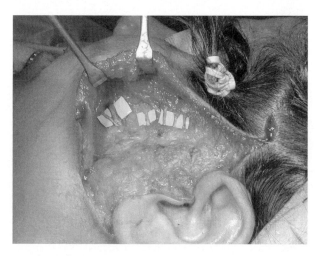

FIGURE 40.4. The branches of the facial nerve can be seen where they exit from the anterior margin of the parotid. They have been separated from the surrounding tissue in preparation for stimulation and functional identification. (Manktelow R. Facial paralysis. In: Mathes SJ, ed. *Plastic Surgery*, 2nd ed. Philadelphia: Saunders, 2006:899, with permission.)

among branches and frequent duplication of branches providing the same function.

There are two to five branches in the temporal division. These branches run deep to temporoparietal fascia after they pass over the zygomatic arch. They innervate the frontalis muscle, corrugator supercilious, and upper orbicularis oculi. A paucity of subcutaneous fat at the lateral border of the frontalis muscle makes the nerves subject to injury from lacerations. Each of the divisions (frontal, zygomatic, buccal, and marginal mandibular) consist of multiple branches, except the cervical division, which usually consists of a single branch.

FACIAL MUSCULATURE

There are 18 paired muscles of the face, including the orbicularis oris, which can be considered as a paired muscle (see Fig. 40.2). Freilinger et al. demonstrated that the facial muscles are arranged in layers about the mouth (2). The most superficial are the depressor anguli oris, zygomaticus minor, and the orbicularis oris. The deepest layer consists of the buccinator, mentalis, and the depressor anguli oris. Except for these three deep muscles, all of the facial muscles receive their innervation via their deep surfaces. A detailed discussion of each of these muscles is available elsewhere (3).

PREOPERATIVE APPRAISAL

Those aspects of the preoperative evaluation that are specific for facial paralysis will be highlighted. The cause and time course of the paralysis is important because they determine the outcome of the paralysis and determine which procedures might be effective. For example, the patient who has had a recent Bell's palsy has an 80% to 90% chance of a complete recovery. However, the same patient seen at 1 year with no recovery has a very slim chance of useful recovery.

The history includes symptoms relating to the eye including dryness, discomfort, tearing, and inability to close the eye and the use of artificial tears or ointments. The complaints related to the lower face may include lack of oral continence, difficulties with speech, nasal airway difficulties, and problems with psychosocial functioning and social interactions. For most patients, the goal is to smile.

Evaluation of facial movements and spontaneous expressions is initiated during the history taking when the surgeon is carefully watching the patient's face. This is a good time for light socialization to occur between the patient and the surgeon and for the surgeon to take the opportunity to see the patient as he or she is likely to be seen by others. Physical examination begins by asking the patient to raise the brow, close the eyes, smile, and pucker the lips.

The eye is examined in detail. The height of the palpebral aperture on the paralyzed side is compared with that of the normal side, and the aperture is measured with eye closure. The effectiveness of a Bell's reflex will affect the amount of corneal exposure. Lower eyelid position is assessed by comparing the two sides relative to the cornea. Tone in the lower eyelid is assessed by the snap test. The location of the inferior canalicular punctum is assessed. Normally it is applied to the globe. It is very important to assess corneal sensibility because the eye that lacks sensation and also has orbicularis oculi paralysis is at risk for corneal damage, ulceration, and scarring.

The lower face is observed at rest and with animation. The asymmetry of the nose and mouth is documented. With the help of a transparent handheld ruler, the surgeon can mark the various points on the vermilion margin and at the base of the nose and nasolabial fold and measure these with respect to the dental midline and the horizontal plane. More sophisticated systems using a video camera and computer provide the surgeon an alternative tool for measuring facial asymmetry and facial movements (4). The measurements provide the surgeon with a quantitative assessment of the facial asymmetry at rest. In unilateral paralysis, there is usually weakening or loss of the nasolabial fold, deviation of the philtrum toward the normal side, commissure depression on the paralyzed side, and deviation of the entire oral sphincter toward the normal side. The sagging is due to gravity, and the deviation to the normal side is due to unopposed muscle action on the normal side. Movements of the commissure and the mid upper and mid lower lip are measured during animation. This gives the surgeon some information regarding the amount and direction of movement that is required for smile reconstruction.

Synkinesis is the simultaneous contraction of two or more muscles that normally do not contract at the same time and is thought to be due to a misdirected sprouting of regenerating axons. A common synkinesis is eye closure with smiling. A particularly frustrating synkinesis occurs when there is simultaneous contraction of the orbicularis oris and the retractors of the mouth. This grimacing appearance is brought on by attempts to smile or to purse the lips.

NONSURGICAL MANAGEMENT

Most patients require some degree of protection and/or lubrication for the eye. Drops containing hydroxypropyl cellulose, hydroxypropyl methylcellulose, or polyvinyl alcohol are effective lubricating agents for preventing eye drying and last much longer than normal tears. Some patients require them hourly and others once or twice a day. A thicker ointment that contains petrolatum, mineral oil, or lanolin alcohol is used at night to prevent drying of the eye. Patients who present with excessive tearing may achieve improvement by using artificial tears. With coating of the eye, the reflex tearing that is initiated by the sense of eye dryness is turned off.

Neuromuscular retraining supervised by an experienced therapist may be beneficial for the patient who has a partial paralysis. Biofeedback exercises frequently provide significant benefit.

SURGICAL MANAGEMENT

The large number of available operations for the forehead, eye, mouth, nose, and cheek suggests that there is no one operation that will be successful in all patients. There are many procedures, however, that can be of benefit depending on the patient's particular problem.

The Brow

A brow lift by direct excision of tissue through an incision just above the eyebrow is the most effective technique. A coronal or endoscopic lift is another option.

With a unilateral frontalis paralysis the drooping of the brow will vary depending on the patient's tissues and age. In an elderly patient the droop may be as much as 12 mm. However, a droop of 3 to 4 mm is quite apparent in most persons. A direct brow lift through a superciliary lift is best able to correct large discrepancies. The important features of this operation are that the incision be placed just along the main line of hair follicles. It should not be placed above every follicle or it will be in a visible position. Thus, a few hairs will be excised. An ellipse of skin and frontalis muscle is excised and the paralyzed frontalis muscle repaired. Care is taken to evert the skin edges. The disadvantage is a visible scar, frequently because the incision is too high or because the scar is indented.

A coronal approach leaves an inconspicuous scar, but the amount of lifting that can be achieved is much less. Similarly, it is difficult to obtain a large lift through an endoscopic brow lift. When doing a coronal incision it may be helpful to put in a sling of fascia lata from the subcutaneous tissues of the brow to the periosteum or bone of the skull. Our approach in recent years has been to do a direct lift through a supraciliary incision. A large proportion of patients will complain of some numbness despite extremely meticulous dissection of the supraorbital nerves. Usually this numbness is of little concern to the patient unless a major branch has been divided. Another option is frontal branch neurectomy on the normal side. If there is marked wrinkling of the forehead on the normal side, a normal-side frontal nerve resection with or without a frontalis muscle resection will help to correct forehead asymmetry. Because a simple resection of the frontal branches often results in reinnervation, the surgeon should consider resecting the entire lateral margin of the frontalis to obtain a permanent paralysis.

The Upper Eyelid

The simplest effective procedure is lid loading with a gold prosthesis. The goal is to provide improved but not complete closure. The amount of weight required for complete closure is frequently too large, and a large weight is more likely to detach and erode through the skin. **The lightest weight that will bring the eyelid within 2 to 4 mm of the lower lid and cover the cornea is quite adequate.** The effectiveness of a gold weight placement can be determined preoperatively by taping the test weight with double-sided tape to the upper eyelid. The operative procedure consists in suturing the gold weight to the tarsal plate with permanent sutures (5) (Fig. 40.5). Care must be taken that the sutures do not pass through the lid conjunctiva. The gold weight should be placed high enough above the lid margin that it is not visible when the eye is open. If the patient has a large amount of exposed eyelid skin above the eyelashes, it may not be possible to use the gold weight without producing a visible bulge. Great care should be taken in placing the weight in order that the levator mechanism is not

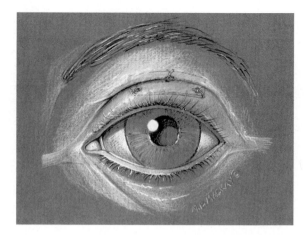

FIGURE 40.5. A gold weight is sutured to the tarsal plate and placed far enough above the tarsal plate that it is not visible with the eye open. (Manktelow R. Facial paralysis. In: Mathes SJ, ed. *Plastic Surgery*, 2nd ed. Philadelphia: Saunders, 2006:893, with permission.)

disturbed. The patient should be carefully examined prior to surgery. If there is any tendency to upper lid ptosis, this will likely be exacerbated by inserting a lid weight. The patient should be advised to practice lid closure whenever the eye feels uncomfortable and to realize that the lid closure (levator relaxation) is a "slow blink" and should be held for 1 to 2 seconds to allow the full descent of the weighted lid. Complications and side effects of the procedure are a visible lump, extrusion of the weight, capsule formation that causes a visible lump, and occasionally irritation of the eyelid by the weight.

An alternative to the weight is the use of a palpebral spring as described by Morel-Fatio (6). This consists of a piece of spring wire shaped by the surgeon like an open safety pin. The upper arm is fixed to the inner aspect of the orbital rim, and the lower arm is attached to the lid margin. When the eye is open, the two arms are brought close to each other, and when the eyelid is relaxed, the force of the wire spring moves the arms apart and thus closes the eye. This procedure is not gravity dependent; however there is a long learning curve, and the results depend up the experience of the operator. Our preference is to use the gold weight.

Transfer of a strip of temporalis muscle provides a dynamic closure of the eyelid using autogenous tissue. A 1.5- to 2-cm-wide strip of temporalis muscle based inferiorly is extended with two strips of fascia or tendon, passed through the upper and lower eyelids, and fastened to the medial canthal ligament (Fig. 40.6) (7). Traditionally, two strips are used for each eyelid. However, most of the requirement for eyelid movement is for the upper eyelid. Our preference is to place a static sling in the lower lid and a temporalis transfer in only the upper lid. The critical aspects of this procedure are setting the tension of the transfer and placing the transfer without deforming the upper lid and lateral lid margins. Closure of the lid may produce a slit-like shape, and there may be lateral movement and skin wrinkling of the lateral lid region. Frequently there is also an obvious muscle bulge over the lateral orbital margin, and there will be some eyelid closure movement when chewing (Fig. 40.7). Advantages of this procedure are that it can provide a forceful and full eyelid closure. Frequent biting movements throughout the day will result in frequent closing of the eyelid, which will facilitate corneal lubrication. This may be the procedure of choice if sensibility in the cornea has been lost.

A tarsorrhaphy is one of the simplest treatments for the paralyzed eyelid and results in support of the lower lid and decreases the amount of exposure by lowering the upper lid. The

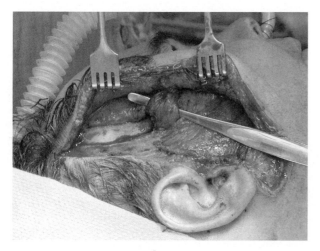

FIGURE 40.6. A strip of the right temporalis muscle has been transferred toward the right upper eyelid.

procedure involves resecting the margins of the adjacent eyelid and suturing the adjacent raw surfaces together. If a tarsorrhaphy involves a sufficiently large area of the eyelid, it almost always produces a good functional result; patients dislike it, however, because of the appearance of a small eye and the difficulty when looking laterally.

Another alternative for dynamic eyelid reconstruction is use of a free platysma transfer. This is a difficult reconstruction and the results are very much dependent on the skill of the surgeon as well as his or her experience with the procedure. Innervation of this muscle transfer requires a separate cross-facial nerve transfer to which the cervical branch of the facial nerve contained in the platysma transfer is attached. The vascular pedicle

of this transfer is very small, usually about 0.5 mm in diameter, and is a branch of the facial artery. The anterior branch of the superficial temporal vascular system is used to vascularize the platysma.

The Lower Eyelid

The lower eyelid may not be a problem in the younger patient; with the passage of time, however, and the normal loss of tone of the lower lid tissues, gravity will produce sagging of the lid, resulting in scleral show. Eventually the inferior canalicular punctum and lid margin will roll out away from the globe and an ectropion will occur. The management should be directed toward repositioning the lid vertically against the globe and apposing the punctum to the globe. The most successful procedure in our hands is to insert a sling in the lower lid using a 1.5-mm-wide strip of tendon (8). This is sutured to the lateral orbital margin in the region of the zygomaticofrontal suture and is tunneled subcutaneously along the lid margin just anterior to the tarsal plate. The placement in the lower lid is crucial. It must be only 1 to 2 mm below the lid margin. If it is too low, it will evert the lid margin and exacerbate the ectropion. If it is too superficial, which is easy in an elderly patient with very thin skin, it may result in an entropion. The sling is passed deep to the anterior portion of the medial canthal ligament and sutured back on itself. Passage of the tendon graft is facilitated in the pretarsal tunnel by threading it onto a curved Keith needle (Fig. 40.8). This procedure is not suitable for the patient with prominent eyes, in whom this type of sling will oppose the lid to the globe but will not raise the lid on the globe.

Various techniques of canthoplasty have been described including tarsal strip, dermal pennant, and inferior retinacular canthoplasty (9). These methods are useful in the aesthetic or posttraumatic situation but stretch over the long term in a patient with facial paralysis. Similarly, lid shortening through a

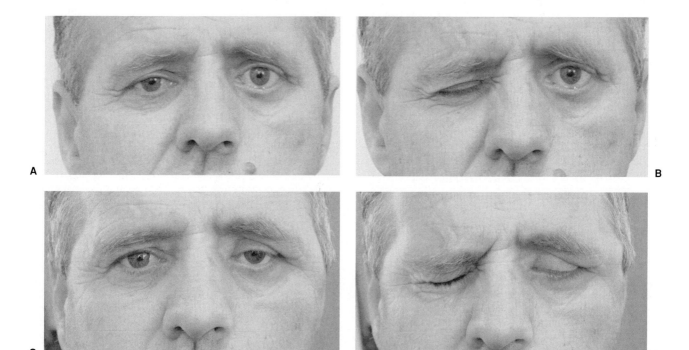

FIGURE 40.7. Temporalis transfer to eyelids. **A:** Preoperative left facial paralysis with eyes open. **B:** Preoperative left facial paralysis with attempted eye closure. The left eye does not close and there is no protective Bell's phenomenon. **C:** Postoperative eyes open. **D:** Postoperative eyes closed. The left eye is effectively closed by biting.

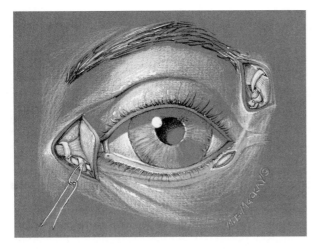

FIGURE 40.8. Placement of a tendon sling in the lower eyelid. It is more reliable to pass the sling through a drill hole in the bone of the lateral orbital margin than to pass it through periosteum as shown here. (Manktelow R. Facial paralysis. In: Mathes SJ, ed. *Plastic Surgery*, 2nd ed. Philadelphia: Saunders, 2006:897, with permission.)

triangular incision such as in the Kuhnt-Szymanowski procedure will give a good initial result but does not provide a lasting correction. Cartilage grafts have also been used to prop up the tarsal plate. The cartilage, usually conchal, sits on the inferior orbital margin. We have been unsuccessful with this procedure. The cartilage tends to rotate outward rather than sit in a vertical position, thus producing a visible bulge and poor eyelid support.

Nasal Reconstruction

The nasal problem is frequently airway obstruction on the side of the paralysis. The intact musculature on the normal side of the face will pull the lower portion of the nose away from the paralyzed side, and gravity will cause drooping of the nasal base on this side. This results in a visual asymmetry and significant breathing problems due to collapse of the right nostril, particularly when sleeping. Correction of airway collapse can be obtained by a spreader graft or a sling of tendon from the lateral aspect of the alar base up to the orbital margin. However, correction of the lower face and lips with either a static or dynamic procedure will usually reposition the nasal base and correct the nasal obstruction.

Lip and Cheek Reconstruction

The dominant complaints are usually facial asymmetry at rest and the inability to smile. Additional concerns are drooling, difficulty managing the food bolus, and labial speech. If the concern is primarily for asymmetry at rest, then a static procedure with slings can be quite beneficial. The sling can be made of fascia such as tensor fascia lata or a tendon, preferably the plantaris. Our experience with prosthetic material such as Gore-Tex (polytetrafluoroethylene) is that it produces an undesirable inflammatory reaction. Plantaris tendon can be usually harvested through a single incision at the ankle. The tendon is present in approximately 85% of patients. If this tendon is not available, the extensor of the second or third toe can be used. Placement of a static sling is a difficult procedure. The objective is to provide symmetry at rest. A slight overcorrection is more acceptable than an undercorrection because the patient is more symmetric when smiling The important technical issues are the following: What tissues should the sling be attached to

about the mouth, in what direction should the sling lie, how much tension should be applied, where should it be attached laterally and superiorly, and what should be used for the sling? Placing a sling when the patient is asleep and lying supine is difficult.

Our technique is as follows: Multiple grafts should be inserted or the one long tendon can be woven back and forth between points about the mouth and the point of origin. Usually three points of attachment are used about the mouth to provide an even lift to the corner of the mouth and upper lip. The graft should be placed through the orbicularis oris simulating the normal attachments of the zygomaticus major and the levator labii. The graft should not be placed circumoral as has been shown in textbooks in the past. This placement prevents the patient from putting anything but small bites in the mouth and makes it impossible for dental care. Because there will be some stretching of the tissues, the position and shape of the mouth as seen 1 day postoperatively will not be the same as it will be a few months later. Overcorrection is required. Although it sounds like an easy procedure, it is technically demanding and requires excellent judgment to obtain symmetry in unilateral facial paralysis.

Dynamic Reconstructions

Dynamic reconstructions can be accomplished with regional muscle transfers using the masseter muscle or the temporalis muscle or with microneurovascular muscle transfers. The goal is to support the mouth at rest and provide animation of the mouth and cheek. The majority of dynamic reconstructions involve the microneurovascular transfer. This transfer is preferred because of the freedom of placement of the muscle within the cheek. The origin, insertion, tension, and location of the muscle can be anywhere the surgeon feels will effectively create a smile. The temporalis and masseter origins, on the other hand, are fixed. There is also some deformity created by the temporalis transfer, with a bulge over the orbital margin, and with a masseter transfer, with a hollow at the angle of the mandible from where the muscle has been removed. However, a microneurovascular muscle transfer also provides some fullness to the face depending on the amount of muscle that was used.

Microneurovascular muscle transfer is a technically demanding procedure and should only be done by surgeons who do a significant volume of facial paralysis reconstruction. Many muscles have been used including the gracilis, the pectoralis minor, rectus abdominis, latissimus dorsi, extensor carpal radialis brevis, serratus anterior, tensor fascia lata, and abductor hallucis. Most muscles need to be cut to the desired length for the reconstruction, which is about 10 to 12 cm. Our preference is to use the gracilis muscle and to custom cut a piece of muscle based on the dominant pedicle (10,11). For a large face and strong movement of the mouth on the normal side and a total paralysis, a larger piece of muscle will be required than for the opposite conditions—small face, weak smile on normal side, and partial paralysis. The gracilis has the advantage that it is easily expendable, the incision is not readily visible, there is no functional problem when it is removed, and it is distant from the facial site so that two surgeons can work simultaneously. Usually 20 to 35 g of muscle is used in an adult and 10 to 20 g in a 5-year-old child. The muscle should be spread out to thin it and minimize bulk. We frequently remove a small slice of cheek fat directly over the muscle. Initially there is some fullness to the cheek. However, this largely disappears over time with muscle atrophy. The muscle after innervation is about 3 mm thick (Fig. 40.9).

Attaching the muscle to the mouth is a critical part of the procedure. It is inserted into the fibers of the orbicularis oris at

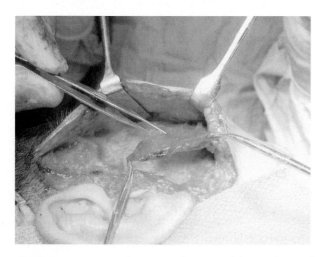

FIGURE 40.9. One year after surgery the origin of the gracilis muscle has been elevated for tension adjustment. The muscle belly is 3 to 4 mm thick.

the same location as the zygomaticus major and levator labia are inserted. The only exposure is a preauricular incision with a small extension inferiorly. No incisions should be placed elsewhere on the face because they are usually unattractive. Usually the facial artery and vein are used for the anastomosis (Fig. 40.10).

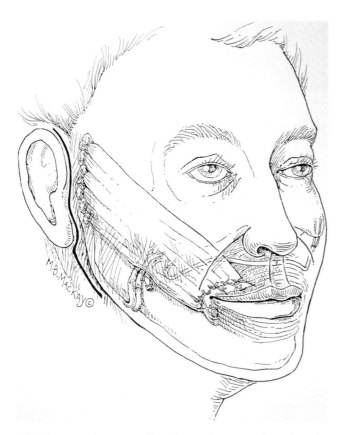

FIGURE 40.10. A segment of gracilis muscle is inserted into the right cheek. It is inserted into the paralyzed orbicularis oris with heavy dissolving figure-of-eight sutures. The origin is the temporalis and the parotid fascia. Revascularization is with the facial artery and vein and reinnervation with a cross-facial nerve graft. (Manktelow R. Facial paralysis. In: Mathes SJ, ed. *Plastic Surgery*, 2nd ed. Philadelphia: Saunders, 2006:906, with permission.)

Innervation of the muscle is with either a nerve graft placed across the face and attached to branches of the facial nerve on the normal side or with a local nerve, usually the masseter motor nerve.

Initially we used a cross-facial nerve graft prior to the muscle transfer for all unilateral paralyses. Certain technical aspects of cross-face nerve grafting deserve mention. It is important that a micro bipolar nerve stimulator be used, which allows the surgeon clearly to identify the function of each branch of the facial nerve. Disposable nerve stimulators are ineffective because the stimulus is not as discretely focused on the nerve. Furthermore, they produce a single jerk rather than a steady tetanic contraction, which can be easily analyzed visually and by palpation. Branches of the facial nerve are identified anterior to the margin of the parotid. Some of these branches will control buccinator, orbicularis oris, or orbicularis oculi function as well as smile function. All of the branches that create a smile are identified, and then approximately one half of them are divided and coapted to the nerve graft. Only branches that have smile function should be used. There should be no orbicularis oris function present in any of these branches. Usually one or two branches are used. The nerve graft is passed across the face, and the end is banked in the upper buccal sulcus just past the midline (Fig. 40.11). This allows a shorter and, if desired, smaller cross section of nerve graft to be used. The sural nerve is gently removed with a nerve stripper to minimize calf scarring. If the sural nerve is significantly larger than the donor nerve on the normal side of the face, the nerve will be split longitudinally into two components using the operating microscope. When only a 10- to 12-cm length of nerve graft is required it is usually possible to split this length of the sural nerve without dividing any nerve fiber crossovers between fascicles.

The muscle transfer is performed 6 to 9 months later. When the muscle is transferred the gracilis motor nerve is passed through a tunnel to the buccal sulcus, where the nerve is attached to the end of the cross-facial sural nerve graft (Fig. 40.12).

Each person has a unique smile. The variables are the presence, extent, and position of the nasolabial fold, the shape of

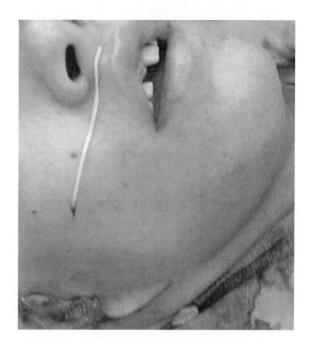

FIGURE 40.11. A "short" cross-facial nerve graft is seen lying on the cheek in the position that it will be in when inserted.

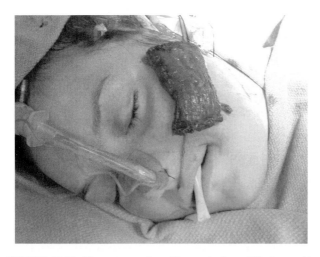

FIGURE 40.12. The segment of gracilis muscle that will be inserted is seen lying on the cheek. It appears thicker than it will be on insertion because it has contracted. The nerve graft passes across to the upper lip. (Manktelow R. Facial paralysis. In: Mathes SJ, ed. *Plastic Surgery*, 2nd ed. Philadelphia: Saunders, 2006:905, with permission.)

the smile as revealed by the shape and exposure of the red lip, the amount of teeth showing, the direction and amount of movement of the commissure and mid upper lip, and the presence or absence of depressor labii function pulling the lower lip downward. It is important to carefully analyze and measure the

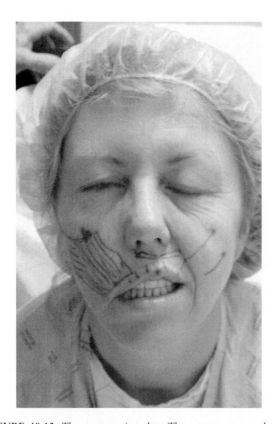

FIGURE 40.13. The preoperative plan. The two arrows on the left cheek illustrate the direction of movement of the left commissure and upper lip when smiling. The location of the cross-facial nerve graft is outlined in the upper lip. On the right side of the face is the intended location of the transferred muscle. Although a short segment on the upper margin of the muscle is shown to the body of the zygoma as a levator replacement, it is difficult to get effective movement with short segments.

patient's smile on the nonparalyzed side with and without finger support of the paralyzed corner of the mouth. This analysis (Fig. 40.13) gives the surgeon a chance to evaluate the shape of smile that is required on the paralyzed side and evaluate the strength of the smile. The muscle transfer is then designed for the individual patient.

Single-stage muscle transfers are an alternative. Based on use of a latissimus dorsi with a long nerve segment, Harii recommended a one-stage procedure. We are reluctant to use this approach because we find it difficult to perform a good facial nerve mapping on the normal side and perform the neurorrhaphy to a branch whose function can be clearly identified. We have used the masseter motor nerve for muscle transfer innervation since 1983, mostly for bilateral muscle transfers but occasionally for unilateral transfers when a cross-facial nerve graft was not feasible. Recently we have been using the masseter motor nerve more frequently in unilateral paralysis. The nerve can be found on the deep surface of the origin of the deep head of the masseter muscle (Fig. 40.14). In our initial experience we used this nerve for bilateral facial paralysis when the seventh nerve was not available as a cross-facial nerve graft. Our finding with the masseter motor nerve innervation was that the amount of movement obtained in the transferred muscle was usually greater than that with a cross-facial nerve graft and the onset of movement occurred sooner and was more reliable. With the cross-facial nerve graft, there was a great variability in the amount of muscle excursion from very little to moderate. It would be rare to obtain more than 60% to 70% of the movement of the normal side. Using the masseter motor nerve, we could obtain as much movement as on the normal side (Figs. 40.15 and 40.16).

Our concern with the use of the masseter motor nerve was that the patient would not be able to use it spontaneously. In a series of 44 muscles in 28 patients, we assessed the ability of the patient to contract the muscles spontaneously without thinking about it and to contract them without using a biting motion. Greater than 80% of patients were able to smile without a biting motion and 60% were able to smile spontaneously. We use a training process in which the patient works in front of a mirror a number of times a day observing himself or herself when biting and learns how to make various types of smiles including

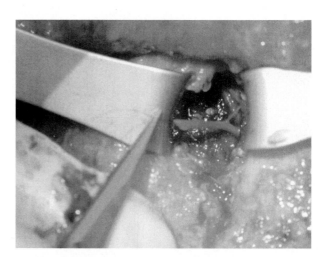

FIGURE 40.14. The masseter motor nerve is identified by releasing a portion of the origin of the masseter muscle to reveal the nerve in or on the deep surface of the muscle and passing inferiorly and anteriorly. The forceps holds the end of the left masseter motor nerve, which has been divided distally. The right-hand retractor is on the arch of the zygoma. By dividing the nerve as far distally as possible one can transpose the deeply placed nerve to the surface to facilitate nerve coadaptation.

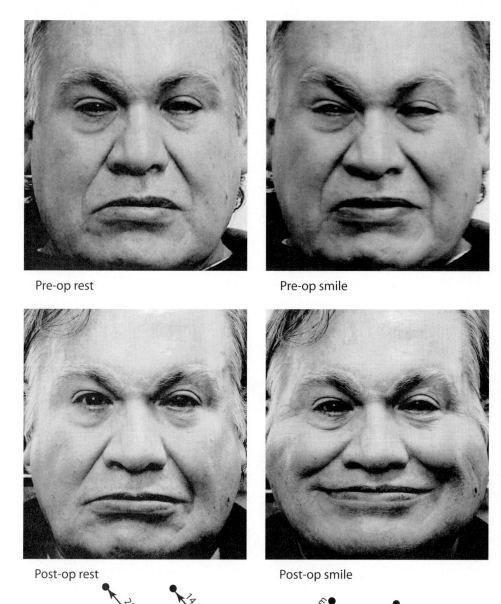

Pre-op rest

Pre-op smile

Post-op rest

Post-op smile

Post-op smile vectors

FIGURE 40.15. A 61-year-old man with bilateral facial paralysis secondary to Ramsay Hunt syndrome 7 years previously. *(Upper left)* Preoperative appearance at rest. *(Upper right)* When the patient attempts to smile preoperatively, synkinesis is present, which gives a grimacing appearance. *(Lower left)* Postoperatively after bilateral 40-g muscle transfers. Nothing else was done to control synkinesis. Face is at rest. *(Lower right)* Postoperatively showing the patient's smile. Smile is not spontaneous. Note that the synkinesis about the mouth is not apparent, probably due to the overpowering effect of the transferred muscles. *(Bottom)* Postoperative movement vectors with maximum smile.

little smiles and big smiles, rapid smiles and slow smiles. The patient is also encouraged to use his or her smile with everyone he or she meets. With time, usually within the first 6 months, the patient develops the ability to separate the muscle movement from biting and develops some spontaneity. Interestingly these adaptations, likely examples of cerebral plasticity, have occurred as frequently in the 50-year-old patients as they have in the younger patients. We are offering many of our unilateral patients either a cross-facial nerve graft or masseter motor nerve for innervation of their muscle transfer. The indications are evolving for the use of the masseter motor nerve. Currently they are the patient who frequently needs to smile when meeting or talking to people such as a teacher or

sales person, a heavy face that requires a large force of muscle, age greater than 40 years, when a good result is not expected with a cross-facial nerve graft, and a preference for a one-stage procedure. All patients must be prepared to do some training. Nevertheless this is a very early stage in the use of the masseter motor nerve for unilateral paralysis, and with the passage of time the indications will become clearer.

The Lower Lip

Lower lip deformity is caused primarily by the depressor labii inferioris. In the normal resting position the deformity is not

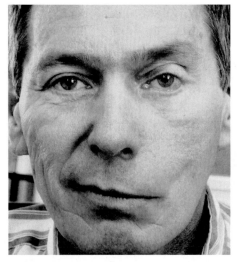

Pre-op rest

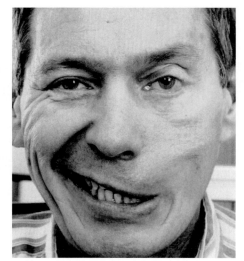

Pre-op smile

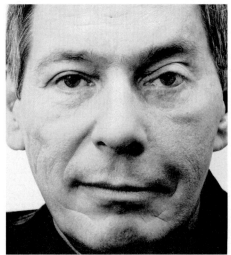

Post-op rest

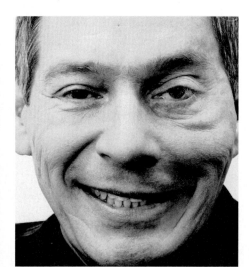

Post-op smile

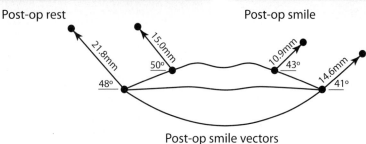

Post-op smile vectors

FIGURE 40.16. A 58-year-old man with partial left facial paralysis secondary to Bell's palsy and present for 20 years. (*Upper left*) Preoperative appearance at rest. (*Upper right*) Preoperative attempt to smile. When the right facial nerve was explored with the intention of doing a cross-facial nerve graft it was judged that there were no suitable nerves that could be sacrificed for the graft (there was one small nerve that contained zygomaticus function and two nerves that contained levator and orbicularis oris function). (*Lower left*) At rest after insertion of a 20-g segment of gracilis muscle into the left lower face with innervation by the left masseter motor nerve. (*Lower right*) Postoperatively, with maximum smile there is a 14.6 mm of commissure movement and 10.9 mm of mid upper lip movement. Smile and laugh are spontaneous. (*Bottom*) Postoperative movement vectors with maximum smile.

usually noticeable because the lips are closed and the depressor on the normal side is relaxed. With speech the paralyzed side remains elevated while the nonparalyzed side moves inferiorly and away from the teeth. This deformity is particularly accentuated when the patient attempts a full smile. The most effective procedure for this has been to resect the depressor labii inferioris on the normal side through a buccal sulcus incision (12). This procedure can be preceded by an injection into the normal depressor labii inferioris muscle of local anesthetic or botulinum toxin to give the patient a chance to evaluate what the effectiveness would be of a depressor resection (13). The surgeon should be well versed in the overlapping anatomy of the lower lip muscles before attempting this procedure. Because the resection is done through the buccal surface of the lip, the

tissues are distorted by the retraction, and it can be difficult to have a clear view of the anatomy.

Moebius Syndrome

Moebius syndrome as originally described was a bilateral seventh and sixth nerve paralysis. However, patients with combined seventh and sixth nerve paralysis may have a unilateral paralysis or they may be only partially paralyzed on one side or the other. For muscle innervation, we have used the masseter motor nerve, as well as the eleventh and the twelfth cranial nerves; our preference is now the masseter motor nerve (14). For bilateral paralysis, muscle transfers are done on separate occasions, usually 3 to 6 months apart. The usual age to commence surgery is about 5 years of age or whenever the child is starting to become aware of his or her "difference." These patients are very gratifying to treat (15). They develop the ability to smile spontaneously and they obtain good support for the drooping lower lip.

References

1. Davis RA, Anson BJ, Budinger JM, Kurth LE. Surgical anatomy of the facial nerve and parotid gland based upon a study of 350 cervico-facial halves. *Surg Gynaecol Obstet.* 1956;102:385.
2. Freilinger G, Gruber H, Happak W, Pechmann U. Surgical anatomy of the mimic muscle system and the facial nerve: importance for reconstructive and aesthetic surgery. *Plast Reconstr Surg.* 1987;80:686.
3. Freilinger G, Gruber H, Happak W, Pechmann U. Surgical anatomy of the mimic muscle system and the facial nerve: importance for reconstructive and aesthetic surgery. *Plast Reconstr Surg.* 1987;80:686.
4. Tomat L, Manktelow R. Evaluation of a new measurement tool for facial paralysis reconstruction. *Plast Reconstr Surg.* 2005;115:696.
5. Manktelow RT. Use of the gold weight for lagopthalmos. *Oper Tech Plast Reconstr Surg.* 1999;6:157.
6. Levine RE. The enhanced palpebral spring. *Oper Tech Plast Reconstr Surg.* 1999;6:152.
7. Salimbeni G. Eyelid reanimation in facial paralysis by temporalis muscle transfer. *Oper Tech Plast Reconstr Surg.* 1999;6:159.
8. Carraway JH, Manktelow RT. Static sling reconstruction of the lower eyelid. *Oper Tech Plast Reconstr Surg.* 1999;6:163.
9. Jelks GW, Glat PM, Jelks EB, et al. Evolution of the lateral canthoplasty: techniques and indications. *Plast Reconstr Surg.* 1997;100:1396.
10. Manktelow RT, Zuker RM. Muscle transplantation by fascicular territory. *Plast Reconstr Surg.* 1984;73:32.
11. Manktelow RT. *Microvascular Reconstruction: Anatomy, Applications and Surgical Technique.* Berlin: Springer-Verlag, 1986.
12. Hussain G, Manktelow RT, Tomat LR. Depressor labii inferioris resection: an effective treatment for facial asymmetry caused by facial paralysis. *Br J Plast Surg.* 2004;57:502.
13. Godwin Y, Tomat L, Manktelow RT. The use of local anesthetic motor block to demonstrate the potential outcome of depressor labii inferiors resection in patients with facial paralysis. *Plast Reconstr Surg.* 2005;116:957.
14. Zuker RM, Goldberg CS, Manktelow RTM. Facial animation in children with Moebius syndrome after segmental gracilis muscle transplant. *Plast Reconstr Surg.* 2000;106:1.
15. Jugenburg M, Hubley P, Yandell H, et al. Self-esteem in children with facial paralysis: a review of measures. *Can J Plast Surg.* 2001;9:146.

CHAPTER 41 ■ MANDIBLE RECONSTRUCTION

JOSEPH J. DISA AND DAVID A. HIDALGO

The mandible contributes to airway stability, is important in speech, deglutition, and mastication, and largely determines the shape of the lower face. Consequently, functional and aesthetic goals are equally important considerations in mandible reconstruction. Specific functional goals include preservation of tandem temporomandibular joint action with maximal opening ability and maintenance of occlusion. In more severe cases in which many teeth are missing, restoration of normal interarch distance and alignment is critical for facilitation of subsequent dental rehabilitation. Key aesthetic goals include symmetry, preservation of lower facial height and anterior chin projection, and correction of submandibular soft-tissue neck defects.

The vast majority of segmental mandible defects are caused by cancer. Epidermoid carcinoma is the etiology in the majority of cases. Osteogenic sarcoma is the second most common cause overall and the most common bone tumor. Mucoepidermoid carcinoma, adenoid cystic carcinoma, leiomyosarcoma, and fibrous histiocytoma are examples of other tumors. A small number of segmental mandibular defects result from extensive benign cystic or fibrotic bone disease. Gunshot wounds are the most common traumatic cause, but their number is very small compared to tumors. Segmental loss because of infection is rare.

Mandible defects requiring reconstruction are sometimes caused by segmental bone loss alone. However, the majority usually include adjacent intraoral soft tissue as well as submandibular neck soft tissue. Some bone defects include external skin loss instead of mucosa, and the most complex include bone, mucosa, and skin.

Two classification schemes have been proposed for mandible defects. The more practical one describes the bone loss in terms of central segments (designated C and defined as lying between the two canine teeth), lateral segments (L), and hemimandible segments (H) (1). Hemimandible and lateral segments are similar except that the former includes the condyle, whereas lateral segments do not. A defect commonly is a combination of more than one segment, for example, LC, HC, or LCL. Although this description may appear tedious, it is actually useful as a common language to standardize the variable reconstructive problems posed by these entities (Fig. 41.1).

METHODS OF RECONSTRUCTION

Mandible reconstruction can be accomplished by a variety of means, including nonvascularized bone grafts, metal plates, pedicled flaps, and free flaps. Nonvascularized grafts, such as an iliac crest segment, can be used for a short bone gap (<3 cm) in a setting of benign disease. This is a rare application. Although conceptually and technically simple, this method relies on creeping substitution for long-term mandible stability.

Pedicled flaps include the trapezius and pectoralis osteomyocutaneous flaps. The primary attraction of these donor sites is that they lie adjacent to the head, thus permitting their movement into this area without disconnecting their blood supply. Although this is an attractive concept, there are several important drawbacks. First, use of these flaps enlarges the size of the primary wound considerably compared to harvesting tissue from a distant donor site. This increases the potential for morbidity at the site of the reconstruction. More importantly, a significant portion of flap volume is used up just to reach the recipient site. The distal portion of the flap, which is used for the actual reconstruction, often has a marginal blood supply and is at risk for ischemic necrosis. Perhaps the greatest limitation of these flaps is that they do not provide enough tissue in the proper configuration to be useful. The bone available with the pectoralis major muscle (rib) and the trapezius (spine of the scapula) is limited compared to free-flap alternatives. Although the pectoralis has been used to reconstruct the anterior mandible and the trapezius to reconstruct the lateral mandible, these flaps generally are not recommended as a primary method of mandible reconstruction.

Prosthetic mandible replacement has evolved as an alternative method of reconstruction that still has legitimate, but limited, application today. Mesh trays made of Dacron or metal were introduced in the 1970s as scaffolds that were filled with bone graft chips and used for segmental bone defects. Long-term follow-up has shown this method to be ineffective. Problems with extrusion and bone graft dissolution commonly occurred. Metal reconstruction plates developed as a result of orthopedic hardware advances in other areas. These plates are available today in a variety of lengths and styles.

Metal reconstruction plates offer advantages of decreased operating time and avoidance of a bone graft donor site. They have important disadvantages: risk of exposure or infection; risk of plate fracture; preclusion of dental reconstruction; and a thin shape that does not provide adequate bulk for reconstruction (Fig. 41.2). Another important drawback is the functional limitation seen with the use of metal plates for hemimandible defects that include the condyle. The prosthetic condyle is a poor substitute for the native structure. The long-term effects of a metal condyle in the native glenoid fossa are unknown, and occlusion is often poorly maintained with a metal plate that includes a condyle.

Reconstruction plates require adequate soft tissue coverage. Plates that are not supplemented with a soft-tissue flap are prone to failure. The pectoralis major myocutaneous flap is commonly used to provide soft-tissue coverage. However, plate exposure still occurs, particularly with anterior reconstructions, in which the tension on the flap is greatest. **One in three plate reconstructions fail when a pedicled flap is used for coverage.**

The most reliable soft-tissue coverage for a reconstruction plate is provided by a free flap, which provides abundant tissue and can be inset without tension. The forearm donor site is commonly used for this purpose because of its ideal tissue

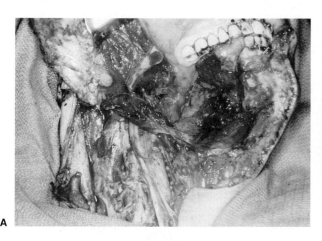

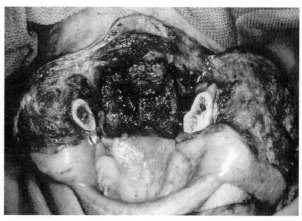

FIGURE 41.1. Examples of mandibular defects. A: A typical lateral defect of the L type. Note how intermaxillary fixation maintains occlusion for later flap insetting. B: An LCL anterior defect showing the free-floating lateral mandibular segments, submental soft-tissue defect, and the lack of reference points to guide accurate flap insetting.

characteristics and its convenient location (2). The sole advantage of this approach (reconstruction plate plus forearm flap) is that it is somewhat quicker to perform than an osteocutaneous free flap. The disadvantage is that it combines the worst features of its two component parts: the risks of infection and exposure from a foreign body, and the risk of free-flap failure. The combination of a soft-tissue free flap and a reconstruction plate is probably best reserved for lateral defects in those patients who are poor candidates for an osteocutaneous free flap. Elderly patients with multiple medical comorbidities may benefit from a shorter operative procedure and are more likely to accept the permanent dentition defect than are young patients (3).

Osteocutaneous free-flap reconstruction is often the most effective method of mandible repair. These flaps have both soft tissue and bone components, which are available in an optimal configuration for solving specific composite tissue problems. This technique is ultimately dependent on the integrity of the microvascular anastomoses for success. Fortunately, the favored donor sites all have excellent flap pedicle qualities (vessel diameter and length), and the head and neck area generally has excellent recipient vessels available, despite previous surgical treatment and radiation. Free flap survival rates are generally approximately 95% (4).

FREE-FLAP DONOR-SITE SELECTION

Since early in the development of free-flap mandible reconstruction there have been multiple donor sites from which to choose. Rib, metatarsal, and ilium were among the first flaps developed (5). The ilium has been the most popular of the three owing to its abundant bone, which even resembles a hemimandible when harvested in a particular way. The ilium has been the workhorse free flap for the first decade of free flap mandible reconstruction (6). Further evolution has led to the development of the radius, scapula, and fibula donor sites (7). These additional options have increased the flexibility and precision of the technique as the specific assets and limitations of each donor site have become clearer.

A review of 155 free-flap mandible reconstructions at Memorial Sloan-Kettering Cancer Center has shown that the fibula is currently the donor site of choice for most patients (Table 41.1) (8). The radius, the scapula, and the ilium (to a diminishing extent) are better choices in a few specific settings. Each has unique advantages and disadvantages. A comparison of the donor sites is helpful in selecting the proper one for a particular problem (Table 41.2). Some have better bone qualities, some have better skin, and some have significant disadvantages that make them seldom the flap of choice despite their good qualities (Fig. 41.3).

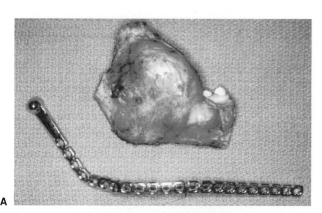

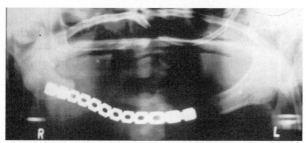

FIGURE 41.2. A: A reconstruction plate containing a prosthetic condyle is shown below the surgical specimen it will replace. Note how the plate is a poor three-dimensional substitute. B: Panorex demonstrating reconstruction plate in place.

Ilium

The ilium has abundant bone but has a predetermined shape that makes graft shaping inherently less precise than in other donor-site options. It may be ideal in some hemimandible

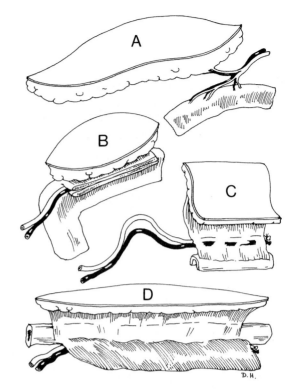

TABLE 41.1

FREE-FLAP DONOR SITE SELECTION IN MANDIBLE RECONSTRUCTION[a]

Donor Site	Number (%)
Fibula	120 (77.4)
Radius	17 (11.0)
Scapula	8 (5.2)
Rectus	5 (3.2)
Ilium	3 (1.9)
Other	2 (1.3)

[a]Used in 155 consecutive cases at Memorial Sloan-Kettering Cancer Center.

reconstructions because its shape resembles most closely this portion of the mandible. The ilium is claimed to have a segmental blood supply from the deep circumflex iliac artery, although this is debatable on a practical level. This type of vascular anatomy is preferred when it occurs because it allows segmental osteotomies to be performed with survival of each portion of the graft. However, long ilium grafts tend to have less robust, even marginal, circulation at the distal end of a multiply osteotomized graft.

The skin island available with the ilium does not have a reliable circulation in many patients. In addition, the soft-tissue component of the flap is often bulky and lacks mobility with respect to the bone. This makes insetting difficult and limits the usefulness of the soft-tissue component of the flap. Some authors propose including a portion of the internal oblique muscle with the flap as an alternative source of flap soft tissue. The muscle is covered with a skin graft when used inside the oral cavity.

Closure of the ilium donor site is arduous and there is a possibility of hernia formation or late attenuation of the lateral abdominal wall. This donor site is painful and limits early mobilization of the patient. Splitting the ilium and leaving its outer rim intact is proposed as a means of facilitating the closure process, but this makes graft harvest more tedious.

Today, the indications for use of the ilium are limited. Perhaps the best indication is a short lateral or hemimandible segment not requiring mucosal lining replacement. The problems with the ilium described above often make other donor sites preferable, even for this type of defect (Fig. 41.4).

Radius

The radius has the best quality skin island compared to other donor-site alternatives. It is thin, pliable, and abundant. The

FIGURE 41.3. The free-flap donor sites for mandible reconstruction. **A:** Scapula. **B:** Ilium. **C:** Radius. **D:** Fibula. Note the relative amounts of skin, the relationship of the pedicle to the bone, and the bone configurations available.

vascular pedicle is also ideal, with long, large-diameter vessels capable of reaching the opposite side of the neck for difficult recipient vessel problems. **The bone, in contrast, is the worst compared to other choices.** The radius must be carefully split during harvest to prevent postoperative fracture at the donor site. Length is generally limited to a segment located between the insertion of the pronator teres and the brachioradialis muscles (approximately 10 cm), although some authors describe taking longer pieces. The bone thickness is marginal for later placement of osseointegrated implants for dental rehabilitation.

There is insufficient soft tissue available with this flap to provide the necessary bulk to fill submandibular neck defects. The donor site appearance is often poor postoperatively owing to a need for skin graft closure and the additional proximal

TABLE 41.2

FREE-FLAP DONOR-SITE COMPARISON FOR MANDIBLE RECONSTRUCTION [a]

Donor Site	Tissue Characterstics			Donor Site Characteristics	
	Bone	Skin	Pedicle	Location	Morbidity
Fibula	A	C	B	A	A
Ilium	B	D	D	B	C
Scapula	C	B	C	D	B
Radius	D	A	A	C	D

[a] Ranked in each category from best (A) to worst (D).
Source: Hidalgo DA, Rekow A. A Review of 60 consecutive fibula free flap mandible reconstructions. *Plast Reconstr Surg.* 1995;96:585.

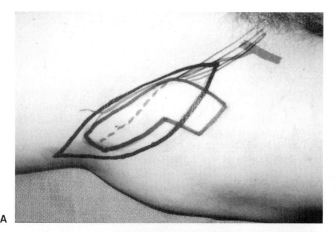

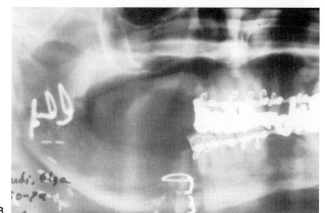

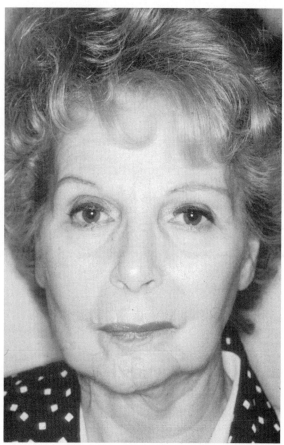

FIGURE 41.4. **A:** Design of osteocutaneous iliac crest flap. Note design of the lateral mandible reconstruction and position of skin island. **B:** Panographic radiograph of iliac crest in place. **C:** Postoperative appearance.

forearm scar necessary for obtaining adequate pedicle length (Fig. 41.5).

The best indication for a radius free flap is a bone defect that is limited to the ramus and the proximal body with a large associated intraoral soft-tissue defect. The split radius is adequate to restore mandibular continuity. Dental rehabilitation is usually superfluous posteriorly, and so the thin nature of the bone is not a factor. The cheek soft tissues are thick and maintain facial contour despite this flap's inherent lack of bulk. The skin island is ideal for resurfacing a large posterior mucosal defect. The radius is contraindicated for most anterior defects because adequate soft tissue and bony volume are essential in this area for the best functional and aesthetic reconstruction. The forearm donor site is probably most useful as a soft-tissue free flap without bone for coverage of a metal plate when this method is chosen for reconstruction.

Scapula

The scapula offers the greatest amount of soft tissue compared to other donor sites. It is possible to include a skin island as long as 30 cm and to include the entire latissimus dorsi muscle if needed. The skin island is somewhat thick compared to the forearm donor site. A useful feature of this flap is that the bone and the soft-tissue components (skin, latissimus dorsi) are independent of each other except for a common vascular pedicle. Approximately 14 cm of bone is available from the lateral scapula. The bone does not have a segmental blood supply, and therefore multiple osteotomies can be hazardous to the viability

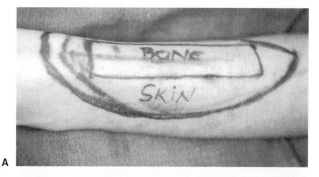

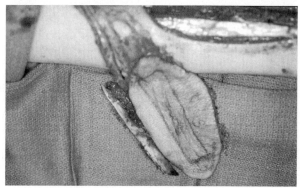

FIGURE 41.5. **A:** Design of osteocutaneous forearm flap. **B:** Note limited diameter of bone relative to available skin.

of some portions of the graft. The primary disadvantage of this flap is its donor site location, requiring delay in flap harvest until the resection is complete. The patient typically has to be repositioned several times throughout the course of the operation. Shoulder function is sometimes compromised following harvest of a scapula flap. Patients can exhibit weakness and a decreased range of shoulder motion (Fig. 41.6).

The best indication for a scapula free flap in mandible reconstruction is for repair of a bone gap associated with a large soft-tissue defect. This applies most to patients who require simultaneous intraoral and external soft-tissue replacement. The priority in these cases of advanced local disease is to achieve uncomplicated primary wound healing. The precision of the bony reconstruction is often a secondary concern. The result is compromised whenever a skin island is placed externally on the face owing to color mismatch and partial facial nerve paralysis associated with the defect. Although rarely indicated, a combined scapula and latissimus dorsi flap is useful for large defects, including those resulting from a radical neck dissection. The latissimus dorsi restores neck contour and protects the exposed vessels. This can actually produce an elegant result, but constitutes a massive effort when performed in conjunction with a mandible reconstruction.

Fibula

The fibula donor site has many advantages (7). The bone is available with enough length to reconstruct any mandible defect. The straight quality of the bone with adequate height and thickness constitutes the ideal bone stock for precisely shaping a mandible graft. Unlike with the ilium, there are no nuances of shape that limit the graft contouring process. Also unlike other donor sites, the periosteal blood supply is functionally of a segmental type. Osteotomies can be planned wherever necessary and can be placed as close as 1 cm apart without concern for bone viability. The vascular pedicle has sufficient length and is of large diameter. The flexor hallucis longus muscle is conveniently located along the posterior border of the bone. This muscle is ideal for filling in adjacent soft-tissue defects in the submandibular portion of the upper neck. The skin island available with the fibula is reliable in approximately 91% of patients. It is thicker than the forearm skin, but thinner than the scapula skin. A large skin paddle can be harvested for complex defects, but the donor site will require a skin graft closure. Of all potential donor sites, the fibula is the most convenient because it is located farthest from the head and neck area.

The main disadvantage is the unreliability of the skin blood supply in 9% of cases (7). There are no reliable preoperative tests to identify the patients who are at risk for an inadequate skin blood supply. Despite this problem, it is uncommon to be faced with a need for skin and to have none available. The forearm skin can be used as a second free flap, should the need for extra skin unexpectedly arise, combining the best features of both flaps. This practice is actually preferable to using a single flap such as the scapula in which neither the bone nor the skin is in the ideal configuration.

The fibula is indicated for all anterior defects and most lateral defects. It is the flap of choice for the majority of mandible defects except for a few special situations in which the radius or scapula may constitute a better choice (8). It is particularly well suited to anterior defects because the skin island can be rotated over it to reconstruct the floor of the mouth. The flexor hallucis longus muscle is perfectly situated to fill in the dead space within the anterior arch of the mandible and restore upper neck contour.

PREOPERATIVE PLANNING

The most serious postoperative problems in patients undergoing mandible reconstruction are cardiopulmonary in origin. Pneumonia, arrhythmias, and myocardial infarction are life-threatening problems for which this patient population is at risk. Patients older than age 40 years should be considered for pulmonary function studies and cardiac stress testing prior to surgery to identify asymptomatic cardiopulmonary disease. A more expeditious type of reconstruction should be considered for those patients found to be at serious risk for a prolonged operative procedure.

Preoperative consultation with the dental service is valuable in the management of mandible reconstruction patients. Intermaxillary fixation, intraoperative tooth extraction, custom fabrication of various splints, and other ancillary procedures are best performed with forethought and the help of interested colleagues. This also sets the stage for the patient's postoperative dental rehabilitation with either conventional dentures or osseointegrated implant technology.

Two specific preoperative studies contribute to improved aesthetic results (9). A 1:1 ratio computed tomography (CT) or magnetic resonance imaging (MRI) scan of the mandible taken in the transverse plane at a level just below the tooth roots is the basis for fabrication of a template showing the full-size shape of the mandible. A lateral cephalogram will allow fabrication of a second template showing the shape of the mandible in the sagittal plane. These images can be transferred to acrylic plastic or used directly as radiographic film cut-outs to assist in the graft-shaping process. Together with the surgical specimen as a reference, this permits the bone to be completely shaped at the donor site while the vascular pedicle remains intact (Fig. 41.7), and contributes to improved accuracy in reconstruction while minimizing graft ischemia time.

The routine use of preoperative angiography is not recommended for the fibula donor site. Although a rare vascular anomaly consisting of a dominant peroneal artery (peroneal arteria magna) exists, in which harvesting of the fibula could lead to leg ischemia. The precise incidence of this congenital variation is not well established. When considering the fibula donor site, the main indications for preoperative angiography are signs and symptoms of peripheral vascular disease or an abnormal pedal pulse exam. However, because fibula reconstruction has been successful even in the presence of overt disease in the peroneal artery, the presence of disease does not always rule out use of this donor site (10).

SURGICAL TECHNIQUE

With rare exception, all patients should have a tracheostomy for safety. It is often possible to begin donor-site dissection at the same time as the ablative portion of the procedure. If there is significant doubt as to the extent of the disease, it is better to wait until the situation is clarified before beginning. The precise method of dissection for each donor site is described in detail elsewhere.

Graft shaping can be done while ablation is in progress with the aid of the templates described previously. The surgical specimen is also a valuable visual aid. Measurements of total graft length can be obtained, as well as measurements to identify where osteotomies are best made to duplicate mandible shape (9). Subtle nuances in shape can be appreciated by direct examination of the specimen. Typical locations or fibula osteotomies include the paraesophageal, midbody, and mandibular angle regions.

Bony fixation is best accomplished with the use of miniplate fixation (Fig. 41.8) (11). This method is efficient, safe, and

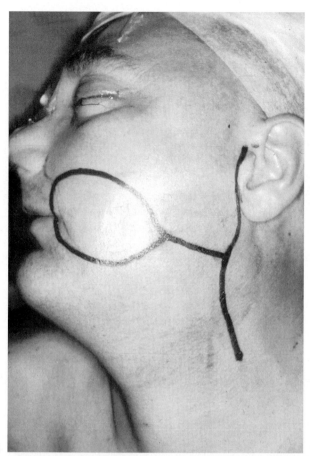

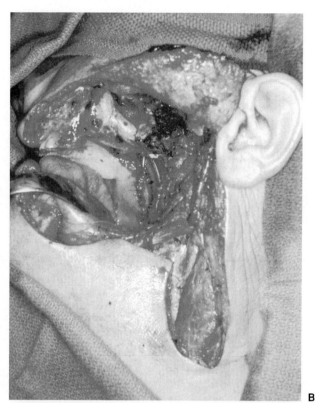

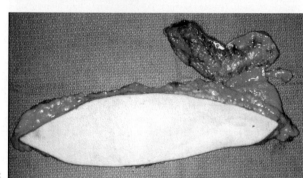

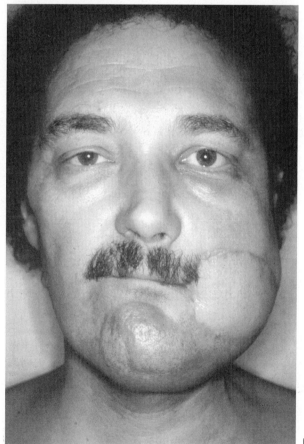

FIGURE 41.6. A: Planned resection of cheek and mandible. B: Full-thickness defect including skin, mandible, mucosa, and associated soft tissues. C: Osteocutaneous scapula flap. D: Postoperative appearance.

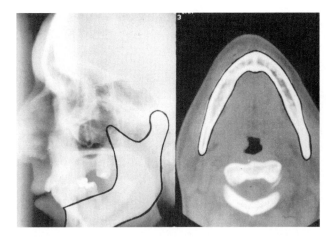

FIGURE 41.7. Templates are fashioned from tracings of a lateral cephalogram (*left*) and a 1:1 scale transverse plane CT scan of the mandible (*right*). These templates serve as valuable references during the graft shaping process. (From Hidalgo DA. Aesthetic improvements in free-flap mandible reconstruction. *Plast Reconstr Surg.* 1991;88:574, with permission.)

strong. Preformed reconstruction plates have been preferred by others, but this method does not allow subtle nuances of mandible shape to show through when a bulky plate is applied to the outer surface of the graft. When hardware requires removal to facilitate osseointegrated dental implants, the miniplate technique limits the exposure necessary by allowing for removal of only the hardware in the region of the implants. Other methods, such as interosseous wires, do not provide enough resistance to torsional stress in a multiply osteotomized bone graft. Intermaxillary fixation is used only as an adjunctive form of fixation. Its primary role is to maintain occlusion during the insetting of lateral grafts (Fig. 41.1A). External fixators, previously popular for stabilizing the lateral segments when reconstruction was deferred, no longer play a role in mandible reconstruction.

Lateral defects differ from anterior defects in terms of the approach to shaping the graft. In the case of the fibula, ilium, and scapula, the angle of the mandible is generally planned where the vascular pedicle enters the bone (Fig. 41.9). This provides maximum pedicle length to reach the recipient vessels in the neck. This is where the first osteotomy is made in the bone, with the second osteotomy made to form the curve in the midbody. The ramus height is determined by measurements taken from the specimen. The condyle can often be harvested

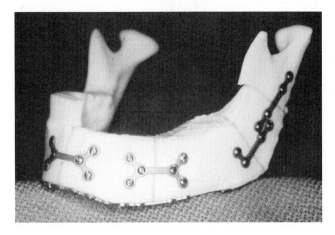

FIGURE 41.8. A mandible model with miniplate fixation in place. The cut-down portion represents the bone graft. Note that plates are also placed along the inferior border of the bone.

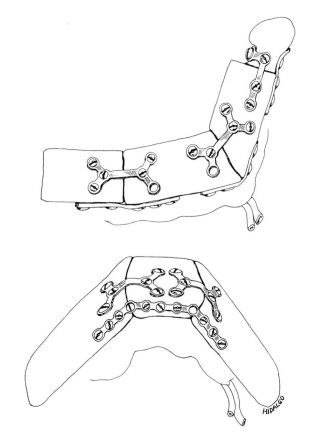

FIGURE 41.9. A typical lateral graft (with transplanted condyle) is shown *above* and an anterior graft *below*. Note the location of the pedicle in each. (From Hidalgo, DA. Fibula free flap mandible reconstruction. *Clin Plast Surg.* 1994;21:25, with permission.)

from the surgical specimen and then mounted directly onto the graft. The condyle must first be proven to be free of disease by frozen-section examination of bone scrapings. It must not be used if doubt exists. This method is better than the alternative of transecting the ramus high and leaving the condyle in situ. It is difficult to fix the graft to it in this situation (12).

Anterior graft shaping begins by planning the location of the central segment so as to maximize flap pedicle length (Fig. 41.9). The central segment usually measures 2 cm. An osteotomy is made on each end in two planes. The body segments curve away from the central segment in both a posterior and superior direction. The body segments are usually of unequal length. It is important to use the transverse template to accurately reproduce the splay of the body segments away from the central segment and each other. As in the case of lateral grafts, it is best to leave the ends of the graft long and make the final osteotomies, which determine overall graft length, at the time of graft insetting.

The recipient site is prepared prior to dividing the flap pedicle. The ends of the mandible segments are dissected in a subperiosteal plane for approximately 2 cm to allow room for miniplate fixation. Recipient vessels are identified, and the intraoral wound closed as much as possible. Intermaxillary fixation is placed in the case of lateral grafts, and the remaining portion of the mandible is placed in fixation to maintain occlusion during graft insetting.

Lateral grafts containing a condyle are inset by seating the condyle first and then finalizing overall graft length. An additional osteotomy is often required near the midline to recreate the curve of the mandible in this area. The transverse template is useful during the insetting process as an aid to achieving symmetry. To avoid the cheek appearing either "bowed-out" or "caved-in," depending on the type of error (Fig. 41.10), the

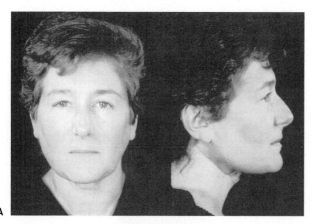

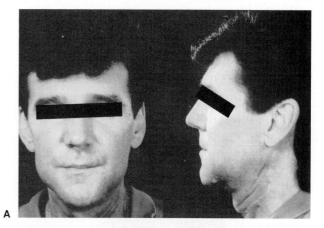

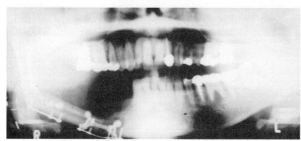

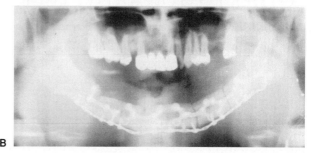

FIGURE 41.10. A: A postoperative view of a lateral reconstruction is shown. Note the symmetry. **B:** The Panorex radiograph for this patient shows the graft and miniplate fixation. (From Hidalgo DA. Aesthetic improvements in free-flap mandible reconstruction. *Plast Reconstr Surg.* 1991;88:574, with permission.)

FIGURE 41.11. A: Postoperative view of an anterior reconstruction. **B:** The Panorex radiograph for this patient shows the graft and miniplate fixation. (From Hidalgo DA. Fibula free flap mandible reconstruction. *Clin Plast Surg.* 1994;21:25, with permission.)

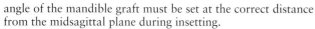

angle of the mandible graft must be set at the correct distance from the midsagittal plane during insetting.

Anterior grafts are more difficult to inset correctly. Often the only visual guides are the maxillary arch and the midline (Fig. 41.1B). The lateral segments usually cannot be stabilized because of a lack of dentition. It is easy to make errors that can result in prognathism, retrognathia, increased or decreased lower facial height, asymmetry caused by a twist in the graft, or a shift in the midline to one side as a result of unequal lengths of the mandible body (9). It is also important to establish the correct interarch distance in anticipation of later dental reconstruction (Fig. 41.11).

After the bone is inset, the microvascular anastomoses are performed. The facial artery is usually selected as a recipient vessel, although the external carotid (end-to-side) and the superior thyroid artery are also good choices. The lingual artery is not preferred, particularly if partial glossectomy has been performed. In some cases, tongue necrosis is possible when the lingual artery is used. The external jugular vein can be used as the recipient vein if it is suitable for use. An end-to-end anastomosis is easily performed. The internal jugular vein can also be used, but an end-to-side anastomosis deeper in the wound is technically more challenging.

Final wound closure follows completion of the microvascular anastomoses. **Watertight closure of the intraoral wound is absolutely mandatory.** A leak will often lead to contamination of the miniplates, which can develop into an orocutaneous fistula that results in considerable morbidity. Fortunately the viability of the graft usually is not threatened. Suction drains are always placed as the neck flaps are closed, but they are carefully positioned away from the microvascular anastomoses. A feeding tube is routinely placed at the conclusion of the procedure.

POSTOPERATIVE CARE

Early patient mobilization is encouraged. Ambulation is possible within the first postoperative week even when the fibula is used. Tube feedings are begun within 48 hours of the conclusion of the procedure. Irrigation of the oral cavity for hygiene is generally begun after 1 week. The tracheostomy is left in place for 10 to 14 days, or until wound healing is assured and it is clear that additional surgery is not needed.

Free-flap monitoring is not precise in most cases of free-flap mandible reconstruction because the bone is buried and the skin island, if present, usually lies within the oral cavity. A conventional or implantable Doppler ultrasonography device often can be used to monitor the vascular pedicle of the flap. A clear arterial signal usually can be obtained over the mandible away from the neck vessels. Frequently, a venous hum also can be heard. Surface temperature probes are not useful unless there is an external skin island. Skin island bleeding response to pinprick is a useful confirmatory test to perform when there is some doubt as to flap viability.

Physical therapy to address donor site problems is rarely necessary. Follow-up studies of the mandible are limited to periodic Panorex radiographs. Radionuclide scans are not necessary.

COMPLICATIONS

There are three categories of potential complications in mandible reconstruction: general medical problems, head and neck wound problems, and donor-site problems. Pulmonary and cardiac problems are the most common source of general medical complications. Free-flap failure is the single most important complication pertaining to the head and neck area.

Fortunately, most failing flaps can be salvaged, and the actual incidence of total flap loss is generally less than 5%. Reconstruction plate exposure and intraoral wound dehiscence (which may lead to orocutaneous fistula formation) constitute other serious problems. Donor-site complications are uncommon and rarely require additional surgery. They include abdominal wall attenuation (ilium donor site), seroma (scapula), exposed tendons or fracture (radius), and delayed skin graft healing (fibula). Cellulitis can occur at the donor site or in the head and neck area. Despite the complexity of mandible reconstruction cases, the incidence and severity of postoperative complications is low.

OTHER POSTOPERATIVE ISSUES

Many patients undergoing mandible reconstruction require postoperative radiation therapy. **The presence of microvascular anastomoses does not affect the timing of radiotherapy.** Radiation can begin as soon as complete wound healing is assured and the patient has recovered sufficiently. This usually requires at least 4 weeks.

Mandible reconstruction is functionally incomplete without dental restoration. A small percentage of patients can be fitted with conventional dentures if there is dentition present on each side of the defect. Patients with reconstruction plates cannot have dentition restored over the plate.

Osseointegrated implant reconstruction is the method of choice for dental restoration when conventional dentures are not feasible. These implants are placed into the bone graft and serve as a permanent foundation upon which a dental prosthesis is mounted with screws (13). These implants are usually placed at a later date when the patient has proven to be free of disease, usually no sooner than 6 months, and more appropriately 1 year, after mandible reconstruction. Three to four implants are usually sufficient for a long dental defect.

Implant placement is usually an office procedure. Preparation of the site of implantation usually requires a preliminary procedure to remove bone graft miniplates, which may interfere with implant placement. Sometimes the skin island overlying the bone must be thinned at the same time. The implants must be correctly aligned during placement. They are uncovered after osseointegration has occurred, usually about 4 months later. The implants are lengthened by the placement of abutment collars, after which the dental prosthesis is mounted on top of the collars (Fig. 41.12).

Osseointegrated implants are unsuitable for placement in irradiated bone grafts. There is concern that the implants will not integrate into irradiated bone or, if they do, that they may not remain stable once loaded. It has been proposed that implants be placed immediately at the time of mandible reconstruction. Although they are more likely to integrate prior to irradiation, their long-term fate will not necessarily be better once the bone is irradiated. Moreover, there are issues of threatened graft viability and proper implant alignment when they are placed immediately. This practice would add more time to an already lengthy procedure. For these reasons, immediate implant placement is not widely practiced.

CONCLUSION

Mandible reconstruction is most commonly performed for tumors, of which epidermoid carcinoma and osteogenic sarcomas are the most common types. Lateral and anterior defects constitute two distinct types of reconstructive problems. Reconstruction is most commonly performed either with reconstruction plates and regional flaps or with microvascular free flaps.

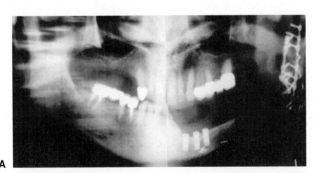

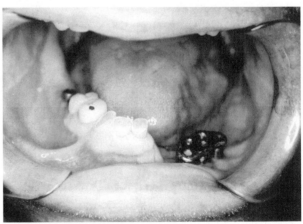

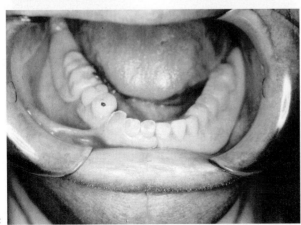

FIGURE 41.12. A: Postoperative Panorex radiograph shows three osseointegrated implants in a previously placed fibula graft. **B:** The abutment collars are shown with the dental superstructure screwed in place. **C:** The completed dental prosthesis is shown after it has been bonded to the superstructure.

Free flaps usually yield the best functional and aesthetic results. These lengthy procedures consist of multiple subcomponents, including bone harvesting, shaping, and fixation; insetting; microvascular anastomoses; and soft-tissue closure. Proper preoperative planning includes cardiopulmonary screening and the fabrication of shaping templates, which increases safety and improves the aesthetic and functional results that are possible with free flaps. Among the most important complications in mandible reconstruction are reconstruction plate exposure, free-flap failure, and serious cardiopulmonary problems.

References

1. Boyd JB, Gullane PJ, Rotstein LE, et al. Classification of mandibular defects. *Plast Reconstr Surg.* 1993;92:1266.
2. Davidson J, Boyd B, Gullane P, et al. A comparison of the results following oromandibular reconstruction using a radial forearm flap with either radial bone or reconstruction plate. *Plast Reconstr Surg.* 1991;88:201.
3. Singh B, Cordeiro PG, Santamaria E, et al. Factors associated with complications in microvascular reconstruction of head and neck defects. *Plast Reconstr Surg.* 1999;103:403.
4. Hidalgo DA, Disa JJ, Cordeiro PG, et al. A review of 716 consecutive free flaps for oncologic surgical defects: refinement in donor-site selection and technique. *Plast Reconstr Surg.* 1998;102:722.
5. Taylor GI. Reconstruction of the mandible with free composite iliac bone grafts. *Ann Plast Surg.* 1982;9:361.
6. Boyd JB, Rosen I, Rotstein L, et al. The iliac crest and the radial forearm flap in vascularized oromandibular reconstruction. *Am J Surg.* 1990;159:301.
7. Hidalgo DA. Fibula free flap: a new method of mandible reconstruction. *Plast Reconstr Surg.* 1989;84:71.
8. Cordeiro PG, Disa JJ, Hidalgo DA, et al. Reconstruction of the mandible with osseous free flaps: a 10-year experience with 150 consecutive patients. *Plast Reconstr Surg.* 1999;104:1314.
9. Hidalgo DA. Aesthetic improvements in free-flap mandible reconstruction. *Plast Reconstr Surg.* 1991;88:574.
10. Disa J J, Cordeiro PG. The current role of preoperative arteriography in fibula free flaps. *Plast Reconstr Surg.* 1998;102:1083.
11. Hidalgo DA. Titanium miniplate fixation in free flap mandible reconstruction. *Ann Plast Surg.* 1989;23:498.
12. Hidalgo DA. Condyle transplantation in free flap mandible reconstruction. *Plast Reconstr Surg.* 1994;93:770.
13. Frodel JL Jr, Funk GF, Capper DT, et al. Osseointegrated implants: a comparative study of bone thickness in four vascularized bone flaps. *Plast Reconstr Surg.* 1993;92:449.

CHAPTER 42 ■ RECONSTRUCTION OF DEFECTS OF THE MAXILLA AND SKULL BASE

DUC T. BUI AND PETER G. CORDEIRO

RECONSTRUCTION OF MAXILLARY DEFECTS

The maxilla is an essential component of the midface that has both functional and aesthetic roles. It contributes to facial appearance, including the orbit, cheek, nose, and upper lip, as well as supports critical functions, such as mastication, speech, and deglutition. Most maxillary defects result from the surgical ablation of maxillary tumors or tumors arising from adjacent structures, including the paranasal sinuses, palate, nasal cavity, orbital contents, overlying skin, and intraoral cavity. Another cause of maxillary defects involves traumatic injuries resulting from gunshot wounds to the midface. Because of its close relationship to crucial components of the midface and unique three-dimensional structure, reconstruction of maxillary defects can be a formidable challenge for the reconstructive surgeon.

Loss of key midfacial structures leads to significant functional and cosmetic deficits. Large oronasal and oromaxillary fistulae, loss of significant alveolar arch segments, loss of lip, cheek, and eye support, and loss of midface projection are disfiguring. In addition, functional sequelae from maxillectomy include masticatory difficulty and speech impairment.

The goals of maxillary defect reconstruction are to

1. reconstruct the orbital floor, maintain the ocular globe position and function, and/or fill the orbital cavity following orbital exenteration;
2. reconstruct the intraoral, cheek, palatal, and nasal lining to restore speech, mastication, and oral continence;
3. separate the oral and nasal cavity from the skull base and orbit;
4. restore external skin and three-dimensional facial contour; and
5. obliterate the maxillectomy defect.

Traditionally, prosthetic appliances were used to reconstruct maxillary defects and are still a reasonable option in some patients (see Chapter 34). This method of reconstruction relies on adequate support from the remaining tissues and split-thickness skin grafting to line the defect cavity to prevent contractures. Despite successes in many cases, there are several disadvantages to the use of prostheses. Leakage and oronasal regurgitation because of bulky dentures, inadequate dentition, and poor retentive surfaces, the need for cleaning, and repeated prosthetic refinements are common problems.

Another method of reconstruction used autogenous tissues. Small defects of the maxilla can be primarily reconstructed with local soft-tissue flaps with or without supplemental bone grafting. Prior to the advent of free-tissue transfer, larger maxillary defects were repaired with a variety of pedicled flaps including the deltopectoral, pectoralis major, latissimus dorsi, temporalis, sternomastoid, and trapezius myocutaneous flaps. These flaps were limited by the length of vascular pedicle, inadequate tissue to fill the defect, or required multiple stages to achieve a final result. More recently, microvascular free tissue transfer has significantly expanded the reconstructive surgeon's armamentarium for maxillary reconstruction. There are many different composite flaps that can be transferred to the midface without limitations of vascular pedicle length or flap geometry.

Although free flap reconstruction now is the preferred method for the vast majority of extensive maxillary defects, flap selection is complex. An initial step to reconstruction is to define the maxillary defect in terms of bony and soft-tissue components. Adjacent critical structures, such as the eye, nose, and lips, are assessed. A history of radiotherapy or previous neck dissection is noted. The necessary length of the vascular pedicle and donor-site morbidity are assessed. The amount, location, and quality of residual bone, dentition, or denture-bearing alveolar arch largely determine whether a bone-containing flap is necessary.

Visualizing the maxilla as a six-sided box with the roof being the orbital floor and the floor being the palate is helpful in determining which walls are missing (Fig. 42.1). The three walls that require reconstruction are the superior (orbital floor), floor (palatal), and anterior (cheek) walls. Bone replacement for the orbital floor is essential to maintain orbital globe position. The orbital floor can be reconstructed with autogenous bone grafts because this area requires minimal supportive strength. The maxillary arch of the midface should be reconstructed to provide anterior projection and dental support. **Any bony replacement of the maxillary arch must have adequate bone stock for osteointegrated dental implants. Hence, vascularized bone is required for reconstructing the maxillary arch.** The palate can be repaired with the skin island of the free flap or replaced with an obturator. The anterior wall of this hypothetical box requires reconstruction but does not require bony reconstruction. The maxillary sinus in the center of the hexahedron can be filled with soft tissue (muscle or fat). The nasal lining may or may not be restored.

A difficulty in midface reconstruction with free flaps is the lack of an available donor site. The closest site for available donor vessels is the ipsilateral neck. The ideal free flap, therefore, must have a pedicle length of 10 to 13 cm to reach the neck without vein grafting.

Although a variety of free flaps, including fibula, scapula, and iliac crest flap, can be used to reconstruct maxillary defects, the two flaps most commonly used that have large and long pedicles are the rectus abdominis myocutaneous and radial forearm flaps. The rectus flap provides reliable skin and a

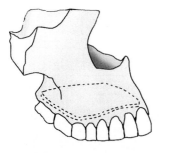

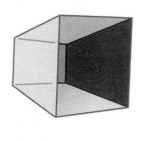

FIGURE 42.1. The maxilla compared with a hexahedron. The roof of the maxilla is the floor of the orbit. The floor of the maxilla is the hard palate. The anterior, posterior, medial, and lateral walls are the vertical buttresses, and the maxillary antrum is contained within the six walls of the bone.

large soft-tissue bulk. The radial forearm flap provides a large surface area of pliable skin with minimal soft tissue and can be combined with a vascularized bone segment. Both flaps can provide multiple skin islands that can be oriented in different three-dimensional positions.

Reconstruction of the highly complex three-dimensional nature of the maxillary defect can be simplified by combining bone grafts with soft-tissue flap. Bone grafts can be rigidly fixed irrespective of the insetting of the soft-tissue flap. Because there is minimal stress on midface bone, vascularized bone is essential only in the maxillary arch.

Many classifications systems have been developed to describe the extent of resection of maxillary and midfacial tumors to provide algorithms for reconstruction. A simple classification system we have previously described subdivides maxillary defects into four types.

Classification System for Maxillary and Midfacial Defects

Type I (limited maxillary) defects involve resection of one or two walls of the maxilla, excluding the palate (Fig. 42.2). These defects usually include the anterior and medial walls of the

maxilla, and occasionally the orbital rim, in combination with the soft tissues and skin of the neck. Hence, the defect has a high surface-area-to-volume ratio. The radial forearm flap is an ideal flap because it has a good surface-area-to-volume ratio, that is, a small amount of soft-tissue volume and large skin surface area. Defects of the orbital rim or orbital floor are reconstructed with calvarial or split-rib bone grafts.

Type II (subtotal maxillary) defects include resection of the maxillary arch, palate, and anterior and lateral walls with preservation of the orbital floor (Fig. 42.3). Resection of these defects include the classic hemimaxillectomy, or "infrastructure maxillectomy," procedure that involves the lower five walls of the maxilla with a medium surface-area-to-volume ratio (large surface area and medium volume). An osteocutaneous radial forearm flap folded into a "sandwich" is ideal for maxillary arch and palate reconstruction because it provides anterior projection and vascularized bone for dental implant osteointegration. Additionally, the bone provides support for the upper lip. The folded-skin surfaces restore the palatal mucosal lining and nasal floor lining. This flap has a "moderate" amount of volume when folded over and still maintains an adequate surface area to resurface the nasal floor and palate. Anterior bilateral subtotal maxillae defects are ideally suited for an osteocutaneous sandwich flap. Patients with these defects and intact upper external lip structures can be reconstructed with excellent aesthetic and functional results (Fig. 42.4).

Type III (total maxillary) defects include resection of all six walls of the maxilla. This type of defect is further subdivided into type IIIA, where the orbital contents are preserved and orbital floor is resected (Fig. 42.5), and type IIIB, which is a total maxillary defect combined with orbital exenteration (Fig. 42.6).

Type IIIA defects have medium-large volume and medium-large surface area requirements. Reconstruction of the orbital floor is required to maintain a functional eye. The floor is restored with nonvascularized bone graft, which must be supported by a well-vascularized flap. The rectus flap provides muscle coverage for bone grafts and adequate subcutaneous fat that can be contoured to fill the dead space. It can provide multiple skin islands for the palate and/or external skin and/or nasal lining as needed. A temporalis muscle flap can also cover

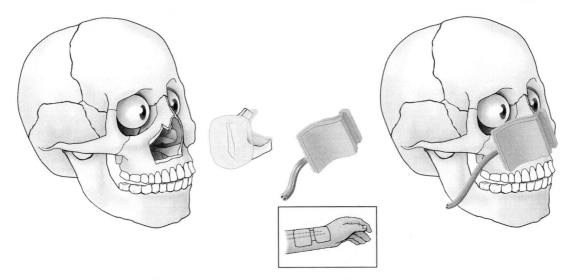

FIGURE 42.2. Type I (limited maxillary) defect. The anterior and medial walls of the maxilla (*left*) have been resected. The illustration demonstrates skin/soft-tissue resection in combination with bony resection (*center, left*) creating a large-surface-area/low-volume defect. The radial forearm fasciocutaneous flap (donor site depicted in *inset*) provides multiple large skin surface areas with minimal volume (*center, right*). The flap is shown in place, demonstrating skin islands to resurface anterior cheek and medial nasal lining (*right*).

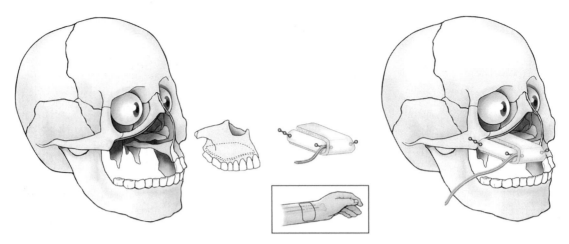

FIGURE 42.3. Type II (subtotal maxillary) defect. The lower five walls of maxilla have been resected, including the palate, but sparing the orbital floor (roof of the maxilla) (*left*). The illustration demonstrates palatal/nasal floor lining and bony resection. This creates a large-surface-area/medium-volume defect (*center, left*). The radial forearm osteocutaneous "sandwich" flap (donor site depicted in *inset*) provides a large skin surface area with vascularized bone and moderate volume (*center, right*). The flap is shown in place, demonstrating a strut of vascularized bone to reconstruct the anterior maxillary arch deficit sandwiched between two skin islands that replace palatal and nasal lining (*right*).

the bone grafts for the orbital floor; however, it cannot replace the palate. Consequently, an obturator is required for palate reconstruction. Temporalis flaps are indicated in older patients who are not candidates for free tissue transfer. Preservation of the malar eminence is helpful to maintain upper midface projection. Primary bone grafting in this area can be challenging because it can compress the flap pedicle.

Type IIIB defects are extensive and have a large volume and large surface area requirement. The palate and nasal lining often require closure to obviate oronasal fistulae. The external defect usually comprises the eyelids and cheek, and occasionally the lip. In addition, the anterior skull base is often exposed. A rectus abdominis flap is the flap of choice. If the external skin of the cheek is present, the skin island of the rectus flap can be used to close the palate. If the flap is not too bulky, then a second skin paddle can be used to reconstruct the lateral nasal wall. A third skin island can even be used to restore the external skin. The aesthetic outcome for patients with reconstructed external skin is fair to good because of the variability of skin color and contour. The contour abnormality can be revised at a later time using liposuction and/or skin excision.

Palatal closure can be accomplished with an obturator or the flap skin island. The palatal skin island often bulges downward, making denture fitting difficult. Despite this, palatal closure with a skin island is preferable because these patients usually are able to speak well and eat soft solids without a denture (Fig. 42.7).

There is a separate group of type IIIB patients who undergo resection of the hemimandible in addition to the maxilla and orbit. These are large volume and large surface area defects. Reconstruction of the bony defect would require a vascularized fibula flap, but this would not provide adequate soft tissue or skin for the external and intraoral defect. The rectus flap can provide multiple skin islands to replace the cheek lining, palate, lateral nasal wall, and external skin. In addition, the flap's significant bulk allows contouring of the cheek. Remarkably good function and reasonable aesthetic result with a single free flap reconstruction can be accomplished.

Type IV (orbitomaxillary) defects include resection of the orbital contents and the upper five walls of the maxilla, sparing the palate (Fig. 42.8). The reconstructive goal consists primarily of filling the dead space and resurfacing the external skin. The rectus flap is the ideal flap for this goal. Conceptually simple from a reconstructive standpoint, achieving this goal can be technically challenging. The temporal and facial

donor vessels are usually resected or unreliable. The flap pedicle can be lengthened by intramuscular dissection up to 20 cm to reach the neck vessels. A superficial tunnel can be created in the facelift plane or medial to the mandible by a parapharyngeal approach to gain access to the neck vessels without vein grafts.

An algorithm for reconstruction based on the above classification system is shown (Fig. 42.9).

A unique challenge of maxillary reconstruction involves repair of not only the maxillary defect but also of adjacent important structures of the face, such as the lip and oral commissure, eyelids, and nose that may be resected during the tumor extirpation. Reconstruction of a functioning lip is extremely difficult, and involves restoring a competent oral sphincter. The primary restoration of the lips with local lip-switch procedure prior to maxillary reconstruction with a free flap is advocated. **The free flap should not be attached directly into the sphincter, or used to reconstruct any portion of the lips, unless more than 80% of either the lower or upper lip is missing. The disadvantage of microstomia is less debilitating than constant drooling.**

Eyelid reconstruction may be necessary in types I and III defects. Ectropion is the most common postoperative problem. This can usually be corrected with a variety of secondary procedures, including tarsal strip procedure, skin grafting, and canthopexy. Type IIIB defects involve orbital exenteration, making eyelid restoration less important. **Because the results of functional eyelid reconstruction are usually unsatisfactory, a patch, dark eyeglasses, or an external glue-on type of prosthesis (cosmetic patch) is preferable to reconstruction.**

Large maxillary resections may involve the nose. Although the nose is aesthetically important, it is not essential from a functional standpoint. Usually local tissues (septum, nasal lining flaps, nasolabial flaps) are unavailable or irradiated. Reconstruction using local tissues, or even a second free flap, is usually difficult and yields poor aesthetic results. **Consequently, delayed nasal reconstruction is advocated in all cases.** Although prosthetic nasal reconstruction is preferable, delayed autogenous reconstruction is also an option.

Summary

Maxillectomy and midfacial defects are classified into four types of defects based on the extent of maxillary resection.

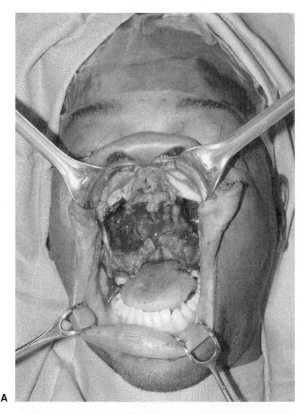

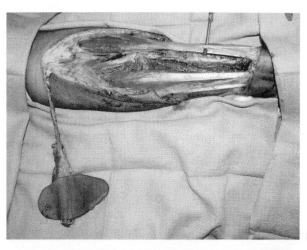

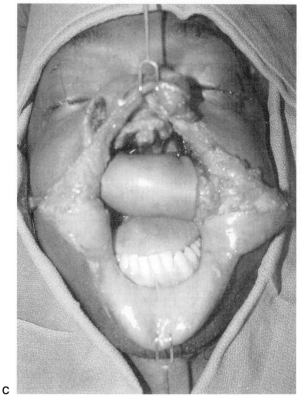

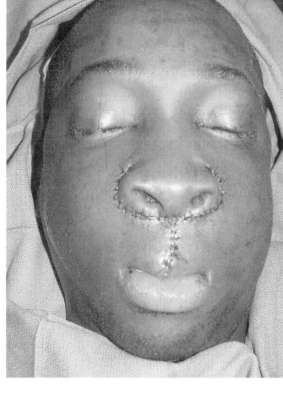

FIGURE 42.4. Bilateral subtotal maxillectomy (type II maxillary defect) and partial upper lip resection in a 30-year-old man with osteosarcoma of the maxilla extending into the oral and nasal cavity. **A:** Intraoperative defect. **B:** The radial forearm osteocutaneous flap harvested with segment of the distal radius bone and long vascular pedicle. **C:** Vascularized bone graft rigidly fixed to remaining maxillary tubercles. The skin island has been folded over the bone and fixed to resurface the floor of the nose and the palate. **D:** Postoperative photograph of patient after inset of the flap and closure of the lip defect.

This classification allows for a simplified approach to midface reconstruction. The algorithm is based on the type of maxillary defect, which will usually have specific skin, soft-tissue, palatal, orbital floor, and bony structure deficits. Bone reconstruction is best accomplished with bone grafts for the floor of the orbit and vascularized bone flap for the maxillary arch. Soft-tissue and skin coverage is commonly provided by free flaps. The choice of flap is determined by the surface area and tissue volume requirements. Large surface area and small- to medium-volume defects are best reconstructed with radial forearm fasciocutaneous or osteocutaneous flaps. Large-volume and medium- to large-surface area defects are best reconstructed with rectus

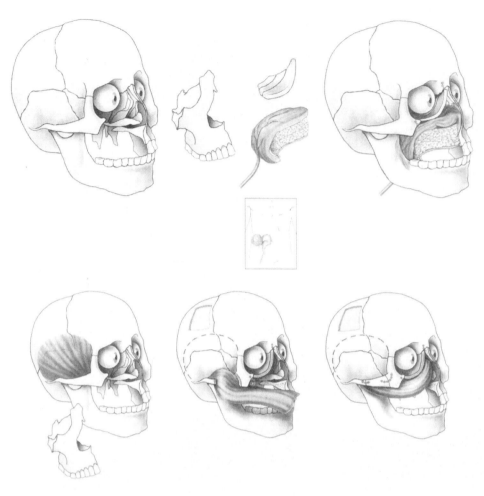

FIGURE 42.5. Type IIIA defect. All six walls of the maxilla, including the floor of orbit and hard palate have been resected. The orbital contents have been preserved (*left*). The illustration demonstrates the orbital floor, vertical maxillary buttresses, and palatal resection (*center, left*). This creates a medium-surface-area–medium-volume defect. Cranial or rib bone graft is used to reconstruct the orbital floor and is covered with a single-skin-island rectus abdominis myocutaneous flap (*center, right*). The rectus abdominis myocutaneous flap (donor site depicted *inset*) provides medium surface area with medium volume. The bone graft is rigidly fixed to reconstruct the orbital floor. The rectus abdominis myocutaneous flap with the skin island is used to close the roof of the palate, soft tissue is used to fill in the midfacial defect, and muscle is used to cover the bone graft. Note the extended length of the deep inferior epigastric vessels to neck (*right*). (*Below*) Patients who are not free-flap candidates can be reconstructed with split calvarial bone grafts, covered with the temporalis muscle, transposed anteriorly. The zygomatic arch should be osteotomized and temporarily removed to increase excursion of the temporalis muscle.

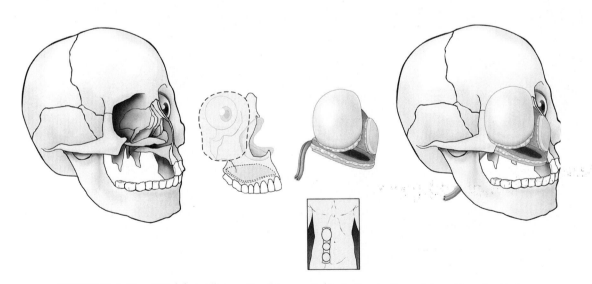

FIGURE 42.6. Type IIIB defect. All six walls of the maxilla, including the floor of the orbit and orbital contents (*left*) have been resected. The illustration demonstrates resection of external eyelid, cheek skin, and orbital contents, in combination with the entire maxilla and palate (*center, left*). This creates a large-surface-area–large-volume defect. A three-skin-island rectus abdominis myocutaneous flap design (*inset*) provides multiple large surface areas with a large volume of soft tissue and muscle to fill in the defect (*center, right*).

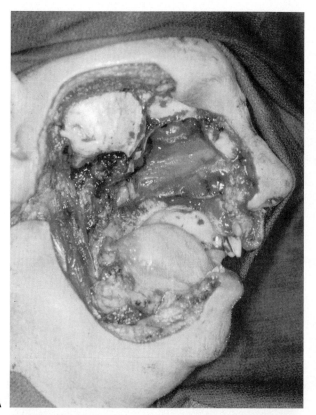

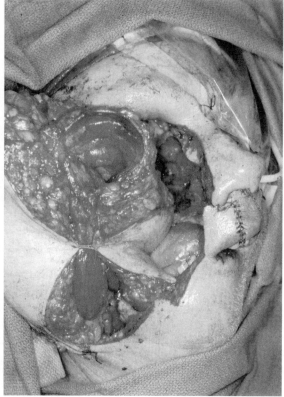

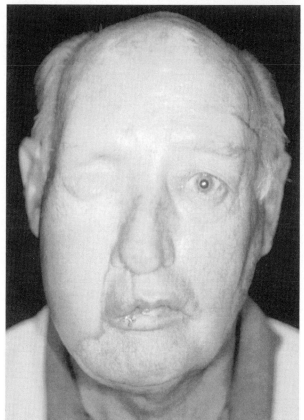

FIGURE 42.7. A 65-year-old man who underwent total maxillectomy with orbital exenteration and segmental mandibulectomy (type IIIB defect) for excision of a recurrent squamous cell cancer of the cheek skin invading maxilla, orbit, and oral cavity. **A:** Intraoperative defect. **B:** Reconstruction of the defect was performed using a two-skin-island rectus abdominis free flap for intraoral/palatal lining and external skin. **C:** Final appearance after two revisions of the flap to decrease bulk.

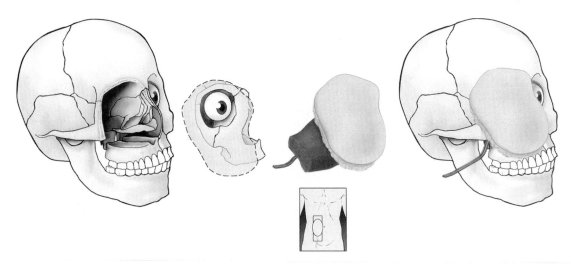

FIGURE 42.8. Type IV (orbitomaxillary) defect. The upper five walls of the maxilla have been resected, including the orbital contents, but sparing the palate (*left*). The specimen demonstrates resection of orbital contents, eyelid, and cheek skin in continuity with bone (*center, left*). This creates a large-surface-area–large volume defect. Note the design of the single-skin-island rectus abdominis myocutaneous flap (*inset*). This flap provides large surface area with large volume to reconstruct the defect (*center, right*). Rectus abdominis myocutaneous flap in place, demonstrating skin island to resurface the external skin defect with muscle and subcutaneous fat used to fill in the soft-tissue deficit (*right*).

abdominis free flaps. Critical midfacial structures, such as the lips, eyelids, and nose, should be addressed separately, using local flaps if possible. The majority of patients whose maxillary defects are reconstructed by using free tissue transfers have remarkably good function. Aesthetic results are mainly dependent on whether the orbital contents are removed and on the extent of external skin resection.

RECONSTRUCTION OF SKULL BASE DEFECTS

The most common cause of skull base defect is from tumor resection. Other etiologies of skull base defects include trauma,

late post-traumatic cerebrospinal fluid leak, craniofacial deformity, recurrent frontal mucocele, and midline dermoid cyst with intracranial extension. Surgical ablation of skull base tumors can result in an extensive defect with exposed brain, dura, cranial bone, and associated defects of adjacent structures, requiring composite tissue reconstruction to restore a combination of skin, soft tissue, bone, and mucosa. The goals of skull base reconstructions are to

1. repair and seal the dura;
2. separate the intracranial contents from the aerodigestive tract;
3. re-establish orbital and oropharyngeal cavities and function;

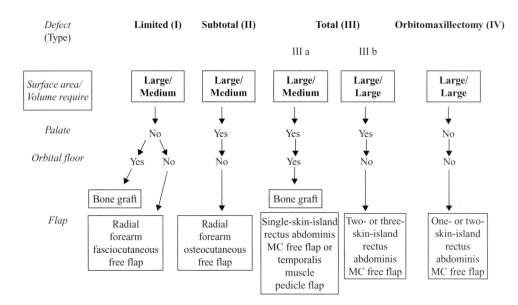

FIGURE 42.9. Algorithm for maxillary reconstruction. MC, myocutaneous.

4. restore form by providing structural support, adequate soft-tissue bulk, and external skin coverage; and
5. obliterate dead space.

Repair of skull base defects is challenging because an unsuccessful reconstruction can lead to life-threatening complications. Early complications following skull base surgery include dural exposure, cerebrospinal fluid leak, pneumocranium, wound infection, meningitis, epidural abscess, brain abscess, hemorrhage, and neurologic injury. Late complications include globe malposition, diplopia, malocclusion, nasopharyngeal stenosis, trismus, chronic sinusitis, nasal obstruction, and facial deformity. Thus, to avoid potentially devastating postoperative complications, the ideal reconstruction for skull base defect needs to be reliable regardless of technical difficulty.

Prior to the 1960s, skull base surgery was limited because of the associated high morbidity and mortality and the paucity of reliable reconstructive techniques. During this period, repair of skull base defects was performed using skin grafts and local available tissue such as scalp, galeal, pericranial, and temporalis flaps. The application of local flaps is limited by their small size, short arc of rotation, and donor site defect. In addition, these local flaps are unreliable in patients who had previous radiation therapy, multiple craniotomies, or a larger skull base resection. With the advent of the combined extracranial–intracranial approach by Ketcham et al., in 1963, and improved reconstructive techniques, the number of skull base surgeries has increased and resulted in larger defects requiring bigger flaps. In the 1970s, regional flaps, such as latissimus dorsi, pectoralis major, sternocleidomastoid, and trapezius flaps, were used to reconstruct these larger defects. These regional flaps are limited by pedicle location located below the clavicle, which restricts the arc of rotation in the superior direction. The development of free tissue transfer in 1980s provided a highly reliable method for repairing large, complex wounds in the skull base. Free flaps are well-vascularized and can be used in irradiated sites or in patients who will receive adjuvant radiotherapy. They provide enough tissue bulk and ease of insetting to obliterate dead space and seal the intracranial contents from the external environment and oropharyngeal cavity. In addition adequate composite tissue can be harvested to replace external skin, mucosa, soft tissue, and bone in large skull base defects in a single stage.

Although either pedicled flaps or free tissue transfer can be used to reconstruct large skull base defects, several authors have compared outcomes using free flaps versus local or regional flaps to repair difficult skull base wounds. They have all demonstrated that free tissue transfer is associated with fewer complications than local or regional flap for large difficult wounds. In addition, a steady decline in the complication rate of skull base surgery in the last 10 years has been observed. Consequently, free tissue transfer is frequently used for reconstruction of extensive, difficult skull base defects. Although skull base surgery has become less invasive (see Chapter 33), the need to reconstruct large defects still arises.

When determining the most appropriate technique for reconstruction, it is useful to identify the location of the skull base resection and the type of defect. Most skull base defects can be categorized as either an anterior or lateral skull base defect. The defect is assessed for extent of dural defect, exposure to the aerodigestive tract, and skin, soft tissue, bone, and mucosal lining deficits. Furthermore, resection of key adjacent structures, specifically, the orbit, ear, maxilla, palate, and mandible, are considered in the flap selection process. Finally, radiation, prior surgery, and availability of local tissues for repair must be weighed.

The first priority in skull base reconstruction is to repair the dural defect in a watertight fashion through either direct closure or patching with autogenous material (pericranium, temporalis fascia, or fascia lata) or alloplastic material. Fibrin glue is an excellent adjunct to prevent cerebrospinal fluid leak. After a watertight dural closure is accomplished, vascularized tissue is interposed between the intracranial contents and the oropharyngeal cavity. This provides a barrier and prevents dural contamination with the oropharyngeal bacterial flora. Usually a flap with extensive soft-tissue bulk is required to obliterate the dead spaces and to restore adequate surface contour of the face. Myocutaneous flaps (latissimus dorsi or rectus abdominis) or fasciocutaneous flaps (radial forearm, parascapular, or lateral thigh) can be used for soft-tissue reconstruction of the skull base.

Often key aesthetic structures, such as the ear, nose, and eyes, are resected during ablative skull base surgery. Definitive reconstruction of these structures is usually not undertaken at the initial stage of reconstruction. Prosthetic reconstruction remains a common and excellent method for replacing unique facial structures. However, simple soft-tissue filler over the anatomic defect and wearing a patch to cover the missing aesthetic structure is another alternative.

The indications for bone reconstruction in skull base surgery include extremely large bony defects of the skull base that will result in gross brain herniation; near-total or complete orbital roof defects that may result in pulsatile exophthalmos; orbital wall or floor defects that carry a high risk of enophthalmos; cranio-orbital defects that will result in inadequate soft-tissue support and deformity; and associated maxillary or mandibular/glenoid fossa defects that will result in facial deformity, malocclusion, and masticatory dysfunction. Alloplastic materials, or nonvascularized bone grafts in conjunction with vascularized tissue can be used for bone reconstruction for most isolated bone defects. Free osseous composite tissue transfer is indicated only in specialized cases where bone grafts combined with soft-tissue flaps are inadequate. Common composite vascularized osseous flaps include fibula, scapula, and radial forearm flaps.

Anterior Skull Base

For small defects of the anterior skull base that do not require obliteration of dead space, the workhorse flap is the pericranial and galea–pericranial flap. This flap provides a thin, well-vascularized sheet of fascia that can easily reach the anterior skull base and reinforce dural repair, separating the dura from the subjacent spaces.

For patients with a history of prior surgery or radiation and large extensive anterior skull base defects, free tissue transfer is required. A variety of different free flaps can be used, including rectus abdominis, latissimus, radial forearm, fibula, and scapular flaps. Flap selection is based on a variety of factors including the size of defect and type of defect, as well as whether adjacent structures such as scalp, orbit, maxilla, and mandible are resected. In general, the surface and volume deficits of the defect are assessed and the flap that best fits the defect is selected. In some cases, the location of the defect may determine the flap selection based on availability of recipient vessels. The superficial temporal vessels can be used for defects high in the skull base involving the scalp or orbit. For defects involving the orbit, maxilla, or lower face, the recipient vessels are usually found in the neck (Fig. 42.7).

Lateral Skull Base

The workhorse for small defects of the lateral skull base is the temporal muscle flap. It has the greatest utility in reconstructing defects of the infratemporal fossa. However, the temporalis is frequently devascularized during the ablative surgery and is not usable. In addition, it is associated with a distinct contour defect in the temporal fossa.

For larger and more complex defects of the lateral skull base, free tissue transfer is indicated. Options include rectus abdominis, latissimus dorsi, anterolateral thigh, and lateral arm flaps. These defects of the lateral skull base usually require filling and resurfacing the defect. Consequently, flap selection is based on the extent of volume and surface area, which is determined by the defect. The rectus abdominus myocutaneous flap is very commonly used because of its location (allowing for simultaneous dissection during resection of tumor), large skin island, and soft-tissue volume, in addition to an excellent vascular pedicle (length and caliber).

CONCLUSION

Local or regional flaps are used for reconstruction of small skull base defects. The morbidity and mortality of aggressive skull base resection has been decreased as a result of a multidisciplinary approach involving neurosurgeon, head and neck surgeon, and plastic surgeon, and of advances in microsurgical techniques. **Free tissue transfer is the preferred method for complex anterior skull base reconstruction involving dura, brain, or other major structures adjacent to the skull base, including the orbit, maxilla, and other structures.** Free flaps are occasionally required for lateral skull base defects as well. Successful reconstruction can be safely achieved, restoring form and function, with adherence to basic principles of reconstruction including watertight dural repair, coverage of dura and separation from nasopharyngeal cavity, and obliteration of dead space.

Selected Readings

Cordeiro PG, Bacilious N, Schantz S, et al. The radial forearm osteocutaneous "sandwich" free flap for reconstruction of the bilateral subtotal maxillectomy defect. *Ann Plast Surg.* 1998;40:397.

Cordeiro PG, Santamaria E, Kraus D, et al. Reconstruction of total maxillectomy defects with preservation of orbital contents. *Plast Reconstr Surg.* 1998;102:1874.

Yamamoto Y, Hawashima K, Sugihara T, et al. Surgical management of maxillectomy defects based on the concept of buttress reconstruction. *Head Neck.* 2004;26:247.

Cordeiro PG, Santamaria E. A classification system and algorithm for reconstruction of maxillectomy and midfacial defects. *Plast Reconstr Surg.* 2000;105:2331.

Cordeiro PG, Wolfe SA. The temporalis muscle flap revisited on its centennial: advantages, newer uses and disadvantages. *Plast Reconstr Surg.* 1996;98:980.

Georgantopoulou A, Hodgkinson PD, Gerber CJ. Cranial-base surgery: a reconstructive algorithm. *Br J Plast Surg.* 2003;56:10.

Chang DW, Langstein HN, Gupta A, et al. Reconstructive management of cranial base defects after tumor ablation. *Plast Reconstr Surg.* 2001;107:1346.

Teknos TN, Smith JC, Day TA, et al. Microvascular free tissue transfer in reconstructing skull base defects: lessons learned. *Laryngoscope.* 2002;112:1871.

Imola MJ, Sciarreta V, Schramm VL. Skull base reconstruction. *Curr Opin Otolaryngol Head Neck Surg.* 2003;11:282.

Neligan PC, Mulholland S, Irish J, et al. Flap selection in cranial base reconstruction. *Plast Reconstr Surg.* 1996;98:1159.

Califano J, Cordeiro PG, Disa JJ, et al. Anterior cranial base reconstruction using free tissue transfer: changing trends. *Head Neck.* 2003;25:89.

Izquierdo R, Leonetti JP, Origitano TC, et al. Refinements using free-tissue transfer for complex cranial base reconstruction. *Plast Reconstr Surg.* 1993;92:567.

Disa J. J, Rodriguez VM, Cordeiro PG. Reconstruction of lateral skull base oncological defects: the role of free tissue transfer. *Ann Plast Surg.* 1998;41:633.

CHAPTER 43 ■ RECONSTRUCTION OF THE ORAL CAVITY, PHARYNX, AND ESOPHAGUS

GIULIO GHERARDINI AND GREGORY R.D. EVANS

SOFT-TISSUE ORAL CAVITY RECONSTRUCTION

Reconstruction the oral cavity is a difficult challenge for the plastic surgeon because of the variety of anatomic structures and complexity of functions involved. The goals of oral reconstruction include the restoration of the anatomy, function, and appearance. It is also important to consider that oral function is required for social function. The ideal reconstruction should provide tissue that resembles in geometry, form, and quality the tissue moved or damaged.

Functional Anatomy of the Oral Cavity

The oral cavity extends from the vermilion of the lips to the junction of the hard and soft palate superiorly. Inferiorly, it extends to the circumvallate papillae of the tongue. It includes the lips, upper and lower alveolar ridges, buccal mucosa, retromolar trigone, hard palate, floor of the mouth, and the anterior two-thirds of the tongue. Each of these structures participates in speech, mastication, bolus preparation, bolus manipulation, and deglutition.

The oral sphincter participates in mastication, speech, and deglutition. It provides a watertight closure during the preparation of the bolus and prevents the escape of saliva. The alveolar ridges are elevated above the floor of the mouth and covered with thin, nonmobile mucosa. Their functions include directing the flow of saliva and collecting the food during the bolus process. The floor of the mouth is important to allow unrestricted mobility of the oral tongue.

The oral tongue, or mobile tongue, has sensory and motor functions, including proprioception, pain, taste, speech, and bolus manipulation. The mobility of the tongue is required for speech. The hard palate is the counterpart to the tongue for speech, bolus preparation, and bolus transit in the oral phase of deglutition. It constitutes a solid separation between the nasal and oral cavities.

The buccal mucosa lines the cheek and is important for mastication and deglutition. During reconstruction, flaps should be mobile enough to expand and allow for mastication, but thin enough to avoid restriction of dental closure. The base of tongue, although technically part of the oropharynx, participates in taste, deglutition, and speech. The final push of the food bolus requires that the base of tongue occlude the oropharynx. The tonsillar pillars can be involved in tumors arising from the lateral part of the tongue or the posterior floor of the mouth. Their function consists in separating the oropharynx from the nasopharynx, thereby preventing nasal regurgitation during speech and swallowing.

Principles of Reconstruction

Although the oral cavity is composed of distinct anatomic elements participating in various functions, including mastication, speech, and deglutition, the accomplishment of a single function often requires the simultaneous participation of each anatomic element.

From a reconstructive point of view, each anatomic area is considered individually to define the characteristics needed to restore the oral lining. It is important to consider the health status of the patient, as well as the overall defect, when considering options for reconstruction. **Carcinoma of the oral cavity tends to occur in patients with other medical problems.**

Available Methods

In the case of small defects, primary closure can be used with recruitable tissue. In selected cases, this technique gives a rapid and uncomplicated reconstruction, and it is particularly suitable for small defects of the floor of the mouth and tongue.

Local flaps provide the best match for color and texture. Often the quality of the reconstruction obtainable is high and may bring sensate cover into the defect. The limitation in the use of local tissue is frequently the size of the defect. **Previous irradiation of the area may render local flaps impractical.**

Skin grafts are used when only skin or oral lining is required. The technical advantage of the method is that it is simple and rapid, although it cannot be used in previously irradiated recipient sites. Regional myocutaneous flaps are an option in reconstruction of larger defects of the oral cavity. They are not complex and technically do not require microsurgical equipment or skills. **Pedicled myocutaneous flaps, however, tend to distort the intraoral reconstruction or leave unsightly external bulges (e.g., the pectoral flap).** Donor-site deformities must also be considered in these regional flaps. Vascular perfusion is frequently not robust, leading to increased complications. Free tissue transfer allows the reconstruction of complex defects of the oral cavity, involving a combination of different composite structures such as bone, mucosa, and muscle. Today, free flaps are used routinely because of a superior blood supply, the improvement in equipment and technique, and a lower complication rate.

Reconstruction of the Floor of Mouth

The floor of mouth requires soft, mobile, and, if possible, sensate tissue, allowing for free mobility of the oral tongue. There are many options for reconstructing the floor of mouth, and the tissue used depends on the size and extent of the defect. Small defects may be resurfaced with a split-thickness skin graft, allowing the preservation of the epithelium necessary for a watertight closure. The graft is sutured into the oral cavity and is stabilized with a bolster. Unfortunately, the tethering and scarring from the use of split-thickness skin grafts can be problematic.

The nasolabial flap is a reliable flap based on the angular artery, which can be used for defects of the anterior floor of mouth. The advantage of this flap is its relative technical ease. It is best used in older patients with skin laxity. The disadvantage is that it requires two stages and creates a temporary orocutaneous fistula.

Historically, regional flaps were useful for anterior floor of the mouth reconstruction and included the forehead flap, the facial artery musculomucosal flap (FAMM), and the deltopectoral flap. As a consequence of advances in microsurgery, these flaps are rarely used today. Their main disadvantages are their tenuous blood supply, their unavailability in irradiated patients, the obvious donor-site defects, and the distortion of structures from their harvest. Some of these flaps require the creation of a temporary orocutaneous fistula.

Free tissue transfer is preferred. The radial forearm flap is a pliable flap based on the radial artery, which is particularly advantageous, especially in previously irradiated patients. The thin nature of the flap provides for tongue mobility and allows for free movement of food during oral deglutition. The flap can become sensate through neurorrhaphy of the medial or lateral cutaneous nerve to the lingual or other sensory nerves in the neck.

The anterolateral thigh can be also be used, with or without a sensory nerve reinnervation. This flap can be adapted for reconstruction of many defects in the head and neck area. The vascular anatomy of the thigh flap may vary but is usually based on the descending branch of the lateral circumflex femoral artery and its comitant veins. Usually the defect can be closed directly with sutures and patients can be mobilized on the first postoperative day. This flap is used less frequently in the Western patient population because of the extent of excess adipose tissue bulk within the thigh.

Alternatively, the temporalis fascial flap allows thin pliable coverage for partial glossectomy and floor of mouth defects. Although the dissection is fairly straightforward, the limitation of vessel size and the potential need for skin grafting the fascia for more durable coverage have limited its use. Furthermore, the necessity of dissecting this flap within the head and neck area frequently precludes the use of two operating teams and makes the procedure less efficient.

Reconstruction of the Tongue

The tongue is the most difficult structure of the oral cavity to reconstruct because of the complex intrinsic musculature and its participation in oral function. In general, the needs for tongue reconstruction include the restoration of speech and swallowing, and, secondarily, a good cosmetic result. Thanks to the redundancy in the tongue musculature, a near hemiglossectomy, leaving more than 20% to 30% of the original structures, allows maintenance of some function. In this case, the reconstruction should employ a thin and pliable flap to ensure mobility of the remaining tongue segment. The radial forearm free flap is an ideal choice.

Some reconstructive surgeons like to use the anterior lateral thigh for partial glossectomy defects. Ultimately, the amount of bulk in the thigh determines the availability of this donor site for use. If the glossectomy leaves less than 20% to 30% of the original structure, the reconstruction focuses on the restoration of the bulk of the tongue in order to direct secretions laterally

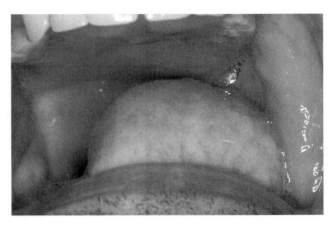

FIGURE 43.1. Free flap reconstruction of glossectomy defect. A rectus abdominis flap was used to provide bulk to the oral cavity.

toward the oropharynx and provide contact of the neotongue with the palate to assist in deglutition.

The rectus abdominis myocutaneous flap, the anterior lateral thigh, and the scapula/parascapular flap are preferred in glossectomies.

The rectus abdominis can be harvested in the vertical, oblique, or transverse direction, depending on the orientation of the defect and the amount of tissue needed. This is true for the anterior lateral thigh, as well as the scapula/parascapular flap. The rectus abdominis flap is based on the deep inferior epigastric vessels and is harvested with the patient in the supine position, allowing for a two-team approach. The rectus flap provides more bulk than other myocutaneous flaps, and has acceptable morbidity at the donor site (Fig. 43.1). The lateral arm free flap, based on the posterior radial collateral artery, is sometimes used for the same defect. It has a thick proximal paddle and thinner distal paddle, which allows for extra bulk at the posterior tongue defect. The main disadvantage of the flap is the appearance of the donor site.

Alternatives to the rectus abdominis flap for tongue reconstruction include the anterior lateral thigh and the scapula flaps. Patient positioning and turning may limit the use of the scapular flap. The vessel size of the scapular flap allows a good match to the recipient vessels in the neck. This flap may be ideal for those patients in whom the donor site of the radial forearm is unacceptable. The anterior lateral thigh also offers a large amount of tissue for restoration of bulk. The perforating vessels, however, can have some variability, and dissection is more technically demanding.

Reconstruction of the Buccal Cavity

Small defects of the buccal cavity can be excised and repaired with direct approximation. Larger defects of the buccal mucosa can be repaired with split-thickness skin grafts or mucosal grafts. Fascial flaps like the temporoparietal flap based on the superficial temporal artery are another option. This thin flap can be skin grafted to provide intraoral lining. The flap is harvested and tunneled under the zygomatic arch and delivered into the oral cavity. Frequently, however, this flap may not reach the oral cavity, necessitating alternative flap selection or use as a free tissue transfer. Large defects of the buccal cavity can be repaired using distant flaps like the pectoralis major. The undersurface of the muscle may support a skin graft for intraoral lining. Alternatively, the flap can be harvested with the skin paddle de-epithelized and placed into the defect. The radial forearm flap is ideal for buccal defects.

Principles of Microvascular Surgery in the Oral Cavity Reconstruction

Because of the complexity of the defects and the damage of the tissue following radiotherapy, microvascular surgery is often the only option in cancer reconstruction of the oral cavity. However, free tissue transfer deserves some consideration in regards to planning, timing, technique, and postoperative management.

Careful planning and a multidisciplinary team approach are essential. An early examination of the patient and an opportunity to plan the reconstruction in conjunction with the extirpation is vital. It is important that the reconstructive surgeon be consulted in advance of the ablative procedure so that treatment options can be adequately explained to the patient.

Preoperative assessment includes evaluation of the patient's overall health with particular attention to the patient's cardiopulmonary, renal, and nutritional status. Many patients are tobacco smokers, and it has been demonstrated that cigarette smoking increases the risk of thrombosis in microvascular surgery. Flaps with the best blood supply are used in these patients to avoid wound-healing complications. Although frequently not possible, it is preferred that smoking cease for 2 weeks before and 2 weeks following surgery.

During examination of the patient, the extent of the surgical resection is estimated and the anticipated tissue needs are assessed. The reconstruction is planned by taking into account the availability of local and regional tissues and possible donor sites for free tissue transfers. If tissue will be harvested from an extremity, a clinical assessment of the vascular supply is performed. Angiography is rarely needed. If a radial forearm flap is planned, the surgeon must confirm that there is adequate filling of the hand through the ulnar artery (the Allen test). If a lower extremity flap is planned (fibula), the presence of a normal pulse at the ankle is usually sufficient evidence that flap harvest will not result in postoperative vascular complications (see Chapter 41).

Routine preoperative laboratory tests should include a complete blood count and blood chemistry profile, clotting studies, a chest radiograph, and an electrocardiogram. If the patient is elderly or has a smoking history, it is advisable to also obtain pulmonary function tests, a cardiac stress test, and a nutritional assessment, including a determination of total serum protein, albumin, and transferrin concentrations. The incidence of malnutrition in head and neck cancer patients ranges from 30% to 50%, although the incidence is probably lower in patients with cancers that do not involve the aerodigestive tract. Poorly nourished patients have a higher risk of complications with surgery and radiotherapy. If a patient is severely malnourished, preoperative nutritional therapy may be indicated. Cardiopulmonary status should be optimized prior to surgery.

Defects are ideally repaired at the time of the resection. The advantages of immediate reconstruction are numerous. The defect is widely exposed, and recipient vessels require little additional dissection. Soft-tissue contractures are not present, and tissue requirements are readily defined. There is less chance of cervical or central nervous system infection. Single-stage treatment maximizes the time of "normal" living without need of repeated hospitalizations or special care, a factor especially important for patients with a poor prognosis and limited life expectancy. Finally, the patient's attitude is greatly improved when form and function are promptly restored.

Procedure

The following practical steps facilitate the free flap procedure. In the operating room, the patient's position is usually reversed such that the patient's head rests at the foot of the table. This facilitates the microsurgery by allowing the surgeon to sit at the patient's head. Skin incisions should be designed taking into account the subsequent reconstruction as well as the need for tumor ablation. When possible, lip-splitting incisions are avoided. This makes flap inset more difficult, but the long-term results are improved. If a neck dissection is necessary, care should be taken to avoid injury to vessels that may later be required for revascularization of the free tissue flap. If branches of the internal jugular vein and the external carotid artery must be ligated, preserving 1 to 2 cm of length may facilitate the microvascular portion of the procedure later.

At times, depending on the location of the donor site, it may be possible for both surgical teams to work simultaneously, significantly reducing the total operating time. Frequently, however, mobilization of the flap must be delayed until the exact dimensions of the defect are known.

After completion of the ablative portion of the procedure, the reconstruction is begun. The first step is to prepare the defect. Those portions that may be closed primarily are approximated first. If local flaps are to be used in addition to the free flap, they are mobilized and transferred, thus defining the final dimensions of the defect that will actually require free tissue. Next, the recipient vessels selected to revascularize the free flap are carefully dissected using loupe magnification. Recipient vessels must demonstrate pulsatile arterial inflow and unobstructed venous outflow. Care must be taken to avoid atherosclerotic plaques, which frequently involve the bifurcations of the arteries. Vascular control is accomplished using latex vessel loops, which occlude the vessels atraumatically and lift them out of the wound for easier access during the microsurgery. Anastomoses may be done end-to-end to branches of the external carotid artery and the internal jugular vein, or end-to-side directly to the large vessels. It is critical to choose a vessel that is the appropriate size for the recipient–donor anastomosis. Frequently, the multitude of branches from these vessels allows a variety of selections to choose the appropriate size. The distance between the defect and the recipient vessels is carefully measured to ensure that the pedicle harvested with the flap is long enough. A vein graft is sometimes necessary if the location of the defect is far from the recipient vessels. Vein grafts can be placed as an arteriovenous loop or, alternatively, the vein grafts can be attached on the back table prior to the anastomosis. Previously irradiated patients deserve special consideration because irradiated tissue is prone to wound complications and vessel changes such as carotid artery stenosis and rupture.

Free flaps provide tissues with the most reliable blood supply and are usually preferred in irradiated patients. The decision to select a specific recipient artery for the microvascular anastomosis depends on the anatomic aspect of the vessel and blood flow.

With the recipient site prepared, the flap is ready for transfer. The vascular pedicle is divided, and the amount of time that the tissue is without a blood supply is carefully monitored. Depending on the type of transfer, revascularization can usually be accomplished in 1 to 3 hours, and special techniques to protect the flap from ischemic injury are rarely necessary. Cooling the flap can extend the ischemic time if dissection has been delayed or recipient vessels not reasonably accessible. **The amount of time a particular tissue can tolerate ischemia varies, but generally, skin and bone tolerate longer periods of ischemia than do more metabolically active tissues such as muscle or viscera.**

It is our practice to partially inset the flap prior to performing the microvascular anastomoses. This technique has two advantages: First, it secures the flap to the bed and ensures the pedicle is oriented properly prior to completing the microsurgery. Second, it reduces the chance that the microvascular anastomoses will be disrupted by subsequent manipulation of the flap as it is inset into the defect.

An operating microscope is used to perform the microvascular anastomoses (see Chapter 8). It provides the best visualization and facilitates the procedure by ensuring that the surgeon and assistant, seated opposite each other, have the same view. Fine microsuture (9-0 or 10-0) material is used. The venous anastomosis is usually completed first, followed by the arterial anastomosis; however, the exact order depends on the location of the vessels. It is easier to proceed with the deeper vessel first, allowing the more superficial vessel to be anastomosed without the interference of the other completed anastomosis. Whether to perform an end-to-end or end-to-side anastomosis depends on the size of the donor and recipient vessels. When possible, an end-to-side anastomosis into the internal carotid artery and internal jugular vein is preferred. Alternatively, branches to these vessels allow a good end-to-end anastomosis. Frequently, the venous anastomosis can be performed using a coupling device. With release of the vascular clamps, the flap should show evidence of perfusion throughout. Signs of adequate perfusion include a return of normal (or hyperemic) color, normal capillary refill (2 seconds), and brisk filling of the pedicle vein.

Clinical and experimental vasospasm may be relieved by irrigating the vessels with topical local anesthetics (lidocaine 2%) or papaverine. Systemic anticoagulants are rarely required to maintain microvascular patency if there are no deficiencies in the microvascular technique and should be avoided if possible because of the risk of hematoma. Local irrigation with heparinized saline, however, is recommended.

With the tissue revascularized, the inset is completed. The tissue is sculpted to the proper contour without compromising its viability. Residual deformity may be revised after the flap has healed in its new location. Care must be taken to avoid compression of the vascular pedicle during final wound closure. If the flap is designed with the vascular pedicle passing through a subcutaneous tunnel to the recipient vessels, the tunnel must be wide enough to allow for postoperative swelling. When a muscle flap is used to close a cutaneous defect, the final step of the reconstruction is usually to harvest and apply a skin graft to the surface of the muscle. Bolsters or other constricting dressings should not be used to secure the skin graft in place because of the potential compromise to the flap by compression.

Postoperative Management

In addition to the routine care provided to any patient after a major operation, special precautions must be taken to properly care for and monitor the free flap. It is important that the patient's head be maintained in a neutral position to avoid mechanical compression of the vascular pedicle in the immediate postoperative period. Avoid tracheotomy tube ties or oxygen masks with elastic bands that encircle the neck. Because these patients frequently have had previous radiation therapy, the ability of keeping the patient well hydrated to avoid collapse and thrombosis of the neck vessels is essential, particularly the internal jugular vein. The flaps should be fully exposed, without dressings, to allow regular inspection.

Flap perfusion must be monitored hourly for 3 to 5 days, with decreased monitoring as time progresses; free flaps rarely fail after that. The clinical signs to assess are color, capillary refill, and turgor. Flaps that appear pale and have prolonged capillary refill may have arterial obstruction. Blue discoloration and more rapid capillary refill suggest venous occlusion. Additional information on the condition of the flap can be obtained by listening to the pedicle of the flap with a percutaneous ultrasonic Doppler device.

Various other monitoring devices, such as laser Doppler and implantable-pulsed ultrasonic Doppler devices, may also be helpful. With most cutaneous reconstructions, however, a large amount of the flap is exposed for clinical assessment, and sophisticated adjuncts are not usually needed.

Excessive bleeding or swelling postoperatively may be a clue that venous outflow is obstructed. If pedicle thrombosis is suspected, the flap requires immediate surgical exploration to confirm that it is adequately vascularized. In the event of thrombosis and occlusion, it is possible to salvage the flap if the blood supply is restored rapidly.

The postoperative feeding is ensured via a jejunal or nasogastric tube and started as soon as active bowel sounds are present. Usually a fluoroscopic study of the esophagus is obtained between the seventh and the tenth day, and if no abnormalities are seen, an oral liquid diet is started immediately and the patient is discharged home following feeding. In patients where a "leak" is detected from the flap suture line, feeding is withheld and a follow-up radiographic swallowing study is done 4 to 6 weeks prior to initiating feeding. With the advent of insurance oversight and cost containment, many of these procedures are now done as an outpatient.

Radial Forearm Flap

This thin flap is particularly suitable when pliable soft tissue is required to repair a contour deformity, partial tongue, and soft tissue loss. An osteocutaneous flap is also available for reconstruction of soft- or hard-tissue defects.

Pertinent Anatomy

The territory of this flap may extend from the wrist flexion crease to the lower third of the arm. The flap is based on the radial vessel, which courses through the anterior lateral intermuscular septum, with drainage from the venae comitantes or a superficial vein such as the cephalic. The skin is supported by small multiple perforators through the fascial septum. The radial artery courses deeply between the pronator teres muscle and the brachioradialis muscle in the upper forearm and between the brachioradialis muscle and the flexor carpi radialis in the lower forearm. Distally, it contributes to the deep palmar arch passing through the anatomic "snuff box" between the tendons of the abductor pollicis longus and extensor pollicis brevis muscles. A rich vascular network is derived from the radial artery in the forearm. The venous drainage is based on superficial and deep veins. The deep system is composed by the venae comitantes accompanying the radial artery and has an average diameter of 1.3 mm. When possible, the superficial system should be included in the flap (the cephalic and the basilic veins). The cephalic vein arises from the radial border of the forearm and receives tributaries from both sides of the forearm. It is our preferred vein in transferring this flap. The basilic vein ascends along the ulnar border of the forearm and then travels forward toward the medial bicipital groove where it joins the cephalic vein.

Technique of Dissection

Patency of the ulnar and radial arteries should be assessed preoperatively via an Allen test. If delay or poor perfusion through the ulnar artery is noted, the radial forearm flap should not be used. The size of the defect to be reconstructed, three-dimensional architecture in complex defects, and the recipient vessels should be evaluated. A tourniquet is placed on the upper arm once the limb is exsanguinated. Skin markings are then performed on the dorsovolar aspect of the forearm. This allows harvest of the cephalic vein during dissection. The flap should be designed as distal as possible in the forearm, but no further than the wrist flexion crease. This allows for the incorporation of as many perforators from the radial artery as possible to perfuse the skin and fascia.

The flexor tendons, radial artery and venae comitantes, cephalic vein, brachioradialis muscle, and median nerve are all noted, and the distal vascular pedicle (radial artery and venae comitantes) is ligated. Elevation can now begin on either radial or ulnar side of the forearm. The plane of dissection is below the antebrachial fascia and above the flexor tendons. To allow skin grafting of the donor site, the paratenon should not be removed. Care is taken not to damage the fasciocutaneous branches emerging from the intermuscular septum. The superficial branches (usually three) of the radial sensory nerve are identified and preserved. The cephalic (and basilic) vein is divided distally when located within the skin paddle. The dissection proceeds from distal to proximal to the bifurcation of the brachial artery. This can be done with a curvilinear or inverted V pattern, if there is skin laxity. The inverted V pattern allows split- or full-thickness skin harvesting for grafting the forearm donor area. The dissection should take about 1 hour. After this time the tourniquet is released, vascularity of the hand is assessed and meticulous hemostasis achieved.

Attention is then directed to the recipient vessel. The vascular pedicle is ligated and divided, the flap is transferred to the reconstruction area and partially inset using 3-0 Vicryl sutures. It is critical to conform the radial forearm flap to the defect, including the creation of a sulcus for food movement. Frequently, additional procedures are necessary in 6 months to revise and reshape the flap. The blood flow in the vessels is then assessed using a transonic Doppler. The inset of the flap is then completed and the head and neck area drained.

The head and neck defect is closed primarily with interrupted 2-0, and 3-0 Vicryl sutures and staples if enough skin laxity is present. Split- or full-thickness skin grafts are placed on the distal donor defect, and the forearm is dressed in a volar splint for 5 days to provide stabilization until neovascularization of the skin graft occurs.

Osteofasciocutaneous Radial Forearm Flap

An anterolateral segment of the radial bone (10 cm) can be harvested in the flap. This bone is particularly suitable for reconstruction of the midface involving the orbit and maxilla and for bony contour defects. The blood supply to the bone is derived from fascioperiosteal branches through the intermuscular septum and musculoperiosteal branches through the flexor pollicis longus and pronator quadratus muscles from the radial artery. The flap is harvested as described. The periosteum of the radius is reached by dividing the muscle bellies of the flexor pollicis longus and pronator quadratus muscles. The bone is then cut in a beveled fashion approximately 0.5 cm on either side of the radial vessels. The excision should not be greater than one-third of the diameter of the radius. Because the radius is thin, a titanium plate is placed on the native radius to prevent fractures and prolonged cast placement.

Rectus Abdominis Flap

The rectus abdominis flap can provide a large amount of tissue with a long vascular pedicle with good-sized vessels. The flap is suitable for filling of deep defects and for covering large surfaces and even the entire floor of the month. It is an ideal reconstruction for total glossectomy defects allowing bulk to assist with food bolus movements and speech. Frequently, 6 months are required for edema in the flap to decrease allowing a more aesthetic reconstruction. The major advantage is that the patient's position for flap harvesting does not require to be altered, and there is enough space for two surgical teams to work simultaneously.

Pertinent Anatomy

The rectus abdominis muscle originates from the symphysis pubis and pubic crest and inserts in the fifth, sixth, and seventh costal cartilages. It measures about 30 cm in length and 0.6 cm in width. The blood supply is provided by the superior and inferior epigastric arteries. The superior epigastric artery originates from the internal mammary artery at the level of the six intercostal space, where it gives off the musculophrenic artery. This vessel is generally accompanied by two venae comitantes and communicates with the inferior epigastric artery at the level of the umbilicus. Several perforators are provided to the muscle and skin. The inferior epigastric artery is the vascular pedicle used for free tissue transfer of the rectus flap.

Technique of Dissection

The patient is placed supine and the skin markings are performed. If a skin flap is required, it is outlined vertically, on one side of the abdomen. The rectus also allows positioning of the skin paddle in horizontal and oblique directions. The superior and inferior extensions of the markings may cover the entire length of the muscle, but generally the proximal marking is placed at the level of the ninth rib, and the distal marking is placed inferior to the paraumbilical area.

The skin incision is performed with the knife, but the dissection proceeds with electrocautery to minimize blood loss. The anterior rectus fascia is visualized laterally and medially, and the flap is elevated to visualize the medial and lateral rows of perforators. The fascia is incised medial to lateral, taking care to preserve the perforators.

Once the lateral and medial borders of the flap are dissected the vascular pedicle is dissected to reach the external iliac vessels. Small branches of the vessel are ligated with bipolar or vascular clips. The flap elevation is completed with the division of the proximal part of the rectus muscle.

Attention is then directed to the recipient vessel. The vascular pedicle of the rectus flap is ligated and divided, and the flap is transferred to the reconstruction area and partially inset using 3-0 Vicryl sutures. The fascia in the donor defect is closed in the standard fashion. Care is taken to include the internal oblique muscle in the closure. Not observing this precaution increases the risk of developing an abdominal bulge. In some cases, alloplastic mesh may be required to reinforce the fascial closure.

Other free flaps have been used successfully to provide soft-tissue reconstruction of the head and neck; they are known as perforator artery flaps. The technique involves the harvesting of free flaps based on dissection of the myocutaneous perforators, using fat and skin alone, while avoiding the use of muscle that can result in functional deficits. These perforator and muscle-sparing flaps can be based on the deep inferior epigastric perforator (DIEP) or the superficial inferior epigastric artery (SIEA).

There are fewer donor-site complications with the perforator flaps, especially complications involving abdominal hernias, bulges, and muscle weakness, when compared to the traditional rectus flaps. Care must be taken, however, with the amount of flap perfusion and the potential for fat necrosis.

Anterior Lateral Thigh Flap

The anterolateral thigh free flap has been used for coverage and reconstruction of full-thickness defects of the mandible or cheek, and for pharyngoesophageal defects after radical resection of malignancy. It is also excellent for total glossectomy defects. The flap has a long vascular pedicle, moderate thickness, and a large cutaneous area. The donor site can be closed primarily or covered with a split-thickness skin. As stated before, this flap may be more versatile in the Asian population where excess adipose tissue is not usually encountered.

Pertinent Anatomy

In most cases, the descending branch of the lateral circumflex femoral artery (LCFA) supplies the anterolateral thigh flap. A Doppler probe can delineate the surface projection of the perforating artery from the lateral circumflex femoral artery. This area of projection is estimated to be within a 3-cm diameter of the midpoint of a line linking the anterior superior iliac spine and the superolateral border of the patella. The descending branch runs downward through the intermuscular space between the rectus femoris and the vastus lateralis, and terminates in the vastus lateralis muscle near the knee joint. The cutaneous branches supply the skin overlying the vastus lateralis.

The cutaneous branches are classified into the following four types: (a) musculocutaneous perforators, which are most common; (b) septocutaneous perforators; (c) direct cutaneous branches that arise from the transverse branch of the lateral circumflex femoral artery; and (d) tiny cutaneous branches found on the surface of the vastus lateralis.

If a sensate flap is desired, the lateral femoral cutaneous nerve (L2–L3) must be included within the harvested flap. The largest branch of this nerve traverses downward along the previously mentioned line that extends from the anterior superior iliac spine down to the lateral border of the patella.

Scapular Flap

The scapular flap affords one of the best color and texture matches compared to other fasciocutaneous donor sites. Its vascular supply is based on the cutaneous branches of the circumflex scapular artery (CSA). This vessel is the terminal branch of the subscapular artery along with the thoracodorsal artery. The circumflex scapular artery splits into two skin branches: the transverse, or scapular, branch and the descending, or parascapular, branch. The two vessels allow the harvesting of two separate skin paddles. Because of the vascular cutaneous system, the skin paddle can be oriented in a vertical, horizontal, or oblique pattern.

Technique of Dissection

The scapular landmarks are marked with the patient in the sitting position. The medial and lateral border and tip of the scapula are noted. The triangular space is identified by palpation and marked. For flap harvesting, the patient is placed in the lateral position and the ipsilateral arm is prepped into the field.

It is possible to elevate the flap starting from the vascular pedicle (prograde) or raising the skin paddle first (retrograde). If the vascular pedicle is dissected first, an incision is made along the upper lateral skin markings, and it is deepened to the thoracodorsal fascia, which is raised with the flap. The posterior margin of the deltoid is identified and retracted, exposing the teres minor. The dissection proceeds along the surface of the teres minor and the cutaneous branches of the circumflex scapular artery are exposed. At this point, the skin incision is lengthened superomedially and inferiorly, and the flap elevation is performed in the space between the thoracodorsal fascia and the muscle fascia. If the skin marking is oriented horizontally, the parascapular artery is ligated and divided; if a larger skin extension is needed, this branch is conserved to supply the inferior part of the flap.

Once the flap has been freed from the chest wall, the long head of the triceps, the teres major, and teres minor muscles are retracted to facilitate the exposure of the vascular pedicle. The vascular branches directed to the teres major and teres minor muscles and the infrascapular branch are ligated and divided, allowing 6 cm of pedicle. If a longer pedicle is needed, a small incision is made in the axilla, exposing the subscapular and the thoracodorsal artery. A tunnel is dissected under the teres minor muscle to connect with the triangular space; the thoracodorsal artery is then ligated and divided. With this technique, a pedicle of 12 cm is obtained. Inset is performed as outlined above. One or two No. 15 French drains are left in place. The donor site is closed primarily.

Temporoparietal Flap

The temporoparietal fascia free flap is a thin, highly vascularized tissue with a reliable vascular pedicle. Although more useful in hand reconstruction, it can be used within the head and neck and oral cavity. The drawbacks of this flap are its lack of skin, alopecia at the donor site, and tedious elevation of the scalp flaps for exposure. The flap is supported by the superficial temporal artery and vein along with the auriculotemporal nerve for sensation.

Technique of Dissection

This vascular fascia is a component of the superficial musculoaponeurotic system and is continuous with the galea aponeurotica. It lies immediately beneath the hair follicles. The superficial temporal fascia overlies the deep temporal fascia and is separated from it by a loose areolar plane, known as the innominate fascia. Dissection begins by identifying the artery in the preauricular region. Elevation of the scalp flaps begins inferiorly where the plane between the dermis and superficial temporal fascia is more easily identified. As dissection proceeds in the cranial direction, separation becomes more tedious and care must be taken not to injure the hair follicles. Following scalp flap elevation, a template is outlined for the required geometry of the flap. The fascia is incised and elevated along with the vascular pedicle.

Outcomes

Speech and the ability to articulate words intelligibly is greatly dependent on oropharyngeal competence and tongue mobility. In addition to its obvious role in speech, the oral tongue is important for propulsion of food and liquid through the mouth. Adequate soft-tissue bulk is necessary to prevent pooling in the lateral buccal recess as well as to decrease intraoral volume. The base of the tongue has been specifically identified as a major generator of pressure in the pharynx and is responsible for transit of food into the esophagus. During the oral preparatory stage of swallowing, the tongue, in combination with the rotary action of the jaw, moves the food onto the teeth for chewing. Subsequently, it pulls the food into a semi cohesive bolus or ball prior to the initiation of the oral phase. Sensory receptors in the oropharynx and tongue itself are stimulated and trigger the swallow reflex to initiate the pharyngeal stage of the swallow. The tongue base retraction and contraction of the posterior pharyngeal wall contribute to the inferior propulsion of the material through the pharynx. **Any reconstruction that tethers or limits the movement of the tongue will be associated with a poorer functional outcome than those in which no tongue is used.** When tongue involvement is minimal, swallowing difficulties are usually temporary. Sensory innervation to these reconstructed structures remains controversial as to the efficacy in restoration of function.

Conclusion

Although a variety of options are available for soft-tissue oral reconstruction, the technique chosen depends on the extent and functional characteristics of the tissue involved, the health of the patient, expectations, and overall motivation.

Microvascular surgery and free tissue transfer have introduced a new dimension in intraoral reconstruction. This technique has a high success rate with low complications and little donor site morbidity. It allows an immediate reconstruction of large defects in one stage.

RECONSTRUCTION OF THE PHARYNX AND CERVICAL ESOPHAGUS

Reconstruction the pharynx and cervical esophagus is a challenging task and an integral part of the treatment of the laryngopharynx and cervical esophagus following trauma, cancer, benign strictures, and other conditions. Usually the resection of tumors requires removal of the larynx, pharynx, and part of the cervical esophagus, leaving the patient with a permanent tracheotomy and the inability to speak, breath, and swallow. The goals of these complex reconstructions are to restore the normal anatomy, allowing the patient to breath and swallow without a permanent tracheotomy, and with acceptable phonation. Frequently, however, the extent of resection requires a permanent stoma for breathing and mechanical devices or tracheoesophageal puncture for speech. As with the oral cavity, these reconstructions are associated with several disturbing issues including a poor 5-year survival rate of 25% to 35%, the need for multimodality therapy that often includes radiation, and the loss of vital social functions such as natural speech and oral feeding.

Functional Anatomy of the Hypopharynx

The hypopharynx is the longest of the three segments of the pharynx, extending from the tip of the epiglottis to the lower edge of the cricoid cartilage. It is widest superiorly and becomes progressively narrower toward the level of the cricopharyngeus muscle, where it merges with the cervical esophagus. It is composed of three distinct regions: (a) The pyriform sinuses, located laterally, are pear-shaped funnels bound superiorly by the oropharynx and glossoepiglottic fold, anterolaterally by the medial aspect of the thyroid lamina, posteriorly by the lateral pharyngeal wall, and medially by the lateral surface of the arytenoids and cricoid cartilage. They open posteriorly into the pharynx and their apex usually extends inferiorly to the level of the laryngeal ventricle. (b) The posterior pharyngeal wall, continues superiorly with the wall of the oropharynx and inferiorly with the esophagus. It extends from a plane drawn through the tip of the epiglottis to a plane drawn through the lower part of the cricoid cartilage, corresponding to the third through sixth cervical vertebrae. (c) The postcricoid area, which is the posterior surface to the arytenoids and cricoid cartilages.

The hypopharynx is a myofascial skeleton covered by mucosa made up of stratified squamous epithelium that contains lymphoid nodules and secretory glands. The pharyngobasilar fascia and the middle and inferior constrictor muscles are innervated by the laryngeal nerves (superior and recurrent) and the pharyngeal plexus (X, IX, and possibly XI). The lower fibers of the inferior constrictors run horizontally, forming the cricopharyngeus muscle. The buccopharyngeal fascia is a thin covering on the external surfaces of the muscles. The muscles of the hypopharynx telescope past each other, creating lateral deficiencies that give passage to the glossopharyngeal nerve, the glossopharyngeal muscle and styloid ligament, the lingual artery before it enters the tongue, the thyroid membrane, and the superior laryngeal vessels and nerves.

The hypopharynx is a dynamic conduit between the oropharynx and the esophagus that allow separation of the digestive and respiratory pathways preventing aspiration. The primary function of the pharynx is deglutition and swallowing of oral secretions.

Functional Anatomy of the Cervical Esophagus

The cervical esophagus is that area of the esophagus situated superior to the sternum. The superior margin is the lower edge to the cricoid cartilage, while the inferior limit is the suprasternal notch. The esophageal wall is composed of a mucosal layer with a stratified squamous epithelium and a deeper layer of muscle called the muscularis mucosa. The submucosa is composed of areolar tissue containing nerves and blood vessels. A muscular layer is organized in inner circular and outer longitudinal fibers.

Principles of Reconstruction

Although the pharynx and the larynx are attached and act in a coordinated fashion, they have different reconstructive requirements. The ideal reconstruction would restore normal anatomy, and enable normal deglutition without aspiration, development of speech, and breathing without a tracheotomy. Despite the advances in reconstructive surgery, this type of reconstruction cannot be achieved with present skills and technologies and reconstructive surgery for these patients should be considered primarily palliative, preserving the quality of life for the duration of survival (Table 43.1).

Frequent removal of the epiglottis occurs with cancer extirpation. These patients often require a permanent tracheotomy and voice prostheses, because there is currently no method for reconstructing the vocal cords. General considerations on the choice of the technique to reconstruct the pharyngoesophageal tract must include the overall general health of the patient and the size of the defect. The technique used for the reconstruction of circumferential defects should simulate the normal anatomy, thus preferring thin-walled tubes, able to relax and/or stretch

TABLE 43.1

GOALS OF PHARYNGOESOPHAGEAL RECONSTRUCTION

Features	Goals
Single-stage reconstruction	Wound closure
Low mortality	Best quality of life
Low morbidity	Swallowing
Short hospitalization	No tracheostomy
Short interval to successful oral alimentation	Speech
High rate of speech development	
Tolerate postoperative radiation of ~6,000 Gy	

TABLE 43.2

RECONSTRUCTIVE OPTIONS FOR PHARYNGOESOPHAGEAL RECONSTRUCTIONS

Technique	Options
Local tissue	Primary closure, laryngeal flaps
Skin grafts	
Cutaneous flaps	Cervical, deltopectoral
Myocutaneous flaps	Pectoralis major, latissimus dorsi
Visceral transposition	Gastric "pull-up," jejunal autograft (free flap)
Fasciocutaneous free flaps	Radial forearm, lateral thigh, scapular/parascapular
Myocutaneous free flaps	Rectus abdominis

to allow the passage of the food bolus. The lumen should be approximately 3 cm in diameter. For partial circumference defects, reconstruction should be directed primarily at "patching the hole" and preventing deterioration of the various functions. Table 43.2 lists these reconstructive options.

Available Methods

Early methods of cervical esophagus reconstruction included the cervical flaps and the use of local cervical tissues. Cervical flaps could be partially folded on themselves and sutured to the pharyngeal and esophageal ends to form a tube that was open laterally. The tubing of the flap was completed later and the neck defect was covered with a split-thickness skin graft. Another popular method of reconstruction of the pharyngoesophagus was the deltopectoral flap, which was described by Bakamjian in the 1960s. This method was replaced by a more, and still, reliable method, the pectoralis major myocutaneous flap (PMMCF). Other types of reconstruction included the stomach "pull-up" to the pharynx and the transverse colon transposition.

Microvascular surgery has greatly expanded the options available for pharyngoesophageal reconstruction. The most popular and versatile free flaps used in this area include the jejunal flap and the tubed radial forearm flap.

Jejunal Free Flap

The jejunal free flap is a standard technique in the reconstruction of complex defects of the head and neck. The jejunal flap is tolerant to external beam irradiation, and provides a conduit for swallowing. Harvesting of the flap can be achieved through conventional open laparotomy or laparoscopic techniques, with decreased morbidity.

Technique of Dissection

Conventional Flap Harvesting. The flap is preferably harvested at the time of the tumor resection in order to decrease the total operative time. The patient is positioned supine and an upper abdominal incision is performed. Transillumination of the mesentery allows the visualization of the nutrient vessels from the mesenteric border back to the superior mesenteric artery and vein. The vascular arcade of the proximal jejunum has the most favorable anatomy with larger branches off the superior mesenteric artery giving rise to primary and sometimes secondary arcades. After selecting the vascular arcade, approxi-

mately 40 to 70 cm from the ligament of Treitz, the length of the jejunum required is established by measuring the neck defect. An additional 1 to 2 cm is taken for a monitored segment. The flap should be planned so that the vascular pedicle is located at the level of the recipient vessels in the neck. It is preferable to begin flap dissection on both sides of the mesentery at the base of the vascular pedicle. Dissection continues toward the proximal and distal ends of the flap, the latter being marked with a silk suture in order to maintain an isoperistaltic orientation of the flap at the time of insetting. After the removal of the tumor the recipient vessels are isolated and prepared for the anastomoses; the flap is transferred, inset, and revascularized. Continuity of the jejunal segments is re-established at the donor site. Jejunostomy and/or gastrostomy tubes are placed as necessary, based on the assumption of prolonged feedings.

Laparoscopic Flap Harvesting. In addition to the standard equipment required for laparoscopy (video monitor, camera, light source, and CO_2 insufflators), a second camera, light source, and video monitor are needed. The second camera, connected only to the light source, is used to provide a source of transillumination. The first percutaneous port is placed, using the open technique, in the right upper quadrant 2 cm below the costal margin centered over the lateral edge of the rectus sheath. The incision is carried down to the peritoneal cavity, under direct vision. Prolene sutures are placed on opposite sides of the deep fascia and a Hassan cannula is secured using these sutures. The abdominal cavity is inflated to 12 cm and a camera is introduced by way of the Hassan cannula to inspect the abdomen. The rest of the cannulas are then placed under visual inspection. The ligament of Treitz is located by tracing the small bowel. At this time, the second light source is introduced into the abdomen through the port in the left upper quadrant and used to transilluminate the small bowel mesentery and trace the vascular anatomy. Using the transillumination a portion of the jejunum with its corresponding feeding vessel is selected (approximately 40 cm from the ligament of Treitz). To visualize and dissect its mesentery, the jejunum is suspended from the abdominal wall with 2-0 nylon sutures wedged onto Keith needles and elevated. The dissection of the vascular arcade is performed by electrocautery and the transverse vessels of the distal arcade are controlled with hemoclips, and divided.

After the complete isolation of the vascular pedicle, the intestinal loop is reduced outside the abdominal cavity. Once externalized, the visceral portion is divided using a conventional gastrointestinal stapling device. The complete jejunal segment is passed to the neck for inset and revascularization. Revascularization is performed via techniques previously described. A portion of the flap is externalized through the skin incision to monitor tissue perfusion during the postoperative period.

Flap insetting is accomplished respecting the isoperistaltic orientation of the flap. The proximal enteric anastomosis is performed before the flap revascularization. This technique allows bowel approximation to be performed without disruption of the microvascular anastomoses and without the peristalsis, mucous production, and bleeding that can occur after revascularization. Usually two layers of interrupted polyglactin sutures are used for the mucosal and serosal closures; however, one-layer closures also can be used. Silk sutures are often used to incorporate the prevertebral fascia and a portion of the tongue musculature. Because the lumen of the pharyngeal defect is usually larger than that of the jejunum, the proximal end of the jejunum should be enlarged. This assists with the decreased incidence in stricture formation. During the insetting care must be taken to adapt the length of the flap to the anatomic defect. The head should be flexed in the neutral position and flap redundancy is to be avoided by gentle traction of the flap in the caudal direction. To avoid strictures, the distal bowel anastomosis is performed by incising the anterior side of the

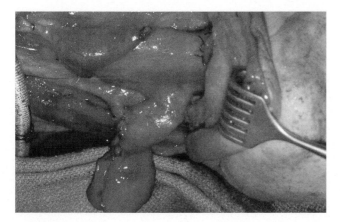

FIGURE 43.2. Jejunal flap. The distal anastomosis and the extra 1 to 2 cm of jejunum that is used as a monitored segment are demonstrated.

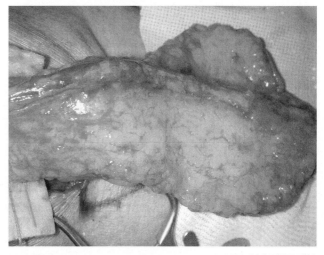

FIGURE 43.3. The tubed radial forearm flap. This flap can replace the pharynx and cervical esophagus for resection of cancer of the larynx. This photograph demonstrates the radial forearm flap tubed on the arm prior to ligation of the vessels and transfer to the neck.

esophagus for 1 to 2 cm caudally, and insetting the distal jejunal segment in the created defect (Fig. 43.2).

A monitor flap is created with a 2-cm segment of bowel. This segment is sutured to the skin of the neck, away from the tracheotomy. This monitored segment is split open to expose the mucosa.

Tubed Radial Forearm Flap

The tubed radial forearm flap is particularly suitable for the reconstruction of circumferential defects of the pharyngoesophagus. Its low morbidity, high reliability, and potential for maintenance of swallowing and prosthetic voice restoration make it one of the best of the reconstructive options.

Although the technique of dissection of the radial forearm flap was previously described, there are few technical aspects on the use of the forearm flap for pharyngoesophageal reconstruction that deserve discussion.

The skin island for circumferential reconstructions should guarantee a final lumen diameter of approximately 3 cm. If possible, the proximal end of the flap should be slightly larger to match the pharyngeal lumen. After the flap is raised the tourniquet is released and the flap is allowed to perfuse. If a circumferential defect is to be reconstructed, the ulnar and radial edges of the skin paddle are sutured together (Fig. 43.3). At the time of flap transfer, it is preferable to proceed to flap inset prior to the revascularization. Both upper and lower pharyngoesophageal anastomoses are completed using one or two layers with 3-0 or 4-0 absorbable closure. To prevent postoperative strictures, the pharyngoesophageal wall may be cut longer on one of the two sides, providing an oblique suture line.

Outcomes

The three major contemporary approaches used to restore oral communication following laryngectomy are the artificial larynx, esophageal speech production, and surgical prosthetic alternatives such as tracheoesophageal voice restoration. Although the final choice for laryngeal speech production should always be the patient's, experience demonstrates that the artificial larynx and surgical prosthetic choice restoration are truly viable alternatives. Several authors suggest that the functional problem with the jejunal autograft has been the failure to develop adequate neoesophageal speech. Although the artificial larynx has the advantage of providing immediate verbal communication with relative ease and little, if any, medical compli-

cations, many patients find it unacceptable because of its mechanical sound quality. Tracheojejunal or tracheoesophageal forearm puncture are popular alternatives. It appears that the quality of the voice restoration is improved by using a component of skin (such as the radial forearm flap) instead of jejunum. It is probably better to wait until healing has occurred and consider tracheoesophageal puncture as a secondary procedure.

Although there are numerous reports regarding reconstructive methods for the oral cavity, pharynx, and larynx, there are few reports that objectively assess and compare the functional results of each. Most are subjective with little objective data, making comparisons difficult. Imaging and nonimaging instrumentation procedures such as videofluoroscopic examination or modified barium swallow can be used to evaluate swallow physiology. Fiberoptic endoscopic examination is increasingly popular. Furthermore, a variety of quality-of-life assessments are available, including the Washington Quality of Life Scale, the functional assessment of cancer therapy–head and neck (FACT-HN) scale, and the Performance Status Scale for Head and Neck Cancer. It is critical that there be constant re-evaluation of our techniques for restoration of the oral cavity and pharynx in order to assess the best method for restoration of form and function.

Conclusion

Patients undergoing ablative surgery for cancer of the cervical esophagus, larynx, and pharynx often require extensive and complicated reconstruction of the anatomy and function.

Because the 5-year survival rate is low (25% to 35%), in patients with locally advanced carcinoma of the cervical aerodigestive tract, reconstructive techniques should allow restoration of speech and swallowing in an expeditious manner. The radial forearm free flap offers the advantages of reliability, minimal morbidity, and maximization of functional rehabilitation. The jejunal free flap offers other advantages such as the abundance of tissue and the flexibility of reconstruction of any size defect with a tension-free bowel anastomosis. The facilitation of esophageal speech by tracheoesophageal puncture appears better in patients whose reconstructions used the radial forearm flap. Up to 50% of patients with jejunal flaps may not achieve a good esophageal speech with the Blom-Singer voice prosthesis.

Suggested Readings

Anthony JP, Singer MJ, Mathes SJ. Pharyngoesophageal reconstruction using the tubed free radial forearm flap. *Clin Plast Surg.* 1994;21:137.

Bakamjian VY. A two-stage method of pharyngoesophageal reconstruction with a primary skin flap. *Plast Reconst Surg.* 1965;36:173.

Blair EA, Callender DL. Head and neck cancer. *Clin Plast Surg.* 1994;21:1.

Butler CE, Lewin JS. Reconstruction of large composite oromandibulomaxillary defects with free vertical rectus abdominis myocutaneous flaps. *Plast Reconstr Surg.* 2004;113:499.

Coleman JJ III. Free jejunal autograft for reconstruction of the pharynx and cervical esophagus. In: Kroll SS, ed. *Reconstructive Plastic Surgery for Cancer.* St. Louis: Mosby; 1996: 139–153.

Evans GRD. The radial forearm free flap. In: Kroll SS, ed. *Reconstructive Plastic Surgery for Cancer.* St. Louis: Mosby; 1996: 242–248.

Evans GRD, Gherardini G, Gürlek A, et al. Drug-induced vasodilation: the effects of nicardipine, papaverine and lidocaine on the rabbit carotid artery. In vitro and in vivo study. *Plast Reconst Surg.* 1997;100:1475.

Gallas M, Lewin JS, Evans GRD. Functional outcome considerations in upper aerodigestive tract reconstruction. In: Achauer BM, ed. *Plastic Surgery: Indications, Operations and Outcomes.* St. Louis: Mosby; 2000: 1115–1128.

Gherardini G, Gürlek A, Stanley CA, et al. Laparoscopic harvesting of jejunal free flap for esophageal reconstruction. *Plast Reconst Surg.* 1998;102:540.

Miller MJ, Janjan NA. Treatment of injuries from radiation therapy. In: Kroll SS, ed. *Reconstructive Plastic Surgery for Cancer.* St. Louis: Mosby; 1996: 17–36.

Miller MJ, Robb GL. Endoscopic technique for free flap harvesting.

Reece GP. Pharyngoesophageal reconstructions. In: Schusterman MA, ed. *Microsurgical Reconstruction of the Cancer Patient.* Philadelphia: Lippincott-Raven; 1997: 67–84.

Reece GP, Bengtson BP, Schusterman MA. Reconstruction of the pharynx and cervical esophagus using free jejunal transfer. *Clin Plast Surg.* 1994;21:125.

CHAPTER 44 ■ CUTANEOUS RESURFACING: CHEMICAL PEELING, DERMABRASION, AND LASER RESURFACING

JOHN A. PERROTTI

Lay practitioners initially performed chemical peeling in the late 1940s and dermabrasion was developed in the 1950s. Reports of these techniques appeared in both the plastic surgery and dermatology literature.

The three methods available for resurfacing are chemical, mechanical, and laser. Resurfacing is further characterized as superficial, medium, or deep, based on the depth of injury produced. Surface irregularities of the skin, including actinic damage, pigmentation disorders, and aging changes such as wrinkling, can be ameliorated. All three techniques produce a controlled injury and this injury must be to the appropriate depth in order to treat the targeted pathology and achieve the desired result. **The different resurfacing techniques produce similar injury and thereby similar aesthetic results.**

SKIN LAYERS

The anatomy of the skin is covered in Chapter 13. Figure 44.1 illustrates the skin's histology. **The efficiency of healing and re-epithelialization is related to the concentration of adnexal structures, which decreases as depth of injury increases.** An increased risk of scarring is associated with injury to the deep reticular dermis with resurfacing techniques. Full-thickness injury to the skin cannot heal by re-epithelialization and permanent scarring is inevitable.

AGING

Aging of the skin affects both the epidermis and dermis and is exacerbated by actinic damage. Aging produces atrophy of skin components. The superimposition of actinic damage results in dermal disorganization and elastosis, the presence of thickened, degraded, elastic fibers. Separating the solar elastotic material from the epidermis is a thin zone of normal-appearing dermis largely composed of collagen, called the *grenz zone* (1). Aging also causes loss of dermoepidermal papillae. These histologic changes are responsible for the clinical signs of aging and sun damage, including wrinkling, laxity, and pigment changes. Cutaneous resurfacing is intended to reverse these changes.

Superficial peeling agents such as Jessner solution, Unna paste, salicylic acid, and the alpha-hydroxy acids penetrate to the epidermal–dermal junction. Medium-depth peels penetrate deep to the epidermal–dermal junction and include trichloroacetic acid (35%). Phenol-croton oil peels, dermabrasion, and laser resurfacing may penetrate into the upper to mid reticular dermis. In general, both the aesthetic benefit and the complication rate are directly related to the depth of injury, mandating that the surgeon decide what degree of risk is reasonable in a given patient.

PATIENT SELECTION

The most important factor in patient selection is skin type. Patient lifestyle and acceptable downtime must be considered. Fitzpatrick identifies six skin types based on reaction to sun exposure (Table 44.1). The lower the Fitzpatrick type, the less melanin in the skin. In general, patients with darker skin types have a greater tendency to develop posttreatment hyperpigmentation, whereas patients with light skin are more prone toward posttreatment hypopigmentation. Patients, particularly darker skin patients, benefit from pretreatment with tretinoin and hydroquinone and may require postpeel treatment with bleaching agents because of hyperpigmentation.

CHEMICAL PEELING

Early reports discussed the benefits of trichloroacetic acid in dermatologic disorders. Baker, Gordon, and Litton developed a formula to achieve a deeper and more uniform penetration of phenol that is still popular today (2). Hetter showed that it is actually the croton oil, and not the phenol, that is the critical ingredient in the Baker peel (3).

Retinoids

The retinoids are a group of compounds consisting of vitamin A (retinol), its derivatives, and *trans*-retinoic acid (tretinoin or Retin-A), which are effective in the treatment of actinically damaged skin. Topical application of tretinoin reverses actinic skin damage. The benefits of increased collagen synthesis, fine-wrinkle reduction, and improvement of skin texture have been shown to last after tretinoin use was discontinued. Treatment begins with 0.025% or 0.05% tretinoin cream applied every other night, which can be increased to every night, for 9 to 12 months, followed by a maintenance schedule of twice-weekly applications. The use of full-strength tretinoin (0.1%) is not necessary to achieve maximal results and can be significantly more irritating. The most common side effect of topical tretinoin therapy is characterized by erythema, peeling, and a sensation similar to sunburn ("retinoid dermatitis"). **Tretinoin is the only therapeutic agent proven to repair photodamage. It is also useful as pretreatment for facial resurfacing techniques.**

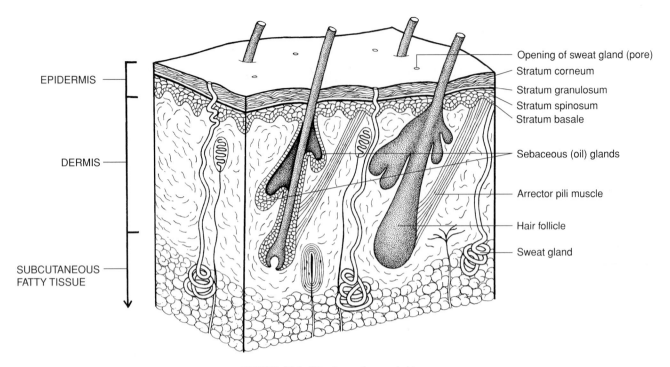

FIGURE 44.1. Histology of normal skin.

Superficial Peels

Superficial peeling agents are used to treat pathology that is localized to the epidermis, such as keratosis and dyschromias. Superficial peeling agents include Jessner solution (resorcinol, salicylic acid, and lactic acid), Unna paste (resorcinol and zinc oxide), salicylic acid (50%), and the α-hydroxy acids. These penetrate to the epidermal–dermal junction. Superficial peels are performed without anesthesia or sedation and complications are unlikely because depth of penetration is limited.

α-Hydroxy acids (AHAs) are naturally occurring organic acids derived from sugar cane (glycolic acid), sour milk (lactic acid), and other substances. AHA peels and/or daily application of AHA products does improve skin texture and reduce fine wrinkling and pigmentation. Glycolic acid is the most commonly used AHA. Skin care formulations contain AHA concentrations of 8% to 14%; peels use concentrations of 30%

to 70%. At low concentrations over extended periods of time, AHAs can aid in normalizing the stratum corneum. Peels can penetrate the dermal junction, noted by appearance of erythema and whitening (epidermolysis). The amount of time that an acid should be left on the skin depends on its concentration. Glycolic acid will continue to penetrate until it is neutralized with water or an alkaline compound, such as sodium bicarbonate. Because a glycolic peel is superficial, the recovery is quick and usually uncomplicated. Multiple glycolic peels separated by at least several weeks are usually required to achieve the desired cosmetic result.

Jessner solution consists of resorcinol (14 g), salicylic acid (14 g), lactic acid (14 mL), and ethanol (100 mL). The depth of peeling is controlled by how many coats of solution are applied. Jessner solution is used as a superficial keratolytic agent to prepare the skin immediately before peeling with trichloroacetic acid (TCA).

Salicylic acid (SA) is a β-hydroxy acid used in 30% concentration for single or multiple peels of moderately photodamaged skin. The SA peel solution causes significantly more desquamation than a 70% glycolic acid peel, but with minimal downtime. An interval of at least 4 weeks is recommended between peels to allow for epidermal regeneration. SA peels volatize in less than 3.5 minutes, after which there is little penetration of the active agent.

Bleaching agents inhibit tyrosinase, the enzyme that converts tyrosine to melanin. Hydroquinone effectively bleaches the skin when applied topically and is available by prescription in 2% and 4% concentrations. Kojic acid, another tyrosinase inhibitor, also has skin-bleaching properties.

Trichloroacetic Acid

TCA is a derivative of acetic acid that has been used in the treatment of aging skin since the early 1960s. It was one of the first agents developed for chemical peeling and still one of the most versatile. TCA ranges in concentration from 10% to 50%. Trichloroacetic acid is most commonly used in 35%

TABLE 44.1

FITZPATRICK SKIN CLASSIFICATION

Type	Color	Reaction to sun exposure
I	White	Always burns/never tans
II	White	Usually burns/tans with difficulty
III	White	Sometimes mild burn/average tan
IV	Moderate Brown	Rarely burns/tans with ease
V	Dark Brown	Very rarely burns/tans very easily
VI	Black	Never burns/tans very easily

Based on data from Fitzpatrick TB. The validity and practicality of sun-reactive skin types I through VI. *Arch Dermatol.* 1988;124:869.

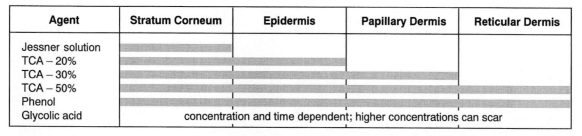

Agent	Stratum Corneum	Epidermis	Papillary Dermis	Reticular Dermis
Jessner solution				
TCA – 20%				
TCA – 30%				
TCA – 50%				
Phenol				
Glycolic acid	concentration and time dependent; higher concentrations can scar			

FIGURE 44.2. Depth of destruction of various peeling agents.

concentration for medium-depth peeling. TCA penetrates the papillary and into the upper reticular dermis and is not absorbed systemically. Depth of penetration is proportional to the concentration. Concentrations of 30% to 40% penetrate the papillary dermis and are considered medium depth. In lower concentrations, TCA affects only the outer layer of the epidermis, and is considered superficial. Once the TCA concentration rises above 40%, it is considered a deep peel. In higher concentrations, TCA can penetrate the reticular dermis, providing deeper treatment but also increasing morbidity and the risk of scarring (Fig. 44.2). TCA is versatile and can be used in a wide range of skin types. TCA is useful for treatment of pigmentation disorders, dysplasias, photoaged skin, and wrinkles. TCA produces limited neocollagen formation and some improvement in facial wrinkling, but is limited in treating deep facial wrinkles, especially in the perioral area. The long-term effects of TCA peels may be more unpredictable than phenol peeling or laser resurfacing. Concentration, pretreatment, skin degreasing, and the number of coats of acid applied affect penetration.

Pretreatment for TCA peels improves the penetration of the acid and provides more consistent results. Pretreatment with tretinoin or AHA should proceed for at least 6 weeks prior to resurfacing. Tretinoin thins the stratum corneum and suppresses melanocyte activity. Hydroquinone should be added as pretreatment for darker skin patients in order to decrease melanin formation and hyperpigmentation. Pretreatment serves to dekeratinize the skin surface, which allows deeper and more even penetration of the peeling agent.

Prior to TCA peeling, the skin is degreased with acetone and/or alcohol to remove surface oils from the skin, which will retard absorption and result in an uneven peel. Sedation is usually unnecessary with 35% TCA. The solution is applied regionally to each facial unit with brushlike strokes. Adequate penetration of the solution usually occurs between 1 and 2 minutes. Trichloroacetic acid is a keratocoagulant and frosting is the key to judging the depth of the peel. Initial frosting is pink or white in color and progresses to more uniform white as penetration proceeds to the papillary dermis. A gray appearance can signal penetration to the reticular dermis and may cause abnormal healing. Once the desired degree of frosting occurs, the acid is washed with water. The water serves to dissipate some of the generated heat, but because trichloroacetic acid is an aqueous solution, it cannot be neutralized, only diluted. If after inspection the frost is not as deep as anticipated, it is appropriate to retouch those areas. During the entire peeling process, a fan can be used to aid in patient comfort.

The concentration of TCA correlates with the depth of destruction but variables such as prepeel preparation, skin type, concentration of sebaceous glands, relative skin thickness, amount of acid applied, and the rigor of application, all must be considered when performing the peel. Using a higher concentration, applying more coats, skin pretreatment, and mechanical abrasion during treatment can increase TCA penetration. Increasing the concentration of TCA increases the depth of destruction correspondingly. Also, chemical peeling is

a technique-dependent procedure. **A 30% TCA solution that is rubbed vigorously into the skin can create a wound comparable to a 45% or 50% solution applied less vigorously.** Patients with thick skin will tolerate higher concentrations of TCA or multiple reapplications of acid. Care must be taken in patients with dry and atrophic skin, as penetration is increased.

Following TCA peel, the skin will feel tight and will darken (Fig. 44.3). After 24 hours, the patient should cleanse the treated areas several times a day with water and/or dilute hydrogen peroxide and apply ointment such as A and D or Aquaphor to hasten re-epithelialization. After several days a moisturizer may be substituted for the ointment. Medium-depth peels produce erythema and desquamation that lasts for 5 to 7 days. Once desquamation is complete, makeup can be applied. After 7 to 10 days, a skin care regimen can be resumed, including use of a broad-spectrum sunscreen against both ultraviolet (UV) A and UVB. Erythema can persist for several months. Histologically, there is collagen remodeling with fibers deposited in more compact parallel arrays.

The most common problem after TCA peel is hyperpigmentation, especially in darker-skinned individuals. Hyperpigmentation can be increased by premature sun exposure. Hypertrophic scarring can occur if the peel reaches the reticular dermis and is often seen in the perioral and mandibular areas. Also, previous use of isotretinoin (Accutane) may lead to hypertrophic scarring. Hypertrophic scarring can be treated with silicone pressure dressings and corticosteroid injections. In severe cases, surgical revision may be necessary. In patients with a history of herpes infection, peeling may cause a herpes outbreak in the chemically damaged skin. These patients should be treated prophylactically with antiviral agents such as acyclovir or valacyclovir. Because many patients are unaware that "cold sores" are herpes infections, surgeons should have a low threshold for prescribing these medications.

TCA has many applications but the learning curve can be prolonged because of the numerous factors that affect penetration. TCA is less toxic than phenol and its effects are milder. The peel can be repeated periodically to maintain youthful-looking skin.

Phenol

Phenol, also known as carbolic acid, is a protein precipitant that causes extremely rapid denaturation and coagulation of surface keratin. Croton oil is added in minute amounts as a skin irritant. A soap (glycerin or Septisol) acts as a surfactant to lower surface tension and as an emulsifier to aid in the penetration. Addition of tap water prepares a solution of 50% phenol concentration. Chemical peeling with phenol-croton oil is used to improve significant actinic damage and moderate wrinkling of the skin. It provides a relatively deep and predictable injury to the dermis, penetrating to the level of the upper reticular dermis. It has become a standard to which other resurfacing methods are compared. It treats both coarse and fine wrinkles

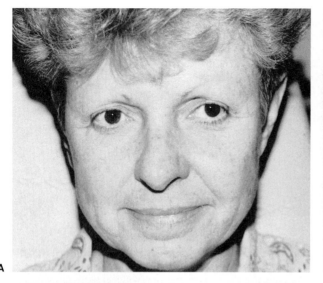

A

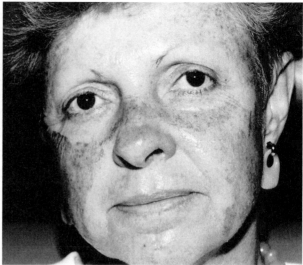

B

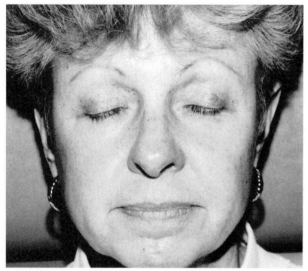

C

FIGURE 44.3. Example of a 35% trichloroacetic acid (TCA) peel. **A:** Pre-TCA peel. **B:** Skin peeling 5 days after TCA peel. **C:** Two months following TCA peel.

and irregular pigmentation. Because of the depth of treatment, phenol peeling has a longer recovery period and increased morbidity.

Phenol is detoxified in the liver and excreted by the kidney. Toxic doses of phenol can injure both the liver and the kidney and may depress respiration and the myocardium. Atrial and other arrhythmias can be seen after rapid phenol absorption. To avoid these complications, cardiac monitoring is recommended if the entire face is peeled.

The Baker-Gordon formula was the standard phenol formula (2). It consists of 3 mL USP liquid phenol, 2 mL tap

TABLE 44.2

BAKER-GORDON FORMULA

3 mL USP liquid phenol
2 mL Tap water
8 Drops liquid soap
3 Drops croton oil

Based on data from Baker TJ, Stuzin JM, Baker TM. *Facial Skin Resurfacing.* St. Louis: Quality Medical Publishing; 1998.

water, 8 drops liquid soap, and 3 drops croton oil (Table 44.2). Soap lowers the surface tension of the mixture and croton oil is thought to act as a vesicant, increasing local inflammation and penetration of phenol. Histologic studies show that the Baker-Gordon formula penetrates deeper than pure phenol (4). The skin is cleansed in a fashion similar to that discussed for TCA peels. The solution is applied with a contact tip applicator, with care being taken to avoid dripping. Missed spots must be avoided. After phenol application, the skin frosts a grayish white color and a burning sensation is experienced. Areas are peeled at 15- to 20-minute intervals with a full-face peel being completed in about 1 to 2 hours. An occlusive dressing applied to the treated area prevents evaporation and increases phenol penetration and depth of the peel. Either tape or a petroleum-based ointment dressing can provide occlusion, although the former may be more painful and morbid for the patient. A further advantage of treatment with ointment allows visualization of the wound. If used, tape is removed within 48 hours and gentle washing is permitted. The skin is kept moist with ointments to speed re-epithelialization, which is usually complete within 10 to 14 days. **Erythema, however, persists for several months.** Sunscreen must be used and bleaching agents are helpful to treat increased pigmentation. Histologically, there is neocollagen formation. A study by Kligman et al. (5) recorded tissue changes in 11 women who underwent phenol peel and subsequently had rhytidectomy. The authors noted that "a new band of connective tissue 2 to 3 mm in width was laid down in the subepidermal region. Fine elastic fibers formed a dense network in the band of regenerated collagen."

Complications of phenol peeling include skin depigmentation caused by a reduction in melanin-producing cells, which is almost unavoidable. Many experienced peelers believe that these peels result in more hypopigmentation for a given depth of injury than other agents and techniques. Postpeel hyperpigmentation is also seen, especially in darker-skinned patients. Prolonged erythema may need treatment with topical corticosteroids and patients will experience sensitivity to sunlight so sunscreen must be used regularly. Patients should receive prophylaxis with antiviral agents to prevent herpes virus infections.

Recently, much has been written regarding the safety of the Baker-Gordon formula. As mentioned above, croton oil appears to be the critical peeling agent, rather than the phenol, as traditionally thought. Hetter varied the concentration of croton oil and demonstrated that it was the concentration of croton oil and not the concentration of phenol that was the factor that controlled depth of penetration (3). He asserted that phenol is simply the carrier. Minute variations in the concentration of croton oil are critical to the outcome of the peel. The different proportions according to depth of peel desired and anatomic site are summarized in what Hetter calls "the heresy phenol formulas." As a result of this work, phenol peels are probably more properly referred to as "phenol-croton oil" peels.

Complications of Chemical Peeling

The goals of chemical peeling are the controlled creation of a partial-thickness wound and to minimize complications. Pigmentary problems are the most common complications. Hypopigmentation is seen with peels that destroy tissue through the entire epidermis. Pigment-producing melanocytes are located at the dermal–epidermal junction, and if destroyed, it is possible for permanent hypopigmentation to occur.

Hyperpigmentation is inflammatory in nature and results from melanocyte overstimulation secondary to trauma. Although hyperpigmentation can be treated and even reversed, patients at risk should be treated aggressively, both before and after chemical peeling, with agents such as retinoic acid, glycolic acid, hydroquinone, and/or kojic acid. Sun avoidance is mandatory in these patients.

Wound infections can occur, most of which are caused by *Staphylococcus* and *Streptococcus*, but can include yeast (*Candida*), *Pseudomonas*, or herpes viruses. The most serious complication of chemical peeling is scarring. In general, the deeper the peel, the higher the risk of scarring. Scars are usually preceded by persistent erythema, and areas of redness should be treated with topical corticosteroids, which can often reverse the process and prevent a scar from forming. If this is not effective, intralesional corticosteroids can be used.

Overall, chemical peeling is a time-tested, safe, and efficacious modality for the treatment of facial aging.

DERMABRASION

Dermabrasion, which was developed in the 1950s, mechanically abrades the epidermis and upper portion of the dermis. It is technique dependent and the depth can be precisely controlled. The epidermis is entirely obliterated and there is partial removal of the dermis, which undergoes incomplete regeneration. Both coarse and fine wrinkling can be treated with dermabrasion. Although dermabrasion has become less popular as the use of laser resurfacing has increased, it is still an effective, convenient treatment with broad application. It is inexpensive and portable, and produces less erythema than other techniques. Wrinkles can be lowered and smoothed mechanically. For resurfacing, dermabrasion is most useful for perioral lines, particularly those of the upper lip. Baker (6) classified perioral rhytides according to depth and number. Type I are superficial, are of limited number, originate from the vermillion border, and cover no more than half of the upper lip. Type II are of moderate depth and extend up to two-thirds of the upper lip. Lower-lip involvement is common. Type III rhytides are coarse and deep and involve the full upper lip with similar involvement of the lower lip.

Dermabrasion patients may receive premedication and/or regional nerve blocks. The hand-held dermabrader is motor driven and operates at 12,000 to 15,000 rpm. There are a wide variety of diamond-tipped burrs, differing in shape, size, and coarseness. Protection against aerosolized particular matter must be taken. Wrinkles are marked before infiltration of anesthesia and regions are treated according to anatomic subunits. The handpiece should be kept moving, with light pressure applied. The edges of treated areas are feathered to blend with those not treated. Providing treatment to the proper depth is important. After the epidermis is removed, the pink epidermal–dermal junction is encountered. As treatment continues, fine punctate bleeding indicates the level of the papillary dermis. At the papillary–reticular junction, bleeding is increased and the surface becomes rougher, indicating the end point of treatment for most patients. Following treatment, the entire face is covered with gauze soaked in lidocaine with epinephrine to provide both anesthesia and hemostasis. Once bleeding has stopped, ointment is applied and the treated area either covered with petroleum or Xeroform gauze or is left uncovered. The patient may clean the areas and apply more ointment as needed. Re-epithelialization is usually completed within 7 to 10 days. All patients are treated prophylactically with antiviral agents to minimize the risk of disseminated herpes simplex. Avoidance of sun exposure and use of sunscreens is important. Dermabrasion presents complications similar to those presented by chemical peeling, including hyperpigmentation, hypertrophic scarring, and milia, although pigmentation changes are less of a problem. Undertreatment may lead to inadequate results whereas overtreatment may lead to hypopigmentation and scarring.

There appears to be neocollagen formation following dermabrasion. Baker and Gordon (7) had found no histologic changes following dermabrasion, but merely a removal of a portion of the dermis that did not regenerate. This was in direct contrast to the deep dermal homogenization of collagen stimulated by a chemical peel. Stegman (4) noted that similar dermal scarring occurs with both dermabrasion and phenol face peeling, a finding that seems logical.

LASER RESURFACING

Chapter 20 has an introduction to laser. The effect of the laser on skin is heat generation that causes photocoagulation of tissue. Laser treatment produces histologic effects similar to those produced by phenol peeling. Laser resurfacing is dose dependent and based on pulse energy and number of passes; treatment can be as deep as the upper reticular dermis. Laser treatment produces visible dermal contraction. Laser treatment may prove more precise than other resurfacing modalities. Reports indicate that laser resurfacing has less effect on melanocytes and pigmentation than do other resurfacing modalities. Lasers are versatile but are significantly more expensive to use than other resurfacing tools. The two lasers that are commonly used for cosmetic resurfacing are the CO_2 and erbium:YAG (yttrium-aluminum-garnet) lasers. Chapter 20 discusses other laser applications and laser safety.

TABLE 44.3

LASER TERMINOLOGY

Laser term	Definition	Units
Pulse width	Duration of action (time tissues are exposed to the laser)	msec
Energy	Power times application time	J
Power	Energy delivered divided by the time	W (J/s)
Power density	Rate of energy delivered per unit area	W/cm^2
Fluence	Total laser energy per unit area	J/cm^2
Pulse energy	Energy of 1 pulse	mJ
Thermal relaxation time	Time required for lased tissue to lose 50% of its heat	msec
Wavelength	Specific to the active medium of the laser	nm

Laser Terminology

Laser treatment is controlled by four variables: power, wavelength, spot size, and duration of action. The duration of action (pulse width) refers to the total amount of time the tissues are exposed to the laser light. Energy is measured in joules (J), which equals power times the application time. Power, in turn, is the energy delivered divided by the time, measured in watts (1 watt [W] = 1 J/s). The power density is defined as the rate of energy delivered per unit area (W/cm^2). Fluence equals total laser energy per unit area (J/cm^2). Pulse energy is the energy of one pulse, measured in millijoules (mJ). The thermal relaxation time is the time required for treated tissue to lose 50% of its heat. The wavelength, measured in nanometers (nm), is specific to the active medium of the laser. Different wavelengths are selectively absorbed by target tissue chromophores. Table 44.3 summarizes laser terminology. The spot size of a laser affects depth of tissue penetration because larger spot sizes have less scatter and penetrate deeper.

Lasers used in skin resurfacing are either ablative or nonablative. Ablation refers to destruction of the epidermis and upper papillary dermis. As healing occurs, collagen is reorganized and remodeled. Ideally, laser treatment targets a specific tissue while minimizing damage to nontarget tissue (collateral damage). This is accomplished by using the highest appropriate wattage over the shortest possible time. During laser resurfacing, energy is absorbed, the tissue is heated, and vaporization and coagulation occurs. Absorption is a function of the tissue's affinity for laser light. The light is preferentially absorbed by a tissue target chromophore, which is water for skin resurfacing. The tissues contain approximately 70% water, which absorbs the majority of the energy. The ideal effect of laser treatment results from vaporization of tissue, not from conductive thermal injury. The goal is minimal conduction of heat to adjacent tissues and minimal collateral damage. Lasers emit energy in short pulses of high energy, which permits intervals of thermal relaxation. To determine laser dosage, thickness of rhytides, skin quality, and the particular area of the face to be treated must be considered.

CO_2 Laser

The CO_2 laser was the first laser used for ablative skin resurfacing and became increasingly popular as pulse widths were shortened, minimizing residual thermal injury. Early CO_2 lasers were continuous-wave lasers, but newer short-pulsed and scanned systems with decreased collateral thermal damage have been developed. The active laser medium consists of carbon dioxide, nitrogen, and helium gases. Because the CO_2 light is invisible, a helium ion light is coaxially transmitted to serve as the aiming beam. Water is the primary chromophore. The amount of thermal energy determines whether cutting, vaporization/ablation, or coagulation occurs. Altering the power, density, and duration of exposure controls the depth of penetration. Enlarging the spot size defocuses the laser beam and energy is spread over a larger area, causing tissue ablation or coagulation. Following energy absorption, a zone of tissue vaporization forms, surrounded by a zone of thermal injury. An inflammatory reaction is initiated, which mediates wound healing. A controlled region of thermal injury is desirable, as this is what contributes to collagen remodeling (8).

Multiple passes are required for resurfacing and the histologic effects during a pass of an ultrashort-pulsed or scanned CO_2 laser are fairly consistent. The initial pass ablates or vaporizes the epidermis and creates epidermis–dermis separation. The second pass ablates the papillary dermis and penetrates to the upper reticular dermis. The third pass extends deeper into the papillary dermis and there is little further penetration with the fourth pass. CO_2 lasers have a high ablation threshold, which results in thermal heating and ablation. This is true for the first pass, but with each subsequent pass there is less ablation and more thermal injury. Additional passes or increased energy of CO_2 lasers lead primarily to thermal coagulation, with minimal additional ablation. Each pass of CO_2 leaves behind coagulated necrotic tissue that must be removed (9).

CO_2 lasers cause skin contraction that is clearly observable (10). Although the exact mechanism of skin shrinkage is unclear, on histologic examination shortened collagen fibers are seen deep in the zone of thermal damage after laser application. These collagen fibers are thought to be responsible for the apparent skin tightening seen clinically. Other studies suggest that skin contraction is a function of collagen remodeling rather than contraction.

The goal of treatment with CO_2 is to ablate (or vaporize) superficial tissues and to coagulate deeper tissues while averting scarring. CO_2 laser ablative and coagulative effects lead to total epidermal regeneration and dermal remodeling. Overall, wound healing is mediated by controlled inflammation, thickening the *grenz zone* over a thinned layer of solar elastosis. This period of inflammation tends to last longer than the typical acute phase of wound healing, and manifests clinically as prolonged erythema. The length of postoperative erythema is directly related to the depth of treatment. The CO_2 laser has been the mainstay of ablative tissue resurfacing (11), although new lasers have been developed that use both CO_2 and erbium:YAG (9).

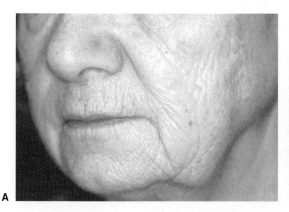
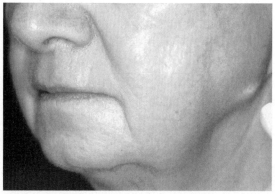

FIGURE 44.4. Erbium laser treatment of perioral area and cheek. **A:** Perioral region pre-erbium laser treatment. **B:** Six months posterbium laser treatment. (From Bass LS. Erbium:YAG laser resurfacing: preliminary clinical evaluation. *Ann Plast Surg.* 1998;40:328–334, with permission.)

Erbium:YAG Laser

The erbium:YAG (Er:YAG) laser emits light whose primary chromophore is also water. The erbium laser has greater specificity for tissue obliteration than does CO_2, as well as a lower depth of penetration per pass and a shorter period of erythema, and it can treat more superficial pathology. The increased affinity for water by the Er:YAG laser results in more absorption of energy, more ablation, and less thermal damage to surrounding tissues than occurs with CO_2 lasers. Erbium's extremely high affinity for water reduces the ablation threshold and creates less thermal injury to the tissue (12). Cutaneous tissue absorbs erbium laser more efficiently than CO_2 light. The effect of the erbium laser is primarily photomechanical whereas that of the CO_2 laser is primarily photothermal.

The tissue effect of the erbium laser is consistent with each pass. The depth of ablation caused by erbium laser does not progressively diminish after multiple passes, in contrast to CO_2, and little necrotic tissue remains after passes (9). The skin contraction and hemostasis seen with CO_2 lasers is not as readily apparent with erbium lasers. By lengthening the pulse width of the erbium laser, the penetration depth can be extended to simulate CO_2 laser effects by creating more thermal effect and less ablation per pass. Long-pulse erbium laser also causes tissue tightening similar to CO_2 as a result of heat-induced collagen formation (13). Variable pulse width erbium lasers are popular for ablative skin resurfacing as they can deliver energy with long pulses relative to the tissues' thermal relaxation time, and can ablate tissue with greater control than CO_2 lasers. Variable-

pulse width lasers have a controllable mix between primary ablation (erbium effect) and primary coagulation (CO_2 effect). With erbium variable-pulse width lasers, a deeper penetration in a controlled fashion can be realized by adjusting pulse widths and making additional passes.

Reduced collateral thermal damage that allows for faster healing and a shorter period of erythema was the impetus for the development of the Er:YAG laser. However, some studies comparing CO_2 and Er:YAG lasers have shown equivalent healing times. More aggressive use of the Er:YAG laser with longer pulses can achieve results comparable to the CO_2 laser, but with little or no residual thermal damage, more rapid healing, and better clinical results (12). Some surgeons prefer initial resurfacing with CO_2 followed by use of erbium (1).

Reported advantages of erbium laser include precision in ablation, less postoperative erythema, and diminished incidence of hypopigmentation. Erbium is limited in its predictability in treatment of coarse facial wrinkles (14). Patients with mild-to-moderate photodamage can achieve excellent cosmetic results with the erbium laser (Fig. 44.4), but those with moderate-to-severe photodamage will achieve the best results with the CO_2 laser (9). Table 44.4 outlines the advantages and disadvantages of CO_2 and Er:YAG lasers.

CO_2 laser resurfacing is associated with increased morbidity, erythema, and hyperpigmentation; a significant risk of scarring; and a high incidence of hypopigmentation (15). The erbium laser has increased affinity for water, does not coagulate blood, and has less effect on the dermis. Combination lasers combine CO_2 with erbium in a single beam, allowing ablation of tissue with erbium and thermal stimulation and coagulation

TABLE 44.4

CO_2 VERSUS ERBIUM LASERS: ADVANTAGES AND DISADVANTAGES

Laser type	Advantages	Disadvantages
CO_2	More tissue contraction Excellent hemostasis Long-lasting results	Prolonged postoperative course Increased hypopigmentation and scarring
Erbium:YAG	Shorter postlaser recovery Potentially fewer complications	Little to no tissue contraction Intraoperative bleeding More passes required Limited collagen remodeling

Based on data from Alster TS. Cutaneous resurfacing with CO_2 and erbium:YAG lasers: preoperative, intraoperative, and postoperative considerations. *Plast Reconstr Surg.* 1999;103:2.

of dermal collagen with CO_2. Combination lasers are indicated for treatment of deep wrinkles, especially in the perioral region (15).

Nonablative Resurfacing

Nonablative techniques are popular although results are variable. Nonablative resurfacing spares the epidermis and denatures dermal collagen, but produces less collagen remodeling. Most of the energy is absorbed in the superficial layers of the dermis, and cooling is required to prevent thermal injury to the epidermis. The reorganization of collagen during the healing process improves skin quality. These lasers have the advantage of shorter recovery time, although less result is achieved.

Patient Selection

The indications for laser treatment are similar to the indications for the other forms of resurfacing. Laser is especially applicable to treat problems localized to the reticular dermis. Laser energy must be optimized to treat pathology and minimize complications (16). Patients with lighter Fitzpatrick skin types are less likely to have postlaser hyperpigmentation than those with darker skin, and patients with darker skin types may have less risk of permanent hypopigmentation. Pretreatment regimens consisting of hydroquinone (4%) and tretinoin (0.05%) can minimize posttreatment pigmentation changes by suppressing melanocyte activity. This treatment can be continued postlaser in high-risk patients. Pretreatment with α-hydroxy acids can also improve the outcome of laser resurfacing. Antiviral prophylaxis with acyclovir (Zovirax), valacyclovir (Valtrex), or famciclovir (Famvir) is indicated.

During laser resurfacing, appropriate safety measures must be taken, especially including ocular protection. The skin must be dry and removal of debris between passes is essential during CO_2 resurfacing. Parameter settings can vary widely and the pulse energy and number of passes must be determined. The initial pass removes the epithelial layer and causes dermal heating and collagen shrinkage. Additional passes cause a mix of ablation, which predominates with the erbium laser, and thermal damage, which predominates with the CO_2 laser. A higher pulse energy causes more vaporization and ablation of tissue. The visual end point is elimination of wrinkles and development of a smooth texture. Entry into the reticular dermis produces a whitish-brown color. Treatment deeper into the reticular dermis produces a tanlike or pale yellow color, and this is an absolute end point for CO_2 resurfacing (18). The variable-pulse width erbium laser has an end point that is less-well defined. Laser resurfacing can be combined with surgical procedures, but care must be taken if undermined skin is to be resurfaced.

Laser wounds may be treated with closed wound dressings or open wound care with ointment with similar results. There is no consensus regarding open or closed wound dressings, but it is known that partial-thickness cutaneous wounds heal more quickly and with a reduced risk of scarring if maintained in a moist environment (9). Meticulous wound care is essential. The average time for skin re-epithelialization after CO_2 laser treatment is about 7 days, and the average time after erbium laser is about 5 days. The time of re-epithelialization with either laser relates directly to the depth of injury created. After re-epithelialization, ointments are replaced with lighter moisturizers and covering cosmetics. The patient's daily skin care regimen may be restarted; the use of sunscreen is mandatory. Clinically, the extent of erythema correlates with the depth of injury and the degree of thermal injury. In general, CO_2 resurfacing produces longer-lasting erythema than does erbium laser resurfacing. Erythema may be regarded as a sign of collagen deposition but may also be a complication of treatment (11). Erythema is more intense and persistent after CO_2 laser treatment, which can last for as long as several months, as compared to that after erbium, which usually lasts for several weeks. Studies comparing the efficacy and postlaser healing of the CO_2 and Er:YAG lasers are ambiguous.

Histologic changes after laser resurfacing are similar to those after phenol peeling. Angiogenesis, neocollagen formation, and regeneration of dermal elastic fibers occurs, but melanocytes retain their ability to function and there is less hypopigmentation. Collagen is remodeled and collagen shrinkage may be responsible for tightening of the dermis (8). Neocollagen formation is secondary not only to the depth of injury, but also to the specific agent used in wounding (14).

Complications of laser resurfacing are similar to those of other resurfacing techniques and include hyperpigmentation, which is the most common; hypopigmentation; herpes infection; hypertrophic scarring; and lid retraction and ectropion. As many as one third of all laser-resurfacing patients experience some degree of hyperpigmentation (9). Laser treatment may cause less pigmentation and textural changes than other resurfacing modalities and can be useful for darker-skinned patients. Lighter-skinned patients are more prone to hypopigmentation because there is less pigment in the dermis. Hypopigmentation after CO_2 laser treatment can occur as late as 1 to 2 years after treatment and its incidence is approximately 10% to 20% (12). Future developments in laser technology will hopefully provide more precise tissue ablation with less risk of excessive thermal damage (9).

There is no perfect resurfacing technique. The choice of treatment must be multifactorial, based on the desired depth of resurfacing, the ease of use and expense of the device, any special features of the modality, and safety and complication profiles. In general, the risk of prolonged erythema or pigment loss is directly proportional to the depth of resurfacing and to the prolongation of wound healing (13). The goal of any resurfacing treatment is removal of abnormal tissue, stimulation of new collagen and elastin, and formation of new epidermis with overall rejuvenation of the skin. The ideal method of skin resurfacing should be judged by long-term wrinkle improvement, predictability, accuracy of depth control, low morbidity, minimal complications, high patient acceptance, and cost-effectiveness (15).

References

1. Bernstein EF, Andersen D, Zelickson BD, et al. Laser resurfacing for dermal photoaging. *Clin Plast Surg*. 2000;27:221–238.
2. Baker TJ, Gordon HL. The ablation of rhytides by chemical means: A preliminary report. *J Fla Med Assoc*. 1961;47:451.
3. Hetter GP. An examination of the phenol-croton oil peel: parts I– IV. *Plast Reconstr Surg*. 2000;105:227–248, 752–763, 1061–1083.
4. Stegman SJ. A study of dermabrasion and chemical peels in an animal model. *J Dermatol Surg Oncol*. 1980;6:490.
5. Kligman AM, Baker TJ, Gordon HL. Long-term histologic follow-up of phenol face peels. *Plast Reconstr Surg*. 1985;75:652.
6. Baker T, Stuzin JM, Baker TM. *Facial Skin Resurfacing*. St. Louis: Quality Medical Publishing; 1998.
7. Baker TJ, Gordon HL. Chemical face peeling and dermabrasion. *Surg Clin North Am*. 1971;51:387.
8. Jacobson D, Bass LS, VanderKam V, et al. Carbon dioxide and Er:YAG laser resurfacing. *Clin Plast Surg*. 2000;27:241.
9. Alster TS. Cutaneous resurfacing with CO_2 and erbium: laser YAG, preoperative, intraoperative and postoperative considerations. *Plast Reconstr Surg*. 1999;103:619–632.
10. Alster TS. Long-term histologic effects of the CO_2 laser [discussion]. *Plast Reconstr Surg*. 1999;104:2245–2246.
11. Schwartz RJ, Burns AJ, Rohrich RJ, et al. Long-term assessment of CO_2

facial laser resurfacing: aesthetic results and complications. *Plast Reconstr Surg*. 1999;103:592–601.

12. Burns AJ. Erbium laser resurfacing: current concepts [discussion]. *Plast Reconstr Surg*. 1999;103:617–618.

13. Fitzpatrick RE. Resurfacing procedures: how do you choose? *Arch Dermatol*. 2000;136:783–784.

14. Stuzin JM, Baker TJ, Baker TM. CO_2 and erbium:YAG laser resurfacing: current status and personal perspective. *Plast Reconstr Surg*. 1999;103:588–591.

15. Weinstein C, Scheflan M. Simultaneously combined Er:YAG and carbon dioxide laser (derma K) for skin resurfacing. *Clin Plast Surg*. 2000;27:273–285.

16. Alster TS, Lupton JR. Prevention and treatment of side effects and complications of cutaneous laser resurfacing. *Plast Reconstr Surg*. 2002;109:308.

17. Fitzpatrick RE. Maximizing benefits and minimizing risk with CO_2 laser resurfacing. *Dermatol Clin*. 2002;20:77.

CHAPTER 45 ■ FILLER MATERIALS

ARNOLD WILLIAM KLEIN

The field of soft-tissue augmentation has a long and colorful history. Soft-tissue augmentation dates back more than 100 years to when Neuber, in Germany, reported on adipose grafts transplanted for reconstruction of a soft-tissue defect on the face. Thus, fat is the oldest material used for tissue augmentation. Over the years, many implantable substances and devices have been used to cosmetically improve soft-tissue defects and deficiencies. Soft-tissue augmentation is increasingly important as an increasing number of patients seek aesthetic improvement without major surgical procedures.

A consequence of time, smoking, sun, and gravity is a loss of dermal collagen and the resulting wrinkles. Age-related changes of the lips and mouth include atrophy of both the upper and lower lips, actinic changes of the mucosal surface and vermilion border and atrophy at the corners of the mouth, causing a downturn of the corners of the mouth and an aged appearance. Subtle improvements in the lips and their surrounding structures can produce astounding results, rebuilding the perioral structure and regaining a more youthful, rested visage. Another of the earliest signs of aging is an increase in prominence of the nasolabial folds. Bovine collagen became approved as an "in-and-out" office procedure in the 1980s and minimally invasive cosmetic enhancement began. Collagen has been used successfully for nearly 25 years to fill in the fine lines and wrinkles associated with aging (1).

Why the increased interest in filling agents? One huge reason is the emergence of Botox (Allergan, Inc., Irvine, CA) (see Chapter 46), which works superbly in the upper face. Of the past 15 years, Botox is the greatest advance in the minimally invasive treatment of the aging face. When used in the upper face in conjunction with fillers in the lower face, remarkable results can be obtained in softening the effects of aging and providing a more youthful and rested appearance of the face. Rejuvenation of the upper face using Botox has awakened a need for agents that work equally well in the lower face. A second reason for the increased interest is the availability of new implants. **A third reason is the recognition that the youthful face has a full look—not a pulled, flat, two-dimensional look. This realization is a central tenet of the field of soft-tissue augmentation. In addition, subtle lip enhancement is a procedure that is here to stay.** In fact, it is the number one indication for injectable fillers. Moreover, affordable outpatient surgery has replaced much of the expensive hospital-based surgery, and the less-invasive techniques provide a new repertoire of therapeutic options. Finally, an increasing number of physicians of all specialties are becoming trained in cosmetic surgery and are offering cosmetic services as part of their office practice. Courses in cosmetic surgery techniques are increasingly popular at medical meetings among nearly all specialties. As a result of all the foregoing developments, physicians have a larger armamentarium of techniques and materials with which to improve facial contours, ameliorate wrinkles, and stall the tell-tale signs of the aging face.

The two basic types of wrinkles (rhytides) are dynamic and static (2). **Dynamic rhytides are caused by muscle action and include glabellar, crow's-feet, nasolabial (in part), and forehead wrinkles. Static rhytides are caused by exogenous sources, such as smoking, gravity, and sun.** Dynamic and static wrinkles can be seen together in areas such as the forehead and cheeks.

Dynamic rhytides are normally best treated by botulinum toxin injections. Botulinum toxin has replaced filler substances as the treatment of choice for crow's-feet, glabellar, and forehead lines. Understanding the anatomy of these wrinkles will help the physician to determine whether botulinum toxin alone will do the job. Combining botulinum toxin therapy with resurfacing or filler substances can often dramatically improve efficacy.

The choice of an appropriate implant, whether solid or injectable, requires a thorough understanding of the materials available and the etiology of the wrinkle. **Fine, superficial rhytides respond best to therapy at the intradermal level. Deeper, more substantial wrinkles typically have a subcutaneous component, with or without a facial-muscular element, and are best approached from the subcutaneous space.** Oftentimes a wrinkle will have both a superficial and deep component, such as the nasolabial fold, and both of these components need to be addressed to obtain optimal results.

Since the earliest experiments with filling substances in the late 1800s, physicians have searched for an ideal bioinjectable material. For a substance or device to be amenable for soft-tissue augmentation by the general medical community, it should possess certain attributes. It must have both a high "use" potential, producing pleasing cosmetic results with a minimum of undesirable reactions, and a low "abuse" potential, in that widespread and possibly incorrect or indiscriminate use would not result in significant morbidity. It must be nonteratogenic, noncarcinogenic, and nonmigratory. In addition, the material must provide predictable, persistent correction through standardized implantation techniques. Finally, if not autologous, the substance, agent, or device must be FDA approved.

The search for the perfect material to eradicate rhytides, smooth scars, and fill traumatic defects continues. **New products appear, sometimes with great fanfare, and often fail to fulfill their promise. Fibrel, Autologen, Dermalogen, and Soft-Form are all no longer available.** Isolagen was withdrawn from the market but is now undergoing clinical trials with the expectation that it will be reintroduced. Although no currently available implant fulfills the criteria for being the perfect material, many options exist that are adequate for a given task, satisfy patients, and offer excellent safety profiles; efforts to develop the perfect soft-tissue augmentation material continue.

It should be noted that autologous and allogeneic products are not FDA approved. Because they are derived from human tissue, they are not required to undergo the FDA approval process.

Physicians must counsel patients as to the risks and benefits of injectable substance therapy, including information about skin testing, the treatment procedure, and treatment expectations.

TABLE 45.1

FILLER SUBSTANCES

AcHyal[a]	Hyacell[a]
AlloDerm	Hyal-System[a]
Amazingel[a]	Hylaform
Aptos threads	Hylan Rofilan Gel[a]
Aquamid 40[a]	Isolagen[a]
Artecoll	Juvederm[a]
Artefill[a]	Kopolymer[a]
Argiform[a]	MacDeermol[a]
Bio-Alcamid[a]	Meta-Crill[a]
Biocell Ultravital[a]	Metrex[a]
Bioformacryl[a]	New-Fill
Bioplastique[a]	Perlane[a]
CosmoDerm NST &	Permacol[a]
CosmoPlast NST	Plasmagel
Cymetra	PMS 350
Dermal Grafting	Procell[a]
DermaLive[a]/DermaDeep[a]	Profill[a]
Dermaplant[a]	Radiance/Radiesse
Dermicol[a]	Resoplast[a]
Endoplast-50[a]	Restylane
Evolution[a]	Restylane-Fine[a]
Fascian	Reviderm Intra[a]
Fat	Rhegecoll[a]
Subcutaneous	Sculptra
microlipoinjection	Silicone[a]
Lipocytic dermal	Silicon1000
augmentation	Surgisis
Formacrill[a]	Ultrasoft & Conform
Gore-Tex	Zyderm Collagen &
Humallagen[a]	Zyplast Collagen

[a]Not approved for use in the United States.

A list of filling substances 10 years ago may have contained five items, but now a veritable encyclopedia of agents is available to the practitioner (Table 45.1).

CURRENT FILLERS

AcHyal is a 1% solution of the sodium salt of hyaluronic acid. It is provided in 2.5-mL prefilled syringes with 30-gauge needles, can be stored at room temperature, and has a shelf-life of 3 years. Indications are wrinkles, scars, and lip and contour deformities. Adverse reactions are listed as reddening, inflammation, or bruising, which dissipate in 2 to 3 days. There is no experience with the material in the United States and it is not FDA approved. AcHyal is manufactured by Tedec Meiji Farma, S.A. Ctra. M-300, KM 30,500 28802 – Alcalá de Henares, Madrid, Spain.

AlloDerm is processed, acellular, freeze-dried human cadaver dermis. This is a decellularized nonimmunogenic human dermal allograft that is inserted through dissected tunnels for soft-tissue augmentation. It contains a protein framework without cells, has been in use since 1992, and has been used in more than 3,500 patients. AlloDerm is available in solid sheets for grafting or implanting. Manufactured by Life Cell Corp., One Millennium Way, Branchburg, NJ 08876-3876. E-mail: custserv@lifecell.com. Phone: 800-367-5737, 908-947-1215; FAX: 908-947-1089. http://www.lifecell.com/healthcare/products/alloderm/index.cfm. It is distributed by Obagi Medical, Chicago, IL.

Aquamid injectable is a hydrophilic polyacrylamide gel that is 97.5% apyrogenic water bound to 2.5% cross-linked polyacrylamide. It has been CE marked since 2001. It is nonresorbable, nonallergenic, biocompatible, physically and chemically stable, immunologically inactive, and migration resistant according to the manufacturer's claims. It is injected subcutaneously with a 27-gauge needle and is indicated for lips, nasolabial folds, mentolabial folds, deep wrinkles, glabellar frowns, cheek augmentation, and aesthetic/reconstructive augmentation of the body. In a European multicenter study, satisfaction exceeded 92% 2 years after treatment. It is not available in the United States, but is available in Europe, Australia, Asia, Canada, and Mexico. It is manufactured by Contura International A/S, Sydmarken 23, 2860 Soeborg, Denmark. Phone: 45-3958-5960. http://www.aquamid.info/ and http://www.contura.com/.

Argiform (aka Argyform) is a hydrophilic polyacrylamide gel manufactured using a silver ion process to help repel bacteria. It has a 0.03% residual unpolymerized acrylamide monomer and is manufactured by Bioform in Russia. It is not available in the United States, but is available in Europe. Bioform Corp., Krasnobogatyrskay Street, 42/1103, Moscow, Russia. Phone: 7(095) 161-0524. E-mail: info@bioform.ru. http://bioform.ru.

Artecoll/Artefill is a suspension of 20% PMMA (polymethylmethacrylate) microspheres of 30 to 42 μm diameter in 80% collagen solution. The collagen is degraded following injection with the resultant permanent deposition of PMMA. Artecoll is supplied in 0.6-mL syringes and designed for implantation into the deep reticular dermis. Clinical trials in the United States have been conducted (3), and it has received FDA approval. It is marketed as Artefill in the United States. **Because of its long-lasting effect, Artecoll is unforgiving. Uneven distribution, long-lasting itching, and redness are common side effects.**

Artecoll was preceded by Resoplast and Arteplast and is basically a combination of these two products. Artecoll is injected deeply with a 27-gauge needle, not in the dermal space, but at the junction between dermis and subcutaneous fat (subdermal) and can be molded with finger-tip pressure. According to the manufacturer, it is indicated for deeper wrinkles and furrows, deep glabellar furrows, nasolabial lines, perioral lines, radial lip lines, lip and philtrum augmentation, scar revision and other dermal, subdermal, and osseous defects. Patients must be skin tested for allergy to bovine collagen prior to use because of the collagen carrier. It is contraindicated in patients who form keloids, have atrophic skin diseases, and those who have very thin, flaccid skin because of the risk of permanent superficial irregularities. The product is manufactured and distributed by Rofil Medical International B.V., Stationstaat 1B, 4815 NC Breda, The Netherlands. Phone: 31-76-531-5670; FAX: 31-76-531-5660. E-mail: RMI@rofil.nl. In the United States: Artes Medical, Inc., 4660 La Jolla Village Drive, Suite 825, San Diego, CA 92122. Phone: 858-550-9999; FAX: 858-550-9997. http://www.artefill.com.

Arteplast (not FDA-approved) is a combination of PMMA beads and Tween 80. Arteplast is basically Plexiglas beads. It was part of the initial research before Artecoll was developed. It is no longer used, its applications having been replaced by Artecoll. The product was manufactured and distributed by Rofil Medical International B.V., Breda, The Netherlands.

Autologen is true autologous collagen. It was a sterile suspension of intact collagen fibers prepared from the patient's own tissue. Host skin from a prior procedure was processed into a suspended, autologous, fibrillar material, usually of a 3.5% concentration. Three square inches of skin produced 1 mL of Autologen at this concentration. It was appropriate for fine lines, wrinkles, depressions, and lip augmentation. It had to be placed as superficially as possible. It was manufactured by Collagenesis, Inc., Beverly, MA. The company has stopped accepting shipments of new skin for processing and Autologen is presently unavailable.

Bio-Alcamid (BioAlcamid) is an injectable hydrophilic polyakylimide gel. It is permanent and used for wasted areas of the face in HIV patients. It is manufactured by Progen, now Polymekon (Italy). It is approved in Europe and in Mexico. It is not available in the United States. http://www.bioalcamid.com/.

Biocell Ultravital is also called Biopolymere III. It is a biopolymer developed in Switzerland by Biocell Ultravital and contains silicium (a derivative of silicon). According to the manufacturer, there is no need for allergy tests prior to treatment and results may be permanent. It is commonly used in South America. It is distributed by Biocell Laboratories, CH 593 Vaduz, Lichtenstein. It is not approved by the FDA for use in the United States.

Bioplastique is a suspension of textured composite silicone polymer of solid, vulcanized methylsiloxane rubber particles from 100 to 400 μm in size in a carrier vehicle (biocompatible plasdone hydrogel) (4). It is an investigational material for soft-tissue augmentation with a controlled foreign-body response. The size of the particles reportedly reduces migration. There are several reports of granulomas requiring excision. It has a CE mark but as a consequence of the controversy and resultant bad press surrounding silicone gel implants, it is unlikely to be FDA approved, thus studies have been largely abandoned.

CosmoDerm and **CosmoPlast** are new products. They are recombinant human collagen with the same consistency and injection properties as Zyderm and Zyplast bovine collagen. They are grown from a single tissue cell line to avoid the possibility of disease transmission. They should eliminate potential allergenicity to collagen injections and do not require skin testing. They are manufactured by Advanced Tissue Sciences, San Diego, CA, and distributed by Inamed Aesthetics, 5540 Ekwill Street, Santa Barbara, CA 93111. Phone: 800-766-0171, 805-683-6761; FAX: 805-967-5839. http://www.inamed.com.

Cymetra is micronized AlloDerm that is cryofractured and rehydrated with 1 mL of Xylocaine. According to the manufacturer, no allergy prescreening or testing is required. Donor screening and viral inactivation is performed. The material is obtained from American Association of Tissue Banks (AATB) guideline-compliant tissue banks. It is implanted with a 26-gauge needle into the subcutaneous space. The treatment area is gently massaged. Clinical studies on 200 patients to date evidenced no allergic or immunologic reactions. Adverse reactions are bruising, redness, swelling and wrinkling of skin. Eye pain with temporary vision loss has been reported. All the adverse reactions are reported as transient and occur at a rate of 2.1%. It is distributed by Life Cell Corp., One Millennium Way, Branchburg, NJ 08876-3876. E-mail: custserv@lifecell.com. Phone: 800-367-5737, 908-947-1215; FAX: 908-947-1089. http://www.lifecell.com/healthcare/products/cymetra/.

DermaLive/DermaDeep are composed of hyaluronic acid/hydrogel solution and acrylic hydrogel (HEMA) fragments. They are nonanimal in origin and are composed of 45- to 65-μm particles. Collagen builds around the particles giving the fillers their volume. Reportedly, skin tests are unnecessary. The material comes in preloaded syringes and is intended for use in the dermal and subdermal planes. DermaLive is used for augmenting lips and smoothing deep wrinkles. DermaDeep is very effective on nasolabial folds and for chin and cheek augmentation. It has a CE mark and has been available in Europe and South America for 5 years. It is produced by Dermatech, 28 Rue de Caumartin, 75009 Paris, France. Phone: 01-42-66-52-00; FAX: 01-42-66-52-24. http://www.dermadeep.com; http://www.dermalive.com.

Dermalogen is a human tissue collagen matrix from the dermal layer of donor skin specimens. It is suspended in a neutral pH buffer and is predominately composed of collagen fibrils and other matrix proteins, such as elastin. It is sterilized and undergoes viral inactivation procedures and a prion inactivation step. HIV and hepatitis tests are performed. The sources of the donor skin are tissue banks accredited by the AATB. It is no longer on the market. It was manufactured and distributed by Collagenesis, Inc., 500 Cummings Center, Beverly, MA 01915. Phone: 508-264-2906; FAX: 508-264-2907.

DermiCol is a uniquely formulated, injectable, cross-linked, collagen-based product. It has the ability to remain stable in the body for a significantly longer period of time than other collagen products. It is not available in the United States. Trials are underway on this product in Europe. It is manufactured by Colbar Life Sciences, Ltd., 9 Haminofim Street, PO Box 12206, Herzliya, Israel 46733. Phone: 09-9718666. E-mail: dorits@colbar.com. http://www.colbar.com.

Endoplast-50 is a product of elastin-solubilized peptides with collagen (bovine, United States) for intradermal injection. Two skin tests are performed at 15-day intervals prior to treatment. Test syringes are available. It is provided in 0.5-mL or 1-mL syringes. A 30-gauge needle is used for injection. It is injected in a serial puncture technique in the reticular dermis and is then massaged. There is a possibility (rare) of hypersensitivity. After treatment, inflammation is expected for 24 to 48 hours. The material influences proliferation of fibroblasts to produce collagen. Duration of correction is said to be 8 to 12 months. It is distributed by Laboratories Filorga, 79 Rue de Miromesnil, 75008 Paris, France. Phone: 01-42-93-94-00; FAX: 01-42-93-79-65. E-mail: filorga@wanadoo.fr.

ePTFE (expanded polytetrafluoroethylene) was developed by Robert W. Gore and William L. Gore as an expanded, fibrillated form of PTFE (Teflon). Gore-Tex (W.L. Gore and Associates, Inc., Flagstaff, AZ) was first introduced in 1971 and approved by the FDA for facial plastic and reconstructive surgery in 1993. As early as 1991, Lassus (5) reported the use of ePTFE for nasolabial fold and rhytide correction. This solid material is inserted under the skin as tied strips, strings, or through a trocar that contains the product. It is marketed as GORE Subcutaneous Augmentation Material (S.A.M.) by W.L. Gore and Associates, Inc., 3300 East Sparrow Drive, Flagstaff, AZ 86004. Phone: 800-528-8763, 928-526-3032; FAX: 800-437-8181. http://www.goremedical.com/English/Products/SAM/Indes.htm.

Maas et al. (6) performed studies in the porcine model comparing the implantation of solid strips, rolled sheets, and tubular implants of ePTFE. This work led to the development of the version of ePTFE marketed as Soft-Form. It is no longer available; it has been replaced by similar materials, such as Conform.

Fascian is preserved, particulate fascia lata derived from screened human cadavers. The material is freeze-dried and typically pre-irradiated. This injectable form of fascia lata can be injected when soft-tissue augmentation is desired. Preserved fascia grafts have proven efficacy and an excellent safety record over the past 73 years. In a clinical trial, Burres followed 81 subjects for 6 to 9 months after implantation without incidence of infection, allergic reaction, or acute rejection (7). Soft-tissue augmentation was evident 3 to 4 months after grafting, or longer, in most cases. Injectable material is supplied in particle sizes of <0.25 mm, <0.5 mm, and <2.0 mm. The Fascian particles are hydrated in 3 to 5 mL of 0.3% lidocaine solution prior to injection. The injected area is pre-undermined with a 20-gauge needle and the material injected into the preformed tunnel with a 16- to 25-gauge needle, depending on the size of the particles used. It is manufactured by Medical Aesthetics International, Inc., Redwood, WA and marketed by Fascia Biosystems, LLC, 465 N. Roxbury Dr., Beverly Hills, CA 90210. Phone: 888-3FASCIA (888-332-7242); FAX: 310-385-8758. http://www.fascian.com.

Fat has been used as an injectable agent since the early 1900s. Its use was reborn with the advent of liposuction in the 1980s (as an answer to the question of what to do with all the stuff they were sucking out). **Fat is used at a much deeper level in the skin than is collagen and is applicable for gross correction. It will not correct fine defects.** There is a vast difference between the use of fresh (recently removed) fat and frozen fat in that the former provides a much longer duration of correction. Fat is one of the most appealing tissues for transplantation. Grafting or transferring autologous fat is attractive because of the relative ease of harvest, as well as the availability of numerous, easily accessed donor sites. The avoidance of allogeneic or alloplastic materials and the potential antigenic and/or inflammatory responses inherent with such agents is also of great benefit. **Nevertheless, whether injected fat actually persists remains an area of controversy.**

The thighs, buttocks, knees, and abdomen appear to be the donor sites most often used. Although many individuals prefer to gently harvest the fat in a syringe, others prefer to remove fat by liposuction, which is then returned to the body. Sites most amenable for correction with microlipoinjection appear to be the dorsal hand, depressed temples, hollow cheeks, deep nasolabial grooves, and defects caused by liposuction or lipodystrophy. Fat implantation has also been advocated for malar and chin augmentation. To place the fat, appropriate anesthesia is used and a 16- to 18-gauge needle is attached to the injecting syringe. An 11-gauge scalpel is employed to prick the skin, and the syringe containing the fat is then inserted at this recipient site and the material injected at the level of the subcutaneous space. Molding after implantation is frequently used.

While swelling and bruising are fairly common and usually minor at the recipient site, occasionally persistent edema, asymmetry, punctate scarring, lumping, and bleeding occur. Infection is a rare occurrence. **There has also been a single case of unilateral blindness reported following autologous fat transplantation.** This is obviously the most serious adverse consequence reported to date (8).

Of all the variables associated with microlipoinjection, longevity of correction achieved with fat transfer remains the strongest area of controversy. The literature suggests that a transplant of fat cells survives best when either cut out and implanted as a small cylinder of tissue, or aspirated and injected through a large-bore needle (14-gauge or larger). Transplanted fat tissue seems to last longest in those areas with the least movement. However, there are many areas on the face where autologous fat is used, including the nasolabial folds, the commissures of the mouth and "marionette lines," submalar depressions, lip augmentation, chin augmentation, malar augmentation, congenital and traumatic defects, surgical defects, wide-based acne scarring, idiopathic lipodystrophy, and facial hemiatrophy. Autologous fat has also been used in nonfacial areas for rejuvenation of the hands and body-contour defects, as well as for depressions caused by liposuction or trauma. Fat has also been used for breast augmentation but this is highly controversial. Some physicians believe that, of all the areas, fat transfer to the hand is the best widespread indication.

Many physicians consider freezing fat for use at a later time as a useful adjunct to autologous fat transfer. Whether the fat cells remain viable after freezing, thawing, manipulation, and reinjection through 18-gauge or smaller needles is open to question. The process of "lipocytic dermal augmentation" was developed in an attempt to use autologous fat to reproducibly correct fine wrinkles. In this technique, centrifuged fat is mechanically manipulated and injected at the level of the dermis through a 25-gauge needle.

Humallagen has poor rheology and cannot get through a 30-gauge needle.

Human placental collagen is gamma-irradiated amnion collagen from human placentae. It has been suggested as an injectable soft-tissue augmentation material and tested in animal studies. This is collagen that is manufactured from human placentae. Placentae are readily available and although there have been clinical trials on the material, it will probably never come to market.

Hyacell is composed of 40% hyaluronic acid and 20% embryonic tissue. It is not an actual filler but it is used in facial and corporal mesotherapy. It stimulates collagen synthesis. Adverse reactions to Hyacell made headlines in the New York area. It is not available in the United States but is undergoing clinical studies in Europe.

Hyal-System is a higher concentration of hyaluronic acid. It has a molecular weight of 10^6 daltons. It comes in preloaded syringes and is manufactured by Fidia S.P., Via ponte della Fabbria 3/A, 35031 Abano Terme (Padua), Italy.

Hylaform (Hylan B), developed in the mid-1980s, is a sterile, nonpyrogenic, viscoelastic, colorless, transparent gel implant composed of sulfonyl cross-linked molecules of hyaluronan polymer. Hyaluronan (hyaluronic acid) is a naturally occurring polysaccharide that is an essential component of the extracellular matrix and has the same chemical structure in all vertebrates. Hylaform is derived from materials of avian origin and contains trace amounts of avian protein. Persons with a sensitivity to avian proteins or eggs should be advised of the potential for an allergic reaction, although there is minimal avian protein present in this product. Although rare, adverse reactions include persistent erythema and ecchymosis. Hylaform has been used in more than 50 countries since 1996. It was approved for use in the United States in 2004.

Hylaform is hydroscopic, giving the implant a natural and soft appearance and feel as a wrinkle filler. It can be injected either by the threading or serial puncture, the latter being the preferred technique. Implantation usually requires topical or local block anesthesia as this product contains no lidocaine.

Hylaform is used for facial augmentation throughout most of the world. It is especially popular for volume augmentation of the lips, although this is an off-label use. There is reportedly no immunologic activity, although there have been some reports of redness that persisted at the sites of implantation. Reported adverse reactions are less than 2% and include erythema, ecchymoses, and acne. Hylaform gel is manufactured by Biomatrix, Inc., Ridgefield, NJ, and is distributed in Europe by Collagen International, Inc., Avenue Gratta-Paille 2CP430, CH-1000 Lausanne 30 Grey, Switzerland. In the United States, it is distributed by Inamed Aesthetics, 5540 Ekwill Street, Santa Barbara, CA 93111. Phone: 800-766-0171, 805-683-6761; FAX: 805-967-5839. http://www.inamed.com.

Hylan Rofilan Gel is a hyaluronic acid cross-linked with a natural acid instead of a chemical compound. The product is manufactured and distributed by Rofil Medical International B.V., Stationstaat 1B, 4815 NC Breda, The Netherlands. Phone: 31-76-531-5670; FAX: 31-76-531-5660. E-mail: RMI@rofil.nl.

Isolagen comes from Isolagen Technologies, Paramus, NJ. It is cultured autologous fibroblasts such as are used for burns, cartilage repair, and marrow transplants. It is applicable for fine lines, depressions, and lip augmentation. There is a temporary halt of the sales of this product because of the growth factors it uses, which might categorize Isolagen as a medical device and not simply a transplant of autologous substance. The product is currently in clinical trials for FDA approval.

Juvederm is a nonallergenic hyaluronic acid derived from a nonanimal source. It comes in three versions: Juvederm 18 for fine lines and crow's-feet, Juvederm 24 for forehead and cheek wrinkles, and Juvederm 30 to fill lips, sculpture cheeks, and fill deep nasolabial folds. Results can last 4 to 6 months after treatment. Juvederm is not yet approved for use in the United States. It is available from Euromedical Systems Ltd., Connaught House, Moorbridge Road, Bingham,

NG138GG, England. Phone: 44-0-1949838111. E-mail: information@euromedicalsystems.co.uk.

Koken Atelocollagen implant is a 2% monomolecular solution of collagen of Japanese origin. It is supplied in cartridges to be injected with a dental syringe through a 30-gauge needle. The indications, contraindications, testing, and injection techniques are the same as those for Zyderm collagen implant. Unlike Zyderm, Koken Atelocollagen does not contain lidocaine. It is an aqueous solution of monomolecular collagen molecules, whereas Zyderm is a suspension containing molecules, fibers, and fibrils of collagen. It is manufactured and distributed by the Koken Co., LTD., 3-14-3 Mejiro, Toshima-KM, Tokyo 171, Japan. Phone: 81-3-3950-6600. It is not available in the United States.

Macrolane is a nonanimal hyaluronic acid manufactured by Q-Med. It is of greater density than Perlane and Restylane, possibly lasting longer than either. It is being studied for body contouring in Europe. It is available from Q-Med AB, Seminariegatan 21, 752 28 Uppsala, Sweden. Phone: 46-18-474-90-00. E-mail: info@q-med.com.

Metacrill is composed of microspheres (20 to 80 μm) of methacrylate in a colloidal suspension without protein. It is similar to Arteplast. It is distributed by Nutricel, Rua Sampaio Viana, 299-Rio Comprido, Rio de Janeiro/RJ, Cep: 20,261-030, Brazil. Phone: 021-502-2314, 021-502-1481; FAX: 021-502-1527. E-mail: metacrill.com.br. http://www.metacrill.com.br.

New-fill (Sculptra) is a polylactic acid from the α-hydroxy acid family; it is not of animal origin. It is provided as freeze-dried material and can be stored at room temperature. After reconstitution with 3.0 mL of water, it is 4.45% polylactic acid and contains 40- to 60-μm microspheres. The material is biocompatible, biodegradable, and immunologically inert. There is no need for skin testing. It is injected either into the superficial dermis or subdermally using a 26-gauge needle. Indications are for nasolabial folds, lips, lipodystrophy of cheeks, acne scars, wrinkles, hands, and liposuction contour deformities. It was approved in Europe in 1999 to increase the volume of depressed areas. In 2004, under the name Sculptra, the product was approved by the FDA specifically for the replacement of fat lost in the cheeks as a result of the effect of antiretroviral therapy in HIV patients. The injections provide a gradual and significant increase in soft-tissue thickness, improving the appearance of folds and sunken areas. Fibroplasia may correct defects for months or longer. In a clinical trial of Sculptra in HIV patients, the treatment results lasted for 2 years after the first treatment session. Repeat injections may be necessary. A possible side effect of Sculptra is the delayed appearance of small bumps or papules under the skin in the treated area. Generally these bumps are not visible and are only noticed when pressing on the treated area. Other possible side effects include injection-related events at the site of injection, such as bleeding, tenderness or discomfort, redness, bruising, or swelling. All patients have some edema and a significant proportion experience pain during the injection procedure. Sculptra is available from Dermik Laboratories Inc., 1050 Westlakes Drive, Berwyn, PA 19312. Phone: 800-633-1610, 484-595-2700. http://www.dermik.com. Dermik Laboratories is a subsidiary of Aventis Pharmaceuticals, 300 Somerset Corporate, Boulevard, PO Box 6977, Bridgewater, NJ 08807.

Outline is made from polyacrylamide copolymer gel that attracts hyaluronic acid and the collagen and elastin precursors toward the injected area, enhancing the quality of skin and allowing the body's own collagen to become incorporated into the gel mass. Longevity is said to be 2 to 3 years. It is manufactured by ProCytech of France. It can be injected into the mid-dermis, deep dermis, and below the dermis. It is not available in the United States, but is used in Europe, Asia, and Australia.

Perlane is a more robust form of Restylane for use with a 27.5-gauge needle. It is placed at the subcutaneous–dermal border. It is manufactured and distributed by Q-Med AB, Seminariegatan 21, SE-752 28 Uppsala, Sweden. Phone: 46-18-50-42-10, 46-18-474-90-00; FAX: 46-18-50-31-35, 46-18-474-90-07. http://www.q-med.com.se; http://www.q-medesthetics.com/indes2.asp?mid=12.

Plasmagel is an autologous, blood-derived augmenting material. Ascorbic acid and lidocaine are added to blood plasma. The material is heated to form a gel, which is injected. It is applicable for wrinkles, contour defects, acne scars, and lip augmentation.

Pro fill (or Profil) is a translucent gel. It is a block copolymer of polyoxyethylene and polyoxypropylene with mineral salts, amino acids, and vitamins. The material contains no animal proteins. It is provided as a liquid that can be refrigerated until used. No skin test is required. The liquid material turns to gel on implantation and thus can be molded after implantation. It is provided in 1-mL syringes and injected with a 30-gauge needle in a serial puncture fashion. Several hours of redness are expected postimplantation. Correction reportedly lasts 6 to 9 months. It is biodegradable but severe reactions have been noted. It is manufactured and distributed by Laboratories Filorga, 79 Rue de Miromesnil, 75008 Paris, France. Phone: 01-42-93-94-00; FAX: 01-42-93-79-65. E-mail: filorga@wanadoo.fr.

Radiance/Radiance FN/Radiesse is composed of 40-μm spheres of calcium hydroxylapatite (CaHA) suspended in a patented pharmaceutical-grade aqueous polysaccharide gel carrier. Because calcium hydroxylapatite is a normal constituent of bone, it should not elicit a chronic inflammatory or immune response. Additionally, the gel carrier does not require allergy testing. Radiance FN is the smaller particle and is the agent that is being used for soft-tissue augmentation in an off-label manner. It is not yet approved by the FDA for aesthetic uses but it is approved for vocal fold insufficiency and radiograph marking. It does not create chronic inflammation, does not migrate, and requires no skin testing. Most patients have minimal to moderate pain and experience some bruising on injection. **Problems have been reported with the formation of submucosal nodules in the lip.** Longevity is 2 to 6 years. The manufacturer is Bioform Medical, Inc., 1875 South Grant Street, Suite 110, San Mateo, CA 94402. Phone: 866-862-1211; FAX: 866-862-1212. E-mail: info@bioformedical.com. http://www.bioforminc.com. There is an ongoing legal battle between Bioform and Artes over the ownership of this product.

Resoplast is bovine monomolecular collagen in solution. Concentrations of 3.5% and 6.5% are available. Indications and techniques of implantation are similar to Zyderm collagen. A skin test is provided. It is available from Rofil Medical International N.V., Breda, The Netherlands. E-mail: RMI@rofil.com. http://www.rofil.com.

Restylane is a stabilized, partially cross-linked hyaluronic acid created via bacterial fermentation from *Streptococci* bacteria and, thus, does not require an animal source. It is biocompatible and biodegradable. It has a higher concentration of hyaluronic acid than does Hylaform gel. This increases the filler's solubility. Although there is a higher concentration, this material has a lower molecular weight. Restylane is provided in 0.7-mL preloaded syringes containing 20 mg/mL of stabilized hyaluronic acid. Initially, a linear threading was recommended, not a serial puncture technique, but now a serial puncture technique is also being used. Restylane is used with a 30-gauge needle and no overcorrection is necessary. The second-generation of this product seems to have eliminated the problems with the intermittent swelling that was associated with the first generation. **Restylane is indicated for rhytides and depressions, but the best indication is for lip augmentation, putting it into the**

potential space and then actually the mucosa itself, thus creating excellent volume lip enhancement. Restylane is FDA approved for injection into the nasolabial folds. Restylane-fine is a less-viscous form of Restylane for use with a 32-gauge needle. Perlane is a more robust form of Restylane for use with a 27.5-gauge needle. It is placed at the subcutaneous–dermal border.

One clinical study involved 113 European patients receiving injection of Restylane to 285 facial wrinkles. Physicians rated the degree of correction to be 82% at 3 months and 66% at 1 year, with similar patient opinion. Side effects were minimal and included erythema when injected too superficially and technique-related unevenness. There were no reported allergic reactions. It is manufactured and distributed by Q-Med AB, Seminariegatan 21, S-752 28 Uppsala, Sweden. Phone: 46-18-50-42-10; FAX: 46-18-50-31-35. http://www.q-med.com.se. In the United States, it is distributed by Medicis Aesthetics, Inc., 8125 North Hayden Road, Scottsdale, AZ 85258-2463. E-mail: restylandquestions@RestylaneUSA.com. http://www.medicis.com.

Reviderm-intra contains 40- to 60-μm dextran beads of the Sephadex type in hylan gel. It is of nonanimal origin. The material is nonimmunogenic, biocompatible, and biodegradable. Intradermal injection is used with a 30-gauge needle. EMLA (eutectic mixture of local anesthetics) or a topical anesthetic can be used. No overcorrection is necessary. The material can be molded after injection to disperse the beads. Usually two injections are required, the second coming 6 weeks after the first. A clinical study of 274 patients showed the material to be resistant to resorption and migration. Results usually last 6 to 9 months. It is not FDA approved. The product is manufactured and distributed by Rofil Medical International B.V., Stationstaat 1B, 4815 NC Breda, The Netherlands. Phone: 31-76-531-5670; FAX: 31-76-531-5660. E-mail: RMI@rofil.nl.

Sculptra. See New-fill.

Silicones are synthetic compounds and do not occur naturally. The liquid silicones used for medical purposes are long polymers of dimethylsiloxane. Siloxane is an acronym used to describe compounds containing repeating units of silicon, oxygen, and methane. **Silicone has a very high use potential, providing pleasing aesthetic results in many patients, but, unfortunately, it also has a high abuse potential. Numerous disastrous complications have resulted from the use of adulterated or impure silicones.** Foreign-body-type silicoma can occur up to 11 years after implantation, even with highly refined, medical-grade silicone and microdroplets. Other reported adverse reactions are movement or drift of the implant, peau d'orange, beading, discoloration, site reactions in 12% to 14% of patients, and immunologic reactions (9). Although injectable silicone has a long history of use in the United States, it has never been approved for use by the FDA.

Nevertheless, two forms of silicone—AdatoSil-5000 and Silikon-1000—were approved as ophthalmic devices for injection into the eye for use as a prolonged retinal tamponade in selected cases of complicated retinal detachment. These are highly viscous agents. Before considering these materials for use, discuss it with your malpractice carrier as to specific laws in your state. AdatoSil is not available except on a case-by-case basis for retinal detachment. It is available from Bausch & Lomb Surgical, Inc., 180 Via Verde Drive, San Dimas, CA 91773. Phone: 800-338-2020, 813-971-5100. http://www.bausch.com/us/resource/surgical. Silikon-1000 is manufactured by Alcon Laboratories, San Diego, CA. A form of it known as Silskin is being tested in clinical trials by Richard-James Inc. for use in treating lipodystrophy of the face. RJ Development Corp., Centennial Park, 2 Centennial Drive, Peabody, MA 01960. Phone: 978-5932-0666; FAX: 978-532-0034.

PMS-350 achieved CE certification in Europe after 15 years. It is silicone with a viscosity of 350 centistokes. It is indicated for glabellar lines, nasolabial folds, perioral lines, lip augmentation, atrophic disorders, and scars. It is distributed by Vikomed in Germany.

Surgisis is derived from porcine small-intestine submucosa. All cells are removed but the complex acellular matrix is retained. It works as a scaffold for host cells and tissue remodeling. It is available in sheets of various sizes and strengths. No immunologic human rejections or sensitization have been reported, although it is not applicable for patients with a known hypersensitivity to porcine products. The material is available from Cook, Inc., PO Box 489, Bloomington, IN 47402-0489. Phone: 800-468-1379. http://www.cookgroup.com. It is not FDA approved.

Zyderm and **Zyplast Collagen Implants** (ZC-I, ZC-II, and Z-P) are all suspensions of bovine dermal collagen. Processing of the material involves purification, pepsin digestion, and sterilization. Pepsin digestion removes the more antigenic end portions of the bovine collagen molecule (the telopeptides) without disturbing the natural helical structure. The resulting agent is more immunologically compatible with the human host. Zyderm Collagen Implants are all 95% to 98% type I collagen, with the remainder being type III. The products are suspended in phosphate-buffered physiologic saline containing 0.3% lidocaine. ZC-I, the original material, and ZC-II differ only in concentration.

In 1981, after 6.5 years of development, clinical trials, and testing, Zyderm Collagen Implant received FDA approval. This was the first time an injectable xenogenic agent was FDA-approved for soft-tissue augmentation.

It should be noted that these substances are all developed from the skin of a closed American herd, negating the possibility of contamination with the bovine spongiform encephalopathy virus or prion. ZP is the third form of implantable collagen. In ZP, bovine dermal collagen is lightly cross-linked by the addition of 0.0075% glutaraldehyde. As a result of this cross-linkage, ZP is more resistant to proteolytic degradation and less immunogenic. All the products are provided in preloaded syringes, which are stored at low temperature (39.2°F [4°C]) so that the suspended fibrils remain fluid and small. This allows passage of the products through small-gauge needles. Once implanted, the human body temperature causes the products to undergo consolidation into a solid gel as intermolecular cross-linking occurs in the injected suspension with the generation of a high proportion of larger fibrils.

Indications for ZC-I/ZC-II include horizontal forehead lines, glabellar lines, crow's-feet, nasolabial lines, fine lip lines, marionette lines, shallow acne scars, and excisional scars. Soft, distensible, superficial defects and lines are most amenable to ZC-I and ZC-II. Deep nasolabial folds, marionette grooves, deep acne scars, and the like respond best to ZP with or without ZC-I/ZC-II overlay. ZP was developed to correct deeper defects often unresponsive to ZC-I. ZP is also best suited to resurface the vermilion border between the lip and skin for lip enhancement. Additionally, true mucosal injection of ZC-I, ZC-II, and ZP is often employed in the lip-enhancement process, although the mucosa is not an FDA-approved site for collagen implantation. ZP is not recommended for use in the glabellar frown lines.

Proper patient screening and, especially, skin testing are of supreme importance in bovine-collagen therapy. Individuals who have lidocaine sensitivity, a history of an anaphylactoid event, or previous sensitivity to bovine collagen are excluded from testing and treatment. Potential allergenicity to injectable collagen is reliably determined by skin testing. Most authorities now recommend a second test as an additional precaution (10).

Zyderm Collagen is implanted in the superficial dermis by serial punctures of the skin with syringes prefilled with the material. ZP works best when placed at a mid-dermal level using a 30-gauge needle at a 10- to 20-degree angle from the skin's surface.

A review of the procedure of lip augmentation by six investigators revealed that the best results were achieved by first injecting ZP in the potential space between the lip mucosa and skin (along the vermilion border) in the upper and lower lip. This was then followed by injecting ZC-I or ZP directly into the mucosa itself. The major vascular supply to the lips runs in the mucosa and blind injections of ZP into this area occasionally will result in vascular events, especially after the lips are repeatedly treated.

Correction with Zyderm/Zyplast collagen is temporary and requires periodic maintenance at 4- to 12-month intervals (11).

Adverse treatment responses to injectable collagen can be divided into nonhypersensitive and hypersensitive. Nonhypersensitive reactions include bruising, reactivation of herpetic eruptions, and bacterial infection. Additionally, local necrosis as a result of vascular interruption at the treatment site has been noted with ZP, but rarely with ZC-I/ZC-II. Two reports of partial vision loss after Zyderm collagen therapy have been noted (12).

Treatment-associated hypersensitivity reactions to bovine collagen implants are, for the most part, cosmetic and consist of redness and swelling at the treatment site. Rarely, mild systemic symptoms can accompany these reactions. Hypersensitive reactions are almost always associated with anti-Zyderm antibodies. These antibodies do not cross-react with human collagen. Cyst-abscess formation is a rare but severe hypersensitivity response. These reactions are usually associated with ZP, but rarely with ZC-I/ZC-II. Zyderm/Zyplast is available from Inamed Aesthetics, 5540 Ekwill Street, Santa Barbara, CA 93111. Phone: 800-766-0171, 805-683-6761; FAX: 805-967-5839. http://www.inamed.com; http://www.inamed.com/products/facial/us/physician/zz/prodinfo.html.

LOOKING AHEAD

Efforts to develop the perfect soft-tissue augmentation material continue. In the years since approval of the first form of injectable collagen, information regarding materials, technique, and indications has continued to evolve. This process is ongoing and will continue as newer formulations become available and the existing products are re-evaluated. New products and techniques are constantly evolving and appearing. The choice of implant material should be based on the location of the defect, potential for hypersensitivity reaction, desire for permanency, and the patient's feelings about the need for a "natural feel" or the implant. An encyclopedia of substances is available to choose from. Of course, safety should be the primary concern when using any implant material. As newer products develop, the methods of soft-tissue enhancement will continue to change, hopefully bringing improved results to patients.

Cosmetically oriented physicians have developed a greater understanding that to achieve the best aesthetic result, the three-dimensional aspects of the face must be preserved. **However, as physicians and guides for our patients, we must resist jumping on the bandwagon of every new fad or implant material that comes along. Although one must be familiar with all of the techniques, materials, and options, it is preferable to become very proficient with two or three different methods so that our patients can be given options with which we have experience.**

References

1. Knapp TR, Kaplan EN, Daniels JR. Injectable collagen for soft tissue augmentation. *Plast Reconstr Surg.* 1977;60:389.
2. Kaminer M, Krause M. Filler substances in the treatment of facial aging. *Med Surg Dermatol.* 1998;5:215–221.
3. Cohen SR, Holmes RE. Artecoll: a long-lasting injectable wrinkle filler material. Report of a controlled, randomized, multicenter clinical trial of 251 subjects. *Plast Reconstr Surg.* 2004;114(4):964–976.
4. Ersek RA, Beisang AA. Bioplastique: a new textured copolymer microparticle promises permanence in soft-tissue augmentation. *Plast Reconstr Surg.* 1991;87:693–702.
5. Lassus C. Expanded PTFE in the treatment wrinkles. *Aesthetic Plast Surg.* 1991;15:167–174.
6. Maas CS, Eriksson T, McCalmont T, et al. Evaluation of ePTFE as a soft tissue filling substance: an analysis of design-related implant behavior employing the porcine skin model. *Plast Reconstr Surg.* 1998;101:1307–1314.
7. Burres S. Recollagenation of acne scars. *Dermatol Surg.* 1996;22:364–367.
8. Teimourian B. Blindness following fat injections [letter]. *Plast Reconstr Surg.* 1988;82(2):361.
9. Ellenbogen R, Ellenbogen R, Rubin L. Injectable fluid silicone therapy: human morbidity and mortality. *JAMA.* 1975;234:308–309.
10. Klein AW. In favor of double testing. *J Dermatol Surg Oncol.* 1989;15:263.
11. Klein AW. Indications and implantation techniques for the various formulations of injectable collagen. *J Dermatol Surg Oncol.* 1988;14(Suppl 1):27–30.
12. McGraw R, et al. Sudden blindness secondary to injection of common drugs in the head and neck. Part 1: clinical experiences. *Otolaryngology.* 1978;86:147.

CHAPTER 46 ■ BOTULINUM TOXIN

MICHAEL A.C. KANE

Injections of botulinum toxin A are the most frequently performed cosmetic procedure in the United States. The change from little-known specialty drug used by ophthalmologists to the most frequent cosmetic procedure occurred in just over a decade. Despite widespread use, the toxin is still not completely understood and poorly used by many physicians. The paradox is not hard to understand when one considers the time allotted to teaching the various components of plastic surgery during residency training. Whereas years are spent teaching the finer points of rhytidectomy, blepharoplasty, rhinoplasty, and liposuction, only an afternoon, or perhaps 1 or 2 days, is typically spent teaching proper technique for botulinum type A injection. In 2003, more botulinum type A injections were performed than rhytidectomy, blepharoplasty, rhinoplasty, and liposuction *combined*.

Dr. Alan Scott, an ophthalmologist, pioneered the use of botulinum toxin type A in humans. His first publication, detailing the effect on rhesus monkeys appeared in 1973 (1); his first publication concerning the injection of the toxin into humans was published in 1980 (2). For years, the toxin was an effective, although seldom used, medication for blepharospasm and strabismus. Rare anecdotal reports of its use for wrinkle reduction are in existence (3). The first comprehensive report detailing cosmetic applicability was published by the Carruthers, an ophthalmologist/dermatologist team, in 1992 (4). This study reported the effects of the toxin on glabellar rhytides in 18 patients. Although the glabellar muscles are still the most commonly injected muscles for cosmetic reasons, every mimetic muscle of the face has been treated with the toxin, with varying success.

MECHANISM OF ACTION

The mechanism of action of the toxin has been carefully researched, but is often misstated. Because botulism is still a serious health threat throughout undeveloped nations and because sporadic outbreaks still occur in the United States, hundreds of publications by many different specialties are generated each year concerning botulinum toxin. The toxin is a fully sequenced, 1,295 amino acid chain. It consists of a heavy chain of 97 kilodaltons (kDa) connected by a disulfide bond to a light chain of 52 kDa. The heavy chain binds to the neuronal cell membrane, allowing passage of the light chain into the cytoplasm of the nerve. The light chain is a metalloprotease that cleaves the protein known as SNAP-25 (synaptosomal-associated protein 25). SNAP-25 is necessary for the transmitter vesicle containing acetylcholine with the cell membrane. **Without fusion of the vesicle with the cell membrane, the neurotransmitter cannot be released into the synapse and a presynaptic neural blockade is created.** Consequently, the toxin does not directly affect the skin. Clearly, it only indirectly affects the

muscle, which loses its stimulus. Properly stated, it only directly affects the nerve.

Clinically, the beneficial effects of the toxin are apparent for 3 to 6 months. However, when carefully scrutinized, it typically takes 6 to 7 months for all of the clinical effects to fade. As patients continue to have the toxin injected on a regular basis over 2 or more years, many note an increased duration of botulinum toxin (Botox) action (5).

The fact that botulinum toxin A disrupts such a basic pathway leads to its efficacy in treating a wide range of states. Any pathologic condition mediated by acetylcholine release from a peripheral nerve has the potential to be treated. As of this writing, there are more than 200 different conditions reported in the scientific literature that can be treated with the toxin, including blepharospasm, strabismus, cervical dystonia, torticollis, achalasia, spasmodic dysphonia, anal fissure, writer's cramp, parkinsonian tremor, spasm of sphincter of Oddi, synkinesis, hyperhidrosis, migraine headache, tetanus, and cerebral palsy.

APPLIED MECHANISM OF ACTION

Because the toxin acts on presynaptic nerve terminals, it is most commonly injected into the muscle where these terminals reside. It is not an all-or-nothing phenomena. A certain amount of toxin will block a certain number of terminals. Thus, fine control over the amount of denervation desired is possible. Despite the common use of the word paralysis when discussing the toxin, it is rare that this is the desired effect. Rather, a selective weakening of the musculature is performed to achieve a pleasant cosmetic effect.

Facial aging consists of many components. Thinning of the dermis, elastosis, loss of facial volume, genetic factors, gravity, skeletal changes, smoking, and so on all play a part in the aging process. So does facial animation. Certain rhytides are primarily caused by facial movement. **As long as a wrinkle is caused or partially caused by muscular action, it can be treated with botulinum toxin A.** This explains why nearly all facial rhytides are able to be treated by the toxin with varying degrees of success. For instance, a glabellar rhytid is nearly completely caused by the actions of the corrugator and procerus muscles and can be completely eradicated in a young patient. Vertical lip rhytides in an elderly woman with thin skin, sun damage, a history of smoking, and loss of lip volume can only be partially improved by careful injection of the toxin into the orbicularis oris muscle, which contributes to the accordionlike scrunching of the overlying lip skin. How well a rhytid responds to treatment with the toxin depends on how much of the rhytid is a result of factors other than animation. Although this chapter is primarily concerned with alterations in animation, it is the overlying skin's ability to resist these forces that is paramount when discussing rhytides.

BOTULINUM TOXINS AND PREPARATION

The *Clostridium botulinum* bacteria secretes eight distinguishable exotoxins (6). The most potent of these serotypes is A. Both toxins A (Botox, Allergan, Irvine, CA) and B (Myobloc, Elan) are available in the United States. Botox is currently approved for the treatment of glabellar furrows in patients age 65 years and younger. All other applications described in this chapter are off-label uses. Another preparation of botulinum toxin type A, available outside of the United States, is called Reloxin (Medicus, Scottsdale, AZ) and is not currently FDA approved. Myobloc (toxin B) is not approved for cosmetic purposes. It has a relatively minor role for cosmetic, off-label applications. Toxin B also exerts its effect via a presynaptic neural blockade but via a different mechanism. It does not act on SNAP-25; instead it acts on synaptobrevin. **Although the onset of action is faster than that of Botox, the increased pain on injection (it is supplied premixed in a vial with a relatively low pH of 5.6) and decreased duration of action limit its cosmetic usefulness.** I currently use Myobloc in isolated instances such as when a patient has a social event within the 3 to 4 days it takes to see some clinical effect of Botox (Myobloc typically takes 6 to 8 hours for clinical effectiveness), for full-face laser resurfacing, and for lower-face scar revision. In the latter two examples, the shorter duration of action is a benefit as the area is relatively motionless during the early healing phase yet prolonged, unattractive facial weakness is avoided.

Botox injection is contraindicated in disorders of neuromuscular transmission, such as myasthenia gravis and Lambert-Eaton syndrome. It should not be used in patients taking aminoglycoside antibiotics whose use may potentiate the effects of the toxin. Although there is no evidence to suggest teratogenicity, I do not treat pregnant women, women actively attempting to become pregnant, or those who are breast-feeding. The toxin does not cross the blood–brain barrier. Complications may occur from drift of the toxin to adjacent muscles, thereby weakening them. This is especially hazardous when injecting the perioral musculature. Other complications include headache, ecchymosis, and eyelid ptosis.

Botox is supplied as a freeze-dried crystalline complex in a vial containing 100 units. The preparation also contains 0.5 mg of human albumin and 0.9 mg of sodium chloride. The preparation is reconstituted with sodium chloride. According to the labeling of the product, it should be mixed with 2.5 mL of nonpreserved saline. In clinical practice, there is a wide variation of reconstitution formulas based on personal preference. I am aware of practitioners using from 1.0 to 10.0 mL of either preserved or nonpreserved saline. The potential advantage of preserved saline is that the preservative, benzyl alcohol, is a mild local anesthetic. I have used 4 mL of nonpreserved saline since 1991.

DOSAGE

Just as dilution of Botox is a personal choice, so is dosage in most circumstances. Different muscles in different people have different strengths. To have a standard dose per area or muscle group makes about as much sense as having a standard amount of fat to remove during liposuction. Every patient is different and requires a different dose placed differently across the muscle being treated. For example, most practitioners inject about 25 units, on average, per glabella. Some dermatologists advocate as much as 80 units. My median dose is 17.5 units, but some patients have excellent results with as little as 7.5 units and some require as much as 27.5 units. Men typically require higher doses as the muscle mass tends to be greater.

I refer to doses in the following text with the reservation that it is up to each injector to determine the optimum dosage for an individual patient.

FUNCTIONAL ANATOMY

The difference between a proficient Botox injector and a technician is an understanding of the functional anatomy of the face. Anatomy texts demonstrate the location of the facial muscles. Although these texts allow for anatomic variations, they do not prepare us for the overwhelming differences in functional anatomy between individuals. A classic example is Rubin's description of the different smile patterns (7). Even though all individuals have the same mimetic muscles, their smile patterns vary tremendously, depending on which muscles dominate within the group. Even within a single muscle, different portions of that muscle may dominate and alter animation. The key is a careful analysis of each patient's face to discern which muscles cause unaesthetic lines or shaping of the face.

GLABELLA

The glabella was the first area to be treated cosmetically with Botox. As with the other areas of the upper face to be treated with Botox, there was a longstanding surgical procedure upon which this treatment was based. The glabellar musculature is commonly debulked during browlift procedures to ease glabellar furrowing and to reduce downward pull on the brow. Chemodenervation of these muscles has the same effect. My median dose for treating the corrugator and procerus muscles is 17.5 units for women and 20 units for men.

Even in a relatively straightforward area of the face such as the glabella, there is a great deal of variation in functional anatomy. When most people frown, they bring their brows together and down. In some patients, however, the brow's movement is mostly vertical, whereas in others it is mostly horizontal.

After observing a patient through normal animation, I ask the patient to frown, relax, frown again, and then scrunch the nose as if smelling something unpleasant. The injection pattern varies depending on the frowning pattern. Horizontal frowners are not injected in the procerus muscle. Vertical frowners are injected in the medial portion of the corrugator and procerus muscles.

FOREHEAD

The frontalis muscle is injected to weaken the forehead to relieve horizontal forehead rhytides. The frontalis also has highly variable functional anatomy. My dosage range for the frontalis is 3.75 to 35.0 units, although most fall within the range of 5.0 to 7.5 units. **Care must be taken to not overly denervate the frontalis because it can lead to an overly smooth, artificial appearance, brow ptosis, and eyelid ptosis in the patient who has been using his frontalis as an accessory eyelid elevator.** Despite its appearance in most anatomy texts, the frontalis is usually continuous across the forehead, with muscle present even in the midline.

After the patient is observed in normal animation, the patient is asked to raise and lower the brows several times, almost to the point of exhaustion. Upon observation of the motion, the strongest portions of this muscle are targeted, not the rhytides. No standard pattern of injection is used.

CROW'S FEET AND LOWER EYELID

The lateral and inferior orbicularis oculi is weakened to diminish crow's feet and lower eyelid rhytides in selected patients. The effects of surgically weakening the lateral orbicularis had been known for several years prior to the cosmetic use of Botox injections (8). The confluence of the crow's feet and lower-lid rhytides and the fact that they are both created by the same muscle makes concomitant treatment appropriate. The functional anatomy of this area leads to a classification of crow's feet patterns (9). The most common pattern is the full-fan pattern where the lateral orbicularis contracts and wrinkles the overlying skin from the lateral brow to the lower lid–upper cheek junction; yet even this pattern occurs in less than half of all patients. The exact incidence of each pattern is not as important as the recognition that different patterns exist and that asymmetry occurs in individual patients.

This is an area where overzealous injection can yield an unpleasant deer-in-the-headlights appearance and even cheek ptosis. **Although most plastic surgeons are aware that the upper lateral orbicularis oculi is a brow depressor, many fail to realize that the lower lateral portion of the muscle is an important cheek elevator.** If overly denervated in its lower lateral section, malar flattening, as well as an extra "roll" of skin between the lower lid and cheek, can occur. Excessive chemodenervation of the orbicularis oculi across the lower lid can cause ectropion or lower-lid retraction. In the patient with minimal to borderline orbital fat prolapse, weakening the middle lamella can exaggerate and hasten the appearance of fat "bags" of the lower lids. Thus these areas are injected judiciously.

Although there are no standard doses or dosing patterns, most patients receive between 3.75 and 5.0 units per side. The key is to not waste your injection on relatively adynamic sections of the muscle. To do this, one must recognize that the functional anatomy of the lateral periorbita varies widely. I inject the most dynamic area of the muscle first, followed by smaller injections radiating out from this point. The idea is to create a gradient of motion so as not to have an area of no motion directly bordering an area of extreme, compensatory motion. This produces an unattractive line of demarcation.

BROW ELEVATION

Botox can easily and reliably lift the brows in excess of 6 mm. The concept is a simple one. To lift the brows, one concentrates on injecting muscle segments that depress the brows. An additional concept is involved that is not simple. Nonweakened sections of muscle react to weakened sections by increasing their pull in a compensatory fashion. This explains why lateral orbicularis injection can cause lower-lid rhytides to increase. This is not simply an illusion as a result of smoothing of the skin laterally, but a real phenomenon caused by an increase in tone of the noninjected portion of the muscle. When the central frontalis is injected strongly, the lateral brows will often peak in an unattractive "Mr. Spock" appearance, with concomitant worsening of lateral suprabrow rhytides. When portions of the frontalis are weakened, the other portions of the frontalis lift more strongly. To maximize brow lift, injecting the portions of the frontalis not responsible for raising brows will induce the frontalis responsible for brow elevation to pull harder. Usually this means injecting the frontalis strongly centrally, in the zone above and medial to the brows. The frontalis lateral to the brows is also injected, causing the frontalis directly over the brows to lift more strongly. Although the frontalis directly above the brows is responsible for brow elevation, the lower frontalis is more responsible than the upper frontalis. Thus,

occasionally, the upper frontalis above the brows is also weakened to increase the action of the lower frontalis.

There are 11 muscle segments that can depress the medial brow: the procerus, transverse heads of the corrugator, oblique heads of the corrugator, depressor supercilii, medial orbicularis oculi, and in some patients, the nasalis muscles. In most patients, the effect of the nasalis on brow position is negligible. However, in a small number of patients, I have fully injected the other medial brow depressors and been disappointed in the ensuing brow elevation. With the other segments completely nonfunctional, these patients were able to depress their brows by wrinkling their nasalis. Subsequent nasalis injection gave the brows additional elevation.

The lateral brow is depressed by the cephalic portion of the lateral orbicularis oculi. The dynamics of this phenomenon differ greatly among patients, and thus there is no single point that can be injected to reliably elevate the lateral brow. In fact, in some patients, this muscle is not a reliable brow depressor, and injecting it will not raise the brow. The problem is to determine whose brows can be elevated and what portion of the muscle should be injected. With the head in neutral position and primary gaze, the patient is asked to smile repeatedly and forcefully. When doing this, some patients will not depress their lateral brow at all. These patients will not reliably achieve brow elevation by simply injecting the upper lateral orbicularis. Patients who do depress their brows are studied carefully and then injected in the portion of the muscle that is pulling downward on the lateral brow. Sometimes this is at the lateral tail of the brow, sometimes directly beneath the brow more medially. **Treatment is individualized based on each patient's functional anatomy.**

There is no standard pattern of injection for brow elevation. For a more medial brow elevation, the medial depressors are eliminated and the lateral frontalis is weakened, leaving the medial frontalis strong. For a more lateral elevation, the lateral depressor and the medial frontalis are injected. For a peaked and arched brow, the lateral depressor is weakened and the frontalis over the junction of the middle and lateral third of the brow is left strong. For men, a wider band of frontalis is left working to raise the brows while keeping them flat. For a unilateral brow lift, in addition to the zones not directly over the brows, the frontalis is weakened slightly over the higher brow, inducing the frontalis over the lower brow to pull harder.

THE NECK

Botox injections in platysmal bands can yield excellent results. Two articles on neck injection were published simultaneously in 1999 with drastically different dosage, patient populations, results, and complications (10,11). One paper advocated up to 250 units be injected, noted that patients received a lift of the lower face, had better results in patients with greater skin laxity, and reported dysphagia as a complication (10). I would caution against injecting such high doses in the neck. In addition to dysphagia, high doses can also lead to dry mouth by affecting the salivary glands.

The key to evaluating the neck as a potential site for cosmetic improvement lies in the relative contributions of the skin and the platysma to banding. **The best patients have minimal skin excess and relatively strong bands.** Despite the results (based on 1,500 patients) of the aforementioned paper, the patient with lax neck skin is a poor candidate for injection. Even with the bands completely paralyzed, the lax neck skin will continue to hang.

My current dose range is 15 to 35 units for the neck, with most patients receiving around 20 units. The patient is asked to show the lower teeth with teeth clenched. The platysma band becomes apparent and is grasped between the thumb and index finger of the noninjecting hand. The patient is then told to relax and the muscle is injected starting just below the mandibular border and progressing inferiorly to the point at which the band is visible. The horizontal "necklace" rhytides can also be mildly improved by injecting toxin just above and below them.

Good candidates for injection fall into two basic categories. The relatively young (35 to 45 years of age) patient with strong bands and minimal skin laxity is an excellent patient. Likewise the patient of any age who has had a surgical procedure on the neck and has relatively little excess skin and recurrent bands is good candidate. A smaller set of patients, but one that is seen more frequently recently, is the young patient who has had an aggressive fat removal procedure in the neck and now has visible bands.

NASOLABIAL FOLD

Treatment of the nasolabial fold demands appropriate patient selection. In addition, the patient must understand the implications of treatment in this tricky area. The levator labii superioris alaeque nasi muscle is the muscle mainly responsible for the medial nasolabial fold and the final 3 to 4 mm of central upper lip elevation. **Weakening of this muscle results in smoothing of the medial nasolabial fold and a change in the smile pattern of the patient.** Rubin described the three major smiling patterns in 1974. The most common, or "Mona Lisa," smile pattern is dominated by the zygomaticus muscle and elevates the oral commissures to the highest point of the smile. The canine smile pattern is dominated by the levator labii superioris and the highest part of the smile is the central upper lip. This pattern occurs in 35% of the population and they are the potential candidates for this procedure. Because injection of the levator labii superioris alaeque nasi muscle results in a drop of the central upper lip upon smiling, it converts canine smilers into Mona Lisa smilers. Injecting Mona Lisa smile patients results in an exaggerated Mona Lisa smile that most patients find unattractive.

Patients with gummy smiles demonstrate extreme canine smile patterns. This group benefits the most from Botox injection (12). Gummy smilers often smile asymmetrically, requiring asymmetric injection. They also tend to have deeper medial nasolabial folds, which is the area of primary improvement with this technique. The resulting drop of the upper lip hides the gingiva and results in a more pleasing smile.

The technique for this injection is relatively straightforward. Before injection, the patient is given a preview of the proposed change. The patient looks into a mirror at eye level and smiles. Using a cotton applicator stick, I push the upper lip down 3 to 4 mm, giving the patient a rough approximation of the change to be expected to the smile and to the nasolabial fold. For injection, the index finger of the noninjecting hand is pressed firmly against the inferior portion of the nasal bone where it meets the maxilla. Thus, half of the finger is falling into the pyriform aperture while the other half lies in the groove between the nasal bone and maxilla. The patient is then asked to smile strongly. The levator labii superioris alaeque nasi muscle can usually be felt just lateral to this groove. It is injected once on each side, just above the periosteum. My dose range for this muscle is 5.0 to 17.5 units total, with most patients falling in the 5.0 to 7.5 unit range. This technique changes the functional anatomy of the patient by changing their smile pattern.

PERIORAL LINES

The perioral rhytides are a common area of complaint for many patients. The radially oriented rhytides are brought about by

intrinsic aging of the skin (dermal thinning, sun damage, smoking), a loss of volume over time, and forced wrinkling of the skin caused by its densely adherent underlying muscle, the orbicularis oris. The most common rejuvenative procedure for this area is the injection of filler materials. Injection of collagen or hyaluronic acid into the lip improves the rhytides, restores lost volume, and offers immediate results with negligible recovery time. However, Botox is an increasingly effective rejuvenate modality for several different patient populations. First, there is the patient group that is already having Botox injected into other areas of the face and asks if Botox could help their lip lines as well. A second group wants improvement of their wrinkles but is adamant about not increasing the size of their lips at all, for fear of looking "done." The third, and largest group, receives concomitant Botox and filler injection. **The filler material partially obliterates the wrinkles and restores volume while the Botox relieves some of the force applied to the skin from the underlying orbicularis oris.** In this way, combined with skin care, the patient receives the maximal amount of improvement without forced downtime. In the patient with severe perioral rhytides, maximal rhytid improvement using fillers alone would necessitate injecting high volumes, which would be unaesthetic. For combination therapy, the lip is injected with a filler material up to the point where the lip would look "done." Botox is then used to weaken the orbicularis oris. If a filler material containing a local anesthetic is used, the filler is injected first.

The patient is asked to purse the lips, then relax, and purse again, repeatedly. This is done to judge the relative strength of the sphincter muscle. Beware the elderly patient with severe rhytides and decreased muscle mass. **My current dosing range is only 2 to 7 units per lip, with most patients receiving 2.0 to 3.75 units per lip.** As opposed to other areas of the face where precise, small drops of Botox are injected, this area is injected broadly to effect a diffuse, general weakening of the sphincter. The philtrum is rarely injected as it rarely contains strong rhytides. A more dilute solution is used. The extra volume allows more even placement of the Botox. The needle is inserted parallel to the vermilion border, a few millimeters above it, and the Botox is injected as the needle is withdrawn. The upper and lower lips can be treated in the same session. Complications can easily result in this area and are usually a result of overinjection. **Overly weakening the upper lip leads to problems with plosive sounds, then general speech, and, finally, oral competence. Overinjection of the lower lip more readily leads to drooling and competence problems.**

MENTALIS

Patients who have difficulty with oral competence tend to form an unattractive, dimpled pattern on the chin during active speech or when closing the lips. This appearance results from contraction of the underlying mentalis muscle. Dimpling and occasional ridging of the skin in patients with hypertrophy of the mentalis can result. This pattern of mentalis strain is particularly common in patients with vertical maxillary excess (gummy smilers), the same patients who benefit from levator labii superioris injection.

Dosing range for the mentalis is 2.5 to 12.5 units, with most patients in the 5.0 to 7.5 units range. Care is taken to inject the superficial mentalis only, leaving the deep mentalis fully functional. The needle is threaded cephalad, parallel to the skin surface, aiming for the plane between the superficial muscle and its overlying fascia. Care must be taken to leave enough of the deep muscle functional so that lower lip elevation and oral competence is maintained. Injection of the mentalis is often paired with depressor anguli oris injection to maintain the height of the lower lip.

DEPRESSOR ANGULI ORIS

The depressor anguli oris is a triangularly shaped muscle that depresses the oral commissures. This action contributes to the marionette lines and often creates a distinct horizontal rhytid below the commissure. Injection of this muscle raises the oral commissures, decreasing show of the lower dentition when smiling. It also helps to improve marionette lines and the horizontal crease below the commissure.

My current dosage range for this area is between 2.5 and 12.5 units total, with most patients falling in the 5.0 to 7.5 units range. The patient is repeatedly asked to show the lower teeth with the dentition occluded. This usually creates a horizontal rhytid below the commissure. Each muscle is injected twice, with the first injection point at the level of the horizontal rhytid. The second point is midway between the first point and the lower border of the mandible in the direction that the muscle pulls the commissure when contracting. Most patients pull the commissures down and laterally when contracting. Some patients, however, will pull their commissures down and medially. It is along this axis of motion that the second injection is placed. **Care must be taken not to attempt to inject this muscle in its cephalad portion as has been taught previously.** First, there is very little active muscle there as the muscle tapers and becomes aponeurotic. Second, the muscle that is there, the lower orbicularis oris, does not tolerate concentrated injections laterally. This can easily lead to oral incompetence and drooling. When properly injected, the depressor anguli oris is one of the safest muscles to inject in the lower face as even if it is slightly over injected, it does not lead to oral incompetence, but rather, an actual raising of the lower lip. In fact, if a patient has oral competence problems from injection of the lower orbicularis oris or mentalis or facial nerve injury, injection of the depressor anguli oris can give them relief. Injection of the lower lip with a viscous hyaluronic acid product at the same time can also add some static support.

HYPERHIDROSIS

Botox injection can also decrease secretion of the eccrine glands in the axillae, palms, and soles of the feet. Care must be taken to inject the Botox intradermally in the palms and soles to minimize the risk of weakening the muscles of the hands and feet. Results for this application typically last somewhat longer, approximately 6 months.

SURGICAL COMPLICATIONS

Complications from aesthetic surgical procedures can often be treated with Botox. Incomplete corrugator or procerus resection after browlift is an ideal indication. If excessive downward muscle pull on the brows is seen in the early postoperative period, it can be treated aggressively, maintaining brow elevation. Surgical misadventures with chin augmentation can lead to mentalis disinsertion and dimpling of the chin, which can be ameliorated by Botox. Overly elevated brows after browlift can be lowered with aggressive frontalis injection. Prolonged spasm of the pectoralis major after breast augmentation can be treated with injection of the portion of the muscle. Facial nerve injuries after surgery or trauma can often be effectively masked by weakening the unaffected muscle on the contralateral side of the face. Marginal mandibular nerve injury after facelift can be disguised by injection of the contralateral depressor anguli oris muscle.

References

1. Scott AB, Rosenbaum A, Collins CC. Pharmacologic weakening of extraocular muscles. *Invest Ophthalmol Vis Sci.* 1973;12:924–927.
2. Scott AB. Botulinum toxin injection into extraocular muscles as an alternative to strabismus surgery. *Ophthalmology.* 1980;87:1044.
3. Clark RP, Berris CE. Botulinum toxin: a treatment for facial asymmetry caused by facial nerve paralysis. *Plast Reconstr Surg.* 1989;84:353.
4. Carruthers JDA, Carruthers JA. Treatment of glabellar frown lines with *Clostridium botulinum* A exotoxin. *Dermatol Surg.* 1992;18:17–21.
5. Kane MAC. *The Long-term Effects of Botox Injections.* The Aesthetic meeting. Dallas, TX: 1998.
6. Osako M, Keltner JL. Botulinum A toxin in ophthalmology. *Surv Ophthalmol.* 1991;36:28–46.
7. Rubin LR. The anatomy of a smile: its importance in the treatment of facial paralysis. *Plast Reconstr Surg.* 1974;53:384.
8. Aston SJ. Orbicularis oculi muscle flaps: a technique to reduce crow's feet and lateral canthal skin folds. *Plast Reconstr Surg.* 1980;65:206.
9. Kane MAC. Classification of crow's feet patterns among Caucasian women: the key to individualizing treatment. *Plast Reconstr Surg.* 2003;112(Suppl):33s.
10. Matarasso A, Matarasso S, Brandt F, et al. Botulinum A exotoxin for the management of platysma bands. *Plast Reconstr Surg.* 1999;103:645.
11. Kane MAC. Nonsurgical treatment of platysmal bands with injection of botulinum toxin A. *Plast Reconstr Surg.* 1999;103:656.
12. Kane MAC. The effect of botulinum toxin injections on the nasolabial fold. *Plast Reconstr Surg.* 2003;112(Suppl):66s.

CHAPTER 47 ■ STRUCTURAL FAT GRAFTING

SYDNEY R. COLEMAN

With the recent recognition of the importance of soft-tissue fillers, fat grafting has assumed an increasingly important roll as both an adjunctive and a primary procedure in aesthetic and reconstructive surgery. However, fat grafting is not new. Surgeons have been grafting fat since 1893 (1). In 1926, Charles Conrad Miller described his experiences with infiltration of fatty tissue through cannulas (2). He believed depositing fat through a hollow metal cannula resulted in a better long-term correction and a more natural-appearing change in facial and body contours than fat grafting through an open incision. Even though Conrad Miller reported good results with the injected fat, the technique he described never became popular.

It was not until 30 years later that Lyndon Peer took a scientific look at fat grafts (3). Using studies of open incision fat grafting, he concluded that approximately 50% of the fat tissue survived after he cut them into small pieces and transplanted them into donor sites. Peer's reports stimulated surgeons to use dermal fat grafts on a limited basis. Interest in fat grafting increased with the advent of liposuction. Liposuction provided plastic surgeons with a valuable byproduct—semiliquid fat that could be grafted with relative ease using a needle or small cannula. Initial reports of fat grafting were discouraging and claimed that grafted fat had a survival similar to injectable collagen (4,5).

In 1986, I began to transplant fat into iatrogenic liposuction deformities and subsequently into faces. Even some of my earliest attempts at fat grafting yielded long-term structural changes that had every indication of permanence. In 1988, I presented my positive experiences with fat grafting at the American Society of Aesthetic Plastic Surgery annual meeting. By 1995, 7 years after one procedure, these same patients demonstrated continued corrections (6). Transplanted fat has the potential to survive as a permanent living graft.

Plastic surgeons now accept the potential longevity of fat. However, many complain that they cannot obtain consistent results. The survival of free autografts of any human tissue (skin, bone, cartilage, cornea) is extremely dependent on the technique used. Likewise, the dependability of grafting fat is related to the technique used to harvest, refine, and transfer the fat.

It is not enough to graft fat so that it survives. The grafted fat must be placed appropriately to accomplish the desired objectives. The surgeon must become familiar with the levels of placement (subdermal, intramuscular, supraperiosteal), and the amounts necessary at each level to accomplish a desirable change. The amounts vary with each part of the face and body, as well as from patient to patient, and a discussion of the subject is beyond the scope of this chapter. However, the subject has been discussed extensively (7–10).

PREPARATION

Determining the amounts to be placed and the levels in which the fat should be placed to create subtle or gross contour changes of the face and body requires a sophisticated plan. The surgeon must evaluate the patient's appearance and be knowledgeable about the patient's lifestyle, expectations, prior aesthetic procedures, and medical history. Patients should be informed of the details of the planned procedure, the expected outcome, and the postoperative course. Of particular importance for structural fat grafting is preparing the patient for the postoperative swelling and bruising.

Photography documents the preoperative appearance and provides guidance for three-dimensional analysis. Physical examination of the face or body is essential to supplement photographic documentation because photographs cannot capture the relationships of underlying structures and the skin. A surgeon grafting fat should have a strategy for placement in order to predict the volumes required, the levels of placement, and the structural support anticipated.

TECHNIQUE

The technique discussed below emphasizes respect for handling tissues and basic sound surgical technique. Fatty tissue is delicate human tissue and can be injured easily outside the body by mechanical, barometric, and chemical insults. For successful transplantation, fat must survive harvesting, transport, and implantation as an intact parcel of tissue composed of connective tissues as well as adipose cells.

Harvesting

I select harvesting sites that are convenient for access and that enhance the patient's contour. The abdomen and medial thighs are the most commonly chosen donor sites. When abdominal or medial thigh fat is in short supply because of prior liposuction or scarcity of body fat, the other potential sites include the suprapubic region, the anterior or lateral thighs, the knees, the lower back, the hips, or the sacrum.

Whenever possible, harvesting sites are accessed through incisions placed in creases, previous scars, stretch marks, or hirsute areas. Meticulous sterile technique is observed with preoperative preparation using antimicrobial scrubs and prep solutions.

Local anesthesia is most commonly used, but epidural or general anesthesia may be preferred for removal of larger volumes or when multiple sites are used for harvesting. In local anesthesia cases, a blunt Lamis infiltrator attached to a

10-mL syringe is used to infiltrate 0.5% lidocaine with 1:200,000 epinephrine into the desired sites. To ensure hemostasis in general or epidural cases, lactate Ringer solution with 1:400,000 epinephrine is infiltrated. In all situations, about 1 mL of solution is infiltrated for every milliliter of fat to be harvested. Superwet or tumescent techniques of the harvested tissue can disrupt the parcels of fatty tissue and decrease survival.

A 15- or 23-cm two-hole Coleman harvesting cannula with a blunt tip and dull distal openings placed extremely close to the end of the cannula is twisted onto a 10-mL Luer-Lok syringe. The distal openings of the harvesting cannula are of an appropriate size and shape for harvesting the largest intact fatty tissue parcels that can readily pass though the lumen of a Luer-Lok syringe. If the fatty tissue parcel can pass through the lumen of the Luer-Lok syringe, it will usually pass through the much smaller (17-gauge) lumen of the infiltration cannula.

After inserting the cannula tip into the donor site, the surgeon pulls back on the syringe plunger to create a small amount of negative pressure within the barrel of the syringe. A 10-mL syringe is small enough to be manipulated manually without locking devices in order to minimize negative pressure. The surgeon pulls back on the plunger of the syringe to create about 1 or 2 mL of space in the barrel of the syringe while the attached cannula is pushed through the harvest site. The combination of slight negative pressure and the curetting action of the cannula's motion through the tissues allows parcels of fatty tissue to move through the cannula, through the Luer-Lok aperture,

and into the barrel of the syringe with minimal mechanical damage.

When filled, the syringe is then disconnected from the cannula and replaced with a "dual-function Luer-Lok plug for capping." After the syringe is sealed at the Luer-Lok end, the plunger is removed from the proximal end of the syringe and the barrel filled with 10 mL of harvested material is placed into a centrifuge.

Refinement and Transfer

Refinement of the harvested subcutaneous tissue into relatively pure fat is crucial for predictable fat grafting. The amount of nonliving components harvested will depend on the quantity of liquid injected by the surgeon, the amount of blood in the harvested specimen, and the damage to fatty cells that releases lipids. Harvested tissue can have as little as 10% viable fat or as much as 90% viable fat, even when coming from the same site during the same operation. To obtain predictable results, most of the oil, blood, and aqueous components must be removed so that the surgeon can know how much of the specimen is viable fat.

To promote sterility, a centrifuge with a sterilizable central rotor and sleeves that hold a 10-mL syringe should be used. The recommended centrifugation speed is 3,000 revolutions per minute for 3 minutes. This separates the denser components from the less-dense components to create multiple layers. The upper level, or the least-dense layer, is

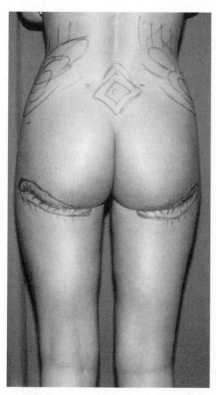 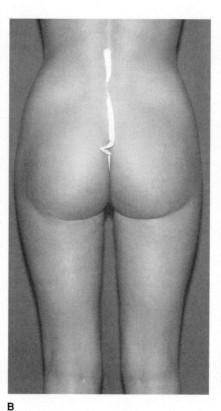 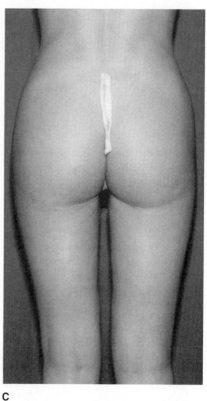

A   B   C

FIGURE 47.1. Fat grafting to correct depressions in buttock creases resulting from liposuction 11 months earlier. The markings in (**A**) demonstrate the areas of removal and placement of fatty tissue. From the love handles and back, 260 mL of fatty tissue was harvested and refined into 183 mL of usable tissue, of which 77 mL was infiltrated into the right buttock crease depression and 105 mL into the left. Comparison of the before (**B**) and 19 months later (**C**) images demonstrates filling of the lateral buttock creases on both sides, as well as expansion of the trochanteric regions.

primarily made up of oil. The middle portion is made up of potentially viable parcels of fatty tissue, and the lowest, most-dense level, is primarily made up of blood, water, and lidocaine.

The oil layer is decanted from the syringe, before the Luer-Lok plug is removed. After the oil is decanted, the Luer-Lok plug can be removed. Neuropads or other highly absorbent materials can be used to wick off the remaining oil from the exposed end of the harvested fat by capillary action. Care should be taken not to allow the material from the wicks to shred off into the refined tissue. After 4 minutes, the wick

can be replaced with another if oil remains. After changing the wick two or three times, the plunger is replaced into the barrel of the 10-mL syringe. This is done by allowing the fat to slide down to the edge of the syringe barrel then advancing the plunger to obliterate the dead space. The fat is then transferred into a 1-mL Luer-Lok syringe. The most efficient manner is to inject the fat directly through the Luer-Lok aperture of the 10-mL syringe into the barrel end of a smaller Luer-Lok syringe. The plunger of the smaller syringe is then replaced. Although 3-mL Luer-Lok syringes can be used for placement into most areas of the body, only 1-mL

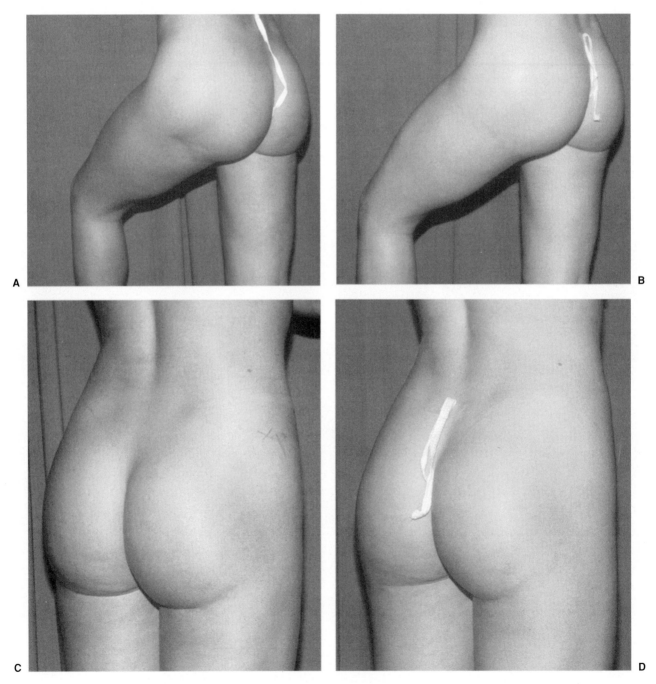

FIGURE 47.2. Lifting the leg in (**A**) demonstrates the depth of the left lateral thigh depression and the correction at 1 year to normal in (**B**). Evaluation of the right buttock crease from the left oblique photo (**C**) demonstrates a significant volume and contour change at 19 months (**D**) with the grafted fat bridging the buttock and thigh.

Luer-Lok syringes should be used for placement into the face and hands.

Placement

The most challenging part of fat grafting is placing the refined fat into a recipient site to encourage uniform survival, stability, and integration into the surrounding tissues. The fatty tissue parcels must be positioned so that they are separated from each other as much as is possible by the host tissues. This creates a larger surface area of contact between the harvested fat and the recipient tissues so that diffusion and respiration can take place.

Anesthesia for placement can be with local anesthesia, regional blocks, and/or general anesthesia. Regardless of which is used, an epinephrine solution is advised for vasoconstriction in the face to minimize the potential for accidental cannulation of arteries or veins (11). The use of a blunt Coleman infiltration cannula is convenient for infiltration of solution into the recipient site and tends to minimize damage to blood vessels and resulting ecchymosis or hematomas.

Placement is best accomplished with a blunt Coleman infiltration cannula with one distal aperture just proximal to the tip. The instruments used for placement of fatty tissue are dramatically different from those used for harvesting—they are of a smaller gauge with only one hole at the distal end. The proximal end of the cannula has a hub, like the harvesting cannula, that fits into a Luer-Lok syringe. The most useful cannula size is 17 gauge. However, larger bore cannulas can be used for corporal fat grafting, and smaller bore cannulas may be appropriate in some instances, such as in the lower eyelids. In the face, 7- and 9-cm cannulas are the most useful; longer cannulas, up to 15 cm, can be useful in the body. For varying situations in the face and body, cannulas with different tip shapes, diameters, lengths, and curves can be used (10).

The use of blunt cannulas is encouraged to allow placement of the fat parcels in a more stable manner. However, less-blunt cannulas give the surgeon more control for placement in the immediately subdermal plane, in fibrous tissue, and in scars. A cannula with pointed or sharp elements can be used to free up adhesions, but care should be taken to avoid damage to nerves and other underlying structures.

Through the same incisions that were used for infiltration of local anesthesia, the infiltration cannula is inserted and advanced through the recipient tissues into the appropriate plane. No fatty tissue should be ejected during the advancement of the cannula. Once the tip of the cannula is placed into the target location, the plunger of the 1-mL syringe is pressed slightly while the cannula is being withdrawn. This deposits fatty tissue in the pathway of the retreating blunt cannula. Unlike the sharp tip of a needle, the blunt tip does not cut a defined channel through the recipient tissues. With the advance of the blunt cannula, the natural tissue planes separate in a somewhat physiologic fashion. As the cannula is withdrawn, the deposited fatty tissue parcels fall into the natural tissue planes as the host tissues collapse around them.

The fatty tissue parcels should be deposited in the desired location, shape, and volume with each pass of the infiltrating cannula so that the surgeon places the fat into the desired shape and volume. Accuracy of this initial placement is important because the infiltrated fatty tissue cannot easily be remodeled afterward. If a cyst or clump forms accidentally, digital manipulation can sometimes flatten minor irregularities. However, the tissue should never be placed with the idea that digital pressure can change the shape after placement.

Separating the parcels of fat one from the other not only increases the chance of survival by placing the newly transplanted fat parcels in greater contact with a source of nutrition and respiration, but also encourages better fat adherence and stability in the new recipient sites. Finally, placing the fat in small parcels and separating every parcel with the donor-site tissues integrates the grafted fat into the tissues. The newly grafted fat feels like the tissue into which it is placed.

Placement of miniscule linear increments is critical to maximizing the surface area of contact and minimizing the potential for irregularities or clumps of tissue. In the face, the largest amount of tissue that should be placed with each withdrawal is 0.1 mL, but in some areas, such as the eyelids, the maximum placed should be closer to 0.03 mL or even 0.02 mL per withdrawal of the cannula.

The end point of placement varies widely between anatomic areas. In the lateral malar cheek and mandibular border, the appearance at the conclusion of infiltration of fat will be similar in shape and size to the final outcome. Conversely, such areas as the lips, eyelids, or hands will be grossly distorted and not resemble the desired outcome for weeks after placement.

Postoperative Care

Placement of fatty tissue as described above will create remarkable swelling in the recipient tissues. The patient should be prepared for a significant recovery period. Even though most patients are presentable at 2 to 4 weeks, they should be prepared for some minimal swelling lasting up to 16 weeks.

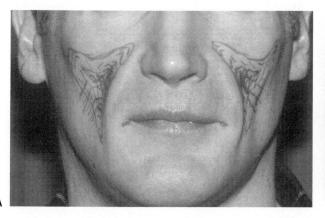
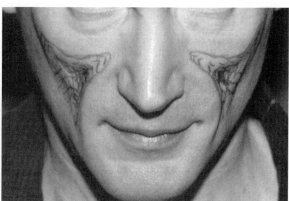

FIGURE 47.3. Markings demonstrate the planned placement of fat into specific areas of facial lipoatrophy without much feathering into the surrounding areas. On the right side of the face, 5.8-mL of fat was placed; 6 mL was placed on the left. (**A**) Anterior view. (**B**) Bird's eye view.

Care after fat transplantation should be aimed at minimizing swelling and stabilizing the area to avoid migration. Elevation, cold therapy, and external pressure with elastic tape help prevent swelling. Other maneuvers, such as holistic medications and electromagnetic therapy, are yet unproven, but may accelerate the resolution of swelling.

COMPLICATIONS

Because structural fat grafting is performed through tiny incisions primarily using blunt cannulas, complications are minimal compared to open aesthetic procedures. Incisions should be placed in a direction and position to minimize the possibility of noticeable scars, and closed with interrupted monofilament sutures. To decrease the possibility of infection, sterile technique should be observed at all times and precautions taken to avoid intraoral or mucosal contamination.

With insertion of even a blunt cannula for removal and placement, it is possible to damage underlying structures such as nerves, muscles, glands, and blood vessels. For that reason sharp needles or cannulas should be used with great caution. Of particular concern with the placement of any filler substance is the cannulation of arteries or veins and intravascular emboli (11). Fortunately, the complication rate with fat grafting is extremely low compared to most open surgical techniques and the incidence of problems decreases dramatically with experience.

The most common complications of fat grafting are related to aesthetic appearance, such as too much or too little fat in a specified area. The next most common problem is the

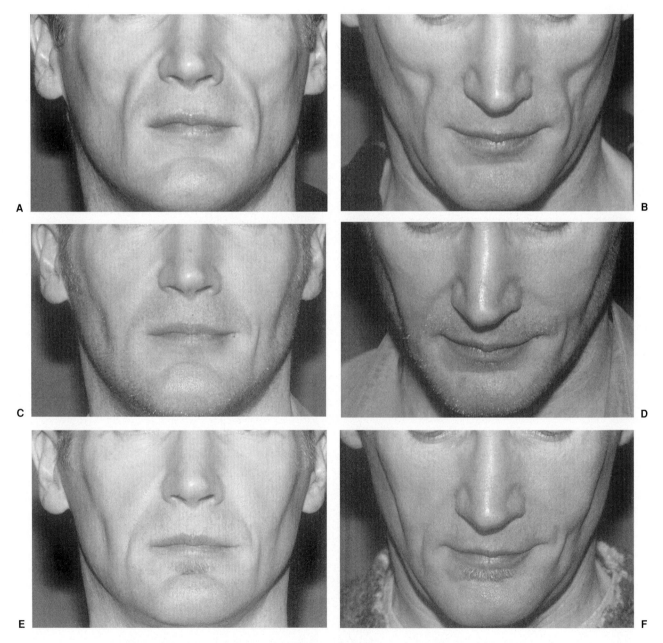

FIGURE 47.4. Same patient as Fig. 47.3 with drug-related lipoatrophy, correction of the anterior malar and buccal regions imparts a much healthier appearance. **A, B:** Before the single procedure. **C, D:** Four months after one treatment. **E, F:** Forty-two months after the procedure with no other treatment. Note that there is almost no difference between the 4-month photographs and the photographs after 42 months. The volume of the fat changes little with this technique after 4 or 5 months.

presence of irregularities, which can be from the intrinsic nature of the patient, from the technique used for placement, and from migration after placement. Irregularities after fat grafting diminish remarkably with experience.

This is a brief summary of some of the more common or noteworthy complications, and a more exhaustive list of potential and experienced complications can be found elsewhere (10).

PATIENT EXAMPLES

The patient examples for this chapter were chosen to represent the simplest application of structural fat grafting: filling a well-defined deficiency to restore a contour to its normal and former appearance.

Patient 1

The first patient is a 22-year-old female who presented 11 months after liposuction to the lateral thighs and buttock creases left her with unnatural-appearing exaggerations of her buttock creases and deep depressions extending into the lateral thighs. Markings (Fig. 47.1A) demonstrate the areas of fat tissue grafting. She is shown before (Fig. 47.1B) and 19 months after one fat grafting procedure (Fig. 47.1C).

In Figure 47.2, note the obvious depression of the lateral thigh and buttock crease that is corrected by placement into the buttock crease. Also note the improvement of the relationship of the lateral buttock with the thigh so that they have a more continuous, flowing, and youthful-appearing relationship. On the oblique view above, the buttock flows smoothly into the thigh in the after photographs. Often the patient will know a maneuver such as lifting the thigh (Fig. 47.2C and D) that best demonstrates the deficiency and resulting correction.

Patient 2

The second example is a 45-year-old healthy male with drug-related facial lipoatrophy of gradual onset. He requested correction of his anterior cheeks only, which were filled with

5.8 mL of fatty tissue on the right and 6 mL on the left in the distribution shown in Figure 47.3. The tissue was harvested from the abdomen, and the refined fat was placed using a Coleman type I cannula from three incisions on each side: a lateral malar incision, an anterior border of the mandible incision, and an incision at the lateral commissure. The volume of the placed fatty tissue seemed to stabilize by about 4 months, and the 4-month appearance appears similar to that at 3.5 years (Fig. 47.4).

CONCLUSION

The key to successful fat grafting is planning and attention to technique. The technique involves the purposeful placement of a specific volume of fat in tiny aliquots that allow a large surface area of contact between the host tissues and the newly grafted tissue. This large surface area of contact not only promotes nutrition and respiration, but also stabilizes the placed fat to deter migration and integrates the fat so that it feels like fullness rather than discrete collections of fatty tissue.

References

1. Neuber F. Fettransplantation. *Bericht uber die Verhandlungen der Dt Ges f Chir Zbl Chir.* 1893;22:66.
2. Miller CC. *Cannula Implants and Review of Implantation Techniques in Esthetic Surgery.* Chicago: The Oak Press; 1926.
3. Peer LA. Loss of weight and volume in human fat grafts. *Plast Reconst Surg.* 1950;5:217.
4. Illouz YG. The fat cell "graft": a new technique to fill depressions [letter]. *Plast Reconstr Surg.* 1986;78:122–123.
5. Ersek RA. Transplantation of purified autologous fat: a 3-year follow-up is disappointing. *Plast Reconstr Surg.* 1991;87:219.
6. Coleman SR. Long-term survival of fat transplants: controlled demonstrations. *Aesth Plast Surg.* 1995;19:421–425.
7. Coleman SR. The technique of periorbital lipoinfiltration. *Oper Tech Plast Reconstr Surg.* 1994;1:120–126.
8. Coleman SR. Structural fat grafts: the ideal filler? *Clin Plast Surg.* 2001;28:111–119.
9. Coleman SR. Hand rejuvenation with structural fat grafting. *Plast Reconstr Surg.* 2002;110(7):1731–1744.
10. Coleman SR. *Structural Fat Grafting.* St. Louis: Quality Medical Publishing; 2004.
11. Coleman SR. Avoidance of arterial occlusion from injection of soft tissue fillers. *Aesth Surg.* 2002;22:555–557.

CHAPTER 48 ■ BLEPHAROPLASTY

MARK A. CODNER AND DEREK T. FORD

The eyes are a focal point in the analysis of upper and midfacial aging. Brow and midfacial rejuvenation have a direct interplay with rejuvenation of the orbital region. For this reason, blepharoplasty is a more complex and challenging procedure than previously thought. It should not be regarded as routine, despite being one of the most commonly performed surgical procedures. Knowledge of periorbital anatomy and the changes associated with aging is paramount. Furthermore, it is required in the correction of complications that may occur after eyelid surgery.

Blepharoplasty is integrated with correction of the brow position and correction of midfacial descent. In the upper lid, the goals include preservation of upper orbital fullness and a defined upper lid crease. In the lower lid, the goals include a smooth transition between the cheek and lid while restoring youthful eye shape. These ideals may require canthal anchoring, periorbital fat preservation or repositioning, and careful anatomical manipulation of the brow and cheek. Less-invasive approaches may be taken in adolescent patients and young adults with fewer age-related anatomical changes.

EYELID ANATOMY

The eyelid is a bilamellar structure (see Chapter 39) comprising an anterior lamella and a posterior lamella. The anterior lamella consists of skin and orbicularis oculi muscle; the posterior lamella includes the tarsoligamentous sling, which is comprised of the tarsal plate and medial and lateral canthal tendons, along with the capsulopalpebral fascia and conjunctiva. The septum originates at the arcus marginalis along the orbital rim and separates the two lamellae (Fig. 48.1).

The Anterior Lamella

The orbicularis oculi muscle lies posterior to the dermis with minimal subcutaneous fat in between. The orbicularis oculi muscle is divided into three components: the pretarsal, preseptal, and orbital divisions (Fig. 48.2). The pretarsal portion of the orbicularis is superficial to the tarsal plate and functions to cause lid closure during involuntary blinking. The pretarsal orbicularis is further subdivided into a superficial and deep head. The preseptal orbicularis also has a superficial and deep component. In addition to voluntary blink, it functions as part of the lacrimal pump for tear drainage. The orbital orbicularis is the largest division of the orbicularis muscle and functions to protect the globe with forced eyelid closure, as well as medial brow depression.

Orbicularis Muscle Innervation

The motor innervation to the orbicularis oculi muscle is quite diffuse with contributions from multiple branches of the facial nerve, including the frontal, zygomatic, and buccal branches (Fig. 48.3). Cadaveric dissection reveals a diffuse network of nerves innervating the orbicularis oculi muscle (Fig. 48.4). Proper lateral canthal anchoring and the preservation of medial buccal branch innervation are important in avoiding lower lid malposition and potential problems with eyelid closure following lower lid blepharoplasty.

The Posterior Lamella and the Tarsoligamentous Structures

While the skin and muscle make up the anterior lamella, the tarsoligamentous sling creates the support structure for the posterior lamella (Fig. 48.5). The tarsal plates constitute the connective tissue framework of the upper and lower eyelids (see Chapter 39). The upper lid tarsal plate is approximately 30 mm horizontally and 10 mm vertically at its widest dimension. Attachments to the upper lid tarsal plate include the pretarsal orbicularis and levator aponeurosis on the anterior surface, the Mueller's muscle on the superior border, and conjunctiva on the posterior surface. The lower lid tarsal plate is approximately 24 mm horizontally and 4 mm vertically. The tarsal plates of the upper and lower eyelid are attached to the orbital rim by the medial and lateral canthal tendons and retinacular support structures.

The lateral canthus also consists of a complex connective tissue framework that functions as an integral fixation point for the lower lid. The lateral canthal tendon, which is approximately 5 mm in length, is formed by the fibrous crura, which connects the tarsal plate to Whitnall's lateral orbital tubercle within the lateral orbital rim. In addition, the lateral retinaculum is formed by ligamentous structures from the lateral horn of the levator aponeurosis, lateral rectus check ligaments, the Whitnall's suspensory ligament, and Lockwood's inferior suspensory ligament, which converge at the lateral canthal tendon (Fig. 48.6).

Retractors of the Upper and Lower Lids

The upper eyelid retractors include the levator palpebrae superioris muscle and Mueller's superior tarsal muscle. The levator muscle is striated muscle and is innervated by the oculomotor nerve (cranial nerve III). The levator muscle originates from the lesser wing of the sphenoid and inserts along the anterior surface of the tarsal plate stabilizing the pretarsal orbicularis muscle. The levator aponeurosis begins at the musculoaponeurotic junction, which is 10 to 14 mm below Whitnall's ligament and 5 to 7 mm above the superior border of the tarsal plate. Mueller's muscle is smooth muscle, which originates from the posterior surface of the levator muscle and inserts into the superior tarsal border. Mueller's muscle is innervated by the sympathetic nervous system. In addition to mechanical dehiscence of the levator aponeurosis, upper lid ptosis can be caused by abnormalities of cranial nerve III causing levator muscle weakness

486

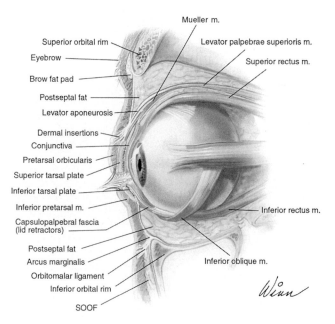

FIGURE 48.1. Cross-sectional anatomy of the eyelids and periorbital region. SOOF, suborbicularis oculi fat.

Labels (Figure 48.1):
Mueller m.
Superior orbital rim
Eyebrow
Brow fat pad
Postseptal fat
Levator aponeurosis
Dermal insertions
Conjunctiva
Pretarsal orbicularis
Superior tarsal plate
Inferior tarsal plate
Inferior pretarsal m.
Capsulopalpebral fascia (lid retractors)
Postseptal fat
Arcus marginalis
Orbitomalar ligament
Inferior orbital rim
SOOF
Levator palpebrae superioris m.
Superior rectus m.
Inferior rectus m.
Inferior oblique m.

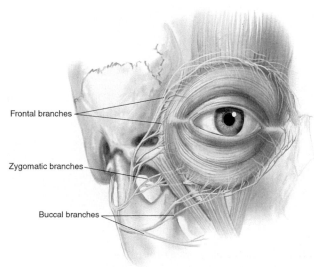

FIGURE 48.3. Innervation of the orbicularis oculi with contributions from the frontal, zygomatic, and buccal branches.

Labels (Figure 48.3):
Frontal branches
Zygomatic branches
Buccal branches

or by loss of sympathetic nerve supply causing Mueller's muscle weakness, resulting in Horner syndrome.

The lower lid retractors include the capsulopalpebral fascia and the inferior tarsal muscle, which are adjacent to each other. The capsulopalpebral fascia originates from the inferior rectus fascia and envelops the inferior oblique muscle. In the lower eyelid, the capsulopalpebral fascia is analogous to the levator aponeurosis in the upper lid, and the inferior tarsal muscle is analogous to Mueller's muscle. Distal to Whitnall's ligament, the levator aponeurosis widens to form lateral and medial horns. The lateral horn divides the lacrimal gland into orbital and palpebral lobes and inserts into the lateral orbital tubercle and lateral retinaculum, as well as the capsulopalpebral fascia of the lower eyelid.

The Orbital Septum

The orbital septum separates the anterior and posterior lamella and helps maintain periorbital fat within the anatomic confines of the orbit. The orbital septum originates from the arcus marginalis of the orbital rim and is discontinuous at the medial canthus. In the upper eyelid, the septum fuses with the levator aponeurosis, approximately 2 to 3 mm above the tarsal plate. In the lower lid, the septum fuses with the capsulopalpebral fascia just below the tarsal plate. There are numerous additional interpad and intrapad septal structures, which

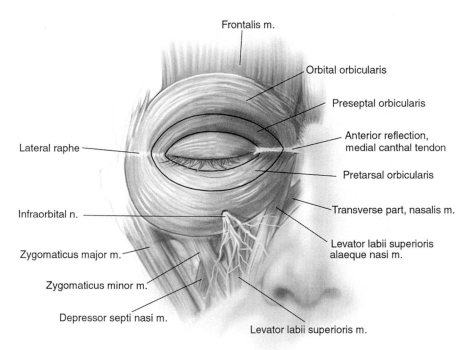

Labels (Figure 48.2):
Frontalis m.
Orbital orbicularis
Preseptal orbicularis
Anterior reflection, medial canthal tendon
Pretarsal orbicularis
Transverse part, nasalis m.
Levator labii superioris alaeque nasi m.
Lateral raphe
Infraorbital n.
Zygomaticus major m.
Zygomaticus minor m.
Depressor septi nasi m.
Levator labii superioris m.

FIGURE 48.2. Anatomy of the orbicularis oculi and surrounding periorbital mimetic muscles.

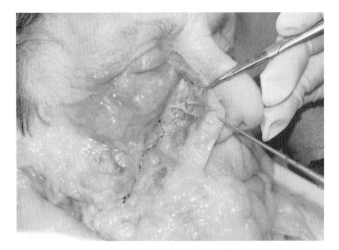

FIGURE 48.4. Cadaver dissection demonstrating buccal branches fusing with the infraorbital nerve with multiple terminal branches to the orbicularis muscle of the upper and lower lid and the procerus.

separate the central from the nasal fat pad in the upper eyelid, and the central from the lateral fat pad in the lower eyelid. Appreciation of the anatomy of the septum is important, particularly when surgical procedures such as resetting, tightening, or excising the septum are considered. Posterior to the orbital septum, the periorbital fat pads play an important role in both upper and lower blepharoplasty (Fig. 48.7). There are two main fat pads in the upper eyelid and three fat pads in the lower eyelid. The two upper fat pads are referred to as the central and nasal fat pads, which are located in the preaponeurotic space just anterior to the levator aponeurosis. The interpad septum separates the central and nasal fat pads and is continuous with a septal fascial connection to the trochlea. The nasal fat pad is more fibrous and is pale in color compared to the central fat pad. The intrapad septum separates the nasal fat into two compartments. The medial palpebral artery is located in the inferior nasal compartment and can contribute to significant

bleeding during blepharoplasty. The central fat pad is superficial to the levator aponeurosis, which is the preaponeurotic space, and contributes to the fullness of the upper lid fold.

The Lacrimal Gland

The lacrimal gland lacks a true capsule and is divided into the orbital and palpebral lobes by the lateral horn of the levator. The orbital lobe is positioned in the fossa glandulae lacrimalis, which is a shallow fossa in the frontal bone at the superolateral orbit. The smaller palpebral lobe is connected to the orbital lobe by an isthmus posterior to the lateral horn of the levator. Lacrimal gland ptosis is caused by dehiscence of the Soemmering ligaments, which are the fibrous interlobular septa that connect the gland to the orbital rim fossa. Fullness in the lateral aspect of the upper eyelid is often caused by lacrimal gland's ptosis. Lateral to the lacrimal gland is a separate compartment just above Whitnall's tubercle. The Eisler fat pad is a small accessory fat pad located in Eisler's pocket, which serves as a useful anatomic landmark for Whitnall's tubercle. The location of this fat pad is clinically useful during placement of the lateral canthoplasty suture.

The Conjunctiva

The most posterior layer of the eyelid is the conjunctival lining, which continues over Tenon's capsule. The palpebral portion of the conjunctiva is closely adherent to the posterior surface of the tarsal plate and the lid retractors. At the fornix, the conjunctiva becomes bulbar conjunctiva overlying the globe to the corneoscleral limbus. Small accessory glands are located within the conjunctiva, creating the aqueous portion of the tear film.

Forehead Anatomy

In the region of the superior and lateral orbit, the forehead is firmly attached to the underlying periosteum (see Chapter 50).

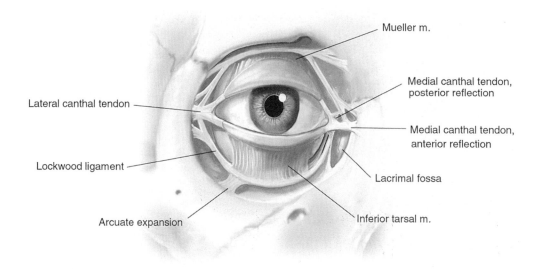

FIGURE 48.5. Anatomy of the deepest structures of the posterior lamella including the tarsoligamentous sling and Mueller's muscle.

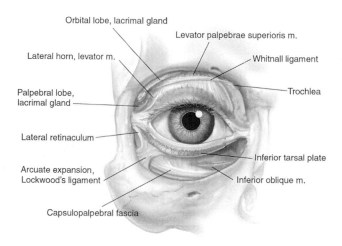

FIGURE 48.6. Anatomy of the more superficial structures of the posterior lamella including the lateral retinaculum and the levator muscle.

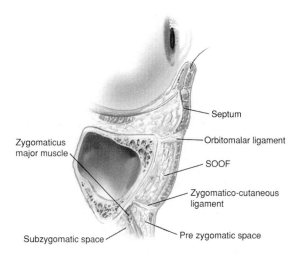

FIGURE 48.8. Cross-sectional anatomy of the midface demonstrating the orbitomalar ligament, the prezygomatic space, and the subzygomatic space. SOOF, suborbicularis oculi fat.

Specifically, in the lateral orbit there is a fibrous fusion between the orbicularis fascia and the underlying periosteum and deep temporal fascia. These attachments must be released and the supraorbital periosteum incised to achieve mobilization of the forehead. The frontalis is a brow elevator and is continuous with the galea aponeurotica. The frontalis inserts into the dermis above the supraorbital rim and upon animation is responsible for transverse forehead furrows.

The orbital orbicularis oculi, depressor supercilii, and the oblique and transverse heads of corrugator and procerus act in synergy to depress the medial brow and produce glabellar furrows. Motor innervation to the frontalis and superior orbicularis oculi is by the frontal branch of the facial nerve. The brow depressors also receive motor innervation from the buccal and zygomatic branches.

Midfacial Anatomy

The anatomy in this region is important to the morphologic changes seen in the lower eyelid–cheek junction with aging. Using cadaveric dissection, Mendelson described the prezygomatic space. The layers of this space include the skin and subcutaneous fat that cover the orbicularis oculi muscle and sub-

orbicularis oculi fat (SOOF). A separate, fixed adipose layer, the preperiosteal fat is found deep to origins of the lip elevator muscles. The upper border of the prezygomatic space is formed by the orbitomalar ligament, a structure that arises from a thickened area of periosteum along the inferior orbital rim and travels through the subcutaneous musculoaponeurotic system (SMAS) and superficial fat to insert into the skin (Fig. 48.8). The orbitomalar ligament along with the levator labii superioris and levator alaeque nasi are responsible for defining the tear trough. With age, there is a herniation of postseptal fat over this ligament. Along with prezygomatic fat ptosis, the region of the tear trough becomes visible as a deep triangular groove between these muscles (Fig. 48.9). The lower border of the prezygomatic space is outlined by the zygomatic ligaments that arise from the origins of the elevator muscles of

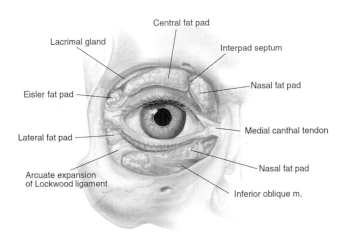

FIGURE 48.7. The orbital fat pads are deep to the septum and are separated by interpad septal extensions.

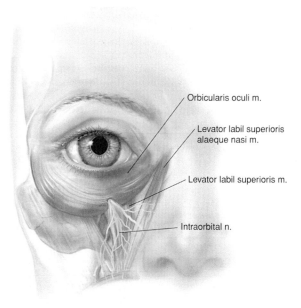

FIGURE 48.9. The tear trough deformity overlies the muscular triangle formed by the orbicularis oculi, the levator labii superioris, and the levator alaeque nasi muscles.

the upper lip. From the skeletal plane, these osteocutaneous ligaments radiate outward to insert into the dermis of the cheek. This prezygomatic space is triangular in shape with the apex being nasal. Malar mounds are the result of edematous fat in the prezygomatic space, which is restricted by the zygomatic ligament. The malar fat pad is a subcutaneous triangular fat pad that contributes to the fullness of the midface and is distinct from the malar mound. Elevation of the malar fat pad and correction of malar mounds require a more aggressive subperiosteal midface lift in order to meet the aesthetic goals.

Surface Orbital Anatomy and Age-Related Changes

The horizontal interpalpebral fissure measures 30 to 31 mm transversely and 8 to 10 mm vertically. The lateral commissure is positioned approximately 2 mm superior to the medial canthal angle, defining an upward lateral canthal tilt. However, the position of the lateral canthus will vary with age, family trait, race, and sex. In primary gaze, the upper eyelid margin forms a smooth arch with the highest point positioned between the medial limbus and the pupil. With age, there is a gradual lateral shift of this point as the tarsal plate migrates laterally as a result of a weakening of the medial levator horn.

The upper eyelid crease is formed by the levator aponeurosis insertion into the dermis after traversing the orbicularis oculi muscle. The fold is formed by excess skin and muscle that overhangs the crease. In the Caucasian upper eyelid, the crease is approximately 7 mm above the lash margin at the midpupillary line in men and 10 mm in women. In the Asian upper eyelid, if a crease is present, it is approximately 4 to 6 mm above the lash margin. The low crease is a result of the low insertion of the orbital septum and levator aponeurosis, allowing preaponeurotic fat to descend into the pretarsal space.

In the youthful orbit, there is a smooth contour from the brow to the upper lid and from the lower lid to the cheek and midface. With aging, numerous changes are observed in the orbital region. Most noticeable is the herniation of postseptal fat presenting as puffy eyes. This is associated with an apparent increase in the vertical length of the lower lid, accentuation of the tear trough, and occasionally the development of malar bags. These findings are seen as the herniated postseptal fat is restricted by the arcus marginalis and the orbitomalar ligament, while midfacial ptosis is restricted by the zygomatic retaining ligaments. The combination of soft-tissue descent and relatively fixed points from the retaining ligaments creates an aged surface contour defined by a series of convexities and concavities.

Brow ptosis is recognized by lateral upper eyelid hooding as well as a narrowed brow-lash distance. Dynamic transverse forehead furrows are often present secondary to subconscious brow elevation using the frontalis muscle. Recognition of the interplay between the lower lid and midface, as well as the upper lid and brow, are critical aspects of designing a surgical plan that can achieve the desired aesthetic goals.

PREOPERATIVE EVALUATION

Visual acuity is determined with the patient wearing eye glasses or contact lenses. This is to document the baseline preoperative vision. Ocular mobility is then assessed by asking the patient to follow an object through the six cardinal positions of gaze. Diplopia can occur as a result of injury to the inferior or superior oblique from prior blepharoplasty. Visual field testing is important in patients with upper eyelid ptosis and upper eyelid skinfolds that interfere with the visual axis. Finally, standard photographs are taken of each patient. These

are helpful in preoperative planning, as an intraoperative reference, and in reviewing the objectives of surgery with the patient postoperatively.

Upper Orbit and Brow

It is important to perform an organized sequential assessment of the orbit, including the upper lid and brow. The brow is evaluated for ptosis, symmetry, and the relationship between the nasal and lateral brows. This is done with the brow under conscious relaxation, with the absence of active furrowing of the forehead. The aesthetic relationships of the brow to other facial features was discussed earlier. In women, the brow should arch above the supraorbital rim with a peak above the lateral limbus. In men, the brow should be more horizontal, traversing the supraorbital rim. Signs of brow ptosis include lateral upper eyelid hooding and descent below the orbital rim. If brow laxity is not corrected or if brow is not stabalized, it will predispose the patient to further descent of the brow following blepharoplasty. Glabellar wrinkling can be treated with botulinum injection or surgically using browlifting techniques. This can be approached endoscopically, using an open approach or via transpalpebral corrugator resection combined with an internal browpexy. An unstable brow will require elevation or stabilization in order to avoid worsening of brow ptosis after upper blepharoplasty.

Upper eyelid fold asymmetry may be caused by several factors, including upper lid ptosis, upper lid retraction, an asymmetry in the amount of tissue in the upper lid, and asymmetrical brow ptosis. In patients presenting with upper lid ptosis, it is important to identify the etiology on history and clinical evaluation. The differential diagnosis includes congenital ptosis, aponeurotic dehiscence, myogenic ptosis including myasthenia gravis, neurogenic ptosis including Horner's syndrome, and mechanical ptosis secondary to a tumor or trauma. On physical examination, the levator function is measured by stabilizing the eyebrow and measuring lid margin excursion. Congenital ptosis is present from birth and characterized by poor levator function. The measured excursion is generally less than 4 mm and often requires correction by means of a frontalis sling procedure. In acquired ptosis, levator function is often normal with an excursion of 10 mm or greater. The eyelid crease is typically high in these patients as the dermal anchor of the levator fibers forming the crease have been disrupted. This can be corrected with tarsolevator advancement at the time of the blepharoplasty procedure. The cover test is recommended in the evaluation of minimal unilateral acquired ptosis. The ptotic lid is covered with an eye pad for 5 minutes. As a result of Hering's law of equal innervation, subclinical ptosis in the "normal" lid will be unmasked after the ptotic lid is covered.

In addition to the evaluation of excess skin and preaponeurotic fat in the upper eyelid, identification of lacrimal gland prolapse is important.

During the upper blepharoplasty dissection, care must be taken to avoid inadvertent removal of the gland, and gland suspension may be necessary. Excess retroorbicularis oculi fat (ROOF) may be removed in a conservative manner lateral to the supraorbital nerve. This procedure may be combined with an internal browpexy in order to raise and suspend the lateral aspect of the brow. Significant bony fullness in the region of the lateral orbital rim can be contoured using a burr. The youthful upper orbit is characterized by fullness. Patients are asked to bring photographs taken approximately 10 years prior to their consultation. These images can be used as a guide to reestablishing the patient's individual orbital contour and volume. This may require the use of free fat grafting, in addition to a fat-conserving blepharoplasty, if the orbit has become skeletonized with age or previous excisional surgery.

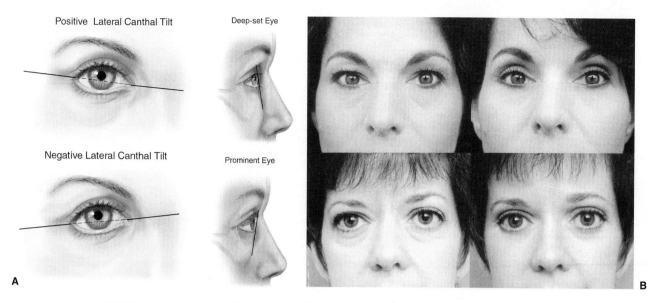

Positive Lateral Canthal Tilt

Deep-set Eye

Negative Lateral Canthal Tilt

Prominent Eye

A   B

FIGURE 48.10. **A:** Preoperative analysis should include defining the canthal tilt, which is determined by the angle of the intercanthal line, and the vector relationship of the globe to the infraorbital rim. **B:** Patient before and after blepharoplasty with positive and negative tilt.

Floppy eyelid syndrome, although uncommon, may be present in large, burly men who present for blepharoplasty. The syndrome is characterized by upper eyelid eversion during forced lid closure and may be addressed by shortening the lid laterally. This requires resection of a portion of the lateral tarsal plate along with a canthoplasty of the upper eyelid. If a floppy upper eyelid is not recognized and corrected, postblepharoplasty complications, including an overriding upper eyelid during eyelid closure, persistent chemosis, and lid separation from the globe, may occur.

Lower Orbit and Midface

Assessment of the lower orbit also can be done using an anatomic sequence. A positive canthal tilt is one where the lateral canthus is positioned superior to the medial canthus. A negative canthal tilt may indicate descent of the lateral canthus from disinsertion, laxity, or the presence of a prominent eye (Fig. 48.10). This orbital morphology may also be present as a hereditary trait. The lower lid is examined for laxity by the amount of distraction attained from the globe, and rate of lid snap back. Anterior lid distraction greater than 6 mm from the globe defines significant lid laxity, which may require lateral lid resection and canthoplasty. In all other cases, canthal anchoring is achieved by means of a canthopexy. With respect to the lower lid, the presence of scleral show, redundant skin and muscle, and evidence of herniated post septal fat is noted. In the midface, elongation of the lower lid, associated midfacial ptosis, a visible tear trough, and malar bags are noted. Of particular note is the presence of scleral show in the preoperative patient. This should serve as a "red flag" sign of caution since it is often associated with a prominent eye, lower lid laxity, and poor infraorbital support, which define patients at high risk for postoperative complications.

The globe is examined to evaluate its position relative to the bony orbital rim (Fig. 48.10). Patients with a negative vector relationship have a prominent eye with poor globe support. This is demonstrated on a lateral view, with the anterior aspect of the globe being anterior to the underlying soft issue of the infraorbital rim. A positive vector is seen where the globe is posterior to the infraorbital rim and overlying soft tissue. These patients have deep-set eyes. A detailed measured analysis is performed using exophthalmometry with a Hertel exophthalmometer. This instrument is used in the assessment of globe prominence by measuring the position of the globe relative to the lateral orbital rim. Normal globe prominence is in the range of 15 to 17 mm. Patients with enophthalmos have a measurement of less than 15 mm; patients with exophthalmos have measurements greater than 17 mm. Both prominent and deepset eyes are at increased risk for complications. Prominent eye lateral canthal anchoring requires supraplacement to avoid inferior lid malposition. Deep-set eyes require no overcorrection but do require internal placement to avoid anterior malposition. Furthermore, primary lower lid spacers and infraorbital rim implants may be considered in patients with prominent eyes to correct the poor globe support.

Dry Eye

Patients at risk for postoperative eye dryness are easily identified with a history of contact lens intolerance. Each patient is then evaluated for the presence of a Bell's phenomenon, as a poor reflex will predispose patients to significant postoperative corneal dryness. These patients are further evaluated using a Shirmer's test. The test is performed by first anesthetizing the conjunctiva in the inferior lateral fornix with tetracaine eyedrops. Any excess tear film is then blotted away and a Shirmer strip is placed in the lateral fornix and the patient is asked to gaze straight ahead. Decreased tear production is identified by less than 10 mm of wetting after a 5-minute period. Patients with dry eyes should have conservative skin excision to minimize lagophthalmos and proper lateral canthal anchoring to prevent ectropion. A temporary tarsorrhaphy suture may also be applied to limit the amount of exposure during the postoperative edematous phase. Liberal use of perioperative lubrication is advocated and postoperative insertion of punctual plugs may be needed in some refractory cases.

Systemic Conditions

In addition to anatomic findings, underlying medical conditions that can increase the risk of complications following blepharoplasty may be present. The first step in a thorough evaluation includes a history directed toward the identification of specific entities, including eyelid inflammatory disorders, Graves disease, benign essential blepharospasm, and dry eye syndrome. All of these medical conditions increase the risk of complications following blepharoplasty, and should be screened prior to surgery.

Blepharoplasty technique should be conservative in order to minimize the risk of corneal dryness or lid malposition. Blepharochalasis is a disorder of eyelid tissue caused by repeated episodes of extreme periorbital edema. This condition is rare and is seen in women who have eyelid edema exacerbated during their menstrual cycle. Chronic stretching of the eyelid skin and septum results in blepharochalasis or chronic puffy eyelids. The most common cutaneous inflammatory disorders that affect the eyelids are rosacea and pemphigus. Patients with rosacea have decreased tear film production, which predisposes them to corneal dryness and possible ulceration from exposure following blepharoplasty. In addition to patients with rosacea and pemphigus, patients with known history of sarcoidosis should be considered to be at increased risk for healing complications following blepharoplasty. Noncaseating granuloma formation in blepharoplasty incisions have been reportedly caused by sarcoidosis of the surgical scar. Pemphigus is an autoimmune disorder that leads to chronic inflammatory changes of the conjunctiva and ocular adnexa. Scar contracture of the conjunctival fornix may occur causing foreshortening and lid malposition.

Patients with puffy eyelids will often present to the plastic surgeon with undiagnosed Graves disease with hyperthyroidism or euthyroid Graves disease. Preoperative evaluation should include screening lab work including free thyroxine (T_4), as well as consideration for endocrine consultation. Ocular manifestation of Graves disease often includes upper and lower lid retraction, increased orbital volume, exophthalmos, and puffy eyelids. Standard blepharoplasty techniques should be modified to correct lid position because of the increased risk of corneal exposure and keratitis. Another periorbital disorder associated with increased risk of complications is benign essential blepharospasm. This is an involuntary spastic disorder of the orbicularis oculi muscle, frequently contributing to redundant upper eyelid skin. Blepharoplasty should be avoided because improvement in symptoms is unlikely. Current management includes a nonoperative approach with periorbital orbicularis oculi muscle injections with botulinum toxin.

Patients who have had recent laser in situ keratomileusis (LASIK) surgery for vision enhancement should avoid blepharoplasty for at least 6 months in order to allow the corneal incision adequate time to heal and to minimize the risk of superinfection in the event lagophthalmos and dryness occur after blepharoplasty.

OPERATIVE TECHNIQUE

Anesthesia

Blepharoplasty can be performed under general anesthesia or under intravenous conscious sedation. Local anesthesia consisting of lidocaine 2% with epinephrine 1:100,000 is injected using a 27-gauge needle into the upper eyelid, lateral canthus, lower eyelid, and inferior orbital rim. If midfacial dissection is planned, the injected area is extended to include the bony malar prominence at the level of the periosteum. Care is taken to avoid injury to the marginal arterial arcades and the deep orbital structures in order to reduce the risk of eyelid or retrobulbar hematoma.

Upper Lid Markings

Preliminary markings are made in the preoperative area to ensure that the scar will be in a crow's foot with the patient smiling in the vertical position, and are completed on the operating room table following the induction of anesthesia. This is done using loupe magnification and calipers to ensure symmetry of markings on both eyelids. A fine, wooden-tip applicator is used to mark the incisions with methylene blue. First, the upper eyelid crease is marked at the level of the midpupillary line. In women, this is 8 to 10 mm superior to the lash margin, and roughly 7 mm above the lash margin in men (Fig. 48.11). The marking is tapered caudally at the nasal and lateral lid margins following the gentle curve of the upper lid crease. The nasal aspect of the marking should not extend medially to the caruncle, so as to avoid webbing or the development of epicanthal folds above the medial canthus. At the lateral canthus, the lateral marking should be 5 to 6 mm above the lash line. The lateral extension should be hidden in a crow's foot skinfold and not extend past the lateral orbital rim. The superior margin of the planned excision is determined by using utility forceps to pinch and identify the quantity of excess skin and muscle. At a minimum, 10 mm of skin should be preserved between the lower border of the eyebrow and the upper lid marking at the level of the lateral canthus. The superior mark is drawn parallel to the contour of the lower marking. Nasally, the amount of tissue to be excised is tapered in a conservative fashion. Overresection of skin and muscle is poorly tolerated nasally resulting in lagophthalmos that can cause corneal dryness in addition to a poor aesthetic result.

Modification of standard technique is required during blepharoplasty on Asian patients. For the Asian eyelid, one must determine if a single eyelid (absent crease) or a double eyelid (single crease) is desired. It is also important to define the desired location of the crease because this is typically lower than in the Caucasian upper eyelid. A distance of 4 to 6 mm above the lid margin is usually used, depending on the patients' desires. A plan is made to limit the amount of skin and preaponeurotic fat excision because this can lead to a high crease and supratarsal hollowness. Furthermore, if present, an epicanthal fold is usually preserved unless change is specifically requested by the patient. Proper communication with the patient regarding the desired outcome is of utmost importance because the aesthetic goals of Asian blepharoplasty are different from those achieved by standard techniques.

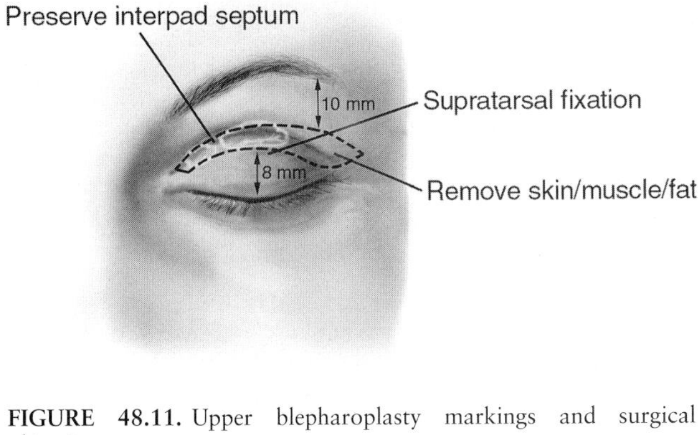

FIGURE 48.11. Upper blepharoplasty markings and surgical objectives.

Lower Lid Markings

From the level of the lateral canthus, a line is extended infer-olaterally for approximately 6 to 10 mm within a prominent crow's foot crease. Roughly 10 mm of skin is preserved between the lateral extension of the upper and lower blepharoplasty incisions. If the incisions are placed too close together, postoperative webbing or distortion can occur. The nasal extension of the marking parallels the lid margin and should be as close to the lash line as possible because the scar becomes more apparent when placed lower.

Upper Lid Blepharoplasty

Using a scalpel, the upper lid markings are incised through the skin and into the orbicularis muscle. A needle-tip cautery is used to incise the orbicularis oculi muscle along the superior incision. This exposes the orbital septum, which is then opened along the length of the incision. The septum is opened first along the upper incision in order to avoid injury to the levator aponeurosis, which is located immediately behind the orbicularis oculi muscle in the lower incision at the lid crease. Care is taken to preserve the interpad septum separating the central and nasal fat pads. Overresection of fat in this area will result in a hollow "A-frame" or peaked arch deformity of the supratarsal crease (Fig. 48.12). Preservation of fat at the interpad septum will maintain a symmetrical gentle arch below the new upper lid fold. When fat excision is indicated, it can be performed by direct sculpting with the needle-tip cautery, which allows greater precision and visualization of the medial palpebral artery. Clamping, resecting, and cauterizing fat should be discouraged because this can result in uncontrolled bleeding. Inadequate cauterization can result in bleeding from the nasal fat pad. Poor visualization and indiscriminate cauterization within the deep nasal orbit has contributed to injury to the trochlea and the superior oblique muscle. Patients with injury to the superior oblique muscle will exhibit diplopia and head tilt toward the side of the superior oblique injury following blepharoplasty. Fat preservation should be considered to avoid creation of a hollow, more aged-appearing orbit.

Excess skin, muscle, and septum are then resected with scissors beveling away from the levator insertion into the upper lid crease. Surgical disinsertion of the levator aponeurosis following upper blepharoplasty is a cause of postoperative acquired ptosis. To minimize this risk, supratarsal fixation of the pretarsal skin muscle to the levator aponeurosis is performed as a routine part of upper blepharoplasty using a horizontal mattress suture of 6-0 Vicryl at the midpupillary line.

The ROOF pad should be evaluated, and conservative resection of the brow fat pad can be performed. Ptosis of the orbital lobe of the lacrimal gland may be present and should be corrected with suspension of the lacrimal gland into the lacrimal sac fossa. The lateral horn is placed on traction and the levator aponeurosis is sutured to the arcus marginalis with 6-0 Vicryl suture just at the level of the lacrimal gland to prevent future lacrimal gland ptosis. The levator aponeurosis needs to be placed on downward stretch to eliminate the risk of postoperative lagophthalmos. Resection of the lacrimal gland can cause postoperative dry eye syndrome and is not recommended.

If lateral brow instability is present, an internal lateral browpexy can be performed through the upper blepharoplasty incision. The orbicularis and ROOF pad are dissected just superficial to the periosteum along the lateral third of the eyebrow, just lateral to the supraorbital nerve along the lateral orbital rim, exposing the temporalis fascia. Dissection cephalic to the orbital rim should be performed bluntly with a cotton-tip applicator to avoid injury by perforating the zygomaticotemporal vein found in this area. Care should be taken to completely release the lateral zone of fixation at the junction of the temporal line of fusion and supraorbital rim. Internal browpexy is performed using 4-0 Prolene interrupted mattress sutures between the orbicularis just deep to the dermis at the level of the inferior brow margin and the underlying temporalis fascia. The inferior margin of the brow at the level of the lateral canthus can be sutured 10 to 15 mm above the lateral orbital rim, depending on the desired position. To achieve the aesthetic goals, the peak of the brow should be placed just above the lateral corneoscleral limbus. Internal browpexy should be considered to correct lateral brow instability and prevent further brow ptosis caused by upper blepharoplasty.

Following removal of excess skin, muscle, and fat, the upper lid incision is generously irrigated with normal saline to remove any residual liquified fat that can result in postoperative granuloma formation. The incision is closed with initial sutures placed superior to the lateral canthus with interrupted 6-0 nylon suture, which aligns the skin and muscle. The incision lateral to the canthus is closed with interrupted 6-0 nylon and the incision medial to the lateral canthus is closed with a running 6-0 nylon suture. While a subcuticular suture is commonly used, including the muscle in the repair may eliminate the fine, white dermal scar often seen following subcuticular closure. Repair of the orbicularis muscle reduces the tension on the dermis, resulting in a less perceptible scar. In addition, the interposed muscle prevents adhesion formation from the dermis to the aponeurosis to the skin, thereby minimizing contour irregularity and lagophthalmos.

Asian Upper Lid Blepharoplasty

A low crease incision, typically 4 to 6 mm above the lash line, is made in an Asian upper lid blepharoplasty. A conservative amount of skin is excised and minimal preaponeurotic fat is removed. To create a dynamic fold, multiple sutures are placed through the junction of the upper tarsal margin, levator insertion, and dermis of the upper skin margin.

Lower Lid Blepharoplasty

The lower lid skin is incised lateral to the canthus with a scalpel exposing the underlying orbicularis oculi muscle. The orbicularis oculi muscle is divided with electrocautery into the submuscular space. Scissors are then used to incise the remainder of the lower lid skin incision along the lid margin with a

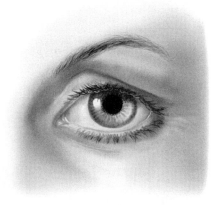

FIGURE 48.12. "A-frame" deformity from overresection of fat at the interpad septum.

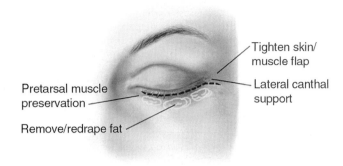

Tighten skin/
muscle flap

Lateral canthal
support

Pretarsal muscle
preservation

Remove/redrape fat

FIGURE 48.13. Lower blepharoplasty diagram and surgical objectives.

second incision through the orbicularis preserving a 5-mm strip of pretarsal orbicularis muscle (Fig. 48.13). Electromyelogram (EMG) analysis has revealed normal function to the pretarsal muscle strip with minimal risk of denervation. The skin muscle flap is dissected anterior to the septum to the infraorbital rim. Dissection continues to the infraorbital rim just superficial to the periosteum separating the orbicularis from periosteal attachments at the lateral orbital rim. The orbitomalar ligament is divided along the entire extent of the infraorbital rim. A tear-through deformity requires a conservative 2- to 3-mm supraperiosteal release of the medial origins of the orbicularis oculi, levator labii superioris, and levator alaeque nasi muscles from the inferior orbital rim. Once the orbitomalar ligament is released, the SOOF becomes visible and dissection superficial to the periosteum is performed approximately 10 mm below the orbital rim preserving the zygomaticofacial nerve. Release of the orbitomalar ligament allows elevation of the SOOF with the skin muscle flap. Fat can be removed in a conservative fashion from all three lower lid compartments, and the orbital septum is resected, along with the excess fat, by a "septectomy." Removal of the septum may reduce the risk of subsequent septal scar formation. Care should be taken to identify and avoid injury to the inferior oblique muscle between the nasal and central fat pads. The inferior oblique muscle is reportedly the most common

extraocular muscle injured during blepharoplasty from indiscriminate cauterization. The arcuate expansion of Lockwood's ligament between the central and lateral fat pads should be preserved for additional support to prevent further herniation of periorbital fat. Alternative procedures could also be considered including arcus marginalis release, septal reset, or septal tightening. Similar to the upper blepharoplasty, the lower lid should be irrigated with normal saline following resection of orbital fat pads.

Transconjunctival Lower Blepharoplasty

The orbital fat can be removed by a transseptal approach that divides the conjunctiva, capsulopalpebral fascia, and septum, or by a retroseptal incision through the conjunctiva and capsulopalpebral fascia that leaves the septum intact. We reserve transconjunctival fat removal for adolescent patients with congenital fat excess and minimal skin laxity, as well as for African American and Asian patients.

Lateral Canthal Anchoring

The degree of lower lid laxity should be further evaluated intraoperatively by placing anterior traction on the lower eyelid away from the globe and using caliper measurement to determine the amount of lid distraction. Lid distraction of 1 to 2 mm indicates minimal lid laxity, requiring minimal lateral canthal support with orbicularis suspension only. Although this subgroup of patients may not need canthopexy, we would include an orbicularis sling to reduce the risk of lid malposition. Laxity measurements of 3 to 6 mm of lid distraction indicates moderate laxity of the lower eyelid. A lateral canthopexy should be used to correct moderate lid laxity (Fig. 48.14). When the lid can be distracted greater than 6 mm away from the globe, significant lid laxity is present and a lateral canthoplasty should be considered.

The objective of lateral canthopexy is to suture the tarsal plate and lateral retinaculum to the periosteum of the lateral orbital rim, thereby tightening the lower lid tarsoligamentous sling. A horizontal mattress suture of 4-0 Mersilene is used to incorporate the tarsal plate and lateral retinaculum. The

Canthopexy

Canthoplasty

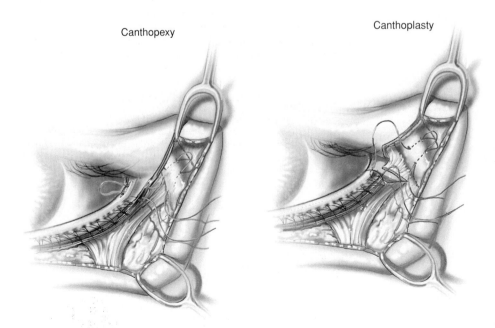

FIGURE 48.14. Lateral canthal anchoring techniques, including canthopexy and canthoplasty.

Mersilene suture is then placed inside the lateral orbital rim periosteum from deep to superficial, allowing the lateral canthus and lower lid to be tightened posteriorly and superiorly to maintain the position of the lower lid margin against the globe. The vertical position of the lateral canthal fixation suture depends on the amount of eye prominence, the amount of lower lid laxity, and the preoperative shape of the lower eyelid. Care should be taken to maintain the preoperative shape of the lower eyelid, avoiding overcorrection or alteration in the preoperative canthal position. The position of the lateral canthal suture is most commonly at the horizontal midpupillary line. However, patients with prominent eyes require supraplacement of the canthal support suture with overcorrection and minimal tightening to avoid "clotheslining" of the lower lid below the inferior limbus, causing scleral show. Conversely, patients with deep-set eyes require more posterior placement of the canthopexy suture, taking care to avoid overcorrection in a superior direction. The downward force of the prominent globe on the lower lid will cause descent of the lid margin following lateral canthopexy; however, this force does not exist in patients who have deep-set eyes.

Patients who have significant lid laxity with lid distraction greater than 6 mm require lateral canthotomy and canthoplasty. Lateral canthoplasty is performed following canthotomy of the inferior limb of the lateral canthal tendon followed by cantholysis, which allows mobilization of the lower lid. The lid is then transposed over the lateral orbital rim and 2 to 3 mm of full-thickness lid margin is resected to correct significant lid laxity. A 4-0 Mersilene suture is used for lateral canthoplasty and is placed through the edge of the tarsal plate from inferior to superior, ensuring vertical alignment while controlling lash rotation. The mattress suture is then placed along the posterior aspect of the lateral orbital rim periosteum at the appropriate level and tied in a surgeon's knot. The desired amount of tension created by the lateral canthoplasty should allow 1 to 2 mm of lid distraction away from the globe, and the lid should be easily mobilized over the cornea. Overtightening of the lateral canthoplasty should be avoided so as to minimize lid malposition. The lateral commissure is then reconstructed with a 6-0 plain catgut suture placed in the gray line to prevent postoperative lateral canthal webbing. To recreate a normal-appearing lateral commissure, the suture is placed in the posterior aspect of the upper lid gray line and the anterior aspect of the lower lid gray line, which allows the upper lid to slightly overlap the lower lid in a normal anatomic relationship.

Following lateral canthal support, the skin–muscle flap is redraped in a superior lateral vector, and a triangle of excess skin and muscle is resected according to the amount that overlaps the lateral extent of the lower blepharoplasty incision. The orbicularis muscle flap is then resuspended to the lateral orbital rim at the level of the lateral canthus using a 4-0 vicryl suture, placed as a three-point quilting suture, from the incised edges of skin and muscle to periosteum along the inner aspect of the lateral orbital rim to recreate the normal concavity associated with the lateral orbital raphe. Similarly, interrupted absorbable sutures are placed in the lateral cut edge of the orbicularis flap to the lateral orbital rim periosteum and temporalis fascia to properly resuspend the orbicularis under appropriate tension. Resuspension of the orbicularis provides additional lower lid support as well as elevation of the SOOF over the inferior orbital rim. If additional elevation of the orbicularis is required, a flap of muscle can be passed into the lateral aspect of the upper blepharoplasty incision and resuspended to the temporalis fascia. Minimal skin and muscle are resected parallel to the lower lid margin to minimize the risk of lid malposition. A small strip of orbicularis is removed from the skin muscle flap to avoid a redundant layer overlying the preserved pretarsal orbicularis. Tension-free closure is then performed in the skin–muscle edges with a 6-0 fast-absorbing catgut suture.

Postoperative Care

Significant periorbital ecchymosis or chemosis of the conjunctiva at the completion of the procedure may indicate signs of delayed healing. In these situations, the use of a Frost suture should be considered. It is placed in the lower lid margin lateral to the lateral limbus and either sutured to the eyebrow or suspended to a Steri-Strip above the eyebrow. To minimize chemosis, a function of both conjunctival dryness and edema, a suture can also be placed as a temporary tarsorrhaphy suture from the lid margin of the upper and lower eyelid along the gray line lateral to the limbus. These techniques minimize corneal exposure in the immediate postoperative period. Head elevation and the application of ice to the periorbital region is used for 48 hours after surgery. Ophthalmic antibiotic ointment is applied along the suture line, as well as on the globe, to prevent or to reduce evaporative tear film loss. Sutures, including the Frost suture, are removed 5 to 7 days after surgery. Patients are asked to avoid the use of eyelid makeup on the suture lines and contact lenses for 2 weeks following surgery. Persistent postoperative chemosis can be treated with liberal ophthalmic ointments and eye drops. Additionally, Voltaren drops and fluorometholone (FML) 0.1% ophthalmic suspension can be used for 2 weeks to minimize the early inflammatory changes that result in chemosis. Severe chemosis that herniates through the palpebral fissure requires more aggressive management with liberal ophthalmic ointment, patching the eye closed for 24 to 48 hours, and applying gentle pressure from an Ace wrap to reduce the swelling. Occasionally the edematous conjunctiva can be surgically drained.

Complications

Given the delicate anatomy of the periorbital region, complications can be common with blepharoplasty surgery. For this reason, it is particularly important to anticipate and prevent such complications by understanding the anatomy and mechanics of the periorbita. The most devastating complication after blepharoplasty is visual loss. Although rare, the estimated incidence is 0.04% and is caused by either retroorbital hemorrhage compromising ocular circulation or direct globe perforation. Rapid surgical decompression and administration of mannitol, acetazolamide, and oxygen is advocated as part of the initial management of retroorbital hematoma. Diplopia can also occur following blepharoplasty and is usually temporary, resulting from edema. Permanent diplopia can occur from thermal injury to the inferior oblique or superior oblique muscles from electrocautery. Strabismus surgery may be required for patients who do not improve with conservative management. In the upper lid, ptosis may occur after surgery from failed preoperative recognition or from levator dehiscence during surgery. To minimize this risk, supratarsal fixation of the pretarsal skin muscle to the levator aponeurosis should be performed.

Signs of corneal irritation or impaired visual acuity require careful ophthalmologic evaluation. This includes a slit-lamp examination with the use of fluorescein eyedrops to evaluate the cornea along with visual acuity testing. Mild lid malposition may contribute to lagophthalmos and corneal exposure. Lagophthalmos may require bandage contact lenses to protect the cornea and conservative massage of the lower lid margin until the patient has passed the critical 6-week postoperative time period, which corresponds with the proliferative phase of healing. Lower lid ectropion or persistent lid malposition following a 2- to 3-month period of conservative management may require surgical intervention, including placement of a posterior lamella spacer graft and lateral canthoplasty.

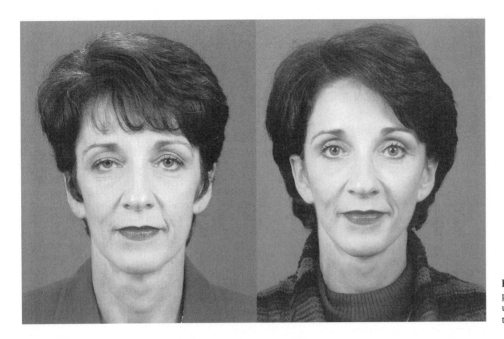

FIGURE 48.15. A patient with upper lid ptosis shown before and after upper and lower blepharoplasty and tarsolevator advancement.

Outcomes

Maintaining the preoperative shape of the palpebral fissure is emphasized, with particular attention to maintaining lower eyelid position (Figs. 48.15, 48.16, and 48.17). Lateral canthal support, most commonly with lateral canthopexy, represents an important step in the technique to maintain lid shape and reduce the risk of lower lid malposition or postoperative round eye syndrome. The tradeoff, which should be discussed with patients prior to surgery, is that the lower lid may appear tight, which may last 2 to 3 weeks after

surgery. The natural S-shape curve to the lower lid and palpebral aperture are preserved following completion of healing process.

Complications associated with lateral canthoplasty include canthal angle webbing or asymmetry, which requires surgical revision. The risk of frank ectropion is reduced when conservative skin excision and lateral canthal support are performed in combination. In addition to minimizing the risk of complications, maximizing the aesthetic result is directly related to safe management of periorbital fat, the orbicularis muscle, and SOOF. Elevation of the skin muscle flap and release of the orbitomalar ligament mobilizes the SOOF, which is elevated with

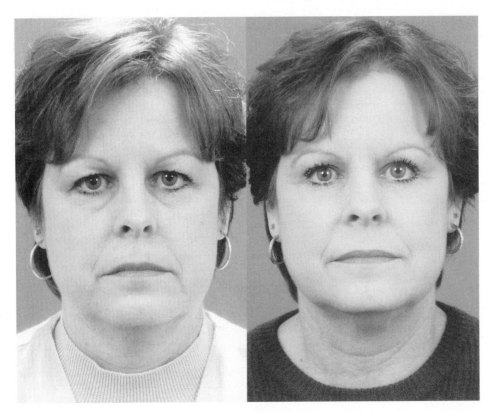

FIGURE 48.16. A patient shown before and after endoscopic browlift and upper and lower blepharoplasty.

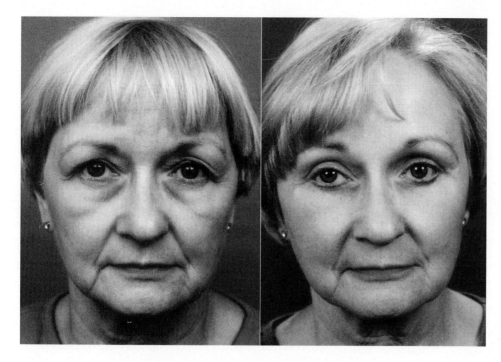

FIGURE 48.17. A patient before and after endoscopic browlift, upper blepharoplasty, and subperiosteal midface lift with correction of malar bags.

the orbicularis muscle. Using the orbicularis muscle as a sling with secure lateral orbital fixation is the key to maximizing the aesthetic appearance of the infraorbital region. This can be performed safely based on the anatomy of the lower eyelid. The posterior lamella (tarsoligamentous sling) has a separate point of periosteal fixation from the anterior lamella (skin–muscle flap). These basic principles, which have an anatomic basis, are the two key points in maximizing the surgical outcome following lower blepharoplasty. Similarly, the two key principles for upper blepharoplasty are fat preservation with conservative removal of skin, muscle, and fat in order to avoid a hollow upper lid sulcus, and supratarsal fixation to avoid acquired postblepharoplasty ptosis. Browlifting procedures should be performed during blepharoplasty when needed. Adherence to these basic principles significantly contributes to achieving the overall goal, which is excellence in blepharoplasty results.

CONCLUSION

The age-related anatomic changes seen in the orbit are closely influenced by those changes seen in the forehead and midface. The interplay between these anatomic regions has allowed blepharoplasty to evolve into a more comprehensive surgical procedure.

Suggested Readings

Carraway JH, Mellow CG. The prevention and treatment of lower lid ectropion following blepharoplasty. *Plast Reconstr Surg.* 1990;85:971–981.

Codner MA, Day CR, Hester TR, et al. Management of moderate to complex blepharoplasty problems. Perspectives in plastic surgery. 15:1, pp. 15–32, 2001.

Codner MA, McCord CD, Hester TR. The lateral canthoplasty. *Operat Tech Plast Reconstr Surg.* 1998;5:90–98.

Flowers RS. Canthopexy as a routine blepharoplasty component. *Clin Plast Surg.* 1993;20:351.

Hamra ST. Arcus marginalis release and orbital fat preservation in midface rejuvenation. *Plast Reconstr Surg.* 1995;96:354.

Hirmand H, Codner MA, McCord CD, et al. Prominent eye: operative management in lower lid and midface rejuvenation and the morphologic classification system. *Plast Reconstr Surg.* 2002;110:620.

Jelks GW, Jelks EB. The influence of orbital and eyelid anatomy on the palpebral aperture. *Clin Plast Surg.* 1991;18:183–195.

Kikkawa DO, Lemke BN, Dortzbach RK. Relations of the superficial musculoaponeurotic system to the orbit and characterization of the orbitomalar ligament. *Ophthalmic Plast Reconstr Surg.* 1996;12:77.

Knize DM. The superficial lateral canthal tendon: anatomic study and clinical application to lateral canthopexy. *Plast Reconstr Surg.* 2002;109:1149.

McCord CD, Codner MA, Hester TR. Redraping the inferior orbicularis arc. *Plast Reconstr Surg.* 1998;102:2471–2479.

Muzaffar AR, Mendelson BC, Adams WP. Surgical anatomy of the ligamentous attachments of the lower lid and lateral canthus. *Plast Reconstr Surg.* 2002;110:873.

Ramirez OM, Santamarina R. Spatial orientation of motor innervation to the lower orbicularis oculi muscle. *Aesthetic Plast Surg.* 2000;20(2):107–113.

CHAPTER 49 ■ FACELIFT

CHARLES H. THORNE

This chapter summarizes my personal approach to facelifting, as well as the most common techniques employed by other plastic surgeons.

STATE OF THE ART

Facelifting was first performed in the early 1900s and for most of the 20th century involved skin undermining and skin excision. A revolution occurred in the 1970s when the public became exponentially more interested in the procedure and Skoog described dissection of the superficial fascia of the face in continuity with the platysma in the neck. Since then techniques have been described that involve every possible skin incision, plane of dissection, extent of tissue manipulation, type of instrumentation, and method of fixation. Many of these "innovations" provide little long-term benefit when compared to skin undermining, and expose the patient to more risk. The trends in facelifting at the present time are best summarized as follows:

1. *Volume versus tension*—Placing tension on the skin is an ineffective way of lifting the face and is responsible for the "facelifted" look and for unsightly scars and distortion of the facial landmarks such as the hairline and ear. The current trend is toward redistributing, or augmenting, facial volume, rather than flattening it with excessive tension.
2. *Less invasive*—That the more "invasive" techniques have not yielded benefits in proportion to their risk combined with the public demand for rapid recovery has led to simplified procedures.
3. *Facial harmony*—The goal is to help a patient look better, not weird or operated on. Excessive tension, radical defatting, exaggerated changes, and attention to one region while ignoring another may result in disharmony. The face is best analyzed and manipulated with the entire face (and the entire body) in mind, not the individual component parts, lest the "forest be lost for the trees."
4. *Recognition of atrophy*—The process of aging involves not only sagging of the tissues and deterioration of the skin itself but atrophy of tissues, especially fat, in certain areas. Most patients are best served with limited defatting and may require addition of fat to areas of atrophy.

BENEFITS AND LIMITATIONS OF FACELIFTING

Facelifting addresses only ptosis and atrophy of facial tissues. It does not address, and has no effect on, the quality of the facial skin itself. Consequently, facelifting is not a treatment for wrinkles, sun damage, creases, or irregular pigmentation. Fine wrinkles and irregular pigmentation are best treated with skin care and resurfacing procedures (see Chapters 13 and 44). Deep creases, such as the labiomental creases, may be im-

proved by facelifting. Other facial creases, however, will not be improved by facelifting (nasolabial creases), and even if improved somewhat, will still require additional treatment in the form of fillers or muscle-weakening agents (see Chapters 45 and 46).

The above disclaimer not withstanding, the facelift is the single most important and beneficial treatment for most patients older than age 40 years who wish to maximally address facial-aging changes.

Patients have individual aging patterns determined by genetics, skeletal support, and environmental influences (Fig. 49.1). Some combination of the following, however, will occur in every patient (those characteristics improved by facelifting are in bold print):

1. Forehead and glabellar creases
2. Ptosis of the lateral eyebrow
3. Redundant upper eyelid skin
4. Hollowing of the upper orbit
5. Lower eyelid laxity and wrinkles
6. Lower eyelid bags
7. Deepening of the nasojugal groove and palpebral-malar groove
8. **Ptosis of the malar tissues**
9. **Generalized skin laxity**
10. Deepening of the nasolabial folds
11. Perioral wrinkles
12. Downturn of the oral commissures
13. **Deepening of the labiomental creases**
14. **Jowls**
15. **Loss of neck definition and excess fat in neck**
16. **Platysmal bands**

A minority of aging characteristics is improved by facelifting. Those that are addressed, however, are of fundamental importance to the attractive, youthful face. The facelift confers another benefit that is more difficult to define. Aging results in jowls and a rectangular lower face. A facelift lifts the jowls back into the face, augmenting the upper face and narrowing the lower face, producing the "inverted cone of youth." **This change in overall facial shape from rectangular to heart-shaped is subtle but real, and is a benefit that no other treatment modality can provide.**

PREOPERATIVE PREPARATION

History

The same compulsive medical history that is indicated before any surgical procedure is obtained when evaluating a patient for aesthetic surgery of the face. Specific inquiry is made regarding medications, allergies, medical problems, previous surgery, and smoking and drinking habits. The most common complication of facelifting is a hematoma and therefore the history focuses on factors that predispose to postoperative bleeding,

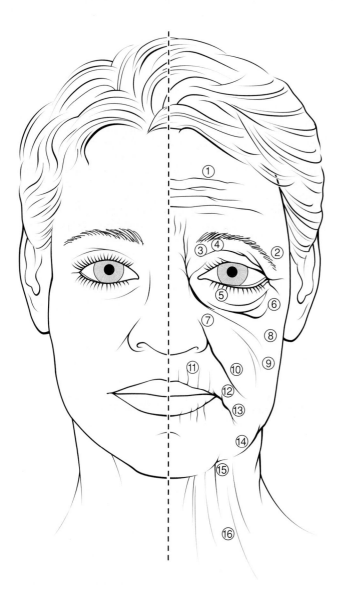

FIGURE 49.1. Aging changes in the face. *1.* Forehead and glabella creases. *2.* Ptosis of the lateral brow. *3.* Redundant upper eyelid skin. *4.* Hollowing of the upper orbit. *5.* Lower eyelid laxity and wrinkles. *6.* Lower eyelid bags. *7.* Deepening of the nasojugal groove. *8.* Ptosis of the malar tissues. *9.* Generalized skin laxity. *10.* Deepening of nasolabial folds. *11.* Perioral wrinkles. *12.* Downturn of oral commissures. *13.* Deepening of labiomental crease *14.* Jowls. *15.* Loss of neck definition and excess fat in neck. *16.* Platysmal bands.

to quit smoking permanently. Cigarette smoking, with all its deleterious effects on health, and having a facelift to feel better about oneself, are fundamentally contradictory. At the very least, patients should cease smoking 2 weeks prior to surgery. It is important that smokers know that they will never become "nonsmokers;" that is, the effects of smoking never totally disappear, and are certainly not gone in 2 weeks.

Because aesthetic surgery is elective, whenever there is a question about a preoperative medical condition, the procedure is postponed until appropriate consultations are obtained and all issues settled.

Preoperative Photographs

Photographs are essential for at least four reasons: (a) assistance in preoperative planning; (b) communication with patients preoperatively and postoperatively; (c) intraoperative decision making; and (d) medicolegal documentation.

Psychological Considerations

One of the most difficult challenges for the plastic surgeon is deciding which patients are not candidates, on an emotional or psychological basis, for elective aesthetic surgery. Studies suggest that patients frequently harbor secret or unconscious motivations for undergoing the procedure. A patient may state that he/she wants to feel better about him- or herself when the real motivation is to recapture a straying mate (unlikely to succeed).

Patients who have difficulty delineating the anatomic alterations desired or in whom the degree of the deformity does not correlate with the degree of personal misfortune ascribed to that deformity, are not candidates for aesthetic surgery. The tough, 50-year-old lawyer who states that she does not like her jowls is a far better candidate than the seemingly docile patient who cannot articulate what bothers her and defers to "whatever you think doctor." The surgeon will regret proceeding with an operation when his or her instincts indicate that the patient is an inappropriate candidate.

Preoperative Counseling

At the time of the preoperative consultation the patient is given written information concerning the planned procedure that reinforces the verbal information provided.

In addition to describing to the patient the anticipated results of the procedure, it is necessary to point out the areas where little or no benefit is expected. As described above, the nasolabial folds that may be softened slightly by a facelift but will reappear when the swelling disappears. Ptotic submandibular glands preclude a totally clean appearance to the neck. Fine wrinkles around the mouth will require a resurfacing procedure.

Preoperative Instructions

Patients are instructed to shower and wash their hair on the night before surgery. On the morning of surgery another shower and shampoo are desirable. At a minimum the face is thoroughly washed. Although patients are not allowed to eat anything after midnight, they are instructed to brush their teeth and rinse their mouths with mouthwash.

Given that the single most important step in avoiding a hematoma is control of the blood pressure, patients with *any* tendency to high blood pressure are given clonidine 0.1 mg by

specifically hypertension and medications that affect clotting. Surgery is not performed until the patient has been off of aspirin for 2 weeks. Facelifting is probably contraindicated in patients on warfarin (Coumadin) or clopidogrel (Plavix), even if they are allowed by their physicians to stop these medications. At the very least, facelifting on such patients is performed with extreme conservatism and only after every possible means of eliminating the effects of these medications has been pursued. **Hypertension is probably the single factor that most closely correlates with postoperative hematomas, thus blood pressure must be under strict control.**

Cigarette Smoking

Smoking increases the risk of skin slough, the second most common complication after facelifting (1). Patients are encouraged mouth preoperatively. Some surgeons administer the drug routinely to all patients. Clonidine is long-acting, however, and may lead to hypotension in healthy patients. Consequently, I prefer to use it selectively.

ANESTHESIA

The subjects of anesthesia and which technique is the safest are poorly understood by patients. A facelift can be safely performed under local anesthesia with sedation provided by the surgeon, or by intravenous sedation or general anesthesia provided by an anesthesiologist. If the surgeon is to perform the procedure without an anesthesiologist, the patient must be completely healthy. The patient is given diazepam (Valium) 10 mg by mouth 2 hours preoperatively and brought to the facility by an escort. Meperidine (Demerol) 75 mg and hydroxyzine pamoate (Vistaril) 75 mg are administered intramuscularly. Once the effect is demonstrable, the patient is moved to the operating room to initiate the procedure. Midazolam (Versed) is given intravenously in 1-mg increments until the patient is sufficiently sedated to tolerate the injections of local anesthetic solution. Additional midazolam (Versed) is given as needed throughout the procedure, also in 1-mg doses.

In most cases, however, facelifts are performed with the help of an anesthesiologist. If the procedure is to be longer than 3 hours because of ancillary procedures, or if the patient has medical problems, then an anesthesiologist is always present.

The anesthesiologist decides where on the spectrum from conscious sedation to general anesthesia the patient is best kept, and it may vary during a procedure. The patient may be under general anesthesia, by any definition, during the injection of the local anesthetic solution, and conscious during other phases of the procedure. In other patients, despite the efforts of the anesthesiologist to provide conscious sedation, the medication will result in loss of the airway, requiring that the anesthesiologist convert the procedure to general anesthesia.

Patients and some other physicians incorrectly believe that patients are safer with "twilight" anesthesia, whatever that is. Local anesthesia is safe and general anesthesia is usually safe, but the *least* safe anesthetic and the one requiring the most skill to administer is the "in between" anesthetic that patients call "twilight." Patients who are sedated but who do not have an endotracheal tube in place to control the airway are more likely to have airway problems than a patient who is completely asleep with the ventilation controlled by the anesthesiologist. Many patients who undergo facelift procedures believe they are receiving "sedation," but they are really receiving intravenous, general anesthesia without an endotracheal tube. There is nothing wrong with the technique in the hands of an expert, but patients should be disabused of the notion that it is safer than general anesthesia.

Blood Pressure Control

An ideal anesthetic for facelifting would be associated with a constant blood pressure and no need for vasoactive medications to either raise or lower it. Dips in blood pressure treated with vasoconstrictors, or spikes in blood pressure treated with vasodilators, are to be avoided if at all possible. Blood pressure is ideally kept at approximately 100 mm Hg systolic, depending on the patient's preoperative blood pressure. Excessive hypotension may obscure bleeding vessels that are best coagulated. Hypertension may be associated with excessive bleeding. The anesthesiologist should inform the surgeon of every medication administered, and the surgeon should inform the

anesthesiologist of any increased tendency for bleeding. There are no secrets in the operating room.

Local Anesthetic Solution

Regardless of the type of sedation/anesthesia chosen, the face is injected with local anesthetic solution prior to the dissection. There is some controversy and little definitive data regarding the maximal amount of local anesthetic that can be used. The package insert in the lidocaine bottle states that no more than 7.5 mg/kg of lidocaine should be administered when given in combination with epinephrine. We know, however, that when dilute solutions are used in liposuction of the *body*, that more than 30 mg/kg of lidocaine is safe. There is evidence that the face differs from the body and that the high lidocaine doses used in the body are not safe in the face. It is reasonable to conclude that doses higher than the 7.5 mg/kg recommended by the manufacturer are *probably* safe in the face, but this is unproven. Until such proof exists, plastic surgeons should limit the total dose to approximately 7.5 mg/kg. In the my practice, I dilute 500 mg lidocaine (one 50 mL vial of 1% lidocaine, which is the approximate maximum dose for a 70-kg patient) to whatever volume is necessary to perform the entire procedure, no matter how dilute that solution is.

The most common solution I use is 50 mL 1% lidocaine plus 1 mL epinephrine 1:1000 plus 250 mL normal saline for a final volume of 301 mL and a final solution concentration of 0.17% lidocaine with epinephrine 1:300,000.

Because of the dilute nature of the solution used and the fact that the total dose of lidocaine does not exceed the manufacturer's recommendation, I inject both sides of the face at the beginning of the procedure, despite recommendations by some that only one side should be injected at a time.

If the patient is adequately anesthetized, the injection of the anesthetic solution is rarely accompanied by *any* change in heart rate or blood pressure. The surgeon must constantly keep the injecting needle moving, however, to avoid a large intravascular injection of the epinephrine-containing solution. If a major change in blood pressure occurs, the surgeon and anesthesiologist must assume that an intravascular injection has occurred and act quickly to limit the extent of hypertension.

FACELIFT ANATOMY

If either skin undermining alone or subperiosteal undermining alone is performed, the surgeon can, to some extent, ignore the anatomy. These two planes of dissection are safe. Manipulation of the tissues between these two planes, however, necessitates an understanding of and constant attention to the anatomy to avoid complications.

Anatomic Layers

There are five layers of critical anatomy: skin; subcutaneous fat; the superficial musculoaponeurotic system (SMAS)–muscle layer; a thin layer of transparent fascia; and the branches of the facial nerve (Fig. 49.2). These five layers are present in all areas of the face, forehead, and neck, but they vary in quality and thickness, depending on the anatomic area.

The first two layers, the skin and subcutaneous fat, are self-explanatory. The third layer (SMAS) is the most heterogeneous (2). It is fibrous, muscular, or fatty, depending on the location in the face. The muscles of facial expression are part of the SMAS layer (e.g., frontalis, orbicularis oculi, zygomaticus major and minor, and platysma). In the temporal region, this layer is not

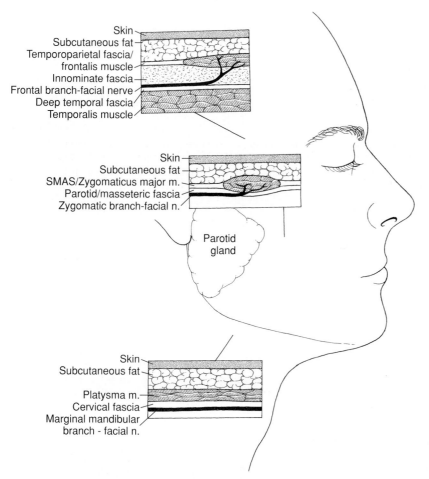

FIGURE 49.2. The anatomic layers of the face. Although the quality of the layers differs in various areas of the face, the arrangement of layers is identical. The facial nerve (cranial nerve [CN] VII) branches innervate their respective muscles via their deep surfaces.

muscular but is fascial in quality and is represented by the superficial temporal fascia (or temporoparietal) fascia.

The fourth layer consists of a layer of areolar tissue that is not impressive in thickness or strength, but is always present and is a key guide to the surgeon as to the location of the facial nerve branches. In the temporal area, this layer is known as the innominate or subgaleal fascia; in the cheek, it is the parotid–masseteric fascia; and in the neck, it is the superficial cervical fascia. Once under the SMAS, the facial nerve branches can be seen through this fourth layer. If the layer is kept intact, it serves as reinforcement to the surgeon that he or she is in the correct plane of dissection. If a nerve branch is encountered without this fascial covering, the surgeon must be aware that the dissection is too deep and nerve branches may have been transected. Just as it is convenient, but not totally accurate, to think of the galea–frontalis–temporoparietal fascia–SMAS–orbicularis oculi–platysma as a single layer, it is useful to think of the subgaleal fascia–innominate fascia–parotid/masseteric fascia–superficial cervical fascia as a single layer.

The fifth layer is the facial nerve, which is discussed in detail below.

Facial Nerve

If the surgeon remembers that the facial nerve branches innervate the respective facial muscles via their deep surfaces, the safe planes of dissection become obvious. Dissection in the subcutaneous plane, superficial to the SMAS–muscle layer, is safely performed anywhere in the face, whether it is the temporal region, cheek, or neck. Dissection deep to the SMAS, superficial to the facial nerve branches, requires care.

There are three to five frontal (or temporal) branches of the facial nerve that cross the zygomatic arch and innervate the frontalis muscle, orbicularis oculi, and corrugator muscles via their deep surfaces (3). Because the layers of anatomy, although present, are compressed over the arch, these branches are vulnerable to injury in this region. Dissection in this region can either be performed superficial to the nerve branches in the subcutaneous plane, or deep to the branches on the surface of the temporalis muscle fascia (deep temporal fascia) (4).

The zygomatic branches innervate the orbicularis oculi and zygomaticus muscles. One must remember that although the facial nerve branches travel deep to the SMAS layer, at some point these branches turn superficially to innervate the overlying muscles. Any dissection in the sub-SMAS plane in the cheek, whether as part of a composite rhytidectomy or standard dissection of the SMAS as a separate layer, necessitates a change of surgical planes at the zygomaticus major muscle to avoid transection of the branch to this muscle. The dissection plane changes from sub-SMAS to subcutaneous by passing over the superficial surface of the zygomaticus major and thereby preserving its innervation.

The buccal branches lie on the masseter muscle and are easily visualized through the parotid–masseteric fascia. Some buccal branches merge with branches of zygomatic origin to innervate the procerus muscle and provide additional innervation of the corrugator muscle. Consequently, the corrugator muscle receives innervation from the frontal, zygomatic, and buccal branches.

Earlier publications indicated that the marginal mandibular branches were located above the inferior border of the mandible in many cases. More recent studies demonstrate that, in fact, these branches are always located caudal to the inferior border of the mandible. The cervical branches innervate the platysma muscle.

Anatomic studies indicate that there are fewer crossover communications between the frontal branches and marginal mandibular branches, which helps to explain why injuries to these nerves are less likely to recover function in their respective muscles than injuries to the zygomatic or buccal branches.

Retaining Ligaments

In at least two areas of the face the anatomic layers are condensed and less mobile with respect to each other. These "ligaments" are areas where the skin and underlying tissues are relatively fixed to the bone (5). The zygomatic ligament (previously known as the McGregor patch) is located in the cheek, anterior and superior to the parotid gland and posteroinferior to the malar eminence. The mandibular ligament is located along the jaw line, near the chin, and forms the anterior border of the jowl.

The retaining ligaments restrain the facial skin against gravitational changes at these points. The descent of tissues adjacent to these points form characteristic aging changes such as the jowl. In addition, some surgeons feel that the ligaments must be released in order to redrape tissues distal to these points.

Platysma Muscle

Although the platysma muscle is a component of the previously discussed SMAS/–muscle layer, it deserves special attention because of its clinical importance. The medial borders of the two muscles decussate to a variable degree in the midline of the neck, helping to explain the variability of aging patterns in the neck (6). The medial borders of the muscles tend to become redundant with age and contribute to the appearance of bands in the submental region.

Malar Fat Pad

The malar fat pad is part of the subcutaneous layer of the face. It is superficial to the SMAS layer represented in this region by the zygomaticus muscles. The malar fat pad appears to descend with age, leaving a hollow infraorbital region behind it and creating larger nasolabial folds and deeper nasolabial creases. Each of the major facelift techniques include a method to mobilize the malar fat pad and restore volume to the upper part of the face and malar region. As is discussed below, the extended SMAS technique involves mobilizing the malar pad in continuity with the SMAS layer. Other techniques involve mobilizing and repositioning the malar pad independent from the SMAS dissection.

Buccal Fat Pad

The buccal fat pad is deep to the buccal branches of the facial nerve, anterior to the masseter muscle, and superficial to the buccinator muscle. Access to the buccal fat pad is achieved by performing a sub-SMAS dissection in the cheek and spreading it between the buccal branches of the facial nerve or through the mouth, by a stab wound in the buccinator muscle. Despite occasional indications to remove the fat pad in patients with very full faces, removal of cheek fat tends to ultimately make the patient look older. As a general rule, rejuvenation of the face involves redistribution, not removal, of fat.

Great Auricular Nerve

The facelift operation inevitably disrupts branches of sensory nerves to the skin. Normal sensibility always returns eventually but numbness may persist for months postoperatively. The only named sensory nerve that is important to preserve is the great auricular nerve. With the head turned toward the contralateral side, the great auricular nerve crosses the superficial surface of the sternocleidomastoid muscle 6 to 7 cm below the external auditory meatus (7). At this point it is 0.5 to 1 cm posterior to the external jugular vein. The vein and nerve are deep to the SMAS–platysma layer, except where the terminal branches of the nerve pass superficially to provide sensibility to the skin of the earlobe. Transection of the great auricular nerve will result in permanent numbness of the lower half of the ear and may result in a troublesome neuroma.

Tear Trough

The tear trough or nasojugal groove is an oblique indentation running inferiorly and laterally from the medial canthus. This groove is a subject of much attention at the present time. Although it is probably better included in a discussion of eyelid surgery, it deepens with age and is a frequent complaint of patients interested in facial aesthetic surgery (see Chapter 48). In general, facelift procedures do not address the tear trough. Redraping of orbital fat or microfat grafting is usually required.

FACELIFT TECHNIQUES AND ALTERNATIVES

The facelift procedure can be performed in the subcutaneous plane, the sub-SMAS (deep) plane, the subperiosteal plane, or a combination of the above. Each of the most commonly used techniques is described in the following sections.

Subcutaneous Facelift

The original facelift consisted of subcutaneous undermining only. The technique is still useful for an occasional patient, but more importantly, it is the basis for other techniques such as the SMAS technique, extended SMAS technique, and the SMASectomy–SMAS plication techniques.

Incisions are designed to avoid distortion of the hairline and ear and to maximally disguise the final scars (Fig. 49.3). The goal is a scar that is so inconspicuous that one has to look for it. Although this is not always the case given the variable and unpredictable nature of wound healing, it is always the goal. If the patient has never had surgery before and has a normal hairline and sideburn, the incision is initiated within the hair, just above the ear. In patients with previous facelifts, the sideburn may already be significantly raised and posteriorly displaced, and an incision within the hair will result in further distortion of the sideburn. These patients are candidates for an incision along the anterior hairline. Patients with thin, sparse hair may be candidates for the hairline incision, even if it is the first procedure they have ever had. A transverse incision is also designed just below the sideburn to allow additional excision of cheek skin without raising the sideburn any higher than desired by the surgeon.

The incision proceeds caudally along the junction of the ascending crus of the helix and the cheek. The eventual scar tends

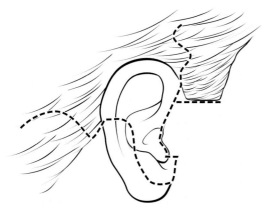

FIGURE 49.3. Standard facelift incision. Regardless of the technique chosen, some form of this incision is employed. In the temporal region the incision is shown within the hair. In patients with extremely thin hair, previous facelifts or if performing the minimal access cranial suspension (MACS) lift, the incision is made along the anterior sideburn and temporal hairline, rather than as shown here. In this illustration, the incision is shown along the posterior margin of the tragus. In men, and in women with oily or hairy preauricular skin, an incision in the preauricular crease may be preferable. In the short scar technique, the incision is terminated at the bottom of the earlobe or just behind it, and the entire retroauricular portion of the incision is eliminated.

to migrate forward slightly and therefore should be placed 1 to 2 mm on the ear side of the ear–cheek junction. My preference is to make the incision in the same location in men. The incision is continued either at the posterior margin of the tragus (retrotragal) or in the pretragal region, usually in a natural skin crease. Patients, and many surgeons, erroneously believe that the incision along the posterior aspect of the tragus is always preferable. In fact, this incision frequently results in distortion of the tragus and is more likely a "tip-off" to a facelift than the preauricular incision. The novice surgeon is encouraged to perfect the pretragal incision prior to tackling retrotragal incisions.

When the retrotragal incision is made, the cheek skin is redraped over the tragus. The normal tragus is covered with thin, shiny, hairless skin (even in most men), and cheek skin is frequently not the ideal covering. I tend to use the retrotragal incisions in young women with thin, hairless cheek skin. In men, and in women with irregular pigmentation in the preauricular region, thick, oily cheek skin, or with furry cheeks, the incision is made in a preauricular crease. **The key to an invisible scar is absolute lack of tension, not its location.** If the retrotragal incision is chosen, the initial undermining is performed slowly and with care to avoid any damage to the tragal cartilage.

The incision passes beneath the earlobe and extends into the retroauricular sulcus. The incision is placed slightly up on the ear because it is also prone to migration and is best hidden if the final scar rests in the depth of the sulcus. The incision traverses the hairless skin in the retroauricular region at a point sufficiently high to be invisible if the patient were to have short hair or be wearing hair in ponytail. The incision then extends along the hairline for a short distance (1.5 cm) and passes back into the occipital scalp in the form of an "S" or an inverted "V." When the neck skin is redraped, it is difficult to completely avoid a step-off in the hairline. If the incision extends too far down the hairline before passing into the scalp, this step-off, however small, is more noticeable. Hence the recommendation to limit the hairline portion to 1.5 cm.

Undermining

Once the incisions are made, undermining is performed. The extent of undermining depends on the degree of aging changes,

the area where these changes exist, the surgeon's instinct about the health and vascularity of the tissues, and the manipulation planned for the deeper tissues. The various options for deep-tissue manipulation are summarized below. Depending on the extent of undermining performed, a fiberoptic retractor may provide useful visualization. Many experienced surgeons undermine using a "blind" technique, gauging the depth of the dissection by feel and by watching the skin as the knife or scissors move beneath it. **I prefer—and strongly recommend—that dissection be performed under direct vision. The tissues involved are thin and it only takes a minor slip of the scissor tip to cut a branch of the facial nerve and result in permanent disability for the patient.** Some surgeons also find that countertraction applied by an assistant facilitates the dissection. The neophyte should be aware that the stronger the countertraction, the thinner the skin flap that is usually dissected. Although one wants to avoid dissection that is too deep, a flap that is too thin is also not desirable.

Redraping

The undermined skin flap is redraped in a cephaloposterior direction. The transverse incision is made below the sideburn. The superior flap, with the sideburn on it, is fixed at the level of the ear–cheek junction—and no higher! The cheek skin is redraped along a line from the chin to the sideburn, overlapping the previously fixed flap. A triangle of hairless, excess cheek skin is excised and the cheek is fixed under some tension with a single suture at the top of the ear, in such a way that there is no dog-ear at the anterior end of the transverse incision. The neck skin is redraped more horizontally, parallel to the neck creases. A second suture is placed under some tension at the apex of the retroauricular incision. Care is taken not to redrape the transverse neck creases up on to the face. This creates another bizarre "facelift look." Once these two tension-bearing sutures have been placed, the flap is incised so that the ear can barely be withdrawn from beneath the flap. The cheek flap is tucked up under the earlobe, leaving no possibility that the scar will be visible. The excess skin in front of and behind the ear is trimmed with extreme conservatism so that there is absolutely no tension on the closure. There should be almost no need for sutures because the coaptation of the skin edges is so precise. If a retrotragal incision is used, the tragal flap is cut so that it is redundant in all directions. The skin over the tragus tends to contract and, if there is not sufficient excess, will pull the tragus foreword, opening the view to the external auditory canal. A closed suction drain is left in the neck in the most dependent portion of the incision.

Regardless of the technique chosen for facelifting, the incisions and the final redraping are critical. If the incisions are performed properly, the redraping is appropriate, and the patient experiences uncomplicated wound healing, it is frequently difficult for the surgeon or the hairdresser to find the scars.

SMAS Dissections

Traditional SMAS Dissection

SMAS dissections vary in extent. The "traditional" SMAS dissection involves a transverse incision in the SMAS at a level just below the zygomatic arch and an intersecting preauricular SMAS incision that extends over the angle of the mandible and along the anterior border of the sternomastoid muscle. The SMAS is elevated off the parotid fascia, a separate anatomic structure, in continuity with the platysma muscle in the neck. The end point of the dissection is just beyond the anterior border of the parotid gland. The SMAS over the parotid gland is relatively immobile, compared to the SMAS beyond the gland.

If dissection is not performed beyond the gland, insufficient re-lease occurs, and tension on the SMAS is less efficiently trans-mitted to the jowls and neck. The SMAS–platysma flap is ro-tated in a cephaloposterior direction, trimmed, and sutured to the immobile SMAS along the original incision lines. The platysma portion of the flap is sutured to the tissues over the mastoid, increasing the definition of the mandibular angle.

The traditional SMAS dissection is effective for minimizing the jowls and highlighting the mandibular angle.

Extended SMAS Dissection

The extended SMAS dissection differs in two ways from the traditional SMAS dissection: the level of the transverse inci-sion and the anterior extent of the dissection. The transverse incision is made above the zygomatic arch. Although concern has been expressed about the safety of this maneuver, it can be performed safely on a consistent basis with appropriate training. The same intersecting incision is made in the preau-ricular region and along the sternocleidomastoid muscle. The flap is elevated well beyond the anterior end of the parotid. The zygomaticus major is visualized. Dissection continues over the superficial surface of this muscle to avoid its denervation (Fig. 49.4). The large SMAS–platysma flap is rotated in a cephaloposterior direction, trimmed, and sutured along the original incision lines. The platysma is sutured to the mastoid periosteum.

The extended SMAS has the advantage of providing malar augmentation as well as an effect on the jowls and neck. It is my opinion, after performing this technique for many years, that there is a trade-off: the benefit of the high dissection is offset somewhat by a less-efficient effect on the jowls. The greater distance between the point of fixation and the jowls in the extended technique accounts for this difference.

SMASectomy and SMAS Plication

SMASectomy

Baker described the lateral SMASectomy procedure (8), and some variation of this technique is probably the most frequently performed facelift technique in the United States today. A strip of SMAS is excised on an oblique line between the angle of the mandible and lateral canthus (Fig. 49.5). The mobile SMAS is sutured to the immobile SMAS, accomplishing all the benefits of both the traditional and extended SMAS procedures. The platysma is sutured to the mastoid in a manner identical to a formal SMAS dissection.

SMAS Plication

In thin patients, the SMAS can be plicated along the same line, without removing any tissue. Although it may be necessary to remove a small amount of redundant SMAS over the angle of the mandible, the rest of the tissue is preserved. With the current trend of fat preservation, this is an appealing alternative. In heavier faces, the SMASectomy alternative is preferable.

The technique has enormous advantages. It is simple in de-sign, can be modified to suit different facial shapes, and is less time-consuming than other techniques. It provides the malar augmentation of the extended SMAS with the more efficient ef-fect on the jowls of the traditional SMAS procedure. It has the theoretical additional benefit that the SMAS is not undermined and thus not subject to the devascularization and atrophy that

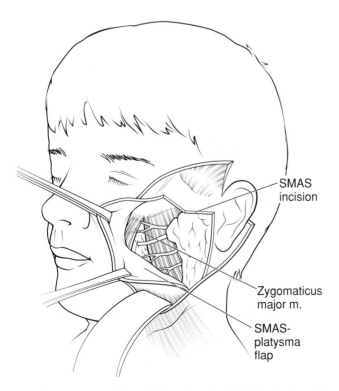

FIGURE 49.4. Extended SMAS dissection. The SMAS flap is elevated, revealing the buccal branches of the facial nerve lying on the surface of the masseter muscle. The dissection passes over the superficial surface of the zygomaticus major, preserving its innervation.

SMAS incision

Zygomaticus major m.

SMAS-platysma flap

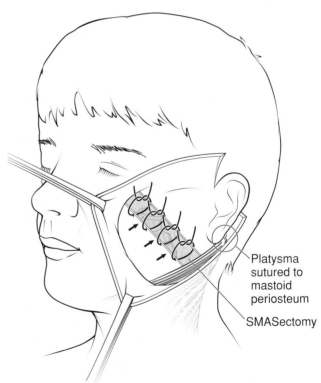

Platysma sutured to mastoid periosteum

SMASectomy

FIGURE 49.5. SMASectomy. The oblique strip of SMAS to be ex-cised is shown, extending from the angle of the mandible to the lateral canthal region. The platysma muscle in the neck is sutured to the mas-toid periosteum. The mobile SMAS anterior to the SMASectomy is advanced to the immobile SMAS. This illustration shows the SMAS being advanced in an oblique cephaloposterior direction. In fact, the oblique SMASectomy defect can be closed in a vertical fashion (imag-ine the *black arrows* pointing vertically). The more vertical the closure, the greater the effect on the neck.

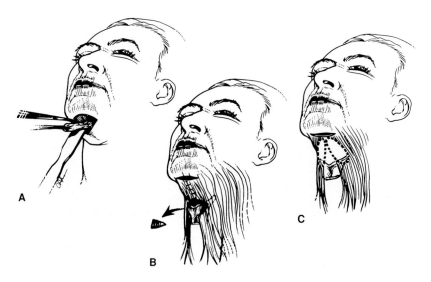

FIGURE 49.6. Treatment of medial platysma and platysma bands. Alternatives include (**A**) defatting of the anterior platysma without muscle modification; (**B**) midline platysmaplasty with wedge excision; and (**C**) resection of platysma bands without midline approximation. If a submental incision is elected, option (**B**) is usually the best alternative.

can occur when SMAS flaps are elevated. The disadvantage is that injury to buccal branches of the facial nerve can occur if sutures are placed too deeply.

Deep Plane or Composite Rhytidectomy

Hamra described the deep plane facelift that he modified to its current iteration, the composite rhytidectomy (9). This brief description does not do the technique justice, but does outline the key points. The SMAS and skin are dissected together as a single flap, rather than independently, as in the techniques described above. The benefit of the procedure is that theoretically the flap is better vascularized and less likely to slough. The technique, as Hamra performs it, includes a superomedial elevation of the malar tissues and orbicularis oculi muscle and a brow lift with a similar superomedial vector. The disadvantage of the technique is the magnitude of the procedure and the prolonged recovery period.

It is my opinion, *never* having performed this procedure myself, that the benefits of the procedure do not justify the invasiveness, risk, and prolonged recovery associated with the procedure.

Rejuvenation of the Neck

The procedures outlined above have a beneficial effect on the neck. In some patients, however, additional procedures are required, in combination with the above, to provide better definition to the neck. Some of these procedures are controversial.

Submental Dissection and Platysmaplasty

The SMASectomy procedure, with its efficient elevation of the jowl and submental tissues, has decreased the need for submental incisions and open-neck procedures. As mentioned above, the closure of the SMAS (or the plication of the SMAS if no tissue is removed) is performed at a shorter distance from the jowls and submental region, and has a profound effect on those areas. There are, however, patients with enough redundant skin, excess fat, and redundant platysma who still require a formal submental dissection.

In these patients, an incision is made just caudal to the submental crease. Subcutaneous undermining is performed. A judgment is made about defatting of the platysma muscle, as mentioned below. An independent decision is made regarding removal of subplatysmal fat. The medial borders of the

platysma muscle are plicated in the midline using buried interrupted sutures (Fig. 49.6). Compulsive attention to both hemostasis and perioperative blood pressure control is essential to prevent a hematoma when this larger dead space is created.

Corset Platysmaplasty

Feldman described the corset platysmaplasty. The medial borders of the platysma are plicated with a continuous monofilament suture that is run up and down the midline of the neck until the desired contour has been achieved. No manipulation of the lateral border of the platysma is performed.

I have had better experience with buried, interrupted sutures, which cause less bunching of the muscle. I also prefer to combine the midline platysmaplasty with lateral tightening of the platysma as described above under "SMAS Techniques" and "SMASectomy."

Defatting of the Neck

A guiding principle is preservation of facial fat. This principle also applies to the neck but less so. Many patients benefit aesthetically from cervical defatting. The surgeon is meticulous about avoiding overdefatting because unsightly adhesions between the skin and platysma can occur. The same applies to removal of subplatysmal fat. Overskeletonization of the neck is one stigmata of an amateurish facelift.

Submandibular Glands

The presence of large and/or ptotic submandibular glands prevents the creation of a clean neck after facelifting. The question of whether excision of the glands is worth the risk of bleeding and nerve injury has not been answered. Sullivan reports an acceptably low complication rate for submandibular gland resection associated with facelifting.

I have not had a complication from submandibular gland resection accompanying a facelift, but no longer believe that the benefits are worth the additional time required or the risk of bleeding and nerve injury.

Digastric Muscle Resection

Connell recommends shaving of the anterior belly of the digastric muscles to further define the cervicomental angle. I believe this creates an excessively sculpted, overdone look in many necks and is best avoided.

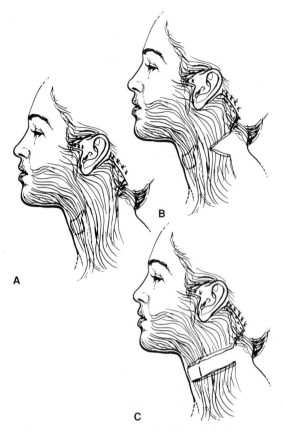

FIGURE 49.7. Lateral platysma modification. Alternatives include (**A**) advancement of lateral platysma parallel to mandibular border with suture fixation to the mastoid periosteum; (**B**) partial transection of lateral platysma with similar fixation; and (**C**) full-width transection of platysma with similar suture fixation. Most SMAS flap and SMAS-ectomy/SMAS plication procedures include tightening of the lateral platysma. The most common alternative is (**A**). Alternative (**B**) may provide additional contouring to the mandibular angle in patients who require increased definition. Alternative (**C**) is the single most powerful technique to increase neck definition, but is associated with a higher incidence of neck irregularities, adhesions between the skin and muscle, and an overcorrected appearance in some patients.

Full-width Platysma Transection

The single most powerful way to create a well-defined neck is to perform full-width transection of the platysma muscle across the neck (Fig. 49.7C). The muscle is divided under direct vision at least 6 cm below the inferior border of the mandible.

I only employ this technique in the most difficult necks, because irregularities and an overoperated look can be created and there is additional risk of hematoma and prolonged induration in the neck.

Short-Scar Technique

Baker described the "short-scar" procedure, in which all the elements of the subcutaneous dissection with SMASectomy and lateral platysma tightening are performed, but the skin incision is limited to the preauricular portion. It is useful in younger patients with minimal excess neck skin. The incision is not extended beyond the earlobe, thereby avoiding the postauricular incision and the extension into the hairline. The technique relies on vertical redraping of the skin. Bunching of skin behind the earlobe often occurs but improves with time. Care is taken, however, to distribute the bunching as much as possible because

patients will complain about it, even if it eventually improves. There is no question that the absence of the retroauricular incision is an advantage. While the retroauricular incision in most patients having traditional facelift incisions heals well and is sometimes virtually invisible, there are patients in whom this is *not* the case and the scar is visible, slightly hypertrophic, and, despite the surgeon's best efforts, there is a slight step-off in the occipital hairline.

MACS Lift

Tonnard described the minimal access cranial suspension (MACS) lift, which employs purse-string sutures in the SMAS structures and malar fat pad with vertical suspension (10). The vertical nature of the lift requires an incision along the anterior sideburn and anterior temporal hairline. The procedure can be performed in combination with midline platysmaplasty to improve the results in the neck. Excess skin may appear below the earlobe, which may require posterior cervicoplasty to correct.

Subperiosteal Facelift

Originally described by Tessier, Heinrichs has reported a large series of subperiosteal facelifts (11). The procedure is designed to rejuvenate the upper and middle thirds of the face. Subperiosteal undermining is performed through the following incisions in various combinations, depending on the surgeon: coronal incision or endobrow approach, subciliary incision, or an upper buccal sulcus incision. Hester has described a subperiosteal midface lift using endoscopic assistance through the lateral aspect of a lower-eyelid incision (12).

I am not impressed with the effectiveness or the longevity of subperiosteal lifts, but surgeons who have extensive experience with the technique probably have better results. Postoperative swelling can be profound after subperiosteal undermining. The author believes that the closer one is to that which is being lifted (i.e., the skin), the more effective the lift and considers subcutaneous undermining the gold standard.

Secondary Facelifting

The goals of secondary facelifting are to (a) relift the face and neck, (b) remove the primary facelift scars, and (c) preserve maximum temporal and sideburn hair. Dissection is usually easier than the primary dissection. Intraoperative bleeding and postoperative hematomas are also less frequent. The amount of skin excised at a secondary lift is much less than at the primary procedure. For this reason pre-excision of skin is never performed for a secondary facelift. The risk of nerve injury may be slightly higher in secondary facelifts, however. The first procedure may have distorted the anatomy and the tissues may be abnormally thin.

Facelifting in Men

The shorter hairstyles of men are less forgiving than the longer hairstyles of women. Male faces tend to be larger and dissection is more time-consuming. Modified incisions have been described for men, but I use the same incision in patients of both sexes. Some men may have a tremendous amount of excess skin in the neck. When this is redraped into the retroauricular area, care is required to avoid a large step-off in the hairline. The previously reported higher incidence of hematomas in men than in women seems to be largely related to blood pressure.

When blood pressure is controlled, the hematoma rates are very similar.

Barbed Sutures

In an effort to make facelifting quicker and less invasive, several authors describe the use of barbed sutures in facelifting. The longevity of the result does not compare favorably with traditional methods. At the present time, the sutures are made of polypropylene and are permanent. Concerns have been raised regarding the safety of permanent barbed sutures in the subcutaneous position. Long-term data are not yet available.

POSTOPERATIVE CARE

Although in most cases the patients do not require hospitalization, ideally they do have an experienced nurse to monitor them closely. Patients are instructed to rest with the head elevated for the first several postoperative days. Blood pressure is monitored and kept under strict control for the first 24 hours. The drains are usually removed on the first postoperative morning and showering and shampooing are encouraged at that point. Pain medication is usually required, especially at night, for several days. Oral antibiotics are generally prescribed, although there is no evidence that they are beneficial. Studies show that steroids are of no benefit in reducing swelling. Sutures are removed progressively beginning on the fourth postoperative day. All the sutures are usually gone by the eighth postoperative day.

Swelling and bruising are variable. Depending on the ancillary procedures performed, patients look reasonably acceptable after 1 week, good with makeup after 2 weeks, and able to attend social functions after 3 weeks. An occasional patient will have prolonged bruising that may limit activity for a longer period of time.

PATIENT SAFETY AND COMPLICATIONS

Despite constant attention to detail, complications do occur. The most common problems and methods to prevent and to treat such complications are summarized in the following sections (13).

Hematoma

Hematomas are by far the most common complication after facelifting and vary from large collections of blood that threaten the survival of the skin flaps (and even compromise the airway) to small collections that are evident only when facial edema has subsided. Most major hematomas occur during the first 10 to 12 hours postoperatively.

The most common presentation of a hematoma is an apprehensive, restless patient experiencing pain insolated to one side of the face or neck. Because localized and worsening pain is unusual following an uncomplicated facelift, it must be regarded as a sign of hematoma until proven otherwise. Rather than provide analgesics for pain relief, the surgeon or nurse removes the dressing immediately to permit examination. In addition to causing skin flap ischemia, a large expanding hematoma under tight skin flaps has the potential to cause respiratory compromise.

The treatment for a hematoma of any degree is evacuation. If the collection is rapidly enlarging or if the flaps appear compromised, then sutures may be removed at the bedside for immediate relief of some of the pressure. Depending on the extent of the bleeding, the emotional state of the patient, and the availability of an operating room, the hematoma is either evacuated at the bedside or in the operating room. The important thing is to get the blood out. If formally explored, a specific bleeding point will rarely be found. If evacuated at the bedside, the patient must be sedated and the blood pressure reduced. Catheters are inserted and the hematoma is evacuated. The region is irrigated with saline until clear, and then with a 0.25% solution of lidocaine containing epinephrine 1:400,000. Gentle pressure is placed on the flap for 20 minutes. If this method does not result in complete removal of the hematomas, then the facelift wound is formally explored under adequate anesthesia to permit visualization and precise control of any bleeding.

The reported incidence of hematomas requiring evacuation ranges from 0.9% to 8.0%, but is approximately 3% to 4% when all studies are combined. Because most patients in the reported studies were women, this 3% to 4% range represents the incidence in female patients. Early studies demonstrated a hematoma rate in men of 7% to 9%, or twice that of women. More recent studies suggest that this difference between the two sexes is at least partly a consequence of blood pressure. When blood pressure in male patients is compulsively controlled, the incidence falls precipitously, approaching that of women.

As mentioned in the "Preoperative Preparation" and "Anesthesia" sections, blood pressure control is the single most important preventative measure. Ranking next in importance is the avoidance of medications that interfere with clotting or coagulation. Finally, every attempt is made to prevent vomiting, coughing, anxiety, or pain.

Small hematomas of 2 to 20 mL that are not apparent until edema begins to subside are a totally different entity and occur in 10% to 15% of patients. Initially, an area of firmness is palpable followed by ecchymosis in the overlying skin. Although somewhat controversial, it is my opinion that every effort should be made to evacuate even the small hematomas. A syringe and large-bore needle are used. Aspiration is repeated every few days until the collection is completely gone or no further liquid can be withdrawn. Repeated aspiration attempts are especially important in the neck where larger collections can be hiding. If the blood is not evacuated, the patient may develop a firm, woody, wrinkled mass that takes months to resolve, and in some cases leaves permanent changes in the skin. Compulsive attention to hemostasis, blood pressure control, drain placement, and postoperative management is required to obtain the best possible results in the neck. Rest-on foam applied to neck as the original dressing may also be of benefit.

Neck hematomas are more common when submental dissections are included in the facelift procedure. This fact, combined with the beneficial effect on the neck that accompanies the SMASectomy/SMAS plication techniques, has led to a smaller percentage of patients having submental incisions and midline platysmaplasties. The cost-to-benefit analysis between opening the neck to improve neck definition and avoiding submental dissections to prevent complications is a judgment that must be made for each patient, with the knowledge that neither choice may be perfect.

Triamcinolone (Kenalog) injections to small hematomas and areas of firmness are discouraged. They probably offer no benefit over watchful waiting and hematoma aspiration, and can result in subcutaneous atrophy and a depression when the hematoma resolves.

Skin Slough

Luckily for the patient and the surgeon, the most common location for skin slough is in the retroauricular area where the scarring is less visible. The bad news is that full-thickness skin loss will inevitably result in less-favorable scarring, which can be distressing to the patient and prevent the patient from wearing certain hairstyles. If the skin necrosis occurs in the preauricular area, it is a devastating complication.

The incidence of skin necrosis is 1% to 3%. The most likely causes of skin slough are (a) unrecognized hematomas, (b) a skin flap that is too thin or is damaged during flap dissection or burned with electrocautery, (c) excessive tension on wound closure, (d) cigarette smoking, and, possibly, (e) dehydration. There is no question that smoking increases the risk of skin slough. It is my impression that patients who are well hydrated tend to heal faster with a lower incidence of skin slough.

If the skin appears compromised at any point in the post-operative period, antibiotic ointment or silver sulfadiazine (Silvadene) cream is applied. The surgeon would much rather apply ointment to an area that turns out to be a partial-thickness injury than miss an area that is dying where some of the damage could be limited by aggressive wound care.

The treatment of skin slough is not surgical; it is conservative wound care. Areas of necrosis will contract dramatically and eventually epithelialize. The final scar, although permanent, is almost always better than would be anticipated from the initial wound appearance. If a secondary facelift is performed in an attempt to remove the scars, minimal excess skin will be present, and it may not be possible to remove scar that is more than 1 cm from the previous incision.

Nerve Injury

Injury to a branch of the facial nerve (cranial nerve [CN] VII) is the complication most dreaded by patients. Motor nerve injury occurs in 0.9% of patients who receive subcutaneous undermining only, but is more common with dissection of the SMAS, either as an independent layer or in a composite rhytidectomy. Many nerve injuries are temporary, presumably the result of traction or cautery. A nerve that has been transected will not recover function. If the surgeon is aware that a branch has been cut, then immediate intraoperative microsurgical repair is mandated. It is more likely, however, that nerve injury is not recognized during surgery, and the surgeon and patient are placed in the difficult position of waiting for return of function. Injuries to buccal branches tend to improve more than those in the frontal and marginal mandibular territories, presumably because of greater degrees of connections between branches in those areas.

Transient numbness of the cheeks and neck skin is a result of interruption of the small sensory branches during skin undermining and is unavoidable. Sensibility always recovers although it may take months to do so. Injury to the great auricular nerve is another matter. It is a large sensory nerve, as described under "Facelift Anatomy," and transection will result in permanent numbness of half of the ear and, in some cases, a painful neuroma. The nerve is quite superficial on the surface of the sternomastoid muscle, especially in thin patients, and is easily transected. If such a transection occurs, the nerve should be approximated with appropriate microsurgical suture.

Hypertrophic Scarring

Hypertrophic scarring is most often attributable to excessive tension on the incision closure. Some patients, however, develop hypertrophic scars despite the best efforts of the surgeon. As with skin slough, this usually involves the retroauricular area, which is less visible, but can occur in the preauricular area where it is a bad complication. Small volumes of dilute triamcinolone are injected into the scars (not the adjacent normal tissue), sometimes more than once, and this usually improves the appearance of the scar significantly. An occasional patient will get true keloids of the facelift incisions, which are difficult to treat. Scar revision with immediate treatment with radiation is the best option is these difficult situations.

References

1. Rees JD, Liverett DM, Guy CL. The effect of cigarette smoking on skin-flap survival in the face-lift patient. *Plast Reconstr Surg.* 1984;73:911.
2. Mitz V, Peyronie M. The superficial musculoaponeurotic system (SMAS) in the parotid and cheek area. *Plast Reconstr Surg.* 1976;58:80.
3. Gosain A, Yousif NJ, Madiedo G, et al. Surgical anatomy of the SMAS: A reinvestigation. *Plast Reconstr Surg.* 1993;92:1254.
4. Stuzin J, Wagstrom L, Kawamoto HK, et al. Anatomy of the frontal branch of the facial nerve: The significance of the temporal fat pad. *Plast Reconstr Surg.* 1989;83:265.
5. Furnas D. The retaining ligaments of the cheek. *Plast Reconstr Surg.* 1989; 83:11.
6. Vistnes LM, Souther SG. The anatomic basis for common cosmetic anterior neck deformities. *Ann Plast Surg.* 1979;2:381.
7. McKinney P, Katrana DJ. Prevention of injury to the great auricular nerve during rhytidectomy. *Plast Reconstr Surg.* 1980;66:675.
8. Baker DC. Lateral SMASectomy. *Plast Reconstr Surg.* 1997;100(2):509.
9. Hamra ST. Composite rhytidectomy. *Plast Reconstr Surg.* 1992;90:1.
10. Tonnard PL, Verpaele A, Gaia S. Optimizing results from minimal access cranial suspension lifting (MACS-lift). *Aesth Plast Surg.* 2005;29(4): 213.
11. Heinrichs HL, Kaidi AA. Subperiosteal facelift: A 200-case, 4-year review. *Plast Reconstr Surg.* 1998;102(3):843.
12. Hester TR, Codner MA, McCord CD, et al. Evolution of technique of the direct transblepharoplasty approach for the correction of lower lid and mid-facial aging: Maximizing results and minimizing complications in a 5-year experience. *Plast Reconstr Surg.* 2000;105(1):393.
13. Baker DC. Complications of cervicofacial rhytidectomy. *Clin Plast Surg* 1983;10:543.

CHAPTER 50 ■ FOREHEAD LIFT

DAVID M. KNIZE

HISTORICAL PERSPECTIVE

Although the concept of using the coronal incision approach for elevation of the forehead and eyebrows was introduced in the 1962 (1), brow or forehead lifting was not incorporated into the facelift procedure until 1974 (2). Thereafter, the coronal incision forehead lift technique quickly became a standard component of the facelift procedure. By the mid 1990s, however, this coronal incision technique was challenged by the introduction of the endoscopic technique (3) and of the limited-incision technique (4), each of which produced shorter scars and less scalp sensory loss. **Today, the surgical results that can be obtained from these two newer techniques are comparable to those obtained from the coronal incision technique with far fewer of the undesirable side effects associated with the coronal incision, specifically, long scars, alopecia, and dysesthesias of the scalp.** Although the coronal incision forehead lift is currently the most commonly used technique, the clear trend is toward procedures performed through shorter incisions.

INDICATIONS FOR THE FOREHEAD LIFT

The great majority of the patients who present to their surgeon with concerns about the appearance of their upper face complain that they are often told by family members or friends that they look tired, sad, or even angry when they do not feel those emotions. These patients want the surgeon to remove the appearance of these negative emotional states, and they almost always assume that this can be accomplished with a blepharoplasty procedure. Consequently, they are surprised to hear that they require a more complex operation to accomplish their goal. The surgeon has the delicate and sometimes difficult task of helping the patient understand that their problem involves not only the eyelids, but also the adjacent tissues that "frame" the eyes. This concept becomes easier for the patient to understand if the surgeon can point out on the patient's face the specific physical changes that contribute to their appearance. The characteristic signs of the aging forehead (Fig. 50.1) that are addressed with the forehead lift procedure are

- ptotic eyebrows (especially the lateral eyebrow segments);
- descended eyebrow skin onto the orbit where it appears to be excess eyelid skin;
- transverse forehead skin lines;
- vertical/oblique/transverse glabellar skin lines.

It is helpful for the patient to understand that these changes in their appearance were produced by a cascade of events over time. The patient's eyebrow ptosis resulted from the effects of gravity plus the contraction forces of certain muscles. The glabellar eyebrow depressor muscles both lowered the medial segment and produced vertical, transverse, and oblique glabellar skin lines. Contraction of the lateral orbicularis oculi muscle lowered the lateral eyebrow segment and produced "crows

feet" lines. As the eyebrows descended, eyebrow skin, especially the lateral component flowed into the upper orbit to augment any redundant upper eyelid skin. As this was occurring, transverse forehead lines were produced by reflex action of the frontalis muscles to pull the descended eyebrow skin off of the upper eyelids.

With this information, the patient can appreciate that the appearance the patient dislikes cannot be changed unless the patient's redundant eyelid skin is treated with a concomitant forehead lift procedure. The combined effect of these procedures produces a cosmetic benefit for the patient that cannot be produced by either procedure alone. **In fact, if the usual upper blepharoplasty is done alone, the patient will experience a progressive lowering of the lateral eyebrow level over time, making the orbital area look smaller. The patient may develop the so-called "beady-eye" appearance. Thus, the patient may become dissatisfied with his or her blepharoplasty result and not understand why (see Chapter 48).**

PREOPERATIVE PATIENT EVALUATION

Medical History

The preoperative evaluation is the same as that for the patient undergoing a facelift procedure (see Chapter 49).

Preoperative Photographs

Photographs are an invaluable tool for demonstrating a patient's facial asymmetries preoperatively. Because most patients are unaware that any asymmetries may exist, this is an important exercise. If unusual facial features are not brought to the patient's attention before the patient's surgical procedure, the patient may experience unnecessary anxiety and concern postoperatively when examining his or her face in the mirror for first time. **Without this preemptive measure, many patients will assume that any postoperative facial asymmetries or abnormalities are the result of surgery.**

There are other important uses for photographic material. Photographs of the patient should be present in the operating room for reference during the operative procedure, because they provide visual information such as eyebrow position or fat pad prominence/location for making judgments at surgery. Other reasons to obtain preoperative photographs are operative planning, result evaluation, legal protection, and educational purposes.

PREOPERATIVE PREPARATION FOR THE SURGEON

The first requirement for any surgeon preparing to do a new or infrequently performed procedure is to become familiar

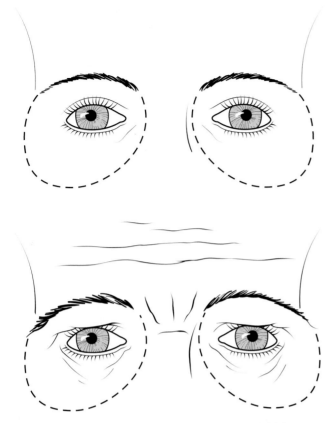

FIGURE 50.1. The aging upper face. Compare the youthful face (top) with the aged face (bottom). Note how the classic appearance of the aged face projects the look of sadness, grief, or tiredness. Removing the appearance of these negative emotional states requires a forehead lift that is usually done in conjunction with a blepharoplasty procedure.

with the local anatomy. The surgeon who understands surgical anatomy is more comfortable and effective at the operating table, and that surgeon's patient benefits from decreased operative risk and better outcomes. The following sections describe the relevant anatomy of the forehead and temporal fossa (5).

Muscles

The paired frontalis muscles (Fig. 50.2) have two parts—a static component and a mobile component. The upper half of each frontalis muscle is relatively static functionally because it is fixed to the underlying deep galea plane that serves as the muscle's origin. The lower half of each frontalis muscle hangs freely and provides the entire range of motion (usually up to 2.5 cm) for the muscle to raise the eyebrows. Thus when the eyebrows are elevated, the lower forehead skin becomes deeply folded or corrugated. The more fixed upper forehead skin is compressed by the mobile lower forehead soft-tissue movement into less deep transverse lines/grooves, whose location is determined by the underlying transverse rows of dermal insertions between skin and frontalis muscle. The mechanism of eyebrow elevation is for the frontalis muscle to pull up the orbicularis oculi muscle, which, in turn, suspends the eyebrow skin through dermal insertions. Thus the frontalis muscle both elevates the eyebrow and unfurrows the orbicularis muscle. Note in Figure 50.2 that the lateral margin of each frontalis muscle typically falls along the clinically palpable temporal fusion line of the skull and its continuation as the superior temporal fusion line. Because the temporal fusion line crosses the eyebrow near the junction of its middle and lateral thirds in the

average patient, **the frontalis muscle can suspend or raise only the medial two-thirds of the eyebrow. Lacking frontalis muscle support in the presence of the lateral orbicularis oculi muscle action to lower the lateral eyebrow, the lateral third of the eyebrow becomes ptotic much earlier in the aging process than the more medial segment.** This unsupported lateral eyebrow segment concept is clinically relevant, because its management must be addressed by any successful forehead lift procedure.

The transverse head of each corrugator supercilii muscle originates from the ipsilateral superior-medial orbital rim and inserts into the dermis immediately cephalad to the middle third of the eyebrow. These bilateral muscles pull the eyebrows medially and produce vertical glabellar skin lines.

Each depressor supercilii muscle originates from the superior-medial orbital rim just caudal to the origin of the corrugator supercilii muscle and, along with the **medial fibers of the orbital portion of the orbicularis oculi muscle and the oblique head of the corrugator supercilii muscle,** acts to depress the medial head of the eyebrow and produce oblique glabellar skin lines.

The procerus muscle originates from the dorsum of the nasal bone and splits into a Y shape to insert into the lower medial edge of each frontalis muscle, and into the midforehead dermis between the frontalis muscles. In this position, the procerus muscle acts as a strong depressor of the medial segment of the eyebrow by antagonizing the frontalis muscle's action to elevate the medial eyebrow. A chronically hyperactive procerus muscle produces transverse dorsal nasal lines.

Fascial Planes

The thick galea plane over the calvarium divides into multiple layers as it flows over the forehead. It forms a superficial and a deep plane at the superior margin of the frontalis muscle on each side of the frontal bone to envelope each muscle. Caudal to the frontalis muscle's origin from the deep galea plane, the deep galea plane splits to envelop the galea fat pad, which lies over the lower half of the forehead. Deep to the galea fat pad, the deepest layer of the deep galea plane fuses to that periosteum that is densely adherent to the lower 2.0 to 2.5 cm of the frontal bone. Elsewhere, periosteum is only loosely adherent to frontal bone, except for a 6-mm wide zone just medial to the superior temporal fusion line of the skull where galea and periosteum are also fused and periosteum is densely fixed to bone (Fig. 50.2). **These two areas of soft-tissue adherence to bone are clinically important, because it is necessary to release the galea tethered to these surfaces before the forehead flap can be adequately mobilized.**

Lateral to the temporal fusion line of the skull, the galea plane extends over the deep temporal fascia of the temporal fossa as the superficial temporal fascia. The deep temporal fascia covers the temporalis muscle. The superficial temporal fascia and the skin of the temporal fossa are firmly bonded together by fibrous dermal insertions such that these two planes move as a unit. Thus suspension of the superficial temporal fascia will support the overlying skin, including the lateral third of the eyebrow. This relationship has clinical relevance to lateral eyebrow elevation with a forehead lift procedure, because it allows the eyebrow to be suspended with tension on the superficial temporal fascia plane instead of the hair-bearing skin plane. Tension-free hair-bearing scalp closure decreases scalp hair loss.

Over the temporal fossa, the superficial temporal fascia and the deep temporal fascia planes are not adherent. However, they form a narrow transverse line of adhesion essentially parallel with and superior to the zygomatic arch. This adhesion line is called the *orbicularis-temporal ligament* (Fig. 50.3). The rami of the temporal branch of the facial nerve reliably pass

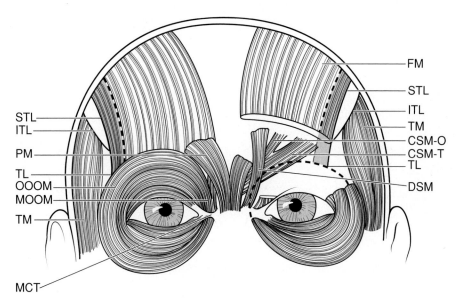

FIGURE 50.2. Muscles of the forehead and glabella. The origin of the paired frontalis muscles (FM) is the deep galea plane. The caudal end of each frontalis muscle interdigitates with the orbital portion of the orbicularis oculi muscle (OOOM), which inserts into the dermis under the eyebrow. The frontalis muscles have no bony attachments. The lateral margin of each frontalis muscle typically falls over the superior temporal fusion line of the skull (STL) and extends just over the 6-mm wide zone (shaded area) within which periosteum and the deep galea plane are densely adherent to bone. The superior temporal fusion line is a continuation of the temporal fusion line of the skull (TL). A strip of periosteum separates the superior from the inferior temporal fusion line of the skull (ITL), which forms the margin of the deep temporal fascia that covers the temporalis muscle. The procerus muscle (PM) takes its origin from the dorsum of the nasal bone and then divides into two heads before interdigitating with the medial margins of the frontalis muscles and inserting into dermis between the frontalis muscles. The depressor supercilii muscle (DSM) is just deep to the lateral edge of the procerus muscle on each side and inserts into dermis under the medial end of the eyebrow. A slip of the orbital portion of the medial orbicularis oculi muscle (MOOM) originates from the medial canthal tendon (MCT) and also inserts into the dermis under the medial eyebrow. This slip of orbicularis muscle lies superficial to the depressor supercilii muscle and the origin of the corrugator supercilii muscle. The corrugator supercilii muscle has two heads—a transverse head (DSM-T) and an oblique (DSM-O) head. The oblique head of the corrugator supercilii muscle inserts into dermis under the medial head of the eyebrow near the insertion of the depressor supercilii muscle. The depressor supercilii muscle, the oblique head of the corrugator supercilii muscle, and the medial slip of the orbicularis oculi muscle all act to depress the medial eyebrow in conjunction with the action of the procerus muscle. Each temporalis muscle originates from the temporal fossa and inserts on the coronoid process of the mandible to act as a muscle of mastication. (Modified from Knize DM. *Forehead and Temporal Fossa, Anatomy and Technique.* Philadelphia: Lippincott-Williams & Wilkins; 2001:12, Fig. 2.1A, with permission.)

immediately caudal to this adhesion line, which makes it a clinically important guide for locating and protecting these nerves.

Sensory Nerves

Sensibility to the forehead is provided by the supratrochlear and the supraorbital nerves (Fig. 50.4). The supratrochlear nerve exits bone within the orbit and passes through the medial head of the corrugator supercilii muscle as six to eight filamentous strands to supply the midforehead skin. The supraorbital nerve trunk can exit bone at any point along the superior orbital rim up to 1.5 cm cephalad to the rim margin. Ninety percent of the time, however, the supraorbital nerve trunk exits bone at the supraorbital notch. The supraorbital nerve trunk divides into a superficial division and a deep division. The superficial division forms filaments that run over the surface of frontalis muscle to supply sensation to the forehead skin and the anterior margin of the frontal scalp. The deep division runs under frontalis muscle between periosteum and galea over the lower 2.0 to 2.5 cm of the frontal bone and then pierces the

overlying galea to run within the layers of the galea, always within an approximately 1.5-cm wide zone immediately medial to the superior temporal fusion line of the skull (Fig. 50.2) en route to the frontoparietal scalp. **It is clinically important to appreciate that this deep division is the primary nerve that provides frontoparietal scalp sensation, and that its transection will result in permanent scalp numbness/dysesthesia.** The deep division's bony exit can be separate from that of the supraorbital trunk. Occasionally, it exits the lateral frontal bone just cephalad to the orbital rim, and the surgeon must watch for this variant.

Motor Nerves

The frontalis muscle is supplied by the three to five temporal branches of the facial nerve that enter the lateral edge of each side of this paired muscle (Fig. 50.5). These temporal branches also supply the lateral end of the corrugator supercilii muscles and the superior end of the procerus muscle. The zygomatic branch of the facial nerve supplies the inferior end of the

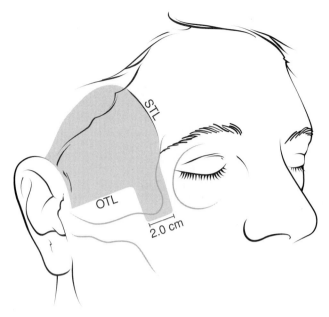

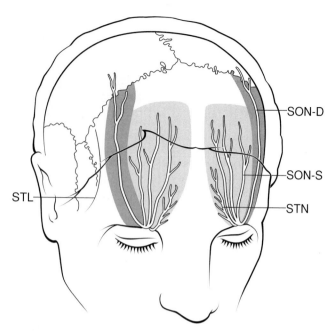

FIGURE 50.3. Safe zone. Dissection in the stripped (*shaded*) area is safe from inadvertent nerve injury if dissection remains on the plane of the deep temporal fascia or periosteum. Over the temporal fossa, the safe zone extends medially to the superior temporal fusion line of the skull (STL) and inferiorly to the orbicularis-temporal ligament (OTL), the transverse zone along which superficial temporal fascia fuses with deep temporal fascia. Lateral to the orbital rim is a 2.0-cm wide extension of the safe zone, as shown, lateral to which the temporal branch of the facial nerve passes as three to five filamentous rami running within the superficial temporal fascia that arches over this area. These overlying rami can be avoided if dissection is performed only on the deep temporal fascia plane, while taking care to avoid a stretch injury to the rami by forceful soft-tissue elevation. (Modified from Knize DM. *Forehead and Temporal Fossa, Anatomy and Technique.* Philadelphia: Lippincott-Williams & Wilkins; 2001:42, Fig. 3.17, with permission.)

FIGURE 50.4. Sensory nerves of the forehead and scalp. The supratrochlear nerve (STN) and the superficial division of the supraorbital nerve (SON-S) provide sensation for the forehead and anterior scalp on each side. The deep division of the supraorbital nerve (SON-D) supplies sensation to the frontoparietal scalp on each side. The deep division has no cutaneous sensory territory on the forehead skin as it passes under the frontalis muscle deep to the galea plane just medial to the superior temporal line of the skull (STL) to reach the frontoparietal scalp. The darker area shown here marks the "danger" zone for injury to the deep division. Within this 1.5-cm zone, the deep division can be transected from any surgical incision or dissection that penetrates the deep galea plane, within which this nerve runs. (Modified from Knize DM. *Forehead and Temporal Fossa, Anatomy and Technique.* Philadelphia: Lippincott-Williams & Wilkins; 2001:32, Fig. 3.5A, with permission.)

procerus muscle and the other medial eyebrow depressor muscles (Fig. 50.2) on each side. The "safe zone" for dissection in the temporal area to avoid injury to the temporal branch of the facial nerve is shown in Figure 50.3. Chapter 48 provides further details on motor innervation of the periorbital muscles.

SURGICAL GOALS OF THE FOREHEADPLASTY PROCEDURE

The specific surgical goals for any foreheadplasty procedure are to

- elevate ptotic eyebrows, especially the lateral eyebrow segment;
- make the transverse forehead lines smoother.
- make the glabellar lines smoother;
- excise excess upper eyelid skin while preserving descended eyebrow skin;
- preserve scalp hair;
- preserve scalp sensation.

The goal of eyebrow elevation deserves special comment. Ellenbogen (6) proposed five criteria for ideal eyebrow position and shape. (a) The brow begins medially at a vertical line drawn perpendicular through the alar base. (b) The brow terminates laterally at an oblique line drawn through the lateral canthus of the eye and the alar base. (c) The medial and lateral ends lie at approximately the same horizontal level. (d) The apex of the brow lies on the vertical line drawn directly through the lateral

limbus of the eye. (e) The brow arches above the supraorbital rim in women and lies at approximately the level of the rim in men.

Although commendable, these criteria may not always be achievable in the clinical setting. For practical purposes, postoperative eyebrow position is almost always satisfactory as long as the lateral eyebrow segment is simply higher than the medial segment in the female patient and level with the medial segment in the male patient.

ANESTHESIA

Although general anesthesia is appropriate, the forehead lift procedure can generally be done comfortably under intravenous sedation and local infiltration or regional blocks. In most cases, anesthesia should be managed by an anesthesiologist or a nurse anesthetist, rather than by the operating surgeon.

TECHNIQUES

Three techniques are used to perform a forehead lift procedure: the coronal, the endoscopic, and the limited-incision foreheadplasty techniques. The following three surgical steps are common to each of these techniques done in conjunction with a bletharoplasty:

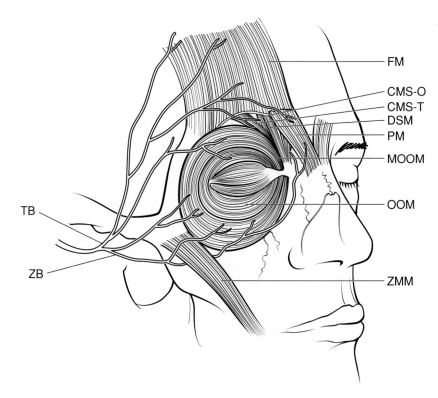

FM
CMS-O
CMS-T
DSM
PM
MOOM
OOM
TB
ZB
ZMM

FIGURE 50.5. Motor nerves of the forehead. The temporal branch (TB) of the facial nerve can be seen supplying the frontalis (FM), the superior orbicularis oculi (OOM), transverse head of the corrugator supercilii (CSM-T), and superior procerus (PM) muscles. The zygomatic branch (ZB) of the facial nerve passes under the zygomaticus major muscle (ZMM) to supply the lower part of the orbicularis oculi and the lower procerus muscle. In addition to supplying the lower procerus muscle, a depressor of the medial eyebrow, the zygomatic branch may also supply the three other depressor muscles of the medial eyebrow, the depressor supercilii (DSM), the medial slip of the orbicularis oculi (MOOM), and the oblique head of the corrugator supercilii (CSM-O) muscles. (Modified from Knize DM. *Forehead and Temporal Fossa, Anatomy and Technique*). Philadelphia: Lippincott-Williams & Wilkins; 2001:39, Fig. 3.13, with permission.)

1. The area of excess upper eyelid skin is measured with a forceps at the start of the procedure. At that time, the surgeon determines how much of this excess upper eyelid skin will be resuspended when the eyebrow is later elevated with transposition of the forehead flap. This resuspended eyelid skin is the eyebrow skin that descended into the orbit, and it should be preserved for the eyebrow. Only the remaining upper eyelid skin is marked for excision.

2. The scalp incision lines are marked, and the forehead/scalp soft tissues are infiltrated with 0.25% to 0.50% lidocaine with 1:400,000 to 1:200,000 epinephrine solution. The first incisions are made after allowing 10 minutes for full epinephrine effect. The incisions are made parallel to the axis of the hair follicles to minimize follicle injury and postsurgical hair loss.

3. Unless a subcutaneous approach is elected, the dense adhesions of galea and periosteum to bone along the 6-mm wide zone just medial to the superior temporal fusion line of the skull and along the supraorbital frontal bone are released to ensure flap mobility for later forehead flap transposition. As soft tissue is dissected from above the orbital rim, the deep division of the supraorbital nerve that runs between galea and periosteum over the lower 2.0 to 2.5 cm of the forehead may be visualized to protect it from inadvertent transection.

Except for these common features, each foreheadplasty technique has unique features, which are described in the following sections.

Coronal Technique (7)

The coronal incision technique requires an incision made 7 to 9 cm posterior to the frontal hairline as shown in Figure 50.6. If the patient wishes to shorten a long forehead, forehead skin can be excised by alternatively placing the coronal incision anterior to the frontal hairline (8). The forehead flap can be

elevated at the subgaleal, subperiosteal, or subcutaneous levels over the frontal bone area and under superficial temporal fascia over the temporal fossa area. Although the deep division of the supraorbital nerve can be spared when dissection is at the subcutaneous plane, it is difficult, if not impossible, to

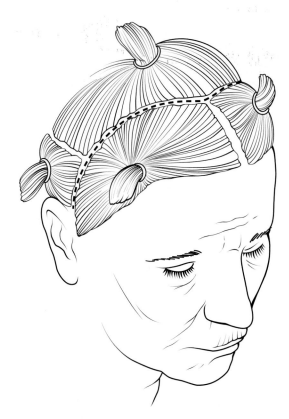

FIGURE 50.6. Incision placement for the coronal incision technique.

avoid transecting the nerve when using the subgaleal dissection plane. **Any incision made through galea across the approximately 1.5-cm zone medial to the palpable superior temporal fusion line can be expected to produce permanent frontoparietal scalp anesthesia, because the deep division of the supraorbital nerve will be transected (Fig. 50.4).**

With the forehead flap elevated, the muscles that act on glabellar skin can be resected or modified under direct vision. **Some surgeons still modify frontalis muscle with cautery ablation or with partial excision to weaken it, but these techniques are generally felt to be unnecessary to obtain smoother forehead transverse lines.** The mobilized forehead flap is transposed in a vertical direction over the posterior scalp incision line until the eyebrows are elevated to the desired level. The overlapping scalp edge of the forehead flap is excised and the wound edges are approximated with 4-0 absorbable sutures at the galeal/superficial temporal fascia level and with staples or nylon sutures at the scalp surface level. This scalp edge reapproximation serves as the fixation mechanism for the forehead flap. **The advantage of the coronal technique is its simplicity and wide exposure. Its disadvantages are the long scar and long-term, usually permanent, changes in scalp sensation, unless the subcutaneous dissection plane is used.**

Endoscopic Technique (9)

Foreheadplasty under endoscopic control is performed using three to five scalp incisions (Fig. 50.7). Initial dissection is performed through the scalp incisions over the upper forehead at either the subperiosteal or subgaleal levels and between superficial temporal fascia and deep temporal fascia in the temporal fossa safe zone areas before the endoscope is inserted. Release of soft-tissue attachments along the superior orbital rim and modification of glabella muscles is performed under endoscopic control. After the released forehead flap is transposed, superficial temporal fascia is fixed to the stable deep temporal fascia with sutures placed through the transverse temporal scalp incisions. These sutures stabilize the lateral eyebrow segment. Through the vertical scalp incisions, screws drilled into bone tunnels made in cortical bone are used as a fixation mechanism to anchor sutures that can suspend the medial eyebrow segment, if desired. Buried absorbable forehead

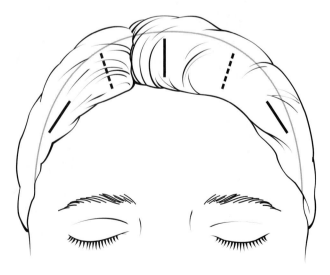

FIGURE 50.7. Incision placement for the endoscopic foreheadplasty technique. One to three vertical frontal scalp incisions and bilateral temporal scalp incisions are used.

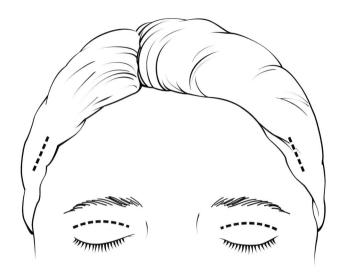

FIGURE 50.8. Incision placement for the limited incision foreheadplasty technique. Bilateral temporal scalp incisions and the usual upper blepharoplasty incisions are used.

anchoring devices were recently introduced into clinical practice. One end of this absorbable device is pressed into a small drill hole made in the skull, and multiple tiny hooks at the other end of the device grasp the undersurface of the forehead flap to support it. With one of these devices in place stabilize the flap, the scalp incisions are closed with staples or sutures. Redundant scalp produced by the forehead flap advancement at the temporal incision closure line may be excised. **The advantages of the endoscopic technique are the limited incisions and controlled dissection. The disadvantages are the expense of purchasing the endoscopic equipment, the learning curve to effectively use the equipment, and the difficulty in stably suspending the transposed forehead flap through small incisions.**

Limited-Incision Foreheadplasty Technique (10)

This technique is a hybrid of the coronal and endoscopic techniques. The forehead soft tissues are elevated at the subperiosteal plane and the temporal fossa soft tissues are raised at a plane between superfical and deep temporal fascia under direct vision using a retractor and a headlight through bilateral, 4.5-cm long, temporal scalp incisions. The muscles that act on glabellar skin are approached through standard upper blepharoplasty incisions (Fig. 50.8). Except for the procerus muscle, all of the muscles that act on glabellar skin can be modified under direct vision through the upper eyelid incisions (Fig. 50.9). The procerus muscle is transected from the medial end of the upper blepharoplasty incisions without direct vision (Fig. 50.10). Simple transection of the procerus muscle is adequate to control its hypertonicity.

After complete release from bone of the soft-tissue attachments just medial to the superior temporal fusion line of the skull and along the superior and lateral orbital rims, the forehead flap is transposed cephalad until the lateral end of the eyebrow is elevated to the level planned preoperatively. Flap position is fixed with 2-0 sutures placed between the superficial temporal fascia of the forehead flap to the underlying stable deep temporal fascia. The scalp redundancy produced by the advancement of the forehead flap is not excised. The scalp incision edges can be simply reapproximated with sutures as a single-layer closure, because closure tension is borne at the

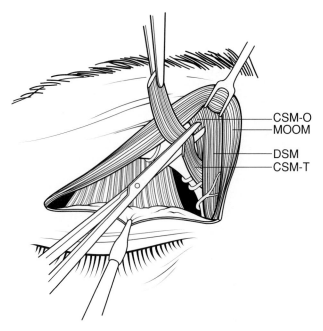

FIGURE 50.9. Transblepharoplasty approach to the glabellar muscles. Resection of the transverse head of the corrugator supercilii muscle through the upper blepharoplasty incision is shown. The oblique head of the corrugator supercilii muscle (CSM-O), the medial slip of the orbicularis oculi muscle (MOOM), and the depressor supercilii muscle (DSM) also can be modified from this approach. (Modified from Knize DM. *Forehead and Temporal Fossa, Anatomy and Technique.* Philadelphia: Lippincott-Williams & Wilkins; 2001:120, Fig. 7.13D with permission.)

deeper superficial temporal fascial level. Tension-free scalp closure markedly lessens the risk of postsurgical hair loss. The roll of scalp this procedure produces is not visible after the hair is washed and groomed, and it flattens progressively over 6 to 8 weeks.

The medial eyebrow segment is "physiologically" elevated by weakening the medial eyebrow depressor muscle group, which allows unopposed frontalis muscle tone to raise the me-

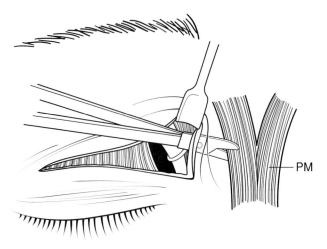

FIGURE 50.10. Transblepharoplasty transaction of the procerus muscle. Procerus muscle transection is accomplished through the medial end of the upper blepharoplasty incision at the level of the radix of the nose. (Modified from Knize DM. *Forehead and Temporal Fossa, Anatomy and Technique.* Philadelphia: Lippincott-Williams & Wilkins; 2001:122, Fig. 7.13G).

dial eyebrow segment approximately 3 to 4 mm. This amount of medial eyebrow elevation is usually adequate. Overelevating the medial eyebrow is a technical error.

Like the endoscopic technique, the advantage of this technique is that it limits scalp incision length and preserves scalp sensation; however, endoscopic equipment is not required. The technique is particularly well suited for treating the patient who has ptotic eyebrows and male pattern baldness. The disadvantage of the technique is that there is less visualization for dissection than with either the coronal incision or the endoscopic techniques, making familiarity with the local anatomy important.

A clinical observation has been that following any type of forehead lift procedure combined with an upper blepharoplasty procedure, the transverse forehead lines will almost always soften without frontalis muscle modification. Both the blepharoplasty and the forehead lift procedures serve to eliminate excess upper eyelid skin that appears to stimulate reflex elevation of the eyebrows and reduce transverse forehead lines.

POSTOPERATIVE CARE

Postoperatively, patients who have undergone a forehead lift usually complain more of "tightness" or a pressure sensation of their forehead and temporal areas than of frank pain. Because a blepharoplasty is usually performed in conjunction with the forehead lift, the eyelids may not close completely for 3 to 4 days. To protect the cornea from exposure and erosion, a lubricating ointment may be placed into the eyes whenever the patient is sleeping, or a temporary lateral tarsorrhaphy may be employed for 5 to 7 days. A laterally placed tarsorrhaphy allows the patient to see through the open medial half of the palpebral fissure, while it protects the cornea and decreases the incidence of developing temporal chemosis.

Dressings are removed on the first postoperative day, if the forehead lift was performed as an isolated procedure. If used, drains are usually removed on the first postoperative day. The patient can begin to shampoo the hair on the second postoperative day. Generally, edema increases over the first 2 to 3 postoperative days, remains stable for the next 2 to 3 days, and then begins to subside. Scalp sutures or staples are removed after 10 to 14 days.

COMPLICATIONS

Scalp scarring and alopecia can occur when the scalp incisions are closed under tension at the hair-bearing scalp level. This complication can be avoided or minimized when the closure is made with tension placed at the deeper galeal/superficial temporal fascial level to allow a tension-free closure at the scalp surface level.

Frontalis muscle palsy from a traction injury to the temporal branch of the facial nerve is almost always transient, but full recovery may require several weeks. **Permanent frontalis muscle palsy is an unusual complication but the possibility of such a complication must be discussed with the patient prior to surgery.**

Long-term or permanent alteration of scalp sensation occurs with the coronal incision approach. While scalp sensory alterations occur following the endoscopic and limited incision techniques, the severity is much less and long-term sensory changes are unusual. Until scalp sensation returns, the patient may experience scalp itching or tingling sensations.

Unlike midface and lower facial aesthetic procedures, hematoma rarely occurs with any of these foreheadplasty techniques.

References

1. Gonzalez-Ulloa M. Facial wrinkles, integral elimination. *Plast Reconstr Surg.* 1962;29:658.
2. Ortiz-Monasterio F. The coronal incision in rhytidectomy: the brow lift. *Clin Plast Surg.* 1978;5:167.
3. Vasconez LO, Core GB, Gamboa-Bobadilla M, et al. Endoscopic techniques in coronal brow lifting. *Plast Reconstr Surg.* 1994;94:788.
4. Knize DM. Limited incision forehead lift for eyebrow elevation to enhance upper blepharoplasty. *Plast Reconstr Surg.* 1996;97:1334.
5. Knize DM. *Forehead and Temporal Fossa, Anatomy and Technique.* Philadelphia: Lippincott-Williams & Wilkins; 2001.
6. Ellenbogen R. Transcoronal eyebrow lift with concomitant upper blepharoplasty. *Plast Reconstr Surg.* 1983;71:490.
7. Marten TJ. Open foreheadplasty. In: Knize DM, ed. *Forehead and Temporal Fossa, Anatomy and Technique.* Philadelphia: Lippincott-Williams & Wilkins; 2001:154.
8. Marten TJ. Hairline lowering foreheadplasty. *Plast Reconstr Surg.* 1999;103:224.
9. Daniel RK, Tirkanits B. Endoscopic forehead lift: an operative technique. *Plast Reconstr Surg.* 1998;98:1148.
10. Knize DM. Limited incision foreheadplasty. In: Knize DM, ed. *Forehead and Temporal Fossa, Anatomy and Technique.* Philadelphia: Lippincott-Williams & Wilkins; 2001:102.

CHAPTER 51 ■ RHINOPLASTY

JEFFREY E. JANIS AND ROD J. ROHRICH

Rhinoplasty is one of the most challenging procedures in plastic surgery. The rhinoplasty surgeon must have an understanding of the underlying anatomy, the ability to perform nasofacial analysis in order to determine the operative plan, and the ability to execute techniques that manipulate bone, cartilage, and soft tissue. These skills are tempered with an aesthetically astute eye in order to produce a result that blends harmoniously with the rest of the face.

ANATOMY

The nose can be divided into external skin and soft tissue, underlying framework (bony and cartilaginous), and ligamentous support. It is crucial that the rhinoplasty surgeon be familiar with the native morphology and potential variations of each structure. Furthermore, the dynamic interplay between these components must be appreciated.

Skin

The nasal skin is not uniform. Rather, its thickness, mobility, and sebaceous character vary along the length of the nose. The upper two-thirds of the nose is thinner, averaging 1,300 μm in thickness versus the lower one-third, which averages 2,400 μm (1). The upper two-thirds of the nose is also more mobile and less sebaceous than the caudal one-third. It is important to note that a straight dorsum is actually produced by the combination of an underlying convexity in the osseocartilaginous framework combined with the aforementioned variation in dorsal skin thickness.

Differences in skin character also exist between different ethnic subpopulations. This difference should be considered during the preoperative planning phase, as thinner skin tends to show even minor alterations of the underlying framework, whereas thicker skin requires more aggressive manipulation to achieve the desired result.

Muscle

Although there are several muscles in the nose, two muscles are particularly important in rhinoplasty—the levator labii alaeque nasi and the depressor septi nasi. The levator labii alaeque nasi assists in maintaining the patency of the external nasal valve, whereas the depressor septi nasi can shorten the upper lip and alter nasal tip projection, if overactive.

The effects of the depressor septi must be evaluated as part of the preoperative nasofacial analysis, and can be recognized by a depressed nasal tip and shortened upper lip upon animation (especially when smiling). In the subgroup of patients in whom this muscle significantly alters the nasal appearance, a dissection and transposition of this muscle can be performed.

Blood Supply

The vascular supply to the nose is derived both from branches of the ophthalmic artery, as well as from branches of the facial artery (Fig. 51.1).

Columellar branches are present 68.2% of the time (2). These branches are transected in the open approach by the transcolumellar incision. This leaves the lateral nasal and dorsal nasal arteries as the remaining blood supply to the tip. Steps must be taken to protect these vessels, especially if the open approach is used. **Therefore, when a transcolumellar incision is used extended alar resections are avoided, as the lateral nasal artery is found 2 to 3 mm above the alar groove. Furthermore, extensive debulking of the nasal tip must be avoided as the subdermal plexus may be injured, which could lead to skin necrosis.**

The veins and lymphatics lie in a subcutaneous plane, which is superficial to the musculoaponeurotic layer in which the arteries travel. In the open technique, the dissection is performed in the submusculoaponeurotic plane just above the perichondrium in order to avoid injury to all of these structures. This minimizes bleeding and postoperative edema.

Osseocartilaginous Framework

The osseocartilaginous nasal framework is comprised of three separate vaults: the bony vault, the upper cartilaginous vault, and the lower cartilaginous vault. The bony vault, which constitutes the upper third to half of the nose, is made up of the paired nasal bones and the ascending frontal process of the maxilla. The thickness of the bones varies, with the thickest portion just above the canthal level. As a result, osteotomies are rarely indicated above this level.

The upper cartilaginous framework, or midvault, is comprised of the paired upper lateral cartilages (ULCs) and dorsal cartilaginous septum. It begins at the "keystone" area, where the nasal bones overlap the ULCs. Normally, this is the widest part of the dorsum, and resembles a "T" shape in cross-section (Fig. 51.2).

The inverted V deformity and/or disruption of the dorsal aesthetic lines may occur if the midvault area is overresected during the dorsal hump reduction. A component dorsal septal reduction, with or without spreader graft placement, is recommended to avoid these complications.

The lower cartilaginous framework is comprised of the medial, middle, and lateral crura, and begins where the lower lateral cartilages (LLCs) overlap the ULCs in what is called the "scroll" area. The LLC's are connected to each other, the ULCs, and the septum by fibrous tissue and ligaments (Fig. 51.3). Disruption of these ligaments during rhinoplasty can result in diminished tip projection, requiring reconstruction to maintain or increase tip support.

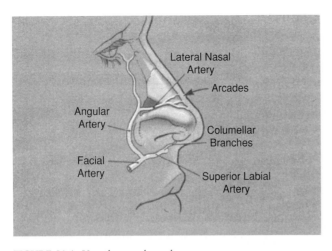

FIGURE 51.1. Vascular supply to the nose.

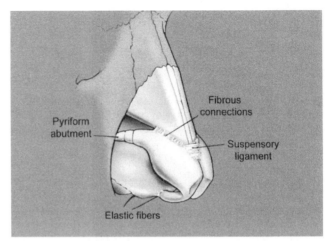

FIGURE 51.3. Ligamentous support of the cartilaginous framework.

Nasal Function

The functions of the nose, specifically respiration, humidification, filtration, temperature regulation, and protection, are regulated by the septum, turbinates, and nasal valves (internal and external).

The constituents of the septum include the septal cartilage, the perpendicular plate of the ethmoid, the nasal crest of the maxilla, and the vomer (Fig. 51.4). Laminar airflow can be al-

tered by septal deformities and can lead to secondary turbinate hypertrophy. It is paramount to analyze and address all portions of the septum when attempting to correct septal deformities. Furthermore, it should be noted that the cribriform plate is contiguous with the perpendicular plate of the ethmoid, so extreme care must be taken when performing a resection of this structure so as not to cause potential devastating consequences, such as anosmia, cerebral spinal fluid (CSF) rhinorrhea, or ascending infection/meningitis.

The turbinates are mucosa-lined extensions of the lateral nasal cavity. They undergo cyclical expansion and contraction mediated by the autonomic nervous system. Their function is to assist in the transport of air during respiration and condition/humidify inspired and expired air. **The inferior turbinate, especially its anterior-most portion, has the greatest impact on airway resistance, providing up to two-thirds of the total airway resistance (3).** Turbinate pathology is frequently addressed via submucosal resection and/or outfracture techniques. One must be careful, however, to avoid overresection as it can lead to adverse effects on regulatory and physiologic functions, and can lead to crust formation, bleeding, and nasal cilia dysfunction.

The internal nasal valve is the angle formed by the junction of the nasal septum and the caudal margin of the upper lateral cartilage, and is usually 10 to 15 degrees (Fig. 51.5). **It can**

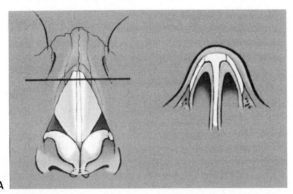

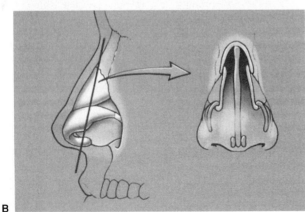

FIGURE 51.2. Upper cartilaginous framework. Note the "keystone area," where the nasal bones overlap the upper lateral cartilages ULCs and the "scroll area" where the lower lateral cartilages overlap the upper lateral cartilages ULCs.

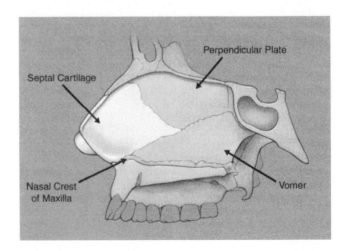

FIGURE 51.4. Constituents of the septum.

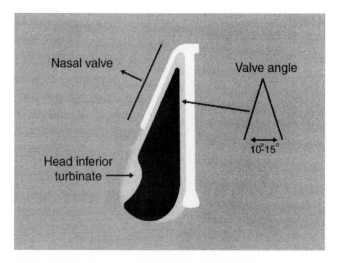

FIGURE 51.5. The internal nasal valve.

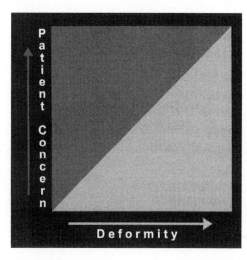

FIGURE 51.6. The "Gorneygram" comparing patient concern with the actual degree of deformity.

be responsible for up to 50% of the total airway resistance, and is the narrowest segment of the nasal airway. Occasionally, the head (anterior-most portion) of the inferior turbinate can be hypertrophied enough to cause further diminishment of the cross-sectional area of this region. Traditionally, a positive Cottle sign (lateral traction on the cheek leading to increased airflow) signals collapse of the internal nasal valve and indicates the need for spreader grafts to increase the valve angle and stent the airway open.

The external nasal valve is caudal to the internal valve, and is the vestibule that serves as the entrance to the nose. This valve may be obstructed by extrinsic factors, such as foreign bodies, or intrinsic factors, such as weak or collapsed lower lateral cartilages, a loss of vestibular skin, or cicatricial narrowing. There are many options to correct these potential problems, including, but not limited to, cartilage grafting (alar batten grafts, lateral crural strut grafts), soft-tissue grafting (mucosal, skin, or composite grafts), lysis of adhesions, or scar revision.

PREOPERATIVE ASSESSMENT

The Initial Consultation

The patient's expectation level must be assessed prior to any operative intervention. Both Gunter and Gorney (4) have commented on "danger signs" that may be exhibited by certain patients. Those patients who fit these criteria should be approached with caution, as surgical intervention may not be in either the patient's or the surgeon's best interest.

Gorney compares the patient's concern to the actual degree of deformity (Fig. 51.6). Patients considered appropriate surgical candidates are ones whose degree of concern is proportionate to their degree of deformity, However, there are some patients with a degree of concern that is not congruent with their degree of deformity. These patients frequently have an expectation level that exceeds the reasonable ability of the operation to gain aesthetic improvement and should be avoided. Furthermore, regardless of the degree of deformity, if the level of skill and expertise required to perform the rhinoplasty exceeds the surgeon's ability, that patient should be referred to another surgeon who possesses the amount of required proficiency.

Computer imaging is useful for providing the patient with a visual level of understanding of the anticipated outcome, al-

though the images are not meant to guarantee surgical results. These images, combined with standardized anterior, oblique, lateral, and basal photographs, serve as helpful adjuncts in the planning of the operation.

Nasofacial Analysis

Accurate, systematic, and thorough nasofacial analysis is critical in determining the subsequent operative plan. The nose must not only be looked at in isolation, but also with respect to the rest of the face, in order to create or preserve overall facial balance and harmony. It is also necessary to evaluate the patient preoperatively for any natural facial asymmetries so that the patient gains a better understanding of exactly what was present before any operative intervention.

The skin type, thickness, and texture are evaluated. **This is important because thicker, more sebaceous skin requires more aggressive modification of the underlying osseocartilaginous framework as changes tend to be camouflaged, whereas thinner skin tends to show even minor changes.**

The nasofacial analysis proceeds in a systematic, methodical fashion. Below are some of the routine relationships and proportions that are used when analyzing the rhinoplasty patient. These are generally for the white female, but can be modified depending on the ethnicity and gender of the patient (5). It is important to remember that these proportions are general guidelines. To achieve optimal nasofacial balance and harmony, each nose should be individualized to the patient.

The face is divided into thirds using horizontal lines tangent to the hairline, brow (at the level of the supraorbital notch), nasal base, and chin (menton). The upper third (between the hairline and the brow) is the most variable, as it depends on the hairline and hairstyle, and therefore is the least important. The middle third lies between the brow and nasal base. The lower third of the face can be subdivided into thirds by visualizing a horizontal line between the oral commissures (stomion). The upper third of this subdivision lies between the nasal base and the oral commissures, and the lower two-thirds between the commissures and the menton (Fig. 51.7). Deviation from these proportions may signal an underlying craniofacial anomaly, such as vertical maxillary excess or maxillary hypoplasia, that may need to be addressed prior to rhinoplasty. The foundation must be sound before the nose that is to be constructed is addressed.

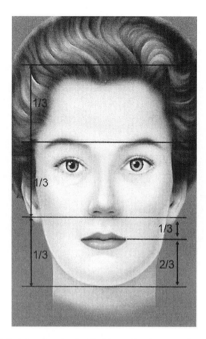

FIGURE 51.7. The face is divided into thirds, using horizontal lines tangent to the hairline, brow, nasal base, and chin.

The nasal length (radix to tip, or R-T) should be equivalent to the stomion-to-menton distance (S-M) (Fig. 51.8).

The lip–chin relationship is assessed by dropping a vertical line from a point one-half the ideal nasal length tangent to the vermilion of the upper lip. The lower lip should lie approximately 2 mm behind this line. **The ideal chin position varies with gender, with the chin lying slightly posterior to the lower lip in women, but equal to the lower lip in men.** Orthodontics, orthognathic surgery, or a chin implant may be necessary to improve overall facial harmony if there is a discrepancy in these relationships (Fig. 51.9).

The nose itself is now addressed from the anteroposterior (AP) view. A vertical line is drawn from the midglabellar area to the menton, bisecting the nasal ridge, upper lip, Cupid's bow,

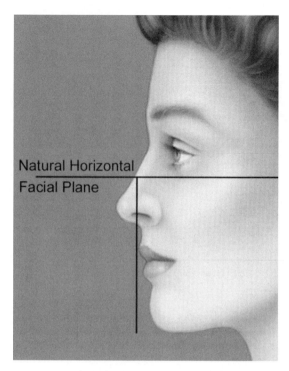

FIGURE 51.9. The ideal lower lip position is 2 mm behind a vertical line dropped from a point half the ideal nasal length along the natural horizontal facial plane.

and central incisors (if the patient has normal occlusion). Any nasal deviation from this line is likely to require septal surgery (Fig. 51.10).

The curvilinear dorsal aesthetic lines are traced from their origin at the supraorbital ridges toward their convergence at the level of the medial canthal ligaments. From here, they flare slightly at the keystone area and then track down to the tip-defining points, slightly diverging from each other along the dorsum during their course. The ideal width of the dorsal aesthetic lines should be approximately equivalent to the width

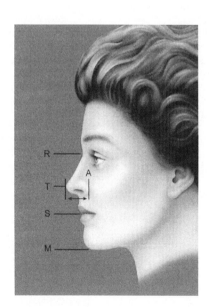

FIGURE 51.8. The ideal nasal length is equivalent to the stomion-to-menton distance. A, ala; M, menton; R, radix; S, stomion; T, tip.

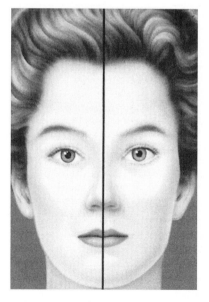

FIGURE 51.10. Symmetry is determined by drawing a vertical line from the midglabellar area to the menton.

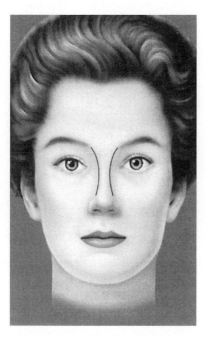

FIGURE 51.11. The curvilinear dorsal aesthetic lines extend from the supraorbital ridges to the tip-defining points.

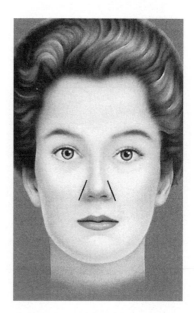

FIGURE 51.13. The alar rims should flare outward inferolaterally.

of either the tip-defining points or the interphiltral distance (Fig. 51.11).

The normal alar base width is equivalent to the intercanthal distance, or the width of one eye. If the alar base width is greater than the intercanthal distance, the underlying etiology should be examined. If the discrepancy is the result of a narrow intercanthal distance, it is better to maintain a slightly wider alar base. If there is true increased interalar width, a nostril sill resection may be indicated. If the increase in width is secondary to alar flaring (>2 to 3 mm outside the alar base), an alar base resection should be considered. The bony base should equal approximately 80% of the alar base width (Fig. 51.12). If the bony base is greater than 80% of the alar base width, osteotomies may be required. Over-narrowing the dorsum should be avoided in males as this can lead to an "over-feminized" look.

The alar rims are examined for symmetry. They normally flare slightly outward in an inferolateral direction (Fig. 51.13).

The tip is assessed by drawing two equilateral triangles with their bases opposed (Fig. 51.14). The supratip break, tip-defining points, and columellar–lobular angle serve as landmarks to draw these triangles. If these triangles are asymmetric, the patient will likely require tip modification.

The final assessment on frontal view is of the outline of the alar rims and the columella. Normally, this outline should resemble a seagull in gentle flight. If the angles are too steep, the patient likely has an increased infratip lobular height. Conversely, if the angle/curve is too flat, it is likely the patient has decreased columellar show, which may require columellar and/or alar rim modification (Fig. 51.15).

The basal view of the nose is addressed next, where both the outline of the nasal base and the nostril itself is analyzed. The outline of the nasal base should describe an equilateral triangle with a lobule-to-nostril ratio of 1:2 (Fig. 51.16). The nostril itself should have a teardroplike geometry, with the long axis oriented in a slight medial direction (from base to apex).

Attention is then turned to the lateral view, beginning with the analysis of the nasofrontal angle. This angle connects the brow and nasal dorsum through a soft concave curve. The apex

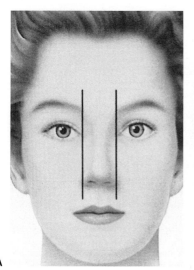

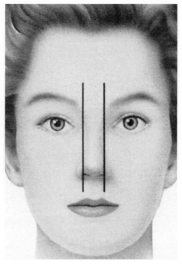

A   **B**

FIGURE 51.12. A: The normal alar base width equals the intercanthal distance, or the width of one eye. **B:** The bony base should be approximately 80% of the alar base width.

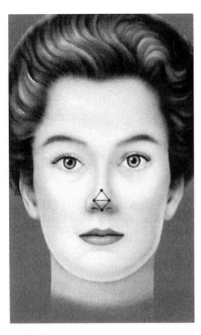

FIGURE 51.14. Tip assessment is performed by analyzing two equilateral triangles with opposing bases.

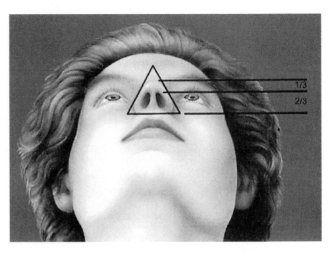

FIGURE 51.16. The outline of the nasal base should describe an equilateral triangle with a lobule-to-nostril ratio of 1:2.

of this angle (radix) should lie between the supratarsal fold and the upper lid lashes, with the eyes in natural horizontal gaze. This angle can vary between 128 and 140 degrees, but is ideally approximately 134 degrees in females and 130 degrees in males.

It is important to note that that the perceived nasal length and tip projection can be altered by the position of the nasofrontal angle. For instance, the nose may appear more elongated if the nasofrontal angle is positioned more anteriorly and superiorly than normal. In this instance, the nasofacial angle (as defined by the junction of the nasal dorsum with the vertical facial plane) is decreased and the tip projection will appear diminished (yellow line). Conversely, the nose can appear shorter if the nasofrontal angle is positioned too far posteriorly and/or inferiorly. In this case, the tip may also appear more projecting (red line) (Fig. 51.17). Ideally, the nasofacial angle should measure between 32 and 37 degrees.

While still analyzing the lateral view, tip projection is addressed. This can be done in two ways. The first is to draw a horizontal line from the alar–cheek junction to the tip of the nose. The distance between these points should equal two things: (a) the alar base width, and (b) $0.67 \times$ R-T (Fig. 51.18). The second way to assess tip projection is to examine how much of the tip lies anterior to a vertical line tangent to the most projecting part of the upper lip vermilion. If 50% to 60% of the tip lies anterior to this line, projection is considered normal. If the tip projection is outside of these proportions, it likely will require tip modification (Fig. 51.19).

The dorsum is analyzed next by drawing a line from the radix to the tip-defining points. **In women, the ideal aesthetic nasal dorsum should lie approximately 2 mm behind and parallel to this line, but in men, it should approach this line to avoid feminizing the nose** (Fig. 51.20).

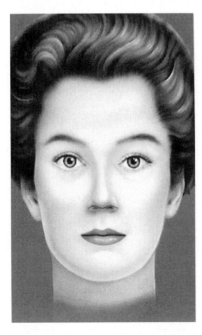

FIGURE 51.15. The outline of the alar rims and columella should resemble a "seagull in gentle flight."

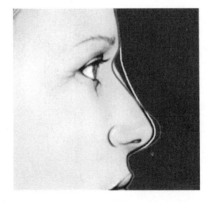

FIGURE 51.17. Perceived nasal length and tip projection can be altered by the position of the nasofrontal angle. Red, A posteriorly and inferiorly positioned nasofrontal angle can make the nose appear shorter with increased tip projection. Yellow, An anteriorly and superiorly positioned nasofrontal angle can make the nose appear longer with diminished tip projection.

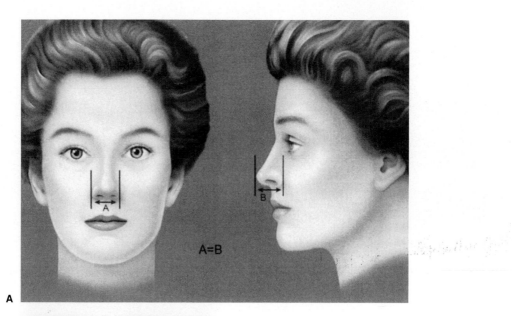

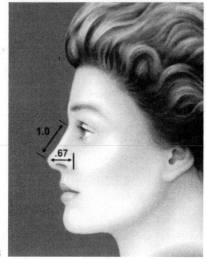

FIGURE 51.18. A: Tip projection should equal alar base width. B: Tip projection should also equal 0.67 × R-T (radix to tip).

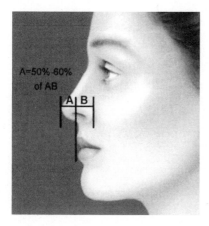

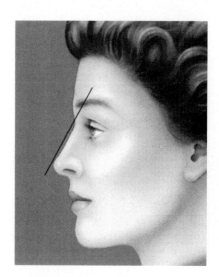

FIGURE 51.19. Fifty to 60% of the tip should lie anterior to a vertical line tangent to the most projecting part of the upper lip vermilion.

FIGURE 51.20. The dorsum is analyzed by drawing a line from the radix to the tip-defining points.

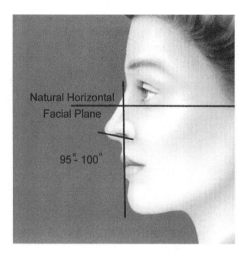

FIGURE 51.21. The nasolabial angle is usually 95 to 100 degrees in females and 90 to 95 degrees in males.

The degree of supratip break is also evaluated on the lateral view. This break helps to define the nose and separate the tip from the dorsum. A slight supratip break is preferred in women but not in men.

The degree of tip rotation is assessed by evaluating the nasolabial angle, which is the angle formed between a line coursing through the most anterior and posterior edges of the nostril and a plumb line dropped perpendicular to the natural horizontal facial plane (Fig. 51.21). This angle is usually between 95 and 100 degrees in women and between 90 and 95 degrees in men.

The nasolabial angle is often confused with the columellar–labial angle, which is formed at the junction of the columella with the infratip lobule (Fig. 51.22). This angle is normally between 30 and 45 degrees. A prominent caudal septum can cause increased fullness in this area, which can give the illusion of increased rotation, despite a normal nasolabial angle.

The alar–columellar relationship is assessed by drawing a line through the long axis of the nostril and a second, perpen-

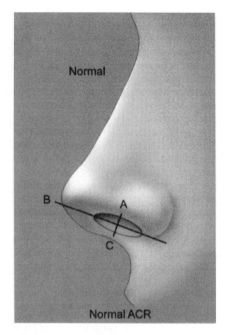

FIGURE 51.23. The alar–columellar relationship is assessed by drawing two perpendicular lines—one through the long axis of the nostril and the other from the alar rim to the columellar rim.

dicular line drawn from alar rim to columellar rim that bisects this axis. If the alar–columellar relationship is normal, the distance from the alar rim ("point A") to the long axis line ("point B") should equal the distance between the long axis line to the columellar rim ("point C") (AB = BC ≈2 mm) (Fig. 51.23). If abnormal, the deformity can be stratified into six classes (6). Classes I to III describe increased columellar show, whereas classes IV to VI demonstrate decreased columellar show. The treatment of the discrepancy varies by class.

The final critical part of the preoperative analysis is the intranasal examination, which is performed with a nasal speculum, headlight, and vasoconstriction. Deformities or abnormalities of the septum, turbinates, and internal nasal valve are

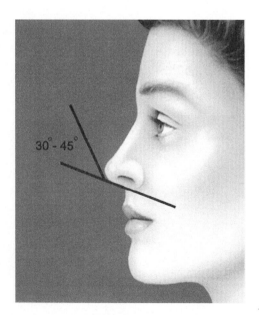

FIGURE 51.22. The columellar–labial angle is normally 30 to 45 degrees.

TABLE 51.1

CAUSES OF AQUIRED INFERIOR TURBINATE HYPERTROPHY

Autonomic
  Vasomotor rhinitis
  Sexual stimulation
  Emotions
Environmental
  Allergic rhinitis
  Dust
  Tobacco
Medical
  Inflammatory
  Hyperthyroidism
  Pregnancy
  Rhinitis medicamentosus
Anatomic
  Associated with deviated nasal septum[a]

[a] Deviation of nasal septum may also be congenital.

evaluated. If turbinate hypertrophy is identified, the underlying etiology should be investigated and a detailed history taken, as the enlargement may be either congenital or acquired. If acquired, it may be the result of autonomic, environmental, medical, or anatomic factors (Table 51.1).

OPERATIVE TECHNIQUE

Type of Approach

There are two schools of approach in modern rhinoplasty—the open approach and the "closed" approach. Although both approaches have their advantages and disadvantages, it is important to be familiar with both. The experienced surgeon tailors the approach to the patient's anatomic deformity. **Regardless of the approach, however, the modifications made to the underlying framework ultimately supersede the choice of incision type used.**

Table 51.2 summarizes the rationale for the open approach. Table 51.3 summarizes the benefits of the endonasal (closed) approach.

Many experienced surgeons prefer the open approach as it affords full exposure of the nasal framework, resulting in an accurate diagnosis of all the potential causes of either the nasal airway obstruction or the etiology of the cosmetic deformity. Furthermore, precise manipulation of the various structures can be performed and the dynamic interplay between these structures appreciated, giving reproducible results. The use of the open approach is strongly encouraged in three particular circumstances: (a) posttraumatic deformities, where complete release of all intrinsic and extrinsic deforming forces is necessary, (b) secondary/revisional surgery, and (c) when complex tip modifications are necessary.

The closed approach lends itself well to patients who have an isolated dorsal hump deformity or where there is minimal change needed to modify the tip structure. In these instances, we prefer access through a marginal incision. This is combined with an intercartilaginous incision in cases of minor tip refinement in order to allow for adequate cartilage delivery and exposure. A hemitransfixion or transfixion incision is used if the caudal septum needs to be addressed.

TABLE 51.2

RATIONALE FOR THE OPEN RHINOPLASTY APPROACH

Distinct advantages	Potential disadvantages
Binocular visualization	External nasal incision (transcolumellar scar)
Evaluation of complete deformity without distortion	Prolonged operative time
Precise diagnosis and correction of deformities	Protracted nasal tip edema
Allows use of both hands	Columellar incision separation
More options with original tissues and cartilage grafts	Delayed wound healing
Direct control of bleeding with electrocautery	
Suture stabilization of grafts (invisible and visible)	

TABLE 51.3

RATIONALE FOR THE CLOSED RHINOPLASTY APPROACH

Advantages

Leaves no external scar
Limits dissection to areas needing modification
Permits creation of precise pocket so graft material fits exactly without need for fixation
Allows percutaneous fixation when large pockets are made
Promotes healing by maintaining vascular bridges
Encourages accurate preoperative diagnosis and planning
Produces minimal postsurgical edema
Reduces operating time
Results in fast patient recovery
Creates intact tip graft pocket
Allows composite grafting to alar rims

Disadvantages

Requires experience and great reliance on accurate preoperative diagnosis
Prohibits simultaneous visualization of surgical field by teaching surgeon and students
Does not allow direct visualization of nasal anatomy
Makes dissection of alar cartilages difficult, particularly in cases of malposition

Anaesthesia—Preoperative Preparation

Either local anaesthesia with intravenous (IV) sedation or general anesthesia may be used. After induction, the nasal vestibules are prepared by clipping the nasal vibrissae and swabbing the entire nostril with Betadine solution. Before injecting local anaesthetic, the line of the anticipated incision is marked (transcolumellar stairstep, if using an open approach) so as not to distort the anatomy. Approximately 10 mL of 1% lidocaine with 1:100,000 epinephrine is injected into the intranasal mucosa, along the septum, and into the soft-tissue envelope. Additional local anaesthetic is used on the inferior turbinates when an inferior turbinoplasty is anticipated.

After injection, cottonoid pledgets soaked with a local vasoconstrictor solution are placed, three per naris to shrink the nasal mucosa, facilitate exposure, and minimize blood loss. Although we prefer oxymetazoline (Afrin), 4% cocaine can be used. A throat pack is carefully placed in the posterior oropharynx to prevent inadvertent digestion of blood during surgery, which helps prevent postoperative nausea and vomiting. At this point, the patient is prepped and draped for surgery.

Incision

Closed Approach

There are two basic techniques—nondelivery and delivery—used for access in endonasal rhinoplasty. The nondelivery approach can be performed using either a cartilage-splitting (transcartilaginous) incision or an eversion (retrograde) incision. The transcartilaginous incision is made by incising several millimeters cephalad to the caudal margin of the lateral middle crura. This preserves a rim strip to support the ala. Exposure is facilitated by double-hook retraction combined with digital alar eversion. The cartilage is exposed for resection by dissecting the vestibular skin off of the cartilage. In the eversion approach, rather than going through the cartilage, the vestibular incision is made at the cephalic-most margin of the lower lateral cartilage. The same exposure technique is used as described above. The theoretical advantage to this incision is that it maintains the caudal alar margins and prevents potential scar contracture deformities in this area.

The delivery approach is used in cases where moderate-complexity tip modifications are necessary. This is especially true where there is significant tip bifidity. Again, the cartilaginous margins are delineated, with double hook retraction in the ala and digital counterpressure, and a no. 15 blade scalpel is used to create an intercartilaginous incision starting just above the cephalic margin of the lateral crus. The incision is carried lateral to medial approximately 2 mm caudal and parallel to the limen vestibule. Subsequently, a marginal incision is created along the caudal margin of the lower lateral cartilage, from lateral crus to medial crus, ending at the columellar–lobular junction (Fig. 51.24). The soft tissue is then dissected off of the cartilage in a plane just above the perichondrium, including over the dorsal cartilaginous septum. The same procedure is repeated on the contralateral side, and the two incisions are connected in the midline over the anterior septal angle, ending in a hemitransfixion incision. Of course, this can be extended to a full transfixion incision, if indicated. The lower lateral cartilage is then dissected free from the surrounding tissues and "delivered" outside the incision. The incisions may be extended and the soft tissue undermined more aggressively if there is difficulty delivering the cartilages. Modifications may be made once the cartilages and domes are delivered.

Open Approach

A transcolumellar stairstep incision across the narrowest portion of the columella is generally preferred. The advantages of the stairstep include the provision of landmarks for accurate closure, the prevention of linear scar contracture, and its ability to camouflage the scar.

Infracartilaginous extensions are then performed bilaterally, from lateral to medial, along the caudal border of the lower lateral cartilage. These incisions meet the transcolumellar incision to complete this approach. Exposure during this dissection is facilitated by double-hook alar eversion and digital counterpressure.

It is important to take your time during this portion of the procedure, as most mistakes are made when trying to obtain exposure. Furthermore, the incisions should be kept superficial and the caudal border of the lower lateral cartilage should be identified prior to cutting to prevent injury to the underlying cartilages.

Skin Envelope Dissection

Extreme care should be taken during the exposure of the nasal framework so as not to injure the cartilages. The dissection should be carried out in the supraperichondrial/submusculoaponeurotic plane in order to avoid injury to the arterial, venous, and lymphatic supply to the nose. If performed properly, there should be no residual soft tissue remaining on the lower lateral cartilages. This dissection is continued superiorly to expose the cartilaginous dorsum and upper lateral cartilages until the bony pyramid is encountered. At this point, a limited subperiosteal dissection is performed over the area of the bony dorsal hump that needs to be addressed. Care is taken to avoid disruption of all of the periosteal attachments to the nasal bones, as this can destabilize the area and lead to prolonged wound healing and potential nasal bone malposition, especially if osteotomies are performed. Care is also taken to assure that the upper lateral cartilages are not detached from the nasal bones by accidental dissection under the nasal bones (rather than on top).

Nasal Dorsum

Our preferred technique is the component dorsal reduction, which includes separation of the ULCs from the septum, separate incremental reduction of both the cartilaginous septum and the bony dorsal deformity, and the verification of acceptable final contour by palpation (7).

Separation of the ULCs from the Septum

The component dorsal reduction technique begins with the creation of bilateral superior subperichondrial tunnels in order to minimize mucosal trauma resulting in potential internal nasal valve stenosis or vestibular webbing. This is done by elevating the mucoperichondrium of the dorsal septum in a caudocephalad direction with a Cottle elevator until the nasal bones are reached. The transverse processes of the ULCs are then sharply separated from the septum using a no. 15 blade scalpel (without damaging the mucosa).

Incremental Component Cartilaginous Dorsal Septal Reduction

At this point, the cartilaginous dorsal septum is separated into three components—the septum centrally, and the transverse portions of the ULC laterally. The cartilaginous dorsum is then reduced in incremental fashion by resecting the dorsal hump deformity with either a sharp scalpel or scissors in serial fashion. This is done under direct vision. Care is taken to avoid damaging the adjacent ULCs. In rare cases, the ULCs may require resection, although this is not routine in our practice. If required, it must be performed cautiously, as overresection of the ULCs can cause internal nasal valve collapse and long-term dorsal irregularity. Maintaining the transverse portions of the ULC also preserves the dorsal aesthetic lines. If the septum and ULCs were taken down en bloc (not in component fashion), a rounded dorsum would result. Furthermore, an inverted V deformity could result if the ULCs were resected to a greater extent than the septum.

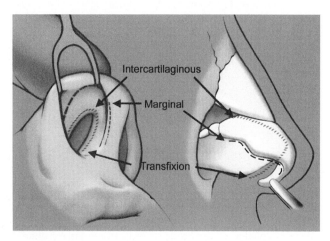

FIGURE 51.24. Intercartilaginous approach to cartilage delivery for closed rhinoplasty.

Component Bony Dorsum Reduction

Large humps (generally >5 mm) are reduced either by a power burr with a dorsal skin protector or a guarded 8-mm osteotome. Smaller humps can be addressed with a sharp rasp (we prefer a downbiting diamond rasp). The rasping is done in a controlled, methodical fashion, proceeding along the left and right dorsal aesthetic lines, and then centrally using the nondominant thumb and index finger for maximal control. It is important to maintain a slightly oblique bias when rasping in order to prevent mechanical avulsion of the ULCs from the nasal bones.

Verification of Final Contour by Palpation

The three-point dorsal palpation test, performed with a saline-moistened dominant index fingertip, is used to gently palpate the left and right dorsal aesthetic lines, as well as centrally, in order to ascertain if there are any residual dorsal irregularities or contour depressions. This maneuver is performed repeatedly throughout this process (after redraping the skin envelope).

Septal Reconstruction and Cartilage Graft Harvest

The septum is harvested if there is a septal deformity or if cartilage is needed for graft construction. Septal cartilage is ideal for cartilage graft harvesting in rhinoplasty because of its minimal donor site morbidity and close geographic proximity to the operating field.

A Killian or hemitransfixion incision is generally used in the closed (endonasal) approach as a complete transfixion incision can lead to decreased tip projection, especially if dissection is carried down over the anterior nasal spine.

In the open approach, the anterior septal angle is exposed by separating the middle crura and incising the interdomal suspensory ligament. The septal perichondrium is incised with a no. 15 blade scalpel exposing the distinctive blue-gray underlying cartilage. A Cottle elevator is then used to carry the dissection in a subperichondrial plane posteriorly to the perpendicular plate of the ethmoid down to the nasal floor and across the face of the septum. This subperichondrial dissection should proceed easily if performed in the correct plane. However, the dissection should proceed with caution at the junction of the cartilaginous and bony septum, as the overlying mucoperichondrium is more adherent, and mucosal perforation is more likely. The same dissection is then performed on the contralateral side, and the entire septum is examined using a Vienna speculum to identify deformities and to help achieve exposure for the septal harvest.

It is important to maintain the stability of the cartilaginous framework by preserving an L-strut with 10 mm of dorsal septum and 10 mm of caudal septum. The harvested cartilage should be preserved in saline to prevent dessication. Residual deviations in the ethmoid or vomer are rongeured or resected and any mucosal perforations are repaired.

Inferior Turbinoplasty

An inferior turbinoplasty is performed in those patients with inferior turbinate hypertrophy that causes symptomatic nasal airway obstruction. There are various ways this can be performed, including turbinate outfracture, submucous morselization of the turbinate bone, and submucous resection of the anterior one-third to one-half of the inferior turbinate. The submucous resection technique begins with the development of medial mucoperiosteal flaps, which exposes the conchal bone. The anterior portion of the conchal bone is resected, as bleeding complications can occur with posterior resection. The flaps are replaced after this resection without the need for suture repair.

Cephalic Trim

Indications for a cephalic trim of the lower lateral cartilages include the need for tip rotation, medialization of the tip-defining points, and when the tip requires better refinement and definition as in the case of the boxy or bulbous tip. A caliper is used to measure out a 6-mm rim strip of the caudal margin of the lower lateral cartilage that is to be preserved. Subsequently, the cephalic portion of the middle and lateral crura is resected and preserved for possible use as a graft later in the case.

Spreader Grafts

Spreader grafts are extraordinarily versatile and can be used to help stent open the internal valve, to stabilize the septum, and to preserve or enhance the dorsal aesthetic lines (Fig. 51.25) (8). These grafts, usually obtained from septal cartilage, are fashioned to measure approximately 25 to 30 mm by 3 mm. They can also be made longer and placed in such a way as to project past the anterior septal angle, effectively lengthening the nose. They can also be positioned more anteriorly ("visible") along the septum to recreate stronger dorsal aesthetic lines or can be positioned lower ("invisible") for septal support or internal valve stenting. The grafts are secured with 5-0 polydioxanone suture (PDS) in horizontal mattress fashion.

Tip Modification

Altering Tip Projection

Tip projection is affected by (9):

- The supporting ligament between the anterior septal angle and the overlying dermis
- The length and strength of the lower lateral cartilages
- The suspensory ligament bridging the anterior septal angle
- The fibrous connections between the upper and lower lateral cartilages (and septum)
- The abutment of the cartilages with the pyriform aperture
- The anterior septal angle

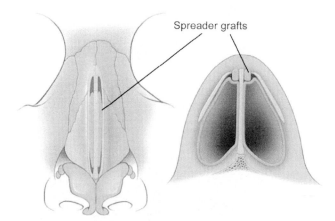

FIGURE 51.25. Spreader grafts can be used to stent open the internal nasal valve, stabilize the septum, or to preserve or enhance the dorsal aesthetic lines.

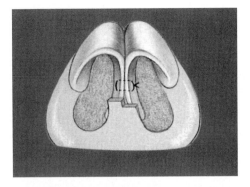

FIGURE 51.26. Medial crural sutures can unify the medial crura and help stabilize the columellar strut.

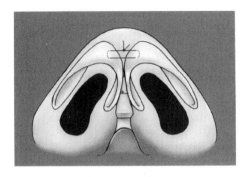

FIGURE 51.28. Interdomal sutures approximate the medial/middle crura and can affect both tip refinement and projection.

Alteration of any of these anatomic structures can result in incremental changes in tip projection.

A graduated algorithm to alter tip projection is used that is based on nondestructive techniques. The algorithm begins with suture techniques, which can reliably deliver an increase of 1 to 2 mm of tip projection. The choice of suture material is surgeon dependent, although the underlying premise is to select a material that will hold the cartilage in its altered position long enough to allow for the natural fibrotic reaction to solidify the result.

The four general types of techniques used to alter projection are

- Medial crural;
- Medial crural septal;
- Interdomal; and
- Transdomal.

Medial crural sutures can be used to unify the medial crura of the lower lateral cartilages and to rectify flaring of the medial/middle crura, thereby effecting a limited increase in projection (Fig. 51.26). They are also frequently used to help stabilize a columellar strut.

Medial crural septal sutures can alter both projection and rotation by anchoring the medial crura to the caudal septum. These sutures are also often used in conjunction with columellar struts (Fig. 51.27).

Interdomal sutures can increase both tip refinement and tip projection. They serve to narrow the interdomal distance by

approximating the medial/middle crura. Sutures are placed in mattress fashion, and can be tightened to a variable degree in order to achieve the desired result (Fig. 51.28).

Transdomal sutures can also affect tip refinement and projection. These mattress-type sutures are placed across the dome of the middle crura after hydrodissection of the underlying mucoperichondrium from the cartilage to help prevent inadvertent incorporation into the suture bite (Fig. 51.29). Knots are left on the medial aspect of the dome and one end may be left long on each side, which can be used to tie the transdomal sutures together (i.e., an interdomal suture) in order to narrow the tip-defining points. It is important, however, to avoid over-tightening of this suture, which will result in an unnaturally sharp tip-defining point. They may be also be placed asymmetrically to correct anatomic differences that may exist from side to side.

The placement of a columellar strut is the second step in the algorithm of tip projection alteration. This strut, usually fashioned from septal cartilage, can be placed in a "fixed" or a

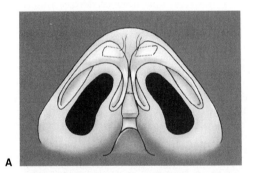

A

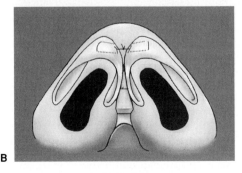

B

FIGURE 51.29. A: Transdomal sutures are mattress-type sutures placed across the dome of the middle crura and can also affect tip refinement and projection. B: Transdomal sutures with the ends left long can be tied together in interdomal fashion, as well.

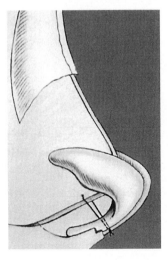

FIGURE 51.27. Medial crural septal sutures anchor the medial crura to the caudal septum and can alter both projection and rotation.

"floating" fashion, depending on whether or not it is secured to the anterior maxilla or not. This strut controls the columellar profile as well as supports tip projection. A pocket is dissected between the medial crura and the strut is inserted. Its final position is set by gently retracting the medial crura anteriorly by a double-hook and gauging the desired amount of tip projection. This configuration is temporarily stabilized with a transversely placed 25-gauge needle and then sutured into position by medial crural sutures (described above). Additional medial crural sutures can then be placed, if necessary, to control medial crural flaring.

Tip grafts are the final step in the algorithm for graduated tip modification if more tip projection or definition is desired after the preceding maneuvers. These grafts may take several forms, but have a tendency to be visible regardless of the specific type used, so their use is reserved only for the patient in which the prior, more predictable, methods do not result in satisfactory tip projection. The three general types of tip grafts are

- Onlay tip grafts;
- Infratip lobular graft; and
- Columellar-tip graft.

The onlay tip graft is usually placed over the dome of the middle crura, and can be fashioned from any type of cartilage, although we find the cartilage obtained from the cephalic trim harvest (if performed) works exceptionally well (Fig. 51.30).

The infratip lobular graft is a shield-shaped graft used to graft increase infratip lobular definition and projection. It is positioned with its superior margin overlying the dome/tip-defining points and extends inferiorly a variable distance (usually 10 to 12 mm). It is fashioned with rounded graft edges in order to avoid a visible and palpable step-off (Fig. 51.31).

The columellar-tip graft is generally used in difficult primary rhinoplasties, thick-skinned patients, and secondary rhinoplasties with inadequate tip projection. It is essentially a "combination" graft of the above-mentioned onlay tip graft and infratip lobular graft. Superiorly, it is anchored to the upper lateral cartilages and inferiorly it is secured to the caudal margin of the medial crura (Fig. 51.32).

A thorough understanding of the anatomic basis of tip support is also required when trying to *decrease* nasal tip projection. For instance, in the open approach where the skin envelope has been undermined and the fibroelastic and ligamentous attachments have been disrupted, the primary means

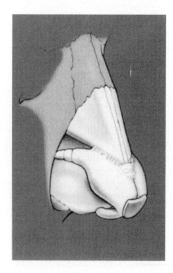

FIGURE 51.31. The infratip lobular graft overlies the dome and extends inferiorly a variable distance.

of decreasing tip projection lies in alteration of the length and strength of the lower lateral cartilages. Several techniques, such as transection, setback, and resuturing of the medial or lateral crura, may be used to obtain the desired result. However, regardless of the technique used, it is important to recognize that if the tip projection is significantly decreased, alar flaring or columellar bowing may result. This, then, would require concomitant correction.

Altering Tip Rotation

To alter tip rotation, the existing extrinsic forces stabilizing the tip at its current position must be released. The first step is usually to perform a cephalic trim, which separates the connection between the upper and lower lateral cartilages. Another technique is to resect a variable amount of the caudal septum. This releases tension on the nasal tip and allows for more cephalad rotation by transecting the fibrous attachments of the medial crura and the caudal septum. This maneuver can also affect tip projection, as well. After the desired amount of tip rotation has been achieved, its position is maintained with suture techniques (medial crural septal sutures) and/or a columellar strut or septal extension graft.

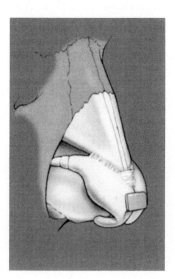

FIGURE 51.30. The onlay tip graft is usually placed over the dome of the middle crura.

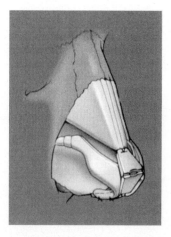

FIGURE 51.32. The columellar tip graft is a combination of the onlay tip graft and the infratip lobular graft.

It may be necessary to perform a limited resection of the nasal mucosa and membranous septum in order to maintain proper nasal balance and harmony, depending on the amount of tip (de)rotation.

Osteotomies

Several techniques exist for performing osteotomies, including medial, lateral, transverse, or a combination of the above. These can be performed via an external or internal approach, depending on surgeon preference.

Osteotomies are generally performed for the following reasons:

- To narrow the lateral walls of the nose;
- To close an open-roof deformity (after dorsal hump reduction); and
- To create symmetry by allowing for straightening of the nasal bony framework.

Contraindications include patients with short nasal bones, elderly patients with thin, fragile nasal bones, and patients with heavy eyeglasses (10).

Lateral osteotomies may be performed as "low-to-high," "low-to-low," or as a "double level" (Fig. 51.33). Furthermore, they may be combined with medial, transverse, or greenstick fractures of the upper bony segment. Regardless of the technique used, however, it is paramount to preserve Webster triangle. This bony triangular area of the caudal aspect of the maxillary frontal process near the internal valve is necessary for internal nasal valve support. Preservation of this triangle prevents functional nasal airway obstruction from internal valve collapse (Fig. 51.34).

It is also vital to prevent a potential step-off deformity by maintaining a smooth fracture line low along the bony vault. The cephalic margin of the osteotomy should not be higher than the medial canthal ligament, as the thick nasal bones above this area increase the technical difficulty, and it is possible to cause iatrogenic injury to the lacrimal system with resultant epiphora.

A "low-to-high" osteotomy begins low at the pyriform aperture and ends "high" medially on the dorsum, and is generally used to correct a small open roof deformity or to mobilize a medium-wide nasal base. The nasal bones are then medialized by a gentle greenstick fracture along predictable fracture patterns obtained based on nasal bone thickness (11). Thicker nasal bones may require a separate superior oblique osteotomy in order to mobilize them enough to be greensticked.

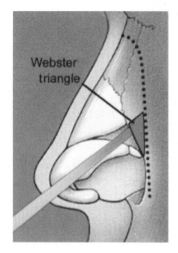

FIGURE 51.34. Preservation of Webster triangle is paramount when performing lateral osteotomies to prevent internal nasal valve collapse.

A "low-to-low" osteotomy starts low along the pyriform aperture and continues low along the base of the bony vault to end up in a lateral position along the dorsum near the intercanthal line. It is generally considered a more powerful technique in that it results in more significant medialization of the nasal bones, and therefore is classically used when there is a large open-roof deformity or if a wide bony base requires correction. This type of osteotomy technique is frequently accompanied by a medial osteotomy in order to better mobilize the nasal bones to achieve the desired result.

Medial osteotomies are used to facilitate medial positioning of the nasal bones and are generally indicated in patients with thick nasal bones or wide bony bases in order to achieve a more predictable fracture pattern. Although medial osteotomies are frequently used in combination with lateral osteotomies, it is not necessary to use both in all cases. If both techniques are performed, however, the medial osteotomy is usually performed first, as this makes it technically easier to perform the subsequent lateral osteotomy. The cant of the medial osteotomy can be oriented in a medial oblique, paramedian, or transverse direction. However, regardless of the cant, the cephalic margin still should not cross the intercanthal line for the reasons stated previously. It is also important to avoid placing the medial osteotomy too far medially as it connects with the lateral osteotomy as this can cause a "rocker deformity," where a

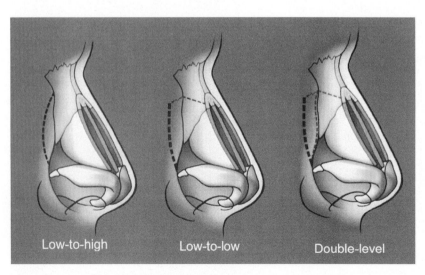

Low-to-high   Low-to-low   Double-level

FIGURE 51.33. The various types of lateral osteotomies.

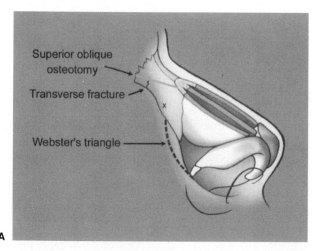

A

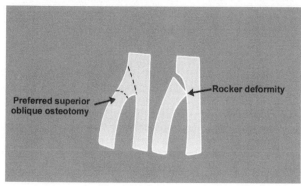

B

FIGURE 51.35. A: The course of a superior oblique medial osteotomy. B: "Rocker deformity" caused by placing the medial osteotomy too far medially.

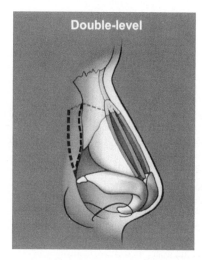

FIGURE 51.36. The double-level osteotomy. The medial-most one is made first.

widened upper dorsum results from the fractured nasal bone "kicking out." This can be avoided by following a superior oblique angle (Fig. 51.35).

A double-level lateral osteotomy is indicated in cases where there is an excessive lateral wall convexity that is too great to be corrected with a standard single-level lateral osteotomy or when significant lateral nasal wall asymmetries exist. The more medial of the two lateral osteotomies is first created along the nasomaxillary suture line. The more lateral of the two is then created in standard low-to-low fashion (Fig. 51.36).

Some of the potential complications that can occur with osteotomies (of any type) have been mentioned above. Table 51.4 has a more complete list (12).

Closure

At the conclusion of the procedure, after meticulous hemostasis has been obtained, the skin envelope is redraped. In some cases a 5-0 Vicryl suture is placed from the underside of the skin envelope to the underlying cartilaginous framework in an attempt to recreate a supratip break, especially if the patient has thick skin or if the patient is a female (males usually do not have a significant supratip break).

The transcolumellar incision is closed in simple interrupted fashion using 6-0 nylon suture, assuring precise reapproximation of the incision. The infracartilaginous incisions are reapproximated using 5-0 chromic suture in simple interrupted fashion. Special care is taken to prevent overbiting with the suture, especially in the soft triangle area, as contour irregularities and notching may result.

The throat pack is removed and the oropharynx and stomach are carefully suctioned to help evacuate any blood which may result in postoperative nausea and vomiting. Antibiotic ointment-coated intranasal silastic splints are placed if septal work has been performed. These splints are secured with a transseptal 3-0 nylon suture. The nasal dorsum is then carefully taped and a malleable metal splint is applied over the dorsum. Finally, a drip pad is fashioned from a 2×2 inch gauze and secured under the nose with 0.5-inch paper tape.

TABLE 51.4

COMPLICATIONS OF LATERAL NASAL OSTEOTOMIES

Infections	Operative trauma	Cosmetic problems
Local	Hemorrhage (hematoma, ecchymosis)	Excessive narrowing or convexity
Abscess		
Cellulitis	Edema	Insufficient mobilization of lateral bony walls
Granuloma	Nasal cyst formation	
Systemic	Anosmia	Unstable bony pyramid
Intracranial	Arteriovenous fistula	Rocker deformity
	Epiphora	Redundant soft tissue
	Canalicular bleeding	Stair-step deformity
	Neuromuscular injury	Nasal bone asymmetry
	Intracranial injury	

POSTOPERATIVE MANAGEMENT

All preoperative and postoperative instructions are reviewed verbally and in writing prior to as well as on the day of surgery. The following are prescribed routinely:

- Cephalexin 500 mg PO q8h × 3 days
- Methylprednisolone Dosepak (Medrol) × 7 days (to minimize postoperative edema)
- Hydrocodone/acetaminophen 5/500 for postoperative pain q4–6h PRN
- Normal nasal saline for postoperative nasal congestion

During the first 48 to 72 hours, the patient is instructed to keep the head of bed elevated at 45 degrees and use a chilled gel eye mask to help minimize postoperative swelling. The drip pad under the nose is changed as often as necessary until the drainage stops, at which time it can be discontinued. Any manipulation of the nose, including rubbing, blotting, or blowing, is discouraged for the first 3 weeks postoperatively. Sneezing should be done through the mouth during this time. It is imperative to keep the nasal splint dry to prevent premature discontinuation of the splint. The hair should be washed as in a beauty salon, with the patient leaning the head backward over the sink.

We prefer to keep our patients on a liquid diet on the day of surgery and then advance them to a soft regular diet the following day. Any foods that require excessive lip movements, such as eating apples or corn on the cob, should be avoided for 2 weeks after surgery.

During the first 2 weeks postoperatively nasal congestion should be treated with the use of normal saline nasal spray and over-the-counter oxymetazoline nasal sprays (Afrin). The patient is encouraged to breathe through the mouth if there is difficulty with air passage through the intranasal splints. Extreme congestion should be treated with office suctioning.

The sutures and nasal splints are removed at the initial visit on postoperative day 5 to 7. The nose (especially the tip) may appear swollen and turned up and the tip may feel numb, but the patient is reassured that both are expected and that both will resolve with time. Normal sensation usually returns within 3 to 6 months. The patient is instructed to avoid letting anything, including eyeglasses, rest on the nose for at least 4 weeks. During this time, glasses should be taped to the forehead. Contacts may be worn as soon as the swelling has diminished enough to allow easy insertion (usually by 7 days postoperatively). The patient is also instructed to avoid direct sunlight and to wear sun protection factor 15 or greater sunscreen to prevent possible hyperpigmentation of the incision.

We restrict the patient's activity for 3 weeks postoperatively, after which the patient can gradually resume normal activity. Any contact sports or activities that may cause direct trauma to the nose are prohibited for at least 4 to 6 weeks after surgery. Although some noses look excellent within 6 to 8 weeks, some may remain swollen for up to 1 year, but after 3 to 4 weeks, it will generally not be obvious to anyone but the patient.

After the first postoperative visit, have the patient return to the clinic at 3 and 8 weeks after the operation. We continue to follow the patient at postoperative months 3, 6, and 12, and then annually thereafter.

SECONDARY RHINOPLASTY

Secondary rhinoplasty offers a unique set of challenges to the rhinoplasty surgeon. Issues such as cicatricial tissue, altered or compromised vascularity, and distorted anatomy can be major factors that alter the planning and execution of a secondary revision. Also, frequently the septal cartilage has already been harvested, which creates the need for remote cartilage harvest from locations such as the conchal bowl or rib.

In the senior author's experience, approximately 1 in 25 primary rhinoplasty patients require revision. The underlying etiology that drives the need for reoperation usually includes one or a combination of the following:

- Displaced anatomic structures
- Undercorrection from an overconservative primary procedure
- Overresection/overcorrection from overzealous surgery

In the lower third of the nose, the most frequent reasons for reoperation include further tip refinement or correction of tip asymmetries. In the middle third, a parrot beak or pinched supratip deformity is responsible for most revisions. In the upper third, it is excessive dorsal reduction or dorsal irregularities that require revision.

Functionally, continued nasal airway obstruction from excessive narrowing of the internal valve (without placement of spreader grafts) is the most common reason for secondary rhinoplasty, although once we adopted the component dorsum reduction technique with preservation of the ULCs, our incidence of internal valve obstruction decreased.

Regardless of the etiology of the deformity, however, we prefer to use an external approach when performing secondary rhinoplasty as it affords excellent exposure of the underlying nasal framework, permits accurate anatomic diagnosis, and facilitates complete correction.

References

1. Gonzalez Ulloa M, et al. [Skin thickness. Report of our microscopic study of the total surface of the face and body]. *Dia Med.* 1961;33:1880–1896.
2. Rohrich RJ, Gunter JP, Friedman RM. Nasal tip blood supply: an anatomic study validating the safety of the transcolumellar incision in rhinoplasty. *Plast Reconstr Surg.* 1995;95(5):795–799; discussion 800–801.
3. Rohrich RJ, et al. Rationale for submucous resection of hypertrophied inferior turbinates in rhinoplasty: an evolution. *Plast Reconstr Surg.* 2001;108(2):536–544; discussion 545–546.
4. Gorney M. Patient selection in rhinoplasty: patient selection. In: Daniel RK, ed. *Aesthetic Plastic Surgery: Rhinoplasty.* Boston: Little, Brown; 1993.
5. Gunter JP, Hackney FL. Clinical assessment and facial analysis. In: Gunter JP, Rohrich RJ, Adams WP Jr, eds. *Dallas Rhinoplasty: Nasal Surgery by the Masters.* St. Louis: Quality Medical Publishing; 2002: 53.
6. Gunter JP, Rohrich RJ, Friedman RM, et al. Importance of the alar–columellar relationship. In: Gunter JP, Rohrich RJ, Adams WP Jr, eds. *Dallas Rhinoplasty: Nasal Surgery by the Masters.* St. Louis: Quality Medical Publishing; 2002: 105.
7. Rohrich RJ, Muzaffar AR, Janis JE. Component dorsal hump reduction: the importance of maintaining dorsal aesthetic lines in rhinoplasty. *Plast Reconstr Surg.* 2004;114(5):1298–1308.
8. Rohrich RJ, Hollier LH. Use of spreader grafts in the external approach to rhinoplasty. *Clin Plast Surg.* 1996;23(2):255–262.
9. Rohrich RJ, Adams WP Jr, Deuber MA. Graduated approach to tip refinement and projection. In: Gunter JP, Rohrich RJ, Adams WP Jr, eds. *Dallas Rhinoplasty: Nasal Surgery by the Masters.* St. Louis: Quality Medical Publishing; 2002: 333.
10. Sullivan PK, Harshbarger RJ, Oneal RM. Nasal Osteotomies. In: Gunter JP, Rohrich RJ, Adams WP Jr, eds. *Dallas Rhinoplasty: Nasal Surgery by the Masters.* St. Louis: Quality Medical Publishing; 2002: 595.
11. Harshbarger RJ, Sullivan PK. Lateral nasal osteotomies: implications of bony thickness on fracture patterns. *Ann Plast Surg.* 1999;42(4):365–370; discussion 370–371.
12. Goldfarb M, Gallups JM, Gerwin JM. Perforating osteotomies in rhinoplasty. *Arch Otolaryngol Head Neck Surg.* 1993;119(6):624–627.

CHAPTER 52 ■ LIPOSUCTION

MARY K. GINGRASS

Liposuction is the surgical aspiration of fat from the subcutaneous plane leaving a more desirable body contour and a smooth transition between the suctioned and the nonsuctioned areas. Liposuction is one of the most popular cosmetic procedures performed by board certified plastic surgeons in the United States. Although liposuction is not a technically difficult procedure to perform, it requires thoughtful planning and careful patient selection to achieve aesthetically pleasing results. **Poor planning or poor execution can result in uncorrectable deformities.**

HISTORY

The aspiration of fat using blunt cannulas and negative-pressure suction was first popularized in Europe in the late 1970s (1). Three French surgeons, Drs. Yves-Gerard Illouz, Pierre Fournier, and Francis Otteni, were the first to present their lipoaspiration experience at the 1982 American Society of Plastic and Reconstructive Surgeons annual meeting in Honolulu, Hawaii. The procedure was initially met with skepticism in the United States. In late 1982, a "blue ribbon committee" was commissioned by The American Society of Plastic and Reconstructive Surgeons to visit Dr. Illouz in Paris and the committee returned with a cautiously optimistic report. American surgeons' interest in liposuction and public demand for minimally invasive body contouring have steadily risen since.

PATIENT SELECTION

Patient selection is a critical determinant of a good aesthetic surgical result, especially in body contouring. Not all patients who request liposuction are good candidates. The consultation begins with an assessment of the patient's goals. What does the patient wish to change about his or her body? What does the patient hope to accomplish with liposuction? The surgeon then provides the patient with a realistic appraisal of what *can* and *cannot* be accomplished with liposuction. Some patients may require alternative procedures (such as an abdominoplasty) or liposuction combined with an open surgical procedure. **An astute surgeon is wary of patients who are particularly poor candidates for liposuction such as (a) perfectionists with imperceptible "deformities," (b) severely depressed patients with eating disorder problems, and (c) significantly overweight patients who are incapable of weight reduction and expect surgery to do it for them.**

A detailed weight history is an important part of any liposuction consultation. Ideal candidates are at a stable weight with a working diet and exercise regimen in place. **Patients who have a history of frequent or significant weight fluctuations are at high risk for weight gain after liposuction. Maintaining a stable weight and practicing a diet and exercise regimen for at least 6 to 12 months indicates the necessary commitment to lifestyle change.**

Liposuction should not be offered as a treatment for obesity. In a perfect world, it is used to remove genetically distributed or diet-resistant fat. In practical terms, however, it is frequently used to remove fat that could be lessened with diet and exercise. Ideal liposuction candidates are within 20% of their ideal body weight (2) or less than 50 pounds above chart weight. Abnormally distributed bulges of fat or fat that is distributed outside the confines of the ideal body shape are the "target" areas that are commonly suctioned.

PATIENT EVALUATION

A thorough physical examination is always performed. Although the focus of the examination should be on "problem areas," it is important to take the entire body shape into consideration. An overall harmonious body contour is desirable. The patient is examined for areas of disproportionate fat, asymmetry between the two sides, dimpling/cellulite, varicosities, and zones of adherence. Asymmetries are noted and, if they are significant, they are brought to the attention of the patient. If the abdomen is being considered as a potential surgical site, the abdomen should be carefully examined for hernia, significant abdominal wall laxity, abdominal scars, history of abdominal radiation, and anything that might affect abdominal wall integrity.

One of the most important physical findings, which will have significant bearing on the final outcome, is the patient's skin tone, or dermal quality. It is important to pinch and palpate the skin, assessing for the degree of laxity and dermal thickness. A thicker dermis is more likely to retract after liposuction and give a desirable result. Thin, stretched skin with striae (indicating dermal breakage) is unlikely to retract and may look worse after liposuction. If it is determined that the skin quality is unsuitable for liposuction, alternative procedures are proposed, such as skin excision, if indicated. **Liposuction does not improve cellulite thus one should not make promises to this effect.**

The quality of the fat should also be assessed because it may affect the outcome. The anatomy of the subcutaneous adipose tissue varies throughout the body. Some areas of the body have both a deep adipose compartment and a superficial adipose compartment, which are separated by a discrete subcutaneous fascia. The superficial fat in the trunk and thigh consists of smaller lobules, tightly organized within vertically oriented, thin, fibrous septa. The deep fat consists of larger lobules arranged more loosely within widely spaced and more irregularly arranged septa (Fig. 52.1) (3). **In these areas, the deep layer of fat is the target for liposuction.** The overlying superficial fat is (usually) relatively thin and will act as a protective layer to hide small contour deformities, especially for the inexperienced liposuction surgeon. In contrast, other areas of the body that are commonly suctioned (arms, lower legs) have only one layer of fat. Suctioning these areas with smaller cannulas will help to avoid contour irregularities.

533

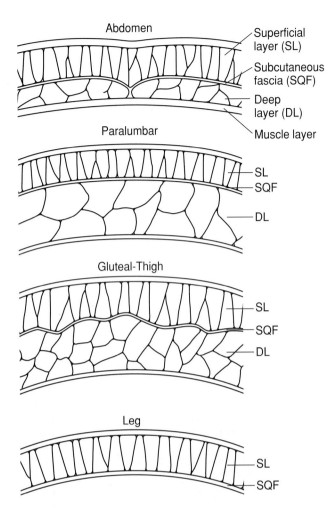

FIGURE 52.1. Superficial and deep fat layers. Markman and Barton studied the subcutaneous tissue of the trunk and lower extremity, finding that the fat lobules in the superficial layer (SL) are small and tightly packed within closely spaced septa, whereas those of the deep layer (DL) are larger, more irregular, and less organized. The arrangement becomes less obvious in the gluteal and thigh area, and disappears as one proceeds from trochanter to knee. There is only one fat layer in the lower leg. (From Markman B, Barton F, Jr. Anatomy of the Subcutaneous Tissue of the Trunk and Lower Extremity. Adapted with permission from *Plast Reconst Surg.* 1987;80:252, with permission.)

Superficial liposuction, a technique popularized by Marco Gasparotti and others, uses small cannulas to aspirate fat from the superficial planes (1–2 mm). Proponents of this technique contend that aspiration in the superficial plane leads to predictable contraction of the overlying skin. **Superficial liposuction leaves very little margin for error and should not be attempted until the liposuction surgeon has gained considerable experience in the deep and intermediate planes. It is my opinion that the superficial plane should be treated with great respect and should be approached with caution until the varsity stage of one's career.**

INFORMED CONSENT

Informed consent should be regarded by the surgeon not only as a legal responsibility, but as a mutually beneficial transaction. The patient is informed of the risks, benefits, and available alternatives to the procedure being considered. A well-informed patient knows what to expect in the postoperative period. If there is a postoperative complication, the patient will recall

that it was a possibility and it is more likely that the doctor–patient relationship will remain intact.

ANESTHESIA

The appropriate type of anesthesia should be chosen based on surgeon preference, patient choice, estimated volume to be removed, and whether other surgical procedures are being combined with liposuction. Liposuction can be performed safely as an outpatient procedure in an office setting or in an outpatient surgery facility as long as strict adherence to patient safety is maintained. Local or regional anesthesia is generally appropriate for aspiration of smaller volumes, and general anesthesia is preferable when larger volumes are removed. **When large-volume liposuction (>5,000 mL of total aspirate) is performed, or when liposuction is combined with a significant open surgical procedure(s), hospital admission or 24-hour observation in a hospital setting is necessary.**

Attention to perioperative fluid management is imperative when significant volumes are suctioned. Approximately 70% of the injected subcutaneous fluid will be absorbed and must therefore be taken into account when calculating intraoperative intravenous (IV) fluid. Anesthesiologists unfamiliar with liposuction may not be aware of this fact and excessive fluids may be administered. When the superwet technique is used (see Wetting Solution below) the following guidelines for fluid resuscitation are recommended: (a) for volumes <5 L of total aspirate, administer maintenance fluid plus subcutaneous wetting solution; (b) for volumes ≥5 liters total aspirate, administer maintenance fluid plus subcutaneous wetting solution plus 0.25 mL of IV crystalloid per mL of aspirate above 5 L (4).

SURGICAL PLANNING AND INSTRUMENTATION

There are a number of tools available to the liposuction surgeon. Each tool has its advantages and disadvantages and some surgeons simply prefer one tool or technique over another. The following discussion is only an introductory comparison, not an in-depth analysis, of the techniques discussed.

Traditional suction-assisted lipoplasty (SAL) became popular in the United States in the 1980s. The technique uses varying diameter, blunt-tip cannulas attached via large-bore tubing to a source of high vacuum, which effectively suctions fat through a hole or holes in the tip of the cannula. Syringe SAL is a variation whereby fat is aspirated with a cannula attached to a syringe. Suction is created when the plunger is withdrawn, collecting the fat into the syringe. This technique is frequently used if fat is to be reinjected in other locations.

SAL has a long track record and is considered the "gold standard" tool for liposuction. Traditional SAL cannulas are typically bendable and come in many sizes and tip configurations, and most hospital operating rooms and surgery centers own this type of equipment. SAL is an excellent technique for smaller-volume cases and removal of soft fat. It is a less-efficient tool for the removal of fat from more fibrous areas, and requires a fair amount of physical effort on the part of the surgeon, which becomes a disadvantage in larger-volume cases. Bruising is expected as a result of disruption of blood vessels by the shearing and suction forces. Cross-tunneling is a necessary step with SAL in order to avoid contour irregularity, which one study reported to be as high as 20% (5). The most frequently reported unsatisfactory results in this study were insufficient fat removal and excessive waviness. Asymmetry, excessive fat removal, and unacceptable scarring occurred with less frequency.

Ultrasound-assisted liposuction (UAL) was introduced in the United States in the mid-1990s to address some of the shortcomings of SAL. Ultrasonic energy is produced in a piezo-electric crystal within the UAL hand piece. The ultrasonic energy is transmitted down the attached probe or cannula to its tip, where the ultrasonic energy causes micromechanical, thermal, and cavitational effects on subcutaneous fat. The intervening fibroconnective tissues remain relatively unharmed and available for postoperative skin retraction. The emulsified fat is suctioned away with low-power suction. UAL requires much less physical effort on the part of the surgeon than does SAL because much of the "work" is done by the ultrasonic energy. UAL is an extremely efficient tool for the removal of fat in fibrous areas such as the upper back, the hypogastrium, and the breast. UAL has been shown to cause less disruption of vasculature than SAL (6), which translates into less bruising. There is energy dissipation in all directions at the tip of the UAL probe or cannula, which gives it a certain "airbrush" effect. Some surgeons believe it is a superior tool for sculpting and find less need for cross-tunneling compared to SAL.

There are also disadvantages to UAL. There is potential for frictional injury at the skin entry site, so constant irrigation at the incision or a skin protector must be used. Seroma rates can be high with prolonged ultrasound treatment times. There is some elevation of tissue temperature with UAL and, if improper technique is used, thermal injury can occur. With proper training these problems rarely occur.

Power-assisted liposuction (PAL) was developed in the late 1990s to address some of the concerns about UAL. PAL is basically traditional SAL powered by a reciprocating cannula. The main advantages of PAL over SAL are its efficiency in fibrous areas and its ease of operation for the surgeon. There is no particular salvage of fibroconnective tissue or neurovascular structures as there is with UAL. The main advantage of PAL over UAL is that there is no heat generation. UAL is safe and effective when the surgeon is properly trained and the procedure is performed properly (7). PAL is an excellent tool for the surgeons who remain uncomfortable with the potential for heat and the more powerful tool.

MARKING AND POSITIONING

Preoperative markings provide an important "topographic map," enabling the surgeon to visualize the targeted convexities, avoid concavities, and address asymmetries when the patient is lying on the operating table. Markings should be made immediately prior to surgery with the patient in a standing position. A permanent marking pen is imperative so that the markings will not wash off when the patient is prepped. Asymmetries should be carefully marked and brought to the attention of the patient. Depressions and indentations should be marked with a different color marker so that these areas can be avoided (Fig. 52.2).

Patient positioning should be planned before the patient enters the operating room. Positioning depends on which areas are being suctioned. Although most body areas can be suctioned from either the prone or supine positions, some surgeons prefer the lateral decubitus position for the hips and lateral thighs. When several body areas are to be suctioned, an intraoperative position change is necessary. If the procedure is performed under local anesthesia, it often makes sense to prep the patient circumferentially while the patient is standing and then have the patient lie down on a sterile drape. The patient can rotate on the operating table as necessary throughout the procedure. When the procedure is performed under general anesthesia, the patient is first prepped in the prone position, which allows easy access to the back, flanks, buttocks, lateral thighs, and the posterior aspect of the entire lower extremity. The patient is then turned to the supine position and reprepped and draped. The abdomen, breasts, arms, and the anterior aspect of the lower extremity can be addressed from this position.

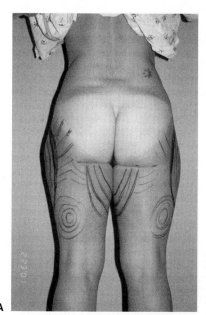 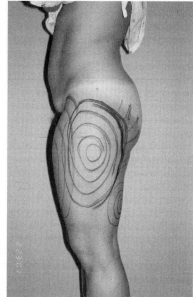 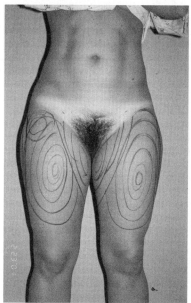

A   B, C

FIGURE 52.2. Preoperative markings before circumferential thigh liposuction. Markings are similar to a topographic map. Lines and circles represent surface features of the body showing the specific shape and size relationships between the component parts. In this case, progressively smaller circles indicate a "higher" point (or more fat) in relation to the surrounding areas. Markings are extremely important to assist the surgeon in getting smooth, even, and predictable results.

Patients are prepped with a 3-minute Betadine scrub, followed by Betadine paint. Bair hugger warming blankets are recommended on unexposed body parts and a Foley catheter should be placed when aspirations >5 L are planned. When liposuction is combined with an open surgical procedure, or when large-volume liposuction is performed, compression hose and/or sequential compression device (SCD) boots for deep vein thrombosis (DVT) prophylaxis are recommended.

WETTING SOLUTION

Liposuction was first practiced as a "dry" technique, meaning that nothing was done to prepare the fat prior to suctioning it from the subcutaneous plane. As one might expect, hemorrhagic complications were common. Illouz is credited for developing the "wet" technique, which he described as a "dissecting hydrotomy," wherein he instilled normal saline, water, and hyaluronidase in the hope of creating a weak hypotonic solution to lyse the adipocyte cell wall (8). Hetter is credited with adding lidocaine and dilute epinephrine to the wetting solution (9). Jeffrey Klein, a dermatologist, developed and coined the term *tumescent technique,* which is now used for the infiltration of large-volume, dilute lidocaine with epinephrine solution for the purpose of performing liposuction with low blood loss (10). The importance of infiltration of wetting solution cannot be overstated. The superwet technique is defined as a 1:1 ratio of the volume of wetting solution infused to the volume of aspirate. The term tumescent technique was classically described as a ratio of 2 or 3:1. Technically, the tumescent and the superwet techniques differ in the ratio of volume infused to volume of aspirate; however, both involve infusion of wetting solution to the point of tissue turgor or a "peau d'orange" of the overlying skin. **Practically, the term tumescent liposuction is used as a generic term for liposuction using wetting solution.**

Wetting solution has a number of advantages. It provides a mechanism for delivery of anesthetic and vasoconstricting agent, thereby providing a component of intraoperative anesthesia, decreasing blood loss and postoperative bruising, and also providing postoperative analgesia. Administration of wetting solution eases the passage of the cannula through the tissue, and minimizes fluid requirements during and after surgery. Some surgeons believe that magnification of the area to be suctioned is an advantage, whereas others believe that distortion of the area is a disadvantage. It is my opinion that "final contour" is an end point that comes with experience, and infiltration of wetting solution is a necessary part of the equation for the student to master.

Table 52.1 describes my standard wetting solution recipes. **The total amount of lidocaine infused per patient should not exceed the maximum recommended subcutaneous dose of 35 mg/kg (Chapter 11) (11). The maximum dose for each patient should be calculated preoperatively and the case should be planned accordingly. If more infiltrate is needed once the maximum dose has been reached, lidocaine can be left out of** the final bags when general anesthesia is used (see the discussion of lidocaine toxicity in Risks and Possible Complications below).

The actual infiltration technique is especially important. An uneven infiltration of wetting solution increases the chances of an uneven final result. Infiltration is begun in the deepest plane of the area to be suctioned and proceeds in a systematic fashion from deep to superficial. Each level, or "plane," should be evenly infiltrated before slowly moving a bit more superficial. The infiltrated fat should be evenly firm, and there should be no disproportionate bulges in the skin at the end of the infiltration process. The wetting solution should be "feathered" at the edges of the target area, just like the suctioned fat is feathered.

ASPIRATION OF FAT

The wetting solution is allowed 7 to 10 minutes for maximal vasoconstrictive effect. Aspiration is performed through various small incisions, the location of which depends on the area being suctioned. Every attempt should be made to hide incisions in anatomic creases or Langer cleavage lines, when appropriate, although most liposuction cannulas are small enough that the eventual scars are almost imperceptible. As a general rule liposuction is performed using the dominant hand, making even strokes in a systematic fashion. For instance, one can approach the lateral thigh through a gluteal crease incision with the patient in a prone position. If the surgeon is right handed, the surgeon may stand on the left side of the patient and insert the appropriate cannula into right or left gluteal crease incision. **The cannula is inserted into the deep plane first.** Using even in-and-out strokes, the cannula is moved back and forth in a fanlike pattern, with the incision as the fulcrum. The cannula is moved more superficially as fat is removed. The nondominant hand is kept over the area being suctioned to provide tactile feedback as to the depth of the underlying cannula and the amount of remaining fat. **Cross-tunneling (suctioning an area from a second incision at right angles from the first incision) is recommended for most areas to avoid contour deformity** (Fig. 52.3).

The end point of aspiration is determined by a number of factors. Contour of the patient is the most important factor, but determining it can sometimes be confusing because of infused wetting solution. The aspirate volume should also be considered. Additionally, a comparison of sides when bilateral areas are suctioned is helpful. When UAL is used, the amount of time that ultrasonic energy is applied should be recorded and considered when determining the end point and can be helpful when attempting to obtain symmetry between sides. The pinch test is also helpful. The *pinch test is* performed by gently pinching the patient's skin and subcutaneous fat between the thumb and forefingers to assess the thickness and smoothness of the underlying subcutaneous tissue and for comparing preoperative with postoperative thickness. Simply pinching or rolling the tissue between one's thumb and index finger helps in the assessment of irregularities. When all is said and done, it doesn't matter what is removed; what matters is what you leave behind!

Final contouring is routinely done at the end of the liposuction procedure. The surgeon may use saline to wet the skin and glide his or her hand over the surface to assist in finding small irregularities. Usually smaller diameter cannulas (2.5 or 3.0 mm) are chosen to do the final contouring and feathering. The old adage "the enemy of good is better" should be kept in mind. **Overresection is more difficult to fix than underresection, so it is better to err on the side of underresection.** Liposuction may not be difficult, but is time-consuming and requires meticulous attention to detail.

TABLE 52.1

STANDARD WETTING SOLUTION

Local anesthesia	General anesthesia
1 L lactated Ringer solution	1 L lactated Ringer solution
1 mL epinephrine	1 mL epinephrine
50 mL 1% Xylocaine	30 mL 1% Xylocaine

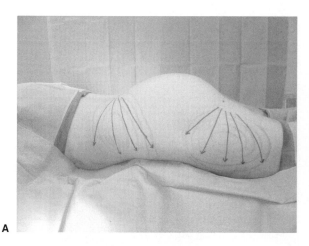 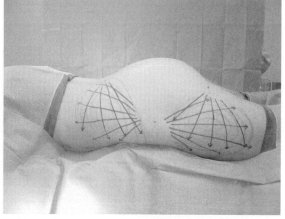

FIGURE 52.3. Cross-tunneling. Cross-tunneling is a technique used to enhance smoothness and to decrease risk of contour irregularity. The patient is in the prone position with her head on the left side of the picture. **A:** The liposuction cannula is inserted into the gluteal crease incision (*black arrow*) to suction the left lateral thigh, and into the parasacral area to suction the left posterior hip. **B:** A second incision is made and the same areas are suctioned from a separate incision in the midaxillary line (at approximately a right angle from the first "line" of suction).

BODY AREAS TREATABLE WITH LIPOSUCTION

Numerous body areas are amenable to liposuction given the plethora of equipment now available. Today's patient can be treated from head to toe (Figs. 52.4–52.7). The face and neck can be successfully treated with liposuction, although fat injection instead of aspiration is increasingly popular. The trunk, including the abdomen, back, breast, and posterior hips (flanks), and the lower extremity, including the knees, calves, and ankles, have all been successfully treated with liposuction. In my experience, treatment of gynecomastia is particularly amenable to UAL (12). The upper arm is also well suited for UAL or SAL when the skin is not too loose. **The buttocks can be successfully treated but should be approached with some degree of caution. Creation of a flat or ptotic buttocks is not only unsightly, but usually requires excisional measures to repair.**

POSTOPERATIVE COURSE

Incisions for cannulas larger than 3.0 mm are generally closed with a 5-0 nylon suture. Some surgeons recommend leaving smaller incisions open to allow wetting solution to drain. The patient is dressed in a compression garment that covers the areas that have been suctioned. I believe that compression foam (e.g., Topi-Foam, Byron Medical, Tucson, AZ) under a garment decreases early bruising and edema, which seems to speed recovery. An abdominal binder can be used when only the hips or abdomen were treated. If thigh suction was also done, a girdle is preferable. **The patient will experience copious serosanguineous drainage from incision sites for approximately 24 to 36 hours, which can be alarming to family and friends if they are not informed in advance.** Showering is permissible on postoperative day 1 or 2 and if the patient is instructed to replace the compression foam over the suctioned areas.

Drains are recommended for gynecomastia and when >2,000 mL lipoaspirate is removed from the abdomen alone. They are left in place until drainage is less than 25 to 30 mL in a 24-hour period. Ideally, foam padding is left in place for 3 to 5 days. Compression garments are generally encouraged

24 hours per day for 4 to 6 weeks if circumferential thigh suctioning is performed. Postoperative follow-up visits are scheduled at 5 days to remove sutures; 2 weeks to make sure that bruising is subsiding normally and to advance the patient's activity; 6 weeks to make sure that edema is subsiding normally and to assess the early result; 3 months to assess early result; and 6 months to assess final result. Maximal swelling can be expected at postoperative days 3 to 5. **In my experience, 60% to 80% of the swelling subsides by 6 weeks postprocedure, and it takes a full 4 to 6 months for 100% of the swelling to resolve, depending on the extent of the procedure.**

Patients should begin ambulating on the day of surgery. Oral fluids and a high protein diet are encouraged. Physical activity should be low for the first week to discourage edema, followed by a gradual increase in activity during the second week, depending on the amount of suction that was done. At the end of the first week, most patients can return to work and should be encouraged to begin light exercise, such as brisk walking on a treadmill (with compression garments on!). At 3 to 4 weeks, if edema and bruising are resolving appropriately, the patient should be advancing to full activity, and may "wean" him- or herself out of the compression garment over the course of a week. These are general guidelines for patients undergoing average volume liposuction (lipoaspirate 2,000–5,000 mL) and must be tailored to the individual patient. Large-volume liposuction and circumferential thigh patients will need a more restrictive postoperative regimen.

RISKS AND POSSIBLE COMPLICATIONS

Any surgical procedure has risks. Fortunately, serious complications are rarely associated with liposuction procedures. **The most common undesirable sequela after liposuction is contour irregularity, which is directly related to inexperience and lack of attention to detail.** Contour irregularities generally fall into four categories: (a) overcorrection, (b) undercorrection, (c) failure of skin retraction or abnormal skin retraction, and (d) complex deformities consisting of combinations of a, b, and c (13). Revisionary procedures should be performed only after all the swelling has completely subsided. Generally, the treatment of undercorrection is removal of more fat; the

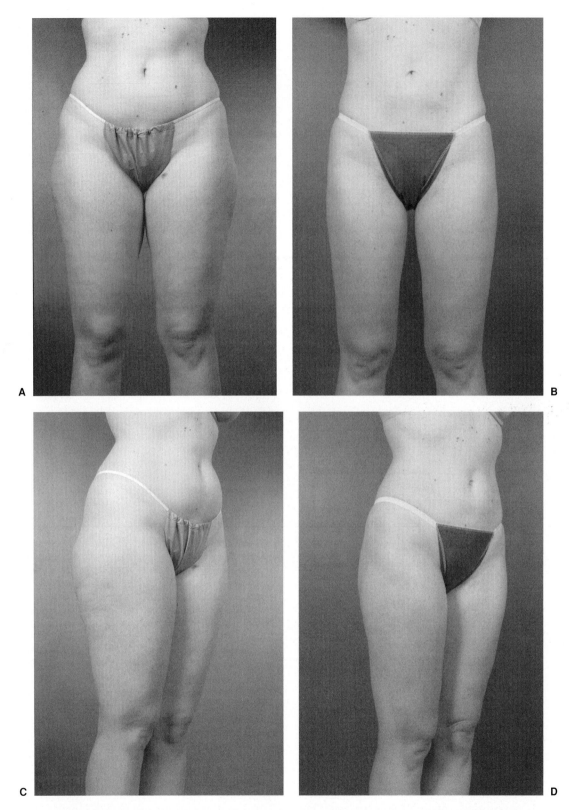

FIGURE 52.4. Ultrasound-assisted liposuction of a 27-year-old woman shown before (**A, C**) and 12 months after (**B, D**) UAL of the abdomen, posterior hips, and circumferential thighs. A total of 4,700 mL of wetting solution was infiltrated and a total of 4,775 mL of lipoaspirate (fluid and fat) was removed: 575 mL from the abdomen, 475 mL from each posterior hip, and 1,625 mL was removed from the each thigh circumferentially.

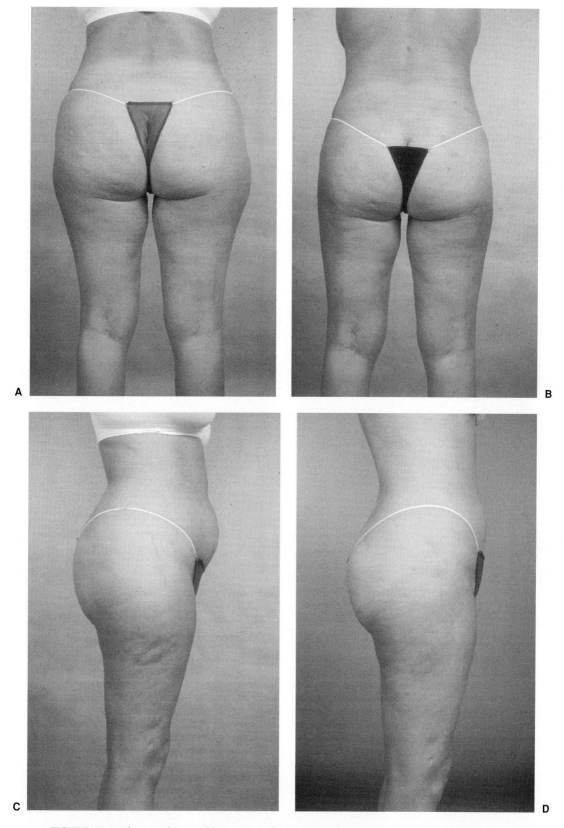

FIGURE 52.5. Ultrasound-assisted liposuction of a 50-year-old woman. She was treated with UAL to the abdomen, posterior hips, and lateral thighs. A total of 1,250 mL, 600 mL, and 700 mL of wetting solution was infiltrated into the abdomen, hips and lateral thighs, respectively. A total of 1,300 mL, 900 mL, and 925 mL of lipoaspirate, respectively, was removed from each area. The total infiltrated was 3,850 mL, and the total aspirated was 4,950 mL.

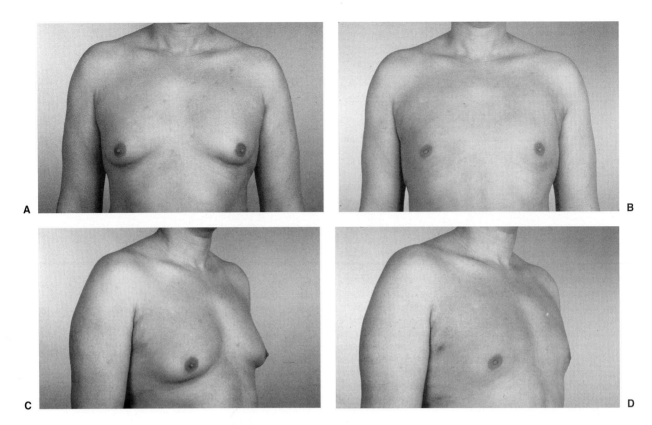

FIGURE 52.6. Power-assistedliposuction of the breast in a 47-year-old man with gynecomastia. The patient is shown before (**A, C**) and 4 months after (**B, D**) PAL of the breast. A total of 650 mL of wetting solution was infiltrated into each breast and 575 mL of lipoaspirate (fluid and fat) was removed from each breast.

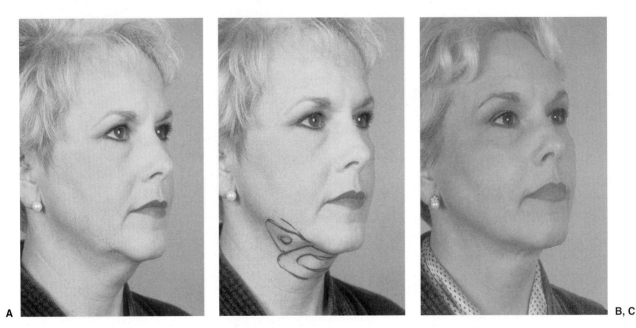

FIGURE 52.7. Suction-assisted lipoplasty of the neck in a 53-year-old woman shown before (**A, B**) and after (**C**) SAL of the neck. Superior results can generally be obtained with liposuction of the neck in the younger population; however, this woman had very good skin retraction for her age. Careful preoperative assessment of skin quality and thorough preoperative counseling with this type of patient is imperative. In this case, incisions were made in the submental area and behind each ear in order to allow contouring along the jawline.

TABLE 52.2

LIDOCAINE TOXICITY

Early signs	Later signs	Late signs
Plasma concentrations 3–6 μg/mL	Plasma concentrations 5–9 μg/mL	Plasma concentration >10 μg/mL
Lightheadedness	Shivering	Convulsions
Restlessness	Muscle twitching	CNS depression
Drowsiness	Tremors	Coma
Tinnitus		
Slurred speech		
Metallic taste in mouth		
Numbness of lips and tongue		

treatment of overcorrection is fat injection; the treatment of loose skin is skin excision; and the treatment of complex deformities is beyond the scope of this chapter. The best way to "treat" contour irregularity is to avoid it.

Other risks, including unusual bleeding, which could result in unusual ecchymosis or permanent skin discoloration, hematoma, seroma, infection, dysesthesia, fat embolism, thromboembolism, fluid imbalance, lidocaine toxicity, skin necrosis, perforation of viscera, and death, fortunately, are rare.

Lidocaine toxicity deserves special mention because according to the *Physicians' Desk Reference*, the maximal recommended dose of subcutaneous lidocaine HCl when used in combination with epinephrine is 7 mg/kg in an adult, yet numerous studies have documented the safety and efficacy of larger doses of lidocaine for the purposes of liposuction (11). Table 52.2 lists the signs and symptoms of lidocaine toxicity.

CONCLUSION

Liposuction is an extremely popular cosmetic procedure in today's body-conscious society. Technically, it is a relatively easy procedure to perform *adequately*; however, it requires strict attention to detail and a keen aesthetic eye to perfect the art of liposuction. Sucking fat is easy, whereas sculpting the human body by removal of the perfect amount of fat, and leaving behind the perfect amount of fat, is an art.

References

1. Fournier P. Popularization of the technique. In: Hetter GP, ed. *Lipoplasty: The Theory and Practice of Blunt Suction Lipectomy.* 2nd ed. Boston: Little Brown; 1990: 35–38.
2. Hughes CE. Patient selection, planning and marking in ultrasound-assisted lipoplasty. *Clin Plast Surg.* 1999;26:279.
3. Markman B, Barton FE. Anatomy of the subcutaneous tissue of the trunk and lower extremity. *Plast Reconst Surg.* 1987;80:248.
4. Rohrich RJ, Kenkel JM, Janis JE, et al. An update on the role of subcutaneous infiltration in suction-assisted lipoplasty. *Plast Reconstr Surg.* 2003;111:926.
5. Pitman GH, Teimourian B. Suction lipectomy: complications and result by survey. *Plast Reconst Surg.* 1985;76:65.
6. Kenkel JM, Robinson J, Beran SJ, et al. The tissue effects of ultrasound assisted lipoplasty. *Plast Reconst Surg.* 1998;102:213.
7. Ablaza VJ, Gingrass MK, Perry LC, et al. Tissue temperatures during ultrasound assisted lipoplasty. *Plast Reconst Surg.* 1998;102:534.
8. The wet technique. In: Illouz YG, DeVillers YT, eds. *Body Sculpturing by Lipoplasty.* New York: Livingstone Churchill; 1989: 124.
9. Hetter GP. The effect of low dose epinephrine on the hematocrit drop following lipolysis. *Aesthetic Plast Surg.* 1984;8(1):19.
10. Klein JA. The tumescent technique for liposuction surgery. *Am J Cosmetic Surg.* 1987;4:263.
11. Klein JA. Tumescent technique for regional anesthesia permits lidocaine doses of 35 mg/kg for liposuction. *J Dermatol Surg Oncol.* 1990;16:248.
12. Gingrass MK, Shermak, MA. The treatment of gyncomasta with ultrasound-assisted lipoplasty. *Persp. Plastic Surgery.* 1999;12(2).
13. Gingrass MK, Hensel JM. Secondary liposuction. In: Mathes SJ, Hentz VR, eds. *Plastic Surgery.* 2nd ed. Philadelphia: Saunders/Elsevier. In press.

CHAPTER 53 ■ ABDOMINOPLASTY AND LOWER TRUNCAL CIRCUMFERENTIAL BODY CONTOURING

AL ALY

Body contouring of the lower trunk region is an integral part of the plastic surgeon's armamentarium. The lower trunk is a circumferential structure that begins at the inferior border of the breasts and ends at the pelvic rim. Although this is a convenient unit, it is difficult to separate from surrounding structures such as the thighs and the upper truncal unit, or thorax. Deformities in the lower truncal region are variable in nature and require different approaches for their treatment. Recent advances in bariatric surgery have resulted in a large population of weight loss patients, which has led to an emphasis on the evaluation and treatment of lower truncal contour deformities. This chapter will focus on excisional procedures, with or without liposuction, in the treatment of lower truncal deformities. Problems that can be ameliorated by liposuction techniques alone are covered in Chapter 52.

PATIENT PRESENTATION

Patients with lower truncal complaints demonstrate a variety of deformities on a continuum from minimal lipodystrophy to circumferential fat and skin excess accompanied by abdominal wall laxity (1) (Table 1).

Weight is the first important factor that affects the presentation of patients with lower truncal deformities. Because absolute weights can be misleading, **body mass index (BMI), which relates weight to height, is the most commonly used parameter.** It is calculated in the following manner:

Body mass index = weight in kilograms/(height in meters)²
Body mass index = weight in pounds/(height in inches)² ×
703

Patients who present for lower truncal contouring span the range of BMI from normal to obese.

The upper limit of normal BMI is 25; 26 to 30 is considered overweight; and 30 and above is considered obese. A variety of surgical approaches is required to treat patients in different BMI ranges.

A second factor that affects the presentation of patients is the fat deposition pattern, which is genetically controlled. Women typically deposit fat in the infraumbilical abdomen, lateral thighs, hips, and medial thighs. Men tend to deposit fat in the flanks, the infraumbilical abdomen, and intra-abdominally (2). **Although these patterns are common, even within the same gender, dramatically different patterns of fat deposition are often present.**

The quality of the skin-fat envelope is a third factor to evaluate. Women who have had one or more pregnancies tend to have abdominal skin laxity and stretch marks. The skin has been stretched beyond its ability to rebound back to its original elasticity. A similar process occurs with massive weight gain

and subsequent weight loss in which the skin is overexpanded, leading to a skin-fat envelope that is loose and inelastic.

HISTORY

Body contouring procedures early in the twentieth century consisted of dermatolipectomies of hanging abdominal panniculi. In these procedures, excess skin and underlying fat were removed to rid the patient of hanging tissues with minimal attention to aesthetic principles. In the second half of the century, advances in abdominoplasty techniques consisted of improved scar placement, abdominal wall plication techniques, and umbilical transposition. In the 1980s, liposuction was introduced, and it became a tremendous tool in the armamentarium of the plastic surgeon for affecting body contour, replacing a number of excisional procedures. Currently plastic surgeons routinely use both excisional and liposuction techniques, alone and in combination, to improve body contour.

RELEVANT ANATOMY

Fat in the lower trunk is organized into superficial and deep layers separated by the superficial fascial system, which pervades the entire body. Anteriorly the superficial fascial system is referred to as the Scarpa fascia (Fig. 53.1).

The blood supply of the abdominal skin and fat is important to understand. The skin overlying the rectus muscles is primarily supplied by arteries that originate from the superior and inferior epigastric vessels that run within the rectus muscles. Branches from these vessels perforate the overlying rectus fascia and traverse through the two layers of abdominal fat, finally reaching the skin. This direct blood supply of abdominal skin is interrupted during the elevation of the abdominal flap in an abdominoplasty. A secondary blood supply is derived from lateral intercostal, subcostal, and lumbar vessels that course anteriorly in the fat superficial to the Scarpa fascia (Fig. 53.2). **These vessels are the only remaining blood supply of central abdominal skin after flap elevation.** Interruption of these vessels by scars such as cholycystectomy incisions can lead to necrosis of inferomedial abdominal flap tissues. The superficial epigastric vessels supply blood to the skin of the lower abdomen but are also divided during abdominoplasty procedures.

The lower trunk has fascial attachments between the skin and underlying muscle fascia that act as anchoring points or zones of adherence (3) (Fig. 53.3). These zones of adherence do not allow overlying skin to move during the processes of aging and/or weight fluctuations. Posteriorly the midline has a zone of adherence that overlies the spine. The anterior midline of the abdomen has a less will defined zone of adherence. Three horizontal zones of adherence are located in the inferior aspects of

542

TABLE 53.1

FACTORS THAT AFFECT THE PRESENTATION OF THE PATIENT REQUESTING LOWER TRUNCAL CONTOURING

Body mass index. (BMI) at presentation
Fat deposition pattern
Quality of the skin–fat envelope

the lower trunk; one is located at the inguinal region bilaterally and extends toward the anterior superior iliac spine (ASIS). Another is located just above the mons pubis and is variable in its adherence properties. The third is located bilaterally between the hip and lateral thigh fat deposits. Truncal tissues become lax due to aging, pregnancy, and/or massive weight loss. They descend the greatest distance laterally, caused by a combination of tissue laxity and central tethering of the midline zones of adherence. As tissues descend around the pelvis they also migrate centrally (see Fig. 53.3).

The inguinal and mons pubis zones of adherence are responsible for holding the final position of abdominoplasty scars in the lower truncal region. Without their effect, the scars would migrate cephalad, possibly above natural underwear lines.

PATIENT SELECTION

Patients who have minimal to moderate subcutaneous fat excess and no abdominal wall laxity are good candidates for liposuction alone. Patients who present with abdominal wall laxity and minimal abdominal skin excess limited to the infraumbilical region are good candidates for mini-abdominoplasty. Patients who present with abdominal wall laxity of both the infra- and supraumbilical regions and generalized skin excess limited to the anterior aspects of the lower trunk are good candidates for a full abdominoplasty. As the deformities increase in magnitude and involve the lateral and posterior aspects of the lower trunk, circumferential truncal liposuction and/or dermatolipectomies become necessary. The indications, goals, and a general description of each procedure are given later.

Lower truncal body contouring procedures are often long and extensive in nature. Medical problems such as heart disease, diabetes, and lung disease must be under control before surgery is contemplated. Cigarette smoking also has a deleterious effect on blood supply and, when combined with the already compromised vascular supply of the abdominal skin, can lead to significant tissue necrosis.

MINI-ABDOMINOPLASTY

Women who present with abdominal wall laxity restricted to the infraumbilical region that is associated with minimal infraumbilical skin and fat excess are candidates for a mini-abdominoplasty. Physical examination of the abdomen in the supine position will demonstrate infraumbilical rectus diastasis, which can be confirmed by the "diver's test" (Fig. 53.4).

These patients are usually young women who have had one or two pregnancies, have good skin elasticity, and are not overweight. They may or may not have localized fat deposits in other areas of the trunk and lower extremity such as the hips and lateral thighs. The goal of surgery in this patient population is to eliminate the infraumbilical abdominal wall laxity and the minimal skin and fat excess.

Technique

An incision is marked in the patient's natural suprapubic crease and angled toward the ASIS. Often the incision can be limited to the width of the pubic hair or just beyond its lateral edges. Intraoperatively the proposed incision is made and the dissection extended to the muscle fascia. An abdominal flap is elevated superiorly to the level of the umbilicus. The infraumbilical rectus muscle diastasis is identified, and rectus fascia plication is performed. Some surgeons prefer a single layer, whereas others favor a two-layer plication (Fig. 53.5). The abdominal flap is advanced inferiorly and tailored to remove the excess skin and underlying fat. This advancement will usually pull the umbilicus down 1 to 3 cm.

The closure of this incision, as in all subsequent incisions discussed in this chapter, is performed in multiple layers, with the most important layer being the reapproximation of the superficial fascial system, or the Scarpa fascia (4). Permanent or long-lasting sutures are used in this layer in an attempt to limit widening of the scar in the long run. I prefer to use interrupted monofilament nonpermanent suture in the subcuticular layer to perfectly approximate skin with an overlying layer of medical-grade skin glue. Drains are inserted to identify hematomas and reduce the seroma rate. A compression garment is used in the postoperative period by most surgeons.

A variation of this technique can be used in patients who have minimal lower abdominal skin excess, no upper abdominal skin excess, and both infra- and supraumbilical rectus diastasis. To allow access to the supraumbilical rectus diastasis, the base of the umbilicus can be amputated. The abdominal flap is then elevated on either side of the midline in the supraumbilical region, and a supraumbilical rectus plication is performed in continuity with the infraumbilical plication. The umbilical stalk is then resutured to the plication at the appropriate level, and the lower aspect of the abdominal flap is tailored appropriately. It is also possible to use a minimal-incision approach to the supraumbilical plication by making an incision in the superior aspect of the umbilicus and using an endoscope to perform a dissection superior to the umbilicus that is wide enough to allow for the desired supraumbilical plication. In any of the

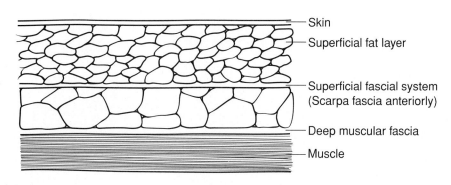

Skin

Superficial fat layer

Superficial fascial system (Scarpa fascia anteriorly)

Deep muscular fascia

Muscle

FIGURE 53.1. Organization of fat and fascia in the anterior abdomen.

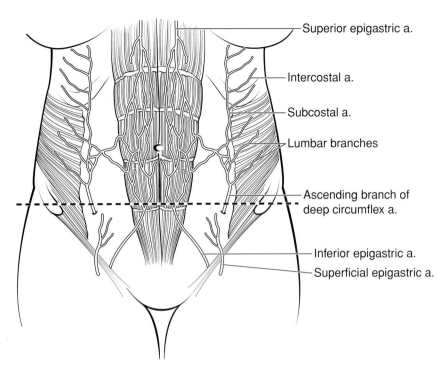

FIGURE 53.2. The abdominal wall vasculature. a., artery.

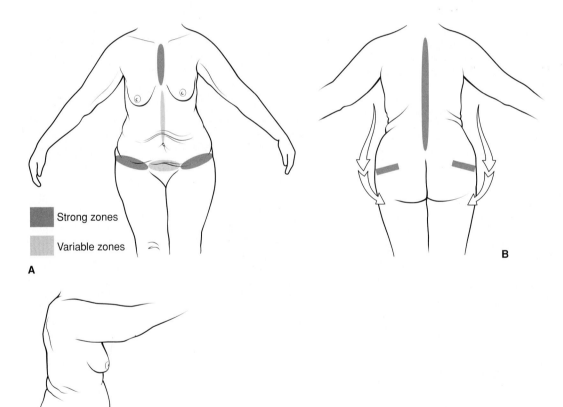

FIGURE 53.3. Fascial zones of adherence. The zones of adherence control the movement of tissue associated with aging and/or massive weight loss. These fascial attachments result in lateral descent of truncal tissues, which rotate toward the midline.

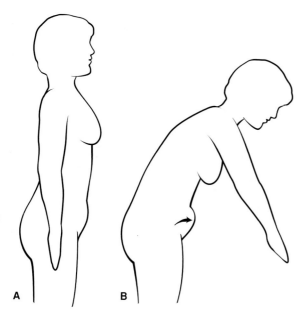

FIGURE 53.4. The classic "diver's test" demonstrates how a bend at the waist will reveal the true extent of abdominal wall laxity.

mini-abdominoplasty techniques discussed, liposuction can be used to decrease the thickness of any part of the abdominal flap that has not been elevated.

One of the most difficult aspects of mini-abdominoplasty is avoiding dog-ears because of the short incision.

ABDOMINOPLASTY

Generally abdominoplasty is indicated in patients whose laxity involves the supra and infraumbilical regions, limited to the an-

terior aspects of the lower trunk. The goals of abdominoplasty depend on the presenting deformities. They include creating a flat abdominal contour, eliminating abdominal wall laxity, enhancing waist definition in some patients, and eradicating mons pubis ptosis if present.

Stretch marks are common and may be limited to the infraumbilical region or may include both the infra- and supraumbilical skin. Rectus diastasis of the entire vertical extent of the abdomen is present in these patients, with the infraumbilical diastasis usually more extensive because of the position of the uterus during pregnancy. Preoperatively abdominal wall laxity can again be detected by the "diver's test" and physical examination. **Massive-weight-loss patients who reach a near-normal BMI may also present with lower truncal excess limited to the anterior abdomen. However, most often they present with circumferential deformities that require more extensive circumferential excisions.**

Patients who present with excess intra-abdominal fat that would prevent flattening of the abdominal wall by plication are not good candidates for abdominoplasty. The outer skin-fat envelope of the belly always conforms to the shape of an inner balloon whose anterior wall is made up of the abdominal muscle wall. If that wall is rendered convex in profile by virtue of overly abundant intra-abdominal contents, then the final profile of the belly will also be convex. Because abdominal contour flattening is one of the major goals of surgery, these patients are better served by weight loss prior to contemplating abdominoplasty-type procedures.

By the nature of an abdominoplasty, where an ellipse of tissue is removed from the lower abdomen, dog-ears can be created at the edges of the ellipse, especially in patients who already have lateral excess. Patients who present with deformities that extend beyond the anterior aspects of the lower trunk may require extending the abdominoplasty excision laterally, liposuction of the lateral and posterior trunk, and/or circumferential dermatolipectomy to attain the best possible contour. Some authors advocate the use of fleur-de-lis or I-type excisions in which an anterior vertical wedge of tissue is resected, as will be discussed later in this chapter. Generally, as circumferential lower truncal dermatolipectomy has become more mainstream in plastic surgery because of the massive-weight-loss population, the indications for isolated abdominoplasty have narrowed.

Technique

The markings for an abdominoplasty are performed prior to surgery. The proposed excision is marked in the lower abdomen. Centrally the inferior incision line is often marked in the natural suprapubic crease and then carried laterally. Recently many surgeons have adopted the use of a "French bikini/thong pattern" in which the lateral aspects of the proposed inferior incision are angled toward the ASIS, but many variations are described in the literature (5). An attempt is made to avoid the incision beyond the ASIS, but it is more important to avoid dog-ears. With the inferior mark in place the patient is slightly flexed at the waist, and the pinch technique is used to approximate the superior extent of the excision. Ideally the patient should have enough excess abdominal skin to allow excision of the skin from just above the umbilicus to the suprapubic crease centrally.

In the operating room a circumumbilical incision is made, and the inferior incision of the proposed excision is made. Abdominal flap is elevated superiorly, around the umbilicus, and up to the xiphoid and costal margins (Fig. 53.6). **This type of wide undermining allows the greatest amount of inferior abdominal flap advancement at the time of flap tailoring, but it also leads to the division of more lateral intercostals, and**

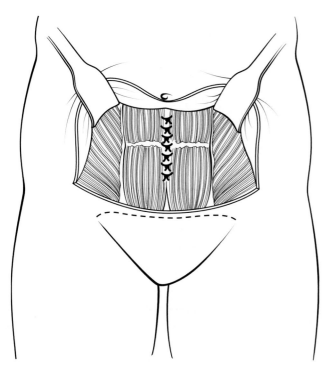

FIGURE 53.5. The abdominal flap elevation and rectus fascia plication in a mini-abdominoplasty.

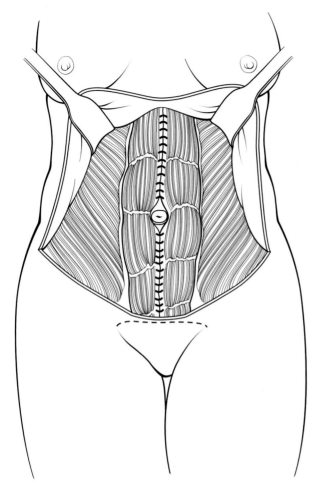

FIGURE 53.6. The extent of abdominal flap elevation and fascial plication in a traditional abdominoplasty.

subcostal and lumbar vessels, which make up the remaining blood supply of the flap. Some surgeons prefer a more limited dissection on either side of the midline above the umbilicus, just enough to allow for supraumbilical rectus fascia plication up to the xiphoid. The benefit of the limited dissection is the increased number of the lateral vessels left intact to support the blood supply of the tailored abdominal flap. In some patients, however, the limited dissection will not allow the appropriate advancement of the abdominal flap and reduce the amount of tissue that may need to be resected to create the best contour. As a general rule, flap elevation should be restricted to just what will allow appropriate rectus fascia plication and appropriate flap advancement. Often it is best to limit the initial elevation and then release the tissues incrementally to allow for appropriate contour.

After flap elevation, rectus fascia plication is performed. Many patterns have been proposed for plication, but a vertical plication in one or two layers is most common. The patient is then flexed at the waist, and the abdominal flap is advanced inferiorly to facilitate the process of flap tailoring. As the abdominal flap is advanced, the surgeon can control where the greatest tension will be at closure—centrally or laterally. Creating the greatest amount of tension centrally is advantageous in limiting the lateral extent of the final scar but may lead to excessive mons pubis elevation and less waist definition. Lockwood, in his "high-lateral-tension" approach to abdominoplasty, has espoused placing the greatest tension on the lateral aspects of the abdominal closure (6). This is based on the fact that the

greatest laxity in the trunk occurs laterally. However, the increased lateral tension often necessitates extensions of the scar laterally to eliminate dog-ears. This approach leads to better waist definition and improvement in anterior thigh contour.

With the tailored abdominal flap approximated to the lower incision, the position of the umbilicus is noted on the flap and a neo-umbilicus is created. The stalk of the umbilicus is brought through the abdominal flap through various types of incisions advocated by different authors. I prefer a simple vertical incision, no defating of the underlying soft tissues, and three, point fixation sutures at 3, 6, and 9 o' clock. Whatever method the surgeon chooses, the umbilicus should be fairly small, vertically oriented, superiorly hooded, and have a slight hollow around it.

The closure of the abdominal incision is accomplished in multiple layers, with the most important layer being the superficial fascial system, or the Scarpa fascia (4). This is accomplished with permanent or long-lasting suture, which, it is hoped, reduces the significant tension that can be generated at closure, prevents acute wound dehiscence, and reduces scar widening in the long run. I prefer to use interrupted monofilament nonpermanent suture in the subcuticular layer to perfectly approximate skin. An overlying layer of medical-grade skin glue is then applied. Drains are placed. A compression garment is used in the postoperative period by most surgeons. Figure 53.7 shows an example of abdominoplasty in an ideal patient.

Combining liposuction with traditional abdominoplasty techniques is controversial and often is left to the surgeon's experience and philosophy (7). Liposuction of the abdominal flap in nonundermined areas is generally considered safe. Liposuction of undermined regions of the flap can potentially lead to flap necrosis because of the compounding effect of liposuction on the already compromised blood supply. Certainly, liposuction of areas outside the bounds of the undermined abdominal flap, such as the hip region or the lateral thighs, can be performed without concern for flap compromise.

CIRCUMFERENTIAL LOWER TRUNCAL DERMATOLIPECTOMY OR CIRCUMFERENTIAL LIPECTOMY

As a basic principle of plastic surgery, it is always better to treat an anatomic unit in its entirety whenever possible. Abdominoplasty treats deformities limited to the anterior lower trunk. When deformities involve more than the anterior abdomen, other procedures are required. If the surrounding areas such as the thighs, buttocks, hip, and lower back regions contain excess fat without ptosis, liposuction can be added to abdominoplasty to create a better overall lower truncal contour. However, for patients who present with generalized laxity and/or ptosis of those areas, circumferential lipectomies are required. Massive-weight-loss patients make up the largest group of such patients who require circumferential excisional procedures. They will continue to grow in numbers, given that obesity has been recognized as a major health care issue in the United States and the world. In addition, women who gain moderate weight, 30 to 40 pounds, usually with childbirth and/or aging, and are not able to lose the weight through normal means of exercise and nutritional changes may be candidates. They often present with a desire to eliminate anterior abdominal excess, but careful examination will demonstrate circumferential excess that is best treated with a circumferential lipectomy. Finally, normal-weight-range patients who desire remarkable improvements in their lower truncal contour may be candidates.

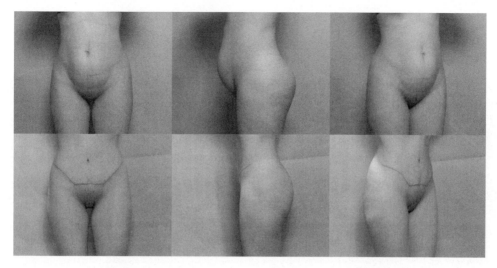

FIGURE 53.7. Traditional abdominoplasty. A young woman who presented after two pregnancies desiring an improvement in her abdominal contour. She complained of loose abdominal skin and protrusion of her belly, despite a regular exercise program. Her abdominal wall laxity was more prominent in the infraumbilical region, consistent with her pregnancies. She underwent an abdominoplasty using a French-bikini pattern of excision and is shown 6 months after surgery. Because her deformities were limited to the anterior abdomen and she was within the normal weight range, there was no need to combine other procedures with her traditional abdominoplasty.

There is a variety of names used to describe circumferential lower truncal dermatolipectomies: extended or circumferential abdominoplasty, central body lift, torsoplasty, and body lift. I prefer to divide these different variations into two general categories based on what they treat and what they accomplish. The first category is made up of centrally based procedures that mainly treat the lower truncal unit, which will be referred to as belt lipectomies, as espoused by Aly and Cram (8,9). The second category includes procedures that treat the lower trunk and thighs as a unit, which will be referred to as lower body lifts, as espoused by Lockwood (10,11). Each procedure has its benefits and drawbacks. Both should be in the armamentarium of the plastic surgeon who performs body contouring surgery. The choice of procedure is based on the patient's desires and presenting deformities. Both procedures eliminate a circumferential wedge of tissue from the lower trunk. **A belt lipectomy removes a wedge that is more superiorly located than that removed in a lower body lift in its lateral and posterior extents (Fig. 53.8).**

The final scar after belt lipectomy is located above the widest aspect of the bony pelvic rim, at the junction between the lower back and buttocks, which maybe visible outside of brief undergarments. Because this allows cinching at waist level, more waist definition can be created by this technique. This is often desired in women but may be less desirable in men. Pelvic rim zones of adherence help to prevent the descent of lower truncal tissues as well as inhibit elevation of lower extremity tissues, (see Fig. 53.4). These fascial attachments are interrupted but not completely eliminated during a belt lipectomy, and they prevent extensive lifting of lower thigh tissues. Thus, overall, a belt lipectomy is capable of creating excellent lower truncal contour by accentuating waist definition, delineating the buttocks from the lower back, and lifting the lateral thighs, but it has limited capability in lifting the distal thighs.

A lower body lift treats the lower trunk and thighs as a unit. The pelvic rim zones of adherence are intentionally interrupted as completely as possible, which allows inferior thigh tissues down to knee level to be lifted, a fact that leads to a significant reduction in anterior and lateral thigh laxity. The final scar is located on the buttocks proper, which can blunt waist definition (see Fig. 53.8). This is often desirable in men but may be less so in women. The resultant scar is easily covered by normal undergarments, and the thighs are dramatically improved down to knee level. However, a lower body lift is less efficient in creating waist narrowing and can result in less than ideal buttocks definition because the scar does not respect the natural junction between the lower back and buttocks.

The majority of patients undergoing a circumferential lipectomy are massive-weight-loss patients. Often they present with a hanging panniculus, mons pubis ptosis, an ill-defined waist, lower back rolls, hip-fat excess, lateral thigh ptosis, and varying types of buttocks deformity. The goals of surgery include elimination of the hanging panniculus, mons pubis elevation, creation of waist definition (especially in women), decrease or elimination of lower back rolls, lifting of the outer thighs, and increase in buttocks definition.

Techniques

Although a circumferential lipectomy is a combination of an abdominoplasty, a lateral thigh lift, and a buttocks lift, the procedure is more complex than simply combining them. The lower trunk of patients who present with circumferential excess has the shape of an inverted cone (Fig. 53.9). A wedge of tissue is marked for proposed excision around the lower trunk. The wedge brings a narrower part of the cone down to the level of a wider part of the cone located at, or near, the pelvic rim (see Fig. 53.9). As previously noted, the wedge to be excised is generally located in a more superior position in belt lipectomy when compared to the wedge to be excised in a lower body lift. In either method, the anterior aspect of the wedge is wider (in vertical distance) than the lateral or posterior aspects. The lateral resection is the next widest aspect so as to reverse the lateral truncal descent (Fig. 53.10).

Because of the circumferential nature of the procedure, more than one position is necessary to accomplish the resection in the operating room. No matter what sequence is preferred by a particular surgeon, the abdominal part of the procedure is performed in the supine position. Surgeons who advocate prone/supine or supine/prone positioning cite the single turn

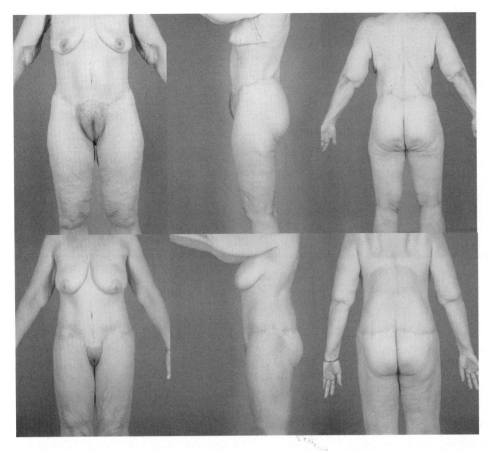

FIGURE 53.8. Belt lipectomy and lower body lift. Two patients who underwent a belt lipectomy *above* and a lower body lift *below*. In a belt lipectomy the scar is placed at the junction between the buttocks and lower back, which helps to frame the natural buttocks contour and accentuate waist narrowing. In a lower body lift the scar is onto the buttocks proper and is overall more inferiorly placed, especially in its lateral and posterior aspects. The combination of eliminating the pelvic zones of adherence and the lower position of the excised wedge allows the lower body lift to elevate the thighs more effectively than in a belt lipectomy.

required in the operating room and the ability to control buttock symmetry as their reasons for choosing the "two-position" sequences. The supine/lateral/lateral or lateral/lateral/supine proponents prefer these "three-position" sequences because they allow for easier lateral thigh liposuction and hip flexion in the lateral decubitus position, which facilitates maximal lateral resections.

The extent of anterior flap elevation in the abdominoplasty portion of the circumferential procedure is based on surgeon preference. The lateral elevation is usually more extensive than

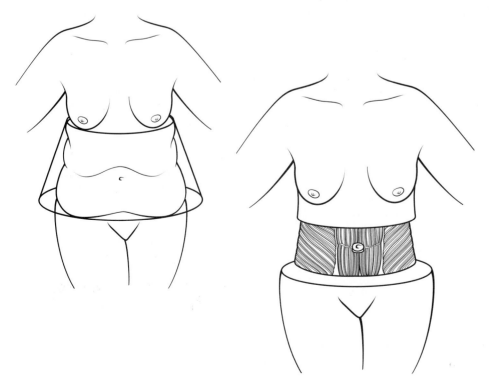

FIGURE 53.9. Truncal deformity in weight loss patients. In the massive-weight-loss patient the presenting lower truncal deformity is in the shape of an inverted cone. In a circumferential lipectomy a wedge of tissue is removed. The diameter of the wedge at its superior edge is smaller than its diameter at the inferior edge.

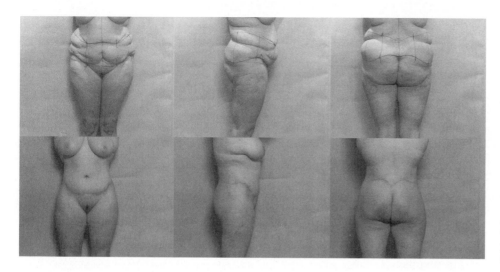

FIGURE 53.10. A 31-year-old woman presented after an 80-pound weight loss to reach a body mass index of 27.31. (*Above*) Shown with preoperative markings for a circumferential belt lipectomy. Note the excision laterally is generally aggressive to counteract the lateral descent that occurs with massive weight loss and/or aging. Vertical marks are placed along the circumference of the proposed resection to help alignment at closure. Surrounding areas of the thigh are also marked for liposuction. (*Below*) The patient 6 months after surgery, demonstrating dramatic waist narrowing, elimination of the panniculus and lower back rolls, and improved buttocks definition.

in an abdominoplasty, which compromises the remaining blood supply to the abdominal flap to a greater extent. Thus it is important that an effort is made to preserve as many lateral feeding vessels as possible. The plication of the rectus fascia is similar to abdominoplasty plication except that it may sometimes require plication distances that far exceed the usual 5 to 7 cm encountered with routine abdominoplasty. Closure of the circumferential wound should include reapproximation of the superficial fascial system with permanent and/or long-lasting suture.

During the lateral and posterior resection aspect of the procedure, some surgeons prefer to incise the superior marks first and dissect an inferior skin–fat flap, which is tailored based on tension, whereas others prefer the opposite. Some surgeons incise both the superior and inferior extents and excise a predetermined marked amount. I prefer to incise on one side and tailor based on tension.

Some surgeons choose to combine extensive liposuction of the surrounding regions, such as the lower back, the upper back, and thighs, whereas others limit their liposuction to the lateral thighs. A major difference between belt lipectomy and a lower body lift is in the treatment of the pelvic rim zones of adherence. In belt lipectomy these attachments are disrupted by liposuction of the lateral thighs, but they are not completely eliminated. In a lower body lift the pelvic rim zones of adherence are intentionally destroyed by discontinuous undermining of the anterior and lateral thighs down to the knee, which allows significant thigh elevation (10).

The results attained from circumferential lipectomies depend to a great extent on the presentation of the patient and the type of procedure chosen (see Fig. 53.10). As a general rule, the lower the BMI of the patient at presentation, the better are the results that can be expected (8,9).

COMPLICATIONS

Table 53.2 lists complications that can occur with lower truncal contouring procedures (12). Circumferential procedures are associated with more complications, but they are often performed on patients with higher BMI. **When complications are stratified by BMI, noncircumferential and circumferential procedures have similar rates.**

Seromas are the most common complications with lower truncal contouring procedures. They are due to large dissection surface areas and can develop anywhere in the surgical field but tend to be located posteriorly in circumferential procedures. Patients who present in the high BMI ranges

are more likely to develop seromas. Measures that are used to reduce their occurrence include the use of suction drains and compression garments, reduction of activity, and use of deep quilting sutures. When they do occur they can most often be treated with serial aspirations. For persistent seromas, sclerosing agents and seroma catheter insertions may be utilized. Occasionally a pseudo-bursa can result from the prolonged presence of a seroma, which may have to be excised surgically.

Seromas are the most common source of infection after lower truncal procedures. Simple cellulitis is fairly uncommon and is usually treated by appropriate antibiotic coverage and close follow-up. Seroma pockets that become infected usually present with overlying cellulitis, fluid collections that may or may not spontaneously drain, fever, and generalized malaise. A diligent effort should be made to find seromas and treat them whenever suspected. Once seromas become infected, aggressive intravenous therapy and appropriate surgical drainage should be instituted.

Toxic shock syndrome can occur with any body contouring procedure. Postoperatively, patients who appear toxic with fever, chills, generalized malaise, and elevated white blood cell counts should be investigated. Although there is often no evidence of frank pus or large fluid collection in the wounds, aggressive surgical drainage is urgently required in this group of patients.

Wound healing problems can occur with any body contouring excisional procedure because of the high tension created at the wound edges. Most often conservative wound care will allow healing with the possible need for subsequent scar revisions. Wound dehiscences, defined as separation of the wound

TABLE 53.2
COMPLICATIONS ASSOCIATED WITH LOWER TRUNCAL BODY CONTOURING PROCEDURES
Seroma
Wound-healing problems/dehiscence
Infections
Tissue necrosis
Bleeding/hematoma
Thrombotic events (deep venous thrombosis pulmonary emboli)
Psychiatric difficulties
Scar and contour asymmetry

at the level of the superficial fascial system, are possible with any of the procedures discussed in this chapter but tend to occur more frequently with circumferential procedures. In procedures limited to anterior resections, mini-abdominoplasty, and abdominoplasty, dehiscences can be prevented by keeping patients flexed at the waist for 5 to 7 days after surgery and educating patients on a slow return to the full upright position over the second week after surgery. Circumferential procedures create competing anterior and posterior tensions, making it difficult to place patients in positions that do not stress at least one aspect of the closure. Avoidance of dehiscences in this patient population entails adjustments of the competing resections to account for opposing tensions, careful ambulation of the patients in the early postoperative period, and education of patients on how to help prevent dehiscences (13).

Vascular compromise can occur with lower truncal body contouring procedures, leading to tissue necrosis. Most commonly the necrosis occurs in the inferomedial aspect of the abdominal flap. A number of factors can contribute to this problem, which include excessive tension on the abdominal closure, aggressive thinning of the abdominal flap, overly aggressive liposuction, and anything that may lead to compromising the lateral feeding vessels of the abdominal flap such as open cholycystectomy incisions. Tissues that appear compromised in the early postoperative period may be treated with nitropaste topical application. Once necrosis occurs the wound is treated conservatively and eventually allowed to heal by secondary intention. Eventually scar revision may need to be performed.

Bleeding after lower truncal contouring procedures can be extensive because of the surface area within which blood can accumulate prior to detection. Although drains do not prevent hematomas, they can often warn the surgeon of a developing hematoma. Small hematomas that are well evacuated by drains in place can be managed expectantly. Large hematomas should be treated by surgical drainage.

Procedures that tighten the abdominal wall can result in an increase of intra-abdominal pressures, leading to a decrease in venous return from the lower extremities. The possible resultant stasis of blood in the deep venous system may cause deep venous thrombosis and/or pulmonary emboli. Measures that are commonly used in the prevention of thrombotic events include early ambulation and sequential compression garments. Some surgeons use subcutaneous low-dose heparin in the perioperative period.

Patients who undergo large excisional procedures of the lower trunk, especially massive-weight-loss patients, can have psychiatric difficulties in the postoperative period that may interfere with their recovery. Although this can occur with any surgery, the long recovery period that is required after circumferential procedures makes it wise for the plastic surgeon to actively investigate a patient's psychiatric reserves and consider obtaining psychiatric clearance prior to surgery. The tendency of massive-weight-loss patients to have life-long psychiatric problems that are not solved by weight loss alone also contributes to the relatively high incidence of these problems.

Although careful marking techniques can help to reduce scar and contour asymmetry, it is not possible to eliminate these problems in many patients because of intrinsic skeletal and soft tissue unevenness. It is best for the surgeon to recognize these natural asymmetries and point them out to patients prior to surgery.

FLEUR-DE-LIS OR T-TYPE PROCEDURES

A fleur-de-lis or T-shaped excision, whether used as an abdominoplasty pattern or in combination with a circumferential lipectomy, is advocated by some authors. The advantage of the vertical wedge is to eliminate horizontal excess, create more waist definition, and decrease lateral fullness. Traditionally this pattern has not been frequently used because it is difficult to justify a vertical midline incision without a pre-existing scar in that position. Recently, however, it has found more use because many bariatric surgeons use open vertical midline incisions. Even with a pre-existing scar, however, there are major disadvantages to the vertical aspect of the T pattern. There is an increased chance of flap necrosis at the T intersection. Waist definition is frequently not increased with this procedure. When used to treat circumferential excess, a fleur-de-lis resection pattern does not eliminate lateral excess or posterior lower truncal deformities. When the pattern is used in conjunction with a circumferential lipectomy it can create a greater mismatch between the upper and lower circumferences of the inverted cone-shaped edges to be reapproximated (see Fig. 53.9). Finally, the vertical wedge excised will often lead to epigastric fullness secondary to the dog-ear effect created by the excision. Due to these disadvantages, I do not recommend this pattern of excision (12).

References

1. Aly AS. Approach to the massive weight loss patient. In: Aly AS, ed. *Body Contouring After Massive Weight Loss*. St. Louis: Quality Medical Publishing; 2006: 49.
2. La Trenta GS. Suction-assisted lipectomy. In: Rees TD, LaTrenta 65, eds. *Aesthetic Plastic Surgery*, 2nd ed. Philadelphia: WB Saunders: 1994: 1180.
3. Aly AS. Options in lower truncal surgery. In: Aly AS, ed. *Body Contouring After Massive Weight Loss*. St. Louis: Quality Medical Publishing; 2006: 59.
4. Lockwood T. Superficial fascial system (SFS) of the trunk and extremities: a new concept. *Plast Reconstr Surg*. 1991;87:1009.
5. La Trenta GS. Abdominoplasty. In Rees TD, La Trenta GS eds. *Aesthetic Plastic Surgery*, 2nd ed. Philadelphia: WB Saunders; 1994: 126.
6. Lockwood T. High-lateral-tension abdominoplasty with superficial fascial system suspension. *Plast Reconstr Surg*. 1995;96:603.
7. Matarasso A. Abdominoplasty: a system of classification and treatment for combined abdominoplasty and suction-assisted lipectomy. *Aesthetic Plast Surg*. 1991;15:111.
8. Aly AS, Cram AF. Body lift: belt lipectomy. In: Nahai F, ed. *The Art of Aesthetic Surgery. Principles and Techniques*. St. Louis: Quality Medical Publishing; 2005: 2302.
9. Aly A, Cram A, Chao M, et al. Belt lipectomy for circumferential truncal excess: the University of Iowa experience. *Plast Reconstr Surg*. 2003;111: 398.
10. Lockwood TE. Thigh and buttock lift. In: Nahai F, ed. *The Art of Aesthetic Surgery. Principles and Techniques*. St. Louis: Quality Medical Publishing; 2005: 2424.
11. Lockwood T. Lower body lift. *Oper Tech Plast Reconstr Surg*. 1996;3: 132.
12. Grazer FM, Goldwyn RM. Abdominplasty assessed by survery, with emphasis on complication. *Plast Reconstr Surg*. 1977;59:513.
13. Aly AS. Belt lipectomy. In: Aly AS, ed. *Body Contouring After Massive Weight Loss*. St. Louis: Quality Medical Publishing; 2006: 7.

CHAPTER 54 ■ FACIAL SKELETAL AUGMENTATION WITH IMPLANTS

MICHAEL J. YAREMCHUK

The morphology of the facial skeleton is a fundamental determinant of facial appearance. Facial skeletal augmentation is usually done with alloplastic materials. Implants can be used to restore symmetry during reconstruction of posttraumatic or postablative deformities. Most often, facial skeletal augmentation is done electively to improve facial aesthetics (Fig. 54.1).

PREOPERATIVE PLANNING

Physical examination is the most important element in preoperative assessment and planning. Reviewing life-size posteroanterior (PA) and lateral photographs with the patient is useful when discussing aesthetic concerns and goals.

Although cephalometric radiograph analysis can be helpful in the planning, the size and position of the implant are largely aesthetic judgments. Although often referenced in texts discussing facial skeletal augmentation, neoclassical canons describing ideal proportions of the head and face have a limited role in surgical evaluation and planning because they are arbitrarily determined. When the dimensions of normal males and females were evaluated objectively and compared to artistic ideals, it was found that some theoretic proportions are never found, and others are one of the many variations found in healthy normals, or those determined more attractive than normals (1,2). For these reasons, we have found it more useful to use the anthropometric measurements of normals to guide our *gestalt* for the selection of implants for facial skeletal augmentation.

In planning facial skeletal augmentation it is important to realize that small increases in skeletal projection can have a powerful impact on facial appearance. It should be emphasized to the patient during the preoperative consultation that all faces are asymmetric. If unrecognized preoperatively, an asymmetric postoperative result usually will be attributed solely to the surgeon.

IMPLANTS

Materials

Virtually all aesthetic facial skeletal augmentation is done with alloplastic implants. The use of synthetic materials avoids donor-site morbidity and vastly simplifies the procedure in terms of time and complexity. Implant materials used for facial skeletal augmentation are biocompatible; that is, they have an acceptable reaction between the material and the host. In general, the host has little or no enzymatic ability to degrade the implant with the result that the implant tends to maintain its volume and shape. Likewise, the implant has a minimal and predictable effect on the host tissue that surrounds it. This type of relationship is an advantage over the use of autogenous bone or cartilage, which, when revascularized, will be remodeled to varying degrees, thereby changing volume and shape (3).

The presently used alloplastic implants used for facial reconstruction do not have a toxic effect on the host (4). The host responds to these materials by forming a fibrous capsule around the implant, which is the body's way of isolating the implant from the host. The most important implant characteristics, those that determine the nature of the encapsulation, are the implant's surface characteristics. Smooth implants result in the formation of smooth-walled capsules. Porous implants allow varying degrees of soft-tissue ingrowth, which results in a less-dense and less-defined capsule. Porous implants, the result of fibrous incorporation rather than encapsulation, have less tendency to erode underlying bone, to migrate because of soft-tissue mechanical forces, and, perhaps, to be less susceptible to infection when challenged with an inoculum of bacteria. The most commonly used and commercially available materials today for facial skeletal augmentation are solid silicone, polytetrafluoroethylene, and porous polyethylene.

Solid silicone or the silicone rubber used for facial implants is a vulcanized form of polysiloxane, which is a polymer created from interlocking silicone and oxygen with methyl side groups. Silicone is derived from silicon, a semimetallic element that in nature combines with oxygen to form silicon dioxide, or silicone. Beach sand, crystals, and quartz are silica.

The advantages of solid silicone are that it is easily sterilizable by steam or irradiation, it can be carved easily with either a scissor or scalpel, and it can be stabilized with a screw or a suture. There are no known clinical or allergic reactions. Because it is smooth, it can be removed quite easily. The disadvantages of silicone implants include their tendency to cause resorption of the bone underlying it, particularly when used to augment the chin, the potential to migrate if not fixed, and the potential for its fibrous capsule to be visible when placed under a thin soft-tissue cover.

Polytetrafluoroethylene

Gore-Tex (W.L. Gore, Flagstaff, AZ) has a carbon-ethylene backbone to which are attached four fluorine molecules. It is very chemically stable, has a nonadherent surface, and, because it is not cross-linked, it is very flexible. There is extensive experience with the use of Gore-Tex for vascular prostheses, soft-tissue patches, and sutures. A variety of preformed implants are available for both subdermal and subperiosteal placement. Preformed implants are made with a pore size between 10 and 30 μm. The porosity allows for some soft-tissue ingrowth, for less fibrous encapsulation, and for less tendency to migrate as compared with smooth-surfaced implants. It is easily sterilizable, smooth enough to be maneuvered easily through soft tissues, and can be fixed to underlying structures with sutures or screws.

551

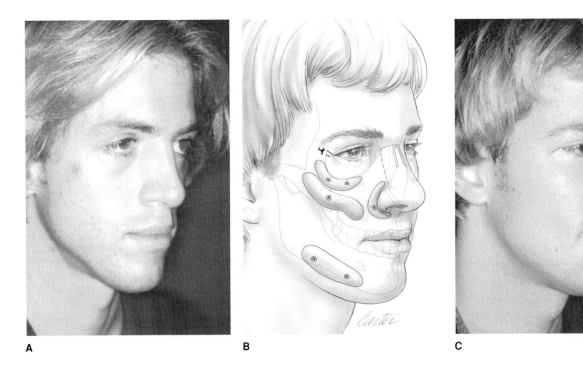

A   **B**   **C**

FIGURE 54.1. A 26-year-old male who in two operations had multiple implants placed. Implant augmentation of the infraorbital rim, paranasal, malar, and mandibular body was performed. In addition, rhinoplasty, midface lift, and lateral canthopexy were also performed. **A:** Preoperative; (**B**) diagrammatic representation of operation; (**C**) postoperative. (From Yaremchuk MJ. Facial skeletal reconstruction using porous polyethylene implants. *Plast Reconstr Surg.* 2003;111:1818, with permission.)

Polyethylene

Polyethylene is a simplex carbon chain of ethylene monomer. The high density variety—Medpor (Porex, Newnan, GA)—is used for facial implants because of its high tensile strength. Although chemically similar to polytetrafluoroethylene, polyethylene has a much firmer consistency that resists material compression yet permits some flexibility. Medpor has an intramaterial porosity between 125 and 250 μm, which allows more extensive fibrous ingrowth than Gore-Tex. Soft-tissue ingrowth lessens the implant's tendency to migrate and to erode underlying bone. Its firm consistency allows it to be easily fixed with screws and to be contoured with a scalpel or power equipment without fragmenting. A disadvantage of Medpor's greater porosity is that it allows soft tissues to adhere to it, making placement more difficult and requiring a larger pocket than is required for smoother implants for its placement. Soft-tissue ingrowth into the larger pores also makes implant removal more difficult than removal of smooth-surfaced implants.

Requisites of Implant Shape, Positioning, and Immobilization

Shape

The external shape of the implant should mimic the shape of the bone it is augmenting. Its posterior surface should mold to the bone to which it is applied. Gaps between the bone and implant result in a relative increase in augmentation and a potential site for seroma and hematoma formation. The implant margins must taper imperceptibly into the bone they are augmenting so that they are neither visible nor palpable.

Positioning

Although some surgeons prefer to place implants in a soft-tissue pocket, clinical experience has led me to adopt a policy of strict subperiosteal placement. Placement in a subperiosteal pocket involves a dissection that is safe to peripheral nerves and relatively bloodless. It allows visualization and more precise augmentation of the skeletal contour desired for augmentation.

The size of the pockets is determined by the type of implant used and its method of immobilization. The longstanding teaching when using smooth silicone implants is to make a pocket just large enough to accommodate the implant so as to guarantee its position. Porous implants require a larger pocket because they adhere to the soft tissue during their placement. When using smooth or porous implants, I dissect widely enough to have a perspective of the skeletal anatomy being augmented, which allows more precise and symmetric implant positioning.

Immobilization

Many surgeons stabilize the position of the implant by suturing it to surrounding soft tissues or by using temporary transcutaneous pullout sutures. Screw fixation of the implant to the skeleton has several benefits. It prevents any movement of the implant and assures application of the implant to the surface of the bone. Because each facial skeleton has a unique and varying surface topography, a nonconforming implant will leave gaps between the implants and the skeleton. Screw fixation also allows for final contouring of the implant in position. This final contouring is particularly important where the implant interfaces with the skeleton (Fig. 54.2). Any step-off between the implant and the skeleton will be palpable and possibly visible in thin-skinned patients.

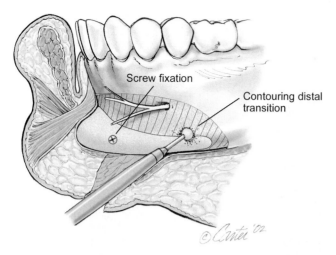

FIGURE 54.2. Representation of a preferred technique for chin augmentation. Through a submental approach a two-piece porous polyethylene implant is fixed to the skeleton with titanium screws. This maneuver immobilizes the implant and obliterates any gaps between the implant and the underlying bone. The implant is being contoured to provide an imperceptible implant-native mandible transition. (From Yaremchuk MJ. Improving aesthetic outcomes after alloplastic chin augmentation. *Plast Reconstr Surg.* 2003;112:1422, with permission.)

ANESTHESIA

Facial skeletal augmentation can be performed under local or general anesthesia. It is routinely done on an outpatient basis. I prefer to perform most facial skeletal surgery under general nasotracheal anesthesia because most facial implants are placed either in the malar midface or along the mandible, usually through a combination of intraoral incisions. Nasotracheal intubation assures protection of the airway and the best possible antiseptic preparation of the oral cavity. Patient positioning and exposure for implant placement are also optimized with nasotracheal control of the airway. The surgical site is infiltrated with a solution containing Marcaine for postoperative pain control and epinephrine to minimize bleeding.

AREAS FOR AUGMENTATION

The mid and lower face are the areas most often altered with implants (Fig. 54.3).

Midface Augmentation

Implants are specifically designed to augment the malar, paranasal, and infraorbital rim areas.

Malar

Patients who seek malar augmentation may have midface hypoplasia or normal anatomy and usually seek greater prominence of their middle malar prominence (5).

Malar augmentation can be performed through intraoral, coronal, or eyelid incisions. I prefer to access the malar midface through an intraoral approach. An upper buccal sulcus incision is made far enough from the apex of the sulcus so that sufficient labial tissue is available on either side for a secure two-layer closure. Division of the lip elevators is avoided. Taking care

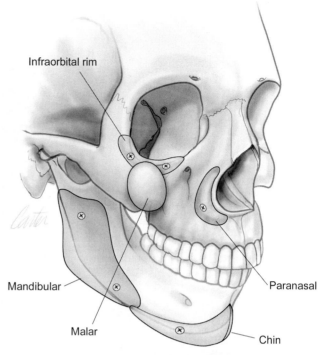

FIGURE 54.3. Representation of commonly used implants designed to augment various areas of facial skeleton. In the midface, these include the malar, paranasal, and infraorbital rim implants. In the lower face, the chin, as well as the mandibular body, ramus, and angle, may be augmented with alloplastic implants.

to identify the infraorbital nerve, subperiosteal dissection is carried over the malar eminence and onto the zygomatic arch, almost up to the zygomaticotemporal suture. The pocket size should enable precise insertion of the implant to the area of the skeleton desired for augmentation.

Surgeons who use smooth silicone implants often assure the position of the implant by using suture suspension fixation. The position of both smooth and porous implants at the time of the placement can be guaranteed with screw fixation of the implant to the skeleton. Patients who are dissatisfied with malar implant surgery frequently complain that the implants are too large, are placed asymmetrically, or are placed too far laterally, increasing midface width.

Paranasal

A relative deficiency in lower midface projection may be congenital or may be acquired, particularly after cleft surgery and trauma. Patients with satisfactory occlusion and midface concavity can have their aesthetic desires satisfied with skeletal augmentation. Implantation of alloplastic material in the paranasal area can simulate the visual effect of LeFort I advancement (Fig. 54.4) (6).

Paranasal augmentation is done through an upper gingival buccal sulcus incision made just lateral to the piriform aperture to avoid placing incisions directly over the implant. An adequate cuff of mucosa is left to allow layered closure.

Infraorbital Rim

Augmentation of this area is useful for patients with severe deficiencies of the midface and infraorbital rim area that result in excessively prominent eyes. Infraorbital rim

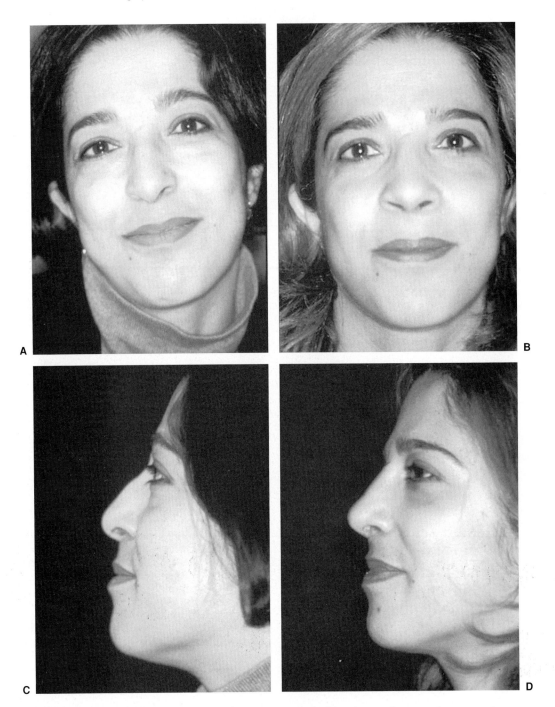

FIGURE 54.4. A 26-year-old woman underwent an aesthetic rhinoplasty and paranasal augmentation. A,C: Preoperative. B,D: Postoperative.

augmentation can effectively reverse the "negative" vector of midface hypoplasia (7).

The infraorbital rim and adjacent anatomy can be exposed sufficiently to assure ideal implant placement, smooth implant facial skeleton transition, and screw fixation. Subciliary skin or skin muscle flap incisions can provide this exposure. A transconjunctival incision alone is inadequate for implant placement or screw stabilization. Use of a transconjunctival retroseptal incision requires its lengthening with a lateral canthotomy or its combining with intraoral or coronal incisions.

Mandibular Augmentation

Each of the anatomic areas of the mandible—the mentum, body, angle, and ramus—can be deficient and is amenable to augmentation with alloplastic materials.

Chin

There is a consensus among surgeons that the ideal profile relation portrays a convex face with the upper lip projecting approximately 2 mm beyond the lower lip and the lower lip projecting approximately 2 mm beyond the chin (8). The projection of the chin should be interpreted in the context of the surrounding facial features, including the projection of the nose, the relationship to the lips, and the depth of the labiomental sulcus.

Implant Design

Early implant designs augmented the mentum only and often created a stuck-on appearance as a result of failure of the lateral aspect of the implant to merge with the anterior aspect of the mandibular body. "Extended" chin implants have tapered lateral extensions that enable the chin implant to better merge with more lateral mandibular contours. Myriad designs are available that give great latitude in the desired effect. Flowers (9) and Terino (10) developed extended chin implants that augmented both the central mentum and the mandibular body. This type of implant widened the anterior jaw line, in addition to increasing the projection of the chin. I prefer a two-piece chin implant (11). A two-piece implant allows the inferior border of the implant to follow the inferior border of the mandible. This is usually not possible with a one-piece chin implant.

Submental Incision

It is my opinion that ideal results from alloplastic augmentation of the chin are not routinely obtained. Problems result from implants that merge poorly with the mandibular body; implants with posterior surfaces that are inappropriate for the tilt of the anterior surface of the chin; asymmetric implant placement; implant migration; and morbidity from surgical exposure. To avoid these problems, I choose to position two-piece extended implants through submental incisions to assure ideal implant placement and to minimize soft-tissue morbidity. The incision is carried onto the mentum and a subperiosteal pocket is created that avoids disturbing the mentalis muscle origin above and allows easy identification of the inferior alveolar nerves (Fig. 54.2).

Intraoral Incision

In patients where a submental scar may be objectionable, an intraoral incision is employed. An approximately 2 cm transverse incision is made 1 cm above the buccal sulcus in the midline. When the mentalis muscles are encountered, these muscles are neither divided nor stripped from the mandible, but are separated in the midline to access the mentum where a subperiosteal pocket is created.

Placement of an extended chin implant through a midline intraoral approach alone is difficult. This intraoral exposure may result in division or damage to the mentalis muscles, damage to the mental nerve, and improper positioning of the lateral tails of the implants. To assure implant placement particularly of the lateral extensions, sulcus incisions 1.5 to 2 cm long are made lateral to the mental nerve. The mental foramen usually lies halfway between the top and the bottom of the mandible and directly between the space between the two premolars.

Once the implant is positioned, it is immobilized with sutures or screws.

Implant Augmentation versus Sliding Genioplasty

Sliding genioplasty involves a horizontal osteotomy of the mandible approximately 4 mm beneath the mental foramen. A now free chin point that can be moved in any direction is positioned as desired, usually anteriorly to increase chin projection. It has two advantages over implant augmentation of the

chin. First, the chin point can be lowered after osteotomy to increase the vertical height of the chin. Vertical elongation may efface the deep labiomental sulcus affecting some patients. Second, the chin point advancement stretches the attached suprahyoid muscles, thereby decreasing submental fullness and improving submental contour.

The major disadvantage intrinsic to sliding genioplasty is the unnatural bony and border contours that accompany the selective movement of the chin point. The contour result is one that has a poor transition, resulting in the stuck-on appearance of the chin—much like a large button chin implant. There are also step-offs at the osteotomy sites along the mandibular body. The notchings or indentations are particularly detrimental to those who have an existing prejowl sulcus. Furthermore, sliding genioplasty requires considerable facility in bone carpentry. Obliquity in a horizontal osteotomy can either lengthen or shorten the vertical height of the chin after advancement.

Ramus and Body

Alloplastic augmentation of the mandibular ramus and body can have a dramatic impact on the appearance of the lower third of the face (12). Two patient populations have had their aesthetic concerns satisfied with mandibular augmentation procedures. One group has mandibular dimensions that relate to the upper and middle thirds of the face within the normal range. These patients perceive a wider lower face with a well-defined mandibular border as an enhancement to their appearance. Patients in this treatment group often present with a desire to emulate the appearance of models, actors, and actresses who have a defined, angular lower face. This patient group benefits from implants designed to augment the ramus and posterior body of the mandible, and, in so doing, increase the bigonial distance. The other major group of patients who benefit from augmentation of the mandibular ramus and body are those patients with skeletal mandibular deficiency. Those patients who have their malocclusion treated with orthodontics alone are left with mandibular skeletal deficiencies that may be deforming. The skeletal anatomy associated with mandibular deficiency that can be camouflaged with implants include the obtuse mandibular angle with steep mandibular plane and decreased vertical and transverse ramus dimensions. The addition of an extended chin implant will camouflage the poorly projecting chin.

Operative Technique

A generous intraoral mucosal incision is made to expose the ramus and body of the mandible. It is made at least 1 cm above the sulcus on its labial side. The anterior ramus and body of the mandible are freed from their soft tissues. The inferior alveolar nerve is visualized as it exits its foramen to avoid its injury. It is important to free both the inferior and posterior borders of the mandible of soft tissue attachments to allow implant placement. As determined by preoperative assessment, the implant is trimmed with a scalpel prior to its placement on the mandible. To assure the desired placement of the implant and its application to the surface of the mandible, the implant is fixed to the mandible with titanium screws. The incision is closed in two layers with absorbable sutures. Care is taken to evert the mucosal edges.

Implants Used to Camouflage Soft-Tissue Depressions

The implants discussed in this chapter are designed to increase the surface projection of the facial skeleton. Certain authors have used implants placed on the facial skeleton to disguise overlying soft-tissue volume inadequacy, usually caused by involutional changes brought on by age. These include the submalar, prejowl, and tear trough implants. Augmentation of the skeleton to compensate for a soft-tissue deficiency should be extremely conservative. Skeletal augmentation does not give the same visual effect as the soft-tissue augmentation. Similarly, soft-tissue augmentation beyond 1 or 2 mm provides a different visual effect than skeletal enlargement. For example, a chin point augmented with fat to increase projection by 5 mm reads as a fatty chin pad, not as a more projecting chin.

COMPLICATIONS

There is no scientific data to document the complication rate related to facial skeletal augmentation. Prospective studies that control for surgical technique, implant site, patient selection, and follow-up time do not exist. Because all the biomaterials commonly used for facial skeletal augmentation are biocompatible, complications are usually technique related—improper implant size, contour, or placement. Infections are unusual when implants are placed through cutaneous incisions. When infection occurs, the most reliable treatment is implant removal.

CONCLUSION

Augmentation of the facial skeleton with alloplastic materials is a powerful way to alter facial appearance. Virtually any area of the facial skeleton can be augmented. Requisites for success include implants of appropriate size and shape, adequate soft-tissue cover, and careful subperiosteal dissection during exposure and implant placement.

References

1. Farkas L, Hreczko TA, Kolar JC, et al. Vertical and horizontal proportions of the face in young adult North American Caucasians: revision of neoclassical canons. *Plast Reconstr Surg.* 1985;75:328.
2. Farkas LG, Kolar JC. Anthropometrics and art in the aesthetics of women's faces. *Clin Plast Surg.* 1987;14:599.
3. Chen NT, Glowacki J, Bucky LP, et al. The role of revascularization and resorption on endurance of craniofacial onlay bone grafts in the rabbit. *Plast Reconstr Surg.* 1994;93:714.
4. Rubin JP, Yaremchuk MJ. Complications and toxicities of implantable biomaterials used in facial reconstructive and aesthetic surgery: a comprehensive review of the literature. *Plast Reconstr Surg.* 1997;100:1346.
5. Whitaker LA. Aesthetic augmentation of the malar midface structures. *Plast Reconstr Surg.* 1987;80:337.
6. Yaremchuk MJ, Israeli D. Paranasal implants for correction of midface concavity. *Plast Reconstr Surg.* 1998;102:51.
7. Yaremchuk MJ. Infraorbital rim augmentation. *Plast Reconstr Surg.* 2001;107:1585.
8. McCarthy JG, Ruff JG. The chin. *Clin Plast Surg.* 1988;15:125.
9. Flowers RS. Alloplastic augmentation of the anterior mandible. *Clin Plast Surg.* 1991;18:137.
10. Terino EO. Facial contouring with alloplastic implants. *Facial Plast Surg Clin North Am.* 1999;7:55.
11. Yaremchuk MJ. Improving aesthetic outcomes after alloplastic chin augmentation. *Plast Reconstr Surg.* 2003;112:1422.
12. Yaremchuk MJ. Mandibular augmentation. *Plast Reconstr Surg.* 2000;106:697.

CHAPTER 55 ■ OSSEOUS GENIOPLASTY

HARVEY M. ROSEN

Osseous genioplasty is an autogenous method for changing the size, or shape, or both of the mandibular symphysis. Although by strict definition it may involve merely recontouring the chin by burring away bone or by adding bone graft material, the term generally refers to an osteotomy of the anterior mandible in the horizontal (transverse) direction below the mental foramina (Fig. 55.1A). The osteotomy was first described in 1942 by Hofer (1). The procedure remained rather obscure until 1964 when it was popularized by Converse and Wood-Smith (2). It is now the second most commonly performed osteotomy of the facial skeleton for both reconstructive and aesthetic reasons (second only to rhinoplasty).

Osseous genioplasty is frequently performed for two reasons: (a) versatility; chin can be moved in any direction— sagittally, vertically, or transversely (Fig. 55.1B-D); and (b) a receding chin or small mandible, or both, are common problems among white North Americans, occurring in approximately 5% of the population (2). When these factors are coupled with the emphasis that Western culture places on aesthetics and the belief that a well-defined jaw line characterizes an aggressive, self-confident individual, it is little wonder that this operation has grown in popularity. The ready availability of alloplastic material such as silastic, however, has prevented osseous genioplasty from becoming an operation that large numbers of plastic surgeons currently employ.

ALLOPLASTIC VERSUS AUTOGENOUS

The choice between alloplastic augmentation (chin implants) and osseous genioplasty for correction of the weak chin remains hotly debated among plastic surgeons. The proponents of alloplastic augmentation cite the technical ease, the relatively low risk of complications, and the ability to perform the procedure under a local anesthetic. Those who favor osseous genioplasty point out the extreme versatility of an osteotomy in correcting three-dimensional deformity.

In an effort to select the correct procedure, one should simply ask which procedure will provide the best correction for the particular patient. **Certain factors are indisputable:** (1) Chin implants can adequately correct mild to moderate volume deficiencies of the mandible at the level of the pogonion in the sagittal dimension (2). Chin implants cannot correct vertical excess of the anterior mandible (3). Chin implants are unreliable in correcting asymmetries of the anterior mandible in any plane of space (4). Although chin implants can modestly increase the vertical dimension of the anterior mandible by covering its inferior border, this has significant potential for complications as the soft tissue in this area is relatively thin (5). Provided that chin implants are positioned directly over the symphysis, as they should be, and not over the dental alveolus, the labiomental fold will increase in depth following chin implant placement.

Given these factors, the only appropriate candidates for chin implantation are those with a mild to moderate sagittal deficiency of the chin accompanied by a shallow labiomental fold. All other patients who request surgical alteration of the chin should be considered for osseous genioplasty.

One of the least mentioned, yet compelling, reasons to choose osseous genioplasty instead of alloplastic chin augmentation occurs when surgical revision is indicated. Osseous genioplasty is more amenable to revision because the soft-tissue chin has not been degloved and there is no scar capsule (as occurs in smooth implants) with which to contend. As a result, soft-tissue displacement closely follows skeletal displacement. Conversely, the soft-tissue response to removing a smooth implant, or to reducing its size, or to changing its position is unpredictable because the soft tissues have been degloved from the bone. In addition, the dead space created by the implant capsule, which does not fully collapse, fills with blood, creating more scar. Surgical excision of the capsule may cause mentalis muscle disfunction with subsequent lower lip ptosis. Accordingly, the aesthetic consequences of removing or changing smooth chin implants are frequently undesirable.

Although a scar capsule may not form with porous implants, these implants can be very difficult to remove because of the soft-tissue ingrowth.

TREATMENT-PLANNING CONSIDERATIONS

Preoperative evaluation of the osseous genioplasty patient includes a history and physical examination. The surgeon should ascertain the patient's specific aesthetic complaints and objectives as they relate to the lower face, including any concerns about the height, the projection, and the symmetry in this area. Specific inquiries should be made into any history of orthodontic therapy, because such therapy may have been used to disguise an underlying class II malocclusion caused by a small mandible.

Physical examination should note the following five items:

1. The sagittal position of the pogonion relative to the lower lip and the remainder of the mid and upper face. **The lower lip, not the mid or upper facial structures, determines the extent to which the chin should be brought forward** (6). Consequently, the chin should not be brought forward any further than a vertical line dropped from the lower lip. **When advancing the chin, the ratio of soft tissue to skeletal displacement is generally 1:1.** If the lower lip is recessive, as it may be in many individuals with small mandibles who are seeking chin enlargement, one must be willing to accept a residual degree of sagittal weakness of the lower face relative to the mid and upper face. **This is aesthetically preferable to a chin that is advanced beyond the lower lip, which invariably results in a bizarre, artificial appearance.** Undercorrection

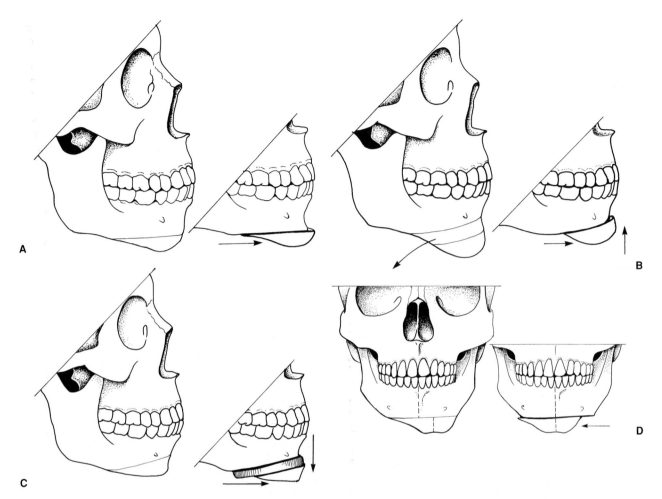

FIGURE 55.1. A: Standard location and orientation of the advancement osseous genioplasty. Note that the osteotomy is placed well below the mental foramina to avoid injury to the inferior alveolar nerve. The osteotomy extends well posterior to the vicinity of the molar teeth. The angulation of this osteotomy allows forward advancement of the chin without any vertical changes. **B:** Simultaneous advancement and vertical reduction of the chin. Note that two parallel osteotomies are performed with an intervening ostectomy. **C:** Simultaneous advancement and vertical elongation of the chin. The interpositional material typically employed are blocks of porous hydroxyapatite. **D:** Lateral shifting of the symphyseal segment to restore lower-face symmetry.

in the sagittal dimension is always preferable to overcorrection.

2. A qualitative assessment of the height of the lower face as it relates to the midface. In a patient with vertical excess of the lower face, one has the option to reduce the vertical height of the chin. This can be accomplished by two parallel osteotomies with an intervening ostectomy or a steeply oblique bone cut that allows the chin to be advanced and superiorly repositioned.

3. The symmetry of the lower face. Osseous genioplasty presents the surgeon with the perfect opportunity to laterally shift the symphyseal segment either to the right or the left to achieve a symmetric lower face. Similarly, the chin can be vertically elongated or shortened in an asymmetric fashion to correct vertical asymmetry.

4. The depth of the labiomental fold. Sagittal advancement or vertical shortening, or both, of the symphyseal segment results in deepening of the labiomental fold (5). Conversely, vertical lengthening of the chin tends to efface or soften the fold. Accordingly, individuals with a normal or exceedingly deep fold who undergo advancement of the chin also should be evaluated for vertical elongation. This should be considered in a person with

a short lower face and in a patient with normal height of the lower face, but never in a patient with excessive height in the lower face. The individual who has a combination of a long lower face and a deep labiomental fold is never a candidate for chin surgery, and such a patient should be offered a more extensive orthognathic correction (5).

5. Examination of the occlusion. The majority of individuals who request aesthetic enlargement of the chin have class II skeletal deformities secondary to a small mandible (5). This is a tip-off that coexisting problems such as abnormalities of lower face height and labiomental fold depth may be present in addition to a "weak" chin. It is important to remember that prior orthodontic treatment can convert a class II malocclusion into a class I occlusion but this does not correct the underlying skeletal problems.

Although the extent of soft-tissue movement closely follows that of skeletal displacement when advancing, shortening, or lengthening the chin, soft-tissue response to posteriorly repositioning of the chin is, at best, 0.5 to 1. **Surgical efforts to correct** an excessively prominent chin are not as predictable as those performed to correct a small chin.

Radiographic evaluation of the chin should include a Panorex radiograph if periapical pathology of the anterior mandibular teeth is suspected. Any preexisting dental pathology in this area is an absolute contraindication to chin surgery. In addition, one may want to evaluate the vertical dimension between the apices of the incisor roots and the inferior border of the mandible when correcting a short chin. It is important that enough room exists both to perform the osteotomy and to apply fixation devices without risk to the roots of these teeth.

SURGICAL TECHNIQUE

Although reports exist describing osseous genioplasty under local anesthesia with intravenous sedation (7), it is best under-taken under general anesthesia with orotracheal or nasotracheal intubation and full protection of the airway. Hemostasis is facilitated by infiltration with a dilute epinephrine solution. The soft-tissue incision is placed at least 1 cm away from the depth of the mandibular buccal sulcus onto the lower lip and is 2 to 3 cm in length. The mucosa and submucosa are incised, bringing the mentalis muscle and its median raphe into view. Once these muscles are very superficially incised, the angle of the soft-tissue incision changes so that it is parallel to the mucosa of the lip. This direction is maintained until the anterior mandibular surface is reached, **leaving a large amount of mentalis muscle attached to the mandible for later muscle reapproximation.** A subperiosteal dissection of the symphysis is performed. The dissection is continued inferiorly only far enough to allow exposure for performing the osteotomy and for applying fixation devises. Complete degloving of the symphysis is not recommended because of the unpredictable

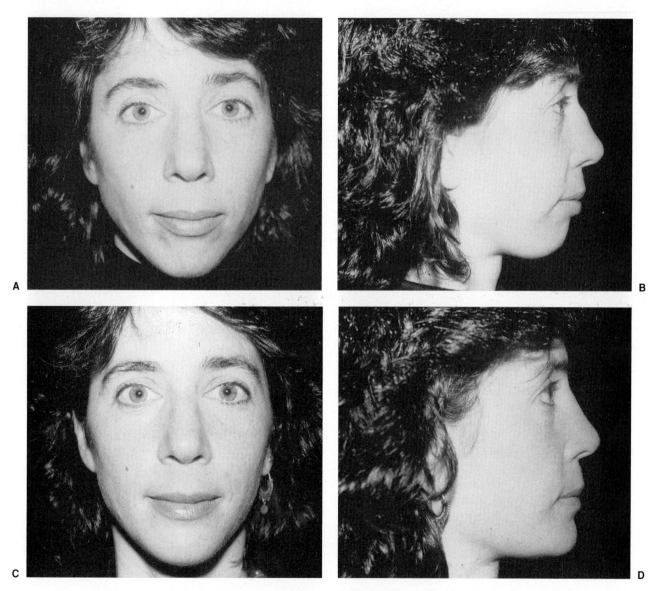

FIGURE 55.2. A 35-year-old woman with a small mandible and increased lower face height. **A,B:** There is lip strain, with superior dislocation of the soft-tissue chin pad and a shallow labiomental fold. Surgical correction will effect an 8-mm advancement of the chin and a 5-mm reduction in its height. Simultaneous rhinoplasty will be performed. **C,D:** Postoperatively, the lip strain has been eliminated and the labiomental fold has been deepened. Note that the chin has been advanced no further that the most anterior position of the lower lip. (From Rosen HM. Aesthetic refinements in genioplasty: the role of the labiomental fold. *Plast Reconstr Surg.* 1991;88:760, with permission.)

reattachment of the soft tissues to the bone and the potential risk for development of soft-tissue ptosis, that is, a witch's chin (8). Exposure is continued laterally so that both mental nerves are identified. Posterior dissection is carried to the inferior border of the mandible directly below the molar roots.

Once the soft-tissue dissection is completed, a fissure burr scores a vertical mark in the midline chin, allowing it to be appropriately positioned in the transverse dimension. The reciprocating saw is used to perform the horizontal osteotomy at least 4 mm below the mental foramina to protect the inferior alveolar nerves. As previously mentioned, the osteotomy is carried as far posteriorly as possible to allow for a generous volume of skeletal displacement. This provides for natural-looking results and avoids waist lining and excessive visibility of the inevitable step in the inferior border of the mandible.

Cortical cuts should be completed with the reciprocating saw, avoiding unnecessary prying downward of the symphyseal segment, which may cause fracturing. Following mobilization of the symphysis, it might be necessary to detach the anterior belly of the digastric muscles from the lingual surface if extensive anterior dislocation is anticipated. After full mobilization is achieved, fixation devices are applied to hold the chin segment in the desired location. Although plate and screws are popular, it is perfectly acceptable to use wire fixation.

If vertical shortening of the chin is desired, it is usually accomplished by performing two parallel horizontal osteotomies and removing the intervening segment of bone. **If vertical elongation is desired, it is most often done by interposing blocks of hydroxyapatite into the osteotomy gaps created by inferior repositioning of the symphysis.**

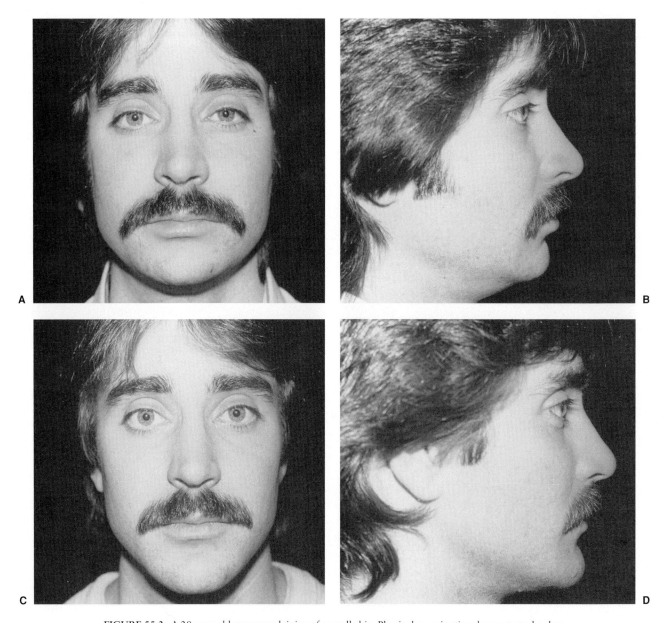

FIGURE 55.3. A 28-year-old man complaining of a small chin. Physical examination demonstrated a class II malocclusion with deficient sagittal projection of the chin as well as decreased height of the lower face. **A,B:** In addition, there is a deepened labiomental fold. Surgical planning included a 6-mm advancement and 6-mm elongation of the chin. **C,D:** The postoperative views demonstrate an increase in the height of the lower face and an apparent decrease in the depth of the labiomental fold. Again, the chin was advanced no further than the most anterior position of the lower lip. (From Rosen HM. Aesthetic refinements in genioplasty: the role of the labiomental fold. *Plast Reconstr Surg.* 1991;88:760, with permission.)

Following fixation, the wound is copiously irrigated with diluted povidone-iodine (Betadine) solution and closed in layers. The mentalis muscle is repaired using interrupted sutures to help avoid soft-tissue ptosis and subsequent development of a witch's chin (8). The mucosa is repaired using interrupted 3-0 chromic sutures. By placing the incision well out onto the lower lip, there is sufficient soft tissue to close without tearing the tissues. This helps to minimize subsequent wound contamination and possible infection. No dressings are applied.

PATIENT EXAMPLES

The following patient examples illustrate the versatility of the osseous genioplasty.

Patient 1

The patient (Fig. 55.2) is a 35-year-old women with a small mandible, increased lower face height, and a modest component of lip strain. As a result, the soft-tissue chin pad is superiorly dislocated, causing effacement and shallowness of the labiomental fold. Surgical correction involves advancement and vertical shortening of the chin. The segment was advanced 8 mm and shortened 5 mm. A rhinoplasty was also performed. **Note that as the chin is advanced the labiomental fold deepens with improved definition.** The lip strain has been eliminated. The chin has been advanced no further than the lower lip.

Patient 2

This 28-year-old man (Fig. 55.3) complained of having a small chin. Physical examination demonstrated that he had a small mandible and a class II, deep bite malocclusion. In addition to a lack of projection of the chin, there was decreased height of the lower face relative to the midface and an exaggerated, deepened labiomental fold. Surgical planning involved a 6-mm advancement and 6-mm lengthening of the chin. In the postoperative views, note the softening of the labiomental fold and apparent decrease in its depth. Note again that the chin is advanced no further than the most anterior position of the lower lip.

COMPLICATIONS

In a recent report of a large series of patients undergoing osseous genioplasty by three experienced craniomaxillofacial surgeons, the complication rate was low (3). Lower-lip paresthesia occurred in 5.5% of the patients. Soft-tissue infection was reported in 3% of patients.

Although not reported as a complication, the most frequent problem associated with osseous genioplasty is the undesirable aesthetic result. Such an outcome is caused by errors in both treatment planning and technique. **The most commonly committed error in treatment planning is overadvancement of the symphyseal segment, resulting in an unnatural, bizarre appearance, with the chin well in advance of the lower lip.** It bears repeating that the osseous genioplasty is a powerful tool and that modest advancement of the chin goes a long way. **When in doubt about the extent of advancement, one should err on the side of conservatism and undercorrect in the sagittal dimension.**

The most commonly encountered aesthetic problem relative to surgical technique is failure to extend the osteotomy cut far enough posteriorly. This can result in an hourglass deformity with excessive tapering of the mandible in the area immediately posterior to the osteotomy. This can be largely avoided if the osteotomy cut is extended back to the molar teeth, as it is placed in an area where abundant soft tissue is present to mask any notching of the inferior mandibular border.

CONCLUSION

The osseous genioplasty represents the most versatile procedure that the plastic surgeon has available to enhance the balance and proportion of the lower face. It is a powerful tool that can yield dramatic results if the surgeon performing the procedure knows that it cannot change the sagittal position of the lower lip. It behooves plastic surgeons to become familiar and comfortable with the procedure so that the alternative—alloplastic chin augmentation—will not be used in patients who would benefit more from a skeletal correction.

References

1. Greenberg ST, Pan FS, Bartlett SP, et al. Complications of osseous genioplasty. *Proc Northeastern Soc Plastic Surg* 1985;92.
2. Converse JM, Wood-Smith D. Horizontal osteotomy of the mandible. *Plast Reconstr Surg.* 1964;34:464.
3. Hofer D. Die osteoplastiche verlaegerund des unterkiefers nach von Eiselberg bie mikrogenie. *Dtsch Zahn Mund Kieferheilkd.* 1957;27:81.
4. Bell WH, Proffit WR, White P, eds. *Surgical Correction of Dentofacial Deformities.* Philadelphia: WB Saunders; 1980:685.
5. Rosen HM. Aesthetic refinements in genioplasty: the role of the labiomental fold. *Plast Reconstr Surg.* 1991;88:760.
6. Rosen HM. Aesthetic guidelines in genioplasty: the role of facial disproportion. *Plast Reconstr Surg.* 1995;95:463.
7. Spear SL, Mausner ME, Kawamoto HK. Sliding genioplasty as a local aesthetic outpatient procedure: a prospective two center trial. *Plast Reconstr Surg.* 1987;80:55.
8. Zide BM, McCarthy JG. The mentalis muscle: an associated component of chin and lower lip position. *Plast Reconstr Surg.* 1989;83:413.

CHAPTER 56 ■ HAIR TRANSPLANTATION

MICHAEL L. REED

State-of-the-art surgical hair replacement using whole donor-dominant hair follicles from areas of nonbalding scalp to replace lost hair on the crown probably reached its zenith in 2004. Further refinements in ergonomics are likely, but better results await research breakthroughs in tissue-engineering technology using follicular stem cells (1).

Modern-day hair transplantation began in the United States in 1959, although micrografting of human scalp hair had been reported in the Japanese medical literature in 1939, and autografting of hair had been done in Germany in the 19th century. Improvements in surgical techniques and instrumentation occurred sporadically until 1993 when surgeons formed The International Society for Hair Restoration Surgery (ISHRS) to share knowledge and advance the field.

Much smaller grafts in much greater numbers placed very close together resulted in much more natural-looking transplants. As early as 1984, basic histologic studies of horizontal sections of scalp had revealed that human scalp hairs grow naturally in small compartments (follicular units) containing clusters of one to four follicles surrounded by concentric layers of collagen fibers (Fig. 56.1) (3). Peripheral areas such as the hairline have one and two-hair follicular units (FU), whereas the more dense central regions have more three and four-hair FU (and coarser hair shafts). Toward the end of the 1990s, transplant surgeons realized the significance of the follicular unit as it applied to hair replacement, which has given birth to the follicular unit transplant (FUT) era.

The older terms of "micrograft" (one to two hairs) and "minigraft" (three to six hairs) have been replaced by single FU (one to two or three to four hair) and multi FU (two to three unit/two to six hair) grafts. However, some surgeons still use the older terminology and restrict the use of the term follicular unit to the procedure known as the single-FU-only transplant (SFUT).

More efficient donor-harvesting methods and better quantitative distribution of hair in the recipient site with adjunctive medical treatment has greatly reduced the use of (and need for) other types of surgery in the treatment of baldness. For these reasons this chapter is restricted to hair transplantation. The reader is referred elsewhere for a discussion of procedures such as alopecia reduction (4).

INITIAL CONSULTATION/SCREENING SESSION

The first step in the consultation is to determine whether or not the donor site is adequate to accomplish the patient's transplant goals. Next, is to give the patient a detailed explanation of the procedure that is optimal based on the patient's hair and scalp tissue characteristics. Realistic short- and long-term goals should be carefully outlined. Because the balding process is progressive and the final results unpredictable, there is always some degree of calculated risk. **Over time, the transplanted hair may have to "stand alone."** This end point transplant pattern should be reasonably natural-looking and resemble some variation of either male- or female-pattern hair loss.

Patients who appear to be good candidates for surgery based on the findings of the initial exam and discussion of achievable goals must determine for themselves when they are ready and must never be pressured to undergo a procedure. Patients usually like to see before-and-after photos of the results they might expect in one or several sessions. Ideally, they like to speak to, or even meet with, someone like themselves who has had a transplant. However, it must be emphasized that the exact outcome cannot be predicted and patient satisfaction cannot be guaranteed. Despite these caveats, the reality is that the overwhelming majority of patients are pleased with the results of transplantation procedures.

THE PREOPERATIVE PERIOD

Prior to the procedure, further communication is essential to optimize the outcome. There should be a specially trained staff member—a "patient care coordinator"—who works closely with the surgeon and is readily available to answer patient questions and address special problems and needs. Many patients experience anxieties, especially with regard to postoperation down time. Patients also receive gratuitous misinformation and misguided counsel from friends and relatives, as well as from other physicians. The coordinator is trained to deal with such problems and assure compliance with preoperation instructions. Patients should be instructed to discontinue medications and diet supplements that can cause bleeding problems such as aspirin, anticoagulants, ibuprofen-type anti-inflammatories, vitamin E, garlic pills, fish oil capsules, and herbal supplements, starting 2 weeks prior to surgery. Topical minoxidil (a vasodilator) should be stopped 3 days prior to surgery, and alcohol and caffeine should be minimized 1 day before surgery. Cigarette smoking should be stopped or at least minimized. A written informed consent needs to be read, discussed, and signed, and written pre-/postoperation instruction sheets provided to every patient. Finally, a photo consent is obtained.

A planning session with the surgeon is conducted 1 to 2 weeks before the procedure to determine or review and confirm the final surgical plan. The entire procedure, from the time the patient arrives until the patient leaves after the procedure, should be reviewed in detail. In addition, patient plans for activity during the 2 week postoperation period should be discussed. A diagram of the pattern and distribution of grafts, including location and shape of a new hairline, can be given to certain patients. Prescriptions for perioperative medications typically include an oral antibiotic (cefadroxil most commonly)

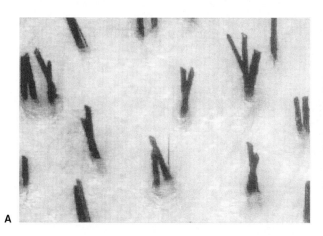
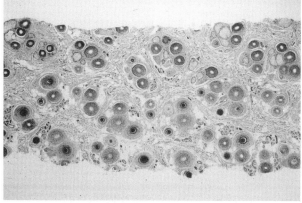

FIGURE 56.1. Follicular units. **A:** Video microscopic view of single follicular units showing one- to four-hair units. **B:** Photomicrograph of horizontal section of human scalp showing follicular units with light microscopy.

for 5 to 7 days starting the day of or the day before surgery, a painkiller such as acetaminophen with or without a narcotic analgesic (codeine or hydrocodone) and a 5-day prednisone taper (e.g., a taper protocol of 50 to 40 to 30 to 20 to 10 mg) to reduce postoperation swelling. Because clinical studies have not established a single regimen, there is great variability among medication protocols. Many surgeons do not routinely use prophylactic antibiotics because they believe the risk of an adverse reaction to the drugs is greater than the risk of infection.

THE OPERATION

Preanesthesia, Anesthesia, and Photography

This is an office-based outpatient procedure that most commonly employs levels I and II sedation. Ativan 2 mg p.o. or Valium 10 mg p.o. are the most commonly used premedications. Some anesthetists also use nitrous oxide, whereas others use intramuscular (or, less often, intravenous) Versed with or without an analgesic such as Demerol or fentanyl. The donor site is shaved to leave 2 to 3 mm of hair shaft for directionality purposes during implantation. The perimeters of the excision site are outlined with a marking pen followed by a Betadine-Povidine preparation. Local anesthesia of the donor site is produced initially with plain buffered 1% Xylocaine followed by longer acting 0.25% to 0.5% Marcaine with epinephrine (1:100,000). Normal saline is used to tumesce the donor site to prevent tissue deformation during the excision and to create a fluid-filled space between the hair follicles located in the subcutaneous fat and the underlying galea aponeurotica to minimize blood vessel and nerve transection during excision. An alternative is to use tumescent anesthesia (0.1% Xylocaine with 1:1,000,000 epinephrine). The discomfort associated with local anesthetic injections can be significantly diminished by the use of a mechanical vibrator placed just inferior to the injection site. The recipient site is anesthetized using a local ring block with 1% Xylocaine with 1:100,000 epinephrine followed by infiltration of the recipient site with normal saline with 1:100,000 to 1:150,000 epinephrine. Regional nerve blocks of the supraorbital and supratrochlear nerves in their respective foramina located above the eyebrow can also reduce discomfort at the recipient site. Preoperation photos demonstrating

the intended recipient area(s) from several different views are taken prior to starting the procedure.

THE DONOR SITE

The ideal donor site is the region containing hair follicles that are not subject to the gradual miniaturization process that causes baldness (invisible hair). The perimeters of this area are variable, but it is generally described as having an anterior border starting at a line that extends perpendicular to the external auditory canal. The inferior border is typically 4 cm above the hairline at the nape of the neck. The superior border varies according to the final location of the posterior border of the balding zone. This border has been described as typically being 7 cm above the inferior border at the occipital midline, increasing to 8 cm toward the midlateral occiput and narrowing to 5 cm above the ears. Hair density is greatest at the midline and diminishes laterally above the ears and again below the inferior border approaching the nape of the neck.

The size of the donor site along with the hair density (hair/cm²) and diameter (microns) are the key factors in deciding whether or not the patient is a good candidate, as well as what kind of results should be anticipated. Most experienced surgeons can inspect the donor site and integrate these variables to make a determination. However, it is desirable to have the ability to perform a more quantitative evaluation using a device such as the Russman densitometer, which has a viewing area of 10 mm². Hair density and follicular unit density can be calculated at different locations along the donor site. Because hair density and FU density, as well as hair diameter, vary, it is necessary to measure at several points. The three commonly chosen sites are the midocciput over the protuberance, the supra-auricular point above the external auditory meatus, and a spot halfway between over the mastoid. The numbers can be averaged. If only one measurement is done, the midmastoid tends to be intermediate with higher and lower densities at the midocciput and supra-auricular spots respectively. Table 56.1 shows the predicted available hair for transplantation in the average straight-haired patient, assuming that 50% of hair can be harvested before the donor site becomes noticeably depleted. These calculations are useful as a reference point, but it is important to remember that there is great variation among individuals.

Hair diameter is the other major factor in determining the coverage achievable with a transplant. The major goal behind

TABLE 56.1

DONOR DENSITY: THE EFFECT OF CHANGES IN DONOR AREA HAIR DENSITY ON MOVABLE HAIR

Donor Density (hairs/mm^2)	Total Hair in Permanent Zone	Hair Must Remain in Permanent Zone	Movable Hair	Change in Density	Change in Movable Hair
1.0	12,500	12,500	0	−50%	−100%
1.3	16,250	12,500	3750	−35%	−70%
1.5	18,750	12,500	6250	−25%	−50%
1.8	22,500	12,500	10,000	−10%	−20%
2.0	25,000	12,500	12,500	0	0
2.2	27,500	12,500	15,000	+10%	+20%
2.5	31,250	12,500	18,750	+25%	+50%
2.7	33,750	12,500	21,250	+35%	+70%
3.0	37,500	12,500	25,000	+50%	+100%

Data from Bernsein R, Russman W. The logic of follicular unit transplantation. *Dermatol Clin.* 1999;17:277–295, with permission.

the frontal zone, especially in the mid postfrontal region, is to see hair rather than scalp. Besides density (hairs/cm^2), hair volume plays a critical role. Hair volume (hv) is defined in the following formula:

$$hv = \pi(r)^2 (h)(d)(a)$$

In this equation, *r* is the radius of the hair shaft, *h* is the hair length, *d* is the hair density (hairs/cm^2), and *a* is the total area covered (cm^2). **It is key to note that a doubling of the radius results in a quadrupling of hair volume, making hair diameter the most important single variable in the coverage achievable in a transplant.** It is also the variable that is most beyond our control, at least in male patients.

Other factors that affect the final coverage include hair texture and hair/scalp color contrast. Wavy, curly, helical, and spiral hairs improve coverage. A lesser contrast between hair color and scalp color improves the illusion of density. Gray hair on fair skin looks considerably denser than dark hair.

The most common technique to harvest donor hair follicles is the single-blade method in which the surgeon uses a no. 10 (or no. 15) blade to remove a long section of scalp that varies in width from 0.5 to 1.5 cm, and in length from 10 to 25 cm (Fig. 56.2A). Optimal hemostasis is achieved with the Redfield infrared coagulator. Simple running or interlocking 3-0 or 4-0 nylon sutures placed close together and close to the wound edge in the deep dermis/subcutis, which are left in for 10 to 14 days, will usually heal with a fine scar that is not noticeable (Fig. 56.2B). It may be necessary to undermine the galea and place buried absorbable sutures to reduce excessive tension on the wound edges in patients with very fibrotic scalps or with scar tissue from multiple procedures. In ideal circumstances, it is desirable to excise the scar from a previous procedure in a subsequent procedure. However, an attempt to do so may reduce the amount of new donor follicles in the strip or require such a wide excision that the resulting scar becomes unacceptably noticeable. Multiple narrow (2- to 3-mm) scars may be less noticeable than one 1.5-cm scar. Some operators use staples instead of sutures. These can be placed faster, but are more painful to remove. It is also possible to close the wound with surface and/or buried absorbable sutures (Vicryl, Monocryl, cat gut). This method eliminates a visit for suture removal. However, more tissue reaction from absorption may result in a wider scar.

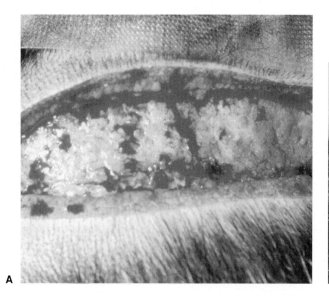

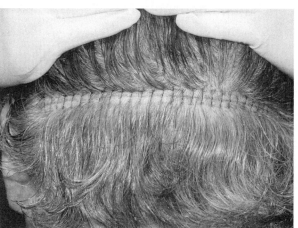

A   **B**

FIGURE 56.2. Scalp donor site for single-strip technique. **A:** Donor site after excision of scalp using the single-strip technique showing the underlying galea aponeurotica. **B:** Donor site after closure with a running 3-0 nylon suture. The suture will be removed after 14 days and the site will heal with a pencil-line surgical scar.

The most common alternative to the single-blade method is the multibladed knife, which can be adjusted to remove one or multiple (two to five) "strips" of donor tissue of variable width (1 to 4 mm). These thin strips are then easily microdissected into grafts. However, the ergonomic advantages of a multi-bladed knife may be offset by loss of viable follicles as a result of follicular transection that occasionally occur even with the most skilled surgeon. The single-blade method allows much better control of the excision when there are multidirectional hairs and when the excision site has unexpected areas of tissue deformation because of incomplete (or lost) tumescence during the harvesting procedure.

The newest technique for harvesting is an attempt to improve on the original Orentreich procedure in which a circular punch was used to remove a small cylinder of hair-bearing donor scalp containing multiple follicular units consisting of 10 to 20 hairs per graft. However, instead of using the 4-mm-diameter punch, the surgeon uses a 1-mm punch and attempts to excise individual follicular units. To minimize transection, the punch incision is down to the deep dermis, but not into the subcutaneous tissue as the follicular stem and bulb are located there and tend to splay out in a manner that puts them in a non-parallel position to the cutting edge of the punch. Instead, the punch is removed and tissue-grasping forceps (with or without a tiny, blunt microdissector) is used to "extract" the individual (one- to four-hair) unit.

This method is called follicular unit extraction (FUE) (5). The major benefit of FUE is avoiding the linear scar(s) associated with a strip excision. The major disadvantages are (a) follicular bulb "decapitation" caused either by transection during the initial incision or by traction while attempting to dissect or "pluck out" each follicular unit, and (b) a significant increase in time and effort for both patient and operators resulting in considerably smaller transplants than what is achieved with the conventional excision methods.

In addition, because not all patients have scalp tissue that will allow extraction without significant traumatic loss, it is recommended to perform a FUE test to determine who is a potential candidate for this method. This test is basically a miniprocedure in which five to ten 1.0-mm grafts are extracted and scored on a 5-point scale for intact tissue. A score of 1 to 2 indicates a potential candidate. In its initial use, the scores obtained found that approximately 60% of patients qualified. More recently, it has been claimed that up to 90% of patients can qualify, probably as a function of increasing surgical expertise (5). Even though transection at the level of the follicular stem leaving the follicular "bulge" region intact may allow survival rates of up to 50%, the new follicles do not achieve their full pretranssection diameters. Nevertheless, FUE with improvements in methodology should be useful in the subset of patients whose donor sites are inadequate for strip excision and in the patient who wishes to avoid potentially visible donor scars if he has to undergo multiple procedures or decides to shave his head.

The Microdissection Procedure (Graft Production)

The harvested donor strip obtained using the single-blade excision method is cut into tiny slices that vary from 1 to 3 mm in width, which translates into one to three FU in a typical white/Asian scalp with an average follicular unit density of one FU/mm^2 (Fig. 56.3). A typical strip is 1×20-cm (20 cm^2) and contains 2,000 units. There are an average of two to three hairs per FU. A dissecting microscope and/or magnification loupes ($4\times$) with backlighting is used for close-up visualization. Single- and double-edge razor blades or no. 11/no. 15

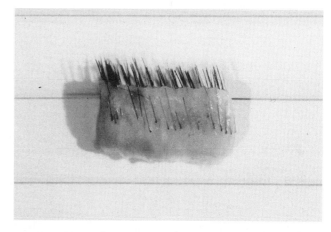

FIGURE 56.3. A "sliver" produced by sectioning of the donor strip obtained with the single-blade technique showing how the follicular bulbs extend into the subcutaneous fat.

Teflon-coated scalpel blades are employed to cut these sections into grafts. In strictly single follicular unit procedures, it is considered ideal to use a dissecting scope exclusively for best visualization so that the technician can attempt to actually cut around (and then cut out) individual units, a process called *slivering*. This technique is in contrast to simple straight-cut sectioning, which might have a greater probability of breaking up some follicular units. Depending on the area being transplanted and the color/texture/density of the donor hair, the technician may cut single-only, single and multiple (two to three FU), or multiple-only grafts. There may be an occasional individual with mostly large (three- to four-hair) units and very coarse dark hair who needs a new frontal hairline where an exception must be made to the dictum to avoid breaking up follicular units. Even a single-hair graft may appear unnatural in a frontal line if it is very coarse. For such cases it has been proposed to not only break up large units, but to intentionally injure (transect) follicular bulbs based on the belief that the 30% to 50% of hairs that survive such injury will have a finer texture and thus more natural appearance along the frontal line. The grafts are kept in gauze-lined, chilled, normal saline-filled petri dishes to prevent rapid dehydration (the primary cause of nonviable grafts). The grafts are separated into 10 to 50 graft clusters according to size (one to two hairs, three to four hairs, etc.).

If a multibladed knife has been used, it is possible to perform graft preparation using a device called the Mangubat graft cutter. This is a rectangular-shaped, stainless steel base containing a series of parallel, closely spaced (1- to 2-mm) blades. The strip is stretched and placed over these blades so that the hair follicles are parallel to the cutting edges. Next, a wooden tongue blade ("force spreader") is laid on top of the strip and a rubber mallet is employed to strike ("impulsive force") the wood surface with several rapid strokes. The entire strip is cut into grafts instantly. This saves a great deal of time for microdissection, but carries an increased risk of splitting follicular units and transecting follicles.

THE RECIPIENT SITE

The area to be transplanted, having been anesthetized and prepped with Betadine-Povidine solution that has dried, is carefully marked with a marking pen according to the preoperation plan. The best long-term results are obtained by transplanting from front to back rather than back to front. The frontal line should be as high as the patient finds acceptable.

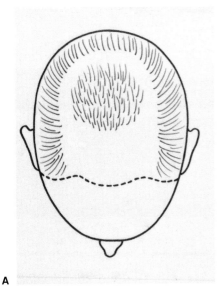
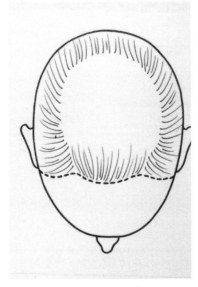

A   **B**

FIGURE 56.4. **A:** "Halo head" hair pattern produced by transplanting the vertex area followed by loss of hair in the peripheral regions. **B:** "Monk's head" hairline produced by placing the hairline too low in the forehead.

Transplanting the vertex area may eventually result in a "halo head" pattern if the donor site is depleted and hair continues to thin out around the posterior and lateral borders (Fig. 56.4A). A low frontal hairline may over time turn into a "monk's head" look if the patient has only one procedure or runs out of donor hair prematurely (Fig. 56.4B). It is always best to perform each transplant as if it will be the last one. Ideally, the transplanted hair should be able to stand alone and resemble a variation of naturally occurring male- or female-pattern hair loss.

A new hairline will typically have a midline low point 7 to 8 cm above the midglabella in male patients, and 6 to 7 cm above the midglabella in females, although there is a wide range of acceptable hairline shapes and locations. It is better to err on the side of a higher line as it is much easier to move the line forward in the future than to move it backward. The so-called hairline is really a transition zone approximately 0.5 to 1 cm at the midline and 1 to 2 cm in the temporal triangle. Depending on the side to side distance, it takes 200 to 500 single/double hair grafts placed 0.75 to 1.0 mm apart to get an acceptable result. A best result may take two or three sessions, especially in patients with straight, coarse, dark hair and fair skin.

Transplanting behind the frontal line is a quantitative challenge because it is theoretically an attempt (at least in the long-term) to use a portion of the estimated 30% of the permanent hairs that reside in the nonbalding areas of the occipitoparietal region to replace the estimated 70% of hairs on the top of the head that are destined to be lost over time. The highest density requirement is in the central postfrontal region. The midscalp and vertex are intermediate in density needs. If the patient has a particular hair style, it can help the plan for density distribution. For example, if the patient combs left to right, it is desirable to place larger grafts closer together on the left side. The donor site density varies from 50 to 350 hairs/cm^2. In most patients 1 cm^2 of donor scalp can provide adequate hair for 2 to 4 cm^2 of recipient site. A clear plastic baggie can be laid over the marked recipient site and the area outlined with a marking pen. The baggie is then laid on a paper with a large grid marked in 1-cm squares, and the squares inside the perimeter are marked and counted. This gives the total cm^2 that need to be covered. In a typical procedure, a frontal/midscalp transplant region of 60 cm^2 can be transplanted adequately using a 1×20-cm (20 cm^2) strip of donor scalp. If the donor site contains an average of 2.3 hairs/FU (range: 1 to 4 hairs/FU) and a total of 2,000 FU (1 FU/mm^2) it will give the patient 4,600 hairs in 60 cm^2, or an average density of 77 hairs/cm^2 (4,600/60).

Incisional instruments used to make the recipient site openings include a wide array of needles, miniblades, and micropunches (Fig. 56.5). For one to two hair grafts, the most commonly used instruments are probably an 18-gauge hypodermic needle for coarse hairs and a 19-gauge hypodermic needle for finer hairs. Spearpoint sp90 (1.5 mm) and sp91 (2.0 mm) miniblades are also popular for single- or double-follicular unit grafts, respectively. Nokor needles (16/18 gauge) and 1.5-mm tribevel (Rossati Starr) punches can be used for large (three- to four-hair) single-unit and small (three- to five-hair) double-unit grafts. For larger (two- to three-unit/four- to seven-hair) grafts, 2-mm tribevel (Rossati Starr) punches work very well.

Excisional devices, such as round and elliptical/slot (Redfield and Butterfield) punches, are less commonly employed than are incisional devices because they cause more tissue injury and, consequently, more scarring (Fig. 56.5). Also, the grafts must be "cut to fit" the site, which may necessitate breaking up follicular units, causing increased follicular transection. If the grafts are of smaller diameter than the site, there will be a gap between the sides of the graft and the walls of the recipient well. Healing will then occur by secondary intention, which may reduce graft survival. It may also result in "pitting" or even epidermoid cyst formation if the graft "sinks" below the surface and gets "buried alive." However, it may be necessary to employ these instruments in very fibrotic/inelastic scalps, where it is necessary to remove some tissue in order to place grafts with more than one to two hairs. Elliptical punches have largely replaced circular ones because of superior graft fitting that gives a more natural-looking result.

Recipient site incisions are made 0.5 to 2.0 mm apart, depending on the size and location of the grafts. They are put as close as possible along the frontal line and in the central postfrontal areas (so-called dense packing). Most procedures are done with incisional rather than excisional devices to reduce scarring and to avoid having to cut the donor tissue to fit the excision sites (Fig. 56.6). The donor tissue characteristics (density, texture, and color) should determine the type of grafts that are used. Recipient site openings should comfortably accommodate what is inserted with a "snug fit." This is not a problem for the popular SFUT. However, in patients with lower-density donor sites and finer hair texture with minimal hair/skin color contrast (e.g., women and gray-haired older men), larger grafts may be needed to achieve optimal density with fewer sessions. In such cases, the 1.5- and 2.0-mm tribevel punches are ideal. A small triangular opening that can

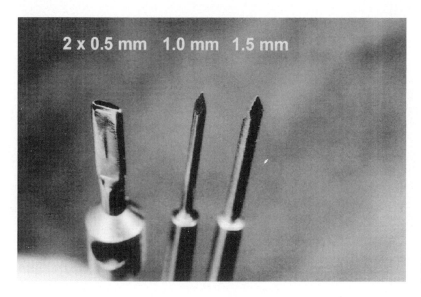

FIGURE 56.5. Excisional and incisional instruments. **Left:** A Redfield excisional slot punch. **Right:** One-mm and 1.5-mm tribevel incisional punches.

be oriented for hair directionality and that is expandable in all directions (360 degrees) is created. The site is able to accommodate variable-sized grafts with the same snug fit up to a maximum diameter of either 1.5 mm or 2.0 mm (Fig. 56.7). Wounds heal by primary intention; if for some reason no graft is placed in the incision site, there is no significant scar tissue generated.

Laser-generated (carbon dioxide or Erbium:YAG) recipient sites enjoyed some popularity during the 1990s, but have declined in use because of problems with delayed wound healing, reduced graft survival, and lateral damage to existing hair follicles in thin-haired (or previously transplanted) recipient sites (6). The only advantage they enjoy over a skilled surgeon using cold-steel devices is that patients are easily

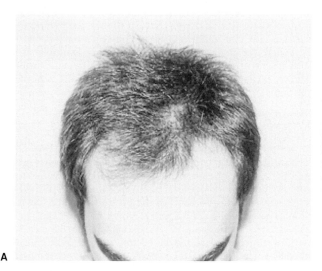

A

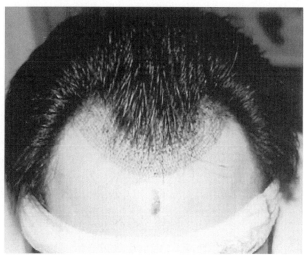

B

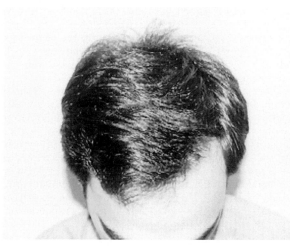

C

FIGURE 56.6. **A:** Preoperative view of patient with frontal resection and thin frontal forelock region. **B:** Intraoperative view showing a series of microincisions. The first two rows were made with 132 incisions using a 1.0-mm tribevel punch; the third to fifth rows were made with 300 incisions using an 18-gauge needle; in the postfrontal region, 263 incisions were made using a 1.5-mm tribevel punch. Single units were placed in the 1.0-mm tribevel punch and the 18-gauge needle incisions, with one to two hairs per graft; two FU grafts containing four to six hairs were placed in the 1.5-mm tribevel punch incisions. **C:** The patient 7 months postoperation showing the advanced frontal hairline and increased density in the postfrontal area.

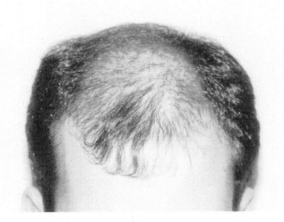

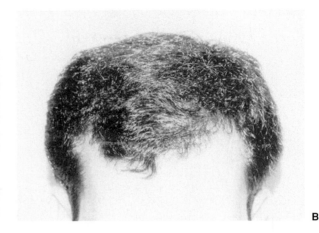

A

B

FIGURE 56.7. A: Patient preoperatively showing extensive frontal hair loss. **B:** Same patient 7 months postoperation, with 700 two follicular units (four to seven hair grafts, dense packed, in the postfrontal region).

impressed by the high-tech perception associated with laser procedures.

The two most common methods for graft placement are (a) simultaneous cut and place and (b) separated cut and place. In the former method, the surgeon makes the incision and an assistant using special, fine-tipped jeweler's forceps slides the graft into the site either while the instrument is still in the site, using it as a guide, or immediately after removal of the device. In the latter method, all (or most) of the incisions are made before graft placement begins. Both methods achieve the same end result, although each has advantages and disadvantages (7).

THE POSTOPERATIVE PERIOD

Postoperation Dressings

The traditional dressing is a bilayered protective and absorptive affair with the first layer made from several nonstick Telfa pads covered with a thin layer of an antibiotic such as mupirocin (Bactroban/Centany) cream or ointment. Micropore tape attaches this underdressing to the patient's forehead. A turban-style overdressing made from a Kerlix bandage wrapped over several layers of 4×4-inch gauze pads is constructed and finished off with elastic retainer netting (Surgilast no. gl-705). Some patients greatly prefer a more minimal dressing, or no dressing at all. This is feasible if the patient is able to wait 2 to 3 hours in the office after the surgery before going home. However, the need to prevent graft dislodgement and bleeding must be weighed against the needs of a self-consciousness patient.

Postoperation Sequelae

There are a number of expected events that are a normal, albeit unpleasant, part of the transplant experience, such as discomfort/pain lasting several days to a week (primarily at the donor site); forehead/periorbital swelling beginning 2 days after the operation and lasting 3 to 4 days; redness/scab formation (recipient site) that lasts 7 to 14 days; variable degrees of telogen effluvium (shock loss) of native hair (recipient and donor sites) that begins to regrow in 8 to 12 weeks; numbness/paresthesias of the donor region that persists for several months, but (rarely)

may take up to a year to resolve. Very rarely some loss of sensation may persist indefinitely.

The transplanted hairs go into a telogen (resting) phase for 2 to 4 months and then begin to regrow. Noticeable regrowth is present by 4 months, but the final results may take as long as a year to be fully manifest. The patient, already self-conscious about hair loss, may look worse for up to 4 months. Women have more difficulty getting through this time period, and in addition to using a variety of cosmetic coverups and styling tricks, may need to use a hair prosthesis (wig/weft) for a time. There will be a linear scar at the site of the donor tissue excision that varies from a fine (1- to 2-mm) pencil line to pencil eraser (4- to 5-mm) width. With multiple procedures, scarring may eventually become visible and problematic, requiring scar revision, transplantation, or camouflage tattooing.

Postoperation Complications

The most common complication is the occurrence of variable numbers of inflammatory and noninflammatory lesions (pustules, papules, nodules, and cysts) caused by transplanted tissue becoming trapped beneath the surface in the recipient region. These lesions are usually ingrown hairs or epidermoid cysts formed by buried grafts. They appear 8 to 12 weeks after the surgery and at the same time that normal regrowth occurs. Some lesions resolve spontaneously, some require intralesional Kenalog or incision and drainage. Rarely, a lesion may need to be excised. It is also fairly common to have a small number of grafts extruded in first 24 hours after surgery, with some associated localized bleeding in the recipient site, especially on the vertex. Finally, although most patients heal with 2- to 3-mm scars, some patients heal with wider scars (3 to 4 mm).

Other complications are uncommon or rare. Donor-site complications include (a) infection (0.1%) treated with antibiotics and incision and drainage; (b) keloid/hypertrophic scarring treated with intralesional corticosteroids and/or excision; (c) hematoma formation treated by aspiration or incision and drainage; (d) wound dehiscence/necrosis treated with debridement and antibiotic prophylaxis; (e) persistent neuralgia/neuroma formation treated with intralesional corticosteroids (neuralgia) or excision (neuroma); and (f) arteriovenous fistula formation, which usually resolves spontaneously, but may occasionally require surgical ligation of the feeding vessel.

Recipient site complications include (a) change in hair texture usually characterized as being coarser or "frizzy," which gradually resolves over time; (b) poor graft survival, usually related to problems in tissue handling that cause follicular bulb transection; (c) elevated ("cobblestoning") or depressed ("pitting") grafts that occur when grafts do not fit well into excisional recipient sites or are placed below the surface during implantation. This complication is not seen with smaller grafts placed into incisional recipient sites or is minimal and resolves over time; (d) chronic folliculitis caused by bacterial infection or foreign-body type reaction to "spicules" of transected hair shafts left on/in some grafts; (e) postfrontal tissue/graft necrosis caused by inadequate blood supply to the postfrontal region where "dense packing" of grafts is commonly performed to achieve maximum density; (f) hyperfibrotic frontal ridging caused by an overreaction to larger grafts or, perhaps, spicules of transected hairs associated with these grafts. This reaction has not been reported with single (one- to two-hair) FU grafting in the frontal line.

Postoperation Follow-up Visits

Patients are seen 1 day after the operation for dressing change to a smaller, lighter bandage (or to no bandage at all). Sutures are removed at 14 days. Typical follow-up visits are scheduled for 8 weeks (wound-healing check), 16 weeks (early regrowth check), and 6 to 12 months (variable final visit for photography). Unscheduled visits are usually for ingrown hairs/cysts that need to be incised or excised.

Postoperation Adjunctive Therapy

Most male patients should be on 1 mg of finasteride (Propecia) to slow or prevent further hair loss and thus prevent or delay the need to "chase baldness" with multiple procedures. Sexual side effects (decreased libido/performance) occur in 2% to 4% of patients and are totally reversible if the medication is discontinued. Topical minoxidil (Rogaine) 2% or 5% is also useful to retard hair loss and can be used alone or in combination with finasteride. Even if a patient chooses not to use these medications on a long-term basis, they may be useful in the 6-month postoperation period to assure better recovery from "shock loss"

and as an aid to earlier regrowth of the transplanted hairs. Finally, these medications may prolong the survival of donor hairs taken from the upper border region that could be subject to miniaturization over time. Female patients may be destined to gradually lose hair diffusely throughout their donor areas. This loss may be at least delayed, if not prevented, with long-term medical treatment. Women who may become pregnant should not receive finasteride, but may use minoxidil prior to pregnancy.

TRANSPLANTATION FOR SPIRAL/HELICAL HAIR TEXTURE

Patients of African ancestry with spiral/helical hair texture have generally lower follicular unit densities (0.6 FU/mm^2 vs. 1.0 FU/mm^2). Acute angulation of the follicular stem and bulb make microdissection somewhat more difficult and avoiding bulb transection is more difficult. Leaving more nonfollicular tissue around the follicular unit will usually correct this problem. However, this also means that larger recipient sites may be needed. In addition, many female patients with this hair texture have fibrotic recipient sites as a result of traction alopecia caused by prolonged use of mechanical and/or chemical hair control measures. Excisional instruments are often needed for recipient site preparation in these type of scalps (Fig. 56.8). Although it is more difficult to obtain high density in a single transplant session in such patients, the multidirectionality of the transplanted hairs compensates to some extent for the lower density.

RECONSTRUCTIVE AND CORRECTIVE HAIR TRANSPLANTATION

Although the majority of transplants are performed for patients with male- and female-pattern hair loss, the improved transplantation techniques increasingly find application in the field of reconstructive and corrective surgery.

Scarring alopecia resulting from many different causes, such as trauma (e.g., burns, automobile accidents), cosmetic surgery

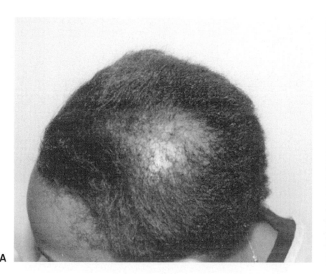
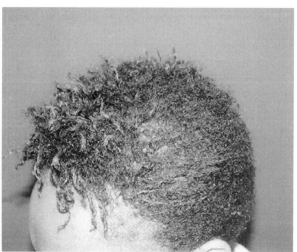

FIGURE 56.8. A: Preoperative patient with helical/spiral hair texture with a 6×8 cm area of traction alopecia. **B:** Same patient, seven months postoperative, after a transplant using the 2.5 mm. Redfield excisional slot punch with 350 grafts.

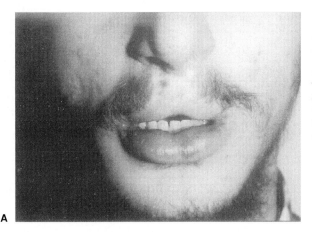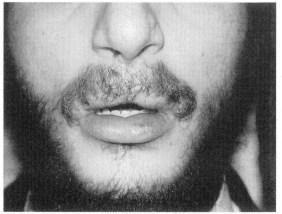

FIGURE 56.9. A: Preoperation photo of patient with cleft lip repair scar resulting in alopecia of the moustache area. **B:** Same patient 7 months after surgery with single-hair grafting from donor hair obtained in the submental region.

(e.g., brow, face lift), inflammatory disease (e.g., lichen planopilaris, discoid lupus), and congenital malformations (e.g., cleft lip repair scars), is correctable by transplantation (Fig. 56.9). In addition, old, large-plug transplants that have become unnatural looking can be "finished" by transplanting follicular units in front and between the larger grafts to disguise them (Fig. 56.10) (8,9). If the old grafts are too low on the forehead they can be punch excised and reimplanted in a better location after being bi- or quadrisected (Fig. 56.11).

Scar tissue is less vascular, more inelastic, and thinner than normal balding scalp. Despite these potential disadvantages, properly placed grafts survive and grow well in scars. It may be advisable to leave slightly larger spaces between the grafts to compensate for the reduced blood supply. In cases where the scar is very thin and "bound down" to the underlying periosteum, the graft may be too long to fit in the thin scar tissue. In this case, an extra step is required prior to graft placement. After making the incision, the operator uses a pair of curved microforceps to bluntly dissect a small "pocket" or "tunnel" extending from the posterior edge of the incision site. This is achieved by inserting the instrument into the incision and pushing the tips between the dermis and the periosteum. The separation is associated with a "popping" sound and the addi-

tional space created allows the graft to be placed deep enough to stay in and survive (Fig. 56.12).

FUTURE HAIR TRANSPLANTATION SURGERY

The idea of obtaining follicular stem cells and using them to create new hair follicles has been around for at least 20 years. The concept is rather simple. First, harvest a small amount of nonbalding scalp normally used in a transplant procedure. Second, microdissect out the stem cells that are responsible for regenerating hair follicles from the telogen (resting) to anagen (growing) phase. Third, multiply these cells in large numbers in vitro (tissue culture). Finally, implant these cells into the balding scalp where they will create new hair follicles that are not subject to the miniaturization process that results in baldness. This procedure would overcome several of the drawbacks that are associated with traditional transplantation, primarily the limited donor supply and scarring from large and multiple donor excisions.

The cells responsible for hair follicle induction are generally believed to be the mesenchymal cells located in either the

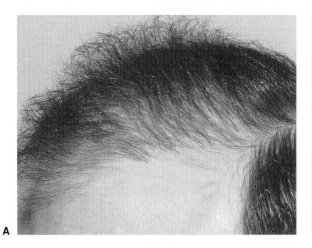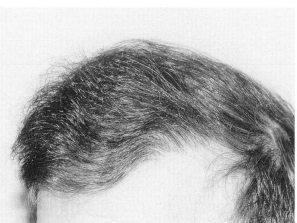

FIGURE 56.10. A: Preoperative patient with unnatural-looking old plug graft transplant. **B:** Postoperative view of patient after correction with single unit micrografting.

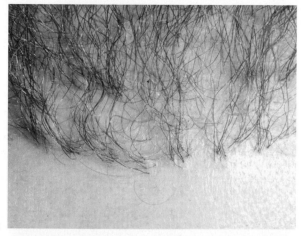

A

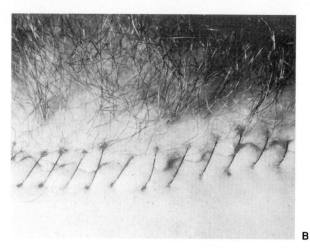

B

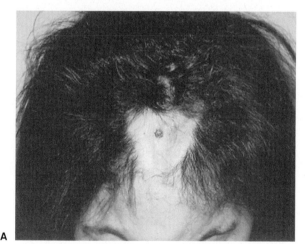

C

FIGURE 56.11. A: Hairline from old, large-plug graft procedure located too low on the forehead prior to repair. **B:** Same patient after excision of plug grafts followed by transverse incisions of scalp between the excisions and a 5-0 running nylon suture. **C:** Same patient after suture removal and reimplantation of plug graft hairs to a better location.

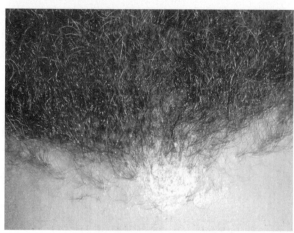

A

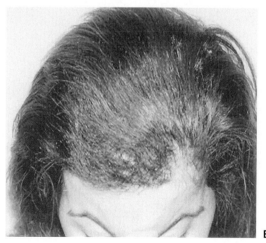

B

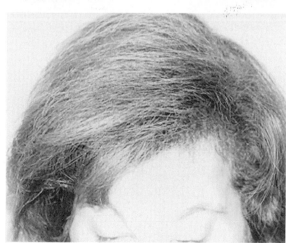

C

FIGURE 56.12. A: Preoperative view of severe scarring alopecia resulting from complication after plastic surgery correction of a congenital defect. **B:** Same patient 6 months after surgery after transplantation with 600 1.5-mm tribevel Starr punch incisions with three to five hairs per graft. **C:** Same patient 6 months after second procedure to increase density.

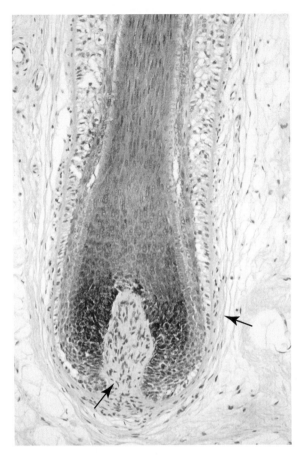

FIGURE 56.13. Photomicrograph of follicular bulb area showing the spade-shaped dermal papilla, which is continuous with the dermal sheath surrounding the lower portion of the bulb area.

by exposing the cells to epithelial germinative cells from the follicular bulb (11). Dermal sheath cells were shown to induce hair follicles when implanted into forearm skin of a female subject using tissue from an unrelated male donor (12). This use of allogeneic (nonself) cells rather than autologous (self) material reveals that mesenchymal stem cells probably lack surface markers that would cause an immunologic response. Thus, they may be "immunologically privileged." If this is true, it may be possible (if not desirable) to obtain stem cells from one individual for use in another.

Other concerns include whether or not the hair produced by this technology will be cosmetically acceptable and whether such "biologic therapy" will be safe and able to pass the rigorous standards required by the U.S. Food and Drug Administration. Much of the present research is being conducted in a clandestine manner to protect "intellectual property" (i.e., profitability). Nevertheless, it seems likely that the "breakthrough" will occur in this generation, which could make present transplantation methods suddenly obsolete.

References

1. Cooley J. Follicular cell implantation: an update on "hair follicle cloning." *Hair Transpl Forum Int.* 2004;14:51–52.
2. Headington JP. Transverse microscopic anatomy of the human scalp. *Arch Dermatol.* 1984;120:449–456.
3. Alopecia reduction and flaps. In: Unger AP, Shapiro R, eds. *Hair Transplantation,* 4th ed. 709–830.
4. Rassman W, et al. *Dermatol Surg.* 2002;28(8):720–728.
5. Rassman W. Follicular unit extraction. *Hair Transpl Forum Int.* 2004;14(1):9.
6. Unger W. Whatever happened to lasers? *Hair Transpl Forum Int.* 2003;13(2):285, 292–293.
7. Stough D. Methodology of follicular unit hair transplantation. *Dermatol Clin.* 1999;17(2):297–306.
8. Bernstein R, et al. The art of repair in surgical hair restoration. Part I: basic repair strategies. *Dermatol Surg.* 2002;28:783–794.
9. Bernstein R, et al. The art of repair in surgical hair restoration. Part II: the tactics of repair. *Dermatol Surg.* 2002;28:873–893.
10. Jahoda, CAB, Reynolds, AJ, Oliver RF. Induction hair growth in ear wounds by cultured dermal papilla cells. *J Invest Dermatol.* 1993;101:584–590.
11. Jahoda CAB, Reynolds AJ. Hair matrix germinative epidermal cells confer follicle-inducing capabilities on dermal sheaths and high passage papilla cells. *Development.* 1996;122:3085–3094.
12. Reynolds AJ, Lawrence. Trans-gender induction of hair follicles. *Nature.* 1999;402:33–34.

dermal papilla or the dermal sheath that is continuous with it (Fig. 56.13). Hair follicles have been induced in rats using cultured dermal papillae (10). However, a major problem has been that cultured cells seem to lose their ability to induce follicles after several passages in vitro. This problem may be overcome

CHAPTER 57 ■ AUGMENTATION MAMMOPLASTY AND ITS COMPLICATIONS

SUMNER A. SLAVIN AND ARIN K. GREENE

No procedure in plastic surgery has been the subject of greater scrutiny and controversy, both scientific and political, than breast augmentation. More than 2 million American women, or 1% of the adult female population, have breast implants. Augmentation mammoplasty is the second most commonly performed cosmetic surgical procedure in the United States, after suction-assisted lipectomy. In 2004, 264,041 patients underwent augmentation mammoplasty. The annual number of breast augmentations has grown exponentially, increasing 676% between 1992 and 2004. Women between the ages of 19 and 34 years old are the largest consumers of cosmetic breast implants (50%), followed by women ages 35 to 50 years (42%).

The history of augmentation mammoplasty reflects the search for the ideal implantable material, commencing with 19th century attempts to transplant lipomas into breast defects, followed by the modern era of polymer-based devices. Medical-grade silicone implants became popular after the earlier success of polyvinyl sponge-based implants, known by the trade name Ivalon. Liquid silicone injections were popularized during World War II and afterward in the Far East, but were later banned in the United States because of a high complication rate characterized by recurrent infections, chronic drainage, and granuloma formation.

When Cronin and Gerow introduced new, "natural feel" prostheses in 1963, their innovative solid-shell elastomeric device with a gel-filled interior became the prototype for all future devices, including the saline-filled implants. The modern mammary prosthesis is actually a mixture of polymers comprised principally of polydimethylsiloxane that can exist in the form of a solid, liquid, or gel. With the exception of substituting saline for the original silicone gel component, the only attempted modification of the silicone implant elastomeric shell was the addition of an exterior polyurethane coating. However, reports of the carcinogenic breakdown products of polyurethane raised serious health concerns, especially when two specific compounds—toluene 2,4-diisocyanate and toluene 2,6-diisocyanate diamine—were subsequently linked to sarcoma formation in rats. Despite an absence of epidemiologic data connecting polyurethane to an increased incidence of cancer (and to breast cancer in particular) in humans, the Food and Drug Administration (FDA) moved to ban all polyurethane-coated implants from the marketplace in 1991. This edict affected approximately 10% of all breast implant patients (about 200,000 women).

GOVERNMENT REGULATION

Few areas of surgery have received greater focus from the government than augmentation mammoplasty. Over the last several years, the FDA hearings regarding the approval of saline and silicone breast implants have received extensive media attention. In 1976, the United States Congress passed the Federal Safe Devices Act, which empowered the FDA to regulate medical devices. Because breast implants were developed prior to 1976, they were "grandfathered" and thus not subjected to FDA approval. However, after reports appeared in the literature in the 1980s describing women with breast implants and connective tissue disorders, the government actively began to investigate the safety of breast implants. Specific concerns of carcinogenicity, autoimmune diseases, product failure, and impaired mammographic evaluation led to a moratorium on the use of all silicone gel implants by the FDA in 1992 (1). Since then saline implants have been available without restriction, and were officially approved by the FDA in 2000. Silicone gel-filled implants, however, have been limited to clinical studies involving both postmastectomy reconstruction and breast augmentation.

After banning silicone breast implants in 1992, the government urged plastic surgeons to produce studies validating both the safety and patient satisfaction with breast implants. In response, one study of 112 women demonstrated improved self-image, decreased self-consciousness, and heightened self-confidence. Overall satisfaction rates approached 86% (2). **Since the moratorium on silicone breast implants, several studies have proved that these devices are safe and do not cause connective tissue disease, malignancy, or risk to breast-feeding infants.**

Although an association between breast implants and systemic disease was disproved, concerns about local complications of silicone implants remained. Specifically, silicone implants were felt to have high rates of capsular contracture, rupture, and infection. However, in April 2005, the results of the prospective Core Study, with a 3-year follow-up of 551 patients after breast augmentation, showed that silicone breast implants do not cause significant local complications. As a result, 13 years after the moratorium on silicone breast implants, the FDA advisory panel recommended approval for Mentor Corporation's silicone breast prosthesis. The FDA has accepted the recommendations of its advisory panel with conditions that had not yet been made public at the time of this writing.

ANATOMIC CONSIDERATIONS

The breast is supplied by a vascular network consisting of perforating branches of the intercostal, internal mammary, lateral thoracic, and thoracoacromial arterial trunks. As a result, devascularization of breast glandular or cutaneous tissues during augmentation mammoplasty is improbable, regardless of incisional site or whether a subglandular or subpectoral position has been chosen.

Sensory supply of the breast is far more vulnerable because there are fewer sources of innervation. Sensation is provided chiefly by branches of the fourth (and sometimes the fifth) anterolateral intercostal nerve. To a lesser extent, anteromedial branches of the fourth and fifth intercostal nerves also contribute to sensation of the breast. **Inframammary and periareolar incisions are more likely to result in injury to these intercostal nerves, especially in the area outside the lateral border of the pectoralis major muscle, whereas transaxillary placement can injure the intercostobrachial nerve (second intercostal nerve) as it traverses the axilla posterior to the usual site of incision.** Loss of intercostal innervation of the nipple produces hypoesthesia of varying degrees, or hyperesthesia, depending on the severity of the injury to the nerve. Axillary and posteromedial anesthesia of the upper arm can develop after trauma to the intercostobrachial nerve.

SURGICAL TECHNIQUE

Four separate incisional sites—inframammary, periareolar, axillary, and transumbilical—have been used for placement of breast prostheses (Fig. 57.1). Each location has its advantages and disadvantages, depending on the individual surgeon's experience and the positioning of the implant in either a subglandular, subpectoral, or the more recently described "dual-plane" position (3). Inframammary crease incisions are preferred for patients with a well-developed crease that conceals the scar, particularly when it is placed slightly above the crease on the breast surface. This approach may be suboptimal when the integrity of the inframammary crease ligament has been compromised.

In general, the periareolar incision provides excellent access to all portions of the breast. For patients willing to accept a scar on the breast surface, this approach permits meticulous positioning of the implant, particularly along the lower pole. Exposure of the inframammary ligament is excellent with this incision when either lowering of the inframammary crease or reconstruction of supporting ligaments is necessary. Transection of breast ductal tissues is required, however, before the pectoralis major muscle is identified. If subpectoral augmentation is chosen, the pectoralis major muscle is either divided along the obliquity of its fibers or the lateral border of the muscle is elevated. Although unfavorable healing can occur at any operative site, the periareolar incision tends to heal with minimal scarring. The periareolar incision facilitates revisional procedures because it allows easier access to all portions of the breast for capsulorrhaphy or capsulectomy. In addition, the incision may be incorporated into future periareolar mastopexy designs for ptosis as the patient ages.

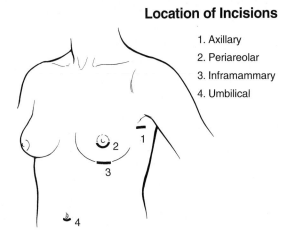

Location of Incisions

1. Axillary
2. Periareolar
3. Inframammary
4. Umbilical

FIGURE 57.1. Four different incisional sites have been used for breast augmentation. The transaxillary approach has gained in popularity with the introduction of endoscopically guided placement.

ENDOSCOPIC APPLICATIONS IN AUGMENTATION MAMMOPLASTY

Although the transaxillary technique of subpectoral augmentation has been available for many years, critics have observed difficulty in attaining precise positioning of the implant in the lower pole of the breast. Major advantages have been the absence of any scar on the breast surface, an avoidance of breast ductal transection, and a low probability of sensory nerve injury. One disadvantage of this technique is a minor risk of trauma to the intercostobrachial nerve. Just as minimally invasive surgical techniques have revolutionized the performance of many procedures, endoscopic assistance has enhanced the transaxillary approach by allowing a more accurate placement of the breast implant inferiorly and improved control of the inframammary crease. For the majority of patients, the procedure can be performed through a 2.5- to 3.0-cm incision along the lower axillary crease at the junction of hair-bearing and non–hair-bearing skin (Fig. 57.2). Following blunt dissection at the lateral border of the pectoralis major muscle, the subpectoral space is dissected digitally and with specialized curved retractors similar to a uterine sound. Introduction of a 10-mm 30-degree endoscope expedites division of fibers of the origin of the pectoralis major muscle along the medial and inferior borders of the breast. Scrupulous avoidance of muscle division laterally (at the 6 o'clock to 9 o'clock position on the right and from 3 o'clock to 6 o'clock on the left) protects the intercostal sensory nerve branches.

Because of the short length of the axillary incision and its distance from the inframammary crease, it is necessary to deflate and fold the saline implant envelope to create a more rigid and tubular structure before insertion, maintaining the fill tube within the plug-and-strap mechanism of the valve. As the device is filled, it can be positioned bluntly. Hemorrhage that cannot be controlled with specialized endoscopic cautery instruments necessitates conversion to a periareolar incision for more direct open access. Endoscopic transaxillary augmentation mammoplasty usually is performed under general anesthesia because of the necessary blunt elevation and sharp separation of the pectoralis major muscle from its attachments. Meticulous preoperative marking of the breasts is extremely important for accuracy of implant placement and breast symmetry. Implant exchange, capsulorrhaphy, and capsulotomy to treat implant-related complications also can be performed with this technique.

Consistent with the concept of minimal scarring, transumbilical augmentation mammoplasty offers an alternate site for placement of saline implants. Using a single infraumbilical incision, this technique uses endoscopic visualization to create a long, subcutaneous tunnel up to the inferior border of the breast, followed by subglandular dissection. Circuitous as it may seem, the technique appears to achieve an accurate subglandular placement of a mammary prosthesis. Although subpectoral placement has been reported with this technique, this approach has not gained wider acceptance because it is more difficult to place implants submuscularly using this incision compared to other approaches. This is a major disadvantage given the preference to place saline implants subpectorally because of their tendency to ripple.

SALINE IMPLANTS

Since silicone gel implants were banned by the FDA in 1992, saline implants have been available for both cosmetic and reconstructive breast surgery. In 1989, the FDA classified saline

Technique of Endoscopic Transaxillary Subpectoral Augmentation Mammaplasty

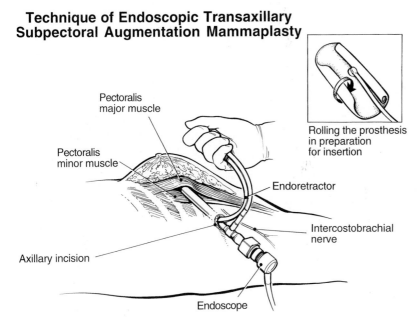

FIGURE 57.2. Endoscopic elevation and division of pectoralis major muscle fibers assist the accuracy of positioning near the lower pole and inframammary crease areas of the breast.

breast prostheses as a class III device, the category designated for implantable devices that lack sufficient data to demonstrate safety and efficacy. As a result of this ruling, saline implants underwent extensive governmental and scientific scrutiny. Satisfied that study enrollment levels were met by organized plastic surgery in 1995, the FDA allowed the continued unrestricted use of saline implants until they were formally approved in 2000.

An elastomeric solid shell of silicone surrounding a hollow interior is the principal design of current models. **Textured implants have been added in an effort to diminish encapsulation, but all available data indicates that smooth-walled saline implants are as efficacious as textured devices in reducing capsular contracture.**

Because of numerous reports documenting the frequency and severity of encapsulation associated with the use of silicone gel devices, saline implants became an alternative choice with a purported benefit of a lower encapsulation rate. However, an unacceptably high incidence of deflation (approaching 78%) was observed in earlier model devices. Manufacturers altered the design of the implant contour, shell thickness, and valve in an effort to produce a safer device with a low deflation rate. Possible causes of deflation include manufacturing defects, fold flaw failure, encapsulation, capsulectomy, and iatrogenic errors. Fold flaw failure may be the most common mechanism of product failure because most of the defects in the structural integrity of saline implants have been identified adjacent to a fold in the elastomeric shell. Presumably, friction at the fold produces a small opening that allows saline to leak. Valvular failure has been attributed to fibrous tissue ingrowth, resulting in incontinence and subclinical or total deflation. Like any water-filled device, saline implants manifest surface irregularities characterized by waves and ripples. These surface features can be visible clinically, particularly when soft-tissue coverage is inadequate. To avoid this problem, subpectoral placement has been promoted, along with complete filling of the implant. Still newer models have anatomic designs that mimic the lower pole curvature and upper pole fullness of normal breast anatomy and may cause less rippling.

Current saline breast implants have a very low spontaneous deflation rate. **A multicenter retrospective review used for premarket approval of saline breast implants showed an overall spontaneous deflation rate of 4.3% after 13 years (4).** The actu-arial implant survival, excluding trauma, was 97.9% to 99.5% at 10 years. A risk factor for implant deflation was implant size greater than 450 cm^3. Implant position and underfilling did not influence the deflation rate. **Other studies, however, have found that underfilling the implant by more than 25 cm^3 significantly increases the risk of implant rupture.** Although intraluminal antibiotics and steroids reduce capsular contracture, they also increase the risk of implant deflation and are associated with atrophy of overlying soft tissues.

SILICONE GEL IMPLANTS

Silicone, a polymer of dimethylsiloxane, is present throughout nature. Silicone is also found in medications, syringes, heart valves, instruments, and numerous types of implantable devices. The longer the polymer chain of silicone, the greater the viscosity. Both saline implants and silicone implants have an outer shell made of silicone. The first-generation of silicone implants had thick walls and viscous gel, and suffered from high rates of contracture. To reduce the incidence of contracture, second-generation silicone implants developed during the 1970s were designed with thinner shells and a gel of lower viscosity. These implants, however, were found to have high rupture and bleed rates. Third-generation silicone gel implants, developed in the late 1980s, used a thicker shell, a gel of higher viscosity, and a silicone barrier coating on the inner surface of the envelope to decrease silicone bleed and capsule formation. Current fourth-generation silicone implants were developed in the mid 1990s and are similar to the third-generation implants but have high gel cohesiveness that limits silicone leak in the event of implant rupture. Although available in other parts of the world, fourth-generation silicone implants may only be used in the United States under FDA-approved experimental protocols.

In contrast to saline implants, rupture of silicone breast implants is often silent because most ruptures are intracapsular. Mentor Corporation's Core Study presentation to the FDA in April 2005 showed a low rupture rate with current-generation gel implants used in the United States. **Using magnetic resonance imaging (MRI), Mentor found a silent rupture rate of 0.5% 3 years after augmentation.** Because the rupture rate increases significantly with age, current-generation gel implants imaged prospectively by serial MRI in Danish women have an estimated 15% risk of rupture at 10 years (5). **Although closed capsulotomy significantly increases the risk of gel rupture and should not be performed, implant position does not affect the rupture rate.**

AUTOLOGOUS AUGMENTATION

Although much attention has been directed toward the FDA approval process for silicone gel breast implants, several authors have recently described autologous breast augmentation. Autologous tissue eliminates the risk of implant deflation, contracture, infection, exposure, and, ultimately, exchange or removal. However, autologous augmentation has not yet gained wide popularity because of increased operative complexity, donor-site complications and scarring, prolonged recovery, and risk of flap failure.

Potential candidates for autologous augmentation include patients unable to have a breast implant, patients after explantation of implants because of complications, or women desiring either abdominal or gluteal contouring in addition to breast augmentation. De-epithelialized pedicled transverse rectus abdominis musculocutaneous (TRAM) flaps have been used for breast augmentation following abdominoplasty. Local perforator flaps from the lateral chest wall also can be used to augment the breasts, which is particularly advantageous when combined with contour surgery in the bariatric patient. Free perforator flaps have been described as potential donors for autologous augmentation. Specifically, deep inferior epigastric perforator (DIEP), superior gluteal artery perforator (S-GAP), and superficial inferior epigastric artery (SIEA) perforator flaps have been used to augment the breast in patients who desired simultaneous excision of abdominal or gluteal tissue.

OVERVIEW OF LOCAL COMPLICATIONS

Although much interest has been focused on controversial complications associated with breast augmentation such as capsular contracture or autoimmune diseases, it is important not to ignore the ordinary problems that can occur, including hypertrophic scarring (6.3%), infection (0.5%), hematoma (2% to 3%), and seroma (0% to 1%) (4). **Hematoma increases infection rates and frequently leads to capsular contracture. Changes in nipple sensation are estimated to occur in 10% of women after augmentation mammoplasty.** Injury to the lateral branch of the fourth intercostal nerve may be reduced with submuscular implant placement.

Infection may cause the loss of an implant, either because the device extrudes through a dehisced wound or because removal is necessary for treatment of the infection. Rates of infection for both saline and silicone breast implants are low, ranging from 0.5% to 2.0% (4). Because the lactiferous ducts are in continuity with the skin, they contain bacteria. The most common normal inhabitant is *Staphylococcus epidermidis; Propionibacterium acnes* is the most frequent nonpathogenic anaerobe; and **Staphylococcus aureus is the pathogen usually responsible for implant infection.** A consensus does not exist regarding the influence of open versus closed filling systems on the infection rate of saline implants.

Management of infection depends on severity and the presence of exposure. Mild infections without implant exposure sometimes can be successfully treated with antibiotics alone.

The most conservative approach for more severe infections or threatened exposure is antibiotic therapy and explantation. However, successful salvage of infected or exposed implants has been described; that is, antibiotic therapy, debridement, capsulectomy, device exchange, primary closure, or flap coverage. In cases of severe infection, the implants cannot be salvaged.

Uncommon complications of augmentation mammoplasty include galactorrhea and Mondor disease. Galactorrhea appears to be activated by injury or irritation of thoracic nerves, and in rare instances, can cause a galactocele. Treatment of galactorrhea includes bromocriptine or intercostal blocks. Mondor disease can occur after many types of breast operations. It is caused by thrombosis of veins along the inferior aspect of the breast, resulting in firm cords that are palpable and tender. This problem resolves spontaneously but can be treated on a symptomatic basis with warm compresses and salicylates.

CAPSULAR CONTRACTURE

Encapsulation of any breast prosthesis resulting in a firm fibrous periprosthetic shell, or capsular contracture, is the most common complication reported after breast enlargement, occurring in 50% or more patients, depending on the system of grading and the clinical experience of the surgeon (Fig. 57.3). **Baker's classification of capsular contracture, modified to include the results of prosthetic breast reconstruction, is used widely for assessment of clinical firmness following breast enlargement (Table 57.1). This system of classification is subjective, but it identifies both ideal and unfavorable results (6).**

Multiple causes of clinically evident capsular contracture have been suggested, including migration of silicone gel molecules across the elastomeric outer envelope, foreign-body reaction, autoimmune–connective tissue disorders, a genetic predisposition to form encapsulation, infection or contamination by bacteria, hematoma, and the surface characteristics of the prosthesis. At the cellular level, abnormal fibroblast activity stimulated by a foreign body and a ubiquitous presence of *S. epidermidis* are popular explanations but unproven causes of fibrous contracture. A prospective, blinded study showed that *S. epidermidis* was significantly associated with capsular contracture. *S. epidermidis* was present in 90% of implants removed for Baker grade III or IV contracture, compared to 12% of implants removed for reasons other than contracture (7).

Recent multicenter data showed a 20.4% rate of significant capsular contracture (Baker grade III or IV) 13 years after placement of saline implants (4). Although silicone gel implants have historically had higher capsular contracture rates than saline implants, current-generation silicone implants appear to have a similar risk of contracture compared to saline implants. Several studies suggest that submuscular placement, implant size smaller than 350 cm^3, and no drainage of the implant cavity reduce the risk of capsular contracture.

Textured implants have shown no advantage. There is no difference in the incidence of contracture between textured and smooth implants. Textured implants do have disadvantages, however, as they are associated with higher rates of rupture, rippling, and malposition.

Although the use of textured versus smooth implants remains controversial, there is general agreement that the incidence of severe capsular contracture is reduced by subpectoral placement, regardless of implant texture. Submuscular placement may protect against capsular contracture because the pectoralis muscle moves the implant in the pocket during regular

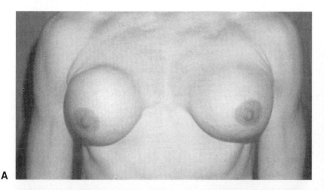

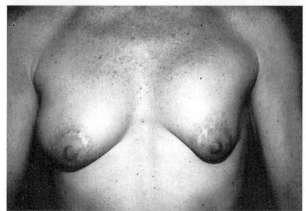

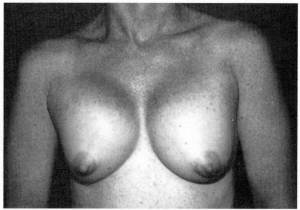

FIGURE 57.3. Capsular contracture. **A:** Bilateral Baker IV contracture, worse on right side, with marked upper pole fullness in a patient with silicone gel implants. **B:** Bilateral capsular contractures with superiorly retracted implants causing upper pole fullness and lack of inferior pole contour. **C:** Capsular contracture of a ruptured left silicone breast implant. Intracapsular versus extracapsular rupture may be difficult to determine from either the appearance of the breast or the physical findings.

activity. A second hypothesis is that the pectoralis major muscle serves as a protective barrier to bacterial contamination from the nipple and is more resistant to infection compared to skin flaps. It may be the muscle simply disguises the capsule because it is one more tissue layer covering the implant.

In a rare consensus, antibiotic therapy in the form of systemic administration and local irrigation is emphasized as a method of encapsulation prevention. In 2000, the FDA warned against breast implant contact with Betadine because of concerns about shell weakening. In response, washing the implant and pocket with a combination of bacitracin, cefazolin, and gentamicin was recommended as a substitute for Betadine (8). A second commonly used strategy to reduce capsular contracture involves moving the implant each day to maintain the pocket size and prevent the developing capsule from tightening around the implant.

Calcification can occur within the fibrous capsule of both silicone and saline breast implants, and is related to the du-

ration of implantation. Calcification is rare before 10 years, but 100% of implant capsules will have calcification after 23 years (9). Calcium adds to implant firmness and complicates the interpretation of mammography. Most mammographers, however, can distinguish accurately between the malignant calcifications of breast cancer and the benign calcifications in the scar tissue surrounding an implant. As a result, pericapsular calcifications do not increase the risk of having a false-positive mammogram (10).

Treatment of Capsular Contracture

Women with Baker grade III or IV capsular contracture often require treatment. Closed capsulotomy can improve capsular contracture, even to a Baker grade I contracture. However, several authors have noted a high recurrence rate following closed capsulotomy. In addition, a significant risk of implant rupture, displacement, or hematoma with this technique exists. **Because of the high recurrence and complication rates following closed capsulotomy, the Institute of Medicine of the National Academies of Science does not recommend closed capsulotomy to treat capsular contracture.**

Open capsulotomy or capsulectomy is the treatment of choice for symptomatic capsular contracture. However, a consensus does not exist about the role for capsulotomy versus capsulectomy. Although capsulectomy has a lower recurrence rate compared to capsulotomy, capsulectomy is a more difficult procedure and thus more likely to be associated with complications. Reasonable indications for capsulectomy include a calcified capsule, removal of a ruptured silicone implant, implant infection, explantation, severe contracture (Baker grades III or IV), or implant placement in another location (11).

TABLE 57.1

ORIGINAL BAKER CLASSIFICATION OF CAPSULAR
CONTRACTURE AFTER AUGMENTATION
MAMMOPLASTY

Class I	Breast absolutely natural; no one could tell breast was augmented
Class II	Minimal contracture; I can tell surgery was performed, but patient has no complaint
Class III	Moderate contracture; patient feels some firmness
Class IV	Severe contracture; obvious just from observation

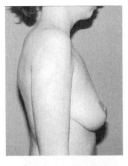

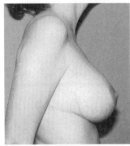

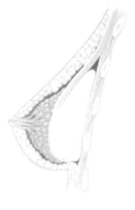

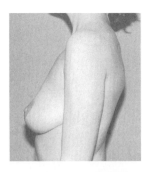

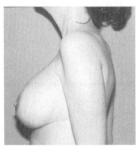

FIGURE 57.4. Moderate pseudoptosis corrected by augmentation mammoplasty using a dual-plane approach.

A more recent method of correcting capsular contracture involves repositioning the implant in a dual plane. In this technique, a capsulectomy is performed followed by elevation of the inferior border of the pectoralis major muscle. Approximately the superior two-thirds of the implant is placed submuscularly, while the inferior one-third of the implant is located in a subglandular position (Fig. 57.4).

AUTOIMMUNE AND CONNECTIVE TISSUES DISORDERS

Numerous case reports in the 1980s appeared to suggest a linkage between silicone gel implants and connective tissue diseases and symptoms. The principal connective tissue disorders included scleroderma, rheumatoid arthritis, systemic lupus erythematosus, Sjögren syndrome, dermatomyositis, polymyositis, and polymyalgia rheumatica. In response to these reports, a number of large, population-based retrospective studies were conducted to test the association between silicone breast implants and connective tissue disorders. Although the details of these studies are beyond the scope of this chapter, all studies have concluded that there is no association between silicone breast implants and any connective tissue disease (12).

SILICONE EFFECTS ON PREGNANCY, LACTATION, AND BREAST-FED CHILDREN

Currently, there is no scientific evidence that silicone is a mutagen or teratogen. Implants do not interfere with lactation or increase the amount of silicone in breast milk over baseline levels present in women without implants. In fact, cow's milk and infant formulas contain much greater amounts of silicone than an augmented mother's milk. Clinical studies conducted by the British Department of Health and the Institute of Medicine of the National Academy of Sciences both demonstrate that silicone breast implants are safe for pregnancy, lactation, and breast-feeding.

CARCINOGENESIS

Two large epidemiologic studies have examined the subsequent risk of breast cancer following augmentation: one based on an implant cohort of 11,676 women in Alberta, Canada, who were followed for 13 years, and a second study in Los Angeles with patients who had had a median of 15.5 years of silicone implant exposure (13,14). These studies concluded that a *lower* incidence of breast carcinoma was found in augmented patients than in nonimplanted control subjects. Similarly, animal studies also have failed to document an increased incidence of carcinoma after silicone implantation.

One possible explanation for the lower risk of breast cancer in augmented women is that augmented women have less volume in which to develop cancer compared to nonaugmented women. A second hypothesis for low rates of breast cancer in augmented women is that silicone may mediate a biologic protective effect against breast cancer.

DETECTION OF BREAST CANCER AND SURVIVAL IN AUGMENTED WOMEN

Do women with breast implants who are subsequently diagnosed with breast cancer suffer any delay in diagnosis or have a worse prognosis as compared to breast cancer patients without implants? This important question was raised because implants can obscure mammary lesions on mammography or make physical examination of the breast more difficult. These concerns about mammographic accuracy are especially serious in view of the 13.5% lifetime breast cancer rate observed among white patients in the United States, who also constitute the majority of implant patients. Similar concerns have been cited repeatedly by the FDA during its investigation into the safety of breast implants.

Because saline implants also are relatively radiopaque on mammographic examination (although more radiotransparent than gel devices), these concerns have not abated with the widespread use of saline breast prostheses. The possibility of a missed lesion, hidden by an implant, could lead to a delay in diagnosis and a less-favorable survival. **As an outgrowth of these concerns, the American College of Radiology recommends that women with breast implants should not only follow the same screening schedule as those without implants, but also should be evaluated only at accredited mammographic facilities experienced with the special needs of this patient group. In addition, mammography is recommended for women older than 30 years of age before and after augmentation.**

Although it has been demonstrated that standard mammography shows 56% and 75% of breast parenchyma in subglandular and subpectoral implants, respectively, Eklund et al. recommended four additional "push-back" or displacement views be taken to improve visualization of the entire mammary glandular tissues (15). The Eklund views increased the amount of breast tissue capable of visualization to 64% and 85% in subglandular and submuscular implants, respectively. In asymptomatic women, screening mammography using Eklund views has a lower sensitivity in augmented women (45%) compared to nonaugmented women (66%) (10). Specificity, however, is approximately the same for asymptomatic augmented and nonaugmented women (96% to 97%). Similar trends are found with mammography among symptomatic women. Mammogram sensitivity and specificity for symptomatic women is 73% and 86%, respectively, for women with breast implants, compared to 81% and 87%, respectively, for women without breast implants (10). In addition to mammography technique, the severity of encapsulation and location of the implant also influence the amount of breast tissue visualized by mammography. A Baker III or IV capsular contracture reduces the amount of breast tissue to be evaluated by mammography by 50%. Subglandular implant placement increases the amount of obscured breast tissue with the Eklund technique from 15% in submuscular implants to 36%.

Despite the potential interference of breast cancer detection posed by implants, breast implants do not adversely affect breast cancer detection, stage of diagnosis, or survival. A large study in Alberta, Canada investigated 13,246 patients with breast cancer (16). The authors found no difference in the 5- and 10-year survival rates of augmented and nonaugmented patients. Although the tumors were smaller in the augmented group, nodal and distant metastases were similar, as were histologic types of the tumors. Of special interest, all of the breast cancers diagnosed in the augmented population were carcinomas rather than the sarcomas observed previously in implanted animals. A study of the Danish Cancer Registry also concluded that women with and without silicone breast implants were diagnosed with breast cancer at the same stage and had similar survival rates.

A recent prospective study showed that in asymptomatic augmented women, cancer stage, tumor size, nodal status, and estrogen-receptor status were the same as for nonaugmented women (10). In symptomatic women, the augmentation cohort had *smaller* tumor size, lower grade, and greater estrogen receptor-positive status than the nonaugmented group. Augmented women with breast cancer may have superior prognostic factors because of their reduced autologous breast volume. In addition, augmented patients may be more aware of their breast composition or more compliant with breast screening than nonaugmented women. Finally, breast implants may facilitate physical exam detection of breast masses by providing a firm background for palpation (10).

MANAGEMENT OF AUGMENTED WOMEN WITH BREAST CANCER

Because 50% of breast cancer affects women older than 65 years of age, the prevalence of breast cancer will continue to increase as the population of the United States ages. Because the rate of breast augmentation is also rapidly rising, an exponential increase in the diagnosis of breast cancer in augmented women will occur in the future. **For those women who develop breast cancer in a breast that contains an implant, breast-conservation therapy is not recommended.** The majority of women with implants treated with lumpectomy and radiation will develop complications. Capsular contracture alone has been documented in as many as 65% of augmented women who received conservation therapy for breast cancer. Fifty percent of augmented women after conservation therapy ultimately have completion mastectomy and explantation as a consequence of complications, inability to obtain negative margins, or local recurrence. Although the overall local recurrence rate for breast cancer is 1% per year, some studies suggest that it may be higher in augmented women after conservation therapy.

Conservation therapy in augmented women is also problematic for future tumor surveillance. Women with breast cancer are not only at risk for local recurrence, but they have a significantly higher likelihood of developing a second cancer in the same breast or a tumor in the opposite breast. Screening mammography in augmented women after conservation therapy is difficult because it is known that the implant reduces the amount of breast parenchyma visualized on mammogram. In addition, the resulting capsular contracture from the radiation treatment further reduces the accuracy of mammography. **Thus conservation therapy in augmented women creates a cohort with a high risk of future breast cancer and serious handicaps to adequate mammography.**

In addition to radiation complications, difficulty obtaining clear margins, and a high recurrence rate, breast conservation in augmented women also is a poor choice because these women have a higher likelihood of a poor aesthetic outcome compared to nonaugmented patients. Patients with breast implants have small native breast volume and thin skin as a result of implant expansion. Consequently, lumpectomy in these women is more likely to result in significant breast deformity. In addition to the low lumpectomy-to-breast-volume ratio in augmented women, radiation therapy also contributes to a poor aesthetic outcome. The high rate of capsular contracture has caused as many as 100% of patients to end their treatment with a fair or poor cosmetic result. Women with a large amount of breast parenchyma may achieve a satisfactory outcome with explantation, mastopexy, and conservation therapy. **However, the safest and most aesthetically acceptable treatment of breast cancer in the majority of augmented women is mastectomy with immediate or delayed reconstruction.**

IMAGING OF BREAST IMPLANTS

Three modalities—mammography, sonography, and MRI—have been used to detect abnormalities of either the implant or its surrounding capsule. MRI is the most accurate and expensive study, with a sensitivity greater than 95% for a ruptured implant. Shell folding ("linguine sign") on MRI indicates a rupture implant (Fig. 57.5). Sonographic signs of implant rupture include the "snowstorm" appearance of free silicone in the breast tissue or the "stepladder" sign of linear echoes. Because significant contracture reduces the sensitivity of ultrasonography, MRI is the radiographic study of choice to determine implant rupture in patients with Baker III or IV contracture.

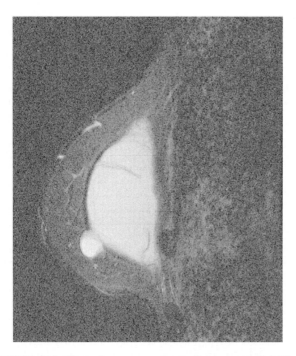

FIGURE 57.5. Magnetic resonance image illustrating shell folding ("linguine sign") and extracapsular rupture of a silicone implant.

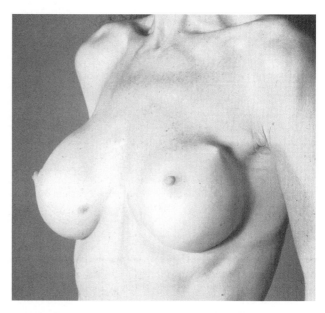

FIGURE 57.6. Saline implant protruding through the capsule. This condition can be confused with a breast mass.

AESTHETIC COMPLICATIONS

Implant malposition and an unfavorable shape are the second most common cause, after capsular contracture, of patient dissatisfaction following augmentation mammoplasty (Fig. 57.6). Correction of these types of problems usually involves a combination of techniques, including removal of the implant, capsulotomy, capsulectomy, alteration of the inframammary crease, or selection of a different location. Sometimes, a different size or shape of implant is required. The current availability of both round and more anatomically constructed devices has improved the aesthetic results.

Two problems that have been more refractory to correction are residual ptosis and the double-bubble deformity. Resid-

ual ptosis is best treated by recognition of the relationship of the nipple to the inframammary crease and placement of the implant in a subglandular position. When excess skin is observed, a combined mastopexy and augmentation procedure may be indicated. The double-bubble deformity results from distortion or disruption of the inframammary crease (Fig. 57.7). It is commonly noted after attempted correction of a constricted, tubular breast, but it might also occur after subpectoral placement with elevation of the crease or after disruption of the inframammary ligament and inferior displacement of the prosthesis. Surgical correction involves varying combinations of inframammary crease reconstruction, pectoralis major muscle release, and replacement with a smaller implant. Avoiding an unfavorable cosmetic result requires that special attention be directed at preoperative assessment of breast anatomy because even modest differences in position of the inframammary crease or nipples can be magnified after augmentation.

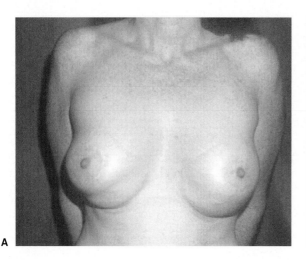

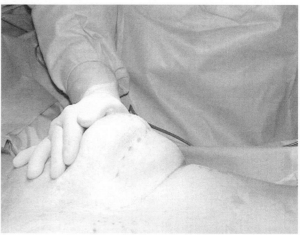

FIGURE 57.7. Double-bubble deformity. **A:** Severe deformity in a patient with saline implants. **B:** Demonstration of deformity at operation, illustrating that the implant transgressed the inframammary crease. **C:** Oblique views of following open repair through a periareolar incision. **D:** Lateral views of postoperative result.

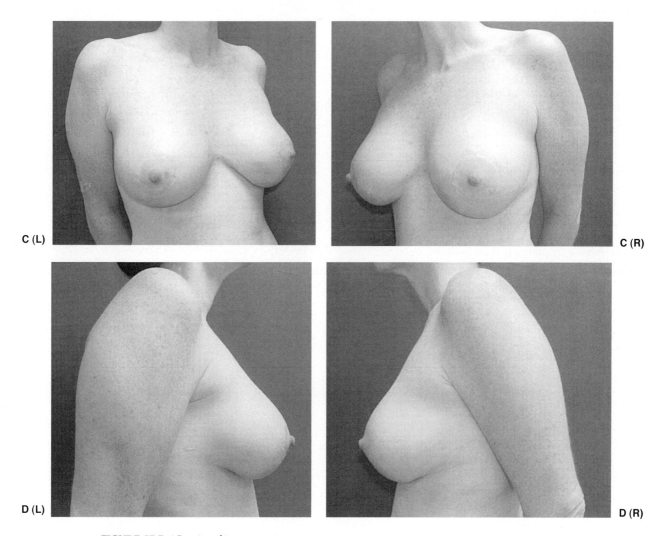

C (L) C (R)

D (L) D (R)

FIGURE 57.7. (*Continued.*)

Rippling is almost always a complication of saline implants, primarily affecting the upper pole. **Risk factors for rippling include underfilling and textured implants.** Textured implants have a greater likelihood of causing traction on the skin because of their increased adherent properties. Prophylactic measures to avoid rippling include using a smooth implant, subpectoral placement, and overfilling the implant. First-line treatment of rippling includes conversion to subpectoral placement if previously subglandular, overfilling the implant, changing from a textured to a smooth implant, or converting a saline to a gel implant. Second-line treatment of rippling includes capsulorrhaphy to suture the ripples or partial capsulectomy to tighten the capsule. Other maneuvers include folding the pectoralis major muscle cephalad to add tissue to the upper pole, placing external bolsters, or using allogenic acellular dermal grafts. Allogenic acellular dermal grafts (AlloDerm), when placed between the implant and skin, can improve rippling. Third-line treatment for severe, refractory rippling necessitates the transfer of healthy, well-vascularized tissue to cover the implant. Local pedicled sources of tissue include muscle or myocutaneous latissimus dorsi or rectus abdominus flaps.

ever, like all cosmetic surgery patients, patients seeking breast augmentation have a higher likelihood of impaired body image compared to the general population. Women interested in augmentation mammoplasty, compared to physically similar women, are more concerned about their appearance, report more frequent teasing, and feel that larger breasts are the ideal breast size. In addition, women interested in breast augmentation are more likely to have used psychotherapy compared to control women with similar-sized breasts (17).

Although augmentation candidates are more likely to have received psychiatric counseling compared to age- and size-matched controls, some reports have found a higher suicide rate among augmented women. However, a link between implants and suicide cannot be substantiated because augmented women, and cosmetic surgery patients in general, have a greater prevalence of psychiatric disease compared to the general population. In addition, several studies have found that women have a significant improvement in body image after breast augmentation. **One interesting report cited an increase in weight among anorexic augmented women, possibly as a consequence of an improved body image after receiving breast implants.**

PSYCHOLOGICAL ISSUES

Patient satisfaction with both saline and silicone breast implants is very high, ranging from 93% to 97% (4). How-

MEDICOLEGAL CONSIDERATIONS

Despite a class action settlement and a corporate agreement to provide $4.2 billion to compensate women who claim that their health was harmed by silicone implants, litigation related to these devices has not spared plastic surgeons from being named as defendants in suits. Surgeons must navigate between product liability and informed consent laws that hold them accountable for a wide array of health issues, proven and alleged. Consequently, one prerequisite for approval of silicone breast implants set forth by the FDA is a strict, standardized, patient education and consent program.

Implant failure or complications create a burden to the patient and thus a potential stimulus for litigation. Currently, both Mentor Corporation and Inamed Corporation will replace deflated implants for the life of the implant with any size or model. In addition, implants from both companies come with either a 5- or 10-year limited warranty that provides $1,200 for surgical expenses not covered by insurance. Extended warranties may be purchased by the patient to cover $2,400 of operating room costs not covered by insurance for 10 years from the time of the augmentation. In addition, these extended warranties also will replace a contralateral implant at no cost.

References

1. Angell M. Breast implants—protection or paternalism? *N Engl Med J.* 1992; 326:1695.
2. Young VL, Nemecek JR, Nemecek DA. The efficacy of breast augmentation: breast size increase, patient satisfaction, and psychological effects. *Plast Reconstr Surg.* 1994;94:959.
3. Tebbetts JB. Dual plane breast augmentation: optimizing implant-soft-tissue relationships in a wide range of breast types. *Plast Reconstr Surg.* 2001;107:1255.
4. Cunningham BL, Lokeh A, Gutowski KA. Saline-filled breast implant safety and efficacy: a multicenter retrospective review. *Plast Reconstr Surg.* 2000;105:2143.
5. Holmich LR, Friis S, Fryzek JP, et al. Incidence of silicone breast implant rupture. *Arch Surg.* 2003;138:801.
6. Spear SL, Baker JL. Classification of capsular contracture after prosthetic breast reconstruction. *Plast Reconstr Surg.* 1995;96:1119.
7. Pajkos A, Deva AK, Vickery K, et al. Detection of subclinical infection in significant breast implant capsules. *Plast Reconstr Surg.* 2003;111:1605.
8. Adams WP, Conner WCH, Barton FE, et al. Optimizing breast-pocket irrigation: the post-Betadine era. *Plast Reconstr Surg.* 2001;107:1596.
9. Peters W, Smith D. Calcification of breast implant capsules: incidence, diagnosis, and contributing factors. *Ann Plast Surg.* 1995;8:34.
10. Miglioretti DL, Rutter CM, Geller BM, et al. Effect of breast augmentation on the accuracy of mammography and cancer characteristics. *JAMA* 2004;291:442.
11. Young VL. Guidelines and indications for breast implant capsulectomy. *Plast Reconstr Surg.* 1998;102:884.
12. Janowsky EC, Kupper LL, Hulka BS. Meta-analysis of the relation between silicone breast implants and the risk of connective tissue diseases. *N Engl Med J.* 2000;342:781.
13. Berkel H, Birdsell DC, Jenkins M. Breast augmentation: a risk factor for breast cancer? *N Engl Med J.* 1992;326:1649.
14. Brody G. Silicone implants and the inhibition of cancer [discussion]. *Plast Reconstr Surg.* 1995;96:519.
15. Eklund GW, Busby RC, Miller SH, et al. Improved imaging of the augmented breast. *AJR Am J Roentgenol.* 1988;151:469.
16. Birdsell DC, Jenkins H, Berkel H. Breast cancer diagnosis and survival in women with and without breast implants. *Plast Reconstr Surg.* 1993;92:795.
17. Sarwer DB, LaRossa D, Bartlett SP, et al. Body image concerns of breast augmentation patients. *Plast Reconstr Surg.* 2003;112:83.

CHAPTER 58 ■ MASTOPEXY AND MASTOPEXY AUGMENTATION

NOLAN S. KARP

Mastopexy is a procedure designed to elevate breast tissue and the nipple–areola complex to correct breast ptosis. Mastopexy procedures are derived from breast-reduction procedures except that only skin is removed with little or no parenchymal resection. Breast-reduction surgery is often performed to relieve neck, back, shoulder, and arm pain. The patient receives significant medical and quality-of-life benefits. Although the appearance of the breast is a factor, the medical benefits are often the primary concern of the patient. Mastopexy is almost always a cosmetic procedure. **Consequently, the trade-offs (i.e., scars) are less well tolerated by the mastopexy patient than by the breast-reduction patient.** Until recently, the predominant scar after breast reduction was the "inverted T" anchor scar. In most cases, breast-reduction patients will tolerate this degree of scarring. The mastopexy patient, for the most part, will not accept this incision and desires as much benefit as possible with the least amount of scarring. Many patients presenting for mastopexy can be treated with breast augmentation alone or in combination with mastopexy. The most common patient seeking mastopexy alone is happy with her breast size or does not want breast augmentation. The best patients for mastopexy alone have fairly large breasts and ptosis. Usually, these patients desire nipple elevation and correction of glandular ptosis. The best operation for this group of patients is a vertical mastopexy similar in design to a vertical breast reduction. **Patients with small (often deflated or empty appearing) breasts, who refuse breast augmentation, are often the worst candidates for mastopexy.** The scars in these patients are frequently not worth the benefit of the operation.

Breast ptosis was originally staged by Regnault (Fig. 58.1). Minor ptosis (first degree) occurs when the nipple is at the level of the inframammary fold (IMF). Moderate ptosis (second degree) is when the nipple is below the IMF but above the lowest breast contour. Severe ptosis (third degree) is when the nipple is at the lowest breast contour and below the level of the IMF. Glandular ptosis is characterized by a nipple above the IMF with breast tissue hanging below the fold.

MASTOPEXY PROCEDURES

The type of mastopexy procedure performed is dictated by the nature of the deformity. Patients with minor degrees of ptosis are frequently treated with periareolar mastopexy procedures. Periareolar mastopexy is also often the procedure of choice when breast augmentation is combined with mastopexy. As the volume of the breast is increased by the implant, the need and degree of the mastopexy procedure becomes less. As the ptosis worsens, vertical mastopexy with a lollipop-type incision or conventional mastopexy with an inverted-T–type incision might be indicated.

Inverted-T Mastopexy Procedures

The original procedures for mastopexy involved skin resection using an inverted-T–type incision. There was extensive skin undermining and minimal parenchymal resection. In 1956, Wise described a series of mechanical aids to help mark and plan a skin mastopexy procedure. In 1971, Goulian described a mastopexy procedure designed to reshape the breast by removing excess skin with no undermining. The dermis was folded on the dermis to reshape the breast. There was no surgery on the breast tissue or the chest wall resulting in less postoperative pain. The final scar was an inverted-T. The theory behind this procedure was that keeping the skin and breast in continuity contributed to a longer-lasting result.

Whidden was the first to introduce the concept of the tailor-tack mastopexy. The operation was similar to the Goulian procedure, but rather than mark the breast based on a preconceived pattern, the skin was invaginated and the operation simulated with sutures. The sutures were modified until the desired breast shape was achieved, and a pattern was individually made to guide the de-epithelialization of the skin. After de-epithelialization the breast was closed without undermining or resecting glandular tissue.

The "skin-only" mastopexy is frequently followed by recurrent ptosis. Several authors have suggested repositioning and suturing of the breast parenchyma in addition to skin resection as a solution to this problem. These operations were based on the pedicle breast reduction procedures that were becoming popular at the time. Ship et al (1). were the first to describe the creation of double superior pedicle flaps that were sutured over each other and then sutured to the pectoralis fascia. The scar pattern was the standard inverted-T. The authors noted that ptosis and bottoming out of the breast occurred more slowly than in the skin only methods of mastopexy.

Concentric Mastopexy Procedures

Because mastopexy is a cosmetic procedure, patient acceptance of the scars has always been a limiting factor. Bartels described the first attempt at concentric mastopexy in 1976. Rees and Aston reported a similar procedure for tuberous breasts at about the same time. These procedures were complicated by poorly shaped breasts, wide scars, and enlarged areola. They never really caught on. The use of purse-string sutures to close a circular wound was first described in plastic surgery in 1985 (2). In 1990, Spear et al. (3) described three rules to mark the patient having concentric mastopexy that seemed to produce more predictable aesthetic results (Fig. 58.2). The three rules are as follows:

1. The outer concentric circle must be drawn not to exceed the original areola diameter by more than the original

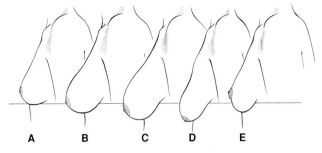

FIGURE 58.1. Breast ptosis classification. **A:** Normal. **B:** Minor or first degree. **C:** Moderate or second degree. **D:** Severe or third degree. **E:** Glandular ptosis.

areola diameter exceeds the inner concentric circle diameter.

2. The diameter of the outer circle should never be more than twice the diameter of the inner circle.
3. The final areola size should be an average of the inner and outer concentric circles.

Periareolar "Round-Block" Mastopexy Procedures

Periareolar mastopexy inevitably flattens the breast. Benelli (4) was one of the first to note that to create an excellent long-

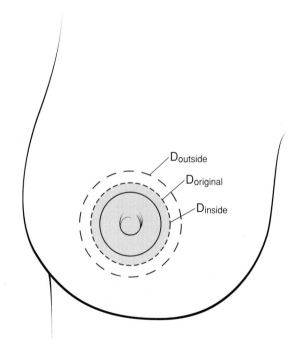

Rule #1
$D_{outside} \leq D_{original} + (D_{original} - D_{inside})$

Rule #2
$D_{outside} \leq 2x\ D_{inside}$

Rule #3
$D_{final} = \frac{1}{2}\ (D_{outside} + D_{inside})$

FIGURE 58.2. Spear rules. Illustrative markings of the three concentric circles for the Spear rules in mastopexy design. D refers to the diameter of the labeled circles.

lasting breast shape, the surgery on the gland must be separated from the surgery on the breast skin. Similar to older procedures that sutured the breast parenchyma to create better breast contour, Benelli shaped the breast parenchyma by creating multiple flaps within the breast gland that were then criss-crossed and sutured together to create a conical breast shape (Fig. 58.3A–C). The breast was then "laced" with a permanent suture (Fig. 58.3D). The round-block permanent periareolar suture (Fig. 58.3E) was placed in the dermis of the skin and then tied down so that the size of the cutaneous areola matched the size of the actual areola. The breast was sometimes sutured to the chest wall to maintain its shape and location. The skin was allowed to redrape over the newly shaped breast. The best patient for this technique had moderately sized breasts with some hypertrophy. Patients with very loose or very large ptotic breasts were difficult to treat. Patients with tubular breast deformity were also considered good candidates for round-block mastopexy. Brink (5) further defined the round-block periareolar mastopexy. He found the ideal patient to be someone with true ptosis, lower breast pole hypoplasia, or tubular breast deformity. These patients are characterized by normal to high inframammary fold position, normal to short nipple-to-inframammary-fold distance, and downward-pointing nipples. Brink found surgical manipulation of the lower pole breast skin was unnecessary. The patients were treated with purse-string round-block mastopexy without parenchymal manipulation. **Spear (6) reevaluated his indications for periareolar mastopexy in 2001 and found that the best patients included those with tuberous breast deformity, small-to-moderate-size breasts with mild to moderate ptosis, and gynecomastia, as well as those having implant explantation.** He emphasized the importance of a permanent periareolar blocking suture, particularly when the outer circle of skin resection is oversized.

Goes (7) also believed that skin-only mastopexy would not prevent early recurrent ptosis. He performed a periareolar mastopexy that supported the glandular elements of the breast by wrapping the tissue with mesh and suturing the mesh to the chest wall fascia. The periareolar dermis was placed underneath the mesh and the external skin was closed in a blocked manner with permanent sutures over the mesh (Fig. 58.4). Goes found that mixed mesh (absorbable and permanent components) worked better than absorbable mesh alone. His results were longer lasting in patients with mild to moderate ptosis.

Vertical-Incision Mastopexy

The periareolar mastopexy techniques are limited by the amount of tissue manipulation and nipple/areola movement that is possible. Some patients require more tissue rearrangement or skin resection than can be achieved with concentric mastopexy techniques.

The vertical mastopexy is performed with a periareolar scar and a vertical limb. The vertical limb is on a barely visible part of the breast, usually heals well, and is rarely an issue with the patient. Unlike the inframammary incision, which can often be seen medially or laterally, the vertical is never seen in bathing suits or clothing as long as it is kept above the inframammary fold. Vertical mastopexy procedures are not new; Lassus (8) and Lejour (9) have been performing these procedures since the 1960s. The Lejour and Lassus mastopexy procedures are similar in many ways. In both cases, the blood supply to the nipple is based on a superior pedicle. Skin is resected in the lower portion of the breast, and a central pedicle of tissue is developed based on the superior blood supply. This central tissue is sutured in an elevated fashion to the pectoralis fascia (Fig. 58.5). This process creates medial and lateral pillars that are then sutured together. The procedures only differ in that Lejour undermines the skin flaps more than Lassus. The result

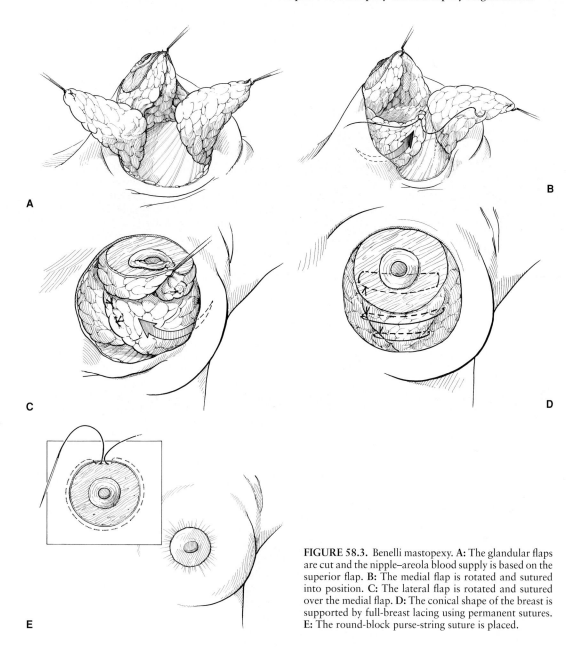

FIGURE 58.3. Benelli mastopexy. **A:** The glandular flaps are cut and the nipple–areola blood supply is based on the superior flap. **B:** The medial flap is rotated and sutured into position. **C:** The lateral flap is rotated and sutured over the medial flap. **D:** The conical shape of the breast is supported by full-breast lacing using permanent sutures. **E:** The round-block purse-string suture is placed.

at the end of the procedure tends to have an overcorrected look that settles down over the first few months after surgery. In the United States, these procedures never really caught on because American patients and physicians have trouble accepting results that are not immediately satisfactory. These procedures do, however, have a role in mastopexy surgery. The result is longer lasting because the breast shape is based on tissue rearrangement and suturing, and not on skin resection alone.

Daniel Marchac (10) developed a technique that is similar to that of Lejour and Lassus except that he places a small transverse scar at the bottom of the breast at the end of the case. This scar eliminates some of the excess skin associated with the Lassus and Lejour techniques. The patient's breast shape is better at the end of the case, but the price is a short transverse scar. **In mastopexy surgery, the most difficult problem is maintaining upper pole fullness and preventing recurrent ptosis.** Biggs and Graf (11) developed a procedure that creates an inferior chest wall flap that is repositioned in the upper part of the breast. This flap is passed under a loop of pectoralis muscle and sutured in place in the elevated position. The Biggs-Graf technique is performed most commonly with a vertical incision,

but an L-shaped incision or an inverted-T incision can also be used.

The blood supply to the nipple-areola is based on a superior dermal pedicle. The inferior chest wall flap blood supply is through the chest wall. The nipple/areola position is marked at the level of the inframammary fold and the superior pedicle is designed. The skin resection is marked as for any other type of vertical breast reduction. The skin is de-epithelialized, and the superior and inferior pedicles are developed (Fig. 58.6A–C). The bottom of the breast is mobilized so that the area is empty when the inferior flap is relocated to the upper part of the breast. The nipple-areola is inset, after which the inferior flap is passed under a loop of pectoralis major muscle. The inferior flap is sutured in place to the pectoralis fascia, and the resulting medial and lateral pillars are sutured together. The skin can usually be closed without tension or gathering. The shape at the end of the case usually looks good with minimal to no overcorrection (Fig. 58.6D, E). The shape of the breast is again based on tissue rearrangement and suturing, not skin resection. The mastopexy techniques that incorporate tissue rearrangement and suturing seem to have longer-lasting

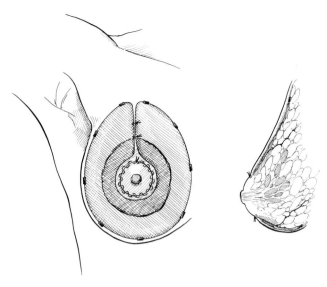

FIGURE 58.4. Goes technique. Diagram shows the position of the mesh and purse-string suture.

results than skin resection mastopexy procedures. The principle is to empty the bottom of the breast, and then reposition the tissue in the upper pole of the breast. An empty space is created in the lower pole of the breast that allows pillar sutures to be applied and the breast narrowed and reshaped. The skin

is allowed to redrape and has no role in the ultimate shape of the breast (Fig. 58.7).

AUGMENTATION MASTOPEXY

Breast ptosis is caused by a relative excess of skin envelope for the amount of breast tissue that is present. The procedures to decrease the skin envelope and rearrange and reposition the breast volume have been discussed above. Another option is to increase the breast volume with breast augmentation. This will often help to correct the skin–breast volume disparity. Breast augmentation is frequently combined with mastopexy. The augmentation procedure usually decreases the size and scope of the mastopexy procedure.

In an augmentation mastopexy procedure, the mastopexy may be as small as a periareolar skin excision to reposition the nipple/areola, or as large as an anchor scar mastopexy with glandular rearrangement. The extent of the procedure depends on the needs of the particular patient. A complete history and physical examination is important in this group of patients. The patients tend to be older than breast-augmentation patients. Prior mammography and personal and family history of breast cancer are discussed. The patient's goals and desires are clearly delineated. Important issues to be determined are size and shape of the breast desired, the position of the breast on the chest wall, and the amount of upper pole fullness. Patients with Regnault grade 1 ptosis who desire enlargement are frequently treated with breast augmentation alone. Patients with Regnault grade 2 or 3 ptosis usually require mastopexy in

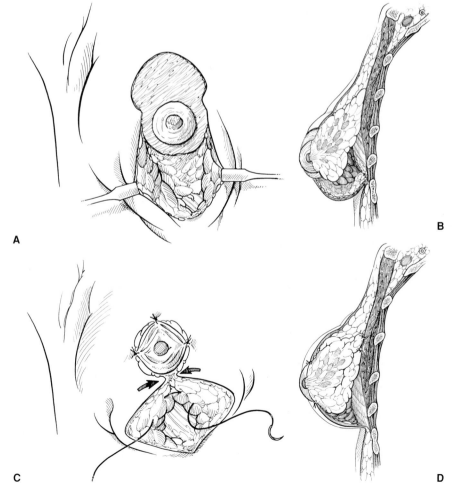

FIGURE 58.5. Lejour and Lassus method. **A:** Mobilization of the central pedicle. **B:** Central pedicle rotated into elevated position. **C:** Glandular pillars sutured together. **D:** Configuration of the breast at the end of the case.

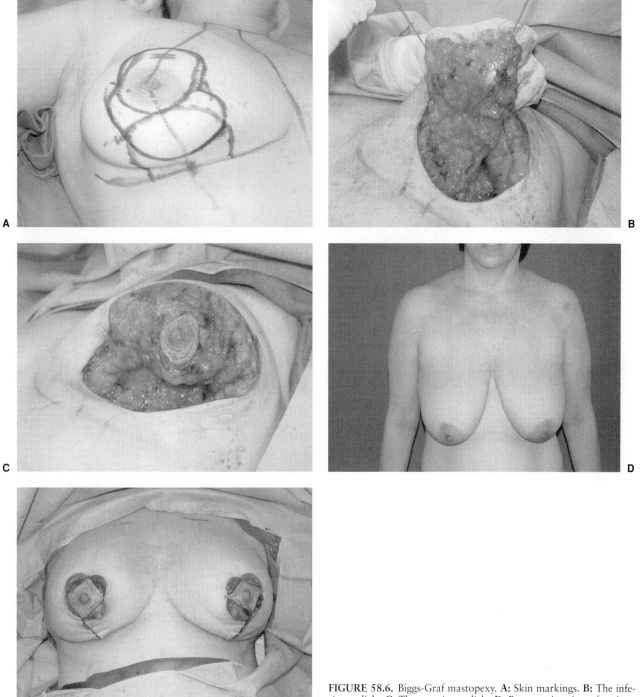

FIGURE 58.6. Biggs-Graf mastopexy. **A:** Skin markings. **B:** The inferior pedicle. **C:** The superior pedicle. **D:** Preoperative view of patient. **E:** View just prior to final closure.

addition to breast augmentation. If the patient is happy with her breast size, then mastopexy alone usually suffices.

The simplest augmentation mastopexy procedure involves resection of an ellipse (also called crescent) of skin above the areola to raise the nipple/areola position relative to the IMF (Fig. 58.8). The most that the nipple/areola can be raised with this type of procedure is about 2 cm. These patients may have early Regnault grade 2 ptosis. The only real risk to this procedure is a wide scar or an elliptical-shaped areola. If the areola shape is an issue, then the procedure should be converted to a concentric mastopexy to redistribute the tension around the entire areola circumference (12).

When modest skin tightening or repositioning of the nipple/areola is required, the full concentric mastopexy might be indicated. If the two circles of the mastopexy are truly concentric, then there will be no nipple elevation. To elevate the nipple, the outer circle must encompass more skin above than below the nipple (Fig. 58.9). In all augmentation mastopexy cases, the markings are planned preoperatively with the patient standing. In the operating room the nipple areola is cut out with a cookie cutter that is usually between 40 and 45 mm in diameter. The pocket for the implant is created either through the periareolar cut or through part of the mastopexy incision, and the implant is usually placed in the subpectoral

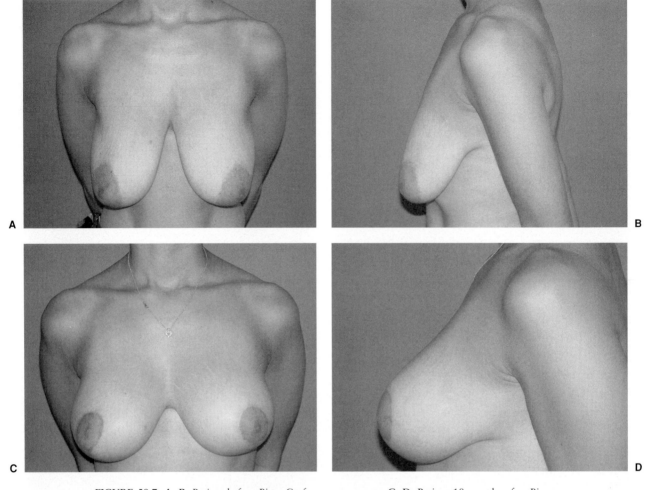

FIGURE 58.7. A, B: Patient before Biggs-Graf–type mastopexy. C, D: Patient 18 months after Biggs-Graf–type mastopexy. Note maintenance of upper pole fullness.

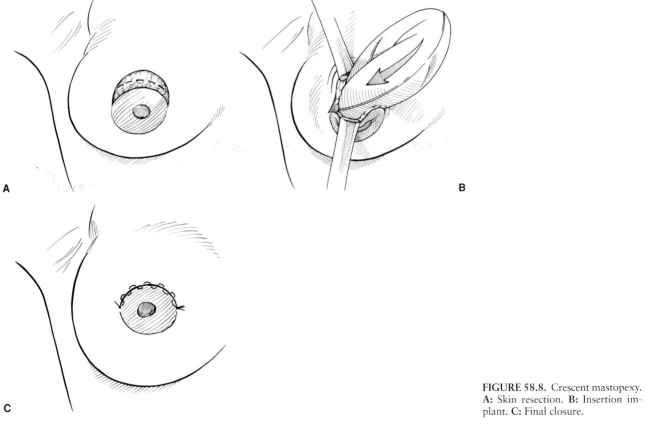

FIGURE 58.8. Crescent mastopexy. A: Skin resection. B: Insertion implant. C: Final closure.

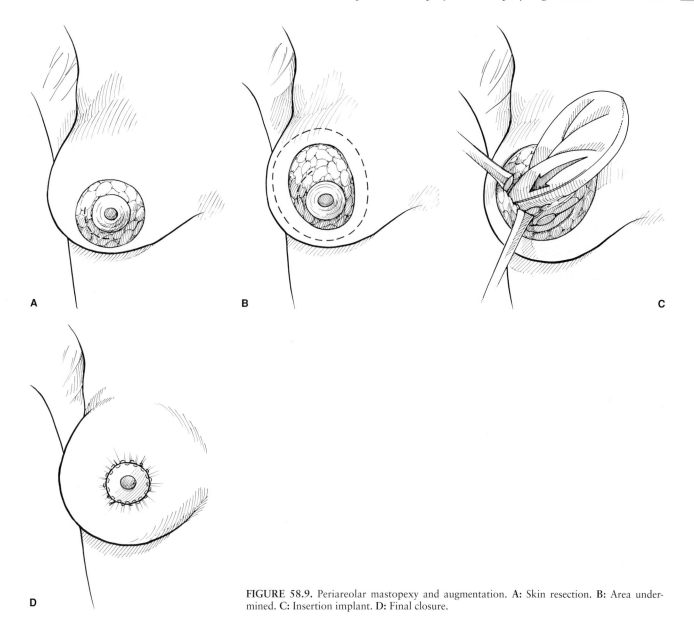

FIGURE 58.9. Periareolar mastopexy and augmentation. **A:** Skin resection. **B:** Area undermined. **C:** Insertion implant. **D:** Final closure.

position. After implant placement, the marks are re-evaluated in the sitting position. Only then are the final incisions opened and the mastopexy performed.

In the case of concentric mastopexy, the outer circle markings are confirmed and incised. The guideline for marking concentric mastopexies were established by Spear and discussed above. A nonabsorbable purse-string suture is placed in the dermis of the outer circle. There is usually some pleating in the incision that resolves within 1 to 2 months. The permanent suture helps keep the scar narrow and the areola from enlarging.

Vertical-scar augmentation mastopexy is usually used to correct moderate degrees of breast ptosis and allows greater ability to move the nipple areola complex and remove excess skin. Occasionally, a small piece of breast tissue at the bottom of the breast is excised to correct ptosis. Relocation of tissue at the bottom of the breast to the top of the breast is less important than in mastopexy alone because the implant is being used. **Vertical mastopexy is more predictable than periareolar mastopexy.** The operation offers the ability to better correct asymmetric nipples and wide breasts (Fig. 58.10).

Inverted-T-scar augmentation mastopexy is rarely indicated. In rare cases, the ptosis is so severe and the implant size is not enough to allow adequate skin resection using the vertical or periareolar techniques. This procedure allows maximal control of the nipple/areola position, skin removal, and breast shaping. The major drawback is the scarring. Augmentation mastopexy patients are no different from other aesthetic patients. They desire maximal improvement with minimal scarring. Some patients will accept a lesser result to avoid longer scars.

Nipple blood supply is an important consideration in augmentation mastopexy patients. There is rarely a problem with nipple viability in patients undergoing mastopexy alone. In augmentation mastopexy, the effect of the implant position on nipple blood supply must be considered. If the implant is placed in the submammary position and there is substantial soft-tissue dissection, nipple blood supply could be compromised. Subpectoral placement of the implant is less likely to interfere with nipple blood supply.

There is a common misconception in augmentation mastopexy patients that the implant should be placed in the

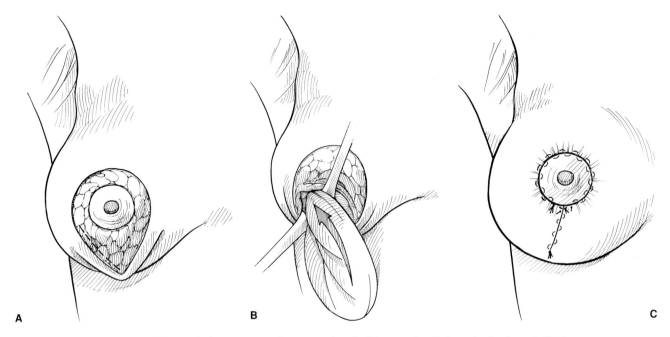

FIGURE 58.10. Vertical mastopexy and augmentation. **A:** Skin resection. **B:** Insertion implant. **C:** Final closure.

submammary position. This offers the patient less surgery and less postoperative pain. Although subpectoral implant placement is associated with more postoperative pain, the incidence of capsular contracture, implant palpability, and excess upper pole fullness is less. Currently, in this country, augmentation mastopexy patients are allowed to have either saline- or silicone-filled breast implants. Silicone implants placed in the submuscular position have a lower incidence of capsular contracture than those placed in the submammary position.

When the implant is placed in the subpectoral position, approximately 50% of the implant is covered with muscle. The partial muscle coverage allows as much flexibility in shaping as does subglandular implant placement. At the same time, mammography is more accurate and the chance of upper pole visibility is less. The augmentation mastopexy population tends to be older and have thinner soft tissue than the breast augmentation population. The ability to perform mammograms and the issues of upper pole fullness are real issues in this group.

Augmentation mastopexy is much more challenging than either breast augmentation or mastopexy alone. The patient's goals and desires need to be carefully addressed, and the scars and limitations of the procedures discussed.

References

1. Ship AG, Weiss PR, Engler AM. Dual-pedicle dermoparenchymal mastopexy. *Plast Reconstr Surg.* 1989;83:281.
2. Peled IJ, Zagher U, Wexler MR. Purse-string suture for reduction and closure of skin defects. *Ann Plast Surg.* 1985;14:465.
3. Spear SL, Kassan M, Little JW. Guidelines in concentric mastopexy. *Plast Reconstr Surg.* 1990;85:961.
4. Benelli L. A new periareolar mammaplasty: the "round block" technique. *Aesthetic Plast Surg.* 1990;14:93.
5. Brink RR. Management of true ptosis of the breast. *Plast Reconstr Surg.* 1993;91:657.
6. Spear SL, Giese SY, Ducic I. Concentric mastopexy revisited. *Plast Reconstr Surg.* 2001;107:1294.
7. Goes JCS. Periareolar mammaplasty: double skin technique with application of Polyglactin 910 mesh. *Rev Soc Bras Cir Plast.* 1992;7:1.
8. Lassus C. Update on vertical mammaplasty. *Plast Reconstr Surg.* 1999;104:2289.
9. Lejour M. *Vertical Mammaplasty and Liposuction of the Breast.* St. Louis: Quality Medical Publishing; 1993.
10. Marchac D, de Olarte G. Reduction mammaplasty and correction of ptosis with a short inframammary scar. *Plast Reconstr Surg.* 1982;69:45.
11. Graf R, Biggs TM. In search of better shape in mastopexy and reduction mammaplasty. *Plast Reconstr Surg.* 2002;110:309.
12. Puckett CL, Meyer VH, Reinisch JF. Crescent mastopexy and augmentation. *Plast Reconstr Surg.* 1985;75:533.

CHAPTER 59 ■ BREAST REDUCTION: INVERTED-T TECHNIQUE

SCOTT L. SPEAR

Reduction mammoplasty represents the clearest example of the interface between reconstructive and aesthetic plastic surgery. Although the avowed goals of this procedure are weight and volume reduction of the breast, aesthetic enhancement is often equally important. Excellent procedures have been described and emphasis has shifted to technical refinements for improved safety and predictable aesthetic results. At the same time, greater importance has been placed on preservation of both sensation and physiologic function. Although there is a fundamental difference between reduction mammoplasty and mastopexy, both operations can follow the design of the techniques to be described for reduction mammoplasty alone (Chapter 58).

ANATOMY AND PHYSIOLOGY

Sensory innervation to the superior portion of the breast is supplied by the supraclavicular nerves formed from the third and fourth branches of the cervical plexus. The medial breast skin is supplied by the anterior cutaneous divisions of the second through seventh intercostal nerves. The dominant innervation to the nipple is derived from the lateral cutaneous branch of the fourth intercostal nerve, whereas lateral cutaneous branches of other intercostal nerves travel subcutaneously to and beyond the midclavicular line of the areola and the skin of the breast. Independent confirmation of the importance of the lateral cutaneous branch of the fourth intercostal nerve has led to greater acceptance of techniques that include its course in the vascular pedicle to the nipple.

There are three chief sources of blood supply to the breast. The internal mammary artery supplies the medial portion through medial perforators near the sternal border. The variable lateral thoracic artery supplies the lateral portion. The anterior and lateral branches of the intercostal vessels supply the remainder. Although there is a substantial degree of collateralization among these vessels in the breast parenchyma, it has been estimated that the internal mammary artery provides approximately 60% of the total. The lateral thoracic artery is thought to supply an additional 30%, primarily to the upper, outer, and lateral portions. The anterior and lateral branches of the third, fourth, and fifth posterior intercostal arteries supply the remaining lower outer breast quadrant. The variability and overlap between these vascular networks account for the remarkable safety of nipple-bearing pedicles of diverse design based on different vascular supplies.

The breast has two major venous drainage systems: one superficial, the other deep. The superficial drainage system is divided into two types: transverse and longitudinal. The transverse veins run medially in the subcutaneous space and empty into the internal mammary veins by multiple perforating vessels. The longitudinal drainage ascends to the suprasternal area to connect with the superficial veins of the lower neck. There

are anastomotic connections across the midline, but only between the superficial systems. The major portion of the deep drainage is through perforating branches of the internal mammary vein. Additional venous drainage is in the direction of the axillary vein. A remaining route of drainage is posteriorly through perforators into the intercostal veins, which carry blood posteriorly to the vertebral veins.

The lymphatic pathways draining the breast parallel closely the venous pathways and include cutaneous, internal mammary, posterior intercostal, and axillary routes. Although most lymph flow is through the axillary region, the internal thoracic channels may carry 3% to 20% of the total. **Despite an extensive search for underlying metabolic causes of breast hypertrophy and gigantomastia, these conditions remain poorly understood phenomena, the products of end-organ hormonal sensitivity, genetic background, and overall body weight.**

REDUCTION MAMMOPLASTY

Indications

Women seek to reduce the size of their breasts for reasons both physical and psychological. Heavy, pendulous breasts cause neck and back pain as well as grooves from the pressure of brassiere straps. The breasts themselves may be chronically painful, and the skin in the inframammary region is subject to maceration and dermatoses. From a psychological point of view, excessively large breasts can be a troublesome focus of embarrassment for the teenager as well as the woman in her senior years. Unilateral hypertrophy with asymmetry heightens embarrassment.

Inverted-T Techniques

Two decisions confront the surgeon: (a) choice of incision (scar) pattern, and (b) choice of pedicle type. **The inverted-T scar pattern can be applied to virtually any pedicle, including a superior pedicle, an inferior pedicle, a vertical bipedicle, a central mound pedicle, and a superomedial pedicle. The scar pattern and the pedicle type used in breast reduction are, for the most part, independent variables. Furthermore, there is no absolute cutoff regarding when an inverted-T scar pattern approach is appropriate instead of a vertical technique that avoids attempts to avoid a transverse inframammary scar.** At Georgetown University Hospital, we use both vertical techniques as well as inverted-T techniques, depending on (a) the size of the breast, (b) the degree of ptosis, and the (c) patient's goals. Even when opting for an inverted-T technique, we shorten the transverse scar component because of increasing experience with vertical scar techniques. The distinction, therefore, between vertical and inverted-T techniques has become less clear as surgeons add a short transverse scar to their vertical techniques or shorten the transverse scar in their inverted-T techniques.

The majority of American plastic surgeons still use an inverted-T scar pattern, most commonly with an inferior pedicle. There are several major advantages to this technique. To begin with, it is reproducible, straightforward, and easily taught. To a large extent, the skin incisions correspond to the glandular incisions that are made on the breast parenchyma itself. In this way, once the lines are drawn on the skin preoperatively, the cutting of the tissues and the closure of the wound proceed along the preoperatively planned lines. This has great advantage in terms of predictability and reliability. **In contrast, vertical scar techniques often involve a significant disparity between the skin incisions and glandular incisions beneath the skin.** A significant amount of intraoperative adjustment is required both in terms of removing tissue and reshaping tissue to obtain an acceptable result. Finally, the closure of the skin may require adjustment to deal with the excess skin at the caudal end of the vertical incision.

Once the decision has been made to perform a breast reduction, the surgeon must choose the orientation of the pedi-cle. This chapter describes the vertical bipedicle technique, the inferior pedicle technique, a central mound technique, and a superomedial pedicle technique, which is my current preferred technique.

Vertical Pedicle Technique

McKissock first described his vertical bipedicle technique for nipple transposition during reduction mammoplasty in 1972. With this technique the central breast is reduced to a vertically oriented bipedicle flap based superiorly on the upper margin of the new areolar window and inferiorly on the inframammary line and chest wall musculature. The flap carries the nipple–areola and, although de-epithelialized, depends primarily on inferior parenchyma for blood supply.

With the patient erect, the markings are made in a fashion similar in all breast reductions (Fig. 59.1). The midline is drawn and the breast meridian is established by dropping a line from the midclavicle through the nipple and continuing inferiorly across the inframammary line. The inframammary fold is marked and a tangent to the fold is drawn across the lower thorax and transposed to the anterior breast and marked

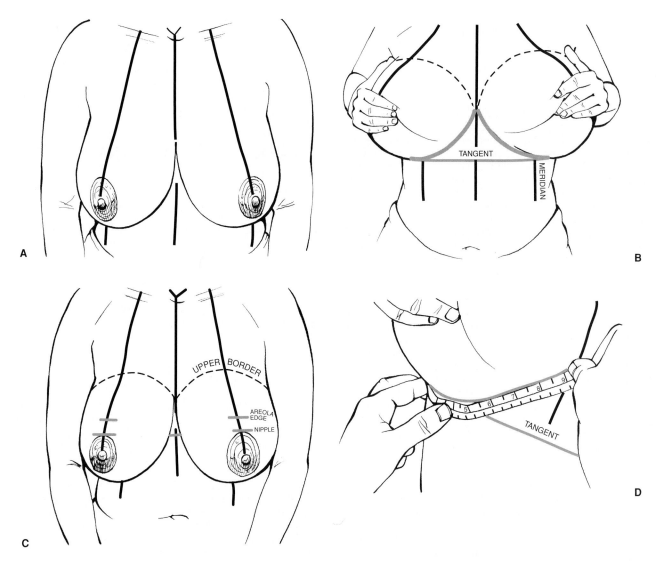

FIGURE 59.1. Preoperative markings. **A:** Drawing the basic landmarks, including the midline and breast meridian, for most breast procedures. **B:** A tangent is drawn from the lower-most portion of the inframammary fold across the midline. **C:** This tangent is then superimposed onto the surface of the breast. **D:** The length of the fold is then measured. It is often between 20 and 24 cm long. *(Continued)*

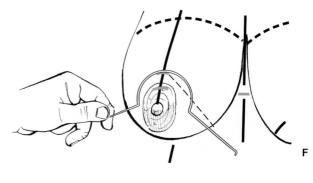

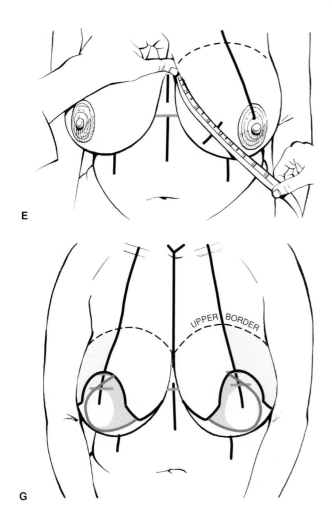

FIGURE 59.1. *(Continued)* **E:** An arc that is just over one-half the length of the fold is transposed onto the surface of the breast medially. **F:** A wire keyhole pattern (which is centered around the nipple site) can then be superimposed on the breast such that it crosses the arc line drawn in Figure 59.4. **G:** The keyhole pattern is completed by making the limbs the desired length, anywhere from 5 to 8 cm long, depending on the size of the breast. It is important to double-check that the length of these proposed superiorly based lateral and medial flaps along their cut, free, inferior edge match the length of the fold to which they are to be approximated.

on the breast meridian. **Whereas the initial descriptions set the nipple some 2 cm higher, the best location for the new nipple position is at the inframammary fold level.** The entire length of the inframammary fold is measured with a tape measure. In most cases, it is between 20 and 24 cm long. Using a tape, a mark is made in the shape of a short arc on the surface of the breast that measures just over one-half the length of the fold (e.g., for a 22-cm fold, the distance would be 12 to 13 cm). Diverging lines are drawn from the nipple point; they pass as tangents to either side of the dilated areola and meet the arc line drawn from the ends of the inframammary fold. A wire keyhole pattern is then adjusted to a similar angle of divergence and superimposed on the lines, indicating the proper size and location of the new areolar window. A distance of 5 to 6 cm is measured from the window to establish the length of the limbs of the pattern. From these extremities, lines are directed medially and laterally to intersect the inframammary fold.

The areola is circumscribed at a diameter of between 42 and 48 mm. The vertical pedicle is outlined by extending the lines of the vertical limbs inferiorly as two parallel lines straddling the breast meridian to the inframammary fold. The entire pedicle, except the reduced nipple-areola, is de-epithelialized. The vertical pedicle is then incised along its medial and lateral margins to the fascia of the underlying musculature, and medial and lateral dermoglandular wedges are resected (Fig. 59.2). **A thin layer of breast over the lateral musculature is retained to favor preservation of sensation to the nipple–areola complex.** Additional breast tissue is resected from the remaining medial and lateral elements: little to none medially, but a considerable amount, including the axillary tail, laterally. A window of

breast tissue is removed from the upper portion of the bipedicle flap, from the level of the nipple to the height of the keyhole pattern, creating a bucket-handle (Fig. 59.3). This resection must not extend above the upper limit of the areolar window in order to avoid loss of superior breast volume. The flap is folded superiorly on itself, bringing the areola into position within the keyhole pattern. The medial and lateral flaps are brought together over the pedicle, and closure is begun, working from the extremities toward the center (Fig. 59.4). Any central excess of skin is either excised at the vertical closure, or "worked-in" to the closure.

Inferior Pedicle Technique

The inferior pedicle technique is the most popular technique among plastic surgeons today. The planning of the inferior pedicle technique is essentially the same as for the McKissock bipedicle procedure, with the desired nipple location determined in the same manner. An inferiorly based dermoglandular pedicle is planned with a base of 4 to 9 cm at the inframammary line that gradually tapers as it ascends to encompass the nipple–areola complex. De-epithelialization with this technique is limited to the zone immediately about and inferior to the nipple–areola (Fig. 59.5). Skin and parenchymal resections are performed medial and lateral to the pedicle, as described above, but also superior to the nipple–areola, up to the level of the keyhole pattern. These excisions are performed leaving a beveled carpet of breast tissue over the muscular fascia, especially laterally. Immediately superior to the 1-cm de-epithelialized cuff about the nipple–areola, the pedicle is

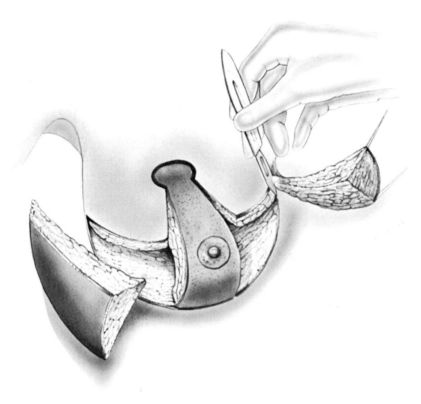

FIGURE 59.2. McKissock technique. Medial and lateral dermoglandular resections.

terminated and incised down to muscle fascia, taking care not to undercut the inferior vascular base (Fig. 59.6). A pyramidal pedicle of dermis and parenchyma is thus left deep to and inferior to the nipple–areola, based on the chest wall musculature and inframammary line. In the vicinity of the areola, it measures 2 to 4 cm in thickness, and near the base it is 4 to 10 cm. After completion of the breast resection, the nipple–areola is brought to the desired position in the keyhole pattern, and the medial and lateral flaps are brought together as with the McKissock technique (Fig. 59.7).

Central Mound Technique

The central mound technique is a further evolution of the prior two designs. The pedicle is based on central chest wall musculature alone and is not contiguous with any skin boundary. Hence it has no directional base in the sense of traditional skin

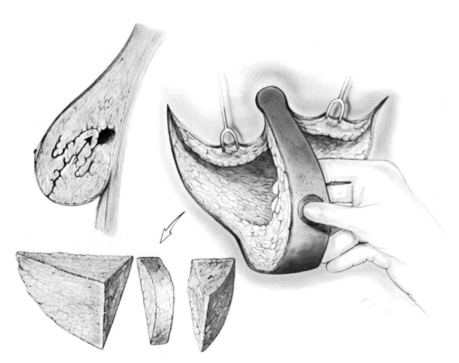

FIGURE 59.3. McKissock technique. Central glandular resection produces bucket-handle flap for infolding.

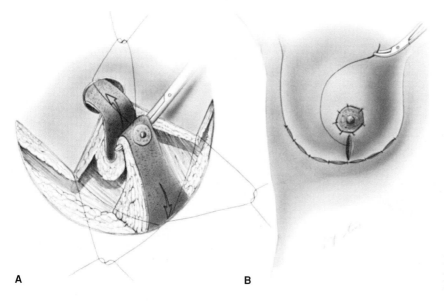

A   **B**

FIGURE 59.4. McKissock technique. **A:** Vertical bipedicle folded on itself as key sutures tied. **B:** Closure.

pedicles that may be classified as superior, inferior, or transverse.

Preoperative marking is again performed as for the McKissock technique. The skin is de-epithelialized within the entire keyhole pattern, a process continued inferiorly to include the reduced nipple–areola complex (Fig. 59.8). An incision is placed in the inframammary crease and is carried down perpendicularly to the pectoralis fascia. Incisions are now made and beveled around the margins of the keyhole pattern at its medial and lateral limbs. This incision is continued below the level of the limbs to circumscribe the de-epithelialized pattern, including the nipple–areola, and is beveled in a caudal direction toward the inframammary fold. The limb incisions, both medial and lateral, are made in the standard fashion, developing flaps of thickness similar to those in other techniques. Now the medial and lateral inferior quadrants of skin and breast, as well as the central inferior tissue intervening between the nipple–areola and the inframammary fold, are excised as a single curvilinear, ellipsoid unit that includes the axillary tail (Fig. 59.9). A skin incision at the superior aspect of the keyhole is deepened only enough to allow comfortable transposition of the central mound pedicle with its nipple–areola into the keyhole position. The skin flaps are brought about the pedicle as in other techniques, and closure is performed (Fig. 59.10).

AUTHOR'S TECHNIQUE

The patient is marked in the standing position in the exam room or in the office the day prior to surgery; the markings are made as described above. I often mark the upper border of the breast to give some perspective as to where the breast will lie at the end of the breast reduction procedure. This allows a better appreciation of where the nipple might sit after the breast reduction.

The ideal limbs of the keyhole pattern vary between 5 and 8 cm, depending on the size of the breast currently and the size of the planned breast after reduction. The larger the breast and the larger the breast that is to remain after the procedure, the longer these limbs should be. Five centimeters is the minimum length of the vertical limb of the keyhole, and I will often go to 6, 7, or even 8 cm, depending on how big the breasts will be left postoperatively. I am well aware that when the breast is made too large for the skin flaps, the skin flaps will often stretch, and that when the skin flaps are larger than the breast, the skin flaps will often shrink postoperatively. A fairly straight line is then drawn from the lowest-most point of the vertical limb of the keyhole to the medial-most extent of the inframammary fold mark. The same is done laterally to the

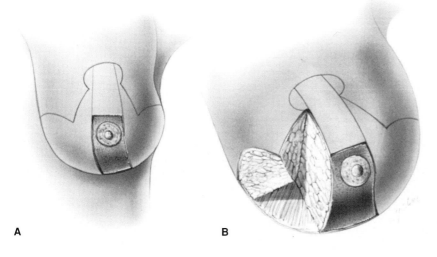

A   **B**

FIGURE 59.5. Inferior pedicle technique. **A:** Preoperative markings with inferior pedicle de-epithelialized. **B:** Medial dermoglandular resection.

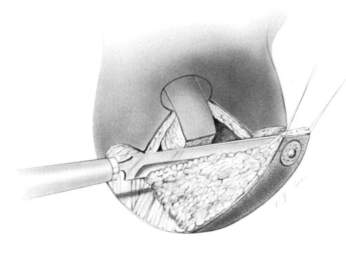

FIGURE 59.6. Inferior pedicle technique. Pedicle developed.

lateral-most extent of the inframammary fold. Having drawn the keyhole and the planned incisions, the pedicle can now be drawn.

I am particularly impressed with the versatility and speed of the superomedial pedicle and now use this approach in a large majority of my breast-reduction procedures, regardless of whether they are inverted-T scar patterns or vertical scar patterns. The design for the superomedial pedicle is drawn so that it starts superiorly, along the arch of the previously drawn keyhole, and ends either at or near the bottom of the vertical limb of the keyhole (Fig. 59.11). The planned areola is circumscribed, leaving several centimeters around the areolar margins as the pedicle is drawn.

At this point, the patient is observed critically for symmetry of the plan. Particular key points for symmetry include the upper border of the planned areola, as well as the location and length of the vertical limb of the keyhole pattern and the line joining the bottom of the keyhole pattern to the medial-most border of the inframammary fold. As mentioned earlier, because of the preexisting asymmetry that is often found in breast-reduction patients, it is acceptable to have more tissue planned for excision in the larger breast.

I like to photograph the patient at this point for reference both intraoperatively and postoperatively. With the advent of digital photography, it is relatively simple to print out these photographs for referencing during the actual surgical procedure.

I often have the patient lie down at this point and shorten the incisions both medially and laterally by at least 2 cm (Fig. 59.12). This shortening is done in such a way that the medial-most extent of the incision is brought lateral by 2 cm and this new end point is drawn midway between the upper and lower previously planned incisions. The same is done laterally, so that the scars or incisions that will be made will curve somewhat off the inframammary fold as compared to the original plan. Thus, even preoperatively, the planned length of the incision will be 4 cm or more shorter than the preoperative length of the inframammary fold.

To be certain that the lines that I have drawn are not lost during the preparation of the patient, I lightly score these lines just prior to surgery using an 18- or 21-gauge needle.

One of the most remarkable things with this procedure is the speed of de-epithelializing. Because the pedicle is almost always quite small and substantially smaller than with other techniques, de-epithelialization is brief and is all within the keyhole pattern itself. The incisions are then scored around the margins of the keyhole and from the keyhole to the inframammary fold and along the inframammary fold. I prefer to dissect the lateral flap first, and this is done by incising the dermis along the edge of the skin incision down to a depth of 1 to 2 cm of breast tissue. A lateral-based flap is created that goes out to the axillary tail, leaving sufficient soft tissue to ensure viability of the lateral skin flap (Fig. 59.13). The medial and inferior incisions are made through the dermis down to or near the muscle

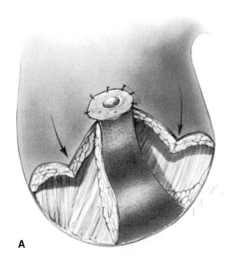

A

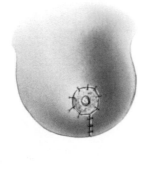

B

FIGURE 59.7. Inferior pedicle technique. A: Nipple–areola positioned. B: Closure.

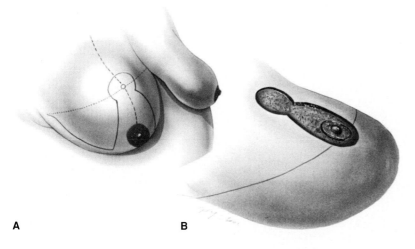

A   **B**

FIGURE 59.8. Central mound technique. **A:** Preoperative markings. **B:** Limited central de-epithelialization.

fascia. Once all these incisions have been made, the pedicle is held using hooks or atraumatic clamps, and incisions are made straight down along the margins of the pedicle superiorly, laterally, and inferiorly, taking care not to undermine the pedicle (Fig. 59.14). In particular, as the dissection is carried laterally, some beveling is done to leave soft tissue along the chest wall in the anticipated path of the neurovascular supply to the nipple–areolar complex. The breast tissue itself is removed in a C, or inverted-C pattern from either breast (Fig. 59.15). The key elements of this resection are to leave adequate blood supply to the nipple–areola pedicle by not undermining the pedicle and leaving it fully attached to the chest wall. The breast tissue is aggressively removed in the medial wedge area, as well as inferiorly and laterally. The area of greatest risk in this operation is the circulation to the lateral skin flap and, therefore, that flap must not be made too thin or be traumatized in the dissection.

I then incise just the dermis of the pedicle itself, where it joins the keyhole medially, to allow for easier rotation of the dermoglandular pedicle. After rotation of the nipple–areola, the areola is attached at the meridian of the keyhole aperture. The keyhole pattern is then closed around the pedicle both at the 6 o'clock location of the areolar window and at the 6 o'clock position of the vertical limbs of the keyhole. The pedicle itself may be tacked to the chest wall to prevent malposition. The incisions are approximated with a few staples. Because the flap lengths have been measured preoperatively to approximate one-half of the inframammary fold length, there are rarely any dog-ears to deal with. A small suction drain is usually placed in the inframammary fold and brought out through a stab incision laterally to help facilitate drainage. The final closure is accomplished and the staples removed.

The technique is easy to perform and to teach. The same pedicle can also be used as part of a vertical reduction technique. The creation of the pedicle is virtually the same. The only difference is that the skin is tailored to the breast at the end of the operation and excess skin can be removed as

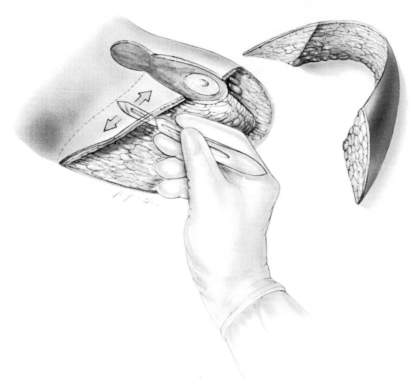

FIGURE 59.9. Central mound technique. Dermoglandular resection.

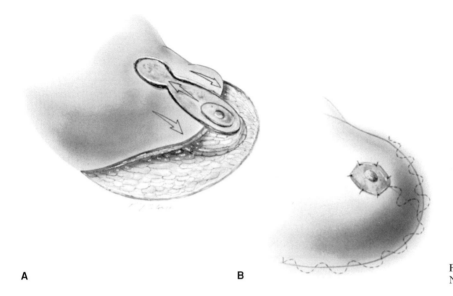

FIGURE 59.10. Central mound technique. **A:** Nipple–areola advanced superiorly. **B:** Closure.

necessary either in a vertical or a combined vertical and short T pattern (Fig. 59.16).

BREAST AMPUTATION WITH FREE NIPPLE GRAFT: AUTHOR'S TECHNIQUE

An excellent, if often maligned, alternative to reduction mammoplasty with a nipple-bearing pedicle remains breast amputation with free nipple graft. This technique consistently produces well-shaped breasts. In large women, in particular, an attractive breast contour is more easily accomplished with this technique than with conventional approaches. The disadvantage is the relatively unnatural appearance and function of the nipple–areola complex: Specialized sensation is certainly lost,

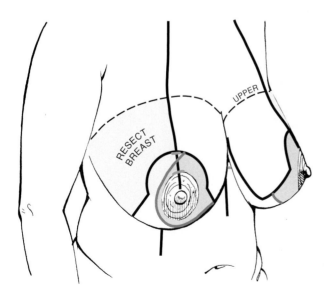

FIGURE 59.11. The base of superomedial pedicle should be drawn so that it connects to the keyhole pattern somewhere along the areola window superiorly and along the vertical limb inferiorly. The precise attachment is not critical, but it should be drawn so as to facilitate rotation.

as well as some degree of nipple projection, especially erectile nipple projection; lactation is similarly sacrificed; and occasional spotty survival of the grafted areola produces areas of depigmentation that can be troublesome in dark-skinned individuals.

This rapid technique is especially indicated for women with gigantomastia, presenting 2,500 g or more of breast tissue per side, as well as for patients with other complicating factors, such as increased age or systemic disease where significant reduction in blood loss and operating time is desired. It remains the preferred alternative for many elderly patients who present for reduction mammoplasty because of increasing symptoms involving a demineralized skeletal system. **With respect to the patient with extremely large breasts, I consider this alternative whenever the nipple–areola complex is to be elevated more than 15 cm.** This guideline is modified by other factors, especially the age of the patient. I am reluctant to use this alternative in young or unmarried patients, for example. Although concern for ischemic injury to the retained nipple–areola complex in such greatly enlarged breasts remains a major indication for this alternative, it may not be the sole reason to recommend it. Rather, the technical reality of breast reduction for such large breasts may prove unwieldy when a pedicle is maintained.

Preoperative Marking

The breast markings remain similar to those for the previously described inverted-T techniques (Fig. 59.17). The wire keyhole pattern is not used for this technique, however. Instead, two diverging arms are drawn from the selected nipple point at an angle approximating 90 degrees. Limb length is measured at 7.5 to 8.5 cm (average 8 cm). The inframammary line is marked, and the medial and lateral extensions from the limbs are indicated as for the standard technique. The areola is marked for reduction with the areolar marker.

Technique

The procedure is begun by removing the nipple–areola complex rapidly with attached subjacent breast tissue and setting it aside in a moist saline sponge, clearly indicating the side of origin, right or left. I do not follow the skin markings as some have suggested when performing the glandular resection,

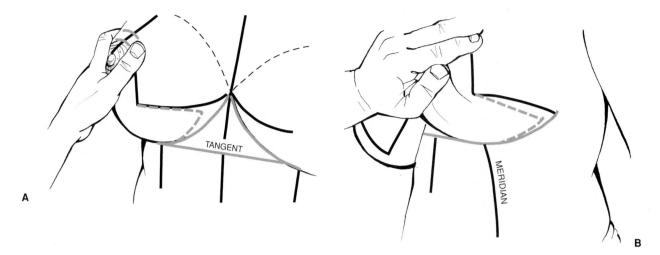

FIGURE 59.12. Even when performing an inverted-T–type reduction, the planned incisions can be several centimeters shorter than the pre-existing inframammary fold, so long as care is taken to resect the breast tissue that would otherwise remain in that area.

because I find it too often results in inadequate central projection of the breast. Far better is Rubin's alternative of retaining inferior parenchyma at the inframammary line to be covered by the superior skin flaps. I prefer, however, to retain superiorly based parenchyma between the diverging limbs of the pattern, as well as an additional amount dropping below this area if needed. This retained tissue is designated with a single curvilinear line placed below the diverging arms, and the enclosed area is rapidly deskinned. Clearly, the greatest pitfall in this otherwise straightforward procedure is the amputation of excessive breast tissue, leaving only superior flaps with subcutaneous tissue and little breast. **If the breast is allowed to hang pendulously, gravity pulls virtually the entire gland below the level of the amputating blade, presenting the surgeon with a regrettable surprise when refashioning an inadequate breast from the remaining superior flaps.** On the other hand, when the gland is gathered and presented in a spherical fashion by an assistant, the amputating blade leaves a significant amount of parenchyma superiorly. The dictum that more can always be removed later prevails.

The amputating incision is carried perpendicularly to the chest wall musculature. The inframammary incision is similarly carried perpendicularly to the musculature. The large intervening wedge of gland is then dissected progressively from medial to lateral away from the muscle fascia, maintaining exact hemostasis as the resection progresses. The central portion of the remaining superior gland, including the deskinned portion between and below the diverging limbs, is now dissected from the underlying muscle fascia superiorly to the apex of the inverted-V pattern. The dermal edges of the inverted-V are incised to allow infolding of the superiorly bases dermal flap. The most inferior points of the inverted-V are then approximated, thus effectively coning and infolding the breast. Closure is completed in the standard fashion working both vertically and from the extremities centrally.

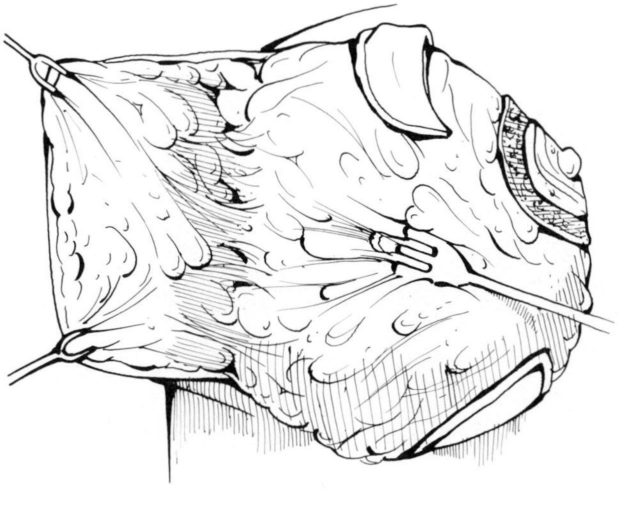

FIGURE 59.13. A laterally based flap of some safe thickness is dissected to allow access to the lateral breast tissue.

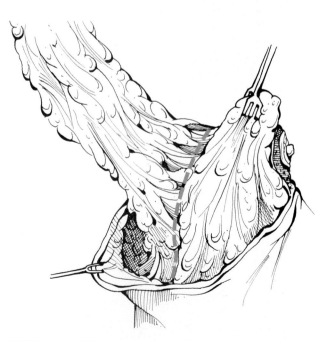

FIGURE 59.14. The superomedial pedicle is developed by cutting around the previously marked pedicle straight down toward the chest wall, without undermining and with some feathering laterally to protect the neurovascular supply.

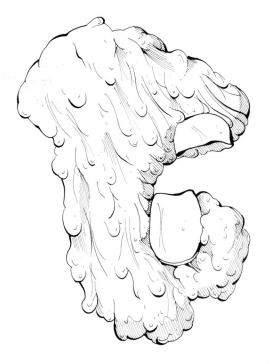

FIGURE 59.15. The resulting specimen is an inverted-C or C shape, depending on which breast.

Finally, the site for the nipple–areola complex is determined and measured upward from the inframammary fold on either side. It may or may not fall precisely at the superior extent of the vertical closure. The area is marked with the areolar marker and is de-epithelialized. The defatted nipple–areola complex is sutured in place and secured with a tie-over dressing. It is important not to thin the areolar portion of the graft excessively during the defatting process, so that the resulting areolar graft has a more natural appearance. Similarly, ductal tissue is left within the papilla, to favor nipple projection. A greasy dressing with wet cotton bolus is then tied in place over the complex and is removed at 4 days.

CONCLUSION

Despite the many recent advances in breast reduction surgery, the inverted-T scar technique remains a comfortable and predictable technique for the surgeon who performs breast surgery. Although there is appropriate increasing interest in short scar or vertical scar techniques, the inverted-T option has proven reliable and safe, which may be as important to the patient as the length of the scar in the inframammary fold.

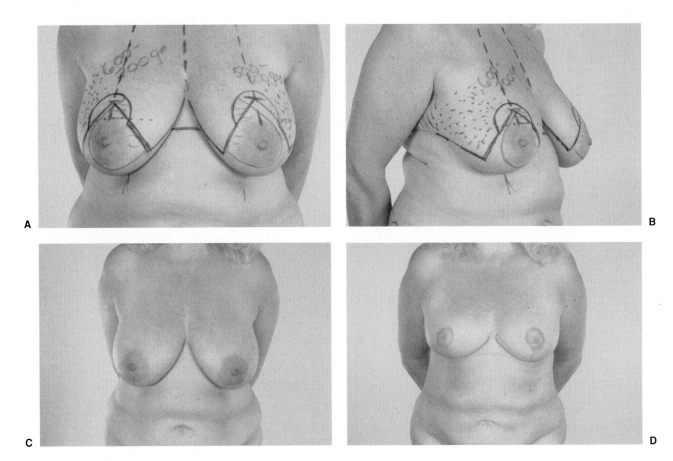

FIGURE 59.16. A: Frontal view of plan for breast reduction using superomedial pedicle and inverted-T scar pattern. **B:** Lateral view of plan. **C** and **D:** Before and 3 months after 575-g reduction using the author's technique.

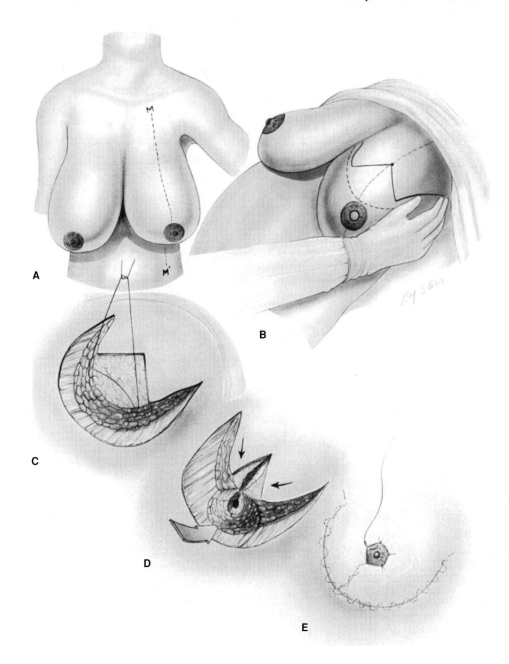

FIGURE 59.17. Author's breast amputation with free nipple-areola graft, technique. **A:** Breast meridian marked. **B:** Preoperative markings completed. **C:** Amputation completed. **D:** Central tissue coned and rotated into retromammary space. **E:** Free nipple–areolar graft added at closure.

Suggested Readings

Balch C. The central mound technique for reduction mammoplasty. *Plast Reconstr Surg.* 1981;67:305.

Courtiss E, Goldwyn RM. Reduction mammoplasty by the inferior pedicle technique. *Plast Reconstr Surg.* 1977;59:500.

Georgiade NG, et al. Reduction mammoplasty utilizing an inferior pedicle nipple–areola flap. *Ann Plast Surg.* 1979;3:211.

Hall-Findlay EJ. Pedicles in vertical breast reduction and mastopexy. *Clin Plast Surg.* 2002;29(3):379.

Hammond DC. The SPAIR mammaplasty. *Clin Plast Surg.* 2002;29(3):411.

Hammond DC. Short scar periareolar inferior pedicle reduction (SPAIR) mammaplasty. *Plast Reconstr Surg.* 1999;103(3):890.

Hidalgo DA. Improving safety and aesthetic results in inverted T scar breast reduction. *Plast Reconstr Surg.* 1999;103(3):874.

Marchac D, de Olarte G. Reduction mammoplasty and correction of ptosis with a short inframammary scar. *Plast Reconstr Surg.* 1982;69:45.

McKissock PK. Reduction mammoplasty. *Ann Plast Surg.* 1979;2:321.

McKissock PK. Reduction mammoplasty with a vertical dermal flap. *Plast Reconstr Surg.* 1972;49:245.

Nahabedian MY, McGibbon BM, Manson PN. Medial pedicle reduction mammaplasty for severe mammary hypertrophy. *Plast Reconstr Surg.* 2000;105(3):896.

Nahabeian MY, Mofid MM. Viability and sensation of the nipple–areolar complex after reduction mammaplasty. *Ann Plast Surg.* 2002;49(1):24.

Robbins TH. A reduction mammoplasty with the areola–nipple based on an inferior dermal pedicle. *Plast Reconstr Surg.* 1977;59:64.

CHAPTER 60 ■ VERTICAL REDUCTION MAMMAPLASTY

ELIZABETH J. HALL-FINDLAY

Many options are available to the surgeon for breast reduction. No one technique should be applied to all breasts. Each surgeon must have a few different approaches with which he or she is comfortable. For example, the vertical techniques (1) are ideal for small to medium reductions. The inverted-T techniques (2) may be better for larger reductions or those with considerable skin excess (as occurs in postbariatric patients). Either technique can be used with free nipple grafts (3) for the massive breast. Liposuction only (4) is available as a technique, but is of limited usefulness.

Confusion is generated by equating the choice of the skin resection pattern with the choice of pedicle used to transfer the nipple–areola complex. Because the vertical skin resection pattern is often associated with a superior or superomedial pedicle and because the inverted-T tends to be associated with an inferior or central pedicle, the terms are often used without clear distinction. **Any pedicle can be used with any skin resection pattern.** There are, however, advantages and disadvantages to each.

Anatomy

Blood Supply

To understand the design choices for breast reduction, one must have a clear understanding of the blood supply to the breast parenchyma and to the nipple–areolar complex (Fig. 60.1A). As described by Ian Taylor (5), the blood supply to the breast is superficial, which is logical because the breast is a structure derived from the ectoderm. There is one large, deep perforator that comes through the pectoralis muscle inferiorly. There are venae comitantes accompanying this artery, but otherwise the veins are very superficial and quite separate from the arteries.

Because the arteries are superficial, the design of the pedicle for the nipple–areola complex can be dermal rather than dermoglandular. **Because the veins lie just under the dermis, it is important to maintain a dermal connection to most pedicles.**

The one exception is the inferior or central pedicle, which relies on the artery and vein of the deep perforator. This vessel comes from the internal mammary artery at the level of the fifth or sixth interspace. It usually perforates the pectoralis muscle just medial to the breast meridian, a few centimeters above the inframammary fold. Branching may occur superficial or deep to the muscle.

The rest of the arterial input is relatively superficial. There is a large branch of the internal mammary system that emerges from the second or third interspace and runs obliquely toward the breast meridian. This vessel is only about 1 cm deep to the skin as it enters the breast. The fact that this vessel is so superficial and provides such good blood supply allows the superior pedicle to be long and quite thin. Because large breasts are quite ptotic, this vessel seems to be more obliquely oriented than it

was before puberty—it runs from about the second or third interspace toward the level of the fourth or fifth interspace. There are numerous superficial veins at this level, but they are separate from the arteries.

There are additional branches running medially from the internal mammary system at the level of the third to sixth interspace. These vessels supply a medially based pedicle, which can be either dermal or dermoglandular.

The lateral thoracic system is also relatively superficial, although deeper than the vessels described above, it is usually found 2 or 3 cm deep to the skin at the level of the inframammary fold. There are also prominent veins in this area. It is these vessels that supply a lateral pedicle.

Nerve Supply

Innervation to the nipple–areolar complex is said to be provided by the lateral branch of the fourth intercostal nerve. Although this is true, it does not constitute the only nerve supply (Fig. 60.1B). The Austrians (6) have shown that the lateral branch has both a deep and a superficial branch. The superficial branch supplies a lateral pedicle. The deep branch runs along the surface of the pectoralis fascia and then it turns upwards toward the nipple at the meridian. This is interesting because it means that any full-thickness pedicle designed straight down to the breast meridian (while not exposing pectoralis fascia) should incorporate this deep branch. Clearly, this branch is usually preserved with an inferior or central pedicle as long as the tissue overlying the pectoralis fascia is left intact. **There are also medial branches of the intercostal system that run superficially and supply innervation to a medial pedicle.** Supraclavicular branches run superficially and supply a superior pedicle.

Ductal Preservation

There are approximately 20 to 25 ducts that enter the nipple. Each duct is fed by glandular breast parenchyma. **Although dermal pedicles may preserve arterial, venous, and nerve supply, it is unlikely that dermal pedicles will retain much breast-feeding potential.** There is some potential for ducts to reconnect, but this is speculative. Dermoglandular pedicles will incorporate more glandular and ductal tissue intact.

Design

There has been considerable reluctance to adopt the vertical skin resection patterns in breast reduction surgery (Fig. 60.2). This is based on a lack of understanding that the principles of this technique do not apply to the inverted-T techniques.

The inverted-T relies on the skin brassiere to maintain the shape. The pattern was designed to minimize stretching of the skin. To prevent pseudoptosis, the vertical skin length, from nipple to inframammary fold (IMF), was restricted to about

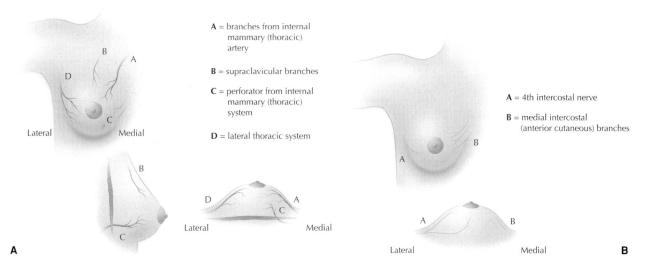

A = branches from internal
mammary (thoracic)
artery

B = supraclavicular branches

C = perforator from internal
mammary (thoracic)
system

D = lateral thoracic system

A = 4th intercostal nerve

B = medial intercostal
(anterior cutaneous) branches

FIGURE 60.1. Anatomy. **A:** Blood supply. The arterial supply is superficial (*A, B, D*) except for the deep perforator (*C*) that comes through the pectoralis muscle. The veins lie just under the dermis and are quite separate from the arteries (except for the venae comitantes which accompany the deep perforator). **B:** Nerve supply. The main innervation to the nipple and areola is from the lateral fourth intercostal nerve. It should be noted that there is a deep branch that courses just above the pectoralis fascia as well as the more superficial branch. This branch can provide sensation in several full-thickness pedicles. There are also medial intercostal branches that supply innervation.

5 cm. Although some coning of the breast tissue occurs, the nature of the resection of the breast parenchyma plays a minor role in shaping. The skin is removed mainly along a horizontally designed ellipse and the dog-ears are chased medially and laterally. Sometimes this pattern results in a boxy breast with definite limitations on the amount of projection achieved.

On the other hand, the vertical skin resection patterns tend to use the breast parenchyma to provide the shape. The skin adapts to the breast shape rather than the other way around. This will vary somewhat with the design of the pedicle chosen. The skin and breast parenchyma are removed mainly along a vertically designed ellipse and the dog-ears are chased up into the new areola and inferiorly toward the inframammary fold. **These breasts have a much longer vertical length, which is needed to accommodate the increased projection that results from this design.**

The choice of pedicle will also influence the resultant breast shape. The superior, superolateral, and superomedial pedicles will rely less on the skin brassiere to hold the shape. The inferior pedicle may respond more to gravity and the pedicle may need to be sutured up to the chest wall in an attempt to prevent bottoming out. With the inferior pedicle, it is important not to violate the inframammary fold for this reason. Large pedicles of any type may be too heavy and may require suturing to the chest wall, or even amputation and free nipple grafts. There remains some controversy about what method of suturing breast tissue to the chest wall is effective in the long-term.

Skin closure will be somewhat determined by the type of pedicle used. A circumvertical skin closure is necessary with an inferior pedicle. Either a straight or circumvertical skin closure can be used with the other pedicles. When there is a considerable amount of loose, inelastic skin, a T or J skin excision

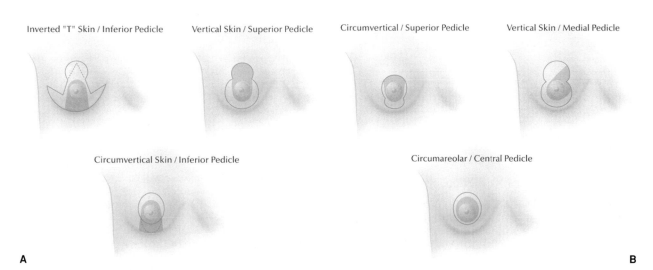

Inverted "T" Skin / Inferior Pedicle

Vertical Skin / Superior Pedicle

Circumvertical / Superior Pedicle

Vertical Skin / Medial Pedicle

Circumvertical Skin / Inferior Pedicle

Circumareolar / Central Pedicle

FIGURE 60.2. Pedicles and skin resection patterns. The skin resection pattern and the pedicle used for the nipple–areolar complex need to be assessed separately. Various combinations are available.

may be needed to remove the excess. This is, however, less frequently necessary than initially thought by those surgeons who have been trained with the inverted-T skin resection patterns.

As with most surgical procedures in plastic surgery, there are variations in the technique and variations in the principles used. Marchac (7) uses parenchymal resection for breast shaping, but he removes some of the excess skin by adding a T excision. Lassus (8) does not undermine the skin or remove breast tissue laterally above the inframammary fold. His pattern maintains the original inframammary fold and relies partly on parenchymal resection and partly on the skin brassiere to hold the shape. Lejour (9) relies on liposuction for volume reduction, and breast sutures to hold the shape of the parenchyma. She uses skin undermining and skin gathering to help the skin adapt to the new shape. All of these surgeons prefer a superiorly based pedicle for the nipple areolar complex and inferior parenchymal resection for breast shaping. Hammond (10) uses an inferior pedicle and a circumvertical skin resection pattern. His procedure relies on both parenchymal suturing and the skin brassiere to maintain the shape.

VERTICAL BREAST REDUCTION USING THE MEDIALLY BASED PEDICLE

The following describes a vertical skin resection pattern and a medially based pedicle for the nipple–areolar complex (11,12).

- *Vertical skin resection pattern:* The skin excision is a vertical ellipse, but the parenchymal resection follows the Wise (13) pattern (vertical plus horizontal). The inferior tissue is removed, the inframammary fold can rise if desired, and the remaining breast tissue is superior, superomedial, and superolateral. **It is believed that this resection pattern best resists the deforming forces of gravity over time.**
- *Medially based pedicle:* The pedicle is full thickness and it maintains sensation equivalent to the other pedicles. The nipple–areolar complex rotates easily into position without kinking or compression. The inferior border of the medial pedicle becomes the medial pillar. The fact that the whole base of the pedicle rotates gives an elegant curve to the inferior aspect of the breast. The superior pedicle can also be used, but it can be more difficult to inset. The superior pedicle can be safely thinned to prevent compression, but some depression can occur inferiorly when closing the pillars.

Markings

The key to marking the breast for breast reduction is to determine the new nipple position. This should be (with some variation; see below) at the intersection of the inframammary fold and the breast meridian.

Determination of New Nipple Position

Inframammary Fold. The IMF varies significantly from person to person. The new nipple needs to be designed according to the patient's anatomy, not an arbitrary distance from the suprasternal notch. Although a finger in the inframammary fold transposed to contact a finger on the breast skin can be used, the best method to determine the actual fold is to place a measuring tape around the chest under the breasts. The true level of the fold can be marked by drawing a line in the midline at the upper border of the tape. (It is interesting that this is often significantly lower than the finger method.) There may be some asymmetry in the levels of the breast folds and this needs to be noted.

Breast and Chest Wall Meridian. The breast may extend so far laterally that the true chest wall meridian may be much more medial. If lateral breast tissue is to be removed, the true chest wall meridian may be the better marking. Otherwise, the breast meridian should be chosen. The meridian is drawn from the midclavicular line down through the breast. Care must be taken to ignore the existing position of the nipple when marking the true meridian, but it is better to err on the side of placing the new nipple too lateral rather than too medial.

The meridian can then be extended on to the chest wall below the inframammary fold. This is usually about 9 to 11 cm from the midline of the body and will obviously vary with different body sizes.

New Nipple Position. The new nipple position will be marked approximately at the intersection of the inframammary fold and the breast meridian. Surgeons who are comfortable with the inferior pedicle inverted-T pattern, should place the new nipple position approximately 2 cm lower than what they are used to; this is needed to accommodate the increased projection that results from this approach. This is especially important when a patient has very little existing upper-pole fullness.

On the other hand, when a patient has significant upper-pole fullness, more flexibility exists and the new nipple position can be placed higher. If the surgeon is going to attempt to raise the inframammary fold (by clearing out tissue along the Wise pattern above the existing inframammary fold) the new nipple position can be raised slightly. **Caution: It is almost impossible to lower a nipple that has been placed too high. It is much easier to raise a nipple that has been placed too low.**

When there is significant size asymmetry, it is important to mark the new nipple position of the larger breast somewhat lower than the new position on the smaller breast. There are two reasons for this. First, the weight of the breast will stretch the skin and make the new marked position rise when the weight is removed. Second, closure of a vertical ellipse will push the upper end upward and the lower end downward. The inverted-T technique involves closure of a horizontal ellipse and the dog-ears are chased medially and laterally. The vertical technique involves closure of a vertical ellipse and the upper dog-ear is chased into the areola. If the vertical ellipse (of skin and parenchyma) is larger on one side, the upper end will be pushed up higher.

Skin Resection Pattern

Areolar Opening. The opening for the areola can be marked preoperatively or intraoperatively. When a surgeon first uses the vertical technique, it is perhaps easier to use the system with which they are familiar. If the areolar opening is made preoperatively, it should be designed so that it becomes a circle when closed. It makes more sense to extend the design vertically than to carry it out laterally in a mosque shape.

If a 4.5-cm diameter is used for the new areola, the exact circumference will be 14 cm; if a 5-cm diameter is used for the new areola, the exact circumference will be 16 cm. It is not actually necessary to match the circumferences exactly, but a significant discrepancy will result in widening of the areola, or the scar, or both. A circumvertical type of suture will be required if there is more than a 4-cm circumferential difference.

Vertical Resection Pattern. In the vertical techniques, the skin is not important in shaping the breast. Only enough skin needs to be removed to avoid skin redundancy. The skin is not being used as a skin brassiere and it is unnecessary—and detrimental—to make the skin closure tight.

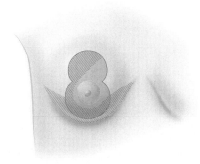

FIGURE 60.3. Design of the skin resection pattern (*outlined in red*), the medially based pedicle (*colored blue*) and the parenchymal resection pattern (*crosshatched*). The parenchymal resection follows a Wise pattern and the skin resection pattern looks like a snowman.

The vertical limbs can be drawn similar to that which would be drawn for a Wise-pattern skin resection. These can also be determined by pushing (and slightly rotating) the breast medially and then laterally to line up the vertical limbs with the previously drawn meridians in the upper and lower chest wall areas.

Instead of extending the vertical limbs laterally and medially as would be done in an inverted-T Wise pattern, the vertical limbs are joined to each other well above the inframammary fold. The final shape of the skin resection pattern with both the areolar opening and the vertical skin resection is much like a child's snowman (Fig. 60.3). The body is round with a smaller round head on top. Some surgeons have made the vertical resection come down as a V in order to limit the skin dog-ear, but, unfortunately, this often does not result in enough redundant lateral skin excision. Instead, the surgeon is forced to add a T or to add further resection and close it as a pursestring.

The skin resection pattern should remain well above the existing inframammary fold. There are two reasons for this. First, the parenchyma and skin are excised as a vertical ellipse and closure results in lengthening of the incision. The closure can push the scar below the fold. Second, when the parenchyma is excised along the Wise pattern horizontally (in addition to the resection along the vertical ellipse), the inframammary fold will often rise. If the fold rises, the scar can fall below the new fold. If these two factors are not taken into account, the scar might end up extending below the inframammary fold onto the chest wall. On average, at least 2 cm of skin must be left above the IMF in a small (300-g) reduction. At least 4 cm must be left in a medium (600-g) reduction, and at least 6 cm of skin must be left in a larger reduction (up to 1,000 g). Larger reductions will benefit from an even larger skin bridge.

Pedicle Design

The medial pedicle can be either dermoglandular or dermal, but breast-feeding is more likely to be preserved if the pedicle is full thickness. The pedicle is carried down directly to the breast meridian. As with all pedicles, it will be quite mobile and may appear to have been undermined.

The medial pedicle is often described as a superomedial pedicle. There is no question that it looks more superior when a patient is standing, but it actually has more of a medial orientation when the patient is lying down. The pedicle can be designed so that it is more superior, but giving the pedicle more of a superior orientation means that it can be sometimes more difficult to inset unless it is thinned.

To allow easy inset of all medially based pedicles, the base should be designed with half of the base into the areolar opening and half of the base into the vertical skin resection opening. When the original nipple position is quite low, the orientation will definitely be oblique. When the nipple does not have to move much higher, a superior pedicle can be chosen. The medial pedicle, however, does allow easy access to resect the redundant lateral breast tissue. This tissue is often very thick and fibrous and is not amenable to liposuction for volume reduction. **The lateral pedicle design was initially chosen because it was presumed to have better sensation (it didn't) and it was easy to inset, but the lateral breast tissue could not be resected because it formed the base of the pedicle. An unsatisfactory shape (with excess lateral fullness) was the result.**

Some tissue will be excised above the pedicle superiorly to allow the pedicle to be inset easily. It may be tempting to leave superior tissue and to push it up with the pedicle in order to achieve more upper-pole fullness, but this is usually doomed to fail. The tissue will drop and pseudoptosis will result. Some tissue can be left superiorly to try to incorporate more arterial input and it can also be used to provide a platform for the medially based pedicle. Although the pedicle is full thickness, it will appear to be undermined (much as the inferior pedicle) and providing a small platform can help prevent inversion of the nipple-areolar complex.

The base of the pedicle averages about 8 cm. The length of the pedicle to the base width is often about a 1:1 ratio, with the smaller reductions (300 g) having a 6-cm base, the medium-size reductions (600 g) having an 8-cm base, and the larger reductions having a 10-cm base. Wider bases are unlikely to improve circulation for very large reductions. Very long, large pedicles may end up causing pseudoptosis with the excess weight and volume, and free nipple grafts should be considered as an alternative. Suturing up the very large pedicles onto the chest wall may be of benefit, but this is unnecessary with most breast reductions up to 1,000 g.

Parenchymal Resection Design

The various types of vertical breast reduction vary. The pedicle chosen will determine to some extent the pattern of the parenchymal resection. For example, using the inferior pedicle means that the breast tissue is removed superiorly. For the other vertical patterns, the breast tissue is removed inferiorly as a vertical ellipse.

The principle that the vertical limbs in an inverted-T should measure only 5 cm does not apply to the skin in the vertical techniques, but it is a useful concept for the parenchyma. Keeping the pillar height at about 7 cm gives an ideal breast shape. To keep the pillars relatively short, the remaining parenchyma is removed horizontally below the pillars along a Wise pattern.

Once the markings are complete, it helps to draw the inverted-T or Wise pattern on the skin to guide the parenchymal resection. The tissue above is maintained to shape the breast and create the breast pillars. The tissue below is removed.

Operative Technique

Figure 60.4 illustrates the operative technique.

Infiltration

Some form of vasoconstriction is helpful. Infiltration along the inferior aspect and the base of the breast of about 40 mL per breast of Xylocaine 0.5% with 1:400,000 epinephrine will reduce bleeding during parenchymal resection. Unfortunately, infiltration along the incision lines can result in small hematomas because of the numerous superficial veins just below the dermis.

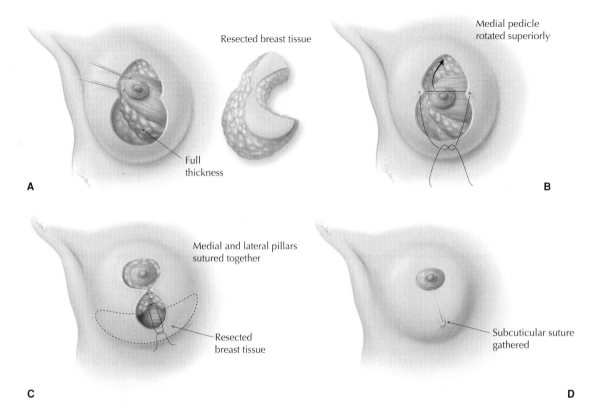

FIGURE 60.4. Operative technique. **A:** Pedicle and skin resection pattern. **B:** Rotation of pedicle. Note that the inferior border of the medial pedicle is now the medial pillar. **C:** Closure of the pillars. The pillar length is only about 5 to 7 cm. The pillar closure starts about half way up the vertical opening because the parenchyma needs to be resected inferiorly as outlined (following the Wise pattern). **D:** Closure of the areola and skin. Originally it was thought that this vertical incision needed to be gathered to allow the skin to retract. It has become increasingly evident that gathering not only interferes with healing but that it also delays resolution of the puckering.

In obese patients it is advisable to infiltrate about 500 to 1,000 mL of a tumescent-type fluid on each side along the lateral chest wall and the preaxillary areas. This reduces bleeding when these areas are suctioned. Some of the tumescent-type fluid can be infiltrated around the base of the breast as well. If too much is used, the breast will become quite "wet" and cutting cautery will be less effective.

Care must be taken to secure accurate hemostasis when using vasoconstrictors for breast reduction. It is especially important to look for and cauterize the perforators that come through the pectoralis fascia. They may remain constricted and not bleed during surgery, but these are usually the vessels that will later open up and cause a postoperative hematoma.

Creation of the Pedicle

The skin of the pedicle is de-epithelialized. Putting the skin on tension by using either a commercial device or a lap pad held at the base of the breast with a Kocher clamp, helps the assistant keep the skin taut. Care is taken to preserve the superficial veins that lie just beneath the dermis.

The pedicle is full thickness. It is incised directly down to the chest wall. Either a scalpel or cutting cautery can be used. Care is taken not to expose pectoralis fascia to both avoid bleeding and preserve the nerves that run just above the fascia. Some tissue cephalad can be left superiorly to leave a platform for the pedicle, but it is important not to try to push that tissue up in an attempt to increase upper-pole fullness.

As with the inferior pedicle, it will be quite mobile and it is important that the assistant not pull excessively to avoid inadvertent undermining of the pedicle.

Parenchymal Resection

Both scalpel and cutting cautery are used to remove breast tissue. The resection is beveled out laterally and medially. The inferior border of the medial pedicle becomes the medial pillar. The whole base of the pedicle rotates as the nipple and areola are inset into position and the pedicle itself gives an elegant curve to the inferior pole of the breast.

The lateral resection will be more aggressive, but some tissue (not much) needs to be left to fashion a lateral pillar. There is often a considerable excess of lateral breast tissue and direct excision is necessary because of its thick fibrous nature. Adipose tissue lateral to the breast (which is actually on the lateral chest wall) can be treated later with liposuction.

It is important to follow the preoperative plan for the amount of tissue to be resected. Because it can be difficult to resect an adequate amount of breast parenchyma with this technique, it may be tempting to remove tissue superiorly. If the patient has very little upper-pole fullness, it is important not to resect superior tissue for a few centimeters on either side of the breast meridian. On the other hand, tissue can be removed superiorly when the patient has a significant amount of upper-pole fullness.

The inferior breast tissue along the Wise pattern is removed by direct excision and then liposuction is used to tailor the resection inferiorly, both laterally and medially. Liposuction is not used for volume reduction, but it is used to correct asymmetry that remains during closure and it is used for cosmetic refinement.

The skin flaps incorporate the breast tissue superiorly and laterally, as well as superiorly and medially. The resection is beveled out laterally and medially and then finished with liposuction. The resection is actually undermined inferiorly so that the inferior breast can now become chest wall (skin and fat) as the inframammary fold rises. The fold will only rise about 1 to 2 cm at the meridian, but it will curve up considerably as it extends laterally and medially. The skin flaps are therefore full thickness superiorly and thinned out (with still a layer of fat to prevent adhesions) inferiorly. Flap thickness is thinnest at the skin margins (about 1 cm) and it gets thicker as one extends laterally and medially. There will be an excess of skin remaining inferiorly compared to breast parenchyma.

Insetting the Pedicle

It is easier to inset the pedicle after the base of the areola is closed. A single 3-0 polydioxanone suture (PDS) or Monocryl suture is used. Some dermis is incorporated with the first bite at the base of the pedicle, but the dermis itself does not need to be undermined. Once this suture is tied, the nipple and areola rotate easily into position. The amount of rotation will vary; only enough rotation is needed to allow a comfortable inset with minimal compression.

Even though the pedicle is carried full thickness down to the chest meridian, it is very mobile and may appear to have been undermined.

The medial and lateral pillars are then closed. Final inset and closure of the areola is performed later.

Closure of the Pillars

The inferior border of the medial pedicle now becomes the medial pillar. The pedicle needs to be completely rotated up so that the first pillar suture is placed at the medial end of the inferior border just next to the base of the pedicle. This suture does not need to be deep. Some lateral pillar tissue at the same level on the other side is also incorporated into this first suture. There is no need to take large bites or to include fatty tissue. It is important to place the suture on either side into fibrous tissue. There is some fibrous tissue in even the fattiest breasts.

Only a few sutures are needed. If the pedicle is long and heavy, it may be wise to suture some of the pedicle up onto the chest wall to help prevent bottoming-out.

Closure of the Dermis

The dermis is closed so that the resultant incision line is vertical. Deep buried 3-0 Monocryl sutures are ideal because they absorb relatively quickly and they are less likely to extrude than are PDS sutures. There is no need to suture the dermis up onto the breast parenchyma (it will delay shape resolution postoperatively). Only enough sutures are used to maintain approximation of the margins.

Liposuction

Before final closure of the skin, it is a good idea to stand back and assess asymmetry and shape. Some surgeons prefer to sit the patient up at this stage. Unless the patient has very thick, fibrous breast tissue (which occurs in many normal-weight teenagers) liposuction can be used to correct asymmetry. **The area that needs to be carefully checked is the area just above the existing inframammary fold. There should be no excess subcutaneous tissue remaining that will result later in a pucker.** The tissue inferiorly at the level of the meridian will often need direct excision (there are definite transverse fibers at the level of the fold) especially if the surgeon wishes the fold to rise. Liposuction can be used medially and (especially) laterally to tailor this region.

Liposuction is also used to reduce excess fat along the lateral chest wall and in the preaxillary areas. If the patient is obese, then tumescent-type infiltration is recommended for the areas to be suctioned. Patients are warned preoperatively that these areas will bruise and that they are often the source of more discomfort postoperatively than the breasts themselves (Fig. 60.5).

Closure of the Skin

The vertical skin closure is best achieved by a running subcuticular 3-0 or 4-0 Monocryl suture. It is important to close this skin relatively loosely. Extra skin does not need to be excised in a lateral or medial direction in order to hold the shape of the breast. Deep bites, tight sutures, and skin tension will only delay wound healing.

This suture can be gathered (only at the inferior end) to help the skin to shrink, but this is far less important than originally thought. In fact, excess skin gathering will actually delay resolution of any skin puckering inferiorly. In the past, surgeons were advised to gather this skin to reduce the vertical length by one-half to one-third. The length should actually be reduced only by 1 to 2 cm at most. Good quality skin will adapt very well to the new breast shape.

It may be tempting to close the skin as an L, or a J, or even a T, but this is usually unnecessary. When there is a large amount of loose, inelastic skin (such as found in a postbariatric patient), excision may be indicated. On the other hand, this is rarely needed in most breast reductions up to 1,000 g. It is not the amount of the parenchymal resection that is important, but the quality of the redundant skin that will make this determination.

The excess skin that remains inferiorly adapts surprisingly well to the new breast shape. It is difficult for surgeons who have been trained to keep the vertical skin length at 5 cm to accept a long (sometimes longer than 12 cm) vertical skin opening. The temptation to excise this extra skin can be difficult to resist.

Closure of the Areola

The skin opening for the areola should be round. In the past, when the vertical skin was gathered significantly, a teardrop shape resulted. This could take several months to settle postoperatively. Now that gathering is not recommended, the problem of distortion of the areola is no longer a concern.

If there is a considerable discrepancy between the circumference of the skin opening and the circumference of the areola (when it is stretched out properly), then consideration should be given to a permanent type of suture to prevent widening. Usually, however, a 4-cm discrepancy is easily tolerated and closure is best achieved by a few interrupted 3-0 or 4-0 Monocryl sutures followed by a running subcuticular suture.

Drains and Antibiotics

The use of both drains and antibiotics is controversial. Drains do not prevent hematoma, but they may reduce the substrate for bacteria. When drains are used postoperatively, they are usually removed on the following day, but some surgeons will leave them in place for several days. Many surgeons do not use drains at all unless there is considerable oozing present (as can occur when patients ignore advice to stop anti-inflammatories for 2 weeks preoperatively). Drains can be brought out through the vertical incision or through a separate stab incision.

Cephalosporins are the most commonly used antibiotics. There is controversy over whether they should be used at all,

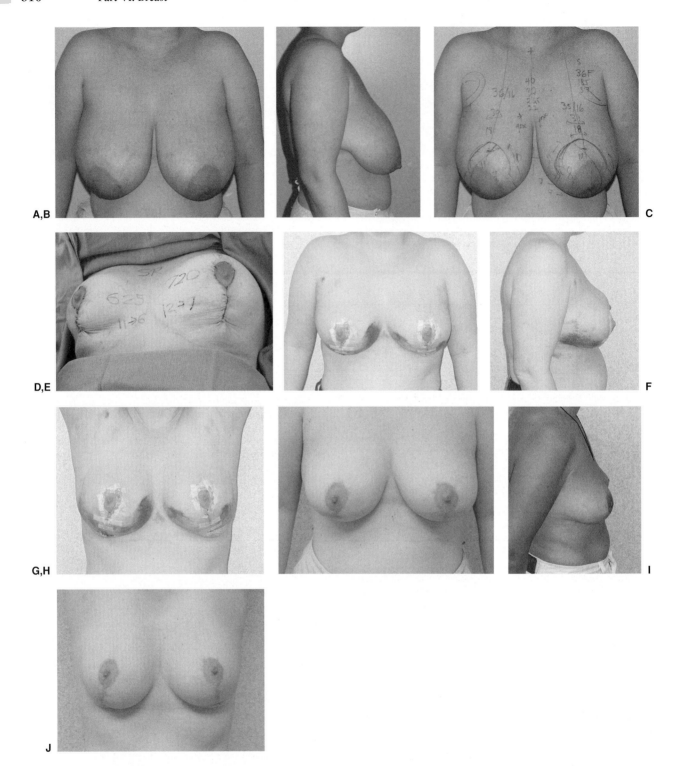

FIGURE 60.5. A 34-year-old, 185-lb, 5'7" patient who wore a 36F brassiere. **A:** Preoperative frontal view of moderate-size breast reduction. **B:** Preoperative lateral view. **C:** Preoperative view with markings (many of these measurements are performed for statistical analysis only). The most important markings note the level of the inframammary fold (and therefore the new nipple position vertically), the breast and chest wall meridian (and therefore the new nipple position horizontally), as well as the areolar opening, the skin resection pattern, and the medial pedicle design. **D:** Intraoperative view at completion of the vertical approach using the medial pedicle. The patient had 625 g of tissue removed from the right breast and 720 g removed from the left breast. She also had 400 cm³ of fat removed from the lateral chest wall and preaxillary areas with some contouring of the lower portion of the breasts. Surgery time was 90 minutes. I now gather this incision far less than shown in this photograph. **E:** Frontal view at 10 days postoperatively. **F:** Lateral view at 10 days postoperatively. **G:** Arms up view at 10 days. The results do not necessarily take a long time to settle postoperatively. **H:** Frontal view at 15 months postoperatively. **I:** Lateral view at 15 months postoperatively. **J:** Arms up view at 15 months postoperatively.

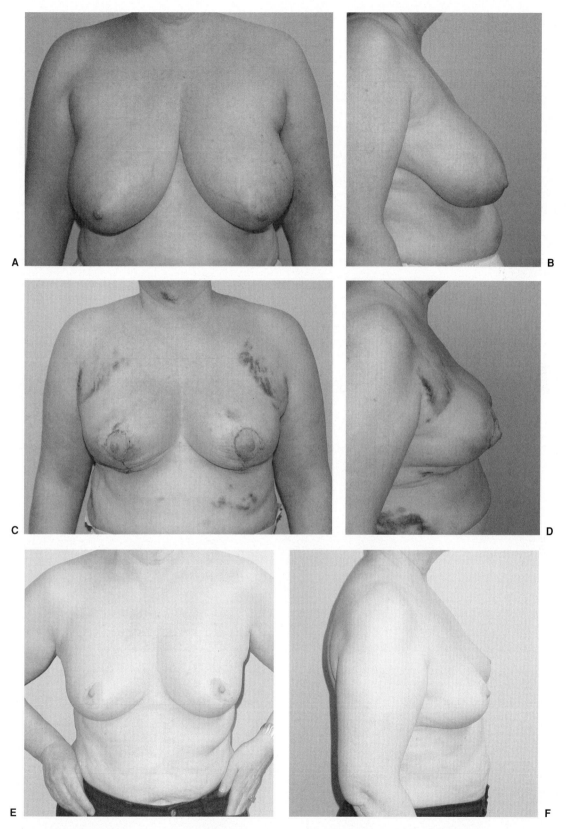

FIGURE 60.6. A 60-year-old patient who was 5′4″ tall, weighed 195 pounds, and wore a 38DD brassiere. She had 680 g of tissue removed from each breast. **A:** Frontal preoperatively. **B:** Lateral preoperatively. **C:** Frontal 10 days postoperatively. **D:** Lateral 10 days postoperatively. **E:** Frontal 4.5 years postoperatively. **F:** Lateral 4.5 years postoperatively.

whether they should be used only perioperatively, or whether they should be used for several days postoperatively.

Postoperative Course

Steri-Strips or Micropore paper tape can be applied to the incisions. If paper tape is used, it can be left in place for about 3 weeks. A couple of horizontal strips can be applied inferiorly to help encourage the redundant inferior skin to settle. Taping of the whole breast is unnecessary. The patient can shower the day after surgery and they wash over the tape and then pat it dry. A brassiere is not used for compression, but can be used to hold gauze bandages (initially) and pantiliners (after a couple of days) in place.

Patients are encouraged to gradually increase their activities. Return to desk work may only take 1 to 2 weeks, whereas return to heavy physical activity may take several weeks. The pucker (dog-ear at the inferior end of the vertical incision) may take several weeks to months to settle. A seroma may occur that makes the pucker look more ominous, but seromas will settle relatively quickly without intervention.

Patients should be warned about the time it takes for resolution of the shape, any asymmetries, or persistent puckers. They should know that revisions may be necessary in a limited number of patients, but that a full year should pass before considering any corrective surgery.

Figures 60.5 to 60.7 show results in three patients.

Complications

Complication rates reported in the literature can be confusing. Care must be taken when comparing complications to determine whether these are "major" or "minor."

Hematoma

Hematomas may develop postoperatively if transected vessels are not apparent because of the vasoconstrictors used for infiltration. Drains will not prevent hematomas and any significant hematoma will require reoperation.

Nipple–Areolar Necrosis

Breast reduction surgery is a blood supply reducing operation. Care must be taken when creating the pedicle to preserve as much blood supply as possible. A clear understanding of anatomy is important, but the actual blood supply in any particular patient is guesswork at best.

Although it has been advised to take a nipple and areola that is compromised and convert it to a free nipple graft, this decision is extremely difficult. It is not uncommon for areolas to look dusky and pale at the end of the procedure. Most surgeons are well aware that recovery is the rule. It would be inappropriate to convert these areolae to free grafts, because grafting results in a lack of sensation, a lack of nipple projec-

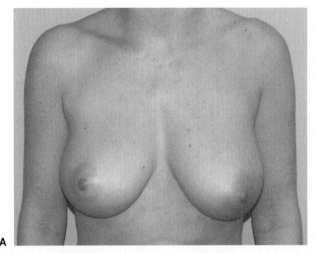
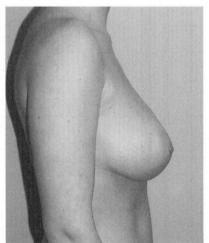
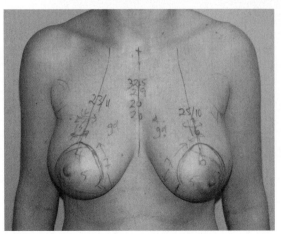
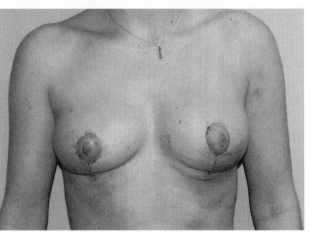

FIGURE 60.7. A 24-year-old woman who had 295 g of tissue removed from her right breast and 315 g from her left breast. **A:** Frontal preoperatively. **B:** Lateral preoperatively. **C:** Frontal markings preoperatively. **D:** Frontal 10 days postoperatively. *(Continued)*

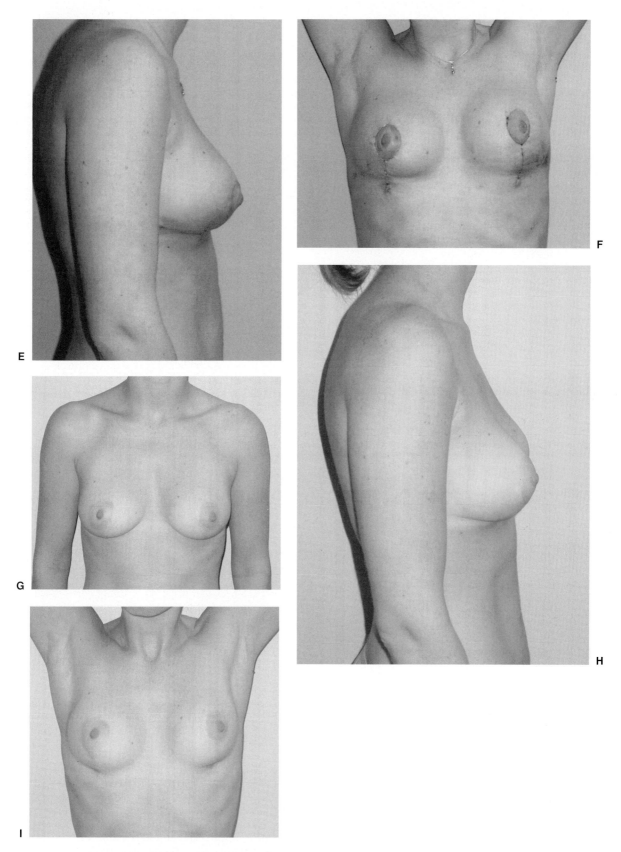

FIGURE 60.8. (*Continued*) **E:** Lateral 10 days postoperatively. **F:** Frontal arms elevated 10 days postoperatively. This view is humbling in that it shows any residual puckering or deformity. **G:** Frontal 18 months postoperatively. **H:** Lateral 18 months postoperatively. **I:** Frontal arms elevated 18 months postoperatively.

tion, and an inability to breast-feed, and grafts can heal with irregular pigmentation.

If it is clear that a nipple and areola are suffering from venous congestion postoperatively, then measures such as removing sutures or taking the patient back to the operating room for exploration may help. Many patients are now being discharged as same-day surgery patients and the opportunity for this type of evaluation is not available. It would make sense to keep patients for observation if this evaluation was clear-cut. But it isn't. Necrosis is most likely a lack of arterial input and this cannot be corrected. Necrosis from correctable venous congestion is much less likely. The risk-to-benefit ratio is such that it is probably best to allow almost all questionable cases to resolve without intervention. Blistering and some loss may occur, but this is often preferable to active intervention, which carries its own risks.

Rarely, complete loss of the nipple and areola will occur. Intervening on the questionable cases is unlikely to decrease this incidence. Each patient will need to be evaluated over time as to whether the necrotic tissue should be allowed to heal by secondary intention, in-office debridement, or intraoperative debridement. Some form of nipple and areolar reconstruction is then considered.

Infection

Infection rates should be no higher with breast-reduction surgery than other clean operations. Many surgeons believe that antibiotics are indicated because the breast ducts are open to the external environment. Some surgeons use no antibiotics, some use perioperative antibiotics, and some use a full course of antibiotics. The most commonly used antibiotics are first- or second-generation cephalosporins.

Wound Healing

All types of breast reduction have problems with wound healing. The inverted-T has more problems with necrosis at the T, and the vertical types can have more problems on the vertical incision line. Both of these can be prevented to some degree by avoiding undue tension on the incision lines. Avoiding tension can be harder with the inverted-T because the procedure relies more on the skin to hold the shape. The vertical is more likely to run into problems if the surgeon causes constriction during closure by excising too much skin or by undue skin gathering. Antibiotics may be helpful in reducing wound-healing problems.

Extensive flap necrosis is rare. It is more likely to occur when the skin is undermined and when excessive tension is applied to the flaps during closure. Debridement may be necessary. Skin grafting may close the wounds earlier, but the cosmetic result is often better if the open areas are allowed to heal secondarily.

Seromas

Seromas can occur with or without the use of drains. Even leaving the drains in for several days does not seem to prevent the development of seromas. Aspiration may be indicated, but the seromas will tend to recur. They can be left to resolve on their own. Although surgeons may be concerned that a pseudobursa may develop, this does not seem to be a problem.

Underresection

It is far more difficult to remove enough breast tissue with the vertical techniques than it is with the inverted-T techniques. At the end of the procedure, the breasts actually look smaller than they are. This can be a problem for surgeons who have been accustomed to assessing size with the inverted-T. The extra

projection can be misleading. It is important to determine the amount of breast tissue to be removed preoperatively and to then follow that plan.

Usually at least 6 to 12 months should elapse before undertaking any re-reduction. This can be achieved through liposuction-only or by re-reducing tissue in the vertical plane. Most of the re-reduction will involve parenchyma. It is important not to take too much skin in the re-reduction or a torpedo-type shape will result. Fortunately, the shape will settle because the skin will inevitably stretch to some degree.

Asymmetry

Correction of asymmetry should follow similar guidelines to re-reduction. The problem may be solved by liposuction-only or it may require parenchymal repositioning, scar release, or excision.

Puckers

The vertical skin pattern approach usually involves excision of skin and parenchyma in a vertical ellipse. This means that there are two dog-ears—one that is chased into the areolar opening and disappears, and one that is chased inferiorly. The skin excision should remain as a U and not be tapered into a V, especially if this would mean that the scar would extend below the inframammary fold. The excess skin will tuck in under the breast as it settles.

It is advisable to wait a full year before performing any revisions. At first glance, the pucker that remains may appear to be a problem of excess skin. But usually the real problem is excess subcutaneous tissue between the original and the new inframammary fold. Very little skin may need excision, and often the skin can be excised by carrying the scar down a bit further vertically, but not below the fold.

Adding a T at the initial procedure may obviate the necessity to revise any puckers, but it has been shown that performing a T resection did not alter the revision rate (14). Fortunately, many of these revisions can be performed in the office under local anesthesia. The need for occasional revisions are an integral part of plastic surgery, and breast reduction is no exception. Revisions do tend to be more common with the vertical approaches, especially during the learning curve. Each surgeon will have a different threshold for revision, but a rate of approximately 5% is not unexpected.

CONCLUSION

It has been repeatedly documented that both physical and psychological outcomes are excellent after breast-reduction surgery. The challenge is to keep scarring to a minimum while giving the breast a pleasing and long-lasting shape.

The vertical approaches are excellent for small- to medium-size reductions. With experience, surgeons also find that the methods are applicable to larger and larger reductions. There is no question that there is an initial learning curve (as there is with the inverted-T), but surgeons eventually feel rewarded by the improved scarring that results and by the improved shape. The procedures take a shorter time to perform, there is less blood loss, and patient recovery time is faster.

The concepts in the vertical techniques involve far more than just a different vector in the skin and parenchymal resection patterns. This vector plus the more superiorly based pedicles give a shape that resists gravity over time. In general, the vertical approaches use the breast to shape the skin, whereas the inverted-T approaches use the skin to shape the breast.

References

1. Spear SL, Howard MA. Evolution of the vertical reduction mammaplasty. *Plast Reconstr Surg.* 2003;112:855.
2. Robbins TH. A reduction mammaplasty with the areola-nipple based on an inferior pedicle. *Plast Reconstr Surg.* 1977;59:64.
3. Gradinger GP. Reduction mammaplasty utilizing nipple–areola transplantation. *Clin Plast Surg.* 1988;15:641.
4. Gray LN. Update on experience with liposuction breast reduction. *Plast Reconstr Surg.* 2001;108:1006.
5. Corduff N, Taylor GI. Subglandular breast reduction: the evolution of a minimal scar approach to breast reduction. *Plast Reconstr Surg.* 2004;113:175.
6. Schlenz I, Kuzbari R, Gruber H, et al. The sensitivity of the nipple–areola complex: An anatomic study. *Plast Reconstr Surg.* 2000;105:905.
7. Lassus C. A 30-year experience with vertical mammaplasty. *Plast Reconstr Surg.* 1996;97:373.
8. Marchac D, de Olarte G. Reduction mammaplasty and correction of ptosis with a short inframammary scar. *Plast Reconstr Surg.* 1982;69:45.
9. Lejour M. *Vertical Mammaplasty and Liposuction of the Breast.* St. Louis, MO: Quality Medical; 1993.
10. Hammond DC. Short scar periareolar inferior pedicle reduction (SPAIR) mammaplasty. *Plast Reconstr Surg.* 1999;103:890.
11. Asplund O, Davies DM. Vertical scar breast reduction with medial flap or glandular transposition of the nipple–areola. *Br J Plast Surg.* 1996;49:507.
12. Hall-Findlay EJ. A simplified vertical reduction mammaplasty: shortening the learning curve. *Plast Reconstr Surg.* 1999;104:748.
13. Wise RJ. A preliminary report on a method of planning the mammaplasty. *Plast Reconstr Surg.* 1956;17:367.
14. Berthe J-V, Massaut J, Greuse M, et al. The vertical mammaplasty: a reappraisal of the technique and its complications. *Plast Reconstr Surg.* 2003;111:2192.

CHAPTER 61 ■ GYNECOMASTIA

NOLAN S. KARP

Gynecomastia is caused by an increase in ductal tissue, stroma, and/or fat in the male breast. Most frequently, the changes occur at the time of hormonal changes: infancy, adolescence, and old age.

The term gynecomastia was introduced by Galen during the second century A.D. and the surgical resection was first described by Paulis of Aegina (1,2) in the seventh century A.D.

ETIOLOGY

The most common cause for gynecomastia is idiopathic; Table 61.1 lists the other common causes. Gynecomastia often appears transiently at birth. The process is thought to be related to an increased level of circulating maternal estrogens. After birth, the estrogen level decreases and the gynecomastia usually resolves. Treatment is rarely necessary.

Gynecomastia is present in almost 66% of adolescent boys (3). This is thought to be the result of an imbalance of estradiol and testosterone. The adolescent gynecomastia resolves in the vast majority of cases (2). In some cases, a degree of gynecomastia remains, but it is not enough to warrant medical attention.

The incidence of gynecomastia rises again in older men (older than age 65 years). This is thought to be the result of a decline in testosterone and a shift in the ratio of testosterone to estrogen.

In all three age groups, gynecomastia appears to be related to either an increase in estrogens, a decrease in androgens, or a deficit in androgen receptors (2). Numerous drugs are associated with gynecomastia (Table 61.1). Systemic causes include adrenal diseases, liver diseases, pituitary tumors, thyroid disease, and renal failure. Tumors of adrenal, pituitary, lung, and testis can be associated with a hormonal imbalance that results in gynecomastia.

In any male patient with breast enlargement, male breast cancer must be considered because 1% of all breast cancers occur in men. There is no increased risk of breast cancer in patients with gynecomastia when compared to the unaffected male population (4). The exception is patients with Klinefelter syndrome. These patients have an approximately 60 times increased risk of breast cancer.

PATHOLOGY

Three types of gynecomastia have been described: florid, fibrous, and intermediate (5). The florid type is characterized by an increase in ductal tissue and vascularity. A variable amount of fat tends to be mixed in with the ductal tissue. The fibrous type has more stromal fibrosis and few ducts. The intermediate type is a mixture of the two. The type of gynecomastia is usually related to the duration of the disorder. Florid gynecomastia is usually seen when the duration is 4 months or less. The fibrous type is usually present after a duration of 1 year. The intermediate type is thought to be a progression from florid to fibrous and is usually seen between 4 and 12 months (5).

DIAGNOSIS

A careful history and physical examination is the most important part of any work-up for gynecomastia. The history must note the time of onset of the gynecomastia, symptoms associated with the gynecomastia, drug use (both medically prescribed and recreational), and careful review of systems. Organ system changes associated with gynecomastia include liver, renal, adrenal, pulmonary, pituitary, testicular, thyroid, and/or prostate.

Physical examination should include assessment of the breast gland. This will include the nature of the tissue, isolated masses, and tenderness. The thyroid should be evaluated for enlargement. The testis should be examined to look for asymmetry, masses, enlargement, or atrophy.

Laboratory evaluation is based on the findings of the history and physical examination. Healthy adults with a normal physical examination (other than gynecomastia) and longstanding gynecomastia do not need further work-up.

Patients with feminizing characteristics should have endocrine testing. In addition, if marfanoid body habitus is associated with the feminization, Klinefelter syndrome must be ruled out. Any other new positive findings on physical examination should be worked up in an appropriate manner.

CLASSIFICATION

Simon et al. (6) divided gynecomastia into four grades as follows:

Grade 1 :   Small enlargement, no skin excess
Grade 2a: Moderate enlargement, no skin excess
Grade 2b: Moderate enlargement with extra skin
Grade 3 :   Marked enlargement with extra skin.

In their opinion, grades 2b and 3 require some skin resection. The need to excise excess skin depends on the shape of the breast. Large breasts with a wide base may be treated without skin excision. Conversely, smaller, but narrow breasts may need skin excision.

Letterman and Schuster (7) created a classification system based on the type of correction as follows:

1:     Intra-areolar incision with no excess skin
2:     Intra-areolar incision with mild redundancy
          corrected with excision of skin through a superior
          periareolar scar
3:     Excision of chest skin with or without shifting the
          nipple

TABLE 61.1

COMMON CAUSES OF GYNECOMASTIA

Idiopathic
Obesity
Physiologic
   Birth
   Puberty
   Old age
Endocrine
   Testis: hypogonadism, Klinefelter syndrome
   Adrenal: Cushing syndrome, congenital adrenal hyperplasia
   Thyroid: hypothyroid, hyperthyroid
   Pituitary: pituitary failure
Neoplasms
   Adrenal
   Testis
   Pituitary
   Bronchogenic
Systemic diseases
   Renal failure
   Cirrhosis
   Adrenal
   Malnutrition
Drug-induced
   Hormones: estrogens, androgens
   Antiandrogens: spironolactone, cimetidine, ketoconazole, ranitidine, flutamide
   Cardiovascular drugs: amiodarone, digoxin, nifedipine, reserpine, verapamil
   Abused drugs: Alcohol, heroin, marijuana

Rohrich (8), in a paper discussing the usefulness of ultrasound-assisted liposuction in the treatment of gynecomastia, developed the following classification:

Grade I :   Minimal hypertrophy (<250 g of breast tissue) without ptosis

Grade II :   Moderate hypertrophy (250 to 500 g of breast tissue) without ptosis

Grade III: Severe hypertrophy (>500 g of breast tissue) with grade I ptosis

Grade IV: Severe hypertrophy with grade II or III ptosis

TREATMENT OF GYNECOMASTIA

If a patient has gynecomastia for less than 1 year and a normal history and physical examination, observation is probably indicated. If there is a possible etiology noted in the patient's history, an attempt should be made to either discontinue the drug believed to be causing the gynecomastia or correct the systemic condition. If an abnormality is found on physical examination, work-up is indicated prior to consideration of surgery for the gynecomastia. If the underlying condition is treated and the gynecomastia persists beyond 1 year, surgical correction is indicated (Fig. 61.1).

The first surgical procedures used to treat gynecomastia were excisional in nature (9). Suction assisted lipectomy was first reported in the early 1980s (10), and more recently ultrasound-assisted liposuction has been used for certain types of gynecomastia (8). The physical deformity requires evaluation and staging to determine the appropriate treatment.

Most fibrous or solid Simon stage 1 or 2a lesions are usually treated with surgical excision or, in some cases, with ultrasonic liposuction. If surgical excision is performed, a periareolar incision is performed as indicated in Figure 61.2A. The

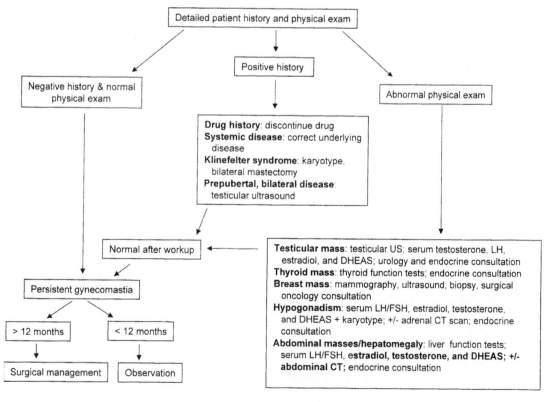

FIGURE 61.1. Algorithm for evaluation and treatment of gynecomastia. (Adapted from Rohrich RJ, Ha RY, Kenkel JM, Adams WP. Classification and management of gynecomastia: defining the role of ultrasound-assisted liposuction. *Plast Reconstr Surg.* 2003;111:909, with permission.)

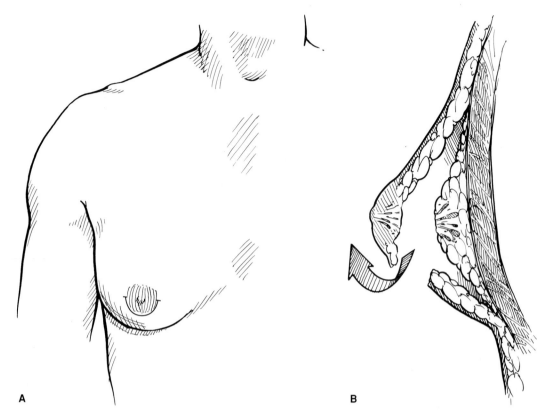

FIGURE 61.2. A: Periareolar incision. Medial and lateral extensions are used only if needed. **B:** Resection of gynecomastia through periareolar incision. Note the cuff of tissue left under areola.

skin incision is placed at the junction of the areola and skin. If placed within the pigmented area, the scar may appear as a white line. The site of the incision should be marked prior to injection of epinephrine-containing solution. If placed properly, the scar may be nearly invisible. After the incision is made, a cuff of tissue 1 to 1.5 cm in thickness is left directly under the nipple areola complex. This maneuver prevents postoperative nipple areola depression and adherence of the nipple areola to the chest wall (Fig. 61.2B). It is always better to leave more tissue than less under the nipple areola. At the end of the case any excess can be trimmed off. The chest skin flaps are developed in a plane between the subcutaneous fat and the breast tissue. To assure a smooth contour, the edges of the breast are trimmed with either scissors or liposuction.

If the patient has a lesion that is glandular, fatty, or mixed in nature and is Simon grade 1 or 2a, the area could be treated with liposuction. Conventional liposuction with sharp-tip cannulas, power-assisted liposuction, or ultrasound-assisted liposuction have all been used in this situation.

The patient is marked in the upright position. All areas of tissue excess are marked, as well as the inframammary fold. The patient is either sedated or placed under general anesthesia. The area is infiltrated with a tumescent solution containing lactated Ringer solution, 1 mL of 1:1,000 epinephrine solution, and 20 mL of 2% lidocaine solution. The infiltration is about 1:1 with the expected aspiration volume, and covers a wide area of the chest—from the clavicle to below the inframammary fold. Whichever method of liposuction is performed, special cannulas, specifically designed for gynecomastia surgery, are used. Figure 61.3A shows typical incisions. There is usually a lateral incision at the level of the inframammary fold and a periareolar incision. Liposuction is performed in all directions through both incisions (Fig. 61.3B). The inframammary fold is disrupted when present. The end point is a

flat, smooth contour with an absence of palpable tissue (Fig. 61.4). In cases of pure fatty gynecomastia no further surgery is necessary.

When liposuction is unsuccessful at removing all of the tissue required to achieve a good result, the pullthrough (11,12) technique may be used. In this technique, either the lateral or periareolar incision is opened slightly longer (about 1.5 cm) and the residual tissue is grasped. The tissue is pulled out through the wound and removed with scissors or electric cautery. The pullthrough resection is performed until the desired contour is achieved. Again, attention must be maintained not to over-resect the subareolar area (Fig. 61.5). Postoperative drainage may be used if the dead space is large. All patients are treated with at least 1 month of a compression garment.

In patients with Simon grade 2b gynecomastia, the initial treatment is similar to that given to patients with grade 1 or 2a gynecomastia. If the lesion is fatty, glandular, or mixed in nature and some type of liposuction is the initial treatment modality, no skin resection is performed at the first surgical session. The patients are treated with compression vests and the chest wall tissue is given time to settle and contract. The patient should wait at least 6 to 12 months before considering skin resection. In the majority of cases, no skin resection is required. When skin resection is performed, the amount of skin removed and the length of the incision are much less than if the resection were performed at the time of the initial surgery.

If the patient has a Simon grade 2b lesion that is very solid or fibrous in nature and an open approach is selected, skin resection might be incorporated into the initial procedure. If the patient desires to keep the visible scar as short as possible, the tissue could be resected with a minimalist periareolar incision and the patient treated with a compression garment. In many cases, no further skin resection is required. Ultrasonic liposuction with the pullthrough technique (if needed) has also

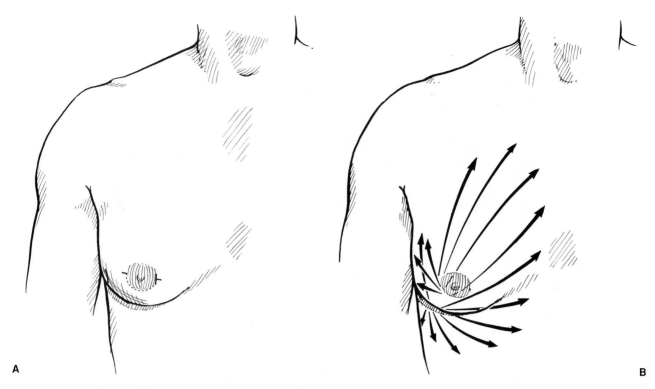

FIGURE 61.3. A: Location of incisions for suction-assisted lipectomy of gynecomastia. **B:** Direction of liposuction through both incisions.

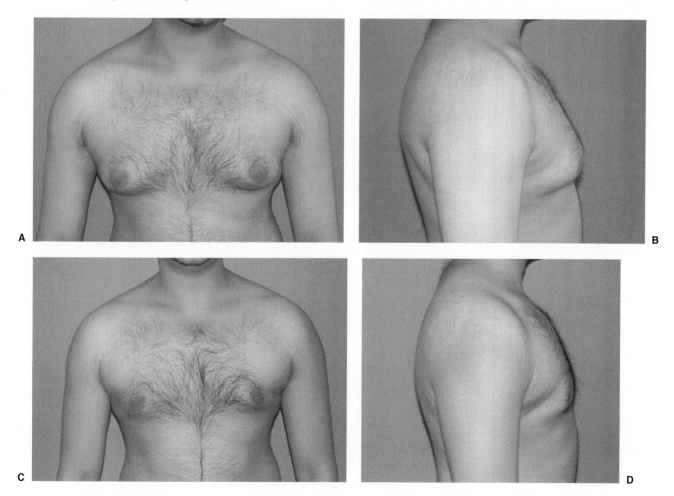

FIGURE 61.4. Patient with Simon 2a gynecomastia who underwent suction-assisted lipectomy of the chest. **A:** and **B:** Preoperative. **C:** and **D:** Postoperative.

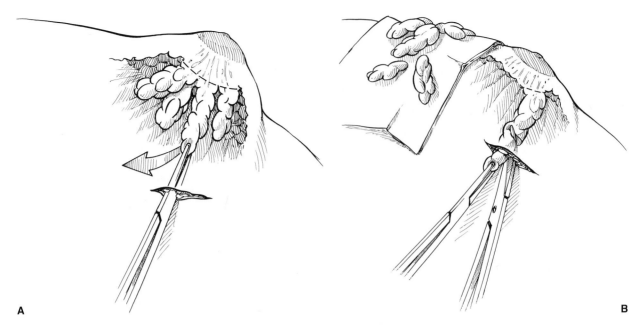

A   B

FIGURE 61.5. Demonstration of pullthrough resection of gynecomastia.

been used in Simon 2b cases without skin resection with good results.

In patients with Simon grade 3 gynecomastia, skin resection is almost always required. Numerous incisions and techniques to resect the skin and keep the nipple viable have been described, including superior and inferior periareolar incisions, omega incisions, nipple transpositions on a variety of pedicles, concentric circle techniques, and any form of liposuction with skin excision. The choice of technique is based on the preference of the surgeon.

COMPLICATIONS

The most common early complication after gynecomastia surgery is hematoma. In an open case, the hematoma should be evacuated if possible. This prevents excessive scarring and distortion of the breast. Postoperative closed suction drainage decreases the incidence of this complication. In liposuction cases, evacuation may not be possible.

Underresection of tissue is the most common long-term complication of gynecomastia surgery. This is particularly common in liposuction cases, when a residual mass of tissue is not removed. This can be avoided by using the pullthrough technique. Underresection at the periphery of the breast can result from poor tapering and causes a noticeable deformity. Overresection in the nipple areola can result in a saucer-type deformity that is difficult to correct. Loose skin is usually not considered a complication if it is part of the operative plan. Occasionally, loose skin occurs in an unexpected manner, and surgical excision is required.

Postoperative wound infection is uncommon. The use of prophylactic antibiotics, particularly in liposuction cases, may account for the low incidence of this complication.

References

1. Goldwyn R. *Plastic and Reconstructive Surgery of the Breast*. Boston: Little Brown; 1976.
2. McGrath MH. Gynecomastia. In: Jurkiewicz MJ, Mathes SJ, Krizek TJ, et al, eds. *Plastic Surgery: Principles and Practice*. St. Louis: Mosby; 1990.
3. Nydick M, Bustos J, Dale JH, et al. Gynecomastia in adolescent boys. *JAMA*. 1961;178:449.
4. Cohen IK, Pozez AL, McKeown JE. Gynecomastia. In: Courtiss EH, ed. *Male Aesthetic Surgery*. St. Louis: Mosby; 1991.
5. Bannayan GA, Hajdu SI. Gynecomastia: clinicopathologic study of 351 cases. 1972;57:431.
6. Simon BE, Hoffman S, Kahn S. Classification and surgical correction of gynecomastia. *Plast Reconstr Surg*. 1973;51:48.
7. Letterman G, Schuster M. The surgical correction of gynecomastia. *A Surg*. 1969;35:322.
8. Rohrich RJ, Ha RY, Kenkel JM, et al. Classification and management of gynecomastia: defining the role of ultrasound-assisted liposuction. *Plast Reconstr Surg*. 2003;111:909.
9. Webster JP. Mastectomy for gynecomastia through a semi-circular incision. *Ann Surg*. 1946;124:557.
10. Courtiss EH. Gynecomastia: analysis of 159 patients and current recommendations for treatment. *Plast Reconstr Surg*. 1987;79:740.
11. Hammond DC, Arnold JF, Simon AM, et al. Combined use of ultrasonic liposuction with the pull-through technique for the treatment of gynecomastia. *Plast Reconstr Surg*. 2003;112:892.
12. Bracaglia R, Fortunato R, Gentileschi S, et al. Our experience with the so-called pull-through technique combined with liposuction for management of gynecomastia. *Ann Plast Surg*. 2004;53:22.

CHAPTER 62 ■ BREAST CANCER FOR THE PLASTIC SURGEON

GRANT W. CARLSON

Cancer of the breast is the second most common cancer in women, skin cancer being the most common. It is the second leading cause of cancer death after lung cancer. There are approximately 180,000 new cases of breast cancer diagnosed each year in the United States, accounting for more than 45,000 deaths a year. The incidence increased dramatically in the 1990s, largely because of increased detection by screening mammography. This is reflected in the fact that noninvasive cancer comprises 30% of new breast cancer cases treated in large medical centers.

The treatment of breast cancer has evolved because of the results of large, prospective, randomized clinical trials organized by the National Surgical Adjunctive Breast and Bowel Project (NSABP) in the United States, and the National Cancer Institute in Milan, Italy. The majority of women with breast cancer today are eligible for breast conservation therapy and receive some form of systemic adjuvant chemotherapy.

RISK FACTORS

It is estimated that one in nine women in the United States who reaches the age of 85 years will develop breast cancer. The etiology is unknown, but is clearly multifactorial, with many exogenous and endogenous risk factors being identified (Table 62.1).

Aside from gender, age is the single most important factor in determining breast cancer risk. The probability that breast cancer will develop increases throughout a woman's life, with half of all cases occurring in women older than age 65 years. Family history is also important because 20% of breast cancer patients have a relative with the disease. The magnitude of breast cancer risk is influenced by several factors pertaining to family history, including number and proximity of affected relatives, their menstrual status, age at diagnosis, and the presence of bilateral cancer.

Hereditary breast cancer accounts for 5% to 10% of breast cancer cases and is caused largely by the presence of BRCA gene mutations. The genes are more common in women of Jewish Ashkenazi ancestry, patients with bilateral breast cancer, cancer diagnosed before age 50 years, and patients with ovarian cancer. The presence of a BRCA gene confers a 60% to 85% risk of developing breast cancer and a 10% to 40% risk of developing ovarian cancer.

Many epidemiologic studies have linked early menarche, late menopause, and late age at first full-term pregnancy to breast cancer. The total duration of menstrual cycles and the number of menstrual cycles before full-term pregnancy appear to be proportional to breast cancer risk. Premalignant histology on breast biopsy may increase breast cancer risk, as is discussed in the following section. A woman with unilateral breast cancer is at increased risk of developing cancer in the opposite breast.

Studies have not shown that the development of contralateral breast cancer impacts adversely on survival.

PATHOLOGY

Screening mammography, by early detection of breast cancers, has increased our understanding of the malignant transformation process. Most cancers arise from the ductal elements of the breast after passing, presumably, through a sequence of premalignant stages as depicted below.

Normal breast → hyperplasia → atypical hyperplasia → ductal carcinoma in situ → invasive cancer

This process can occur over a 10- to 20-year period and orderly progression through the various stages is not obligatory. Ductal carcinoma in situ (DCIS), also known as intraductal carcinoma, is cancer confined by the basement membrane of the ducts. It most commonly presents as mammographic microcalcifications and currently comprises 30% of newly diagnosed cancers in populations following screening mammography guidelines. DCIS occurs in several histologic patterns with varying propensity to progress to invasive cancer. *Comedo DCIS* is characterized by pleomorphic cells, high-grade nuclei, and central areas of necrosis. *Noncomedo DCIS* occurs in several subtypes that are generally not as cytologically malignant as comedo DCIS. It may be difficult to distinguish noncomedo DCIS from atypical hyperplasia.

Invasive ductal carcinoma accounts for the majority of all cases of breast cancer. Grossly, it appears as a gray-white, irregular, speculated mass that is hard and gritty on cut section. It has no specific microscopic features, but can be recognized histologically as an invasive adenocarcinoma involving the ductal elements.

A number of histologic variants arise from ductal epithelium. *Medullary carcinoma* is grossly soft and fleshy and accounts for 6% of invasive cancers. It tends to grow to a large size and is well circumscribed. Histologically, it is characterized by poorly differentiated nuclei and infiltration by lymphocytes. Medullary carcinoma has a favorable prognosis, even in the presence of nodal metastases. *Tubular carcinoma* is a rare histologic variant in its pure form and accounts for 2% of breast cancer. It is characteristically small and is usually found on mammography. It tends to be highly differentiated and has an excellent prognosis. *Mucinous* or *colloid carcinoma* is another well-differentiated variant, which tends to form a well-circumscribed soft, gelatinous mass. Histologically, nests of tumor cells are surrounded by a mucinous matrix.

Although most cancers arise from the ductal elements, malignancies may also arise from the epithelium of the breast lobules. *Lobular carcinoma in situ* (LCIS) has no radiologic or physical manifestations and traditionally has not been

TABLE 62.1

BREAST CANCER RISK FACTORS

Gender
Age
Family history
Reproductive history
   Early menarche
   First birth after age 30 years
   Late menopause
Benign breast disease
   Atypical hyperplasia
   Lobular carcinoma in situ
Personal history
? Exogenous factors
? Dietary factors

regarded as a malignancy. It is usually an incidental finding after a biopsy of a mass or mammographic abnormality. Current evidence suggests that the histologic diagnosis of LCIS confers a 20% risk of developing cancer in either breast by the 20-year follow-up examination.

Five percent to 15% of infiltrating cancers arise from the breast lobules. Once it has become invasive, *lobular carcinoma* has a similar prognosis to the ductal type. It tends to be extensively infiltrative without a distinct tumor mass. Histologically, the cells demonstrate a characteristic single-file pattern. The tumor does not form microcalcifications and mammographic detection may be difficult.

STAGING

The American Joint Committee on Cancer (AJCC) TNM (primary tumor, regional lymph node, remote metastases) staging system is based on clinical and pathologic information. The classification by primary tumor (T), status of axillary lymph nodes (N), and presence of distant metastases (M) places patients in different prognostic groups (Tables 62.2 and 62.3). Stages I and II are considered *early breast cancer* for which surgery plays a primary role in treatment. Stage III disease is also known as *locally advanced breast cancer* (LABC). Despite the absence of metastatic disease, this stage has a poor prognosis and is best treated with a combination of chemotherapy, surgery, and radiation therapy. This stage includes *inflammatory breast cancer*, a clinical entity characterized by breast warmth, erythema, and edema. The orange-peel appearance of the skin, peau de orange, results from dermal lymphatic invasion.

LOCOREGIONAL TREATMENT

The goals of locoregional treatment are to provide optimal local control, adequate disease staging, long-term survival, and preservation or restoration of body form. Total mastectomy and axillary dissection were the standard treatment for more than 50 years, based on the Halsted mechanistic theory of cancer dissemination. Halsted believed that cancer was predominantly a local disease that spread by permeation of lymphatic pathways. He proposed the radical mastectomy to remove the cancer and prevent systemic spread. Numerous prospective randomized trials have refuted this theory of tumor biology. The bloodstream is an important pathway in early tumor dissemination, and more conservative locoregional treatment

TABLE 62.2

AJCC TNM STAGING SYSTEM OF BREAST CANCER

Primary Tumor (T)

TX	Primary tumor cannot be assessed
T0	No evidence of primary tumor
Tis	Carcinoma in situ, intraductal carcinoma, lobular carcinoma in situ
T1	Tumor ≤2 cm in greatest dimension
T1mic	Microinvasion ≤0.1 cm in greatest dimension
T1a	Tumor >0.1 cm but ≤0.5 cm in greatest dimension
T1b	Tumor >0.5 cm but ≤1 cm in greatest dimension
T1c	Tumor >1 cm but ≤2 cm in greatest dimension
T2	Tumor >2 cm but ≤5 cm in greatest dimension
T3	Tumor >5 cm in greatest dimension
T4	Tumor of any size with direct extension to chest wall or skin only
T4a	Extension to chest wall
T4b	Edema (including peau d'orange) or ulceration of the skin of the breast or satellite skin nodules confined to the same breast
T4c	Both T4a and T4b
T4d	Inflammatory carcinoma

Regional Lymph Nodes (N)

NX	Regional lymph nodes cannot be assessed (e.g., were previously removed)
N0	No regional lymph node metastasis
N1	Metastasis to mobile ipsilateral axillary lymph node or nodes
N1a	Micrometastases only, ≤0.2 cm
N1b	Metastasis to node or nodes, >0.2 cm
	N1bi Spread to 1–3 nodes, >0.2 cm, all <2 cm
	N1bii Spread to ≥4 nodes, >0.2 cm, all <2 cm
	N1biii Extracapsular invasion of nodes or nodes <2 cm
	N1biiiv Spread to a node >2.0 cm in greatest dimension
N2	Metastasis to ipsilateral axillary lymph node or nodes fixed to one another or to other structures
N3	Metastasis to ipsilateral internal mammary lymph node or nodes

Distant Metastasis (M)

MX	Distant metastasis cannot be assessed
M0	No distant metastasis
M1	Distant metastasis (including metastasis to ipsilateral supraclavicular lymph nodes)

From American Joint Committee on Cancer (AJCC). *AJCC Cancer Staging Manual.* 6th ed. New York: Springer-Verlag; 2002, with permission.

combined with systemic therapy has proved to provide local disease control with prolonged survival.

Breast Conservation

Breast conservation is the treatment of choice for the majority of stage I and stage II breast cancers. Six prospective randomized trials of more than 4,300 women found breast-conserving treatment to result in survival rates similar to those achieved by total mastectomy. Removal of the cancer with pathologically negative margins is termed a lumpectomy. The remaining

TABLE 62.3

STAGE GROUPING WITH THE AJCC

Stage 0	Tis	N0	M0
Stage I	T1	N0	M0
Stage IIA	T0, T1	N1	M0
	T2	N0	M0
Stage IIB	T2	N1	M0
	T3	N0	M0
Stage IIIA	T0, T1, T2	N2	M0
	T3	N1, N2	M0
Stage IIIB	T4	Any N	M0
	Any T	N3	M0
Stage IV	Any T	Any N	M1

From American Joint Committee on Cancer (AJCC). *AJCC Cancer Staging Manual*. 6th ed. New York: Springer-Verlag; 2002, with permission.

breast is usually treated with 50 Gy of external breast radiation to improve local control. The NSABP B-06 trial compared total mastectomy, lumpectomy, and lumpectomy and radiation in 1,843 women (1). The survival was the same for all three groups but the addition of breast irradiation to lumpectomy reduced the local recurrence from 40% to 8%. Young patients and those with extensive intraductal cancer surrounding the invasive component are at increased risk of local recurrence. Because of the propensity for ductal carcinoma to spread upward toward the nipple along the duct, a quadrantectomy has been proposed to reduce local recurrence. Larger excisions result in slightly improved local control rates at the expense of the cosmetic result but have no impact on ultimate survival. Local recurrences are generally treated by total mastectomy.

There are few absolute contraindications to breast conservation (Table 62.4). The cosmetic outcome of lumpectomy is dependent on both treatment-related factors and patient selection, and is judged to be excellent to good by 60% to 90% of patients.

Total Mastectomy

Removal of the entire breast, nipple-areola, and skin overlying superficial tumors is still the most common local treatment of breast cancer despite the proven results of breast conservation. In continuity removal of the axillary lymph nodes is termed a *modified radical mastectomy*. The pectoralis major and minor muscles are usually preserved. A *skin-sparing mastectomy* preserves the inframammary fold and as much native skin as possible. It is used when immediate breast reconstruction is

TABLE 62.4

CONTRAINDICATIONS TO BREAST CONSERVATION

Absolute
  Multiple ipsilateral lesions
  Diffuse suspicious microcalcifications
  Steroid-dependent collagen vascular disease
Relative
  Small breast–large tumor
  Radiation induced
  Ongoing pregnancy

planned. Its oncological safety has been proven by numerous studies.

Management of the Axilla

The removal of axillary lymph nodes provides pathologic staging as well as regional disease control. Lymph node involvement is the most important prognostic factor in breast cancer. The clinical examination of the axilla is inaccurate, with 25% of clinically normal axillae harboring micrometastatic disease. Spread to a single axillary lymph node implies a reduction in long-term survival from 90% to 60% for a 1-cm cancer (2). An axillary dissection that removes 10 to 20 lymph nodes is adequate staging in clinically uninvolved axillae. Arm stiffness, numbness, and the risk of lymphedema are potential complications.

Axillary sentinel lymph node biopsy is increasingly used to stage the nodal basin and avoid the morbidity of an axillary dissection. Blue dye and radioactive tracers are injected into the breast and are taken up by breast lymphatic system. This allows identification and removal of the lymph node(s) most likely to contain metastases. The false-negative rate for sentinel lymph node biopsy in large series is 0% to 11%.

Treatment of Ductal Carcinoma in Situ

The malignant potential of DCIS depends on the size, tumor grade, and the presence of comedo necrosis. If left untreated, some but not all, DCIS carcinomas will progress to invasive cancer. Local recurrence after surgical excision alone occurs in up to 30% of cases, depending on tumor size and histology. One-half of recurrences will be invasive carcinomas. Radiation therapy reduces local recurrences. The NSABP B-17 trial studied 818 women with DCIS randomly assigned to either lumpectomy alone or lumpectomy followed by breast irradiation (3). With a median follow-up of 43 months, local recurrences developed in 16% treated by lumpectomy alone, and in 7% treated by lumpectomy plus irradiation. The role of tamoxifen in the management of DCIS was addressed in the NSABP B-24 trial, which studied 1,804 women treated with breast conservation therapy (4). After a median follow-up of 74 months, tamoxifen was found to reduce the risk of ipsilateral breast tumors in women younger than age 50 years by 38% and in women age 50 years and older by 22%. There was also a 52% reduction in contralateral breast cancer events. This translates into an absolute reduction in breast cancer events from 13.4% to 8.2%.

To correlate the risk of recurrence with pathologic features and treatment, Silverstein et al. devised an index dependent on major risk factors for local recurrence. The index identified the following risk factors: nuclear grade, size, comedo histology, and surgical margins based on retrospective data analysis (5). The Van Nuys Prognostic Index is based on tumor size, tumor grade, and the presence of comedo necrosis. Small, low-grade tumors without comedo necrosis have a low incidence of recurrence and may be treated with excision alone in select patients.

Postmastectomy Radiotherapy

Postmastectomy radiation therapy is increasingly being administered in patients with early breast cancer. It reduces the risk of locoregional recurrence of breast cancer by approximately 67%, but a survival benefit has been largely offset by an increase in cardiac deaths secondary to radiation. Two recent randomized trials showed a survival benefit for postmastectomy radiotherapy in patients with one to three metastatic lymph nodes (6,7). The National Institutes of Health (NIH) Consensus Statement on the Adjuvant Therapy for Breast Cancer (2000) concluded that women with four or more positive lymph nodes or advanced primary tumor would benefit from postmastectomy radiotherapy (8). It stated that the role of postmastectomy radiotherapy for women with one to three positive lymph nodes remains uncertain.

Chest wall irradiation postimplant reconstructions results in an increase incidence of capsular contraction and implant exposure. Because of this, many authors feel that implant reconstruction is contraindicated when postmastectomy radiation is planned. It also has a deleterious effect on transverse rectus abdominis musculocutaneous (TRAM) flap reconstruction as evidenced by increased incidence of fibrosis, fat necrosis, and revision surgery.

SYSTEMIC THERAPY

Adjuvant chemotherapy and hormonal therapy are used to eliminate occult metastases responsible for later recurrences. Clinical trials have shown that adjuvant therapy can reduce the odds of cancer recurrence by up to 30%. The effect on disease-free interval is generally greater than the effect on overall survival. Obviously, those at higher risk of recurrence and death will obtain a greater benefit. Commonly used chemotherapy regimens include CMF (cyclophosphamide, methotrexate, 5-fluorouracil), FAC (5-fluorouracil, doxorubicin, cyclophosphamide), AC (doxorubicin, cyclophosphamide), and the taxanes (paclitaxel, docetaxel). Tamoxifen, a selective estrogen receptor modulator, and has been the mainstay of hormonal therapy in estrogen-responsive tumors. A new class of agents, the aromatase inhibitors (anastrozole, letrozole), blocks the peripheral conversion of adrenal steroids to estrogen. Recent studies in postmenopausal women show anastrozole to be more effective than tamoxifen in the adjuvant treatment of hormone responsive breast cancer.

The Early Breast Cancer Trialists' Collaborative Group performed an overview of 69 randomized trials of adjuvant combination chemotherapy (9). For recurrence, combination chemotherapy produced significant proportional reductions among women younger than 50 years of age (35% reduction) and among those 50 to 69 years of age (20% reduction). For mortality, the reductions for women younger than 50 years of age (27% reduction) and those 50 to 69 years of age (11%) were significant. Adjuvant tamoxifen administered for 5 years reduces the risk of recurrence at 10 years by 47% and the mortality at 10 years by 26% in estrogen receptor-positive tumors.

Node-Negative Tumors

The risk of recurrence for node-negative breast cancer is related to tumor size and can approach 30%. Clinical trials have proven the benefit the adjuvant therapy in the majority of node-negative cancers. There is a subset of patients, however, with an extremely low risk of recurrence that would not benefit from therapy. This subset includes tumors <1 cm and certain histologic variants (tubular, medullary, mucinous) that have an excellent prognosis.

Neoadjuvant Chemotherapy

Preoperative chemotherapy is indicated in patients with locally advanced breast cancer. It can be considered in patients with operable invasive cancers who would be candidates for adjuvant chemotherapy. The goal is to shrink the tumor to permit breast conservation. Randomized trials of neoadjuvant chemotherapy in operable breast cancer show significant tumor downstaging with a pathologic complete response rate of 12% to 24% (10).

References

1. Fisher B, Redmon C, Poisson R. Eight-year results of a randomized clinical trial comparing total mastectomy and lumpectomy with or without irradiation in the treatment of breast cancer. *N Engl J Med.* 1989;320(13):822–828.
2. Rosen PR, Groshen S, Saigo PE, et al. A long-term follow-up study of survival in stage I (T1N0M0) and stage II (T1N1M0) breast carcinoma. *J Clin Oncol.* 1989;7(3):355–366.
3. Fisher B, Costantino J, Redman C, et al. Lumpectomy compared with lumpectomy and radiation therapy for the treatment of intraductal breast cancer. *N Engl J Med.* 1993;328(22):1581–1586.
4. Fisher B, Dignon J, Wolmark N, et al. Tamoxifen in treatment of intraductal breast cancer: National Surgical Adjuvant Breast and Bowel Project B-24 randomised controlled trial. *Lancet.* 1999;353(9169):1993–2000.
5. Silverstein, MJ, Lagios MD, Craig PH. A prognostic index for ductal carcinoma in situ of the breast. *Cancer.* 1996;77(11):2267–2274.
6. Ragaz J, Jackson SM, Le N, et al. Adjuvant radiotherapy and chemotherapy in node-positive premenopausal women with breast cancer [see comments]. *N Engl J Med.* 1997;337(14):956–962.
7. Overgaard M, Hansen PS, Overgaard J, et al. Postoperative radiotherapy in high-risk premenopausal women with breast cancer who receive adjuvant chemotherapy. Danish Breast Cancer Cooperative Group 82b Trial [see comments]. *N Engl J Med.* 1997;337(14):949–955.
8. *Adjuvant Therapy for Breast Cancer. NIH Consensus Statement.* Bethesda, MD: National Institutes of Health; 2000.
9. Polychemotherapy for early breast cancer: an overview of the randomised trials. Early Breast Cancer Trialists' Collaborative Group. *Lancet.* 1998;352(9132):930–942.
10. Fisher B, et al. Effect of preoperative chemotherapy on the outcome of women with operable breast cancer. *J Clin Oncol.* 1998;16(8):2672–2685.

CHAPTER 63 ■ BREAST RECONSTRUCTION: PROSTHETIC TECHNIQUES

JOSEPH J. DISA

The use of prosthetic devices for breast reconstruction began in the early 1960s with silicone-gel-filled implants. Over the years, implant technology and surgical techniques have evolved, resulting in improvement in the quality of the reconstructed breast. Currently there are multiple methods of prosthetic breast reconstruction and various types of implants with different shapes, textures, and fill materials for the plastic surgeon to choose from.

The popularity of one-stage implant reconstruction has diminished over the years with the development of two-stage expander–implant reconstructions. Early experience with tissue expanders used smooth surface, round devices with remote fill ports. These devices were fraught with problems, including capsular contracture, poor expansion of the mastectomy pocket, and failure of the device as a consequence of mechanical problems with the fill port. The current era of tissue expanders in breast reconstruction uses textured surface and anatomically shaped expanders with integrated valves. These devices have a semirigid back to allow for preferential expansion in the anterior dimension. Device design also allows for preferential expansion in the region of the lower pole of the reconstructed breast so as to create a better match with a natural breast. Finally, the textured surface on the expander reduces the incidence of capsular contracture (Fig. 63.1). Depending on the manufacturer, these expanders are typically made in varying heights, widths, degrees of projection, and shapes, so that the optimal device can be selected for the individual patient's needs (1,2).

PATIENT SELECTION

In general, most patients are candidates for prosthetic breast reconstruction. However, there are limitations with the overall shape of permanent breast implants that dictate the quality of the final result. Factors to consider include whether or not the reconstruction is unilateral or bilateral, the patient's overall body habitus, associated comorbidities, and the patient's psychological profile. The ideal candidate for breast reconstruction with prosthetic implants is a thin patient with bilateral reconstruction, or a thin patient with a normal, nonptotic breast who requires unilateral reconstruction. In this situation, symmetry is relatively straightforward to achieve. As the patient's breast size increases and the degree of ptosis increases, it becomes more difficult to match with a prosthetic reconstruction. In this situation, the patient may be a candidate for a contralateral symmetry procedure such as a mastopexy or a reduction mammoplasty. Even with such procedures, however, exact symmetry out of clothing may not be possible. The patient should be made aware that the goal is to achieve as much symmetry as possible, but that this may only be accomplished when she

is in her brassiere and clothing (3). Although not an absolute contraindication, morbid obesity makes implant reconstruction difficult. In patients with a broad chest wall and a large contralateral breast, the expansion process may fail to achieve a pocket of appropriate volume to achieve a meaningful and symmetric result. In this situation, the addition of autologous tissue to an implant-based reconstruction, or the use of autologous tissue alone, may achieve a more pleasing result. For patients with multiple medical problems, an implant-based reconstruction may be simpler than an autologous tissue reconstruction; however, it must be considered that implant-based reconstructions may require more than one operation and may require revisions over time. Additionally if the patient has a chronic respiratory illness, the pressure from the tissue expander on the chest wall during the expansion process may exacerbate any underlying conditions. Finally, prosthetic-based breast reconstruction often requires multiple steps and multiple visits to the office. The patients must be reliable and stable enough from a psychological standpoint that they can manage the reconstructive process.

TIMING

Breast reconstruction using prosthetic techniques can be accomplished either in the immediate or delayed setting. The advantage of immediate reconstruction is that the first step in breast reconstruction is accomplished at the time of the mastectomy under the same anesthetic. In this setting, maximum amounts of breast skin can be preserved as the prosthetic device will occupy some of the mastectomy space. In the setting of a single-stage breast reconstruction using a permanent implant, immediate reconstruction allows for placement of an optimally sized device. Delayed breast reconstruction using a prosthetic technique is also possible; however, tissue expansion is generally necessary. In this method, the mastectomy skin flaps are re-elevated and expanded postoperatively to re-create a pocket for the ultimate placement of a permanent breast implant. Although delayed breast reconstruction with a tissue expander requires an extraoperative procedure, it benefits from simplification of the initial phase of the patient's management. In the setting of high-risk disease and patients who may require chemotherapy and radiation therapy, delayed reconstruction will not delay the initiation of adjuvant treatment.

TECHNIQUE

With all types of breast reconstruction, the primary goal is to achieve a breast mound that is as symmetrical as possible with the normal breast, or to the contralateral reconstruction in the

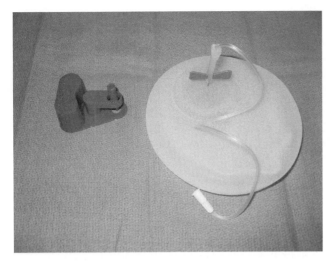

FIGURE 63.1. Textured surface, integrated valve, biodimensional-shaped tissue expander with Magna-Site (Inamed Aesthetics, Santa Barbara, CA) fill port locating device.

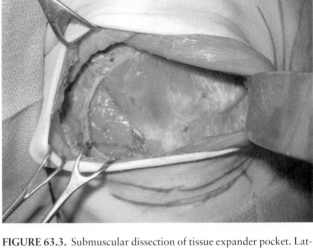

FIGURE 63.3. Submuscular dissection of tissue expander pocket. Lateral border of pectoralis major muscle is retracted medially while the medial border of serratus anterior muscle is retracted laterally.

setting of bilateral mastectomy. Coordination and communication between the surgeon performing the mastectomy and the reconstructive surgeon is paramount. Ideally, mastectomy incisions are planned to minimize their impact on subsequent tissue expansion and their visibility in conventional clothing. Skin flaps should be of adequate thickness to maintain blood supply, and **the site of the inframammary fold should be marked and preserved whenever possible (Fig. 63.2).** The position of the point of maximum projection of the breast should also be noted. At the conclusion of the mastectomy, if the inframammary fold has been detached, it should be repaired. After obtaining hemostasis within the mastectomy pockets, a submuscular pocket for the placement of the tissue expander is prepared. The lateral border of the pectoralis major muscle is elevated from the chest wall and from the underlying pectoralis minor muscle. Care must be taken to adequately coagulate perforating vessels to the muscle to avoid hematoma formation. The surgeon then has two choices as to the placement of the tissue expander. Expanders can be placed in a complete submuscular–subfascial pocket by elevating the medial border

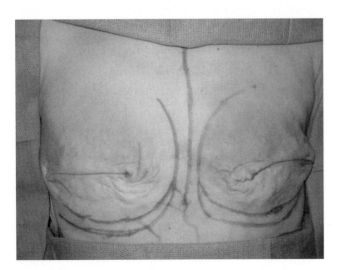

FIGURE 63.2. Intraoperative appearance of bilateral mastectomy defect. Original position of inframammary folds and planned lower position of new inframammary fold are marked.

of the serratus anterior muscle, elevating the pectoralis major from lateral to medial, and bringing both the subserratus and subpectoral pocket into communication at the level of or slightly below the inframammary fold by elevating a small portion of the anterior rectus sheath. Doing so allows for complete submuscular placement of the tissue expander (Fig. 63.3). Final coverage of the expander occurs by suturing the lateral border of the pectoralis major muscle to the serratus anterior muscle. This technique completely separates the tissue expander from the mastectomy space (Fig. 63.4A, B) (4). Another option is simply to elevate the pectoralis muscle, detach it inferiorly, and reattach it to the inferior mastectomy skin flap using either internal sutures or transcutaneous "marionette sutures" (5,6). The potential advantage of the latter technique is that the serratus anterior does not need to be elevated; by not raising the anterior rectus sheath there may be less resistance to expansion and possibly less discomfort. In the setting of a very thin mastectomy skin flap, there may be inadequate soft-tissue coverage over the inferior pole of the expander; thus caution is recommended. Exposure of the expander either through the skin flap or through a poorly healed mastectomy incision can occur. In general, if soft-tissue coverage of the expander is questionable, any mastectomy skin flap necrosis should be treated aggressively with excision of devitalized tissue and closure of the wound. Occasionally saline needs to be temporarily removed from the expander to accomplish this.

Choosing the appropriate expander is based on several factors, including breast volume, breast dimensions (height, width, and projection), breast shape, and the patient's body habitus. **In general, an anatomically designed, textured surface, integrated valve tissue expander is preferred (see Fig. 63.1).** The expander comes in variating heights, widths, and amounts of projection that either can be compared to the contralateral breast or can be matched to another expander if a bilateral procedure is performed. Final considerations include the amount and quality of remaining breast skin after mastectomy and the impact of planned contralateral symmetry procedures (augmentation, mastopexy, reduction) on the shape of the opposite breast. The expander typically comes partially filled with air. The air is evacuated from the expander and a small amount of saline solution is infiltrated into the expander to confirm the functioning of the port. The expander is then placed into the pocket in the appropriate anatomic orientation. The expander can be filled to match the available space in the submuscular/submastectomy pocket. A closed suction drain is placed in

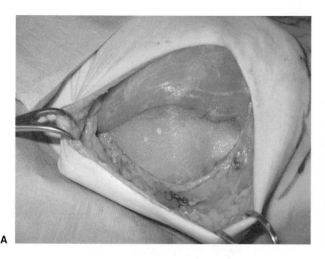

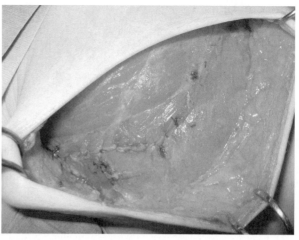

FIGURE 63.4. **A:** Tissue expander in place, covered by the pectoralis major muscle and serratus anterior muscle. **B:** Lateral border of pectoralis major muscle is sutured to medial border of serratus anterior muscle to provide complete submuscular coverage of the tissue expander.

the mastectomy space, and the mastectomy wounds are closed in layers (Figs. 63.5–63.8).

DELAYED TISSUE EXPANDERS

Delayed breast reconstruction with a tissue expander is very similar to immediate reconstruction. Typically, the mastectomy scar is excised and the mastectomy flaps are re-elevated, although not to the extent as was necessary during the original mastectomy. Once adequate pectoralis muscle is exposed, either the lateral border of the pectoralis muscle is identified and elevated from the chest wall, or the muscle is split in the direction of the muscle fibers and a subpectoralis major pocket is created. Similar to immediate expander placement, care is taken to avoid elevation of the pectoralis minor

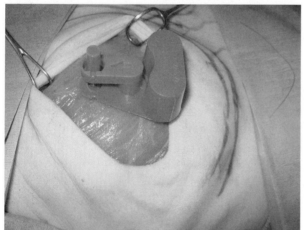

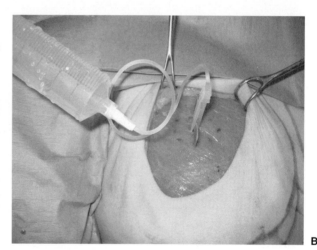

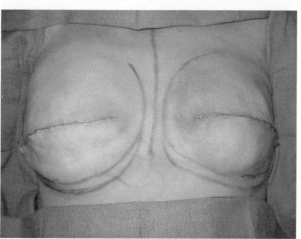

FIGURE 63.5. **A:** Magnasite device is used to locate port intraoperatively. **B:** Saline solution instilled into tissue expander intraoperatively. The expander is filled to match the available space in the submuscular pocket. **C:** Intraoperative appearance of partially filled tissue expanders after wound closure.

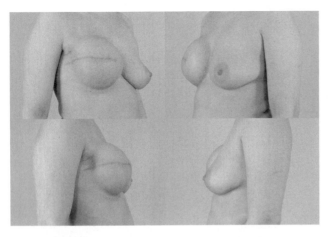

FIGURE 63.6. Unilateral right breast reconstruction with tissue expander. The expander is intentionally overfilled to maximize projection and inferior pole skin.

muscle. From this point, dissection beyond the pectoralis can be extended either into the subcutaneous plane inferiorly and laterally, or into the submuscular/subfascial plane as noted in the description of placement of an immediate tissue expander. Similar to immediate tissue expander placement, the importance of a careful dissection of the tissue expander pocket cannot be overemphasized. It is critical to free any scar tissue that will restrict expansion of the mastectomy flaps. The expander is placed such that the zone of maximum expansion is located in the lower pole of the reconstructed breast, allowing for preferential expansion of the lower pole, for a more natural shape of the reconstructed breast.

Expansion

Intraoperatively, the tissue expander is filled to a volume that optimally obliterates dead space, but does not impart excessive pressure on the mastectomy skin flaps (Fig. 63.5A–C). Because blood supply to the newly created mastectomy skin flap may be tenuous, overfilling the expander intraoperatively can impede circulation. Closed suction drainage tubes left at the time of expander placement are removed when output is ≤30 mL

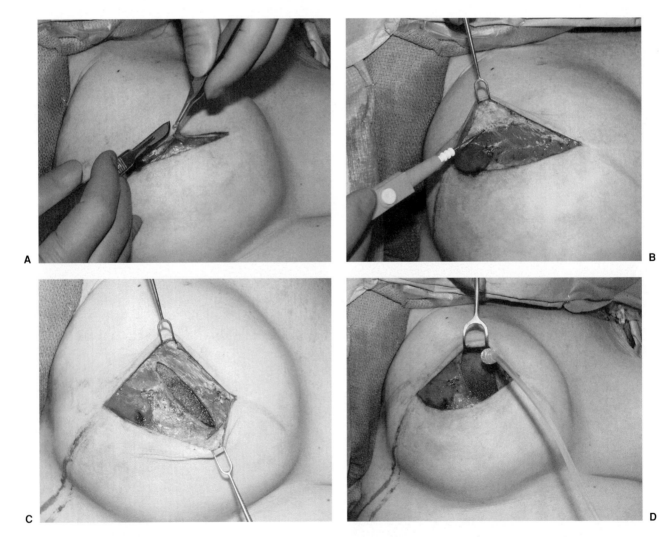

FIGURE 63.7. Exchange of tissue expander to permanent implant. **A:** Excision of mastectomy scar. **B:** Mastectomy skin flaps elevated off pectoralis major muscle. **C:** Pectoralis muscle incised in the direction of its muscle fibers, exposing the tissue expander. **D:** Removal of fluid from tissue expander to estimate planned volume of permanent implant.

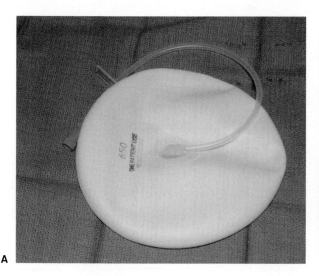
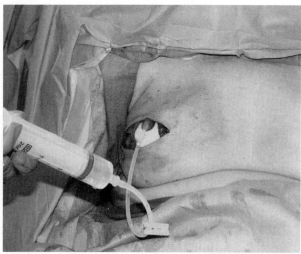

FIGURE 63.8. **A:** Disposable saline-filled sizers can be used to determine appropriate permanent implant. **B:** Intraoperative appearance of sizer in implant pocket.

per 24 hours, which typically occurs by 2 weeks after surgery. Tissue expansion begins in the office approximately 10 to 14 days after surgery. A magnetic expander port finding device is used to identify the site of the integrated fill valve under the patient's skin. The area is cleansed with an antiseptic solution and a butterfly needle is used to gain access to the tissue expander. Approximately 30 to 120 mL of saline is injected into the expander during each expansion session. Expansion sessions can occur as frequently as once per week or as infrequently as once per month, although there is no set criterion to the expansion schedule. **The final goal of the expansion is to achieve a volume that is approximately 25% to 30% greater than the expander volume (Fig. 63.6).** This allows for extra skin to be available at the exchange procedure, which can be used to create maximum breast ptosis and inferior pole projection. Overexpansion also allows for the removal of unsightly mastectomy scars, or scars that have resulted from delayed or poor wound healing. If the patient is to receive postoperative chemotherapy, the onset of this typically coincides with the expansion process. **Patients can be safely expanded during chemotherapy, although it may be necessary to coordinate the expansion schedule with their chemotherapy schedule. Final replacement of the expander to a permanent implant is deferred until the patient's blood counts have returned to normal after the conclusion of chemotherapy.** In general, soft tissues are allowed to rest for at least 1 month between the time of the last expansion and the time of the exchange procedure (7).

EXCHANGE OF TISSUE EXPANDER FOR PERMANENT IMPLANT

The second stage in breast reconstruction using a prosthetic device involves exchanging the tissue expander to a permanent implant. This procedure can be accomplished at any time after the tissue expansion is completed. Typically, patients will wait at least 1 month following the last expansion before undergoing the exchange procedure. If the patient received chemotherapy as part of her management, then at least 3 to 4 weeks after the last chemotherapy session is allowed to pass so that bone marrow suppression induced by chemotherapy can resolve before undergoing an elective surgical procedure. The goals of the exchange procedure are to create a breast mound that has similar shape, volume, and position as the contralateral breast

in a unilateral reconstruction, and to maximize symmetry and position in a bilateral reconstruction.

The patient is positioned in the operating room such that the reconstruction can be accomplished in the sitting position, allowing for maximum ptosis of the natural breast. The permanent implant can then be placed with maximum symmetry. Preoperatively, the decision between the use of a saline or silicone gel implant is discussed and decided with the patient preoperatively. At the time of this writing, silicone implants are available only for use as part of the Adjunct Study sponsored by the U.S. Food and Drug Administration and the implant manufacturers (Inamed Aesthetics, 5540 Ekwill Street, Santa Barbara, CA 93111, and Mentor H/S Inc., 5425 Hollister Avenue, Santa Barbara, CA 93111).

Patients undergoing breast reconstruction are candidates for use of a silicone gel implant as long as they meet the inclusion criteria determined by the manufacturer. Once the type of device is chosen, then the shape of the device is selected. Smooth surface devices are round in shape and have variable projection—including low, medium, and high profile—depending on the type of implant (saline or silicone) and the implant manufacturer. Anatomically shaped devices have textured surfaces to facilitate incorporation of the capsule with the device and to minimize the risk of the device changing position, thereby distorting the reconstruction. The selection of the proper final implant is aided by measuring the dimensions of the normal breast. Specific measurements include base diameter, breast height, and projection. The final goal in choosing the appropriate breast implant is matching the volume of the contralateral breast. There are various techniques that can be used to facilitate this process. One involves comparing the weight of the breast removed at the time of mastectomy to the volume of the tissue expander. This technique will help in approximating the mass and volume needed for the reconstruction. Another technique is to partially empty the expander (which typically is overexpanded so as to maximize inferior pole skin and projection) prior to removing the expander (Fig. 63.7A–D). The expander is emptied to a point where its volume approximates the contralateral breast. The expander can then be removed and emptied of its remaining contents; this amount of saline can be measured. By using this volume of remaining fluid in the expander, the base dimension of the pocket from which the expander came, and the height and projection of the contralateral breast, an implant of the appropriate size and shape can be selected. Disposable sizers corresponding to particular

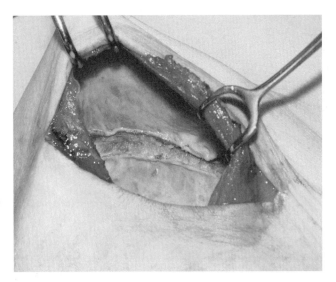

FIGURE 63.9. Releasing an implant capsule aids in maximizing projection and ptosis of permanent implant.

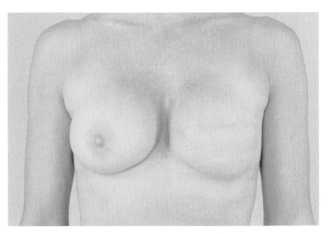

FIGURE 63.11. Unilateral left breast reconstruction with saline implant. Photo taken prior to planned nipple–areola reconstruction.

permanent implants are also available, and can aid in permanent implant selection (Fig. 63.8A, B).

Perhaps the most important step in placement of the permanent implant for breast reconstruction is accurate positioning of the inframammary fold. The placement of the inframammary fold on the breast mound should be marked preoperatively with the patient in the upright position. This marking then can be confirmed with the patient in the supine position. Depending on the degree of ptosis and whether or not a contralateral symmetry procedure will be performed in the opposite breast, this marking will help to determine the final location of the inframammary fold. In general, the position of the inframammary fold of the reconstruction should match the normal side of the contralateral side in the setting of a bilateral reconstruction. If a contralateral symmetry procedure (augmentation, mastopexy, or reduction) is to be performed, care should be taken to match the symmetry procedure to the reconstruction. In the setting of a more ptotic breast, where the breast gland descends below the level of the inframammary fold, it may be desirable to place the bottom of the implant at the level of the bottom of the breast on the natural side. In

this circumstance, the inframammary fold on the reconstructed side may be slightly lower than it is on the contralateral side; however, the overall position of the breast mounds are similar. There are multiple different techniques in recreating the inframammary fold. Some examples of these include internal placement of capsulorrhaphy sutures, external marionette sutures as described by Spear (5), liposuction of the region of the inframammary fold to allow the external skin to stick to the chest wall, and advancement of the an upper abdominal skin flap, suturing this internally to the chest wall to define the fold. The combination of appropriate positioning and definition of the inframammary fold, along with ample inferior pole skin expansion, will create the desired pocket for prosthetic breast reconstruction. Maximizing projection of the reconstructed breast can be further accomplished by performing internal capsulotomies positioned either circumferentially, radially, or both, or by performing a capsulectomy of the capsular tissue (Fig. 63.9). Care must be taken to ensure adequate thickness of the mastectomy skin flaps when performing these procedures in order to avoid injury to the mastectomy skin flaps. An inferior pole capsulectomy or capsulotomy will allow for maximizing inferior pole projection and ptosis in the reconstructed breast (Fig. 63.10).

If the patient desires a contralateral symmetry procedure, this is typically accomplished at the time of the exchange of the tissue expander to the permanent implant (the second stage of breast reconstruction). Contralateral symmetry procedures include augmentation mammoplasty, mastopexy, or reduction mammoplasty. Performance of a contralateral symmetry procedure at the time of the exchange of the tissue expander to the permanent implant, rather than at the time of the mastectomy and placement of the tissue expander, gives the reconstructive surgeon maximum opportunity to obtain symmetry with the reconstruction to the normal breast. In the setting of a bilateral mastectomy and reconstruction, the same principles as noted above are applied; however, the use of capsulotomy, capsulectomy, and repositioning of the inframammary fold is done to maximize the symmetry of the pockets and thus the overall symmetry of the reconstruction (Figs. 63.11–63.15).

BREAST RECONSTRUCTION WITH IMMEDIATE PLACEMENT OF AN IMPLANT

In select cases, immediate breast reconstruction can be accomplished with placement of an implant. The mastectomy skin

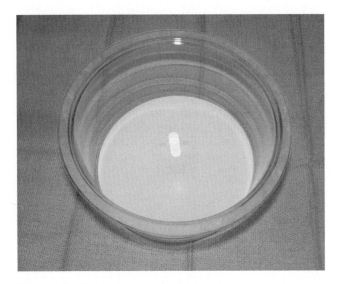

FIGURE 63.10. Permanent saline implant.

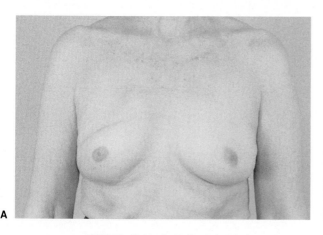
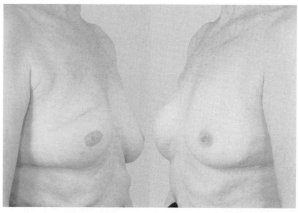

FIGURE 63.12. **A:** Unilateral right breast reconstruction with saline implant after nipple–areola reconstruction. The reconstructed inframammary fold was intentionally lowered so that the lower pole of the reconstructed breast was symmetrical to the natural breast. **B:** Oblique views.

flaps must be completely healthy, the pocket must be of adequate size so as to insert an implant of the appropriate size, and the appropriate implant must be selected. If the pocket is inadequate for a permanent implant of sufficient volume, then an expandable implant, such as an expandable saline device with a remote access port, can be used. The port is removed at a later stage, or an expandable silicone/saline device can be used. The advantage of an expandable device is its adjustability during the postprocedure period prior to final port removal, which generally can be accomplished in the office setting. The disadvantage of immediate reconstruction includes the risk of asymmetry with the contralateral breast, inadequate size and projection of the device, and the need for a secondary revision to improve the quality of the overall reconstruction. **In gen-**

eral, use of a two-staged reconstruction with a tissue expander placed at the first stage, followed by a permanent implant at the second stage, maximizes the control the reconstructive surgeon has over the pocket. Whenever reconstruction in a single stage is performed with an implant, patients should be made aware that there may be a need for a revisional procedure to improve the overall result (8–11).

POSTOPERATIVE CARE

After placement of a tissue expander, or after exchange of an expander for a permanent implant, the patient is placed in a surgical bra, which helps to hold dressings in place and provides

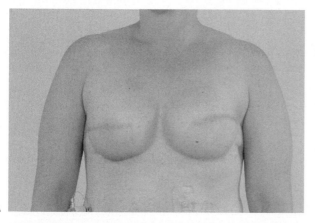
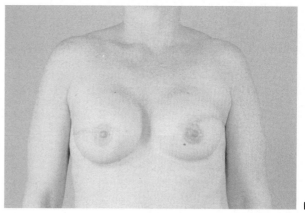
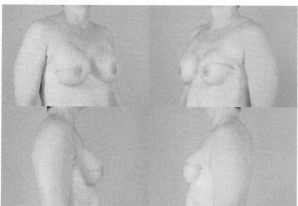

FIGURE 63.13. **A:** Bilateral breast reconstruction with saline implants. **B:** After completion of nipple–areola reconstruction. **C:** Oblique and lateral views.

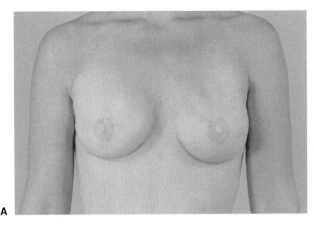
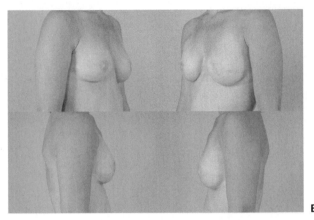

FIGURE 63.14. A: Bilateral breast reconstruction with silicone gel implants after nipple–areola reconstruction. B: Oblique and lateral views.

a place for drains to be fastened. The use of oral antibiotics after surgery is discretionary with the surgeon. The use of a conforming breast binder to hold the implant position might be advantageous. Patients are instructed to avoid the use of an underwire bra for several weeks after surgery and, depending on the type of implant used, may be instructed to massage their implants. Implant massage is usually reserved for patients with smooth implants rather than shaped, anatomic implants where massage may lead to implant malposition. Pain medication is prescribed as needed.

COMPLICATIONS

Complications specific to prosthetic breast reconstruction are similar to those associated with breast implant surgery in general. Bleeding in the immediate postoperative period resulting in hematoma usually warrants re-exploration. Hematomas under the mastectomy skin flap or in the tissue expander or permanent implant space increase the risk of infection and predispose to the development of capsular contracture. Consequently, if a hematoma of significant size is recognized, it should be promptly evacuated. Infection of the prosthetic device can occur early in the immediate postsurgery period, or late, occurring even many years after the placement of the permanent implant. Infections typically present as cellulitis of the skin flaps above

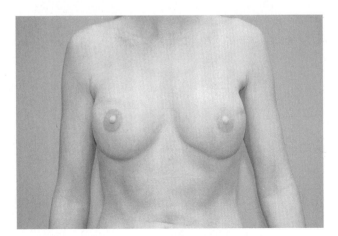

FIGURE 63.15. Bilateral breast reconstruction with silicone gel implants after nipple–areola reconstruction.

the implant. Occasionally a frank abscess is identified. **In a large series of tissue expanders placed at my institution, the incidence of infection requiring expander removal was approximately 2% (7).** Typically, if the patient presents with cellulitis of the mastectomy skin flaps, a course of intravenous antibiotics or, occasionally, oral antibiotics is used. Only in circumstances where cellulitis fails to resolve with antibiotic therapy, or a frank abscess develops, is the removal of the implant indicated (12). In certain circumstances cellulitis of the skin flaps can be adequately managed with antibiotics without implant removal.

Another early complication after mastectomy and expander placement includes mastectomy skin flap necrosis. Factors such as the length of the mastectomy skin flap, the patient's overall medical condition, the thickness of the mastectomy skin flap, and whether or not the patient is a smoker, can contribute to the development of mastectomy skin flap necrosis. Superficial or partial-thickness flap necrosis is usually managed conservatively with local wound care. Occasionally small areas of full-thickness necrosis also can be managed with local wound care, particularly if the expander is in a complete submuscular location, thus having an interface of normal healthy tissue between the device and the area of skin necrosis. When the eschar resolves, the underlying tissue granulates and heals as a scar that can later be revised. However, in the setting of larger areas of mastectomy skin flap necrosis or questionable soft-tissue coverage of the implant, resection of necrotic skin with immediate wound closure is indicated. If a tissue expander that has been partially expanded is in place, fluid can be removed from the device, which might allow for tension-free closure of the remaining mastectomy skin flaps. If mastectomy skin flap closure is not possible after resecting devitalized tissue, either the device can be removed and the skin subsequently closed, or a skin graft can be applied, which later can be expanded along with the skin flaps and eventually resected to allow for closure.

Late complications of prosthetic breast reconstruction include asymmetry, implant wrinkling, implant malposition, implant deflation, capsular contracture, and infection. Infection is discussed above. In almost every case of unilateral breast reconstruction, and even in certain cases of bilateral breast reconstruction, some degree of asymmetry is expected. The development of capsular contracture around a reconstructed breast can lead to implant malposition, changes in projection of the implant, and, occasionally, pain and discomfort. All of these factors may lead to the patient's desire to have a revision of the breast reconstruction (13). Implant wrinkling or ripple formation is common sequelae of breast reconstruction with implants. Unlike the setting of an augmentation mammoplasty, where a breast implant is covered by skin, breast tissue, and often muscle, the reconstructed breast is covered by skin and muscle, or perhaps only skin, subcutaneous tissue, and implant capsule. Normal contour irregularities because of the compliance of the implant are transmitted through the skin and appear as a ripple on the reconstructed breast. As a consequence of gravity, these ripples tend to occur most commonly on the upper pole of the reconstruction, where they are most visible to the patient. Strategies to improve rippling include overfilling of saline implants (although this will lead to a more firm-feeling implant reconstruction) and the use of smooth wall devices. **Textured surface breast implants tend to be associated with rippling more commonly than smooth surface devices.** In the current era of implant reconstruction and with current implant design, it is unknown whether the risk of capsular contracture is any different between smooth surface and textured surface implants. However, the only types of devices that are available in the smooth surface are round devices either in a low, moderate, or high profile. Some authors report on the use of fat injection or the use of dermal substitutes such as acellular human dermis (AlloDerm) to improve ripples. Although this has been reported, experience with these techniques is limited.

IMPACT OF RADIATION ON PROSTHETIC RECONSTRUCTION

The indications and incidence of radiation therapy to the chest wall after mastectomy has increased significantly in the past decade. As a result of studies demonstrating a diminished local recurrence in certain subsets of patients with breast cancer, radiation therapy is now indicated after mastectomy for patients with tumors that are ≥ 5 cm in maximum diameter, three or more lymph nodes with metastatic breast cancer, or skin involvement. Additionally, the indications for radiotherapy seem to be expanding. Consequently, it is controversial in plastic surgery as to whether or not to perform immediate breast reconstruction in the setting of planned postoperative radiation therapy. Another controversial issue is management of the patient who has had a prior lumpectomy and radiation therapy for breast cancer and now for either reasons of local recurrence or prophylaxis, requires a salvage mastectomy on the previously irradiated breast. Radiation therapy, whether it is delivered preoperatively or postoperatively, complicates breast reconstruction. With respect to preoperative radiation therapy, placement of a tissue expander at the time of the mastectomy may lead to failed expansion, poor expansion with lack of projection, poor wound healing, and an inability to achieve the desired result from this method of reconstruction. Careful patient selection is mandatory when attempting to perform an expander-based reconstruction in a patient who has been irradiated. Ideally, the skin should show no evidence of prior radiation therapy and there should be no fibrosis within the pectoral muscle. A slow and careful expansion should be performed and the patient and surgeon should be ready to convert to autologous tissue reconstruction if the expansion process fails.

Another approach to the previously irradiated patient with the use of a tissue expander is immediate placement of a latissimus dorsi myocutaneous transposition flap over the expander. The latissimus flap will have not been previously irradiated and thus is much more likely to expand without resistance. Additionally, the autologous tissue provided by the latissimus flap will increase the volume of skin for the breast reconstruction, thus enabling the reconstruction to have more projection and ptosis.

In patients who require postoperative radiation therapy, radiating the permanent implant leads to a higher incidence of capsular contracture and need for revision. **However, the majority of patients have satisfactory results after radiation of their prosthetic reconstruction (14). In general, whether or not the patient needs postoperative radiation therapy after mastectomy is not known until the final pathology returns. If the tissue expander has been placed at the time of the mastectomy, then the protocol recommended by my institution includes expansion of the tissue expander during chemotherapy, exchange of the tissue expander to the permanent implant as soon as possible after the conclusion of the chemotherapy, and beginning radiation therapy several weeks after the permanent implant is placed.** In the setting where the surgeon and patient are aware that postoperative radiation therapy will be required, a frank discussion must be had regarding the use of delayed reconstruction after the conclusion of chemotherapy and radiation therapy with autologous tissue, the use of autologous tissue primarily, or the use of a prosthetic-based reconstruction, including an understanding of the increased risks and complications that are associated with radiation therapy to prosthetic breast implants.

References

1. Spear SL, Majidian A. Immediate breast reconstruction in two stages using textured, integrated-valve tissue expanders and breast implants: a retrospective review of 171 consecutive breast reconstructions from 1989 to 1996. *Plast Reconstr Surg.* 1998;101(1):53–63.
2. Spear SL, Spittler CJ. Breast reconstruction with implants and expanders. *Plast Reconstr Surg.* 2001;107(1):177–187.
3. Losken A, Carlson GW, Bostwick J, et al. Trends in unilateral breast reconstruction and management of the contralateral breast: the Emory experience. *Plast Reconstr Surg.* 2002;110(1):89–97.
4. Bacilious N, Cordeiro PG, Disa JJ, et al. Breast reconstruction using tissue expanders and implants in Hodgkin's patients with prior mantle irradiation. *Plast Reconstr Surg.* 2002;109(1):102–107.
5. Spear SL, Pelletiere CV. Immediate breast reconstruction in two stages using textured, integrated-valve tissue expanders and breast implants. *Plast Reconstr Surg.* 2004;113(7):2098–2103.
6. Serra-Renom JM, Fontdevila J, Monner J, et al. Mammary reconstruction using tissue expander and partial detachment of the pectoralis major muscle to expand the lower breast quadrants. *Ann Plast Surg.* 2004;53(4):317–321.
7. Disa JJ, Ad-El DD, Cohen SM, et al. The premature removal of tissue expanders in breast reconstruction. *Plast Reconstr Surg.* 1999;104(6):1662–1665.
8. Hunter-Smith DJ, Laurie SW. Breast reconstruction using permanent tissue expanders. *Aust N Z J Surg.* 1995;65(7):492–495.
9. Gui GP, Tan SM, Faliakou EC, et al. Immediate breast reconstruction using biodimensional anatomical permanent expander implants: a prospective analysis of outcome and patient satisfaction. *Plast Reconstr Surg.* 2003;111(1):125–138.
10. Mahdi S, Jones T, Nicklin S, et al. Expandable anatomical implants in breast reconstructions: a prospective study. *Br J Plast Surg.* 1998;51(6):425–430.
11. Camilleri IG, Malata CM, Stavrianos S, et al. Review of 120 Becker permanent tissue expanders in reconstruction of the breast. *Br J Plast Surg.* 1996;49(6):346–351.
12. Nahabedian MY, Tsangaris T, Momen B, et al. Infectious complications following breast reconstruction with expanders and implants. *Plast Reconstr Surg.* 2003;112(2):467–476.
13. Spear SL, Baker JL Jr. Classification of capsular contracture after prosthetic breast reconstruction. *Plast Reconstr Surg.* 1995;96(5):1119–1123.
14. Cordeiro PG, Pusic AL, Disa JJ, et al. Irradiation after immediate tissue expander/implant breast reconstruction: outcomes, complications, aesthetic results, and satisfaction among 156 patients. *Plast Reconstr Surg.* 2004;113(3):877–881.

CHAPTER 64 ■ LATISSIMUS DORSI FLAP BREAST RECONSTRUCTION

DENNIS C. HAMMOND

Reconstruction with autologous tissue provides the patient with a reconstructed breast created with her own tissues, obviating the potential complications associated with a prosthesis. The disadvantage with this strategy is related to the creation of an additional donor site with scarring and potential morbidity. Although reconstruction with tissue expanders and implants eliminates the need for the additional donor site, the potential complications associated with these devices are a concern. Thus the latissimus dorsi musculocutaneous flap (LDF) seems to offer no advantage as, most commonly, tissue expanders and implants are still required, and the additional donor site is created on the back. For this reason, the LDF remains a distant third option for many reconstructive breast surgeons. **With the development of newer and more effective tissue expanders and implants, however, the advantages of combining these devices with the well-vascularized LDF have generated a resurgence of interest in this technique.** This chapter focuses on the technical strategies for optimizing the use of the LDF with tissue expanders and implants.

OPERATIVE STRATEGY

The LDF was originally described in 1906 by Iginio Tansini in Italy (1). It was used to reconstruct mastectomy wounds at the time, but soon fell from favor, to be rediscovered in the late 1970s (2,3). Since its rediscovery, the flap has been used to reconstruct nearly every part of the body, as both a pedicled and a free flap. The LDF is a reliable and richly vascularized flap, and the proximity of the flap to the chest wall makes it an ideal choice for providing muscle, fat, and skin for use in reconstructing the breast after mastectomy. Sacrifice of the muscle creates a negligible functional deficit except in extremely athletic women (4–6). Transposition of the flap from the back to the anterior chest wall provides a healthy layer of soft tissue that can line the mastectomy defect, effectively softening the edges of the wound and thus recreating the gentle soft curves of the normal female breast. By adding any one of the numerous different styles of expanders and implants under the flap, the volume that is inherently lacking in the flap can be provided to restore the breast to its natural size and contour (7,8). Using this as a basic strategy, there are several variables both in flap design and elevation, as well as in expander and implant choice, which can be manipulated to maximize the aesthetic quality of the result, while minimizing the donor site morbidity and potential complications.

Flap Elevation

Historically, use of the LDF has involved transposing only the muscle to the mastectomy defect with an isolated island of skin and fat of varying size positioned on top of the muscle. Although this can effectively provide cutaneous cover for the breast, **a more effective technique for providing volume is to harvest the deep layer of subcutaneous fat with the muscle.** The deep thoracic fascia provides a readily recognizable anatomic landmark that can guide dissection and even allow the deep fatty layer below the fascia to be harvested beyond the borders of the muscle. By increasing the overall volume of the flap and creating a *volume-added latissimus flap*, the ability to fill in and soften the margins of the mastectomy defect is enhanced.

Expander/Implant Choice

Recent developments in expander and implant design have resulted in a wide array of devices available for use in reconstruction. Choosing between round and anatomically shaped devices that are either textured or smooth and filled with either saline or silicone provides a variety of choices, which can be strategically exploited to solve individual reconstructive problems. For instance, a thin patient with stark breast contours may be served best by an anatomically shaped silicone gel textured implant. By combining the volume-added latissimus flap with an appropriately chosen expander or implant, excellent results are possible.

MARKING

With the patient in the standing position, the borders of the latissimus dorsi muscle are delineated. The midline of the back is identified and the tip of the scapula is marked (Fig. 64.1A). With the arm elevated, the anterior border of the muscle is drawn as it extends from the posterior border of the axilla downward toward the iliac crest. The upper border of the muscle is drawn as it extends from the axilla over the tip of the scapula to the midline of the back (Fig. 64.1B). The origin of the muscle is marked inferiorly as it curves from the lower midline of the back to the anterior border of the muscle. The inferior segment of the trapezius is drawn as it overlaps the upper medial border of the latissimus as a reminder of this important anatomic relationship.

Once the limits of the muscle have been identified, the location and orientation of the skin island is identified. The skin island is positioned in the center of the muscle to ensure equal soft-tissue coverage of the expander or implant in all directions once the skin island is inset. When a small, circular skin island is required, as is commonly the case when a skin-sparing mastectomy strategy is used, the skin island is positioned directly in the center of the flap. The relaxed skin tension line is identified as it passes through the center of the skin island, and this line guides the drawing of a gentle ellipse around the

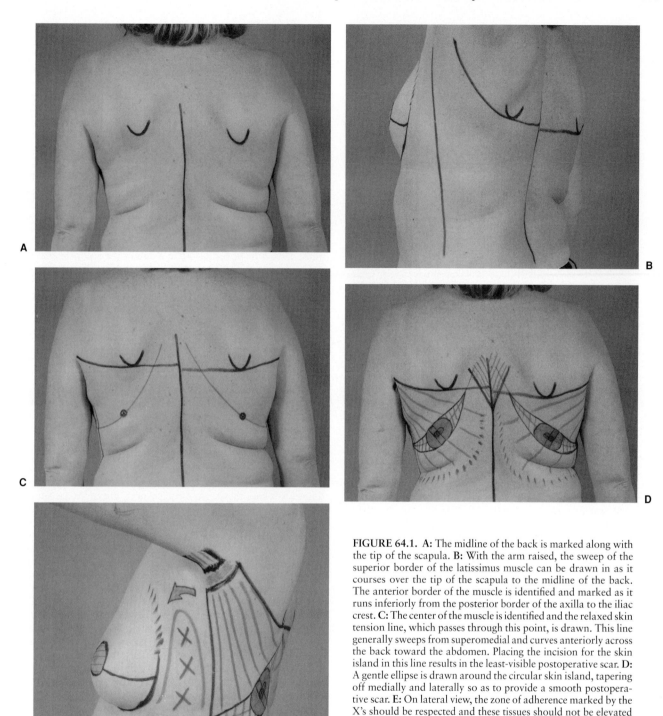

FIGURE 64.1. A: The midline of the back is marked along with the tip of the scapula. **B:** With the arm raised, the sweep of the superior border of the latissimus muscle can be drawn in as it courses over the tip of the scapula to the midline of the back. The anterior border of the muscle is identified and marked as it runs inferiorly from the posterior border of the axilla to the iliac crest. **C:** The center of the muscle is identified and the relaxed skin tension line, which passes through this point, is drawn. This line generally sweeps from superomedial and curves anteriorly across the back toward the abdomen. Placing the incision for the skin island in this line results in the least-visible postoperative scar. **D:** A gentle ellipse is drawn around the circular skin island, tapering off medially and laterally so as to provide a smooth postoperative scar. **E:** On lateral view, the zone of adherence marked by the X's should be respected and these tissues should not be elevated during flap transfer. Instead, the flap is optimally passed through a tunnel created high in the axilla and dropped into the mastectomy defect. This preserves the lateral breast contour, which is a landmark that can be difficult to create with internal sutures.

skin island (Fig. 64.1C). By tapering off around the skin island medially and laterally, adequate exposure for flap dissection is provided, while allowing for direct closure of the skin defect without dog-ear formation at the medial or lateral ends of the incision (Fig. 64.1D).

When a larger skin island is required, as in cases of delayed breast reconstruction, the same strategy is employed, attempting to place the elliptical skin island more or less in the center of the flap and orienting the long axis of the ellipse along the same relaxed skin tension line. The advantage of orienting the

long axis of the skin paddle in this fashion is that, despite the scar sweeping up to the upper back, it heals in an acceptable fashion. This is in contradistinction to other scar orientations, which can be quite unsightly as the orientation of the skin island crosses the relaxed skin tension lines of the back, resulting in widened or hypertrophic scars.

Once the skin island is marked and the limits of the muscle identified, the zone of attachment between the upper anterior border of the muscle and the lateral border of the breast is marked. **If at all possible, avoid dissection in this area as** this preserves the lateral border of the breast. This contour can be difficult to reconstruct with suture plication if it is released during either the mastectomy or in making the tunnel for passage of the LDF. Finally, the tunnel through which the flap is to be passed anteriorly is drawn high in the axilla. This serves to preserve the lateral contour of the breast and limits any potential lateral chest wall fullness or deformity that can occur as a result of overzealous tissue release in this area (Fig. 64.1E).

OPERATIVE TECHNIQUE

Stage 1

After the mastectomy is completed, the viability of the skin flaps is assessed. If there is a question of mastectomy flap ischemia, fluorescein is infused to assess vascular perfusion. **Debridement of all nonperfused areas is performed.** It is helpful at this point to predissect the high axillary tunnel through the mastectomy defect in preparation for subsequent flap transfer. This space is then easily entered during flap dissection on the back, facilitating subsequent transposition of the flap once it is completely released, preventing inadvertent overdissection of the lateral chest wall during creation of the tunnel.

At this point, the wound is temporarily stapled closed and covered with a sterile dressing. The patient is rotated into the prone position for both unilateral and bilateral reconstructions. In the prone position, the anatomic landmarks are more easily identified than in the lateral decubitus position.

The skin island is incised and the thoracic fascia is divided along the line of incision. With division of the fascia, the wound springs open as the loose, deep, fatty layer is exposed to retractive pressure from above. Dissection then proceeds just under the fascia in all directions, keeping the deep layer of fat attached to the muscle. Once the limits of the muscle are reached, dissection proceeds through the deep layer of fat down to the margins of the latissimus muscle in all directions. The trapezius muscle is identified in the upper medial corner of the dissection space and the latissimus is released from under it. The upper border of the latissimus muscle is then identified and released. The fibers of origin are then peeled away from the fascia of the back, extending from the upper medial corner of the dissection space toward the iliac crest. As the muscle is undermined, crossing perforators from the intercostal spaces are controlled. Inferiorly, the muscle is divided from its attachments to the iliac crest. The muscle is released from its attachments to the serratus anterior and the anterior border is identified and released, care being taken to avoid inadvertent elevation of the fibers of origin of the external oblique in the anterior-inferior corner of the dissection space. The muscle is then flipped up toward the axilla and any remaining attachments to the teres major muscle posteriorly are divided.

Communication with the mastectomy wound is then made high in the axilla and the muscle is passed anteriorly to the mastectomy defect. The pedicle is easily identified entering the underside of the muscle and care should be taken to avoid tethering or otherwise injuring the vascular leash. **With full release of the muscular attachments, there is no need to divide the serratus branch, which can become important, as this vascular conduit can support the flap entirely if the main thoracodorsal pedicle was injured during the original mastectomy (9).**

The back wound is then closed over suction drainage. The placement of quilting sutures securing the upper and lower back flaps to the intercostal muscles may assist in preventing or limiting persistent postoperative drainage from the back donor site (10). The patient is rotated back into the supine position. The flap is fully withdrawn into the mastectomy wound and the insertion of the muscle identified. I prefer to divide this insertion completely, just above the entry point of the vascular pedicle, as this facilitates easy rotation of the LDF in any direction required, depending on the dimensions of the mastectomy defect. Alternatively, it is a reasonable compromise to divide the posterior 90% of the insertion, as the remaining attachments protect against inadvertent traction being placed on the pedicle, and yet full transfer of the flap into the mastectomy defect is greatly facilitated.

The vascular pedicle is readily identified. I prefer to divide the thoracodorsal nerve at this point. With division of the nerve, unwanted and distracting motion in the reconstructed breast is greatly diminished or eliminated, a finding that has been a welcome addition to my results over the years. Such denervation has not resulted in enough volume loss in the flap to significantly detract from the aesthetic result of the reconstruction.

The flap is now prepared for insetting. In small- to medium-size breasts, there is no need to elevate the pectoralis major muscle. The edges of the LDF are simply sutured into the medial, superior, and lateral margins of the mastectomy defect, and the tissue expander is placed under the flap. The remaining edge of the LDF is then inset into the inferior margin of the mastectomy wound around the inferior border of the expander, providing a complete muscle cover for the device.

In larger breasts, the surface area provided by the LDF may not be enough to provide sufficient padding for the entire surface area of the mastectomy defect without tethering, and the skin envelope of the breast may not be sufficiently filled out. In these cases, full release of the pectoralis major muscle can enlarge the muscular soft-tissue envelope, allowing the now upwardly retracted pectoralis muscle to cover the upper portion of the defect, and using the LDF to cover the lower portion. Centrally, where these two muscles meet, the edges are simply sutured together in a vest-over-pants fashion, with the latissimus secured on top of the pectoralis major. Whatever strategy is used, it is important to close off the tunnel leading to the back donor site to an opening of only 2 to 3 cm to prevent inadvertent slippage of the expander through the axilla into the back postoperatively.

At this point, the dimensions of the skin island are finalized and inset, discarding redundant skin as needed. In cases of immediate reconstruction, often only a circular skin island is required to fit into the defect created by removal of the nipple and areola (Fig. 64.2). In delayed reconstruction, an ellipse is generally used to fill in the cutaneous defect created at the time of mastectomy. This ellipse of skin can be positioned in one of two ways. Perhaps the most straightforward inset strategy involves opening the mastectomy wound along the scar line and insetting the flap directly into the resulting wound. In this manner, no new scars are created on the breast, and the vascularity of the mastectomy flaps is not compromised. In thin patients, or in patients with mastectomy scars positioned low on the chest, it is possible to resect nearly the entire lower mastectomy flap and replace it with the LDF skin island, placing the lower scar directly in the inframammary fold. However, in patients with larger breasts or high-riding mastectomy scars, not all of the lower mastectomy flap can be removed, and the LDF skin island will create an obvious patch effect once it is inset into the reconstructed breast. To prevent this, many surgeons will ignore the previous mastectomy scar and open the mastectomy wound by making an incision low and lateral along the proposed inframammary fold. Once the LDF skin island is then inset, the lower scar will be hidden in the fold, and the shape of the ellipse will assist in creating a rounded ptotic appearance to the reconstructed breast. This approach can risk compromise of the vascularity of the remaining lower mastectomy flap as

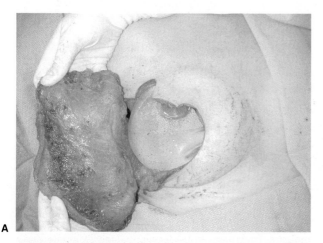

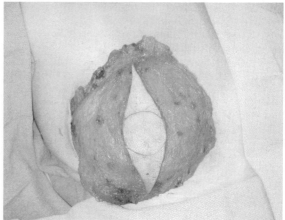

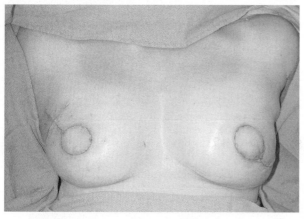

FIGURE 64.2. **A:** The flap has been passed anteriorly through the axilla and the tissue expander positioned centrally within the mastectomy defect. **B:** The muscle is then wrapped around the expander, suturing the edges of the muscle into the margins of the mastectomy defect. This maneuver softens the contours of the mastectomy wound, improving the overall quality of the reconstructive result. **C:** After inset of the skin island in this case of a bilateral reconstruction performed in conjunction with a periareolar skin-sparing mastectomy, an aesthetic result has been created, even at this early stage, with the tissue expanders in place.

a result of the crisscrossing scars; for this reason, many surgeons will keep the remaining upper mastectomy flap attached to the pectoralis major muscle, positioning the expander under the muscle. The disadvantage is that the breast may have unwanted motion postoperatively because of the subpectoral placement.

After positioning the expander and insetting the flap and the skin island, the skin incisions are closed over suction drains. **It should be noted that in cases where adjustment of the opposite breast is planned, that procedure (whether it be breast augmentation, reduction, or mastopexy) is performed at this initial stage.** In this fashion, the breast is allowed to settle until the stage 2 procedure is performed, which enhances the accuracy of the second procedure, as the reconstructed breast is matched to a stable opposite breast size and shape.

Postoperative recovery is generally uneventful, with most patients leaving the hospital within 2 to 3 days. Early motion of the arms and shoulders is encouraged to prevent stiffness. Expander inflation is performed in the office setting as needed to achieve the desired final volume, beginning as early as 2 weeks postoperatively. **Often only one or two expansions are necessary because of the adequacy of the dimensions of the skin surface area created by adding the latissimus skin island.** For this reason, it is also not necessary to overinflate the expander to a significant degree in most cases.

Stage 2

After the postoperative recovery from the stage 1 procedure is complete and all swelling has resolved, the final shaping of

the breast is performed, usually 4 to 6 months after the stage 1 procedure. The procedure is generally performed in the outpatient setting. At this stage, the tissue expander is removed, the breast is reshaped as needed, and the nipple and areola are reconstructed. Additional adjustments to the opposite breast can also be made as needed. Under the best of circumstances, all that will be required to complete the reconstruction will be to remove the tissue expander, replacing it with a permanent implant, and reconstruction of the nipple and areola using one of several different techniques. **It bears noting that, because the back dermis is quite thick, the appearance and longevity of nipples made with latissimus flap skin tends to be excellent.** In selected cases, further modification of the reconstructed breast may be required to obtain the optimal result. These modifications may include contour reconfiguration with elevation or lowering of the inframammary fold, widening of the pocket, or capsulectomy with removal of scar. Breast implant dimensions, volume, and shape are chosen to give the best possible result. Liposuction of the lateral chest wall is occasionally required to treat excess fullness in this area. Using this staged approach, excellent results can be obtained in most cases.

EXPANDER VERSUS IMPLANT

Many surgeons insert the primary implant at the same time the latissimus flap is inset. This is an attractive option, as the need for a second separate procedure to remove the tissue expander is avoided. It can be accomplished, particularly in cases of immediate breast reconstruction, because generally there is no loss of skin envelope surface area to the breast. Consequently, there is no need to "expand" the skin. Despite this, I prefer to use a tissue expander during the stage 1 procedure. When true expansion is not required, I consider the expander to be an intelligently chosen spacer, holding the soft-tissue envelope of the reconstructed breast open while the soft tissues heal around it. This strategy facilitates more accurate implant selection at the stage 2 procedure, allowing changes in implant base diameter, projection, volume, and shape to be made based on how the breast has recovered from the stage 1 procedure. As well, a strategy for manipulation of the soft-tissue pocket at stage 2 is built into the operative plan, which only enhances the overall ultimate result.

RESULTS

The LDF is an excellent option for almost any reconstructive situation. It can be used with ease in cases of immediate or delayed reconstruction (Fig. 64.3). It is a particularly attractive option for patients in need of bilateral reconstruction (Fig. 64.4). In patients who may not have enough volume for a bilateral transverse rectus abdominis musculocutaneous (TRAM) flap and who want more of an expander/implant reconstruction, the bilateral latissimus flap option can be an excellent choice. It is also a very useful flap for reconstruction of the partial mastectomy defect, or for autogenous salvage in cases of significant fat necrosis after TRAM flap recon-

struction. At times, in patients with relatively small opposite breasts, it can be used as a completely autogenous flap, obviating the need for an implant. In these latter circumstances, the "volume-added" strategy becomes a particularly attractive option for increasing the available soft-tissue bulk provided by the flap.

COMPLICATIONS

The most recognized complication of latissimus flap harvest is donor-site seroma formation. It is not uncommon for drains to remain in the back donor site for as long as 6 weeks postoperatively. Occasionally, outpatient aspiration of a persistent seroma is required after drain removal. With time, fluid accumulation eventually stops, leaving behind an empty bursa of varying dimensions. Although isolated arm strength can be diminished after flap transfer, this is rarely a significant finding, as the other muscles of the back compensate for the absent muscle. The vascularity of the LDF itself is robust, and only rarely is there any vascular compromise or fat necrosis noted after LDF transfer. However donor-site marginal skin necrosis can occur particularly in smokers, which might suggest avoiding excessive undermining. After transfer of the flap with placement of a tissue expander or implant, capsular contracture can occur. Treatment generally consists of complete capsulectomy, which alleviates the problem in the vast majority of cases.

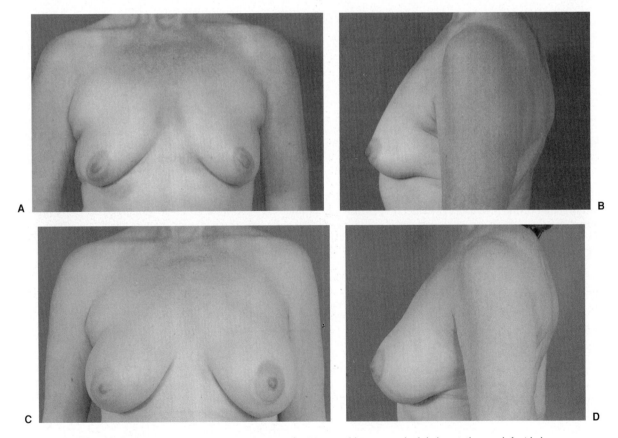

FIGURE 64.3. A, B: Preoperative appearance of a 54-year-old woman scheduled to undergo a left-sided modified radical mastectomy for adenocarcinoma of the breast. **C, D:** One-year postoperative appearance after eventual placement of a 400-cc smooth, round, silicone gel implant on the left, and an augmentation of the right breast with a 375-cc smooth, round, silicone gel implant. The reconstructed nipple and areola has been tattooed.

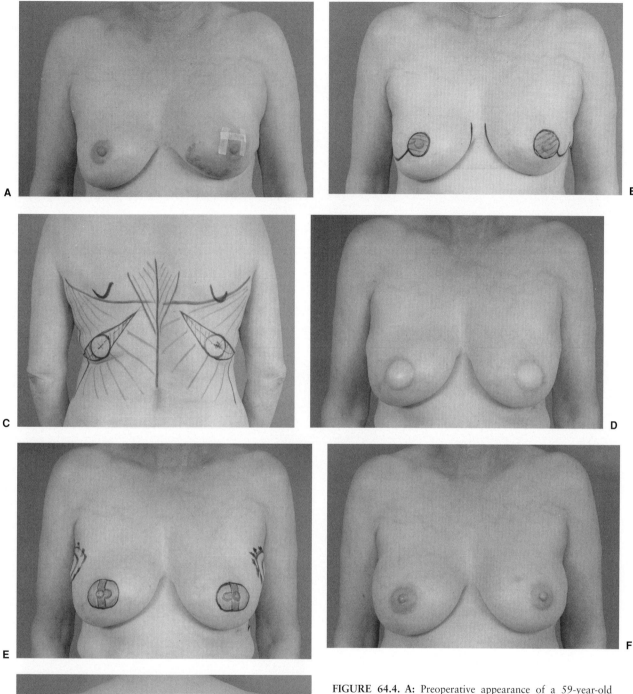

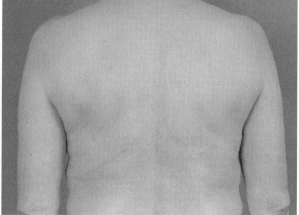

FIGURE 64.4. A: Preoperative appearance of a 59-year-old woman with lobular carcinoma in situ of the left breast. She had undergone subcutaneous mastectomy with implant reconstruction in the remote past. **B:** The preoperative marks outline a periareolar skin-sparing mastectomy that includes a lateral extension for better access to the breast. **C:** The back marks outline the circular skin island used to replace the missing nipple and areola. The position of the ellipse is oriented along the relaxed skin tension lines. **D:** Appearance 6 months after her stage 1 procedure reveals good symmetry and a pleasing overall aesthetic result. **E:** The preoperative marks for her stage 2 procedure outline her bilateral nipple and areola complex reconstruction along with soft-tissue recontouring in the upper outer quadrant of the breast. The tissue expanders will be replaced with silicone gel implants. **F:** Appearance 1 year after placement of a 600-cc smooth, round, silicone gel implant on the right, and a 500-cc implant on the left. **G:** Appearance of the back reveals no contour deformity and a very-well-healed scar with no distortion or bunching.

CONCLUSION

The latissimus dorsi musculocutaneous flap provides a readily available and reliable block of tissue that can be used in breast reconstruction. Because it dramatically enhances the ability of the plastic surgeon to artistically reconstruct the contours of the breast in a wide variety of clinical settings, it is recommended as an essential technique in the armamentarium of the reconstructive breast surgeon.

References

1. Maxwell GP. Iginio Tansini and the origin of the latissimus dorsi musculocutaneous flap. *Plast Reconstr Surg.* 1980;65:686.
2. Olivari N. The latissimus flap. *Br J Plast Surg.* 1976;29:126.
3. Schneider WJ, Hill HL, Brown RG. Latissimus dorsi myocutaneous flap for breast reconstruction. *Br J Plast Surg.* 1977;30:277.
4. Laitung JKG, Peck F. Shoulder function following the loss of the latissimus dorsi muscle. *Br J Plast Surg.* 1985;38:375.
5. Russell RC, Pribaz J, Zook EG, et al. Functional evaluation of latissimus dorsi donor site. *Plast Reconstr Surg.* 1986;78:336.
6. Fraulin FOG, Louie G, Zorrilla L, et al. Functional evaluation of the shoulder following latissimus dorsi muscle transfer. *Ann Plast Surg.* 1995;35:349.
7. Luce PA, Hammond DC. Latissimus dorsi musculocutaneous flaps and tissue expanders/implants in immediate breast reconstruction. *Plast Surg Forum.* 1995;64:133.
8. Fisher J, Hammond DC. The combination of expanders with autogenous tissue in breast reconstruction. *Clin Plast Surg.* 1994;21:309.
9. Fisher J, Bostwick J III, Powell RW. Latissimus dorsi blood supply after thoracodorsal vessel division: the serratus collateral. *Plast Reconstr Surg.* 1983;72:502.
10. Rios J, Adams WP, Pollock T. Progressive tension sutures to decrease latissimus donor site seroma. *Plast Reconstr Surg.* 2003;112:1779.

CHAPTER 65 ■ BREAST RECONSTRUCTION: TRAM FLAP TECHNIQUES

JAMES D. NAMNOUM

The transverse rectus abdominis musculocutaneous (TRAM) flap had its introduction as a technique for breast reconstruction more than 20 years ago. Initially described by Holmstrom as a free flap, it was later popularized by Hartrampf, who independently conceived of its use as an abdominal island flap for breast reconstruction (1,2). Drawing on the work of Esser, Hartrampf theorized that the lower abdominal skin and fat could be transferred to the chest to create a breast mound based on circulation provided from the rectus abdominis muscle (3). The successful outcome following this procedure in a patient with a history of implant failure following radical mastectomy ushered in a new era of breast reconstruction.

INDICATIONS

Both the pedicle and free TRAM procedures may be indicated for patients who desire immediate or delayed breast reconstruction. Although there are no absolute indications for one type of flap over the other, several relative indications merit consideration. As a general rule, selection of one technique over the other must take into account the comfort level of the surgeon with either technique. For the surgeon who infrequently performs microvascular surgery, the free TRAM technique is probably best avoided. Patients in high-risk categories, such as those with a history of heavy cigarette use (>10 pack/years smoking) and those who are overweight or obese, are more suitable for free than for pedicle TRAM reconstruction. This is particularly true for those undergoing bilateral reconstruction. In contrast, patients without significant comorbidity, high body mass index (BMI), or heavy smoking history show no difference in incidence of flap or abdominal complications whether one (unipedicle) or two (bilateral single pedicle or double pedicle) pedicles are used, or whether a free TRAM flap is performed (4).

PEDICLE TRAM

Most surgeons who perform the TRAM flap prefer the pedicle TRAM technique for breast reconstruction. Informal polling of attendees at the annual breast symposium in Atlanta attest to its continued popularity, as it routinely exceeds free TRAM in preference by more than 20 to 1. Despite continued technical refinements, such as the free TRAM and deep inferior epigastric perforator (DIEP) flap, which limit the sacrifice of rectus abdominis muscle and consequent abdominal wall morbidity, interest in the pedicle TRAM may actually be increasing. Advocates for the pedicle TRAM cite its reliability, predictable blood supply, ease and speed of harvest, and avoidance of a requirement for microvascular skills and instrumentation. Declining

reimbursement for breast reconstruction may also play a role in the shift away from microvascular procedures to shorter-duration pedicle TRAM procedures.

Technical Details

The pedicle TRAM is based on the superior epigastric vessels (Fig. 65.1). A split muscle technique is used for flap harvest. This reduces the incidence of abdominal contour deformities and permits a more secure immediate abdominal closure (5). Mesh is used as an onlay only after the best possible primary fascial closure. The indications for mesh include excessive tension on the repair and fascia that tears at closure or appears thin and weak. Mesh is rarely required following single-pedicle TRAM flaps, but is required more frequently in patients undergoing bilateral pedicle or double-pedicle TRAM flaps. A continuous, nonabsorbable suture is used for the fascial repair. Care is taken to ensure that the internal oblique fascia is included in the repair. This is especially important in the lower abdomen where it may retract underneath the external oblique fascia and be inadvertently excluded, with postoperative abdominal bulging or hernia as a result. The pedicle TRAM can be successfully based either on a contralateral or ipsilateral pedicle; whether the flap orientation is vertical or horizontal is at the surgeon's discretion. Adherence to Hartrampf's criteria for flap selection is associated with a low incidence of fat necrosis and partial and total flap loss; abdominal bulge and hernia are rarely encountered with the muscle-sparing technique in normal-risk patients (6).

FREE TRAM

The free TRAM represents an evolution of technique from the pedicle TRAM. First described by Holmstrom and later popularized by Grotting, Elliott, and others, it is the preferred technique for many surgeons performing TRAM flap breast reconstruction (7–9). Advocates for the free TRAM cite its advantages of reduced abdominal dissection and muscle sacrifice, enhanced flap vascularity, ease of flap inset, and avoidance of disturbance of the medial inframammary fold. Patients undergoing free TRAM appear to have less immediate postoperative pain and a quicker initial abdominal recovery.

In contrast to the pedicle TRAM, patients undergoing free TRAM show no increase in incidence of flap or abdominal complications such as total flap loss, fat necrosis, hernia, or bulge despite elevated BMI or a history of heavy tobacco use (4). Thus, the free TRAM is more appropriate for use in these high-risk patients. Patients in high-risk categories are at risk for abdominal or mastectomy skin loss, umbilical loss, seroma, and

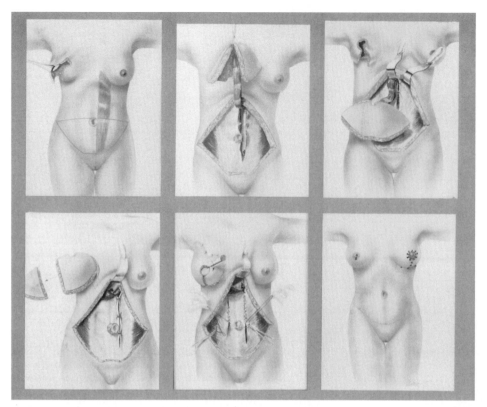

FIGURE 65.1. Pedicle TRAM flap technique. A muscle-sparing flap is harvested preserving medial and lateral rectus muscle. Circulation is based on superior epigastric vessels. Flap is tunneled to mastectomy defect. The fascia is closed with a running nonabsorbable suture. Inset is completed at mastectomy defect.

infection, indicating that TRAM flap surgery in general is not without increased morbidity in these patient populations regardless of the technique used (4,10,11). Besides requiring microvascular skills, and longer operative times, the main disadvantage of the free TRAM is the significantly higher incidence of total flap failure when compared with pedicle TRAM, where total flap failure is virtually nonexistent (4). Consequently, deciding which technique to use should take into consideration a surgeon's personal success rate with the free TRAM before committing a patient to a procedure with a potentially higher rate of failure.

Technical Details

A small segment of muscle and fascia from the lower abdomen is used for harvest of the free TRAM flap, simplifying the abdominal closure (Fig. 65.2). The flap is based on deep inferior epigastric vessels. The thoracodorsal vessels or internal mammary vessels may be used as recipients, depending on the ease of harvest. As more surgeons shift from formal axillary dissections to sentinel node biopsies or very limited axillary dissections, the internal mammary vessels have gained in popularity. Use of these vessels permits more central positioning of the flap, avoids the need for an axillary extension of the skin-sparing incision, and avoids disturbance of the axilla. This must be balanced against the increased difficulty using the internal mammary vein, which is very thin, and the potential disadvantage of sacrificing the left internal mammary artery, which may later be necessary for coronary artery revascularization. The increased flap vascularity permits a more flexible approach to shaping.

AESTHETICS

Both the pedicle and free TRAM techniques can be used to create an attractive breast mound (Figs. 65.3 and 65.4).

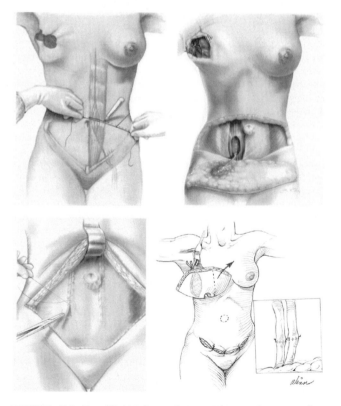

FIGURE 65.2. Free TRAM flap technique. The muscle-sparing flap removes a small, central segment of rectus muscle and fascia from the lower abdomen. Circulation is based on inferior epigastric vessels. The flap is transferred to the chest. Microvascular anastomoses are completed end to end to the thoracodorsal or internal mammary vessels. The fascia is closed with running nonabsorbable suture. The flap is inset at the mastectomy defect.

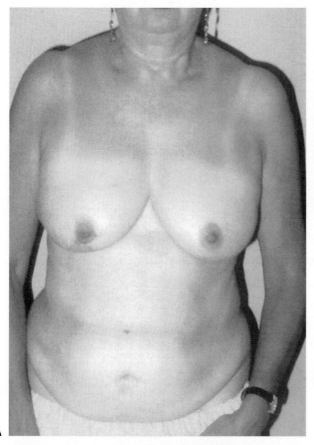

A

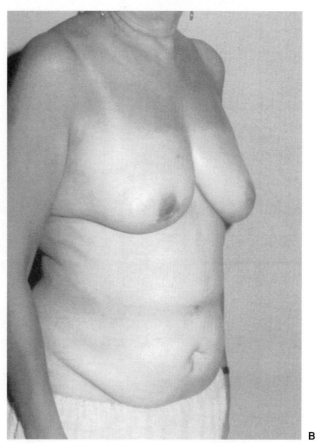

B

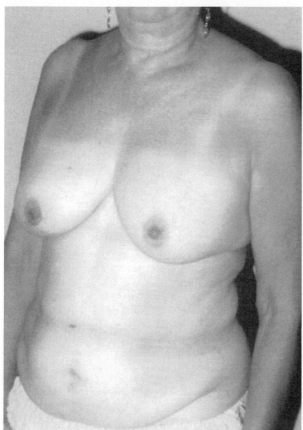

C

FIGURE 65.3. Pedicle TRAM flap reconstruction. A 56-year-old patient with right breast cancer. Figure shows (A–C) preoperative and (*Continued*)

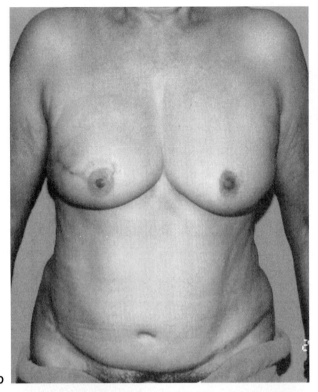

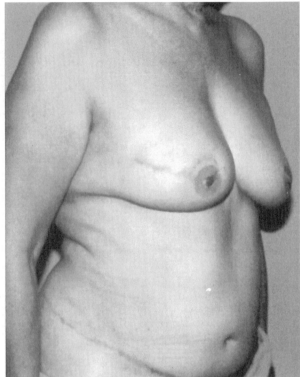

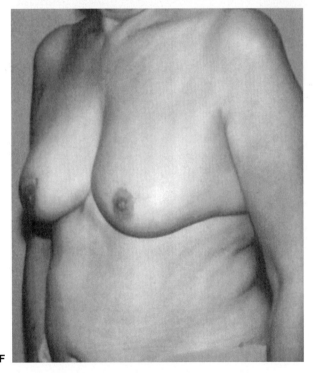

FIGURE 65.3. (*Continued*) (**D–F**) 2-year follow-up after single-pedicle TRAM reconstruction views.

Disturbance of the inframammary fold because of tunneling and of the upper abdominal bulge over the costal margin created by the rectus muscle is a factor that, in the short-term, may give the free technique an advantage. In most cases, the crease disturbance settles down after several months. As long as all the intercostal nerves to the rectus muscle have been divided, the pedicle atrophies and is not noticeable. Abdominal contour disturbances can be minimized by use of a muscle-sparing technique, but are seen from time to time regardless of which technique is used.

Selection of a mastectomy skin pattern generally may be made without regard for the type of flap used. Practically,

however, a skin-sparing pattern requires use of the internal mammary vessels as recipients unless a short axillary extension or vertical incision is added. For surgeons preferring the pedicle TRAM, the skin-sparing incision offers a great opportunity for near anatomic breast reconstruction. Reduction patterns for mastectomy are plagued by problems with mastectomy skin flap compromise, particularly when coupled with pedicled TRAMs, and are best reserved for patients undergoing free TRAM reconstruction, which does not require tunneling. In such instances, use of a vertical skin pattern may reduce the risk of mastectomy skin loss; a transverse incision can be added at the second stage of reconstruction if needed.

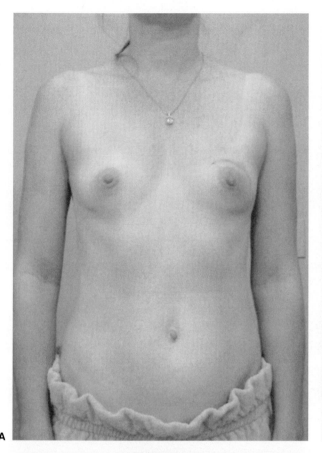

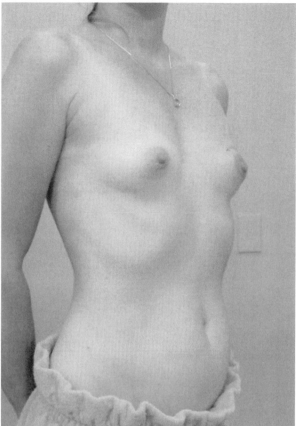

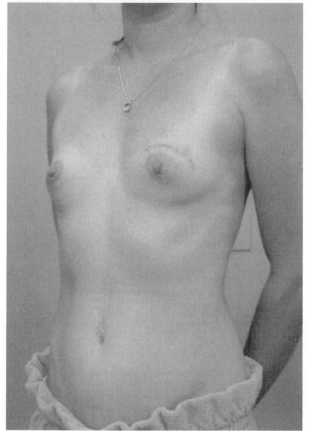

FIGURE 65.4. Free TRAM flap reconstruction. A 38-year-old patient with left breast cancer. Figure shows (**A–C**) preoperative and (*Continued*)

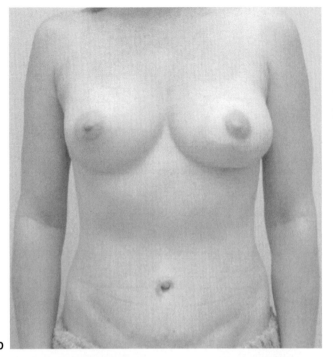

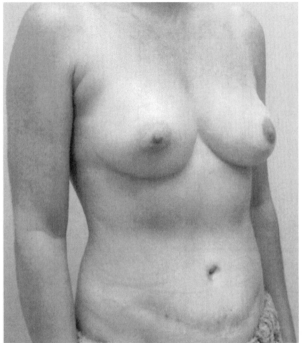

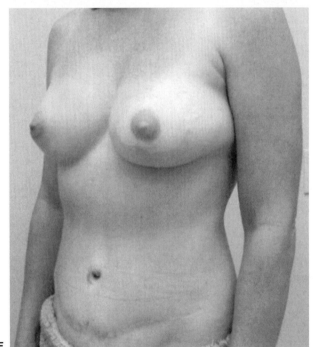

FIGURE 65.4. (*Continued*) (D–F) 3-year follow-up after free TRAM reconstruction and subsequent augmentation of opposite breast and TRAM for symmetry views.

Intraoperative fluorescence can help to distinguish compromise of mastectomy skin flaps but tends to overcall the extent of skin flap ischemia.

DONOR-SITE MORBIDITY

Donor-site issues, such as abdominal bulge and hernia, weakness, and interference with activities of daily living, have been debated since the introduction of TRAM. Sacrifice of muscle is associated with contour disturbances and bulging if the whole muscle is used instead of a muscle-preserving technique (12). The ability to perform sit-ups postoperatively is dependent on the amount of muscle harvested and is more likely to be

preserved in patients undergoing free TRAM than in patients undergoing pedicle TRAM (1,2). Despite this finding, pedicle TRAM harvest rarely affects activities of daily living and most patients return to preoperative athletic pursuits (13).

FLAP MORBIDITY

Fat necrosis and partial and total flap loss can occur with either TRAM technique. Patients who are heavy past smokers, actively smoking at the time of surgery, and are obese or overweight may be at increased risk for flap complications. Direct comparisons between pedicle and free TRAM flaps have not yielded consistent results regarding the incidence of fat necrosis. Although fat necrosis is reported to occur more commonly in pedicled than free TRAM flaps, our series showed a higher incidence of fat necrosis only in heavy past smokers and active smokers (4).

SURGICAL DELAY

For patients in high-risk categories, surgical delay has been suggested as a method to improve flap vascularity. To date, no study has shown a consistent reduction in the incidence of fat necrosis or abdominal morbidity in patients undergoing delay of TRAM, but the experimental data in animals and humans is compelling (14–15).

References

1. Holmstrom H. The free abdominoplasty flap and its use in breast reconstruction: an experimental study and clinical case report. *Scand J Plast Reconstr Surg*. 1979;13:423.
2. Hartrampf CR, Scheflan M, Black P. Breast reconstruction with a transverse abdominal island flap. *Plast Reconstr Surg*. 1982;96:216.
3. Esser JFS. Island flaps. *N Y Med J*. 1917;August:264.
4. Namnoum JD. An analysis of 920 pedicled and 286 free TRAM flap breast reconstructions. Presented at the Annual Meeting of the American Society of Plastic Surgeons. Orlando, FL: November 2001.
5. Nahabedian MY, Dooley W, Singh N, et al. Contour abnormalities of the abdomen after breast reconstruction with abdominal flaps: the role of muscle preservation. *Plast Reconstr Surg*. 2002;109:91.
6. Hartrampf CR Jr, Bennett GK. Autogenous tissue reconstruction in the mastectomy patient. A critical review of 300 patients. *Ann Surg*. 1987;205:508.
7. Grotting JC, Urist MM, Maddox WA, et al. Conventional TRAM flap versus free microsurgical TRAM flap for immediate breast reconstruction. *Plast Reconstr Surg*. 1989;83:828.
8. Elliott LF, Eskenazi L, Beegle PH, et al. Immediate TRAM flap breast reconstruction: 128 consecutive cases. *Plast Reconstr Surg*. 1993;92:217.
9. Schusterman MA, Kroll SS, Weldon ME. Immediate breast reconstruction: why the free TRAM over the conventional TRAM? *Plast Reconstr Surg*. 1992;90:255.
10. Chang DW, Wang B, Robb GL, et al. Effect of obesity on flap and donor-site complications in free transverse rectus abdominis myocutaneous flap breast reconstruction. *Plast Reconstr Surg*. 2000;105:1640–1648.
11. Chang DW, Reece GP, Wang B, et al. Effect of smoking on complications in patients undergoing free TRAM flap breast reconstruction. *Plast Reconstr Surg*. 2000;105:2374.
12. Kroll SS, Schusterman MA, Reece GP, et al. Abdominal wall Strength, bulging, and hernia after TRAM flap breast reconstruction. *Plast Reconstr Surg*. 1995;96:616.
13. Mizgala CL, Hartrampf CR, Bennett GK. Assessment of the abdominal wall after pedicled TRAM flap surgery: 5- to 7-year follow-up of 150 consecutive patients. *Plast Reconstr Surg*. 1994;93:988.
14. Restifo RJ, Ward BA, Scoutt LM, et al. Timing, magnitude, and utility of surgical delay in the TRAM flap: II. Clinical studies. *Plast Reconstr Surg*. 1997;99:1217.
15. Erdmann D, Sundin BM, Moquin KJ, et al. Delay in unipedicled TRAM flap reconstruction of the breast: a review of 76 consecutive cases. *Plast Reconstr Surg*. 2002;110:762.

CHAPTER 66 ■ BREAST RECONSTRUCTION—FREE FLAP TECHNIQUES

L. FRANKLYN ELLIOTT

Breast reconstruction after mastectomy has progressed enormously in the past 20 years. Before 1980, plastic surgeons were chiefly limited to the insertion of a silicone implant either beneath the skin or beneath the skin and a latissimus flap. The early 1980s marked the introduction of the tissue expander (Chapter 63) and the use of the transverse rectus abdominis musculocutaneous (TRAM) flap (Chapter 65). While these events were taking place, the field of microsurgery was developing. A case of breast reconstruction using what was essentially a free TRAM flap was reported by Hans Holstrom in 1979 but was largely overlooked (1). In fact, it was overshadowed by the introduction of the pedicle TRAM flap and the tissue expander. Microsurgery, however, continued to improve, leading inevitably to the application of microsurgical techniques to breast reconstruction.

Although the pedicle TRAM flap (the transverse abdominal island flap [TAIF]), as described by Carl Hartrampf, provided good results around the world, the procedure continued to have a percentage of complications (2). These complications were related to the amount of muscle harvested from the donor site and the vascularity of the tissue transferred to the recipient site. Microsurgeons addressed both these issues with the free TRAM flap (3).

With a free TRAM flap, less muscle is harvested. In addition, a better blood flow is achieved using the inferior epigastric system as opposed to the superior epigastric system upon which the pedicle TRAM is based. Ian Taylor's elegant studies of the venous system of the abdomin demonstrated the relatively unnatural flow from the flap through the superior epigastric veins (4). Flow through the inferior epigastric veins was shown to be more natural, or anatomic, and explained the higher frequency of venous congestion in the pedicle TRAM versus the free TRAM. In addition, the inferior epigastric arteries were found to be larger than the superior epigastric arteries, with a higher pressure and more total blood flow than the superior pedicles.

Although these findings stimulated many microsurgeons to use the free TRAM over the pedicle TRAM, there remained a large number of surgeons who were uncomfortable with microsurgical technique, the close follow-up required after free tissue transfer, or the disquieting prospect of total flap loss. Thus, in the late 1980s and 1990s, the free TRAM flap assumed a more important position in many reconstructive surgeons' practices, but certainly did not displace the pedicle TRAM as the first choice for autogenous tissue breast reconstruction.

It was only natural that developments continued and the free TRAM flap evolved to the DIEP (deep inferior epigastric perforator) flap, which has the advantage of harvesting no muscle. This technique was adopted by some microsurgeons, but not all (5). Elegant clinical and laboratory investigations have continued to refine the DIEP flap, and operating time has been reduced. The opportunity to use essentially all of the abdominal tissue without harvesting any muscle remains an attractive ideal. However, there continues to be an incidence of abdominal wall weakness/hernia that occurs after the DIEP flap, which is similar to that which occurs when the muscle-sparing technique is used for the free TRAM flap (6). Furthermore, there remain the occasional DIEP flaps that do not have the perfusion through one to two perforators that would be expected with the free TRAM flap, where there may be 10 to 15 perforators.

Another refinement that was introduced quite early, and re-introduced recently, is the use of the superficial inferior epigastric artery (SIEA). This technique requires no incision into the muscle and allows the abdominoplasty tissues to be transferred without violation of the muscular fascial abdominal wall. The superficial inferior epigastric vessels, however, demonstrate more variable anatomy than would be ideal. The flap can only be harvested in 40% to 50% of the cases and the operating time is quite long. Recent studies by Nincovich suggest that this flap can be harvested safely and predictably in an increasing number of cases (7). The superficial inferior epigastric artery, however, is definitely smaller than the deep inferior epigastric artery and does not have the blood flow volume one would find in the deep system.

Parallel to the abdominal wall developments for microsurgeons was the development of other donor sites. The gluteal free flap was introduced by Bill Shaw as an adequate source of adipose tissue with a donor site that is relatively well hidden (8). The flap was initially introduced as a myocutaneous flap, which included a plug of underlying gluteus maximus muscle through which perforators from either the superior gluteal or inferior gluteal system passed. A segment of muscle approximately 2 to 3 cm in vertical height by 6 to 8 cm in transverse width was harvested, thus including perforators from either of the underlying vascular systems to the overlying fat. The dissection, however, is extremely difficult and, in order to get adequate length on the vessels, the vein, in particular, became quite large. The vein at times was found to be 6 to 10 mm, which posed a significant problem with size material at the recipient site. In addition, if the inferior gluteal system was used, much of the soft tissue around the sciatic nerve was harvested, occasionally leading to painful donor sites and an unattractive flattening of the lower buttock. For these reasons, the superior gluteal system became increasing attractive in that the harvest of fat and the scar were placed in a less painful and debilitating position. The gluteal flap remains difficult and also requires various remote incisions on the recipient site for access to and the turning down of recipient veins.

Allen introduced the application of perforator techniques to the gluteal flap, which obviated almost all of the above

648

problems (9). No muscle was harvested, leading to a less morbid donor site, and the vessels could be lengthened by dissecting them through the muscle. The blood flow was excellent through one to two perforators, but the technique remains quite demanding.

The lateral transverse thigh flap, the brainchild of Carl Hartrampf, was introduced in 1987 as an alternate donor site (10). The idea was generated by patients requesting that their "saddle bags" be used for a breast. Laboratory injections demonstrated that the lateral circumflex femoral artery was found to have perforators through the tensor fasciae latae muscle and into the overlying fat and skin of the lateral thigh. This flap was more easily harvested than the gluteal flap, but did leave a scar on the lateral thigh; always visible in a bathing suit. In addition, the amount of fat needed for harvest often created an unnatural depression on the lateral thigh.

The Rubens' flap was introduced in 1991 as yet another site for autogenous breast tissue reconstruction (11). This was another idea of Carl Hartrampf; it was a variation of Ian Taylor's iliac crest flap. It was reasoned that if the iliac crest could be elevated on the deep circumflex iliac vessels with an overlying skin and fat island, then it should be possible to elevate the overlying skin and fat island without the underlying bone. Cadaver injections demonstrated musculocutaneous perforators all along the inner table of the iliac crest, extending from the anterior superior iliac spine to the posterior superior iliac spine. This was truly a musculocutaneous flap in which a segment of the full-thickness abdominal wall was required to allow the passage of musculocutaneous perforators from the deep circumflex iliac artery to the overlying skin and fat. Thus, it was necessary to resect full-thickness abdominal wall musculature just inside the iliac crest, which included the periosteum over the iliac crest, as well as segments of the external oblique, internal oblique, and transverse abdominis muscles. The flap was not particularly difficult to harvest, but donor-site closure of the abdominal wall musculature required drilling holes in the iliac crest to which the abdominal musculature was closed. The flap was reliable, even if a previous TRAM or abdominoplasty had been performed, and resulted in shapely, feminine contours of the donor site, especially when applied bilaterally.

Even though microsurgical options were developed, their use continued to be relatively small compared use of pedicle tissue transfer (the pedicle TRAM or latissimus dorsi cutaneous flap) or of the expander/implant. Economic factors have certainly affected surgeon's choices. As reimbursement, particularly in the United States, fell in the latter half of the 1990s, surgeons increasingly were attracted to less time-consuming procedures that provided adequate results. Economic factors continue to affect the surgeons entering practice, who are all trained in microsurgical techniques, and the older surgeons who are extremely accomplished microsurgeons who no longer feel they have the time or stamina for these time-consuming procedures.

INDICATIONS AND CONTRAINDICATIONS

The silicone implant controversy that erupted, particularly in America, but ultimately throughout the world, in 1992 and 1993, had a significant impact on the use of autogenous tissues and microsurgical techniques for breast reconstruction. After the "silicone scare," many women were afraid to use the implants or expanders and specifically requested autogenous breast reconstruction. This led to increased use of the TRAM flap and also to the use of other sites.

TABLE 66.1
TRAM RISK FACTORS
Obesity
Smoking
Diabetes
Abdominal scarring
Thinness
Lupus, vasculitis, etc.
Need absolutely all tissue

The microsurgical options were also found to be an acceptable alternative in patients in whom the pedicle TRAM flap was contraindicated. As defined by Hartrampf and others, the TRAM flap is associated with a consistent list of risk factors (Table 66.1). Chief among these risk factors were obesity, previous scars, and diabetes. The free TRAM flap, with its reduced muscle harvest and better blood flow, was successful in many patients in whom the pedicle TRAM flap would not be successful. Thus the indications for microsurgical breast reconstruction expanded somewhat for these patients, just as it contracted for the use of the pedicle TRAM flap. Nonetheless, the above-mentioned risk factors continue to plague any technique and, at times, place patients out of the acceptable category for breast reconstruction in general.

Radiation either before or after breast reconstruction also continues to plague the ultimate result no matter which technique is performed. Radiation prior to breast reconstruction significantly affects the native skin flaps of the chest wall and leads the surgeon to be extremely careful in preserving any radiation damaged skin. Autogenous tissue techniques offer significant advantages in this difficult clinical situation. While the overlying skin can be significantly affected, there is no evidence that the underlying vascular pedicles are affected; therefore, microsurgical free tissue transfer is generally found to be unaffected by previous radiation. **Although there are a few scattered reports alleging a high level of success with the use of implants after radiation, conventional wisdom does not support this conclusion. Thus, it could be concluded that previous radiation or expected postoperative radiation is a contraindication for the use of the expander/implant and an indication for the use of autogenous tissue** (Chapter 63). However, it has not been proven that free tissue transfer for breast reconstruction is better than the pedicle TRAM flap in the presence of radiation.

Contraindications for free flap techniques for breast reconstruction generally focus on either the surgeon's lack of experience with these techniques or the ability to appropriately follow and monitor the flaps in the acute postoperative period. Other contraindications are few, although it seems that a relatively "silent" contraindication, which is not generally discussed, is the economic one. The realities of current reimbursement patterns make it increasingly difficult for surgeons to dedicate significant time to these operations.

TECHNIQUES

Free TRAM

The pedicle and free TRAM operations were discussed in a previous chapter. However, because the free TRAM remains the most common of free flap techniques in breast reconstruction, this chapter includes some of the most important aspects of the technique.

The surgeon must assess preoperatively the volume of abdominal wall tissue available for breast reconstruction. It is improper to harvest a TRAM flap that has no chance of duplicating the desired breast size. Thin patients, however, can often be successfully reconstructed with the TRAM flap and the free TRAM flap is probably the best option, as there is the best chance of abdominal tissue perfusion (Fig. 66.1).

The breast incision should always be planned with the resecting oncologic surgeon. Obviously, a smaller incision is aesthetically the best; however, it is imperative that oncologic considerations override aesthetic ones. In addition, if free tissue transfer is planned, the incision must be adequate to visualize either the thoracodorsal vessels or the internal mammary vessels. If a counter incision in the axilla is needed, this can certainly be performed. The internal mammary recipient vessels have become the recipient of choice for essentially all free tissue breast reconstruction, either in the immediate or the delayed setting. In the delayed setting, the previously dissected axilla makes it difficult to expose recipient vessels. However, even in the immediate setting, the internal mammary vessels have significant advantages, including better positioning of the TRAM flap on the chest wall, larger vessels with better blood flow, an unscarred and undissected plane deep to the medial third or fourth rib, and a better position for the surgeon's assistant. **The thoracodorsal vessels had been a previous first choice, but the above advantages of the internal mammary vessels and the fact that less axillary dissection is being done, have led to a strong preference for the internal mammary vessels over the past 5 years.** Smaller incisions can also be used on the chest, with excellent visualization of the internal mammary vessels as opposed to inability to visualize the thoracodorsal vessels unless the incision is extended or a counter incision is made in the axilla.

Dissection of the flap is performed almost completely with electrocautery, which speeds the operation and reduces blood

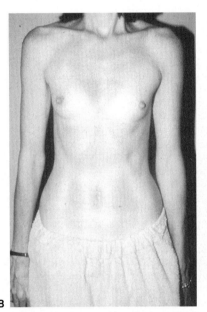
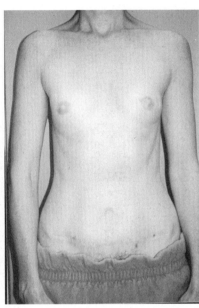
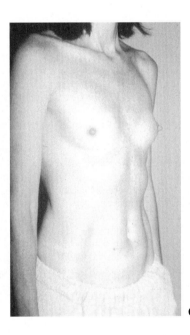

A,B   C

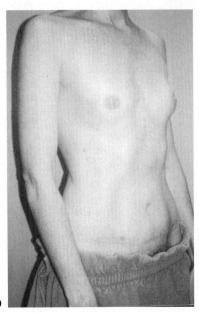

D

FIGURE 66.1. Very thin patient with successful bilateral pedicle TRAM reconstruction A: Preoperation. B: Postoperation. C: Preoperation lateral. D: Postoperation lateral.

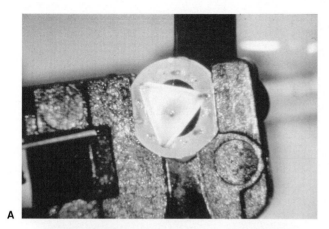

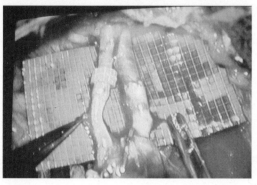

FIGURE 66.2. Microanastomotic coupling device. **A:** Vein end in coupling device. **B:** Intraoperative coupling device on vein, arterial anastomosis sewn.

loss. It is rare that a transfusion is needed today in free TRAM breast reconstruction, which is usually a 3-hour procedure. The vessel-coupling device is used for the venous anastomosis (Fig. 66.2). While using the coupler, one must be careful to avoid twisting the veins, which is, of course, important even if the vessels are sewn in the traditional manner.

Temperature strips aid the monitoring of the flap, particularly for darker-skinned patients (Fig. 66.3). Although color,

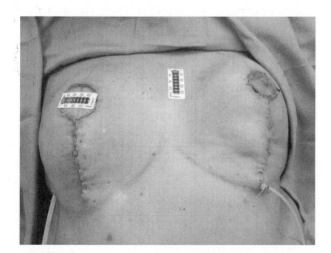

FIGURE 66.3. Temperature strip on free TRAM skin island (right breast) and control temperature strip on presternal area.

distention, and drain output must be followed in all patients, the temperature strip is particularly helpful in the darker-skinned patient in whom color changes cannot be followed as successfully.

Gluteal Flap

When using the gluteal flap, the best option is the perforator technique for the superior gluteal tissues. This technique places the resultant scar and tissue harvest in the upper gluteal area, which is not the area on which one sits. It lies below the usual upper line of a bathing suit and is tolerated aesthetically (Fig. 66.4). The use of the perforator technique obviates the harvest of any underlying musculature and allows for elongation of the vascular pedicle to approximately 5 to 6 cm. With the use of the internal mammary vessels as recipient vessels, a pedicle of this length is almost always adequate. The dissection remains tedious, however, as one dissects the perforator through the gluteus muscle. This dissection is significantly helped via the use of the microbipolar and loupe magnification. We do not find preoperative localization of perforators particularly helpful; instead, we elevate the fat off the underlying musculature, identifying perforators as they are encountered, choosing the largest we find. As the dissection proceeds through the gluteal muscle, one is always faced with the problem of determining when to stop the dissection. As the dissection proceeds deeper, difficulty with visibility and a multitude of vascular branches increases. The size of the recipient vessels dictates when to stop the dissection. If the superior artery and vein achieve a size that is close to those of the internal mammary vessels, no further dissection is necessary.

Lateral Transverse Thigh Flap

The lateral transverse thigh flap (LTTF) should be designed preoperatively on the most prominent part of the lateral thigh, generally centered over the greater trochanter. If the patient has inadequate fullness in this area (popularly known as the saddlebag area), the operation is not indicated. This operation, like the gluteal flap and Rubens' flap, has a limited overlying skin island. The skin island is limited in vertical height by the ability to close it primarily; this is generally no more than 8 cm (Fig. 66.5). Conversely, the skin island can measure from 15 to 20 cm transversely, depending on the length of the scar in the transverse manner. Anteriorly, the scar generally extends to the lateral border of the rectus femoris muscle, as it is at that point that the lateral circumflex femoral vessels dive deep to the rectus femoral muscle. The flap is generally harvested from lateral to medial; the lateral extent being a relative gray zone between the lateral thigh and the gluteal fat. As the flap is developed medially, the tensor fasciae latae muscle is divided superiorly in its muscular aspect and inferiorly in its fascial aspect to reveal a vascular hilum of the lateral circumflex femoral vessels, which is generally 10 cm caudal to the anterior superior iliac spine. Once this hilum is identified and the tensor fascia lata muscle has been divided, the vascular pedicle can be dissected for 6 to 8 cm medially until adequate length is achieved. As in the gluteal flap, the further the pedicle is dissected, the larger the vein can ultimately be, leading to size discrepancies with the recipient vessels.

In closing the donor site, we usually de-epithelialize 1 to 2 cm of the superior skin, which can then be tucked under the inferior flap to bolster the sutures lines and help prevent depression in that location. Nonetheless, liposuction above and

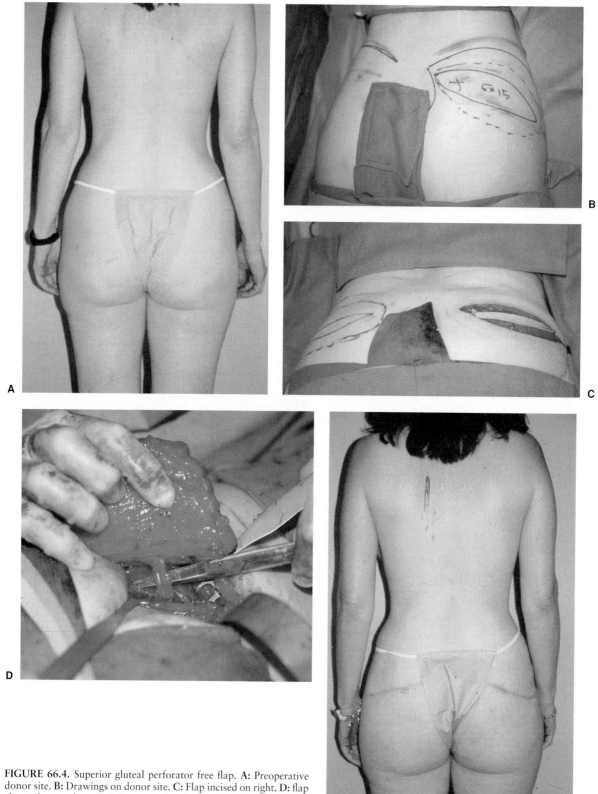

FIGURE 66.4. Superior gluteal perforator free flap. **A:** Preoperative donor site. **B:** Drawings on donor site. **C:** Flap incised on right. **D:** flap elevated on perforator. **E:** Postoperative donor sites.

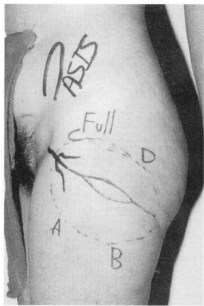
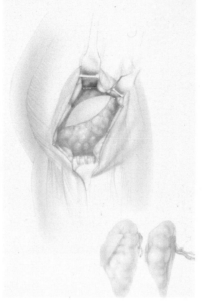
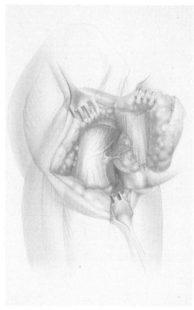

A,B   C

FIGURE 66.5. **A:** Donor site on left lateral thigh. **B:** Drawing of flap elevated. **C:** Flap elevated with vastus lateralis deep.

below the scar is often necessary to ultimately achieve a natural result (Fig. 66.6).

Rubens' Flap

The preoperative design of the Rubens' flap is essentially centered over the iliac crest. The flap then bevels superiorly and inferiorly so as to recruit adequate fat for the flap itself. As in the TRAM flap, it is important for the surgeon to be able to estimate how much tissue is available, as harvesting a flap that is too small is not ideal. The flap can extend anteriorly and posteriorly as far as one wishes, but the skin island is limited in vertical height by the ability to close the donor site. Again, the junction between the posterior limits of the flap and the gluteal fat is a somewhat gray area and should not extend more than 3 to 4 cm past the posterior superior iliac spine. Once the skin incision has been made, it is generally extended toward the pubic tubercle and a dissection is made through the abdominal wall musculature, much as in a hernia repair. The deep circumflex iliac vessels are best located as they arise from the iliac/femoral vessels near or with the origin of the deep inferior epigastric vessels. The vessels run along the pubic ramus laterally and can also be located with a sterile Doppler, as there are essentially no other vessels in this location. Once the vessels have been located, the flap is elevated off the iliac crest by incising through the abdominal wall musculature 1 to 2 cm cephalad to the iliac crest and elevating the periosteum caudally off the iliac crest, completing the soft-tissue elevation (Fig. 66.7). The flap is then liberated, but is generally not transferred until the abdominal wall musculature is repaired to the iliac crest. Although this delays the transfer of the free flap, leaving the abdominal wall musculature retracted "incising" cephalad makes subsequent closing even more difficult. With proper planning, the closure can be done expeditiously by placing 0.54-mm K-wire holes through the iliac crest and suturing the transverse abdominus and internal oblique to the iliac crest using permanent interrupted sutures. The external oblique is then closed over the deep closure to adjacent soft tissue. The free flap transfer is then performed in the usual manner and usually to the internal mammary vessels (Fig. 66.8).

CONTRAST OF TECHNIQUES

The free TRAM flap remains the first choice for free flap breast reconstruction. The donor site is best tolerated, the vascularity is excellent, the muscle harvest is minimized, the patient acceptance is maximized, and breast shaping is relatively straightforward. The free TRAM flap, however, does not always provide as much projection as the other choices, particularly the LTTF or gluteal flaps. Overzealous shaping of the free TRAM flap in order to achieve projection can lead to fat necrosis and should be avoided. Final shaping may be deferred until the time of nipple/areolar reconstruction, but this does not necessarily obviate the difficulty associated with shaping. Projection remains the most elusive aspect of the final breast shape in the use of a free TRAM flap. One must avoid placing the TRAM flap too far laterally. The use of the internal mammary vessels helps to avoid this excessively lateral placement.

The DIEP flap shares essentially all the advantages and disadvantages of the TRAM flap. One must be even more careful to excise zone IV and other more proximal portions of the flap if excellent blood flow is not observed at the time of de-epithelialization. This may lead to shaping needs that cannot be solved. It appears that in most patients, the DIEP flap has good perfusion and the tissue is adequate for breast shaping. Nonetheless, the time required for flap harvest and the relatively decreased blood flow continue to make this option generally secondary to the free TRAM flap.

The gluteal flap is probably second to the abdominal tissues as the best free flap option. The donor site is excellent, although it can generally be improved with liposuction both above and below the scar at the time of secondary nipple/areolar reconstruction. Seromas are few without the harvest of any muscle, and pain is minimal. This is probably the least painful of all the donor sites. Although the technique remains exacting, with

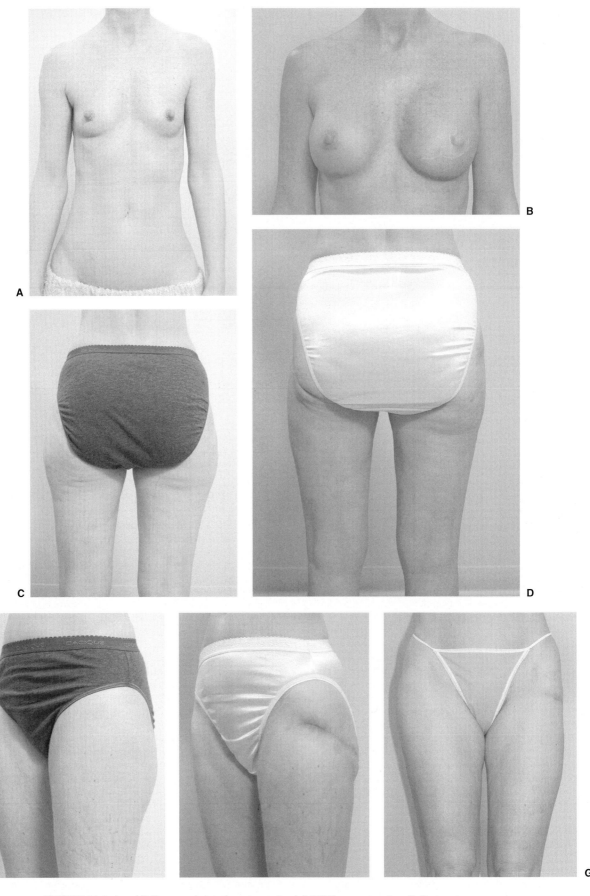

FIGURE 66.6. A and **B:** Preoperation and postoperation left LTTF reconstruction. **C:** Donor site preoperatively. **D:** Postoperatively, donor site on left with liposuction on right lateral thigh for balance. **E:** Donor site on left lateral thigh revised with scar revision and liposuction preoperatively, 4 months postoperation (**F**), and 1 year postoperation after 1 revision (**G**).

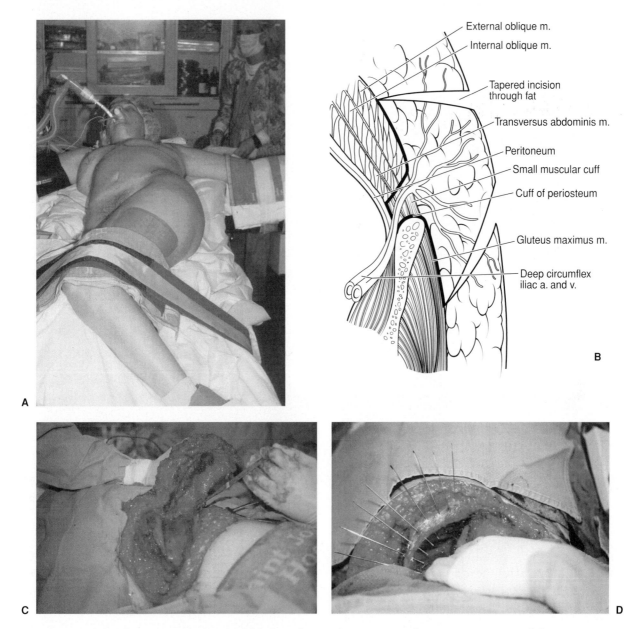

FIGURE 66.7. **A:** Positioning for left Rubens' flap transfer. **B:** Drawing of operative incisions. **C:** Left flap elevated from lateral to medial. **D:** K-wire holes through iliac crest to facilitate muscle closure.

proper experience and training, this operation can flow along in only slightly more time than that needed for a TRAM flap and will generally be as successful. Turning is required for this operation in that the recipient vessels should be dissected first (usually the internal mammary vessels); then the patient turned in a prone position for flap harvest and donor site closure, and, finally, the patient turned back to a supine position for flap anastomosis and breast shaping.

Breast shaping for the gluteal, LTTF, or Rubens' flap is essentially done as the flap is harvested. The surgeon should use his or her artistic ability to predict the needs for fat filling on the chest wall as the flaps are harvested. This is in contrast to the use of abdominal tissues, where the entire flap must be harvested and then carved down as indicated once the tissues are on the chest wall. **The LTTF and Rubens' flap are generally in the last tier of choices because of the scar location with regard to the LTTF flap and the difficulty of abdominal wall closure**

using the Rubens' flap. Nonetheless, these two choices do work and may be indicated for a particular patient.

THE FUTURE

Patients will continue to demand autogenous tissue for breast reconstruction. It is probable that free flap techniques will continue to be refined and perforator techniques take over all these donor sites. On the other hand, small amounts of muscle harvest may always be used in order to recruit additional perforators and speed the operation along. This increases blood flow relative to flaps as opposed to those based on a single perforator and allows the surgeon to perform the operation within acceptable time intervals.

Economic factors cannot be overemphasized in assessing the future for free flap techniques in breast reconstruction. As

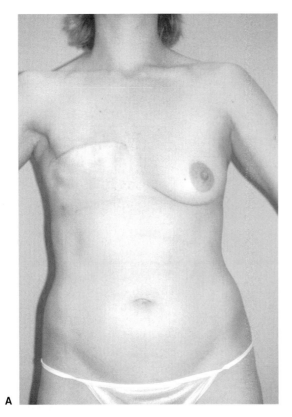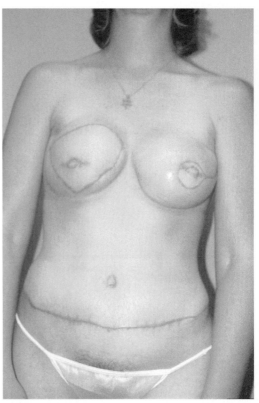

FIGURE 66.8. A: Preoperative for left mastectomy and bilateral breast reconstruction with left Rubens' and right free TRAM flaps. **B:** Rubens' flap 6 months after the operation.

doctors, we tend to remain somewhat altruistic and want to do what is best for our patients. Nonetheless, expander/implant techniques and devices continue to improve and economic factors continue to weigh on us.

References

1. Halstrom H. The free abdominoplasty flap and its use in breast reconstruction. *Scand J Plast Reconstr Surg.* 1979;13:423.
2. Hartrampf CR, Scheflan M, Black PW. Breast reconstruction with a transverse abdominal island flap. *Plast Reconstr Surg.* 1982;69:216.
3. Grotting JC. Immediate breast reconstruction using the free TRAM flap. *Clin Plast Surg.* 1994;21:207.
4. Taylor GI, Caddy CM, Watterson PA, et al. The venous territories (venostomies) of the human body: experimental study and clinical implications. *Plast Reconstr Surg.* 1990;86:185.
5. Kroll SS, Reece GP, Miller MM, et al. Comparison of cost for DIEP and free TRAM flap breast reconstruction. *Plast Reconstr Surg.* 2001;107:881.
6. Nahabedian MY, Trangaris T, Momen B. Breast reconstruction with the DIEP flap or the muscle sparing (MS-2) free TRAM flap: is there a difference? *Plast Reconstr Surg.* 2005;115:436.
7. Ninlrovic M. *SIEA Flap: A Reliable Option.* Presented at Breast Surgery Symposium, January 17–19, 2003, Atlanta, Georgia.
8. Shaw WW. Breast reconstruction by superior gluteal microvascular free flap without silicone implants. *Plast Reconstr Surg.* 1983;72:490.
9. Guerra A, Metzinger SE, Bidros RS, et al. Breast reconstruction with gluteal artery perforator (GAP) flap: a critical analysis of 142 cases. *Ann Plast Surg.* 2004;52:118.
10. Elliott LF. The lateral transverse thigh flap for autogenous tissue breast reconstruction. *Perspect Plast Surg.* 1989;3:80.
11. Elliott LF, Hartrampf CR. The Rubens flap—the deep circumflex iliac flap. *Clin Plast Surg.* 1998;25:283.

CHAPTER 67 ■ NIPPLE RECONSTRUCTION

MICHAEL S. BECKENSTEIN

Nipple reconstruction is an essential component of an attractive breast. When viewing the breasts, the eyes are drawn to the nipple–areola complexes. A surgeon can create aesthetically pleasing breast mounds, but the improper placement of the nipple–areola complexes can compromise the final result. Whereas nipple reconstruction techniques seem minor in the scheme of the breast reconstruction, they play a major role and demand meticulous attention in order to achieve good aesthetic results.

The goal of nipple–areolar reconstruction is to create nipples that are appropriately located on the breast mound and are of appropriate size, shape, color, and texture. It is more challenging to achieve these goals when performing unilateral breast reconstructions, because one has to match the contralateral nipple–areola complex.

MARKING

When performing unilateral breast reconstruction, simply triangulating the distances from the contralateral nipple onto the reconstructed breast mound may not result in an appropriate placement. Because there are usually breast mound asymmetries, the surgeon uses aesthetic judgment to position the nipple. One way to approximate the nipple–areola position is to cover the contralateral breast and carefully study the reconstructed breast mound and place a mark where the nipple location appears appropriate. The contralateral breast is then uncovered and a careful comparison is made. Adjustments are made as deemed necessary. The patient is allowed to have input into the nipple–areola location as well. A round adhesive bandage is placed on this location. The patient can relocate the bandage at home, to where she feels is an appropriate location.

In bilateral reconstructions, covering one breast at a time and placing the nipple position where it appears appropriate is performed first. The covers are removed, and careful inspection of both breasts will allow adjustments to be made to the appropriate locations.

METHODS

The surgeon should become familiar with a variety of techniques to meet the requirements associated with the various forms of breast reconstruction. The more common reconstruction methods consist of local flaps, grafts, or a combination of both. Tattooing can also serve as the sole form of nipple–areola construction in select patients.

Local Flaps

Local flaps are the most frequently performed methods of reconstruction today. A central dermal fat pedicle is wrapped by full-thickness skin flaps, creating a nipple. These procedures employ skin grafts or primary closure to close the donor defects. Examples of the commonly used pedicle flaps are the skate flap, modified skate flap, star flap, cervical visor (CV) flap, wrap flap, and fishtail flap. To be successful in creating nipples of sufficient projection and dimension, the breast mound must provide well-vascularized soft tissue of sufficient thickness. One must keep in mind that these are second-generation flaps, that is, flaps raised from flaps! **These methods may not be suitable for reconstructions in patients with thin skin or irradiated tissue.** Local flaps are best suited for breast mounds composed of autologous tissue where the soft-tissue requirements are met. These flaps often lose volume and contract substantially over time. Consequently, an initial overcorrection is warranted. To accommodate for this, in unilateral reconstruction, the local flap size is made 50% to 75% larger than the contralateral nipple size. If the final dimensions of the reconstructed nipple result in a substantially larger nipple, a reduction can readily be performed as an office procedure. It is easier to reduce the size than to perform a secondary procedure to increase the size of a volume-depleted, contracted nipple.

Technique

All local flap procedures begin by designing the flaps so that the base of the flap is located at the marked position of the nipple. The flap dimensions are drawn within the confines of a 38-mm or 42-mm "cookie cutter." The skin incisions are then made, the lateral flaps are raised as partial-thickness skin grafts, leaving a portion of the dermis on the breast mound. The dermal flap pedicle is incised into the subcutaneous adipose layer, raising the dermal-fat pedicle 90 degrees to the plane of the breast mound. Care is taken to preserve the delicate blood vessels in the adipose tissue to minimize tissue atrophy postoperatively. The dermal fat pedicle must be of sufficient thickness to provide the necessary bulk for the nipple. The donor site is closed in layers, approximating the deep dermis with an absorbable 4-0 suture. The skin is closed with 5-0 absorbable simple mattress sutures. The lateral skin flaps are then rotated around the dermal fat pedicle and sutured with simple mattress sutures. All remaining skin edges are closed in a similar manner. Figure 67.1A–C demonstrate these tenets, using Hartrampf's Penny flap as the example. A dressing is then applied, consisting of the base of a 20-mL syringe, padded by an eye pad with the center cut out. A 1-inch Xeroform strip is placed into the barrel of the syringe after it is placed over the newly reconstructed nipple and a Tegaderm dressing is applied. An alternative dressing consists of an arterial line protector, which is then injected with bacitracin solution, after it is placed over the nipple. The dressings are removed 1 week postoperatively. The patient wears the plastic nipple shields for an additional week, placing them through the center of an adhesive bandage. These dressings are changed twice daily, applying bacitracin ointment to the nipple.

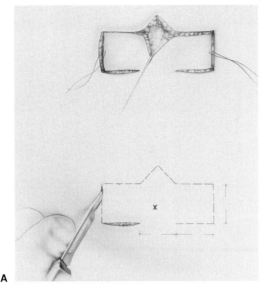

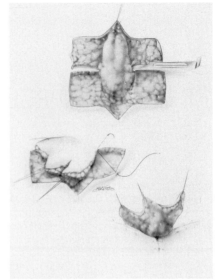

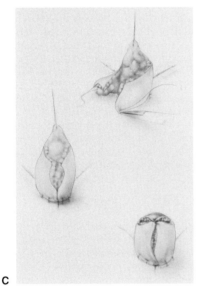

FIGURE 67.1. The "penny flap" demonstrates the basic tenets of dermal fat pedicle reconstruction of the nipple. A central dermal fat pedicle is elevated from the breast mound with partial- or full-thickness lateral "wings" elevated in continuity. The lateral "wings" are wrapped around the dermal fat pedicle and sutured into place. The base of the flap is sutured to the breast mound. The donor defect can be closed primarily or reconstructed with a small skin graft. **A:** Flap design. **B:** Flap elevation. **C:** Formation of the nipple.

Grafts

The use of grafts is another effective method of nipple–areola reconstruction. Grafts are particularly useful in prosthetic reconstructions as there is often a paucity of soft tissue to create nipples with sufficient projection using the local flap techniques. The disadvantage of grafts is that they usually require a donor site. Grafts of tongue, earlobe, toe, and labia have been used, but these donor sites are undesirable and are of mostly historical significance.

One of the best methods in unilateral breast reconstruction is a composite nipple graft from the contralateral nipple. If the patient has sufficient projection of the contralateral nipple and is willing to use it as a donor site, excellent nipple symmetry can be attained. This is an easy technique to perform and can readily be accomplished in the office. The patient must be informed that the donor nipple can suffer loss of sensation and erectile and ductile function. The graft can be harvested in several ways, depending on the nipple size and projection. If there is sufficient donor nipple projection, a simple transection of the distal 30% to 50% of the nipple can be performed. The donor nipple can be closed primarily with 4-0 chromic, interrupted,

vertical mattress sutures. Alternatively, a central vertical wedge can be excised closing the defect in a similar fashion. If the donor nipple does not have a significant projection to accommodate simple transection, a wedge can be excised along the horizontal axis (similar to a pie excision), closing the defect primarily. This will diminish the diameter of the donor nipple but not alter the projection. The appropriate diameter of skin is excised to prepare the recipient site. The graft is then placed duct side down and sutured to the skin with 4-0 chromic mattress sutures. Another method, that increases both the nipple size and projection, raises a small, local skin flap 90 degrees from the plane of the recipient breast mound. The nipple graft is sutured to the base of the recipient site and to the local flap edges creating a hybrid local flap–composite graft nipple reconstruction. Dressings, similar to those used for local flaps, are employed. The donor site is dressed with bacitracin ointment and a bandage. The graft dressings are changed 1 week postoperatively, and they are dressed every other day with Xeroform for an additional week. Although at the first postoperative visit the graft may appear dark and dusky, within 2 to 3 weeks it will appear pink and viable. Over the next 2 to 3 months, the graft may grow approximately 20% to 30% larger, attaining the appearance of the contralateral nipple.

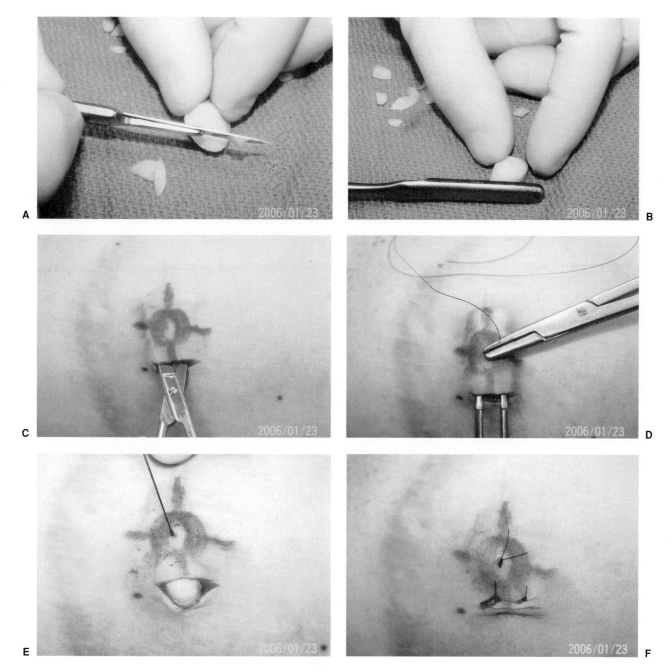

FIGURE 67.2. Nipple reconstruction using costal cartilage. **A:** The grafts are shaped into the patient-specific dimensions of diameter and projection. **B:** The graft is made smooth with a rasp. **C:** After the skin incision is made, the pocket to accommodate the graft is created with the gentle spreading of a tenotomy scissor in the plane between the skin and pectoralis major muscle. **D:** A horizontal mattress suture is placed from the center of the nipple position, through the graft, and back through the same skin location. **E:** The graft is inserted into the pocket employing traction on the suture to guide the graft into position. **F:** The incision is closed.

Skin Grafts

Skin grafts can be used to create the nipple–areola complex, often using an ellipse of medial thigh skin. The graft is placed over the de-epithelialized donor site and sutured into the circular donor site. A separate, central graft is placed to simulate the nipple. Alternately, the skin graft is placed around a local flap or composite graft. Although skin grafting alone may not create significant projection, it may provide a more natural areola than areolar tattooing. These grafts are poor color matches to "normal" areolae and they do not take up the tattooed pig-

ments readily. The medial thigh donor site is also undesirable to most patients.

Donated Cartilage

The use of cartilage is an excellent method of nipple reconstruction, particularly in prosthetic reconstruction where there might be a soft-tissue deficiency. The surgeon has complete control over the dimensions of the nipple. The procedure is applicable to both unilateral and bilateral nipple reconstruction, is an easy procedure to perform, does not involve a donor site, and maintains long-lasting projection. A disadvantage of donated cartilage is that the resulting nipple is firm and unnatural in feel. If the grafts are placed too superficially and do not have a smooth contour, they can extrude through the skin, warranting revision and/or removal. Thin skin flaps or irradiated tissue also make extrusion more likely and extreme caution should be exercised in these patients. The use of simple nipple–areola tattooing may be the best option for these patients. The patient must be aware, during the informed consent, that the cartilage is from an organ donor and there is a minor risk of infectious diseases.

Technique

A pocket is created to accommodate the nipple graft, which is performed by making an incision approximately 2 cm from the position of the nipple. After the skin is incised, a double-hook retractor is placed and the subcutaneous tissue is carefully dissected down to the pectoralis major muscle or capsule. Gentle dissection is performed to the location of the nipple position and then spread for an additional 1 cm around the marked dimensions of the nipple. Extreme care must be taken not to perforate the capsule, as this structure is essential in providing the vascularized tissue for the base of the graft. If the skin flaps are of sufficient thickness, the dissection can proceed into the subcutaneous tissue avoiding the muscle or capsule, provided there is enough soft tissue for the underlying to overlying skin to cushion the graft. Hemostasis is achieved with a needle-tip cautery and the wound is irrigated with antibiotic solution.

The graft is carved carefully with a no. 10 scalpel to create a nipple of the appropriate dimensions. The anterior aspect (or tip) must be completely rounded and devoid of any sharp edges. A no. 5 rhinoplasty rasp can be used to soften and smooth the anterior surface to prevent potential areas of pressure necrosis leading to graft extrusion. The base of the graft should be slightly wider than the tip to create a more natural shape and 4-0 nylon sutures are placed at the center point of the nipple location, through the skin, and into the pocket. The suture is then placed through the tip of the graft, back through the pocket, and out through the center point of the nipple location (essentially a horizontal mattress suture). It is useful to place a forceps into the pocket to prevent inadvertent puncture of the implant. Using the suture as a guide, gentle traction is placed on it while the opposite hand pushes the graft into the pocket

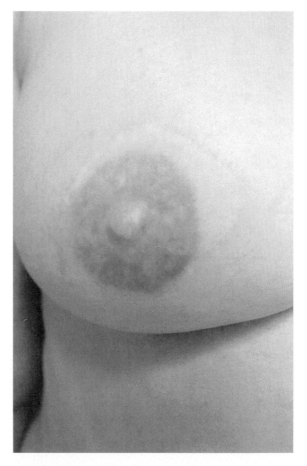

FIGURE 67.3. A 2-year follow-up of a Penny flaps with areolar tattooing in a transverse rectus abdominis musculocutaneous (TRAM) flap reconstruction.

and to the appropriate location. Traction on the suture will assure the graft is upright and the suture is then gently tied. The skin incision is then sutured with 4-0 chromic horizontal mattress sutures. Four or five 5-0 chromic, quilting sutures are then placed around the circumference of the graft to define the base of the reconstructed nipple. The avoidance of overly tight sutures is essential as these can constrict the dermal blood supply,

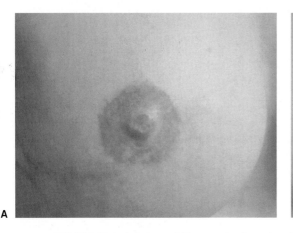
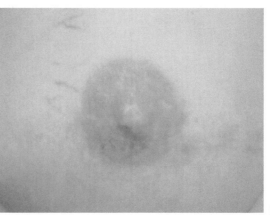

FIGURE 67.4. A: A 1-year follow-up of unilateral cartilage graft nipple reconstruction and areolar tattooing. B: A close-up view of another patient 1 year after cartilage graft reconstruction and areolar tattooing.

leading to graft extrusion. An eye pad and adhesive is placed over the graft and left in place for 3 to 5 days. The central guide structure is removed 2 weeks postoperatively.

Nipple–Areola Tattooing

Nipple–areola tattooing is an excellent adjuvant treatment. Because color choice is unlimited, excellent symmetry is attainable in both unilateral and bilateral reconstructions. With attention to detail, excellent three-dimensional illusions can be created with the use of basic light and shading principles. Nipple–areola tattooing is a two-dimensional entity and results in a flat areola, when compared to a natural areola. This method will not achieve the three-dimensional appearance of a skin-grafted areola. Tattooing should be performed approximately 6 to 8 weeks after nipple reconstruction, to allow for wounds to heal. While this is an easy office procedure, insurance carriers no longer reimburse for this procedure, as it is included into the global CPT (Current Procedural Terminology) code for the nipple–areola reconstruction. As a result surgeons are now delegating this procedure to outside sources, including cosmetologists, salons, and other venues.

For select patients, the entire nipple–areola complex can be created with tattooing. Using basic principles of light and shadowing, a three-dimensional illusion can be created. This is particularly useful in patients with prosthetic reconstructions who have thin, tenuous skin that would not support a local flap or graft. Some patients do not wish to undergo additional surgical procedures and may simply opt for tattooing alone. A nipple can be reconstructed at any time thereafter if the patient desires.

SECONDARY CASES

In cases where a reconstructed nipple has insufficient dimensions and there is disparity with the contralateral nipple, secondary procedures can be performed. Small asymmetries can be rectified with the insertion of a small dermal graft into the base of a local flap. A skin or composite graft can be placed on top or around a portion of the flap or graft. Autologous fat can be injected into the base of a local flap as well. For more significant disparities involving local flaps, a second flap can be raised using the base of the previous flap as the new nipple location. A CV or fishtail flap is particularly useful in this situation. Banked cartilage also can be used by simply inserting the graft beneath the base of the reconstructed nipple. The use of long-term injectable fillers can be used to supplement smaller nipple deficits.

ON THE HORIZON

The use of injectible fillers can be used to create a new nipple as well as augment or improve the contours of an established. Dermal substitutes can also be utilized for this as well. However, the costs of these methods may exceed third party reimbursement, thus limiting their use.

CONCLUSION

Although the techniques of nipple reconstruction seem simplistic compared to those employed in creation of the breast mound, nipple reconstruction is extremely important. Inappropriate position of the nipple–areola complexes on the breast mound leads to an unacceptable result. Careful planning is required and the procedure relies on the aesthetic judgment of the surgeon. Patient input is also useful.

Several methods are available for nipple–areola reconstruction. It is important for the surgeon to become familiar with several techniques to meet the various challenges of breast reconstruction. Local flaps, with or without skin grafts, are best suited for autologous reconstruction as there is adequate subcutaneous fatty tissue to provide sufficient volume and projection. These methods may not be suited for prosthetic reconstructions where the mammary flaps are thin. In these situations, the grafting techniques are indicated. The use of tattooing alone may be an acceptable alternative in select patients.

Suggested Readings

Anton M, Eskenazi LB, Hartrampf CR. Nipple reconstruction with local flaps, star and wrap flaps. *Perspect Plast Surg*. 1991;5(1):67.

Gruber RP. Nipple–areola reconstruction: a review of techniques. *Clin Plast Surg*. 1979;6:71.

Jones G, Bostwick J. Nipple–areola reconstruction. *Oper Tech Plast Surg*. 1994;1:35.

Little JW. Nipple–areola reconstruction. In: Spears SL, ed. *Surgery of the Breast: Principles and Art*. Philadelphia: Lippincott-Raven; 1998.

Little JW, Spear SL. The finishing touches in nipple–areola reconstruction. *Perspect Plast Surg*. 1988;2:1.

Serafin D, Georgiade N. Nipple–areola reconstruction after mastectomy. *Ann Plast Surg*. 1982;8:29.

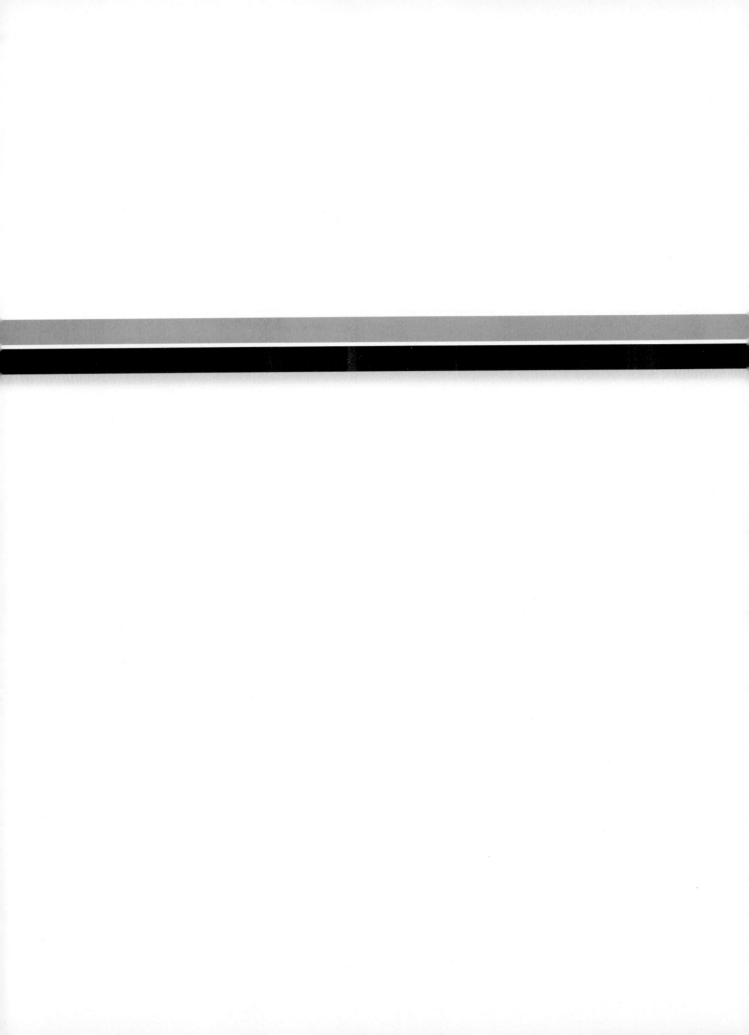

PART VII ■ TRUNK AND LOWER EXTREMITY

CHAPTER 68 ■ THORACIC RECONSTRUCTION

RAYMOND R. CHANG

The chest wall is a stable yet flexible structure that provides the mechanism for ventilation and serves to protect the underlying vital organs of the chest. Various pathologic processes or injuries can affect the integrity of the chest wall. Stability of the thorax is required for normal respiratory function. Reconstruction of the chest wall can involve both skeletal and soft-tissue components. Thoracic defects continue to pose interesting challenges for the reconstructive plastic surgeon.

ANATOMY AND PHYSIOLOGY

The chest wall skeleton consists of the sternum in the anterior midline, the bilateral clavicles, 12 thoracic vertebrae, the paired scapulae posteriorly, 10 pairs of ribs with associated costal cartilages, and two pairs of ribs without cartilage. The ribs extend anteriorly from the vertebrae toward the sternum. The superior seven rib pairs articulate directly with the sternum and are known as "true" ribs (1). The inferior five pairs of ribs are known as "false" ribs because they do not directly articulate with the sternum. Of these, the 8th, 9th, and 10th ribs have indirect cartilaginous attachments to the sternum, whereas the 11th and 12th ribs articulate only with the posterior vertebrae (1). The major function of the anterior chest wall muscles is movement of the upper extremities (1). Three layers of intercostal muscles comprise the intercostal spaces, which expand the chest wall during inspiration. Accessory muscles of respiration include the sternocleidomastoid muscle, which elevates the sternum, and the scalene muscles, which elevate the upper ribs. These accessory muscles are not usually functional in typical respiration, but contribute to chest wall movement in patients with pulmonary incapacity of some degree.

The dynamic elasticity of the skeletal and soft tissue components of the chest wall supports the mechanics of ventilation (1). Changes in the chest wall result in lung inflation and deflation. During inspiration, there is expansion of the thorax, causing negative intrathoracic and intrapulmonary pressures. This results in inflow of atmospheric air into the lungs. Recoil of the chest wall contracts the thorax and increases intrathoracic pressure, resulting in outflow of gas from the lung. As the intrapulmonary and atmospheric pressures equalize, expiration commences.

ETIOLOGY OF CHEST WALL DEFECTS

Chest wall defects can involve skeletal structures, soft tissues, or a combination of both. Wounds can extend partway through the chest wall or involve the full thickness of the chest wall. A variety of pathologic factors can contribute to the development of chest wall defects. The etiologies include infectious pro-

cesses, neoplasms, and trauma (Table 68.1). Perhaps the most common cause of chest wall defects seen by the reconstructive surgeon is the surgical resection of chest wall disease.

Neoplasm

A common cause of chest wall defects is the extirpation of chest wall tumors. Many types of neoplasms affect the chest wall, however the surgical treatment of such pathologic processes is similar. Treatment involves wide resection to extirpate the tumor, with a margin of several centimeters (2). Bone is resected when primarily involved or in the case of high-grade neoplasms. The resection of ribs includes those that are directly involved with tumor, as well as those ribs located superiorly and inferiorly. All attached structures, such as chest wall musculature, lung, pericardium, and thymus, may be included in the wide resection. Tumor ulceration, which may be accompanied by bleeding or infection in advanced stages of disease, is an indication for excision, even if the ultimate goal is palliation only (2). Frequently, these cases are further complicated by a history of irradiation to the affected tissue, and may result in complex composite defects of the chest wall.

Chest wall neoplasms may be primary or metastatic. The sternum, clavicle, and ribs are common areas of metastasis from primary malignant processes of distant structures such as the kidney and thyroid gland (2). Chest wall tumors may also result from malignancies of contiguous structures, such as the lung, pleura, mediastinum, and breast, which locally or regionally invade adjacent tissues. Primary chest wall tumors are rare and encompass only a small percentage of all neoplasms. Most commonly, primary chest wall tumors originate in the soft tissue, and a majority of these processes are malignant (2).

Primary bone tumors of the chest wall are rare and most frequently involve the sternum and ribs. The most common benign bone tumor of the chest wall is an osteochondroma (2). Chondromas are among the most common. Because they are difficult to differentiate from malignant chondrosarcomas, chondromas are treated as if they are malignant. Other benign bone processes that may affect the chest wall include fibrous dysplasia and histiocytosis. The common malignant bone tumors of the chest wall are myeloma, chondrosarcoma, Ewing sarcoma, and osteogenic sarcoma (2). More than 96% of primary bone tumors that occur in the sternum are malignant (2). Primary bone tumors rarely involve the scapula and clavicles. Benign soft-tissue tumors of the chest wall include fibromas, lipomas, giant cell tumors, and vascular tumors such as hemangiomas. **Desmoid tumors originate in muscle and fascia, tend to aggressively invade adjacent structures, and have a high recurrence rate.** Forty percent of desmoid tumors occur in the shoulder and chest wall areas (2). The most common malignant soft-tissue tumors of the chest wall are malignant fibrous histiocytoma and rhabdomyosarcoma (2). Both are associated with

TABLE 68.1

ETIOLOGY OF CHEST WALL DEFECTS

Neoplasm
  Benign
    Primary chest wall bone
    Primary chest wall soft tissue
    Tumor ulceration
  Malignant
    Primary chest wall bone
    Primary chest wall soft tissue
    Locally or regionally advanced disease,
      contiguous structures
    Metastatic disease
    Tumor ulceration
Infection
  Abscess
  Empyema
  Osteomyelitis
  Postoperation
    Median sternotomy wound
    Thoracotomy wound
  Bronchopleural fistula
Radiation therapy
  Soft-tissue radionecrosis
  Osteoradionecrosis
Trauma
Iatrogenic
  Bronchopleural fistula postpneumonectomy
    or lung lobectomy

muscle fibers and have a tendency to grow rapidly. Other malignant neoplasms of the chest wall include liposarcomas and leiomyosarcomas. **In a recent review of chest wall reconstruction cases from the Memorial Sloan-Kettering Cancer Center, the most common pathologic etiologies underlying chest wall defects were breast carcinoma and sarcoma (3). All patients in this series underwent surgical resection for disease, resulting in chest wall defects of varying complexity. Other, less-frequent pathologic neoplasms that were associated with chest wall resections included squamous cell carcinoma and desmoid tumor (3).**

Infection

Plastic surgeons are frequently called upon to assist in cases of sternal wound infection and dehiscence following cardiac surgery. The principles of treatment of sternal wound infections are wide debridement of nonviable tissues, removal of foreign bodies, and obliteration of mediastinal dead space, usually with muscle flap transposition. Pairolero divided sternal wound problems into three types (4): Type I presentations consist of early wound separation with or without sternal instability. Typically, this occurs within a few days after surgery. Treatment consists of debridement, removal of foreign materials, and closure of the wound over closed suction. Fulminant mediastinitis characterizes type II presentations, which occur within the first few weeks after sternotomy. There is frank cellulitis and purulent drainage from the sternotomy wound. Necrotic tissue must be widely debrided and excised. Dressing changes are initiated, with repeat debridement if necessary. Closure of the wound is accomplished in a secondary setting with muscle flaps. Type III

presentations are chronically infected wounds with sinus tracts that drain into the sternum, and which occur several weeks or months after the procedure. Treatment consists of wound exploration, wide debridement of infected and nonviable tissue, and aggressive wound care. When clean, the wound is closed using muscle flaps (4).

Radiation

Radiation therapy continues to play an important role in the treatment of malignant neoplasms that primarily or secondarily involve the chest wall. Neoadjuvant, adjuvant, and primary therapies for breast cancer and lung cancer may incorporate radiation. Some primary chest wall tumors, such as Ewing sarcoma, are radiosensitive and are treated with radiation as a first-line therapy. **In a recent 10-year retrospective review of chest wall reconstruction cases at the Memorial Sloan-Kettering Cancer Center, it was noted that a majority of patients had received radiation therapy in the course of treatment (3).**

The late effects of radiation on tissues are well known (see Chapter 19). Radiation induces detrimental cellular and vascular changes resulting in cell death. Ultimately, compromised wound healing results. Ulceration of the soft tissues and osteoradionecrosis are common in patients who have received prior radiation therapy. Treatment of these ulcers involves wide excision of all devitalized tissue and results in difficult reconstructive problems. Radiation therapy for malignant processes of the chest wall or contiguous structures can induce new primary malignancies such as basal cell carcinoma or squamous cell carcinoma, osteosarcoma of bone, and fibrosarcoma of soft tissues. Treatment of these induced tumors can result in resection of previously resected and reconstructed areas.

SKELETAL RECONSTRUCTION

The skeleton of the chest wall has a central role in the dynamic stability of the chest. Proper pulmonary physiologic function depends on an intact skeletal structure. Furthermore, the bone of the chest wall forms a protective barrier around the vital organs and vascular structures contained within the thorax. This same structure provides the underlying contour of the chest. In cases in which a large portion of the rigid chest wall has been resected, reconstruction of the stable skeleton is paramount. **A chest wall resection comprising a diameter >5 cm or more than four to five ribs may result in chest wall flail (5,6) with paradoxical respiratory motion and abnormal ventilation. Through proper skeletal reconstruction, chest wall flail may be avoided and respiratory function preserved (5).**

One option for reconstruction of the chest wall skeleton is autogenous bone grafts, which avoids the use of foreign materials. Donor sites for bone grafts include the ribs, iliac crest, and fibula. For successful reconstruction, the bone graft must be apposed to a large surface area of trabecular bone around the chest wall defect margins so as to enhance graft survival and osteoconduction (5). Autologous fascia lata graft may also provide a semirigid skeletal substitute. The fascia graft can be combined with bone chips or a bone graft. The use of the fascia lata graft is limited by its inherent flaccidity and susceptibility to infection (5). **Bone defects of the chest wall skeleton that are <5 cm in diameter do not generally require rigid reconstruction because physiologic disturbances will not usually ensue from these smaller defects (5).** In such cases, soft-tissue reconstruction using autologous muscle or musculocutaneous flaps may satisfactorily provide structural stability.

One important development in skeletal reconstruction of the chest wall has been the use of prosthetic materials. These materials have many advantages and they are widely available and easy to use. Furthermore, they have inherent flexibility, allowing conformation to any size or shape of defect (5,6). Synthetic materials such as Gore-Tex, Teflon, Marlex, Vicryl, and Prolene are available for use. Ingrowth of tissue into the mesh material promotes incorporation into the chest wall (5). Marlex mesh can also be used in a "sandwich" to form a composite reconstruction of the chest wall. Marlex mesh is formed to the appropriate size based on a template of the defect. Methyl methacrylate is then prepared and spread over the mesh. A second layer of mesh is added over the methyl methacrylate. While hardening, this Marlex mesh–methyl methacrylate "sandwich" is shaped to replace the contour of the chest wall defect. Among the advantages of this composite replacement are its adaptability, durability, biologic inertness, and radiographic translucency (5).

SOFT-TISSUE RECONSTRUCTION

Vital to complete chest wall reconstruction is the soft-tissue coverage. Well vascularized soft-tissue cover is critical for proper wound healing, protection from infection, and preservation of normal ventilatory function. The success of the soft-tissue reconstruction is particularly crucial in the setting of an irradiated pathologic field, or in the presence of underlying prosthetic materials. Reconstruction of the chest wall soft tissue is most often completed with the use of local and regional muscle or musculocutaneous flaps (7–9). There are a variety of donor sites available. Authors in several clinical series have demonstrated the successful use of flaps to accomplish soft-tissue coverage and full reconstruction of the chest wall (3,7–9). Because of the increasing complexity of chest wall defects that result from wider and more aggressive surgical extirpations, more advanced reconstructive techniques, such as microsurgical free tissue transfer, may be necessary for full coverage.

Trapezius Flap

The trapezius muscle is a triangular-shape muscle that is located at the superior aspect of the posterior chest wall. It lies superficial to the levator scapulae, rhomboid major, and rhomboid minor muscles. The trapezius flap is a Mathes and Nahai type II flap and can be used as a muscle or musculocutaneous flap (10). The dominant vascular pedicle is the transverse cervical artery and vein. Minor pedicles include the posterior intercostal arteries and veins and occipital artery and vein branches. The muscle is supplied by the spinal accessory nerve. The standard arc of rotation of the muscle flap pivots at the posterior base of the neck, which allows coverage of the superior aspect of the posterior chest wall.

Parascapular Flap

The parascapular flap is a fasciocutaneous flap located in the posterior thorax, between the axilla and the midline, over the infraspinous area of the scapula. The fascial portion of the flap overlies the fascia overlying scapular muscles, including the teres major and minor muscles (10). The dominant vascular pedicle is the circumflex scapular artery and venae comitantes, which branch from the subscapular artery and vein. This pedicle is located in the triangular space, which is formed by the borders of the teres major, teres minor, and triceps muscles. The standard arc of rotation of the flap pivots at the entry point of the vascular pedicle. Areas that may be covered include the shoulder, axilla, and lateral chest wall.

Latissimus Dorsi Flap

The latissimus dorsi muscle is a broad muscle that covers the inferior portion of the posterior trunk. The muscle lies superficial to the erector spinae, serratus posterior inferior, and serratus anterior muscles. This flap, which may be used as a muscle or musculocutaneous flap, has a Mathes and Nahai type V circulation (10). The dominant vascular supply is formed by the thoracodorsal artery and vein, with segmental pedicles originating from perforating branches of the posterior intercostal and lumbar arteries and veins. The thoracodorsal nerve is the motor nerve supplying the muscle. This versatile flap can be used to cover both anterior and posterior chest wall defects. The standard point of rotation at the posterior axilla allows transposition of the muscle to the superior aspect of the posterior chest wall, as well as anteriorly to the anterolateral and anterior midline areas of the chest wall. The muscle may be divided at its insertion into the intertubercular groove of the humerus so as to extend the arc of rotation. In addition, the dominant vascular pedicle of the flap may be divided, and a reverse flap can be created, based on the segmental blood supply at the posterior midline. The reverse flap can be used to cover contralateral posterior chest wall wounds.

Pectoralis Major Flap

Like the latissimus dorsi muscle, the broad, fan-shaped pectoralis major muscle is categorized as a Mathes and Nahai type V flap (10). The muscle is a superficial muscle of the anterior chest wall. It can be used as either a muscle or a musculocutaneous flap. The thoracoacromial artery and venae comitantes, branching from the subclavian artery and vein, form the dominant vascular pedicle of the muscle. Perforating intercostal branches from the internal mammary artery and vein and intercostal arteries form the segmental pedicles. In the thorax, the pectoralis major muscle flap is most commonly used to reconstruct midline sternal defects. The muscle may be advanced on its dominant pedicle toward the midline. The muscle insertion at the humerus may also be divided to allow further advancement. A reverse or turnover flap can be created with division of the dominant pedicle and preservation of the segmental midline blood supply. This allows the muscle to be folded over into the areas of the sternum and mediastinum.

Serratus Anterior Flap

The serratus anterior muscle extends over the lateral chest wall, with multiple segments from the upper ribs towards the scapula. The flap can be used as a muscle, musculocutaneous, or fascial flap. The use of the entire muscle is contraindicated as winging of the scapula will result (10). The long thoracic nerve provides the motor nerve supply of the muscle. This Mathes and Nahai type III flap has two dominant vascular pedicles—the lateral thoracic artery and branches from the thoracodorsal artery (10). Because of its two dominant pedicles, which are quite long, this flap has a versatile arc of rotation to both the anterior and posterior chest wall areas. The muscle may also be used to fill intrathoracic cavitary defects.

External Oblique Flap

The external oblique muscle, the most superficial muscle of the lateral abdominal wall, can be used as a muscle or musculocutaneous flap to cover anterior chest wall defects. With major segmental pedicles from the lateral cutaneous branches of the inferior eight posterior intercostal arteries and venae comitantes, Mathes and Nahai characterize the muscle as type IV (10). The standard arc of rotation pivots at the edge of the costal margin along the anterior axillary line, allowing easy coverage of anterior chest wall defects.

arteries and venae comitantes function as minor pedicles. Based on the two dominant vascular pedicles, there are two standard arcs of rotation. For coverage of the anterior chest wall, the superior rotation point at the costal margin is used, allowing transposition of the muscle to the chest.

Rectus Abdominis Flap

The rectus abdominis muscle, located in the midline of the abdomen, can be used as a muscle or musculocutaneous flap for thoracic reconstruction. When used as a musculocutaneous flap, the skin island can be oriented either vertically or transversely. The muscle is noted to have a type III Mathes and Nahai circulation (10). There are two dominant pedicles, the superior epigastric artery and vein, originating from the internal mammary artery and vein, and the inferior epigastric artery and vein, originating from the external iliac artery and vein. Intercostal

Omental Flap

The greater omentum, which is the intraperitoneal structure that extends from the stomach and transverse colon over the peritoneum, may be used as a versatile flap that reaches the anterior chest wall and thoracic cavity (Fig. 68.1). The omental flap has a Mathes and Nahai type III circulation (10). There are two dominant pedicles. The right gastroepiploic artery and vein branch from the gastroduodenal artery and vein. The other dominant pedicle, the left gastroepiploic artery and vein, rises from the splenic artery and vein. There are two standard arcs of

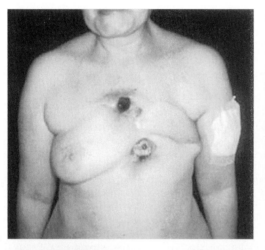

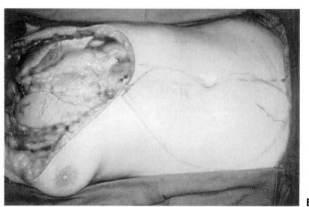

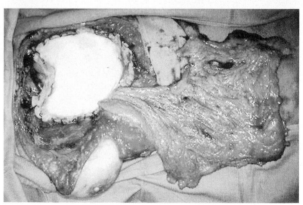

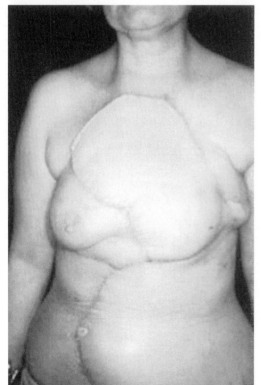

FIGURE 68.1. Chest wall reconstruction after resection of metastatic breast cancer. **A:** Recurrent breast cancer. **B:** Full-thickness resection of chest wall with exposed lungs and pericardium. **C:** Marlex–methyl methacrylate sandwich and omental flap. **D:** Vertical rectus abdominis musculocutaneous flap for skin coverage. Courtesy of and used by permission of Dr. Peter Cordeiro, Memorial Sloan-Kettering Cancer Center.

rotation, which are based on either pedicle. On the right side, the flap rotates at the first portion of the duodenum. On the left side, the pivot point is the splenocolic ligament. In standard flap harvest, the abdomen and peritoneal cavity usually are entered through a midline incision. After the flap is harvested for transposition to the chest wall, a tunnel must be created over the costal margin or through the diaphragm. The use of the omentum for reconstruction of the chest wall has been well described (11). It is a hearty, reliable, well-vascularized flap that can generally be harvested with minimal morbidity, but which does require an abdominal laparotomy (12).

Free Flap

Whereas soft-tissue coverage of chest wall defects is most often accomplished with the use of local and regional muscle or musculocutaneous flaps, wounds of greater complexity may require the use of advanced reconstructive techniques. Microsurgical free-tissue transfer of tissues allows great freedom in reconstruction of chest wall defects and has many advantages when compared to pedicled flaps (13). The use of the free flap obviates concerns about compromised vascular supply, especially in coverage of large defects. Furthermore, constraints in positioning or placement of the tissue flap are avoided, as pedicle attachments are freed. The attendant risks of microvascular surgery and free-tissue transfer are well known. Despite the inherent risk of vascular thrombosis and flap failure, with successful microvascular anastomosis of vessels, a reliable and more robust vascular supply of the flap results, ultimately providing the best vascularized coverage of the defect (13). In a recently reported series of chest wall reconstructions from the Memorial Sloan-Kettering Cancer Center, the most common free flap was the rectus abdominis flap, and the incidence of thrombosis of microvascular anastomoses was 1% over a 10-year period (3).

RECONSTRUCTIVE CHOICES

With a wide variety of etiologies of chest wall defects and varying degrees of complexity, the decision-making in reconstruction can be complicated. Successful reconstruction requires close collaboration between the reconstructive surgeon with the thoracic surgeon. Multiple factors dictate the type of reconstruction undertaken, including the etiology of the defect; the patient's history, physical stability, hemodynamic status, ventilatory capacity, and comorbid conditions; and the ultimate prognosis. The specific chest wall defect should be evaluated in a three-dimensional fashion prior to reconstruction. The missing components of the chest wall are identified in or-der to achieve a reconstruction that is both functional and simultaneously restores form. Skeletal reconstruction is typically coordinated with the thoracic surgeon, who can best advise on maintenance of structural stability and preservation of physiologic function in the setting of bony resection (3). When designing and choosing flaps for soft-tissue reconstruction, factors for consideration include the location, size, and shape of the defect. Specific flap properties, such as anatomy, vascular pedicle patency, and arc of rotation, must also be considered (3,7,9,13). As defects become increasingly complex, more complicated reconstruction is likely required, which can involve the use of multiple flaps in combination. Microvascular free-tissue transfer may also be necessary, especially when vascular pedicles are inadequate or unavailable.

CONCLUSION

Adequate surgical treatment of chest wall disease would not be possible without subsequent definitive reconstruction. Most often, chest wall reconstruction can be safely accomplished in an immediate, single stage with minimal morbidity (3,7–9).

References

1. Blevins CE. Anatomy of the thorax. In: Shields TW, ed. *General Thoracic Surgery.* Vol. 1, 4th ed. Philadelphia: Williams and Wilkins; 1994.
2. Pairolero PC. Chest wall tumors. In: Shields TW, ed. *General Thoracic Surgery.* Vol. 1, 4th ed. Philadelphia: Williams and Wilkins; 1994.
3. Chang RR, Mehrara BJ, Hu QY, et al. Reconstruction of complex oncologic chest wall defects: a 10-year experience. *Ann Plast Surg.* 2004;52(5):471–479.
4. Pairolero PC, Arnold PG. Management of infected median sternotomy wounds. *Ann Thorac Surg.* 1986;42(1):1–2.
5. McCormack PM. Use of prosthetic materials in chest wall reconstruction. Assets and liabilities. *Surg Clin North Am.* 1989;69:965–976.
6. Lardinois D, Muller M, Furrer M, et al. Functional assessment of chest wall integrity after methylmethacrylate reconstruction. *Ann Thorac Surg.* 2000;69(3):919–923.
7. Arnold PG, Pairolero PC. Chest wall reconstruction: an account of 500 consecutive patients. *Plast Reconstr Surg.* 1996;98(5):804–810.
8. Arnold PG, Pairolero PC. Chest wall reconstruction. Experience with 100 consecutive patients. *Ann Surg.* 1984;199(6):725–732.
9. Mansour KA, Thourani VH, Losken A, et al. Chest wall resections and reconstruction: a 25-year experience. *Ann Thorac Surg.* 2002;73:1720–1726.
10. Mathes SJ, Nahai F. *Reconstructive Surgery: Principles, Anatomy, & Technique.* New York: Churchill Livingstone; 1997.
11. Fix RJ, Vasconez LO. Use of the omentum in chest wall reconstruction. *Surg Clin North Am.* 1989;69(5):1029–1046.
12. Hultman CS, Carlson GW, Losken A, et al. Utility of the omentum in the reconstruction of complex extraperitoneal wounds and defects: donor-site complications in 135 patients from 1975 to 2000. *Ann Surg.* 2002;235(6):782–795.
13. Cordeiro PG, Santamaria E, Hidalgo D. The role of microsurgery in reconstruction of oncologic chest wall defects. *Plast Reconstr Surg.* 2001;108(7):1924–1930.

CHAPTER 69 ■ ABDOMINAL WALL RECONSTRUCTION

GREGORY A. DUMANIAN

Why should plastic surgeons perform abdominal wall reconstruction? If the abdomen is thought of as viscera with overlying muscle and skin, who better to deal with issues of soft-tissue cover of the abdominal compartment than plastic surgeons? This chapter provides the reader a framework for the management of all types of abdominal wall situations, including wounds, fistulae, and hernias. Management of the abdominal wall depends on the following:

1. An understanding of the forces on the abdominal wall that lead to hernia formation.
2. Prompt closure of open wounds and the conversion of enteric fistulae into ostomies.
3. Delaying definitive reconstruction until patients are well-nourished and have closed wounds.
4. A realization that abdominal wall reconstruction involves two intertwined decision trees regarding repair of the abdominal wall and treatment of the skin. Maintenance of skin blood supply rather than wide undermining of skin flaps reduces complications.

FORCES ON THE ABDOMINAL WALL

The abdomen is a cylinder with a uniform internal pressure. The posterior third of the cylinder is rigid. With inspiration, the Valsalva maneuver, or body movement, the diaphragms descend and the abdominal wall muscles contract to increase intra-abdominal pressure. This contraction is isometric, thereby increasing muscle fiber tension without shortening. The increased internal abdominal pressure is matched by the increased tone of the abdominal wall muscles. When there is a local imbalance of intra-abdominal pressure and muscle tone, a bulge becomes apparent. Examples of bulges include the lower abdominal area in women after childbirth, and the lateral bulges (with associated muscle denervation) often seen after flank incisions. What is important is the uniformity of the abdominal wall counter pressure. When this uniformity is lost, bulges and hernias emerge. Episodic high peaks of intra-abdominal pressure caused by chronic coughing and episodic lifting of heavy objects further impact areas of the abdominal wall with decreased counterpressure. Obesity plays a role in two ways—first, there is an increased amount of tissue inside the abdominal wall raising baseline intra-abdominal pressure. Second, the abdominal wall must support a greater amount of weight above the diaphragm, increasing both the intensity and number of peaks of high intra-abdominal pressure.

When intra-abdominal pressure is consistently greater than the active and static counterpressure of the abdominal wall, areas of weakness will protrude outward, forming hernias and bulges. The outer covering of hernia sacs is scar, whereas bulges are comprised of some aspects of intact (although weakened, partially resected, or denervated) abdominal wall. Hernias demonstrate "necks" where the abdominal wall is intact, whereas bulges are smoother without abrupt changes. Hernias typically expand with time, because of the tendency of scar to stretch and deform, and therefore do not tend to reach a steady state. Bulges, on the other hand, can reach a steady state in size when the inelasticity of the tissue is matched to the abdominal wall pressure.

As abdominal viscera move into the growing hernia sac, derangements of normal patterns of intra-abdominal pressure occur. As stated earlier, with less viscera in the abdomen, the intra-abdominal pressure decreases. The Valsalva maneuver, used so intuitively to brace the body during exertion, becomes ineffective. The abdominal wall muscles now contract isotonically rather than isometrically. With contractions of the abdominal musculature, the muscles shorten, the hernia increases in size, but intra-abdominal pressure does not increase. Abdominal wall work increases, because isotonic contraction consumes more energy than does isometric contraction.

The goal of a hernia repair is to return uniformity to abdominal wall counterpressure against the viscera, improving the counterpressure where it is weak, and possibly weakening the abdominal wall where it is strong. Mesh repairs and the "separation of parts" hernia repair restore counterpressure in different ways (Fig. 69.1) (1). In mesh repairs, a cap or lid is sutured to replace the weak area of the abdominal wall. The strength of the mesh to resist outward deformation is achieved through the strength of the circumferential attachment of the mesh to the normally innervated abdominal wall. The larger the hernia, the further the unsupported center of the mesh will be from innervated abdominal wall, and the greater will be the bowing. In contradistinction, the separation of parts hernia repair releases the external oblique muscle and fascia from its attachment to the midline rectus abdominis muscles. A direct reapproximation of the rectus muscles in the midline strengthens the counterpressure at the hernia site, while simultaneously weakening the sides.

After repair of massive hernia defects, despite the magnitude of the procedure, patients often claim they feel stronger than they did before surgery. I attribute this sense of well being to a restored ability to raise intra-abdominal pressure, and for a reversion to isometric contraction of the abdominal wall muscles.

CLOSING THE WOUND

After dehiscence of a laparotomy incision, the operative field is inflamed, and the patient is often nutritionally depleted. A

Mesh Repair

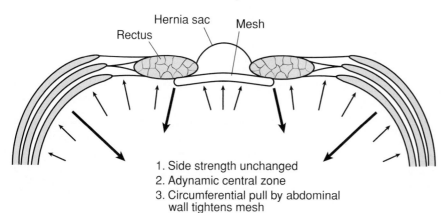

1. Side strength unchanged
2. Adynamic central zone
3. Circumferential pull by abdominal wall tightens mesh

FIGURE 69.1. Diagram of forces on the abdominal wall after a laparoscopic mesh repair. (Redrawn from Dumanian GA, Denham W. Comparison of repair techniques for major incisional hernias. *Am J Surg.* 2003;185:61, with permission.)

good strategy after such a surgical complication, is that the next procedure "had better work." **Early wound closure in the simplest manner possible has multiple benefits, including patient comfort, ease of wound care, and a decreased incidence of enterocutaneous fistulae (2).** When devising a plan to close the wound, the following questions must be answered:

1. Are the viscera "frozen," and what are the chances for an evisceration?
2. Do bowel contents need to be controlled?
3. What are the location, size, and characteristics of the wound? Should the wound be modified to help achieve wound closure?

Evisceration

Little is written about evisceration. Patient management depends on why the abdominal wall lost integrity. Rarely, a purely technical problem of wound closure leads to a disruption of the suture line. Patients at exploration who have pristine wounds with minimal capillary leak, and can simply be reclosed. More commonly, the patient has an ileus, several days have elapsed since surgery, and the evisceration is proceeded by intra-abdominal fluid leaking through the skin suture line. These are contaminated wounds, and prone to further difficulties. Therefore, a minimalist approach to prevent a second evisceration and to control the infected soft tissues should be employed. As alluded to earlier, abdominal wall reconstructive surgery can be broken into two parts—the management of the abdominal wall and the management of the skin. For the abdominal wall, an absorbable polyglycolic acid mesh is placed using a running absorbable monofilament suture to prevent a second evisceration and to keep the viscera in their proper domain. For the skin, we have temporized the situation with a vacuum device, or in relatively clean situations, closed the skin over drains. Eventual skin closure is performed by delayed primary closure, skin grafts, or by secondary intention. When the skin gapes widely and several months are expected before closure by secondary intention, skin grafting provides the simplest and most reliable closure as is discussed below.

Why not try to reclose the abdomen directly or with the aid of bioprosthetic mesh? In an infected field with swollen underlying bowel, the chance for failure is high. It is better to leave the abdominal muscles where they are and to patch the central defect. Mass closures with retention sutures can occasionally be successful, but hernias usually develop, and the sutures cause necrosis of the skin and medial aspects of the rectus muscles.

Open Wounds after Abdominal Surgery

Dehiscence of the abdominal closure is not uncommon after gastrointestinal surgery. Clues for fascial dehiscence include loose abdominal sutures at the base of the wound, a history of a "seroma" drained from underneath the skin (intra-abdominal fluid emerging through the open abdominal wall), and a computed tomography (CT) scan demonstrating bowel loops located anterior to the abdominal fascia. Informed consent at this juncture is important. Patients with open abdominal wounds after a laparotomy have a fairly high incidence of developing hernia formation. Patients with a fascial dehiscence essentially have a hernia already, although it is not yet manifest. If and when the patient develops a hernia, it is not because of improper treatment of the open abdominal wound; rather, it is expected. Another point for informed consent is that patients with fascial dehiscence are at risk for bowel injury during debridement. However, waiting and using dressings to treat the wound *also* risks bowel injury, because the intense local inflammation may cause an opening at a bowel suture line or site of a previous serosal tear. **I believe that early wound closure increases patient comfort, reduces the chances for bowel injury, and is the first step in abdominal wall reconstruction.** The most reliable method of wound closure is with skin grafts. The "two-dimensional" healing of skin grafts is not dependent on the patient's nutrition, unlike the "three-dimensional" healing required of sutured skin flaps. The timing from the most recent laparotomy is critical. Wounds that are grafted 10 to 14 days after the last laparotomy in patients with demonstrated normal wound healing have a low risk for evisceration at the time of skin grafting. A week is added for patients on steroids. The visual clue that the open abdomen is ready for skin grafting is that individual bowel loops are no longer discernible amidst the sea of granulation tissue.

At the time of surgery, the overhanging skin edges are saucerized to present a flat surface for grafting. Skin bridges are divided. Blunt dissection with a large periosteal elevator is used to debride the granulation tissue down to a clean base. So long as only the bowel surface and not individual bowel loops are debrided prior to skin grafting, the loops stay matted to the undersurface of the abdominal wall and to each other. The grafts are stapled to the edges of the base of the defect, and a moist dressing applied. Moist dressing changes on the graft itself are initiated 2 to 3 days after the placement of the graft. Unlike the base of the wound, the sidewalls take skin graft poorly, probably as a result of poor vascularity and significant motion on the sides of the skin flaps.

Fistulae

Every tube placed percutaneously into the bowel is a fistula. The difference between controlled fistulae seen on a general surgery service and the fistulae in the midst of an open abdominal wound is lack of overlying soft tissue. When a percutaneous tube is removed, the overlying integument contracts around the tract. When a fistula occurs in the center of a wound, there is no overlying soft tissue to help the fistula to seal. Bowel rest and octreotide help decrease the flow of succus entericus across the fistula and aid in wound management. The granulation tissue surrounding the fistula prevents adherence of an ostomy device to catch the fluid. The only manner to stop the fistula is to perform a bowel resection and repair, but the patient is usually in no condition for an intra-abdominal procedure. The plan, therefore, is to convert the fistula into an ostomy, allowing for patient comfort and cleanliness, and to delay definitive surgery. Skin grafts stick well to the surrounding tissue, and the key maneuver in the operating room is to temporarily keep the surgical site dry for the first 24 to 48 hours after graft placement. Typically, suction is applied to a rubber drain placed into the fistula to remove succus. Attention to detail is critical to keep this tube functioning early after surgery. After 48 hours, moist dressings are begun to the entire grafted area for cleanliness and to aid epithelialization. After 14 to 21 days, the skin graft is strong enough to withstand placement of an ostomy bag. Three to 6 months must pass for inflammation to subside and the wound to soften before definitive reconstruction (3).

Wound Shape and Position

In the infraumbilical area in the obese patient, some wounds are so deep and with so much fat necrosis that local wound care does not suffice to achieve closure. In these selected patients, a panniculectomy encompassing the necrotic tissue is helpful to change the shape of the wound. Even if part of the wound is left open on dressings, a transversely oriented wound closes much more quickly than a vertically oriented wound. Prior to panniculectomy, a CT scan is obtained to confirm the position of the bowel to avoid an iatrogenic enterocutaneous fistula.

ABDOMINAL WALL AND SOFT-TISSUE RECONSTRUCTION (VENTRAL HERNIA REPAIR)

As mentioned above, successful hernia repair requires a plan for the abdominal wall and for achieving stable skin coverage. The timing for abdominal wall reconstruction is also important. In the ideal case, the patient has a stable, closed wound with soft, pliable tissues over the hernia sac. **An easy rule to remember is that if the hernia is expanding, it is ready to be fixed.** An expanding hernia implies that bowel adhesions and scar attaching the bowel to the abdominal wall has significantly softened and will be straightforward to dissect.

Stable Soft Tissues: Midline Abdominal Wall Defects

When the skin and subcutaneous tissues are pliable, no wounds are present, and no gastrointestinal surgery is planned, many options exist for this hernia repair. For small hernias less than 3 cm across, a direct repair is often performed, although there is still a surprisingly high recurrence rate (4). For hernias larger than 3 cm, a laparoscopic mesh hernia repair is ideal. These la-

paroscopic repairs are shown in the literature to have a recurrence rate in the 3% to 4% range, low incidences of infections, short hospitalizations, and quick recoveries (5). The hernias should not have a neck >10 cm to allow for 3 cm of overlap between the mesh and the posterior aspect of the abdominal wall, while still having room to place and maneuver the trocars. Other options for treatment of hernias with stable soft tissues include open mesh repairs and closure with sliding myofascial rectus abdominis flaps (modified separation of parts procedure, as is discussed below).

Conceptually, mesh repairs are lids attached to the top of an open pot. The quality of the attachment is paramount—when mesh repairs fail, it is typically because of a lack of a durable attachment of the mesh to the abdominal wall. Mesh can be laced on top of the abdominal wall, sewn directly to the edges of the defect, or used as an underlay. The first two methods minimize the amount of bowel in contact with the mesh. Mesh underlays serve to maximize the attachment of the mesh to the abdominal wall, using the pressure of the viscera to push the mesh against the abdominal wall. For mesh underlays, sutures are used to create at least 3 cm of overlap between abdominal wall and the mesh. Enough sutures are needed to prevent the herniation of a bowel loop between stitches, but too many sutures can cause ischemic necrosis of the edge of the abdominal wall, and in turn lead to a poor mesh attachment.

Numerous nonabsorbable mesh alternatives exist. Selection of one versus another depends largely on the complication profile associated with each of the meshes. A brief description of the mesh choices currently available and the associated complications for each follows.

Expanded Polytetrafluoroethylene Mesh

Several formulations of this mesh exist (Gore-Tex, W.L. Gore and Assoc., Flagstaff, AZ). The advantage of this material is the smooth, nonporous surface of the mesh to prevent bowel adhesions. The lack of adhesions to the mesh is both its most favorable characteristic and its major drawback. Placed intraperitoneally during laparoscopic repairs, it is "tacked" or "stapled" to the undersurface of the abdominal wall as an underlay patch, and its smooth surface does, indeed, prevent adhesion formation. However, this lack of incorporation means that the mesh is difficult to salvage in the event of an infection. When infection occurs, antibiotics and drainage are provided for local wound control for several weeks, allowing a rind of granulation tissue to occur on the deep side of the mesh. When the mesh is removed, the granulation tissue is generally strong enough to prevent an evisceration. The skin can be closed over the rind (using several drains) to achieve wound closure. The resultant hernia can be repaired when it begins to expand.

Polypropylene Mesh

Polypropylene mesh is porous, allowing for egress of fluid collections and ingrowth of fibrous tissue for improved incorporation into the tissues. Two types of polypropylene mesh are commonly used to replace full-thickness defects of the abdominal wall. Marlex mesh (C.R. Bard Corp., Cranston, RI) and Prolene mesh (U.S. Surgical Corp., Norwalk, CT) are made of the same material, but differ in how they are weaved. Of the two, Prolene mesh has a lower complication rate of such complications as enterocutaneous fistula and the need for removal after infections (6). Several studies advocate intraperitoneal placement of Prolene mesh, stating that bowel adhesions are minimized if the mesh is placed under tension to avoid wrinkles (7). In those cases when Prolene mesh becomes exposed, wound contraction of the soft tissues can often cover the exposure. The strength and good handling characteristics of Marlex were recently paired with Gore-Tex for a bilaminar mesh. The Gore-Tex is presented on its deep surface to the bowel to avoid adhesions and fistulae, whereas the Marlex is on the superficial side to allow for improved incorporation.

Human Acellular Dermis

Even though the skin of the hernia sac stretches and deforms as a consequence of underlying abdominal pressure, treated acellular human dermis (AlloDerm, LifeCell Corporation, Branchburg, NJ) has shown interesting characteristics when used to replace full-thickness losses of the abdominal wall (8). In animal models, it has incorporated well and shown resistance to infection. Clinically, the mesh has performed well structurally, but size limitations require that pieces of acellular dermis must be patched together. Placement intraperitoneally is possible because of a low rate of visceral adhesions; thus it may be an excellent adjunct to both direct hernia repairs and to separation of parts repairs. Hernia recurrence rates using this substance are being studied.

Porcine Submucosa

Surgisis (Cook Surgical Co., Norwalk, CT), like acellular human dermis, is a biomaterial touted for properties of incorporation and replacement by host tissues. As with AlloDerm, the material is regarded as being more resistant to infection than prosthetic meshes. Surgisis comes in larger sheets than does AlloDerm, and has been used laparoscopically in hernia repairs. No reliable long-term data exists regarding this material.

Fascia Lata

Decades of experience and follow-up exist for use of this autogenous biomaterial. The long-term hernia rate is 30% with this graft, although it is used in some of the most difficult and contaminated cases (8). Sheet grafts up to 22 × 12 cm in size can be harvested through long incisions along the posterolateral aspect of the leg. The donor-site complication rate, including seromas and hematomas, approaches 50%.

Stable Soft Tissues: Lateral Abdominal Wall Defects

In contrast to midline hernias that tend to be large, lateral abdominal wall defects tend to be smaller and with good soft-tissue cover. The hernia can typically be repaired using mesh, placed either laparoscopically or by using the open technique. On occasion, for larger nonmidline hernias where there has been a mild loss of domain, a contralateral release of the *opposite* external oblique (as is described in the next section) is

performed to give the hernia contents room in the abdominal cavity.

More troublesome are the lateral bulges that are associated with some degree of denervation injury to the abdominal musculature. These bulges often occur after flank incisions for exposure of the spine and the retroperitoneum. Informed consent on operative management of these bulges is critical, because surgery generally improves but does not completely resolve the bulge. Exposure of the abdominal bulge with wide elevation of skin flaps, imbrication of the abdominal musculature while flexing the operating table to take tension off the sutures, and a large mesh overlay generally improves the bulge by only 50%.

Unstable Soft Tissues and/or Contaminated Fields: Midline Defects

A large number of possible solutions exist for the repair of complex abdominal wall defects, as has been delineated by treatment algorithms published in the literature (9). A simplified approach to the surgical management of these problems is presented below. **Again, the solution lies in understanding that abdominal wall reconstruction is the interplay of two competing problems: how to repair the abdominal wall and how to achieve cutaneous coverage.**

When both skin and abdominal wall are deficient in the midline, the procedure of choice is abdominal wall reconstruction using bilateral myofascial rectus abdominis flaps. Referred to as "components separation" and as the "separation of parts," the operation described by Ramirez moves the laterally displaced skin and rectus muscles toward the midline (10).

The surgical procedure is a radical removal of tissue between the medial aspects of both rectus abdominis muscles. Thin, atrophic hernia skin cover, wounds, infected mesh, draining stitch abscesses, and fistula are removed en bloc, leaving only unscarred tissue for the eventual closure (11). The releases of the external oblique muscle and fascia are performed through bilateral transverse 6-cm incisions located at the inferior border of the rib cage (Fig. 69.2). Tissues over the semilunar line are elevated by blunt dissection. The external oblique muscle and fascia are then divided under direct vision from above the rib cage to the level near the inguinal ligament. The inferior aspect of the release is completed under a small tunnel that joins the lower aspect of the midline laparotomy incision with the lateral dissection. The external oblique is then bluntly dissected off of the internal oblique, allowing the muscles to slide relative to each other. **Performed in this manner, the skin over the rectus abdominis muscle has a completely preserved blood supply.** After approximation of the fascial edges,

Separation of Parts

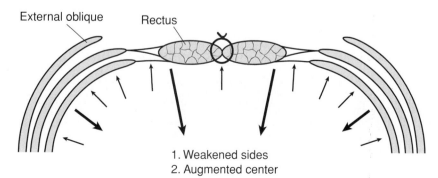

External oblique   Rectus

1. Weakened sides
2. Augmented center

FIGURE 69.2. Diagram of forces on the abdominal wall after bilateral releases of the external oblique muscle and fascia along the semilunar lines. (Redrawn from Dumanian GA, Denham W. Comparison of repair techniques for major incisional hernias. *Am J Surg.* 2003;185:65, with permission.)

the midline closure appears identical to a standard laparotomy incision. As such, without any undermined skin flaps in the midline, mesh cannot be used in overlay fashion. However, a mesh underlay can be used to augment the midline closure and to distribute tension away from the suture line. The operation done in this manner respects the innervation and vascular anatomy of the tissues. The significantly improved soft-tissue vascularity gives the operative team the confidence to perform simultaneous bowel surgery without an increase in soft-tissue infections (12).

Rather than focus on the maximal defect size closeable with releases of the external oblique muscles, an analysis of factors that make hernias easy or difficult to close is helpful. Significant weight loss since the last laparotomy, a hernia centered on the umbilicus, no previous use of retention sutures, and an absence of previous stomas or lateral incisions all make the hernia repair more straightforward. Conversely, an upper abdominal hernia, scarred rectus muscles, stomas, and lateral incisions all make the repair more difficult. Previous mesh repairs cause the dissection to be more difficult, but the repair to be easier, because the mesh typically acts to keep the hernia down to a smaller size. By CT scan measurement, simple releases of the external oblique have allowed each of the rectus muscles to be moved 8 to 9 cm medially. **By external measurements, hernias as large as 40 cm across have been closed successfully without any additional releases.**

Even after external oblique release, there are times when the rectus muscles cannot be closed in the midline without undue tension. The technique, however, still brings well-vascularized skin to the midline, and this good soft-tissue cover allows the use of prosthetic mesh in clean cases, or a biologic mesh in contaminated situations. I have combined the release of the external obliques with a sheet of fascia lata in at least nine instances with no complications. The mesh is a smaller component of the repair after the releases, and the forces on the mesh are decreased because of weakened lateral musculature. Alternatively, releases of additional components of the abdominal wall, including either the transversalis fascia or the internal oblique, can be performed, but this runs the risk of significant weakness along the semilunar line. Consequently, this maneuver is to be avoided.

The infraumbilical midline hernia in the obese patient is another example of how the skin problem and the abdominal wall problem are approached separately. For these patients, a panniculectomy addresses the heavy, thick skin while simultaneously exposing the fascial edges of the hernia. Mesh can be used to patch the abdominal wall defect, but I prefer the autogenous closure provided by the separation of parts procedure (Fig. 69.3) (13). Tunnels are elevated over the semilunar lines bluntly, preserving the perforators extending from the rectus muscle to the upper skin flap. The external oblique muscles are released, and the rectus muscles can be brought to the midline in standard fashion. Increased complications, including hernia recurrence and wound complications, have been encountered with increasing body mass index.

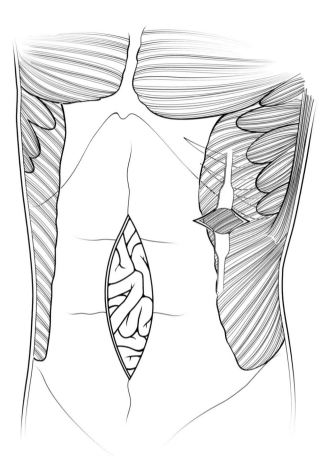

FIGURE 69.3. Separation of parts procedure. Transverse incision located at the inferior aspect of the rib cage facilitates the exposure of the semilunar line. Skin vascularity is intact because of preservation of periumbilical perforators. The external oblique muscle is divided off of the rectus fascia at the anterior extent of the muscle fibers.

and biologic mesh for contaminated situations. Pedicled flaps or even free flaps are needed for larger skin replacement situations. Defects in the infraumbilical area can be treated with unilateral or even bilateral tensor fascia lata (TFL) flaps. A delay procedure is helpful to ensure tip viability of the TFL flap. The TFL flap can also be used for simultaneous structural support, but inset of the tissue when used as a flap is difficult in the inguinal area. When used for structural support, tip viability is a critical issue. **Large, supraumbilical, nonmidline skin deficits are the most problematic situations, with each case requiring a unique solution for closure.** Patients have undergone large adjacent tissue transfers with skin grafts of the donor site, pedicled myocutaneous latissimus flaps, and even free flaps on vein grafts for soft-tissue coverage in this region.

Unstable Soft Tissues and/or Contaminated Fields: Lateral Defects

The skin issues are the most important to solve for lateral defects with poor skin, because mesh can often be used for reconstruction of the abdominal wall. For smaller skin defects, such as those that arise from tumor excisions, an assessment is made of local tissues for closure using the pinch test. Incisions along the dermatome lines, wide undermining, flexion of the patient on the operating table, and closure over drains often solves the skin problem. Prosthetic meshes are selected for clean cases,

References

1. Dumanian GA, Denham W. Comparison of repair techniques for major incisional hernias. *Am J Surg.* 2003;185:61.
2. Sukkar SM, Dumanian GA, Szczerba SM, et al. Challenging abdominal wall defects. *Am J Surg.* 2001;181:115..
3. Dumanian GA, Llull R, Ramasastry SS, et al. Postoperative abdominal wall defects with enterocutaneous fistulae. *Am J Surg.* 1996;172:332.
4. Luijendijk RW, Hop WCJ, van den Tol MP, et al. A comparison of suture repair with mesh repair for incisional hernia. *N Engl J Med.* 2000;343:392.
5. Heniford BT, Park A, Ramshaw BJ, et al. Laparoscopic ventral and incisional hernia repair in 407 patients. *J Am Coll Surg.* 2000;190:645.

6. Stone HH, Fabian TC, Turkleson ML, et al. Management of acute full-thickness losses of the abdominal wall. *Ann Surg*. 1981;193:612.
7. Mathes SJ, Steinwald PM, Foster RD, et al. Complex abdominal wall reconstruction: a comparison of flap and mesh closure. *Ann Surg*. 2000;232:586.
8. Silverman RP, Singh NK, Li EN, et al. Restoring abdominal wall integrity in contaminated tissue-deficient wounds using autologous fascia grafts. *Plast Reconstr Surg*. 2004;113:673.
9. Rohrich RJ, Lowe JB, Hackney FL, et al. An algorithm for abdominal wall reconstruction. *Plast Reconstr Surg*. 2000;105:202.
10. Ramirez OM, Ruas E, Dellon AL. "Components separation" method for closure of abdominal wall defects: an anatomic and clinical study. *Plast Reconstr Surg*. 1990;86:519.
11. Szczerba SR, Dumanian GA. Definitive surgical treatment of infected or exposed ventral hernia mesh. *Ann Surg*. 2003;237:437.
12. Saulis AS, Dumanian GA. Periumbilical rectus abdominis perforator preservation significantly reduces superficial wound complications in "separation of parts" hernia repairs. *Plast Reconstr Surg*. 2002;109:2275.
13. Reid RR, Dumanian GA. Panniculectomy and the separation of parts hernia repair: a solution for the large infraumbilical hernia in the obese patient. *Plast Reconstr Surg*. 2005;116:1006.

CHAPTER 70 ■ LOWER-EXTREMITY RECONSTRUCTION

ARMEN K. KASABIAN AND NOLAN S. KARP

LOWER-EXTREMITY TRAUMA

Treatment of high-energy lower-extremity trauma with soft-tissue and bone injury remains a formidable problem. These injuries often occur in the multiply injured trauma patient, which makes management even more difficult. Current motor vehicle air bag designs have reduced mortality and the incidence of facial fractures, but do not offer adequate protection of the lower extremities in accidents. Pedestrian motor vehicle accidents, falls from heights, and sporting injuries result in open tibial fractures that require the management of complex bone and soft-tissue injuries and may be associated with vascular and nerve injuries.

The management of lower-extremity trauma has evolved over the last two decades to the point that many extremities that would have required amputation are now routinely salvaged. Treatment requires a team approach with the orthopedic, vascular, and plastic surgeons as part of the team. Fracture management has improved techniques of external fixation, intermedullary rodding, and internal plating. Bone grafting now includes vascularized bone grafts, Ilizarov bone lengthening, artificial bone matrix and bone growth factors, and nonvascularized bone grafts. Soft-tissue management includes microvascular free tissue transfers, local muscle flaps, and a better understanding of the role of local fasciocutaneous flaps and skin grafts for treatment of defects. Techniques of vascular and nerve repair have been further refined.

The goal in treatment of open tibial fractures and lower-extremity salvage is to preserve a limb that will be more functional than if it is amputated. If the extremity cannot be salvaged, the goal is to maintain the maximum functional length. The management of these injuries is a topic of debate in the literature. A severely mangled extremity may take multiple operative procedures and months to years before it can be used for weightbearing and the patient can return to employment.

In a review of 72 patients with Gustilo grade IIIB open tibial fractures, Francel et al. found that despite a 93% successful limb salvage rate, a majority of patients had problems with ankle motion or leg edema. Only 28% returned to work after 42 months' mean follow-up compared to 68% of patients who had a below-knee amputation (1). Similarly, Georgiadis et al. compared 27 patients who had attempted limb salvage with 18 patients who had primary below-knee amputation. They found that patients who had limb salvage took longer to achieve full weightbearing, were less willing to return to work, and had higher hospital charges than those who had primary amputation (2). Laughlin et al. reviewed the functional outcome in eight patients with grade IIIB and six with grade IIIC injuries. He found that despite a long recovery period, eight of nine patients returned to work (3).

In a series of 128 patients treated at Bellevue Hospital for open tibial fractures, 66 were available for follow-up for at least 5 years. More than 60% of the patients returned to work after extremity salvage. For some patients, the delay to return to work was as long as 10 years after their original injury. A significant cause for the delay to return to work was social factors, such as pending litigation. No patients required further reconstruction more than 5 years after their microvascular free tissue transfer. All but three patients were satisfied with their reconstructions and would do it again if they had the chance. Of the three who were dissatisfied, none were willing to convert the reconstruction to an amputation (4).

Extremity salvage is a long, complicated process. Patients must be made aware of the expected course and the anticipated functional outcome. Patient selection is an important variable in evaluating the final outcome. Although normal function is rarely achieved, most patients are grateful for their salvaged limb. In comparing amputees with patients with salvaged limbs, psychological factors must be addressed. A patient with an amputation has a fixed loss and more likely learns to cope with his handicap. A patient with a salvaged limb has a constant reminder of the long, arduous reconstructive process and functional deficits. Long-term studies comparing the functional and psychological difference between patients with amputations and patients with salvage of mangled extremities are needed.

History

Amputation was practiced early in the history of humans. One of the earliest writings is that of Hippocrates (460–370 BC), who described amputation as the method of last resort when faced with ischemic gangrene. Celsus (25 BC–50 AD) introduced the rules of wound management, with removal of all foreign bodies and hemostasis. The rules advocated the amputation through viable tissue.

Ambroise Pare (1509–1590) described and performed the basic rules of amputation still followed today. He recommended amputation through viable tissue and closure of amputation stumps to fit prostheses. He went on to describe phantom pain and stump revision.

Pierre-Joseph Desault (1744–1795) coined the word *debridement* in the treatment of traumatic wounds. He recommended primary amputation for injuries with extensive vascular, soft tissue, and bone injuries. He recommended secondary amputation only in infected wounds. The concept of immobilization was introduced by Ollier (1825–1900), who introduced the plaster cast. During the U.S. Civil War, numerous lower-extremity injuries were treated. However, the mortality of these injuries was 50%, secondary to sepsis. The advent of antiseptics and antibiotics decreased this mortality rate through World War I.

The "closed plaster technique" of management of open tibial fractures was introduced by Orr. It was further advanced during the Spanish Civil War by Trueta, who performed surgical debridement prior to placement in plaster.

During World War II, no new techniques were employed. However, improvement in aseptic technique and antibiotics decreased the mortality of wound complications from 8% in World War I to 4.5% in World War II. Nonetheless, the increased destructive capacity of military equipment in World War II resulted in a 5.3% amputation rate compared to 2% in World War I. Earlier amputation may have had a role in the reduced mortality. The incidence of postfracture osteomyelitis decreased from 80% in World War I to 25% in World War II.

The next major advance in lower extremity salvage came during the Korean conflict. Lower-extremity injuries during this war involved injuries to the major arteries in 59% of the cases. The concept of artery repair as opposed to artery ligation was introduced. This practice decreased the amputation rate from 62% at the beginning of the war to 13% at the end of the war, with wound mortality dropping to 2.5%.

In the late 1960s, plastic surgeons discovered the transfer of regional flaps to cover soft-tissue defects of the lower extremity. With the advent of microsurgery in the 1970s, improved techniques of bone coverage with soft tissue and of nerve repair further advanced the ability to salvage traumatic lower-extremity injuries. The free fibular flap also solved the problem of bone gaps in these devastating injuries. The concept of bone lengthening was discovered by Codivilla much earlier and advanced by Ilizarov. It was popularized in the Western world only in the 1980s. This concept provided additional techniques to solve both bone and soft-tissue deficiencies.

The concept of negative pressure dressings was introduced in the 1990s by Argenta et al (5). It was found that negative pressure on a wound would decrease edema, decrease bacterial count, promote contraction of the wound, and, with the help of a sponge dressing, promote granulation. Many wounds that were difficult to manage now were easier to manage and enabled simpler reconstructions.

Anatomy

The leg has several characteristics that make it susceptible to unique problems. The human is a bipedal animal, thus full weightbearing in the erect position is on the two lower extremities. The full force of the weight of the body is transposed through the legs. The muscles of the leg provide predominantly ankle function with plantar flexion, dorsiflexion, eversion, and inversion. Additional leg muscle functions include toe flexion and knee extension and knee flexion. If the ankle were fused, the functional needs of the leg muscles would be greatly unnecessary and generally tolerated. Therefore, a significant functional muscle loss of the leg can be tolerated and bipedal ambulation will be maintained. Consequently, muscle loss of the leg is not a contraindication to reconstruction and salvage.

The hydrostatic pressures imposed on the leg increase the incidence of edema, deep venous thrombosis, and venous stasis problems. These problems are rare in the upper extremity, but common in the lower extremity as a result of its dependent position. The lower extremity is also much more commonly afflicted with atherosclerosis than the upper extremity. These vascular properties of the lower extremity must be considered in the reconstructive procedures of the lower extremity.

The anteromedial portion of the tibia is largely covered by skin and subcutaneous fat. This relatively unprotected anatomy leads to many instances of bone exposure, which require specialized soft-tissue coverage in the event of injury.

Because the full force of the body is transposed to the feet, sensation of the plantar aspect of the foot is necessary for normal ambulation. The normal sensation is required for tactile sensation, position sensation, and protection of the vulnerable

pressure-bearing portion of the body. Loss of the posterior tibial nerve, with loss of sensation of the plantar aspect of the foot, is a relative contraindication for lower-extremity salvage. However, many patients with peripheral neuropathy are able to ambulate. They must remain cognizant of the potential problems; motivated patients can enjoy normal ambulation without soft-tissue breakdown. Thus, in selected patients, loss of sensation of the plantar aspect of the foot may not be a contraindication for lower-extremity salvage.

Bones

The bones of the leg are the tibia and the fibula. **The tibia provides 85% of the weightbearing capacity of the leg, whereas the fibula serves as a structure for muscle and fascial attachments and as a significant structural portion of the ankle joint.**

The tibia is the second longest bone in the body. It articulates with the femur at the knee joint on two condyles and joins the fibula to articulate with the talus to form the ankle joint. It articulates with the fibula proximally at the tibiofibular joint and distally at the tibiofibular syndesmosis. The tibia is connected to the fibula in the midportion with the interosseous membrane. It is a classic long bone with a diaphyseal shaft with a thick cortical bone surrounding a marrow cavity. The tibia is wide proximally where it articulates with the femur and narrows to the shaft. The diaphyseal portion is usually described as three surfaces: medial, lateral, and posterior. The medial border is subcutaneous, and thus most prone to exposure during injury. The lateral surface is one of the origins of the tibialis anterior muscle and is protected by the anterior compartment muscles. The posterior surface is well protected by the soleus and gastrocnemius muscles.

The fibula is the second, smaller bone of the leg. It originates slightly posterior and distal to the tibia and it articulates with the posterolateral tibia. The shaft of the fibula serves as the origin of many of the muscles of the leg. Distally, it articulates with the talus and forms the lateral malleolus. Because the fibula is not weightbearing and is in a relatively protected position, it is of less concern in trauma, except when the lateral malleolus is involved. Because only the proximal and distal portions are important, and because of an independent blood supply from the peroneal artery, the central portion of fibula is an excellent source of vascularized long bone and can be sacrificed readily.

Compartments

The anatomy of the leg is best understood by dividing it into its four muscle compartments. The leg has four muscle groups: anterior, lateral, posterior, and deep posterior. The deep fascia of the leg invests these muscle groups, forming discrete areas or compartments (Table 70.1 and Fig. 70.1).

The anterior compartment is comprised of four muscles: the tibialis anterior, the extensor hallucis longus, the extensor digitorum longus, and the peroneus tertius. All four muscles dorsiflex the foot, but the primary dorsiflexor is the tibialis anterior, which also inverts the foot. The extensor hallucis longus primarily extends the great toe; further contraction causes foot dorsiflexion. The extensor digitorum longus extends the phalanges of the lateral four toes and dorsiflexes the foot. The peroneus tertius dorsiflexes and everts the foot. All four muscles are innervated by the deep peroneal nerve, and their blood supply is from muscular branches of the anterior tibial artery.

The lateral compartment is comprised of the peroneus longus and peroneus brevis muscles. Both muscles plantarflex and evert the foot. They are both innervated by the superficial peroneal nerve. The vascular supply of the peroneus longus is the muscular branches of the anterior tibial and peroneal arteries. The vascular supply of the peroneus brevis is muscular branches from the peroneal artery.

TABLE 70.1

COMPARTMENTS OF THE LEG

Compartment	Muscle function	Nerve	Artery
Anterior tibialis anterior	Dorsiflex foot, invert foot	Deep peroneal nerve	Anterior tibial artery
Extensor hallucis longus	Extend great toe, dorsiflex foot	Deep peroneal nerve	Anterior tibial artery
Extensor digitorum longus	Extend toes II–V, dorsiflex foot	Deep peroneal nerve	Anterior tibial artery
Peroneus tertius	Dorsiflex foot, evert foot	Deep peroneal nerve	Anterior tibial artery
Lateral peroneus longus	Plantarflex and evert foot	Superficial peroneal nerve	Anterior tibial and peroneal artery
Peroneus brevis	Plantarflex and evert foot	Superficial peroneal nerve	Peroneal artery
Superficial posterior Gastrocnemius	Plantarflex foot, flex knee	Tibial nerve	Popliteal artery, sural branches
Soleus	Plantarflex foot	Tibial nerve	Posterior tibial, peroneal, sural
Plantaris	Plantarflex foot	Tibial nerve	Sural
Popliteus	Flex knee, rotate tibia	Tibial nerve	Popliteal, genicular branches
Deep posterior Flexor hallucis longus	Flex great toe, flex foot	Tibial nerve	Peroneal artery
Flexor digitorum profundus	Flex toes II–V, flex foot	Tibial nerve	Posterior tibial artery
Tibialis posterior	Plantarflex, invert foot	Tibial nerve	Peroneal artery

The superficial posterior compartment is comprised of the gastrocnemius, soleus, plantaris, and popliteus muscles. They are all innervated by the tibial nerve. The gastrocnemius muscle plantarflexes the foot and flexes the knee. Its blood supply is from sural branches of the popliteal artery. The soleus muscle plantarflexes the foot and is supplied by the muscular branches of the posterior tibial, peroneal, and sural branches of the popliteal artery. The plantaris muscle plantarflexes the foot and is supplied by the sural branches of the popliteal. The popliteus flexes the knee and rotates the tibia and is supplied by genicular branches of the popliteal.

The deep posterior compartment is comprised of the flexor hallucis longus, flexor digitorum longus, and tibialis posterior muscles. They are all innervated by the tibial nerve. The flexor hallucis longus flexes the great toe and aids in plantarflexion of the foot. It is supplied by muscular branches of the peroneal artery. The flexor digitorum longus flexes the phalanges of the lateral four toes and aids in plantarflexion of the foot. It is sup-

plied by the branches of the posterior tibial artery. The tibialis posterior plantarflexes and inverts the foot. It is supplied by muscular branches from the peroneal artery.

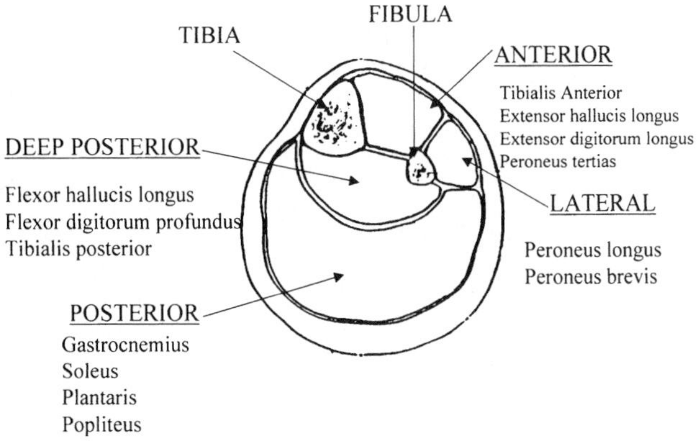

Compartment Syndrome

Compartment syndrome is an increase in interstitial fluid pressure within an osseofascial compartment of sufficient magnitude to cause a compromise of the microcirculation, leading to myoneural necrosis. Any crush injury to a closed compartment may lead to compartment syndrome. The literature indicates an incidence of compartment syndrome of 6% to 9% in open tibial fractures. It is important to realize that a laceration with an open fracture may not adequately decompress a compartment.

The cardinal signs of compartment syndrome are pain disproportionate to the injury, pain on passive flexion or extension, and palpably swollen or tense compartments. Loss of pulses is usually a late sign and the presence of pulses does not rule out compartment syndrome. The definitive diagnosis is made by measuring the compartment pressure.

Various methods have been used to measure the intercompartmental pressure, including slit catheters and saline injection techniques. Although portable, commercially produced units are available, an 18-gauge needle flushed with saline and connected to a transducer is usually adequate. The threshold for fasciotomy is controversial. Some surgeons consider a pressure >30 mm Hg in any compartment an indication for fasciotomy. Allen et al. considered fasciotomy when the compartment pressure was >40 mm Hg for 6 hours or was >50 mm Hg for any length of time (6). Four-compartment fasciotomy should be performed when there is any index of suspicion of compartment syndrome, as the morbidity of a fasciotomy is far less than the morbidity of ischemic necrosis of the lower extremity secondary to compartment syndrome.

FIGURE 70.1. Cross-sectional anatomy of the leg.

TABLE 70.2

GUSTILO CLASSIFICATION OF OPEN FRACTURES OF THE TIBIA

Type	Description
I	Open fracture with a wound <1 cm
II	Open fracture with a wound >1 cm without extensive soft-tissue damage
III	Open fracture with extensive soft-tissue damage
IIIA	III with adequate soft-tissue coverage
IIIB	III with soft-tissue loss with periosteal stripping and bone exposure
IIIB	III with arterial injury requiring repair

Fracture Classification

Classification of open tibial fractures with relation to fracture pattern and soft-tissue injury is useful in describing injuries and prognosis. The most commonly quoted classification for open fractures is that of Gustilo (Table 70.2).

Plastic surgeons are consulted on an open tibial fracture only when the grade is a Gustilo grade IIIB or IIIC. This limits our classification system to two categories.

A grade IIIA injury is an open fracture with extensive soft-tissue damage. However, because it has adequate soft-tissue coverage, it rarely requires plastic surgical consultation. A grade IIIB injury involves an open fracture with periosteal stripping and bone exposure. A grade IIIC injury is an open fracture associated with an arterial injury requiring repair. Although this is the most commonly quoted classification, it remains woefully inadequate to describe the injury or to evaluate the prognosis of an open tibial fracture for which the plastic surgeon is involved. An open tibial fracture with 3 cm of periosteal stripping and exposed bone (Fig. 70.2A) is not the same as an open tibial fracture with an 8-cm bone gap, 12 cm of exposed bone, and necrosis of 16 cm in all four compartment muscles (Fig. 70.2B), though they would be both classified as grade IIIB injuries. Similarly, the phrase "arterial injury requiring repair" in the classification of a grade IIIC injury is ambiguous. Some surgeons may believe it is necessary to repair a second vessel in a one-vessel leg, whereas others may think a single vessel is an adequate blood supply to the foot. In the first case, the injury would be classified as grade IIIC; in the second case, as grade IIIB. The classification also makes no note of nerve injury, which is crucial in the assessment of prognosis.

In an attempt at a better classification, the Mangled Extremity Syndrome Index, Mangled Extremity Severity Score, Predictive Salvage Index, and Limb Salvage Index were created. Even these indices often have proved unhelpful in predicting outcome (7). A more precise classification system needs to be developed to help predict the outcome of salvage efforts for mangled extremities.

MANAGEMENT OF THE MANGLED EXTREMITY

Management of the mangled extremity requires the combined expertise of the trauma, vascular, and plastic surgeons. When approaching such a patient, an algorithm must be used to best manage the complicated aspects of this injury. For the management of the mangled extremity, we use the following protocol at Bellevue Hospital (Fig. 70.3).

Initial Evaluation

High-energy lower-extremity injuries are usually associated with other life-threatening injuries. **The priorities of multisystem injuries are always to salvage the life of the patient, not necessarily the salvage or treatment of the limb.** The advanced trauma and life support guidelines must be adhered to prior to fracture management with the priority being the ABCs of trauma: airway, breathing, and circulation. If the patient has other life-threatening injuries, treatment of the extremity injury should be limited to stabilization of the extremity and control of bleeding. **Amputation of a mangled extremity in a**

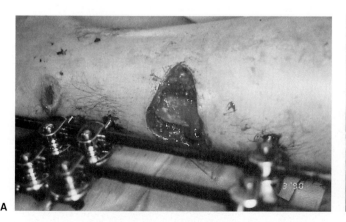

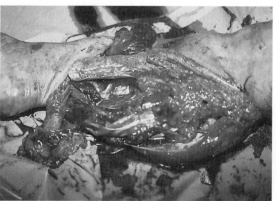

FIGURE 70.2. Grade IIIB fractures can vary tremendously in severity. **A:** Grade IIIB open tibial fracture with periosteal stripping and soft-tissue defect. **B:** Grade IIIB open tibial fracture with extensive bone and soft-tissue loss.

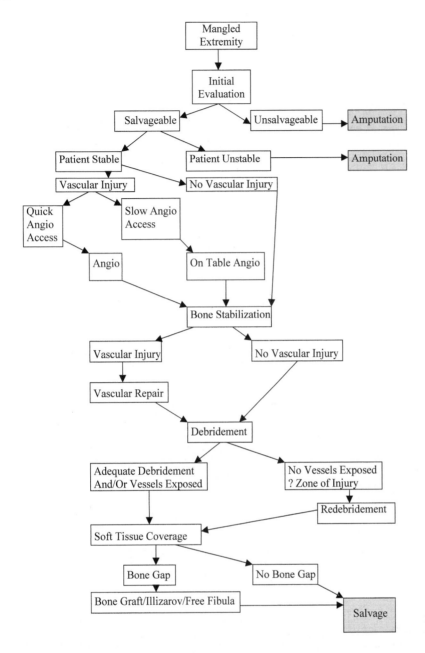

FIGURE 70.3. Algorithm for treatment of lower-extremity trauma.

clinically unstable patient may be more prudent than an extensive reconstructive course and should be considered in the initial evaluation of the patient.

Assuming that the patient's other injuries have been addressed, an initial assessment must be made to determine if the extremity is salvageable. The initial evaluation is by visual and manual examination. An assessment of limb viability is made with obvious examination of the wound. A more careful examination of the vascular, bone, soft-tissue, and nerve injuries is then made to determine if the patient is a candidate for limb salvage.

Examination of the vascular status of the extremity is made, including examination of the pulses, color, temperature, and turgor of the foot. One must realize that an ischemic limb does not imply a vascular injury. The vessels may be in spasm or may be kinked secondary to the injury. Pulses may return after fracture reduction. Questionable manual exams may require Doppler examination of the vessels. Angiograms are usually necessary to evaluate thoroughly the vascular status of a man-

gled extremity that remains ischemic or requires a microvascular free flap for later reconstruction.

Bony evaluation is initially made by visual examination of the open wound. Radiographs are mandatory for evaluation of the fracture. Thorough evaluation of the fracture fragments and accurate assessment of bone loss and devascularization and periosteal stripping of the bone require assessment in the operating room.

Soft-tissue evaluation includes examination of the skin subcutaneous tissue, muscle, and periosteum. Avulsion and crush soft tissues can be assessed in the emergency room, but soft-tissue and muscle viability usually cannot be evaluated except in the operating room on debridement. In complicated cases, even experienced surgeons have difficulty assessing soft-tissue viability and may require serial debridements.

Neurologic evaluation includes motor and sensory evaluation of the peroneal and posterior tibial nerves. A complete injury of the neurologic function of the lower extremity may be a relative contraindication for extremity salvage, as nerve repair in the lower extremity has poor functional results and a below-knee amputation may be preferable to an insensate foot.

The initial assessment is to determine if the limb is salvageable. Does the extremity require revascularization and is this technically possible? Is the soft-tissue defect treatable with local or microvascular free tissue transfer? Is there bone loss and is the bone loss reconstructible? Is there nerve injury and is this repairable or does the nerve injury preclude a functional limb? If the extremity is deemed unsalvageable, an amputation is indicated. If the extremity is salvageable, the reconstructive protocol is followed.

Reconstructive Plan

After the patient is stabilized and a decision is made to salvage the extremity, the first issue to address is whether or not there is a vascular injury. If there is a vascular injury, a decision must be made as to whether an angiogram should be obtained in the angio suite or in the operating room. If there is quick access to a high-quality angiogram, it is preferable to use it rather than an angiogram in the operating room. If there might be a several-hour delay before an angiogram can be obtained in the angio suite, the patient is taken to the operating room and an on-table angiogram is obtained.

The first step in repair is stabilization of the bone injury. If the extremity requires revascularization, the stabilization must be done quickly or consideration be given to the placement of temporary vascular shunts until stabilization is achieved. Once the bone is stabilized, the vascular injury is repaired if indicated. Sometimes posttraumatic ischemia results from spasm, which can be corrected by fracture reduction. If the foot is viable, there may be adequate collateral circulation, or a single intact vessel to the foot may be adequate for extremity viability. **If revascularization is performed, fasciotomy to prevent compartment syndrome should be considered.**

Once bony stability and vascular integrity are established, all nonviable tissue must be debrided. If blood vessels are exposed and an adequate debridement has been performed, immediate soft-tissue coverage is indicated with a microvascular soft-tissue transfer. If there are no vital structures exposed and/or the zone of injury is not clear, the patient should be brought back for a second, or even a third, debridement before definitive soft-tissue coverage is achieved. Most authors agree that early soft-tissue coverage is associated with a lower complication rate. Byrd et al. found that the overall complication rate of wounds closed within the first week of injury was 18% compared to a 50% complication rate for wounds closed in the subacute phase of 1 to 6 weeks (8). In a review of Godina's work, closure of wounds within the first 72 hours after injury was associated with the lowest complication rate and highest success rate (Table 70.3) (9). Yaremchuk et al. believe that serial, complete debridement is more important than abso-

lute timing of soft-tissue coverage (10). **Platelet counts increase nearly fourfold in the subacute phase after injury, which may play a role in the increased complication rate seen during this period (11).** Early complete debridement and early soft-tissue coverage improve the results of extremity salvage.

Special Problems

Soft-Tissue Avulsion

Soft-tissue avulsion must be treated as a special condition. Massive areas of soft tissue may be avulsed that initially appear viable, and it is tempting to suture the avulsed tissue back in place. This avulsed tissue is usually injured much more extensively than is initially appreciated and progressive thrombosis of the subdermal plexus ensues, followed by necrosis of nearly the entire flap of soft tissue. It is usually more prudent to remove the entire avulsed soft tissue, remove the skin as a skin graft, and reapply it to the soft-tissue defect. It may seem radical at the time, especially when the avulsed soft tissue appears viable, but nothing is more disheartening than seeing necrosis of the entire flap with the skin, requiring additional donor defects for later skin grafting.

Vascular Injuries

With the advent of repair of vascular injuries instead of ligation, the amputation rate of 50% during World War II was reduced to 15% during the Korean War and to 8% during the war in Croatia.

Injury to the popliteal vessels or vessels more proximal represent an emergency that requires immediate repair or reconstruction. Posterior dislocations of the knee are prone to disruption of the popliteal vessels and represent a vascular emergency. The best treatment for injuries to the vessels distal to the trifurcation are somewhat more controversial. Certainly if all three vessels distal to the trifurcation are injured, reconstruction of at least one is indicated. If one vessel is injured, then ligation of one vessel may be more prudent than attempted repair. If two vessels are injured, it is perhaps better to repair at least one; **however, there are no studies that demonstrate any difference in outcome whether the leg is a single-vessel leg or a second vessel is reconstructed.** Sound surgical judgment is necessary to determine whether the extremity will benefit from a second distal vessel and whether the morbidity of the additional surgery to reconstruct the second vessel is warranted.

Vascular injury is initially assessed with physical examination of palpable pulses, color, capillary refill, and turgor of the extremity. Doppler examination may be necessary for equivocal physical examinations. An angiogram is indicated for massive injuries, an ischemic injury that will probably require reconstruction, or an injury that may require microvascular

TABLE 70.3

HOW TIMING OF FREE FLAP COVERAGE AFFECTS OUTCOME IN TREATMENT OF OPEN FRACTURES, FROM GODINA

Timing	Failure rate	Infection rate	Bone healing time	Hospital time
<72 hours	1%	2%	68 months	27 days
72 hours–3 weeks	12%	18%	123 months	130 days
>3 weeks	10%	6%	29 months	256 days

reconstruction. In the ischemic extremity, angiography must be done emergently, with reconstruction to follow. If there is a delay in obtaining an angiogram, an angiogram should be obtained in the operating room. Often, if a vascular bypass is required to revascularize the extremity, an immediate microvascular free flap may be required to cover the bypass graft, further complicating the emergent treatment of the wound. If the extremity is not ischemic, angiography may be delayed after initial treatment of fracture fixation and wound debridement followed by delayed soft-tissue coverage. If pulses are palpable, recent studies show that preoperative angiography may not be necessary prior to microvascular free tissue transfer.

Nerve Injury

Injuries to the lower extremity often have associated nerve injuries. Although improved microvascular techniques have allowed for nerve repair and nerve grafting, the results of nerve repair and grafting in the lower extremity have been poor. These poor results are in part a result of the long distance from the spinal cord and the motor endplates, the complex distribution of nerve fascicles, and the long distance required for the nerve to grow to the motor endplate, resulting in end-organ atrophy. Recent experience with nerve grafting shows some promising results. Trumble found an average return of strength of 11% and protective sensation in all of nine patients treated with nerve grafts for repair of the peroneal and sciatic nerves (12). However, most of these patients were in the pediatric age group.

Disruption of the peroneal nerve results in foot drop and loss of sensation of the dorsum of the foot. Although not crippling, lifelong foot splinting or tendon transfers are required to offset the foot drop. The loss of sensation of the dorsum of the foot does not cause much morbidity. The loss of the posterior tibial nerve is more devastating. It results in the loss in plantarflexion of the foot, which facilitates the step off in ambulation. The most devastating loss is the loss of sensation of the plantar aspect of the foot. It results in the loss of some position sense and in chronic injury and wounding of the plantar aspect of the foot. Atrophy and vasomotor changes complicate the injury and often result in amputation. Although not an absolute indication for amputation, as it is not much different from the foot of the patient with diabetic neuropathy, it is a relative contraindication.

Nerve injuries to the lower extremity should be repaired at the time of injury, if primary repair can be achieved. If nerve grafts are necessary to bridge nerve gaps, they are perhaps best delayed until a healthy soft-tissue bed is established. The prognosis of nerve repair is guarded at best, and most patients require tendon transfers or lifetime splinting.

FRACTURE MANAGEMENT

Before vascular or nerve repair can be performed or adequate debridement attempted, a stable framework must be constructed. It is the basis for early fracture management. If a vascular anastomosis is performed prior to fracture fixation, the maneuvering during fracture reduction may disrupt the anastomosis, or the interposition grafts may be found to be too short or redundant after fracture reduction. Consequently, our protocol is to perform fracture fixation first.

The techniques available for fracture fixation include traction, casting/splinting, intramedullary nailing, internal fixation, or external fixation.

Traction fixation is used only rarely, when the patient is too sick to undergo fracture stabilization. It necessitates immobilization of the entire patient and does not rigidly immobilize the fragments. It is used more commonly in the upper leg; however,

it may be used in the lower leg as a temporary measure for the unstable patient until the patient's medical condition allows a more stable fixation.

Cast immobilization is adequate for closed leg injuries or open tibial fractures once wound management results in a stable wound, but it allows poor fracture immobilization and difficulty in wound care if there is an active wound. Although the "closed plaster technique" was introduced by Orr and popularized by Trueta, it is rarely used for the mangled extremity now that newer techniques are available. Occasionally an open technique is used. In these cases, a window must be made in the cast to allow for dressing changes and wound debridement. This open cast technique can be used until wound control is achieved and definitive wound management approached.

Intramedullary nailing is popular because of its many advantages in fracture fixation. There are reamed nails and non-reamed nails. Reamed nails provide rigid fixation by providing a tight fit in the medullary canal after reaming out the canal. There is proximal and distal fixation. With the tight intramedullary fixation, it provides rigid fixation that allows for early ambulation and good fracture reduction and fixation. Intramedullary nails are useful only for minimally comminuted fractures without significant bone loss. The price of the benefits of this technique is the obliteration of the entire endosteal blood supply to the bone by stripping out the medullary canal. In bone that may already have compromised blood supply, devascularization of the injured bone may result, thus the technique may not be indicated for the massively traumatized lower extremity.

Nonreamed nails have been advocated by some surgeons for the advantages of reamed nails without their disadvantages. Because they do not take up the entire intramedullary canal, they do not require complete stripping of the endosteal blood supply. They share the advantage of relatively stable fixation and allow early mobilization. They also only can be used in relatively stable fracture patterns; when used for Gustilo grade IIIB or IIIC injuries, immediate coverage of the exposed bone and hardware is required. Exposure of the hardware runs the risk of a progressive, rapid infection up the intramedullary canal; consequently, serial debridements and delayed soft-tissue coverage are contraindicated with this technique. Although it is generally agreed that nonreamed locked nails are effective in open grades I, II, and IIIA tibial fractures, their use in grade IIIB fractures is less clear. In some cases of grade IIIB tibial fractures, however, Trabulsy (13) and Tornetta (14) showed that nonreamed locked nails combined with early soft-tissue coverage and early bone grafting was more effective than external fixation.

Internal fixation of diaphyseal tibial long bone injuries with plates and screws provides relatively good alignment and relatively rigid fixation. Application of the fixation devices may require extensive soft tissue and periosteal stripping, and introduces a significant amount of foreign body into the wound. Already compromised tissue may further devascularize. In extensive lower-extremity wounds with soft-tissue injury, already compromised tissue may be further compromised. The introduced foreign body must be covered immediately with soft tissue and local or microvascular free flaps if adequate local soft-tissue coverage is not available. Again, serial debridement and delayed flap coverage are not indicated in this type of fracture fixation.

External fixation is the fixation of choice in a severely traumatized lower extremity with massive soft tissue and bone injury. External fixation allows rigid fixation without additional soft-tissue trauma and minimal bone devascularization. It allows easy access to the wound for additional debridement. It may, however, obstruct surgery when performing microvascular free flaps. Such problems can be avoided with proper planning of placement of the pins and rods. External fixation is more difficult to manage in some patients than internal fixation because pins and rods are bulky. Another potential complication is pin tract infections. External fixators can be used with the Ilizarov technique for bone lengthening in situations of bone gaps, or they may be left in place after cancellous or vascularized bone grafting until additional stability of the fracture is obtained. Because of the wide zone of injury in grades IIIB and IIIC injuries and contamination at the fracture site, external fixation is usually the fixation of choice.

Management of Bone Gaps

There are three ways of managing bone gaps: nonvascularized cancellous bone grafts, Ilizarov bone lengthening, and vascularized bone grafts. The timing of bone grafting remains controversial. One may prophylactically graft bone at the time of soft tissue coverage if a bone gap exists or fill the bone gap with antibiotic beads. Early bone grafting relies on adequate debridement and the confidence that the soft tissue coverage will provide adequate vascularity to support the bone grafting. Many surgeons believe it is better to get wound control prior to bone grafting, avoiding the risk of losing valuable limited bone stock for grafting. We prefer to postpone bone grafting until 6 to 12 weeks after soft-tissue wound coverage has been achieved.

Nonvascularized cancellous bone grafts are best used for nonunions or small bone gaps of less than a few centimeters. In well vascularized beds, union rates >90% can be achieved with nonvascularized bone grafts with small gaps.

With larger bone gaps, the success of nonvascularized bone grafts decreases and the need for vascularized bone grafts or Ilizarov bone lengthening is indicated. The Ilizarov technique uses the concept of distraction osteogenesis to lengthen bone segments (see Chapter 12). Bone lengthening with the Ilizarov technique theoretically can bridge gaps of large dimensions, but for practical purposes, is best used for gaps of 4 to 8 cm. Two approaches can be used. If a bone gap exists, the gap can be obliterated and the bone can be lengthened subsequently. The other method of treatment is to leave the bones out to length with a bone gap and use distraction osteogenesis to distract one or both segments to meet at the fracture site. Shortening of the bone and later lengthening offer the advantage of easier soft-tissue management. When the bones are left out to length, soft-tissue coverage by microvascular free flaps followed by distraction osteogenesis is also possible. Complications include leg-length discrepancies, axial deformities, refracture, pin track infections, and incomplete "docking" requiring secondary bone grafting.

Vascularized fibular grafts can theoretically bridge gaps of ≤24 cm. In harvesting the fibula, it is necessary to preserve the proximal and distal 6 cm of fibula in order not to interfere with knee or ankle function; thus, the limit of fibula harvest is the native fibular length minus 12 cm. The use of the fibula assumes the availability of the contralateral fibula as a donor and of a recipient vessel in the injured leg. The fibula cannot achieve the native strength of the original tibia because of the markedly smaller mass of the fibula compared to the tibia. In fact, the fibula is prone to fracture on stress. However, after healing, the fibula hypertrophies and increases in strength. Weiland had an 87.5% success rate in the use of 32 free fibular grafts, and the average time to full weightbearing was 15 months (15). Fyajima et al. reduced time to weightbearing to 6 months by use of a twin-barreled vascularized fibular graft (16).

Soft-Tissue Management

The choice of soft-tissue coverage of open tibial fractures depends on the extent and the location of the injury.

Split-Thickness Skin Grafts

Split-thickness skin grafts are best used to cover exposed muscle or soft tissue, but occasionally they can be used to cover bone with healthy periosteum or tendon with healthy paratenon. In some circumstances, skin graft can also be used to cover small areas of some vessels or nerves, but more substantial soft-tissue coverage with subcutaneous tissue or muscle is recommended to cover vessels, nerves, and—in most situations—bone and tendon, even with healthy periosteum or paratenon. Skin grafts may be adequate to cover Gustilo grade IIIA open tibial fractures, but they are inadequate coverage alone for Gustilo grade IIIB or IIIC injuries.

Local Flaps

Local fasciocutaneous or muscle flaps are useful to cover small to moderate defects of bone or to cover exposed vessels or tendons. It is generally accepted that local flaps can cover defects of the proximal or middle third of the leg, but local flaps to cover these defects in the lower third of the leg do not exist. **The defects of the lower third of the leg nearly always require free tissue transfer.**

Fasciocutaneous flaps may be proximally based and cover small defects of bone, exposed vessels, or tendons; however, general principles of rotation flaps must be considered. A small defect will require a rather large flap to be rotated to cover a small defect, and the donor site will always require a split-thickness skin graft. In a series of 67 fasciocutaneous flaps to the lower extremity, Hallock found an 18.5% complication rate. Distally based flaps had a 37.5% complication rate, although wound closure was ultimately achieved in 97% of patients (17). Local fasciocutaneous flaps are usually not available in Gustilo grade IIIB or IIIC injuries in which the local soft tissue is within the zone of injury and unavailable for transfer.

Local muscle flaps are quite useful to cover defects of exposed bone, artery, nerve, or tendon in the proximal or middle third of the leg. The lateral or medial gastrocnemius flap is useful for defects of the proximal third of the leg (Fig. 70.4). Defects of the knee can be covered easily. The middle third can be covered by the soleus flap (Fig. 70.5). A hemisoleus muscle can be taken, preserving function of the remaining half of the soleus muscle. Again, it is important to note that large flaps are required to cover even small defects because of the arc of rotation. A considerable donor-site defect that requires skin grafting may be encountered. Functional deficits of muscle harvest are real, but have not been adequately studied. Smaller defects may be covered by the tibialis anterior muscle or other muscles of the anterior and lateral compartments; however, these muscles have a less reliable blood supply and may be less readily expendable for small defects. The tibialis anterior is an important muscle for dorsiflexion of the foot and is not readily expendable. It should be transferred as a bipedicle flap for small defects. **The main problem with using local muscle flaps is that they are usually in the zone of injury of high-energy grade IIIB or IIIC injuries.** High-energy injuries may result in bone, soft tissue, arterial, nerve, and significant muscle injury. The muscles in these high-energy injuries with significant associated crush injury may not be available for local transfer.

Free Tissue Transfer

Microvascular free tissue transfer has revolutionized the treatment of high-energy lower-extremity injuries with associated bone, soft tissue, and muscle loss, and with exposure of bone and vital structures. Once the basic principle of debridement of all devitalized tissue is followed, and if an available recipient artery is available, abundant, healthy muscle and soft-tissue

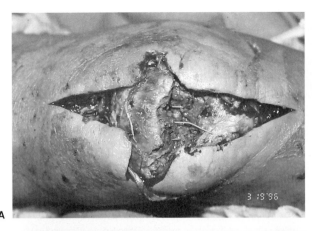

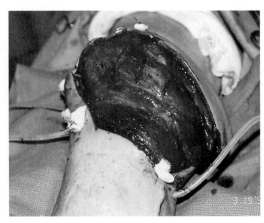

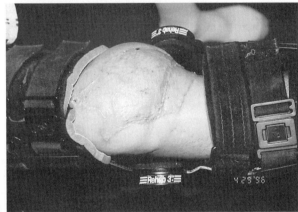

FIGURE 70.4. A: An open knee wound with necrotic patella. B: The wound covered with a gastrocnemius rotation flap. C: The healing wound 6 weeks postoperation.

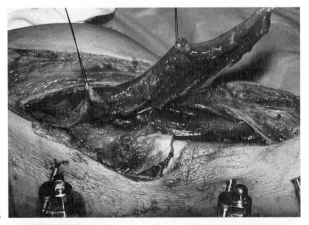

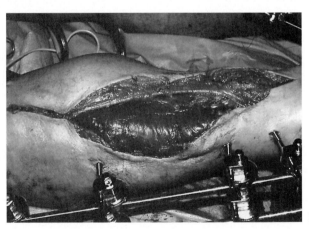

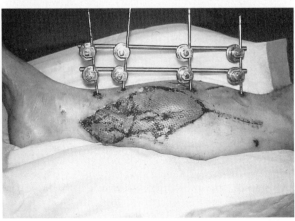

FIGURE 70.5. A: Hemisoleus flap for middle third tibial fracture. B: Insetting of muscle covers a tibial fracture. C: The healing wound 3 weeks postoperation.

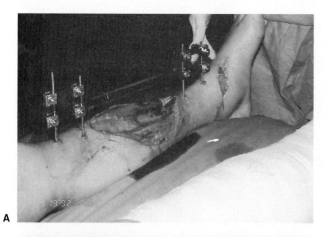

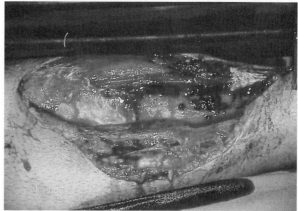

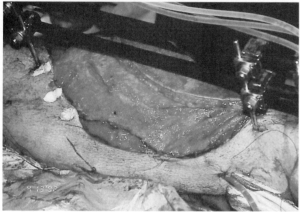

FIGURE 70.6. **A:** A grade IIIB open tibial fracture. **B:** A large area of soft-tissue loss and exposed bone. **C:** An area of exposed bone and fracture site covered with latissimus dorsi microvascular free flap.

coverage can be supplied to cover the exposed vital structures. The rectus muscle or the latissimus dorsi muscle, or the latissimus dorsi combined with the serratus muscle, can cover large defects (Fig. 70.6). In a review of 304 cases of microvascular free flap reconstruction of the lower extremity, Khouri and Shaw reported a 92% success rate (4). Reported success rates by many authors with early wound coverage with microvascular free flaps has been 85% to 95%.

Negative Pressure Dressings

Some wounds may be difficult to manage despite the options of skin grafting, local flaps, or microvascular free tissue transfers. Some patients may not be candidates for these procedures. Chronic wounds may not be amenable to these treatment options because of poor wound beds and inadequate granulation. Argenta et al. described a vacuum-assisted closure using a foam dressing with controlled negative pressure on the dressing sponge and thus the wound. This method of wound care promotes granulation, promotes wound contracture, and decreases bacterial count. The technique has been successful in treating even grade IIIB open tibial fractures that may have required a local muscle flap or a microvascular free tissue transfer (18). Surgical debridements are still necessary as an adjunct to the dressing changes. Though some wounds may be treated with this technique until complete closure has occurred, many wounds require additional surgery, such as a skin graft or flap. The significant improvement in the wound bed, however, makes the reconstructive procedure easier. This technique is ineffective for ischemic wounds.

Chronic Osteomyelitis

Chronic osteomyelitis after grade III tibial fractures occurs in approximately 5% of open tibial fractures. Early debridement of open fractures appears to be the key to prevention of osteomyelitis. Once osteomyelitis occurs, the mainstay of treatment is debridement of all devitalized tissue and necrotic bone (Fig. 70.7) and replacement with healthy, well-vascularized tissue, followed by treatment of the bone defect. Anthony et al. treated 34 patients with chronic osteomyelitis with debridement and immediate muscle flap coverage and antibiotics. They had an overall success rate of 96% (19). May reviewed a 13-year experience with treatment of chronic traumatic bone wounds with microvascular free tissue transfer (20). He had a 95% success rate in his series of 96 patients. The treatment of choice for chronic osteomyelitis remains radical debridement of necrotic tissue and coverage with well-vascularized tissue.

Salvage of Below-Knee Amputation Stumps

In cases of severe open tibial fractures and lower-extremity traumatic amputations, when limb salvage is not possible, every attempt should be made to preserve as much limb length as possible. This is particularly important with respect to the knee joint. If the knee unit is salvageable, a below-knee amputation should be performed. The work of ambulation is significantly reduced in patients with below-knee amputations as compared to patients with above-knee amputations. Patients with below-knee amputations have a more normal gait and a greater ability to perform more physical activities than patients with

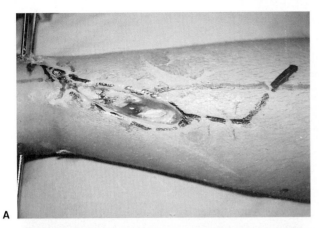

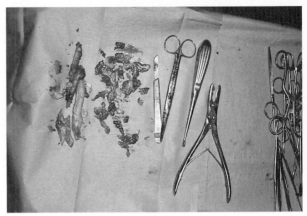

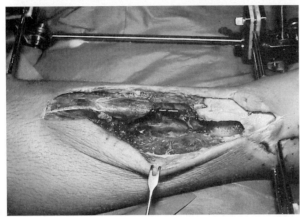

FIGURE 70.7. **A:** A chronic wound with exposed bone. **B:** Radical debridement of all devitalized bone and soft tissue. **C:** The wound after extensive debridement.

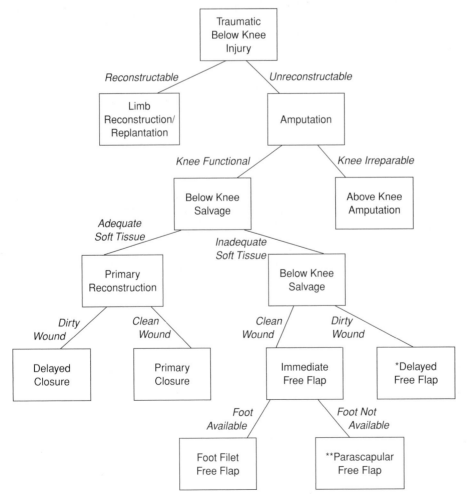

FIGURE 70.8. An algorithm for amputation in lower-extremity injuries.

above-knee amputations. The development of microvascular surgery has allowed salvage of extremities at a more distal level. This is particularly true when the main problem is inadequate soft-tissue coverage.

Advantages of More Distal Amputations

A patient with a below-knee amputation has a 25% increased energy and oxygen consumption requirement with ambulation when compared to a person without an amputation. Patients with above-knee amputations have a 65% increase in the oxygen and energy consumption requirement for ambulation when compared to nonamputees. Patients with bilateral below-knee amputations have a 45% increased oxygen and energy consumption requirement for ambulation when compared to nonamputees. The amputee will walk more slowly to compensate for the increase in energy required. The higher the level of the amputation, the more energy required, and the slower and less effective the ambulation.

Quality of life is also significantly affected by the level of amputation. The daily distance walked is significantly less in above-knee amputation patients as compared to below-knee amputation patients. More above-knee amputation patients walk only in the house or do not walk at all. Above-knee amputation patients have more trouble with stairs and ramps and often require hand controls to drive.

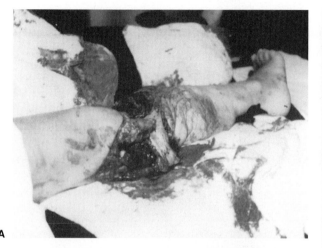

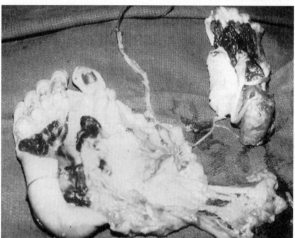

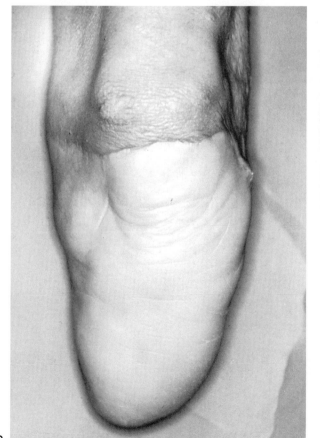

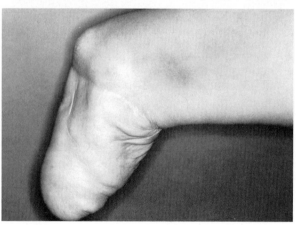

FIGURE 70.9. Foot fillet coverage. **A:** A large zone of injury in proximal tibia area with a long segment of exposed tibia. The foot is relatively uninjured. **B:** Foot fillet dissection performed. **C, D:** The final result.

Free Flap Salvage of Below-Knee Amputation Stumps

If the distal limb is nonsalvageable but the knee joint is functional, every attempt should be made to preserve a below-knee amputation. Although the ideal below-knee amputation stump has >6 cm of tibia below the tubercle, any length of tibia should be preserved as the benefits of a below-knee amputation are great compared to above-knee amputation. If adequate soft-tissue coverage is present, the stump may either be closed primarily or closed in a delayed fashion, if there is significant contamination. If the soft-tissue coverage is inadequate, a skin graft reconstruction may be possible. If insufficient soft tissue exists to cover the bone, free flap reconstruction is considered. In clean wounds, free flap coverage is accomplished as it is for any open tibial fracture. The flap should be performed in the early postinjury period, depending on the patient's overall condition. If the foot on the amputated part is uninjured, an immediate foot fillet free flap is considered. If the foot on the amputated part is not usable, then a parascapular free flap or muscle free flap plus skin graft can be performed shortly thereafter. In dirty wounds, the free flap is delayed until wound conditions are optimized. Figure 70.8 summarizes the decision-making tree.

In a study by Kasabian (21) patients achieved stable coverage of below-knee amputations with free flap coverage. The most common flap was the parascapular flap, used in 11 patients. The parascapular flap allowed for the most accurate reconstruction of the amputation stump. A foot fillet flap was used in six cases. The other free flaps employed were the latissimus dorsi (4), lateral thigh (1), tensor fascia lata (1), and groin (1). The patients in the study required an average of 4.9 operations related to their injury. There were 1.3 operations after the free flap. Most patients had long hospitalizations as a result of the combination of their injuries and their overall situations.

The foot fillet flap offers several advantages over other flaps. It is the only flap available from the amputated part and as such has no donor-site morbidity. In addition, sensory innervation is provided by the tibial nerve, peroneal nerves, and sural nerves. The tibial nerve is used most commonly and provides sensibility to the plantar surface of the foot, which is usually inset at the end of the below-knee amputation stump. Neurorrhaphy may be accomplished to a proximal nerve stump or the nerve may be left in continuity. Finally, the foot fillet has glabrous skin that is durable and not prone to ulceration (Fig. 70.9).

Muscle free flaps with skin graft coverage tend to heal slowly. There are often areas of partial graft survival. In addition, as the muscle atrophies and the flap shrinks, revisions are required to both the stump and the prosthesis. The additional surgical procedures lengthen the time to the fitting of the final prosthesis when compared to patients with fasciocutaneous flaps.

References

1. Francel TJ, Vander Kolk CA, Hoopes JE, et al. Microvascular soft-tissue transplantation for reconstruction of acute open tibial fractures: timing of coverage and long-term functional results. *Plast Reconstr Surg.* 1992;89:478–487.
2. Georgiadis GM, Behrens FF, Joyce MJ, et al. Open tibial fractures with severe soft-tissue loss. Limb salvage compared with below-the-knee amputation. *J Bone Joint Surg Am.* 1993;75:1431–1441.
3. Laughlin RT, Smith KL, Russell RC, et al. Late functional outcome in patients with tibia fractures covered with free muscle flaps. *J Orthop Trauma.* 1993;7:123–129.
4. Khouri RK, Shaw WW. Reconstruction of the lower extremity with microvascular free flaps: a 10-year experience with 304 consecutive cases. *J Trauma.* 1989;29:1086.
5. Argenta LC, Morykwas MJ. Vacuum-assisted closure: a new method for wound control and treatment: clinical experience. *Ann Plast Surg.* 1997;38(6):563–576.
6. Allen MJ, et al. Intracompartmental pressure monitoring of leg injuries. An aid to management. *J Bone Joint Surg.* 1985;67B:53.
7. Bonanni F, Rhodes M, Lucke JF. The futility of predictive scoring of mangled lower extremities. *J Trauma.* 1993;34:99–104.
8. Byrd SH, Spicer ET, Cierny G III. Management of open tibial fractures. *Plast Reconstr Surg.* 1985;76:719.
9. Godina M. Early microsurgical reconstruction of complex trauma of the extremities. *Clin Plast Surg.* 1986;13:619.
10. Yaremchuk MJ, Brumback RJ, Manson PN, et al. Acute and definitive management of traumatic osteocutaneous defects of the lower extremity. *Plast Reconstr Surg.* 1982;80:1–14.
11. Choe IE, Kasabian KA, Kolker RA, et al. Thrombocytosis after major lower extremity trauma: mechanism and possible role in free flap failure. *Ann Plast Surg.* 1996;36:489–494.
12. Trumble T, Vanderhooft E. Nerve grafting for lower-extremity injuries. *J Pediatr Orthop.* 1994;14:161–165.
13. Trabulsy PP, Kerley SM, Hoffman WY. A prospective study of early soft tissue coverage of grade IIIB tibial fractures. *J Trauma.* 1994;36:661–668.
14. Tornetta P III, Bergman M, Watnik N, et al. Treatment of grade IIIB open tibial fractures. A prospective randomized comparison of external fixation and non-reamed locked nailing. *J Bone Joint Surg Br.* 1994;76:13–19.
15. Weiland AJ, Moor JR, Daniel RK. Vascularized bone autografts: experience with 41 cases. *Clin Orthop.* 1983;174:87.
16. Fyajima H, Tamai S. Twin-barreled vascularized fibular grafting to the pelvis and lower extremity. *Clin Orthop.* 1994;303:178–184.
17. Hallock GC. Complications of 100 consecutive local fasciocutaneous flaps. *Plast Reconstr Surg.* 1991;88:264.
18. Greer S, Kasabian A, Thorne C, et al. The use of subatmospheric pressure dressing to salvage a Gustilo grade IIIB open tibial fracture with concomitant osteomyelitis to avert a free flap. *Ann Plast Surg.* 1998;41(6):687.
19. Anthony JP, Mathes SJ, Alpert BS. The muscle flap in the treatment of chronic lower extremity osteomyelitis: results in patients over 5 years after treatment. *Plast Reconstr Surg.* 1991;88:311.
20. May JW, Jupiter JB, Gallico GG, et al. Treatment of chronic traumatic bone wounds. Microvascular free tissue transfer: a 13-year experience in 96 patients. *Ann Surg.* 1991;214:241.
21. Kasabian AK, Colen SR, Shaw WW, et al. The role of microvascular free flap in salvaging below-knee amputation stumps: a review of 22 cases. *J Trauma.* 1991;31:495.

CHAPTER 71 ■ FOOT AND ANKLE RECONSTRUCTION

CHRISTOPHER E. ATTINGER AND IVICA DUCIC

Ambulation subjects the foot to repetitive trauma. On average, an individual takes more than 10,000 steps each day. The foot possesses specialized plantar tissue that can withstand the effects of such repetitive direct and shear stress forces. Blunt and/or penetrating trauma can also cause immediate breakdown of the soft tissue and/or bone. In addition, infection and changes in blood supply, sensation, immune status, and biomechanics renders the foot susceptible to chronic breakdown. Inability to salvage the injured foot leads to amputation, which mandates a lifetime dependence on prosthetic devices. Some patients never wear the prosthesis and lead a wheelchair existence. Major amputation in diabetics is associated with premature death and high likelihood of subsequent contralateral leg amputation.

The foot is a complex body part and salvage requires a team approach, with a team composed of a vascular surgeon skilled in endovascular and distal bypass techniques, a foot and ankle surgeon skilled in bone stabilization techniques including use of the Ilizarov frame, a soft-tissue surgeon familiar with modern wound healing as well as soft-tissue reconstructive techniques, and an infectious disease physician specializing in surgical infections. In addition, a podiatrist skilled in routine foot care and a pedorthotist skilled in orthotics and assisted-foot-orthoses are critical in preventing recurrent breakdown. Medical specialties such as endocrinology, nephrology, hematology, rheumatology, and dermatology are often necessary.

Plastic surgeons are called upon to address the wounds that result from trauma and/or infection. The first task is to convert the existing wound into a healing wound by aggressive debridement as well as application of modern wound-healing techniques. **Most wounds can then be closed using simple soft-tissue techniques, such as delayed primary closure, skin grafts, and local flaps.** Some wounds, however, require more sophisticated techniques that mandate an intimate knowledge of the local angiosomes, arterial blood supply, and flap anatomy. Finally, all reconstructions have to be biomechanically sound to avoid recurrent breakdown.

ANATOMY

Vascular Anatomy

The foot and ankle consists of six angiosomes. The following arteries feed the angiosomes of the foot and ankle (1): (a) the distal anterior tibial artery feeds the anterior ankle while its continuation, the dorsalis pedis artery, supplies the dorsum of the foot; (b) the calcaneal branch of the posterior tibial artery feeds the medial and plantar heel; (c) the calcaneal branch of the peroneal artery feeds the lateral and plantar heel, (d) the anterior perforating branch of the peroneal artery feeds the anterolateral ankle; (e) the medial plantar artery feeds the plantar

instep; and (f) the lateral plantar artery feeds the lateral plantar mid- and forefoot (Fig. 71.1). Note that the plantar heel receives dual blood supply from the calcaneal branches of the posterior tibial and peroneal arteries. **When the heel develops gangrene, this usually implies severe vascular disease involving both the peroneal and posterior tibial artery.**

Because the foot is an end organ, there are many arterial–arterial anastomoses that provide a duplication of inflow. These arterial–arterial anastomoses (Fig. 71.2) provide a margin of safety if one of the main arteries becomes occluded. At the ankle, the anterior perforating branch of the peroneal artery is connected to the anterior tibial artery via the lateral malleolar artery. At the Lisfranc joint, the dorsalis pedis artery dives into the first interspace to connect directly with the lateral plantar artery. This vascular loop is critical in determining the direction of flow within the anterior or posterior tibial arteries, which can be antegrade or retrograde or both. In addition, the plantar and dorsal metatarsal arteries are linked to one another at the Lisfranc joint by proximal perforators and at the web space by distal perforators. Finally, the posterior tibial artery and peroneal artery are directly connected deep to the distal Achilles tendon by one to three connecting arteries. Using a Doppler ultrasound probe and selective occlusion, one can determine the patency of these connections as well as the direction of flow. This is critical in designing local flaps, pedicled flaps, and amputations.

Motor and Sensory Anatomy

The sciatic nerve divides into the tibial and common peroneal nerves proximal to the popliteal fossa. Within the popliteal fossa, it is lateral to the popliteal vessels, while distally it travels in the deep posterior compartment of the leg. The tibial nerve innervates muscles of the deep and superficial posterior compartments (except gastrocnemius muscle), and ends at the distal inner ankle deep to the flexor retinaculum, trifurcating into the calcaneal and medial plantar and lateral plantar nerves. These nerves supply the motor branches to the intrinsic muscles of the foot (except the extensor digitorum brevis [EDB] muscle). The common peroneal nerve passes around the lateral aspect of the fibular head before splitting into the superficial and deep branches. The deep peroneal nerve innervates the extensor muscles in the anterior compartment before exiting the extensor retinaculum to innervate the extensor digitorum brevis muscle. The superficial peroneal branch innervates the everting peroneal muscles of the lateral compartment before it pierces the fascia to become subcutaneous and provide sensibility to the lateral lower leg and dorsum of the foot.

The sensory nerves to the foot and ankle (Fig. 71.3) travel more superficially than the motor nerves, and their degree of function is a useful index to the localization of trauma in the lower extremity. As mentioned above, the superficial peroneal

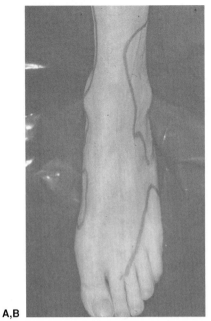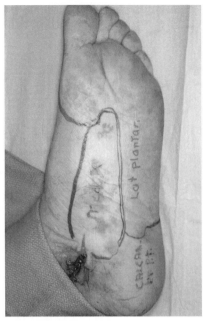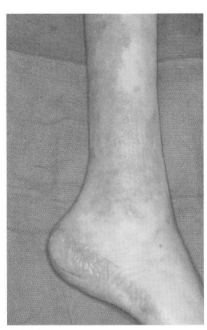

A,B   C

FIGURE 71.1. Angiosomes of the foot and ankle: Angiosomes include (**A**) the anterior ankle fed by the anterior tibial artery and the dorsum of the foot fed by the dorsalis pedis artery; (**B**) the medial and plantar heel fed by the calcaneal branch of the posterior tibial artery, the plantar instep fed by the medial plantar artery, the lateral plantar midfoot and plantar forefoot fed by the lateral plantar artery; and (**C**) the anterolateral ankle fed by the anterior perforating branch of the peroneal artery and the lateral and plantar heel fed by the calcaneal branch of the peroneal artery.

nerve (L4, L5, S1) supplies the anterolateral calf skin while descending within the anterolateral compartment. It exits approximately 10 to 12 cm above the lateral ankle and travels anterior to extensor retinaculum to supply the dorsum of the foot and skin of all the toes except the lateral side of the fifth toe (sural nerve) and the first web space (deep peroneal nerve). The deep peroneal nerve (L4, L5, S1) exits the anterior compartment deep to the extensor retinaculum to supply ankle and midfoot joints, sinus tarsi, and the first web space. The sural nerve (L5, S1), derived from both the tibial and common peroneal nerves, descends distal to the popliteal fossa in the posterior aspect of the calf along the course of the lesser saphenous vein. It provides sensibility to the posterior and lateral skin of the leg's distal third, prior to passing between the anterolateral border of the Achilles tendon and lateral malleolus in order to supply skin of the dorsolateral foot and fifth toe. The skin of the medial half of the lower leg and dorsomedial portion of the foot is innervated by saphenous nerve (L5, S1), a cutaneous branch of the femoral nerve. The dorsum of the foot has communicating branches between saphenous, sural, superficial, and deep peroneal nerves, and thus there is often an overlap in their respective terminal areas of innervation. The posterior tibial nerve at the distal portion of the tarsal tunnel divides into three branches that supply the sole of the foot: the calcaneal branch (S1, S2) supplies the medial aspect of the heel pad; the lateral plantar nerve (S1, S2) supplies the lateral two-thirds of the sole and the fifth and lateral fourth toes; the medial planter nerve (L4, L5) supplies the medial one-third of the sole and the first, second, third, and medial fourth toes. The medial and lateral plantar nerve can have an overlap in their respective zones with the saphenous and sural nerves, respectively.

Lower Leg, Ankle, and Foot: Muscle and Fasciocutaneous Flaps

The following lower leg, ankle, and foot flaps are briefly described, emphasizing their vascular supply and their use in foot and ankle reconstruction. The details of the individual flap dissection are described in several atlases on flaps (2,3). More importantly, repeated cadaver dissection of these flaps, emphasizing the blood supply, is the most reliable way to become facile in their use.

Lower Leg and Ankle Flaps

The lower leg muscles are poor candidates for pedicled flaps because most of them are type 4 muscles with segmental minor arterial pedicles. As a result, only a small portion of the muscle can safely be transferred without applying the delay principle. Even when the minor pedicles are sequentially ligated to delay the muscle flap, the results are disappointing. To successfully transfer a significant portion of the muscle, all the relevant minor perforators have to be preserved with the accompanying major artery. The sacrifice of a major artery should only be considered if all three arteries are open and there is excellent retrograde flow. Although the bulk of these muscles is often disappointing, the distal portion of some of these type 4 muscles (Fig. 71.4) can be used to cover small defects around the ankle medially, anteriorly, laterally. It is important to tenodese the distal end of the severed tendon of the harvested muscle to a muscle with similar function so that the harvested muscle's function is not lost. For example, if the distal extensor hallucis muscle is harvested, the extensor hallucis longus (EHL) tendon distal to the harvest site should be tenodesed to the extensor digitorum longus so that the hallux maintains its position during gait. **Because the loss of the anterior tibial tendon is so debilitating, this muscle should not be harvested unless the ankle has been or is being fused.**

The extensor hallucis longus muscle can cover small defects that are as distal as 2 cm above the medial malleolus. The extensor digitorum longus muscle and peroneus tertius muscle are used for small defects as distal as 2.1 cm above the medial malleolus. The peroneus brevis muscle can be used for small defects as distal as 4 cm above the medial malleolus. The flexor digitorum longus muscle can be used for small defects as distal as 6 cm above the medial malleolus. The soleus muscle is the

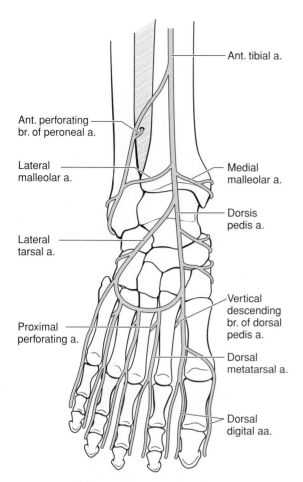

Ant. tibial a.

Ant. perforating
br. of peroneal a.

Lateral
malleolar a.

Medial
malleolar a.

Dorsis
pedis a.

Lateral
tarsal a.

Proximal
perforating a.

Vertical
descending
br. of dorsal
pedis a.

Dorsal
metatarsal a.

Dorsal
digital aa.

FIGURE 71.2. Arterial anatomy of the foot and ankle. At the ankle, the anterior tibial artery gives off the lateral malleolar artery at the level of the lateral malleolus. It anastomoses with the anterior perforating branch of the peroneal artery. At the Lisfranc joint, the dorsalis pedis artery dives down in the first interspace to join the lateral plantar artery. At the second, third, and fourth proximal interspaces, the proximal perforators link the dorsal and plantar metatarsal arteries. Not shown is the direct connection between the peroneal and posterior tibial artery underneath the distal Achilles tendon. (From Attinger C. Vascular anatomy of the foot and ankle. *Oper Tech Plast Reconstr Surg.* 1997;4:183, with permission.)

only type 2 muscle in the distal lower leg where the minor distal pedicles can be detached and the muscle can be rotated with its intact proximal major rotated to cover large (10 × 8 cm) anterior lower-leg defects as distal as 6.6 cm above the medial malleolus. It can be harvested as a hemisoleus for small defects and as an entire soleus for larger defects. These flaps require skin grafting. In addition, the ankle has to be immobilized to avoid dehiscence and ensure adequate skin graft take. External frames are useful for immobilization and vacuum-assisted closure devices (Kinetic Concepts Inc., San Antonio, TX) assist graft take.

Fasciocutaneous flaps had their origin in 1981 when Ponten described the medial calf flap. Fasciocutaneous flaps are useful for reconstruction around the foot and ankle, although the donor site usually requires skin grafting (4). The retrograde peroneal flap is useful for ankle, heel, and proximal dorsal foot defects. Its blood flow is retrograde and depends on an intact distal peroneal arterial–arterial anastomosis with either or both the anterior tibial artery and/or posterior tibial artery. The dissection is tedious and it does sacrifice one of the three major arteries of the leg. A similar retrograde anterior tibial artery fasciocutaneous flap has been described for coverage in young

patients with traumatic wounds over the same areas. Because the anterior compartment is the only compartment of the leg whose muscles depend solely on a single artery, only the lower half of the artery can be safely harvested as a vascular leash. The retrograde sural nerve flap (Fig. 71.5) is a versatile neurofasciocutaneous flap that is useful for ankle and heel defects. The sural artery travels with the sural nerve and receives retrograde flow from a peroneal perforator 5 cm above the lateral malleolus. The artery first courses above the fascia and then penetrates deep to the fascia at midcalf while the accompanying lesser saphenous vein remains above the fascia. The venous congestion often seen with this flap can be minimized if the pedicle is harvested with 3 cm of tissue on either side of the pedicle and with the overlying skin intact. Problems with the venous drainage can be further helped if the flap is delayed, 4 to 10 days earlier, by ligating the proximal lesser saphenous vein and sural artery. The inset of the flap is critical to avoid kinking of the pedicle. Ingenious splinting is necessary to avoid pressure on the pedicle while the flap heals (the Ilizarov external frame can be useful in this regard). The major donor deficit of the flap is the loss of sensibility along the lateral aspect of the foot, while the skin-grafted depression in the posterior calf may pose a problem if the patient subsequently has a below-the-knee amputation. The supramalleolar flap can be used for lateral malleolar, anterior ankle, and dorsal foot defects. It can be either harvested with the overlying skin or as a fascial layer that can be skin grafted. When harvested as a fascial flap, the donor site can be closed primarily. Small local fasciocutaneous flaps based on individual perforators can also be designed over the row of perforators (Fig. 71.6) originating from the posterior tibial artery medially and the peroneal artery laterally. Although the reach and size of these flaps are limited, these can be expanded by applying the delay principle. These local flaps are extremely useful in the closure of soft-tissue defects around the ankle in patients in an Ilizarov frame because accessibility to pedicled flaps or recipient vessels for free flaps is problematic.

Foot Flaps

The muscle flaps in the foot (5) have a type 2 vascular pattern and are useful for coverage of relatively small defects. The abductor digiti minimi muscle (Fig. 71.7A) is very useful for coverage of small mid- and posterior lateral defects of the sole of the foot and lateral distal calcaneus and ankle. The dominant pedicle is medial to the muscle's origin at the calcaneus and it has a thin distal muscular bulk. The abductor hallucis brevis muscle (Fig. 71.7B) is larger and can be used to cover medial defects of the mid- and hindfoot, as well as the medial distal ankle. Its dominant pedicle is at the takeoff of the medial plantar artery. Both of the above muscles can be used together to cover somewhat larger plantar defects in the midfoot and heel. The flexor digiti minimi brevis muscle is a small muscle that can be used to cover defects over the proximal fifth metatarsal bone. It receives its dominant pedicle at the lateral plantar artery takeoff of the digital artery to the fifth toe. The flexor hallucis brevis muscle has similar vascular anatomy, but can be harvested on a much longer vascular pedicle as an island flap on the medial plantar artery to reach defects as far as the proximal ankle.

The extensor digitorum brevis muscle (Fig. 71.8) has disappointingly little bulk but can be used for local defects over the sinus tarsi or lateral calcaneus. The muscle can either be rotated in a limited fashion on its dominant pedicle, the lateral tarsal artery, or in a wider arc if harvested with the dorsalis pedis artery. The flexor digitorum brevis muscle can be used to cover plantar heel defects. Because the muscle bulk is small, it works best if it is used to fill a deep defect that can be covered with plantar tissue.

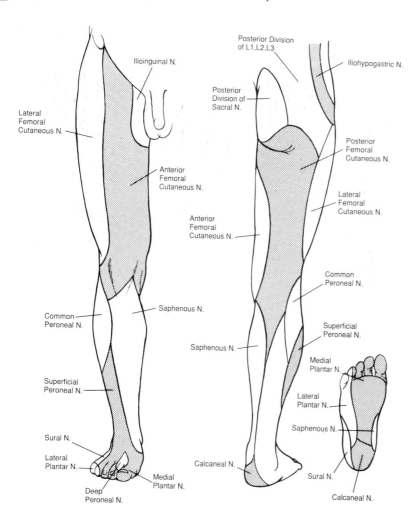

FIGURE 71.3. Sensory innervation of the lower leg. Note that the sensory distribution of the deep peroneal nerve is limited to the first web space, whereas the superficial peroneal nerve runs in the lateral compartment and provides sensibility to the dorsum of the foot. The posterior tibial nerve that runs in the deep posterior compartment supplies the sole of the foot and toes.

The most versatile fasciocutaneous flap of the foot is the medial plantar flap, which is the ideal tissue for the coverage of plantar defects. It can also reach medial ankle defects. The flap can be harvested to a size as large as 6 × 10 cm, has sensibility, and has a wide arc of rotation if it is taken with the proximal part of the medial plantar artery whether distally based on the superficial medial plantar artery or on the deep medial plantar artery (Fig. 71.9). Although easier to harvest on the deep medial plantar branch, it is preferable to harvest the flap based on the superficial branch because there is less disturbance of the inflow to the remaining foot. When harvested with retrograde flow, the flap should be based on the deep branch of the medial plantar artery.

The lateral calcaneal flap (Fig. 71.10) is useful for posterior calcaneal and distal Achilles defects. Its length can be increased by harvesting it as an L-shape posterior to and below the lateral malleolus. It is harvested with the lesser saphenous vein and sural nerve. Because the calcaneal branch of the peroneal artery lies directly on the periosteum, there is great danger of damaging or cutting it during harvest.

The dorsalis pedis flap can be either proximally or distally based for coverage of ankle and dorsal foot defects. A flap wider than 4 cm usually requires skin grafting on top of the extensor tendon paratenon, which deprives the dorsum of the foot of durable coverage. Because the donor site is vulnerable from both a vascular and tissue breakdown perspective, the dorsalis pedis flap is now rarely used.

The filet of toe flap is useful for small forefoot web space ulcers and distal forefoot problems, even though the reach of the flap is always *less* than expected. The technique involves removal of the nail bed, phalangeal bones, extensor tendons, flexor tendons, and volar plates while leaving the two digital arteries intact. An elegant variation is the toe island flap, where a part of the toe pulp is raised directly over the ipsilateral digital neurovascular bundle and then brought over to close a neighboring defect, while its neurovascular pedicle is buried underneath the intervening tissue.

WOUND CARE

The etiology of foot and ankle wounds is usually traumatic, with the underlying pathology complicating the healing process. Significant accompanying disease processes include infection, ischemia, neuropathy, venous hypertension, lymphatic obstruction, immunologic abnormality, hypercoagulability, vasospasm, neoplasm, self-induced wound, or any combination of the preceding. The most frequent systemic comorbidities include diabetes, peripheral vascular disease, venous hypertension, and connective tissue disorders.

Diagnostic Studies

Evaluation of the patient with a foot wound or ulcer begins with a complete history and physical examination. Important points in the history include etiology, duration and previous treatment of the wound(s), comorbid conditions (diabetes, peripheral vascular disease, venous insufficiency, atherosclerotic disease, autoimmune disorders, radiation, coagulopathy, etc.),

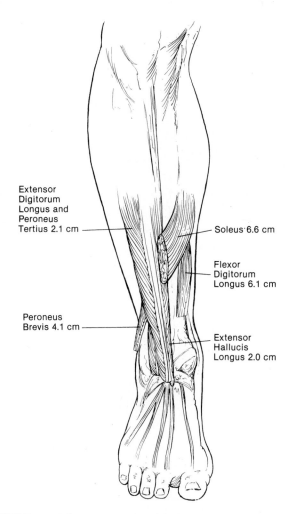

Extensor
Digitorum
Longus and
Peroneus
Tertius 2.1 cm

Soleus 6.6 cm

Flexor
Digitorum
Longus 6.1 cm

Peroneus
Brevis 4.1 cm

Extensor
Hallucis
Longus 2.0 cm

FIGURE 71.4. The type 4 muscles of the lower leg. These muscles are thin and can only be harvested for a distance of two to three segmental pedicles. They provide little bulk to cover lower-leg defects. The figure indicates how far proximal to the medial malleolus each muscle is useful for coverage of lower leg defects. For larger defects, a free flap is almost always a better option. (From Attinger C. Plastic surgery techniques for foot and ankle surgery. In: Myerson M, ed. *Foot and Ankle Disorders.* Philadelphia: WB Saunders; 2000:627, with permission.)

current medications, allergies, and nutritional status. It is also important to assess the patient's current and anticipated level of activity. **If the patient is using the leg in any way, including simple transfers, then salvage, if medically tolerated and technically possible, is usually indicated. However, if the limb is not going to be used, then strong consideration should be given to performing a knee disarticulation or above-knee amputation to cure the problem and minimize the risk of recurrent breakdown.**

The complete physical examination starts with a careful wound measurement (length, width, and depth), as well as the types of tissue involved (i.e., epithelium, dermis, subcutaneous tissue, fascia, tendon, joint capsule, and/or bone). The most accurate way of assessing if bone is involved is if one can directly feel bone with a metal probe, which correlates 85% of the time with the existence of osteomyelitis (6). **Diabetic ulcers with an area >2 cm^2 have a 90% chance of underlying osteomyelitis regardless of whether bone is probed at the base of the wound.** The levels of tissue necrosis and possible avenues of spread of infection via flexor or extensor tendons are then determined. If cellulitis is present, the border of the cellulitis is delineated with a marker and the date and time are noted.

This permits the clinician to immediately monitor the progress of the initial treatment despite the lack of bacterial culture results.

The vascular supply to the foot is then examined. If pulses are palpable (dorsalis pedis or posterior tibial artery), there is usually adequate blood supply for wound healing. If one cannot palpate pulses, a Doppler should be used. The Doppler ultrasound probe also allows the surgeon to evaluate the nonpalpable anterior perforating branch and the calcaneal branch of the peroneal artery. It also helps determine the direction of flow along the major arteries of the foot to accurately assess local blood flow when designing a flap or amputation. **A triphasic Doppler sound indicates excellent blood flow; a biphasic sound indicates adequate blood flow; and a monophasic sound warrants further investigation by the vascular surgeon.** A monophasic tone does not necessarily reflect inadequate blood flow as it may reflect of lack of vascular tone and absent distal resistance.

If the pulses are nonpalpable or monophasic, then noninvasive arterial Doppler studies are indicated. **It is important to obtain PVRs (pulse volume recordings) at each level because arterial brachial indices are unreliable in patients with calcified vessels, that is, in 30% of diabetics.** Ischemia may be present if the PVR amplitude is <10 mm Hg. Obtaining arterial toe pressures yields further information because digital arteries are less likely to be calcified; if the toe pressure is <30 mm Hg, ischemia may be present. Tissue oxygen levels are also helpful in determining whether there is sufficient blood flow to the extremity. Tissue oxygen pressure levels <40 mm Hg suggest insufficient local blood flow. If the noninvasive tests suggest ischemia, an arterial imaging study is obtained to evaluate whether a vascular inflow procedure (absent femoral pulse) and/or vascular outflow procedure (absent distal pulse) is required. The advent of the endovascular techniques allows revascularization with dilation, recanalization, or atherectomy with or without stents of stenosed or obstructed arteries. Combined endovascular and bypass techniques are also effective. Successful distal revascularization using the "in situ" bypasses and short-segment grafts to bypass local obstructions enjoy excellent long-term patency rates.

Sensory exam is performed with a 5.07 Semmes-Weinstein filament that represents 10 g of pressure. If the patient cannot feel the filament, protective sensation is absent, leading to an increased risk of breakdown. Motor function is assessed by looking at the resting position of the foot and the strength and active range of motion of the ankle, foot, and toes.

The bone architecture is evaluated by looking at whether the arch is stable, collapsed, or disjointed. Bone prominence can occur with collapsed midfoot bones (cuboid or navicular bone with Charcot destruction of the midfoot), osteophyte formation, or abnormal biomechanical forces (hallux valgus, hammer toe, etc.). An x-ray series of the foot is critical (anteroposterior, oblique, and lateral). The views of the lateral foot should be weight bearing. Calcaneal, sesamoids, and metatarsal head views may be necessary if local pathology is suspected in those areas. It is important to remember that the x-ray appearance of osteomyelitis lags behind the clinical appearance by up to 3 weeks. A magnetic resonance imaging (MRI) scan can help with earlier detection of osteomyelitis, as well as with differentiation between osteomyelitis and Charcot collapse. **In general, bone scans are of no value in evaluation of osteomyelitis when there is an ulcer present.** The bone under an ulcer will show increased uptake, regardless whether or not osteomyelitis is present. However, if proximal spread of osteomyelitis along a long bone is to be ruled out, then a negative bone scan can be very useful.

Finally, the Achilles tendon should be evaluated. If the ankle cannot be dorsiflexed 10 to 15 degrees above neutral, the Achilles tendon is tight and is placing excessive stress on the

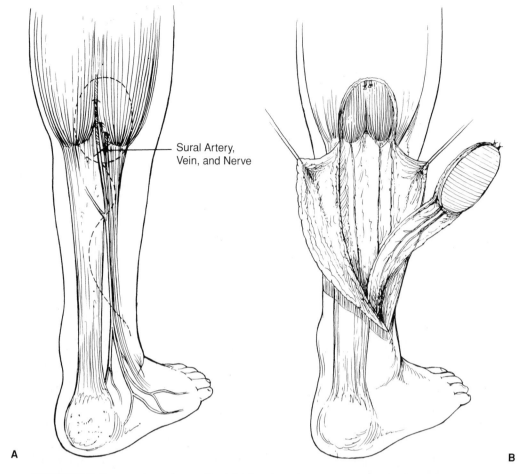

FIGURE 71.5. Retrograde sural artery flap. This flap depends on a peroneal perforator 5 cm proximal to the lateral malleolus. It also includes the lesser saphenous vein. Use of the flap sacrifices the sural nerve, leaving the lateral foot insensate. It is useful in covering lower leg, ankle, and hindfoot defects. **A:** Flap design. **B:** Flap dissection and arc of rotation. (From Attinger C. Soft tissue coverage for lower extremity trauma. *Orthop Clin North Am* 1995;26:3, with permission.)

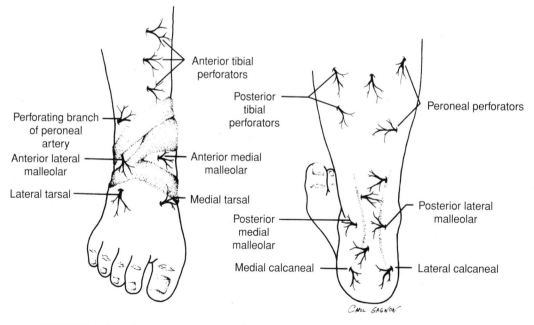

FIGURE 71.6. Location of the cutaneous perforators. Perforators are shown as they emanate from the posterior tibial artery, peroneal artery, and anterior tibial artery. A flap designed with one of these perforators at its base, located by Doppler ultrasound probe, can encompass the territory fed by an adjoining perforator. To extend the flap successfully beyond those boundaries requires a delay procedure. (From Hallock J. Distal lower leg random fasciocutaneous flaps. *Plast Reconstr Surg.* 1990;86:304, with permission.)

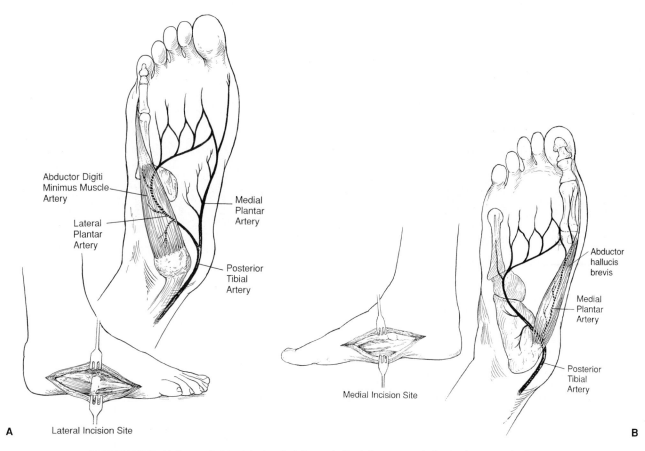

FIGURE 71.7. Abductor digiti minimi and abductor hallucis brevis muscle flaps. These muscles have a type 2 vascular pattern, with the dominant pedicle at the level of the distal calcaneus. They are harvested on their dominant proximal pedicles. The distal muscle bulk is often disappointingly small. However, these muscles are useful to fill small midfoot, rearfoot, and distal ankle defects. **A:** Abductor digiti minimi. **B:** Abductor hallucis brevis.

arch in the midfoot and on the plantar forefoot during gait. This necessitates release so as to avoid excessive pressure that could lead to Charcot collapse or forefoot plantar ulceration.

Preparing the Wound for Reconstruction

The goal of treating any type of wound is to promote healing in a timely fashion. The first step is to establish a clean and healthy wound base. An acute wound is defined as a recent wound that has yet to progress through the sequential stages of wound healing. If the wound is adequately vascularized, a clean base can be established with simple debridement and either immediate closure or covering the wound with a negative-pressure closure device (a vacuum-assisted closure [VAC] device) for subsequent closure. A chronic wound is a wound that is arrested in one of the wound-healing stages (usually the inflammatory stage) and cannot progress further. Converting a chronic wound to an acute one requires correcting medical abnormalities (high blood sugar levels, coagulation abnormalities, changing or modifying drug therapy, etc.), restoring adequate blood flow, administering appropriate antibiotics if any infection is present, and debriding the wound aggressively. If the wound has responded to this aggressive therapy, healthy granulation should appear, edema should decrease, and neo-epithelialization should appear at the wounds edge. The VAC device (7) is a useful postdebridement dressing for the unin-fected, well-vascularized wound because it decreases wound edema, helps to keep the bacterial count down, and promotes the formation of granulation tissue. Measuring the wound area weekly is a useful way to monitor progress, **as the weekly rate of normal healing is a 10% to 15% decrease in surface area per week.** Assuming the underlying abnormalities have been corrected (e.g., infection, ischemia, coagulopathy) and the healing falls below the normal healing rate, topical growth factors, cultured skin, and/or hyperbaric oxygen can be applied alternatively or in combination.

Surgical debridement is the single most underperformed procedure in treating foot and ankle wounds and ulcers because of concerns of how to close the resultant defect. Leaving dead or infected tissue or bone behind because of concerns about wound closure leads to subsequent infection and possible amputation. Tissue with clotted veins or arteries in the dermis or subcutaneous tissue, liquefied fascia or tendon, and nonbleeding bone should all be debrided. Debridement should be considered complete only when normal bleeding tissue remains. By the same token, any viable tissue should be preserved as it may be useful in the final reconstruction. The most effective debridement technique consists of removing thin layers of tissue in a sequential fashion until only normal tissue is left behind. This minimizes the amount of viable tissue sacrificed while ensuring that the tissue left behind is healthy. An effective alternative debriding device is a high-pressure water jet (up to 15,000 lb of pressure per square

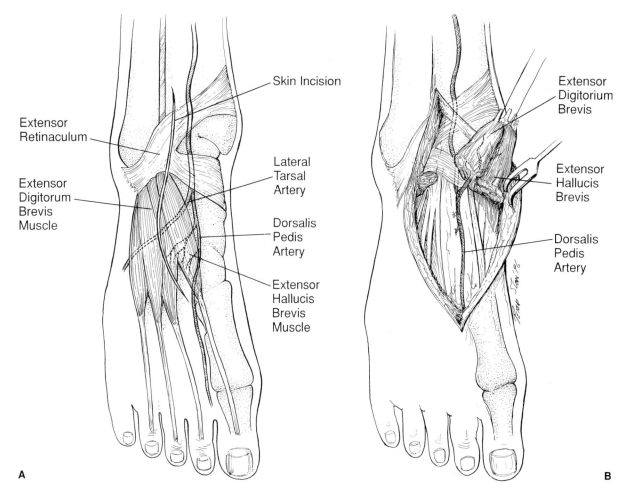

FIGURE 71.8. Flexor digiti minimi muscle flap. This muscle is a type 2 muscle that arises from the base of the proximal fifth metatarsal. Its proximal blood flow arises from the digital artery as it branches off the lateral plantar artery. The muscle can be rotated posteriorly to cover ulcers over the proximal fifth metatarsal bone. (From Attinger C. Soft tissue coverage for lower extremity trauma. *Orthop Clin North Am* 1995;26:3, with permission.)

inch) that removes serial layers of tissue (Smith & Nephew, Largo, FL).

The skeleton can usually be stabilized by splinting or corrected by application of an external fixator (monoplanar frame, Ilizarov frame). The Ilizarov frame provides superior immobilization, allows for bone transport and minimizes the risk for pin track infection because of the thin wire pins.

Deep uncontaminated tissue cultures should be obtained during the initial and subsequent debridements to guide antibiotic therapy (both intravenous and topical). Effective dressings for wounds that may still harbor significant bacteria are an appropriate topical antibiotic, a silver ion sheet, or antibiotic-impregnated methylmethacrylate beads covered with an occlusive dressing. For heavily exudative wounds, an absorbent dressing with bactericidal ingredients (silver or iodine) or VAC should be used. For wounds that are clean and well vascularized, a moist dressing or the VAC can be applied. **Debridement is rescheduled as frequently as necessary if there is progressive tissue necrosis or destruction.**

Biologic debriding agents such as maggots are currently being reintroduced in the United States as a therapeutic agent. They are useful in patients too ill for anesthesia or in patients awaiting revascularization. Maggots consume all bacteria and help sterilize wounds contaminated with antibiotic resistant bacteria such as VRE (vancomycin-resistant *Enterococci*) or MRSA (methicillin-resistant *Staphylococcus aureus*).

After initial debridement to clean tissue, it is important to prevent a subsequent build up of metalloproteases that destroy naturally produced growth factors. **The bacterial biofilm and proteinaceous debris that form on the wound surface must be removed at regular intervals.** This can be done by scrubbing the wound daily or using wet-to-dry dressings. The latter, however, also removes healthy new tissue in the process. The VAC (6), by applying negative pressure to the surface of the wound, helps prevent a build up of proteases and bacteria that inhibit or break down growth factors.

If the wound fails to show signs of healing despite being clean and having adequate blood flow, it can often be converted into a healing wound by providing local wound healing factors to the site. One can either apply a platelet-derived growth factor (Regranex, Ortho-McNeil Pharmaceutical, Raritan, NJ) daily to the wound or place a sheet of cultured skin that produces the entire range of growth factors every 1 to 6 weeks (Apligraf, Organogenesis, Canton, MA; Dermagraft, Advanced Tissue Sciences, La Jolla, CA). The formation of new tissue also can be stimulated by placing a layer of inert dermis (Integra, Integra LifeSciences, Plainsboro, NJ) over a healthy wound bed and allowing it to revascularize over the next 10 to 12 days (with the VAC) or over 3 weeks (without the VAC). The newly vascularized dermis can then be skin grafted with a thin autograft.

Finally, systemic hyperbaric oxygen can also be used to convert a nonhealing wound into a healthy granulating wound. It

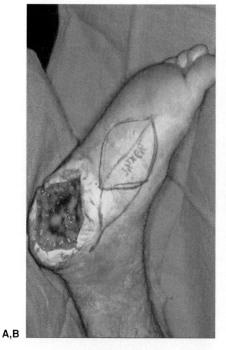
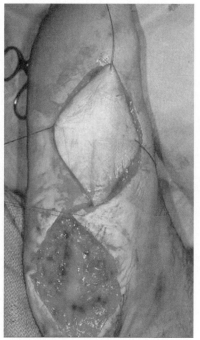
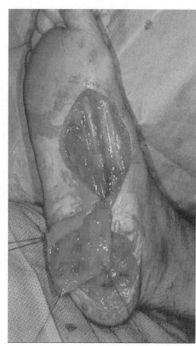

A,B

C

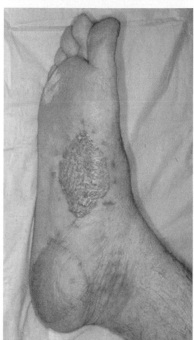

D

FIGURE 71.9. Medial plantar flap. The most versatile fasciocutaneous flap of the foot is the medial plantar flap. It is ideal for the coverage of plantar defects. It can be harvested on the superficial medial plantar artery or on the deep medial plantar artery. The flap shown is based on the deep medial plantar artery.

stimulates local angiogenesis in the wound bed, helps in the formation of collagen (cross-linking and extrusion from the cell), and potentiates the ability of macrophages and granulocytes to kill bacteria. When healthy granulation tissue appears, the wound can then be closed safely. **Failure to wait until the wound has developed signs of healing (healthy granulation tissue, neo-epithelialization at the skin edge, etc.) carries a high risk of failure.**

Treatment Options

Reconstruction is guided by the principle that coverage of a wound should be performed as quickly and efficiently as possible. Once the wound is clean and well vascularized, a reconstructive option is chosen from the reconstructive ladder: (a) allowing the defect to heal by secondary intention; (b) closing the wound primarily; (c) applying a split- or full-thickness skin graft; (d) rotating or advancing a local random flap; (e) rotating a pedicled flap; (f) transferring a microvascular free flap. The solution is guided by the patient's health, the depth of the wound, the location of the wound, and the surgeon's experience. The solution must always include restoration of a biomechanically sound foot to prevent recurrent breakdown.

Useful guidelines suggest simple coverage (secondary intention, delayed primary closure, or simple skin graft) if there is no tendon, joint, or bone involved. Even more complex wounds involving exposed tendon, joint, or bone that mandated flap reconstruction in the past can now be treated with simpler

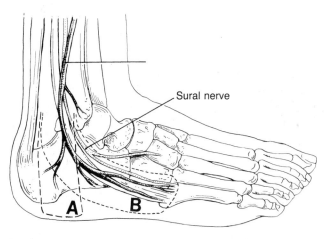

Sural nerve

FIGURE 71.10. Lateral calcaneus flap. This fasciocutaneous flap can be extended into an L shape so that it can cover part of the weight-bearing heel. The donor site is skin grafted. (From Attinger C. Soft tissue coverage for lower extremity trauma. *Orthop Clin North Am* 1995;26:3, with permission.)

methods. For example, wounds over the Achilles tendon easily develop adequate granulation tissue with good wound care that can then be simply covered with a skin graft. With the VAC, granulation tissue can form over tendon, bone, or joints that can then heal either by secondary intention or be skin grafted. With Integra, with or without the VAC, a healthy dermal layer can form over tendon, bone, or joints that can then be skin grafted with a thin autograft (Fig. 71.11). It is critical to immobilize the wound over a moving joint and to offload the wound to prevent shearing forces from disrupting the healing process. Both the VAC and external fixator can be used to minimize motion at the wound site, while the Ilizarov frame can be used to offload the wound (i.e., heel). **Using these methods, more than 85% of all wounds can usually be closed by simple techniques, while less than 15% require flaps.**

RECONSTRUCTION

Biomechanics are a critical part of the reconstructive plan and may involve bone rearrangement, partial joint removal or fusion, or tendon lengthening or transfer. The method of soft-tissue reconstruction chosen hinges on the surgeon's experience, the size of the wound, the vascular status of the foot, the exposed structures (tendon, joint, and/or bone), and the access to the wound (i.e., an Ilizarov frame limits the access to the foot). Wounds can be allowed to heal by secondary intention with daily dressing changes, application of the VAC, and/or correction of the biomechanical abnormality. A tight Achilles tendon is the principal cause of forefoot plantar ulceration in diabetics. By simply lengthening the tendon, the plantar wound usually heals without further treatment over the next 6 weeks (see section on diabetic foot ulcers). The application of growth factor or cultured skin can speed up healing by secondary intention.

Delayed primary closure is easier to accomplish when the edema and induration of the wound edges has resolved. The VAC can be helpful in reducing the edema by absorbing all excess fluid. After primary closure, one should always check that relevant arterial pulses have not diminished because of an excessively tight closure. If the gap is too large to allow for immediate closure of the defect, the wound can be closed serially or the remaining gap can be treated to heal by secondary intention. Adequate soft-tissue envelope can also be created by removing underlying bone. This occurs in partial foot amputa-

tions where just enough bone is removed to develop adequate soft-tissue envelopes for delayed primary closure. Correcting the Charcot collapse of the midfoot arch by removing the arch and re-fusing the metatarsals to the hindfoot with the help of the Ilizarov external fixator usually allows for loose approximation of the plantar soft-tissue ulcer.

Skin grafting can be used to close most foot and ankle wounds. A healthy granulating bed is the necessary prerequisite. This can be achieved by the methods delineated above and include VAC, cultured skin, dermal regeneration template, growth factor, and/or hyperbaric oxygen. Successful skin graft take is aided by removing the granulation bed that contains bacteria before placing the skin graft. The wound is then pulse lavaged and new instruments are used to avoid recontaminating the wound base. The skin graft is meshed at a 1:1 ratio to prevent build up of seroma or hematoma. The use of the VAC on low continuous suction as a temporary dressing for the first 3 to 5 days helps absorb excess fluid and provides excellent fixation of the skin graft to the underlying bed, thereby minimizing possible graft-bed disruption from shear forces (8). If the skin graft is over moving muscle or joint, it is critical to immobilize the foot and ankle by splinting or placement of an external fixator until the skin graft has completely healed.

The ideal graft donor site for a plantar wound is the glabrous skin from the plantar instep because the thicker glabrous skin graft resists the shear forces applied to the plantar foot during ambulation. It is harvested at 30/1000th of an inch, meshed, and covered with a VAC. The donor site is, in turn, covered with a thin skin graft of 10/1000th of an inch. For plantar wounds where the patient is noncompliant either by choice or because of body habitus, consideration is given to placing an Ilizarov frame with a protective footplate until the graft has healed.

The use of any flap requires an accurate assessment of the blood flow. For local flaps, there should be a Dopplerable perforator close to the base of the flap. For pedicled flaps, the dominant branch to the flap should be patent. For free flaps, there should be an adequate recipient artery and vein(s). If there is any question, either a duplex scan, magnetic resonance angiogram, or normal angiogram is obtained.

Local flaps are useful in coverage of foot and ankle wounds because they only need to be large enough to cover the exposed tendon, bone, or joint while the rest of the wound is skin grafted. This frequently obviates the need of larger pedicled or free flaps (Fig. 71.12). In addition, an infinite variation of local flaps can easily be done around or through an Ilizarov external fixator (Fig. 71.13) because the lack of access makes pedicled flaps or free flaps hard to carry out.

Pedicled flaps in the foot and ankle area are often more difficult to dissect and have a higher perioperative complication rate, although equal long-term success, as free flaps. However, pedicled flaps allow the surgeon to perform a rapid operation with a short hospital stay that yields long-lasting results. The anatomy and techniques of dissection are discussed above and in flap anatomy books (9). Free flaps in the foot and ankle carry the highest failure rate in the microsurgical literature and should be planned carefully. One reason for this is that complications arise when the anastomosis is performed at or near the zone of injury. In addition, the arteries are often calcified and special hardened microneedles are often required. Anastomoses should be performed away from the zone of injury, either proximal or distal to the zone of injury providing that the neurovascular bundle is intact. An end-to-side anastomosis to the recipient artery should be employed whenever possible. Two venous anastomoses are performed whenever possible to minimize postoperative flap swelling. The use of a coupling device for vein anastomoses speeds up the procedure.

The choice of free flap depends in large part on the length of pedicle needed. For long pedicles, the serratus, latissimus,

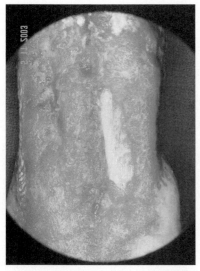
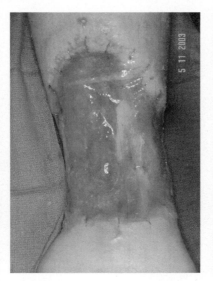
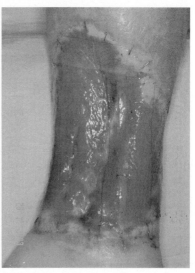

A,B   C

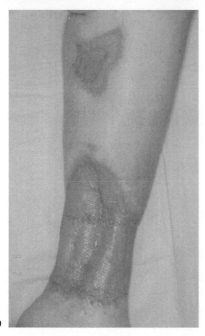

D

FIGURE 71.11. Ankle ulcer. This large ulcer above the medial ankle was debrided to clean bleeding tissue and tibia (**A**). The wound was covered with Integra (**B**) and the VAC for 10 days (**C**). The silicone sheet was then removed off the now vascularized Integra dermal template and a thin autograft was applied (**D**).

vastus lateralis, and the rectus femoris muscles are excellent. It is important to remember that the pedicle can be extended by further dissection within the muscle belly. For the dorsum of the foot and ankle, thin fasciocutaneous or cutaneous flaps work best. For the plantar foot, skin-grafted muscle flaps and skin graft seem to hold up better than fasciocutaneous flaps in the long run.

Postsurgical Care

Patients are generally not allowed to bear weight on the operated foot for 6 weeks if the plantar surface is involved. Appropriate offloading devices can be prescribed to offload specific parts of the plantar foot: heel, forefoot. The help of a pedorthotist should be sought in cases where off-the-shelf offloading devices are not available. For dorsal wounds, patients are allowed to ambulate far sooner, providing they are in a dressing that prevents damage to the reconstruction. Because of these limitations, a patient will often need a course of physical and occupational rehabilitation to gain the strength and mobility to

live independently at home. Patients should be followed closely in clinic during the postoperative period and should be seen by a pedorthotist to get the appropriate shoe to wear once they can bear weight. If diabetic, they should return to the care of a podiatrist for preventive foot care.

RECONSTRUCTIVE OPTIONS BY LOCATION OF DEFECT

Forefoot Coverage

Toe ulcers and gangrene are best treated with limited amputations that preserve any viable tissue so that the amputated toe is as long as possible when closed. Attempts to preserve at least the proximal portion of the proximal phalanx should be made so that it can serve as spacer, preventing the toes on either side from drifting into the empty space. If the hallux is involved, attempts should be made to preserve as much as possible because of its critical role in ambulation.

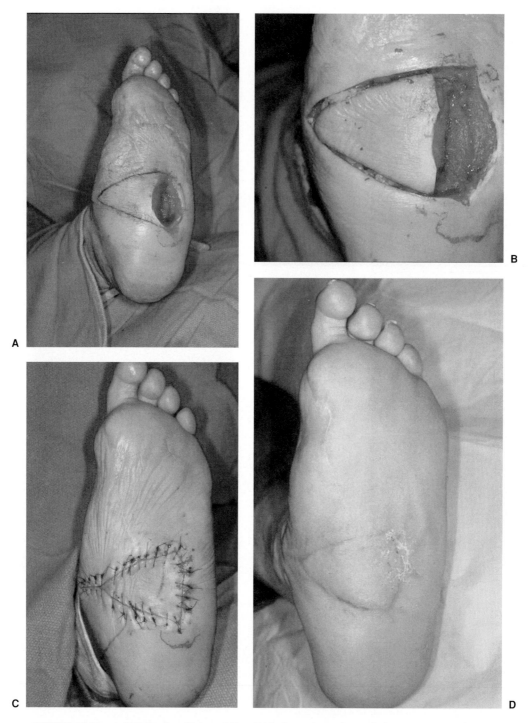

FIGURE 71.12. A *V-Y flap* is a V-shaped flap (**A,B**) that, when advanced, forms a Y (**C**). The V-Y flap depends on direct underlying perforators to stay alive. For that reason, the flap is dissected down through the fascial layer with *no undermining* whatsoever. On the plantar aspect of the foot, the maximum advancement is limited to 1 to 2 cm (**D**).

Ulcers under the metatarsal head(s) occur because biomechanical abnormalities place excessive or extended pressure on the plantar forefoot during the gait cycle. Although hammertoes, long metatarsals, or sesamoids can be contributing factors, the principal abnormal biomechanical force is a tight Achilles tendon that prevents ankle dorsiflexion beyond the neutral position. If the patient cannot dorsiflex his foot with the knee bent or straight, both the gastrocnemius and soleus portions of the tendon are tight. In addition, the posterior capsule of the ankle joint may be tight. A percutaneous release

of the Achilles tendon is performed (Fig. 71.14A, B) and if the foot still does not dorsiflex, then a posterior capsular release is performed. If the patient can dorsiflex his foot only when the knee is bent, then the gastrocnemius portion of the Achilles tendon is tight. A gastrocnemius recession should correct the problem (Fig. 71.14C, D, E). The patient is kept non–weight bearing for 1 week and in a CAM Walker for the next 5 weeks. Because compliance is at best 28%, the CAM Walker may have to be reinforced with casting material so it cannot be removed. With the release of the Achilles tendon,

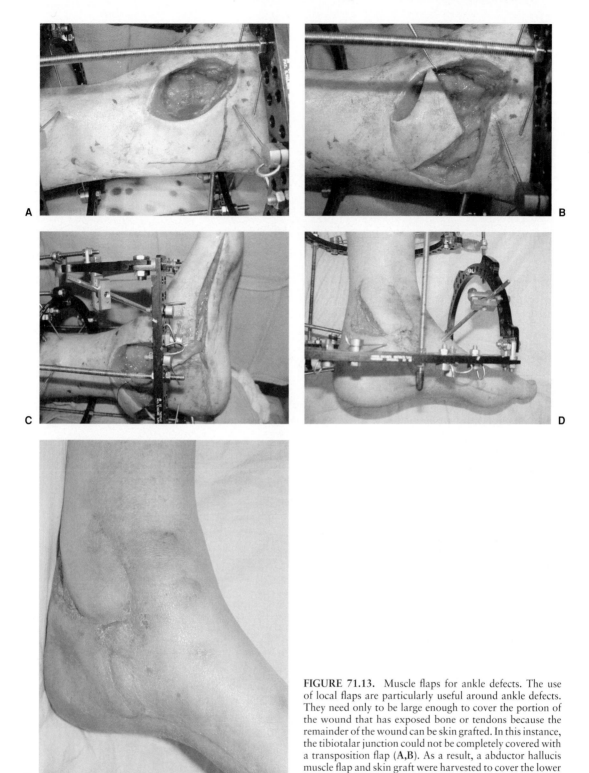

FIGURE 71.13. Muscle flaps for ankle defects. The use of local flaps are particularly useful around ankle defects. They need only to be large enough to cover the portion of the wound that has exposed bone or tendons because the remainder of the wound can be skin grafted. In this instance, the tibiotalar junction could not be completely covered with a transposition flap (**A,B**). As a result, a abductor hallucis muscle flap and skin graft were harvested to cover the lower half of the wound (**C,D,E**).

the forefoot pressure drops dramatically and the ulcer(s), if bone is not involved, heals simply by secondary intention in less than 6 weeks. **The lengthening of a tight Achilles tendon has decreased the ulcer recurrence rate in diabetics by half at 2 years.**

For patients with normal ankle dorsiflexion who have a stage 1 to 3 plantar caused by a plantar-prominent metatarsal head, the affected metatarsal head can be elevated with pre-planned osteotomies and internal fixation. The metatarsal head

is shifted 2 to 3 mm superiorly. Upward movement with its attendant pressure relief is usually sufficient for the underlying ulcer to heal by secondary intention. The small, deep forefoot ulcers, without an obvious bony prominence, can be allowed to heal by secondary intention or with a local flap. For larger ulcers where the metatarsal head and distal shaft are involved, consideration should be given to a partial ray amputation. Resecting the more independent first or fifth metatarsal causes less biomechanical disruption than resecting the second, third, or

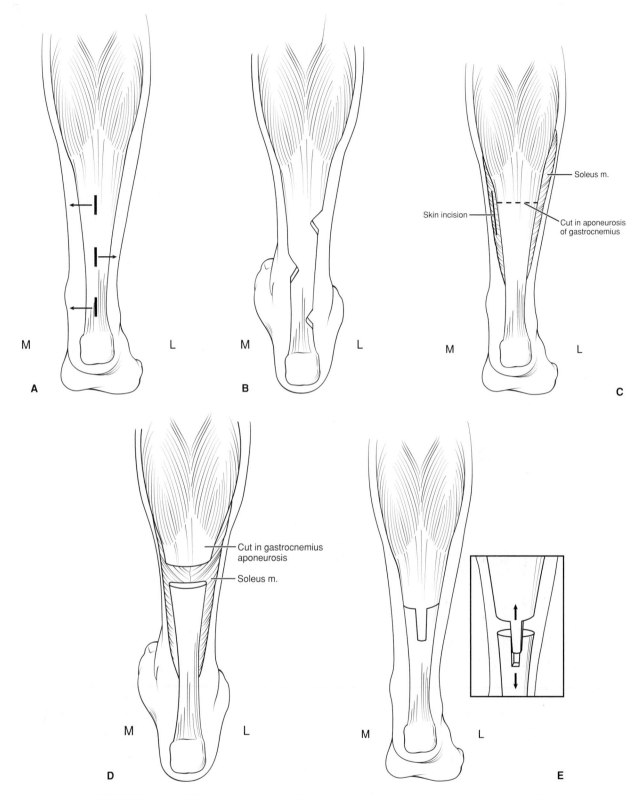

FIGURE 71.14. Achilles tendon lengthening. If both the gastrocnemius and soleus portion of the Achilles tendon are tight, the tendon can be released percutaneously by making three stab wounds at 2, 5, and 8 cm above the insertion of the Achilles into the calcaneus. A no. 15 blade is inserted into the central raphe of the tendon and the blade is turned 90 degrees to cut half of the tendon at each site (**A**). The upper and lower cuts are in the medial direction and the center cut is in the lateral direction. Gentle dorsiflexion pressure is exerted on the foot until the tendon releases (**B**). If only the gastrocnemius portion of the Achilles tendon is tight, then a gastrocnemius recession can be done. The Achilles tendon (**C**) is cut just below the muscle belly of the gastrocnemius muscles in a linear fashion while the soleus muscle remains intact (**D**). If the function of the gastrocnemius muscles is to be spared, then the cut can be made in a tongue-and-groove fashion (**E**).

fourth metatarsal because the central three metatarsals operate as a cohesive central unit.

All efforts should be made to preserve as much of the metatarsals as possible if more than one is compromised because they are important to normal ambulation. Because local tissue is often insufficient to do this in the forefoot, a microsurgical free flap is considered. If ulcers are present under several metatarsal heads, or if a transfer lesion from one of the resected metatarsal heads to a neighboring metatarsal has occurred, a pan-metatarsal head resection should be considered. If more than two toes with the accompanying metatarsal heads have to be resected, then a transmetatarsal amputation should be performed. The normal parabola, with the second metatarsal being the longest, is preserved. To avoid the resultant equinus deformity from the loss of the long and short toe extensors, the extensor and flexor tendons of the fourth and fifth toe should be tenodesed with the ankle in the neutral position and the Achilles tendon lengthened. As much plantar tissue as possible should be preserved to cover as much of the anterior portion of the amputation with healthy plantar tissue

The most proximal forefoot amputation is the Lisfranc amputation where all the metatarsals are removed. The direction of the blood flow along the dorsalis pedis and lateral plantar artery should be evaluated. If both have antegrade flow, then the connection between the two can be sacrificed. However if only one of the two vessels is providing blood flow to the entire foot, the connection has to be preserved. To prevent an equinovarus deformity, the anterior tibial tendon should be split and the lateral aspect inserted into the cuboid bone. In addition, the Achilles tendon should be lengthened. The Lisfranc amputation can be closed with volar or dorsal flaps, if there is sufficient tissue. If there is inadequate tissue for coverage, a free muscle flap with skin graft is used. Postoperatively, the patient's foot is placed in slight dorsiflexion until the wound has healed.

Midfoot Coverage

Defects on the medial aspect of the sole are non–weight bearing and are best treated with a skin graft. Ulcers on the medial and lateral plantar midfoot are usually caused by Charcot collapse of the midfoot plantar arch. If the underlying shattered bone has healed and is stable (Eichenholz stage 3), then the excess bone can be shaved via a medial or lateral approach while the ulcer either can be allowed to heal by secondary intention or can be covered with a glabrous skin graft or a local flap. For small defects, useful local flaps include the V-to-Y flap, the bilobed flap, the rhomboid flap, and the transposition flap. If a muscle flap is needed, a pedicled abductor hallucis flap medially or an abductor digiti minimi flap laterally works well. For slightly larger defects, large V-to-Y flaps, random, large, medially based rotation flaps or pedicled medial plantar fasciocutaneous flap can be successful. Larger defects should be filled with free muscle flaps covered by skin grafts. Great care should be taken to tailor the flap so that it is inset at the same height as the surrounding tissue. If the midfoot bones are unstable (Eichenholz stage 1 or 2), then they can be excised using a wedge excision and the arch is recreated by fusing the proximal metatarsals to the talus and calcaneus via an Ilizarov frame. The shortening of the skeletal midfoot usually leaves enough loose soft tissue to close the wound primarily or with a local flap.

Hindfoot Coverage

Plantar heel defects or ulcers are among the most difficult of all wounds to treat. If they are the result of the patient being in a prolonged decubitus position, they usually also reflect severe vascular disease. A partial calcanectomy may be required to develop enough local soft tissue to cover the resulting defect. Although patients can ambulate with a partially resected calcaneus, they will need orthotics and molded shoes. If there is an underlying collapsed bone or bone spur causing a hindfoot defect, the bone should be shaved. These ulcers are usually closed with a large, distally based V-to-Y flap, or larger medially based rotation flaps. Plantar heel defects can also be closed with pedicled flaps that include the medial plantar fasciocutaneous flap or the flexor digiti minimi muscle flap. Posterior heel defects are better closed with an extended lateral calcaneal fasciocutaneous flap or the retrograde sural artery fasciocutaneous flap. If the defect is large, then a muscle free flap with skin graft should be used. The flap should be carefully tailored so there is no excess tissue and it blends in well with the rest of the heel. Medial or lateral calcaneal defects usually occur after fracture and attempted repair. There is usually associated osteomyelitis of the calcaneus. After debridement of the infected bone and placement of antibiotic beads, the medial defect can usually be covered with the abductor hallucis muscle flap medially or the abductor digiti minimi flap laterally. The exposed muscle is then skin grafted. After 6 or more weeks, the beads can be replaced with bone graft.

The two hindfoot amputations are the Chopart and Symes amputations. The Chopart amputation leaves an intact talus and calcaneus while removing the mid- and forefoot bones of the foot. To avoid going into equinovarus deformity, a minimum of 2 cm of the Achilles tendon has to be resected. When healed, a calcaneal-tibial rod can be used to further stabilize the ankle. The Symes amputation should be considered if there is insufficient tissue to primarily close a Chopart amputation and there is insufficient arterial blood supply for a free flap, or if the talus and calcaneus are involved with osteomyelitis. The tibia and fibula are cut just above the ankle mortise and the deboned heel pad is anchored to the anterior portion of the distal tibia to prevent posterior migration. The large medial and lateral dog-ears can be carefully trimmed at the initial operation or 4 to 6 weeks later to yield a thin, tailored stump that can fit well into a patellar weight-bearing prosthesis.

Dorsum of the Foot

The defects on the dorsum of the foot are often treated with simple skin grafts. If the tissue covering the extensor tendons is thin or nonexistent, a dermal regeneration template (Integra) should be applied, and when vascularized, covered with a thin skin autograft. Local flaps that can be used for small defects include rotation, bilobed, rhomboid, or transposition flaps. The EDB muscle flap works well for sinus tarsi defects and its reach can be increased by cutting the dorsalis pedis artery above or below tarsal artery, depending on the presence of antegrade and retrograde flow and the location of the defect. The supramalleolar flap can be used over the lateral proximal dorsal foot and its reach can be increased by cutting the anterior perforating branch of the peroneal artery before it anastomoses with the lateral malleolar artery. For larger or more distal defects, the most appropriate microsurgical free flap is a thin fasciocutaneous flap to minimize bulk. The radial forearm flap is an excellent choice because it is thin, sensate, and provides a vascularized tendon (palmaris tendon) to reconstruct lost extensor function. Thin muscle or fascial flaps with skin grafts are effective options as well.

Ankle Defects

Soft tissue around the ankle is sparse and has minimal flexibility. If there is sufficient granulation tissue, a skin graft will work well. To encourage the formation of a healthy wound bed, the

VAC, with or without Integra, can be used. The Achilles tendon, if allowed sufficient time to form a granulating bed, will tolerate a skin graft that will hold up well over time. Local flaps only need to cover the critical area of the wound including exposed tendon, bone, or joints while the rest of the wound can be skin grafted (Fig. 71.13). Useful local flaps include rotation or transposition flaps based on posterior tibial and peroneal arterial perforators. Pedicled flaps include the supramalleolar flap, the retrograde sural artery flap, the medial plantar flap, the abductor hallucis muscle flap, the abductor digiti minimi muscle flap, the extensor hallucis longus, and the extensor digitorum brevis muscle flap. Free flaps can either be fasciocutaneous or muscle with skin graft but they should be kept thin. To ensure good healing, the ankle should be temporarily immobilized with an external fixator.

TREATING WOUNDS WITH SIGNIFICANT COMORBIDITIES

Diabetes

Seven percent of all Americans have documented diabetes mellitus, 15% of whom eventually develop a foot ulcer during their lifetime. Almost 15% of the health care budget of the United States goes toward management of diabetes, with a large segment of that used for the treatment of diabetic foot ulcers, gangrene, and Charcot foot collapse. More than half of all the major amputations performed per year in the United States are performed in diabetics (10). **Indeed, a diabetic patient presenting to the emergency room with a foot ulcer faces a 24% risk of immediate major amputation. Major amputation carries significant morbidity for diabetics during the subsequent 5-year period with more than half dying and more than half losing the contralateral limb.** Part of the morbidity of major amputations involves a significant increase in the energy of ambulation (33% increase with below-knee amputation, 46% increase with wheelchair, 86% increase with above-knee amputation, and 100% increase with crutch walking). Combined with the natural psychological depression accompanying a major amputation, this energy increase adds significant stress to an often already compromised cardiac system.

It is well known that diabetes negatively affects many organ systems including joints and tendons. This is especially evident in the Achilles tendon where advanced glycosylated end products (AGEs) cross-link the collagen molecules of the tendon so that it loses its elasticity and eventually shortens. **The resultant inability to adequately dorsiflex the ankle means that the arch and metatarsal heads experience high pressure for a longer portion of the gait cycle than they would otherwise.** Lengthening the Achilles tendon helps relieve the plantar forefoot of excess pressure during gait and decreases the risk of Charcot midfoot collapse. Diabetics have a depressed immune response and hence have increased susceptibility to infection and are especially prone to *Streptococcus* and *Staphylococcus* skin infections. In addition, diabetics with uncontrolled sugars tend to have erythrocytes with stiff cell walls. The use of erythrocyte wall-deforming drugs such as pentoxifylline can help to decrease blood viscosity and increase flow in the microcirculation.

Up to 60% of diabetics with nonhealing ulcers have concurrent macrovascular disease. **The arteries below the popliteal trifurcation are frequently compromised, whereas the smaller arteries of the foot and ankle are often spared.** For this reason, distal bypass in the diabetic patient is frequently possible. Noninvasive arterial studies, especially ankle–brachial indices, can be misleading in the diabetic because vascular calcification decreases the compressibility of the vessels. If there is any question, the patient should be seen by a vascular surgeon who is trained in distal revascularization techniques.

The surgical approach to a diabetic foot ulcer was described earlier and includes diagnosing the components that contributed to the ulceration(s): neuropathy, skeletal and/or tendon pathology, vascular insufficiency, and medical imbalances such as uncontrolled blood glucose levels. The ulcer is measured and a deep tissue culture is obtained. If local signs of infection are present (cellulitis, induration, excessive drainage, odor), broad-spectrum antibiotics are started and then adjusted when culture and sensitivities are available. If wet gangrene is present, the wound is immediately debrided regardless of vascular status. If there is dry gangrene or the ulcer is stable and the leg is ischemic, the leg is first revascularized. If there was adequate blood flow or the blood flow has been restored, then the wound is debrided and the biomechanical abnormalities are addressed. The most appropriate coverage is then selected according to the principles outlined earlier.

Peripheral Neuropathy

Diabetic peripheral polyneuropathy is the major cause of diabetic foot wounds. More than 80% of diabetic foot ulcers have some form of neuropathy present, with the distal, large fiber, symmetrical polyneuropathy being the most common (11). The neuropathy is a consequence of chronically elevated blood sugars that cause vascular and metabolic abnormalities. Elevated intracellular concentrations of sorbitol, a glucose byproduct, causes the nerve to swell and therefore malfunction. Decreased insulin levels, along with altered levels of other neurotrophic peptides, altered fat metabolism, oxidative stress, and altered levels of vasoactive substances such as nitric oxide affect nerve function and repair. Unregulated glucose levels increase AGE levels seen in cross-linked collagen molecules that stiffen anatomically tight spaces in upper or lower extremities (the carpal, cubital, and tarsal tunnels). The combination of nerve swelling caused by any of these pathophysiologic mechanisms and tight anatomic compartments caused by glycosylated collagen lead to the "double-crush syndrome" that can present as autonomic, motor, and/or sensory nerve dysfunction.

Autonomic neuropathy has two effects: anhidrosis and the opening of arteriovenous (AV) shunts. Motor neuropathy most often affects the intrinsic muscles of the foot as a result of compression of the medial and lateral plantar nerves in their respective tunnels. Although it is not completely understood why distal autonomic and sensory neurons are preferentially targeted in diabetic peripheral polyneuropathy, it is well known that the decrease in protective sensation prevents patients from responding appropriately to minor trauma (callous, pebble in the shoe, tight shoe wear, etc.). Inability to feel a 5.07 Semmes-Weinstein filament is indicative of the patient's loss of protective sensation and thus presents a high risk for future foot breakdown. Today's state-of-the-art approach for diagnosis and follow-up of the loss of foot sensibility is being performed with the pressure-specified sensory device (PSSD) using the 99% upper confidence limit to identify abnormal sensibility, and it has a 95% interobserver reliability (12). Its major contribution is that it detects the neuropathy while still in early and reversible phases.

Beside diabetes, hypothyroidism, autoimmune diseases, drug-induced (steroids, certain chemotherapeutics, and anti-HIV medications), and idiopathic causes are among other known common causes of peripheral neuropathy. Regardless of the cause, the patient can present with foot paresthesia, numbness, pain, and/or muscle weakness, as well as balance problems and a history of falls. These symptoms usually precede the occurrence of wounds and are signs of axonal loss because of, at this stage, still reversible peripheral neuropathy.

Several nerve-specific anatomic compression sites responsible for signs and symptoms in diabetic and other patients with symptomatic peripheral neuropathy are identified. When appropriately diagnosed and treated, signs of symptomatic peripheral neuropathy can be partially or fully reversed with nerve release surgery at those compression sites (13). **In the lower extremities, these compression sites include common peroneal nerve at the fibular neck; the superficial peroneal nerve as it exits the deep anterolateral compartment; deep peroneal nerve at the dorsum of the midfoot (Fig. 71.15); tibial nerve at tarsal tunnel; and calcaneal, medial, and lateral plantar nerves within their respective tunnels distal to the tarsal tunnel in the hindfoot (Fig. 71.16).** Thus, symptoms of symptomatic peripheral neuropathy can be reversed in at least 70% of patients who present with a Tinel sign and abnormal PSSD electrophysiologic test. By restoring sensation via nerve decompres-

sive surgery, the incidence of ulcers and thus amputation can be significantly reduced (14).

Ischemia

Atherosclerotic disease is a common cause of nonhealing foot ulcers, especially in combination with diabetes. Hypercholesterolemia, hypertension, and tobacco use are major risk factors for atherosclerosis. Other causes of ischemia in the foot include thromboangiitis obliterans (Buerger disease, generally seen in young smokers), vasculitis, and thromboembolic disease. The etiology of the ischemia has to be accurately diagnosed before treatment is initiated.

When discussing revascularization plans with the vascular surgeon, it is important to consider within which angiosome the ulcer is located. Failure to revascularize the affected angiosome can lead to a 15% or greater limb loss rate despite a patent bypass. If the affected angiosome is directly revascularized, wound healing increases by 50% and the risk of major amputation decreases fourfold. For ulcers on the dorsum of the ankle or foot, the anterior tibial artery or dorsalis pedis should be revascularized if possible. If the connection between the dorsalis pedis and lateral plantar artery is intact, then a bypass to the posterior tibial artery is equally successful. For heel ulcers, revascularizing either the posterior tibial artery or peroneal artery is critical. For mid- and forefoot plantar wounds, the posterior tibial artery should be chosen, although revascularizing the dorsalis pedis can be equally effective if the connection between the dorsalis pedis and the lateral plantar artery is intact. If the ideal option is not available, then revascularization should proceed with the understanding that there is a 15% chance of failure.

When the patient with significant peripheral vascular disease presents with gangrene, the timing of revascularization versus debridement is critical. If there is stable dry gangrene without cellulitis, then the revascularization should proceed promptly but nonurgently. If the patient presents with wet gangrene with or without cellulitis, the wound should immediately be debrided. Revascularization should proceed on an urgent basis as progressive gangrene will occur unless there is new blood flow. After revascularization, no repair should be initiated unless the wound shows signs of healing with the appearance of new healthy granulation tissue and neoepithelialization. It takes anywhere from 4 to 10 days for the wound to develop maximal benefit from the revascularization. To proceed prematurely is to risk failure as the blood flow has not had time to revascularize the periwound area.

Connective Tissue Disorders

The connective tissue disorders (e.g., systemic lupus, rheumatoid arthritis, and scleroderma) are frequently associated with Raynaud disease, which causes distal vasospasm and cutaneous ischemia. The treatment of these connective tissue disorders frequently requires immunosuppressive drugs such as steroids and chemotherapeutic agents to control the autodestruction of the local tissue. Until the optimal immunosuppressive regimen is determined, the wound will not heal. The wound-retarding effects of steroids used in the immunosuppressive therapy can be mitigated with oral vitamin A (20,000 U per day while the wound is open). The use of topical vitamin A is also effective in this setting. Close coordination with the rheumatologist is necessary to heal these most difficult of wounds.

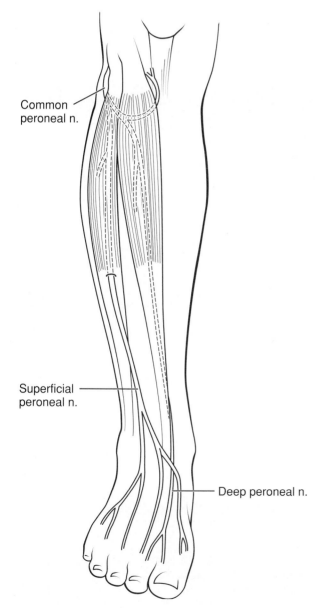

Common peroneal n.

Superficial peroneal n.

Deep peroneal n.

FIGURE 71.15. Compression sites for common, superficial, and deep peroneal nerves.

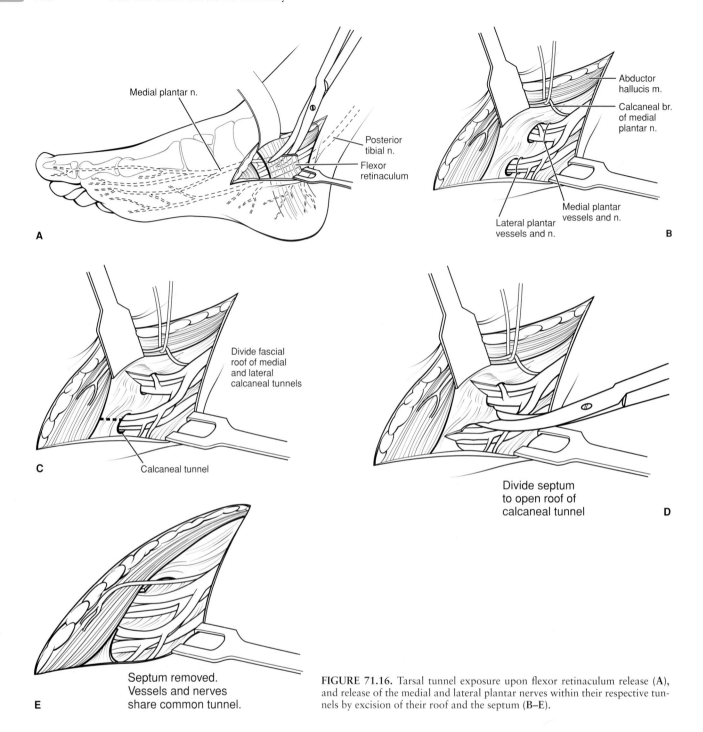

FIGURE 71.16. Tarsal tunnel exposure upon flexor retinaculum release (**A**), and release of the medial and lateral plantar nerves within their respective tunnels by excision of their roof and the septum (**B–E**).

In addition, almost half of patients with vasculitic ulcers also suffer from a coagulopathy leading to a hypercoagulable state. The most frequent abnormalities involve antithrombin III, Leiden factor V, protein C, protein S, and homocysteine. Consequently, a coagulation blood panel should be obtained on these patients and if abnormalities exist, they should be treated with appropriate anticoagulants and/or medications by the hematologist.

The treatment of these ulcers is principally medical. Once the abnormalities are identified and corrected, wound-healing adjuncts can help in healing the wound. The use of cultured skin and hyperbaric oxygen can be used to stimulate the formation of a healthy granulation bed. It is important to be patient in treating these wounds as they can take as long as 18 months to heal.

CONCLUSION

Treatment of foot wounds requires, at a minimum, the presence of adequate blood flow, absence of infection, and an eventually stable skeletal framework. This requires a team approach to limb salvage. One first has to ensure that the extremity has adequate blood flow. Debridement is the platform on which all reconstruction begins. It has to be aggressive and repeated as many times as necessary until the wound is ready for reconstruction. The use of the VAC after debridement is a useful adjunct in preparing the wound for closure. Additional wound adjuncts such as cultured skin, growth factor, and/or hyperbaric oxygen should be used if the wound bed does not respond to modern wound healing care.

Reconstruction should only be performed when the wound shows signs of healing. Most wounds can be closed with simple surgical techniques and only a few require more sophisticated anatomic knowledge to perform the necessary pedicled or free flaps. Biomechanics should be addressed with every reconstruction so that recurrent breakdown can be averted. Finally, when healed, appropriate orthotics and shoes should be ordered to protect the reconstruction.

References

1. Attinger CE, Cooper P, Blume P, et al. The safest surgical incisions and amputations using the angiosome concept and Doppler on arterial–arterial connections of the foot and ankle. *Foot Ankle Clin North Am.* 2001;6:745.
2. Masqualet AC, Gilbert A. *An Atlas of Flaps in Limb Reconstruction.* Philadelphia: JB Lippincott; 1995.
3. Mathes SJ, Nahai F. *Reconstructive Surgery: Principles, Anatomy, & Technique.* New York: Churchill-Livingston; 1997.
4. Cormack GC, Lamberty, BGH. *The Arterial Anatomy of Skin Flaps,* 2nd ed. London, UK: Churchill Livingston, 1994.
5. Attinger CE, Ducik I, Zelen C. The use of local muscle flaps in foot and ankle reconstruction. *Clin Podiatr Med Surg.* 2000;17(4):681.
6. Grayson ML, Gibbons GW, Balogh K, et al. Probing to bone in infected pedal ulcers: a clinical sign of osteomyelitis in diabetic patients. *JAMA.* 1995;273:721.
7. Morykwas MJ, Argenta LC, Shelton-Brown EI, et al. Vacuum-assisted closure: a new method for wound control and treatment: animal studies and basic foundation. *Ann Plast Surg.* 1997;38(6):553.
8. Scherer LA, Shiver S, Chang M, et al. The vacuum assisted closure device: a method of securing skin grafts and improving graft survival. *Arch Surg.* 2002;137:930.
9. Masqualet AC, Gilbert A. *An Atlas of Flaps in Limb Reconstruction.* Philadelphia: JB Lippincott; 1995.
10. Wrobel JS, Mayfield JA, Reiber GE. Geographic variation of lower-extremity major amputation in individuals with and without diabetes in the Medicare population. *Diabetes Care.* 2001;24(5):860.
11. Vinik AI. Diagnosis and management of diabetic neuropathy. *Clin Geriatr Med.* 1999;15:293.
12. Dellon AL, Keller KM. Computer-assisted quantitative sensory testing in carpal and cubital tunnel syndromes. *Ann Plast Surg.* 1997;38:493.
13. Delon AL. Treatment of symptomatic diabetic neuropathy by surgical decompression of multiple peripheral nerves. *Plast Reconstr Surg.* 1992;89:689.

CHAPTER 72 ■ RECONSTRUCTION OF THE PERINEUM

JEFFREY D. FRIEDMAN

Successful reconstructive surgery is dependent on the restoration of both adequate form and adequate function. These concepts are as important for vaginal and perineal reconstruction as for other parts of the body. The perineal region in both males and females is complex because of the multiple functional systems that lie in close proximity to one another, including the lower urinary tract, the organs of sexual function and reproduction, and the lower gastrointestinal tract, which includes the anus, rectum, and pelvic musculature. Reconstructive procedures in the pelvic region must aim to restore sexual function while maintaining the adequacy of micturition and proper evacuation of the fecal stream.

Deformities of the perineal structures result from both congenital and acquired causes. Congenital deformities occur as a result of failure of müllerian or wolffian development. These disorders of urogenital development result in deformities such as bladder exstrophy, congenital absence of the vagina, and imperforate anus. Numerous other congenital conditions also lead to deformities in this region, such as spina bifida and a variety of gender dysphorias. Acquired defects result from the surgical and medical treatment of gynecologic, urologic, and colorectal malignancies. Although much less common in our experience, traumatic injuries and infectious processes of the perineum and genitalia may also require the need for reconstructive procedures that involve the plastic surgeon.

Although there is considerable overlap between the issues faced when dealing with congenital and acquired deformities, patients with acquired defects tend to present more difficult reconstructive challenges because of the size of the associated defects, as well as the influences of conditions that negatively affect wound healing such as prior radiation therapy, previous operative procedures in the region, diabetes mellitus, atherosclerosis, immunosuppression, smoking, and advanced age. All of these conditions, either alone or in combination, tend to result in altered blood supply to the soft tissues of the pelvic region and result in wound-healing delays. Many of these factors, particularly smoking and arteriosclerosis, limit the options for skin grafts and local tissues and may prevent the use of regional muscle and myocutaneous flaps. As a result, one must assess the local blood supply and have knowledge of the radiation portals and dosages prior to reconstruction.

These issues are also important in secondary reconstruction of patients with congenital anomalies because of the numerous operative procedures that these patients have undergone. Consideration must be given to the location of previous incisions, the possibility of absent or inadequate regional musculature (e.g., bladder exstrophy), and the potential contraction of the associated soft tissues. A careful review of the patient's previous operative procedures and examination of the regional soft tissues is mandatory to avoid errors in flap selection.

GENERAL PRINCIPLES

Adequate function of the structures in the pelvic region is a priority. Aesthetics are generally a secondary concern, but should be addressed if proper function can be simultaneously achieved. For instance, functional vaginal reconstruction must satisfy two essential requirements: (a) sufficient length of the vaginal wall and (b) adequate transverse dimension of the introitus and vaginal pouch. Both of these conditions are necessary for adequate, pain-free sexual function. Scars and linear suture lines preferably are limited to the most proximal area of the vagina so that scar contractures, should they occur, can be treated at the level of the perineum, thereby avoiding the difficulty of operating deep within the vaginal vault. The vaginal lining must be durable in order to withstand the forces associated with intercourse and to prevent the inherent difficulty of treating recurrent open wounds in this region. The need to provide, or in some cases, restore, sensation to the vagina is an issue of less importance. Although sensate flaps can be provided to this area, as long as erogenous sensation is maintained, sensory recovery to the vagina is a lesser concern.

The option of maintaining fertility in these patients is a rare circumstance because the uterus has usually been removed or is insufficiently developed to allow for a term pregnancy. In those rare cases with a functional uterus, however, the uterus and cervix should be incorporated into the reconstruction so that the potential for childbearing can be maintained. Such a situation may occur in patients with congenital deformities and in those patients who were treated at an early age for tumors of the vagina.

Reconstructions in male patients also present requirements that must be met to provide adequate functional return. When considering reconstruction of the phallus, providing adequate length and allowing sufficient skin for unrestricted erections is paramount. As with female patients, the skin must also be durable in order to provide for satisfactory intercourse. Sensation must be re-established in order to allow for erogenous sensibility as well as to avoid the problem of chronic skin breakdown. With regard to scrotal reconstruction, ample skin coverage needs to be established to protect against dessication of the testes. In addition, providing for extraperitoneal positioning of the testes avoids exposure to elevated systemic temperatures that can predispose patients to alterations in spermatogenesis and place the organs at risk for malignant degeneration.

708

FUNCTIONAL RESTORATION OF THE FEMALE PATIENT

Congenital Absence of the Vagina

The most common congenital deformity of the female pelvis is absence of the vagina. This condition, commonly referred to as the Meyer-Rokitansky syndrome, results from maldevelopment of the müllerian duct system, which normally gives rise to a portion of the vagina, the uterus, and fallopian tubes. Most patients have normal ovaries and either an absent or a rudimentary uterus. Thus these patients typically present with absence of the vagina and normal-appearing external genitalia. Clinically, they are phenotypic females with an XX genotype.

The frequency of vaginal agenesis ranges from 1 in 4,000 to 1 in 80,000 live births. There are a number of associated deformities found with Meyer-Rokitansky syndrome, including anomalies of the urinary tract and skeletal system (rib, vertebral). Deformities of the urinary tract are common (25% to 50%) and include duplications, agenesis, and renal ectopy. Preoperative evaluation of the lower urinary tract by either an intravenous pyelogram or an abdominal/pelvic ultrasonogram to delineate the presence of any of these conditions is essential in these patients.

The most important issue with regard to the reconstruction of these patients remains the timing of the initial procedure. Most patients present between the ages of 14 and 16 years with complaints of primary amenorrhea. A simple physical examination with findings of an absent vagina with normal external genitalia, suggest the presence of this syndrome. Once the diagnosis of congenital absence is established and diagnostic work-up completed (karyotype, ultrasonography), discussions with both the patient and family are held so that appropriate planning for the reconstruction can be carried out. These procedures require a mature, motivated patient and, ideally, one who is nearing the age for sexual intercourse. Failure to detect certain levels of immaturity can greatly limit the surgical results and lead to a poorly functional or, in some cases, nonfunctional reconstruction.

There are a number of techniques for reconstruction of the absent vagina. The simplest technique is the so-called Frank method. This procedure uses graduated vaginal dilators that, over time, may slowly lengthen the vaginal canal. In essence, this procedure is simply a form of tissue expansion. Most patients, however, find this to be a painful and often inconvenient method of reconstruction. To achieve suitable vaginal depth, dilations must be performed several times a day and continued over several months to a year. Because of these issues, compliance rates are low and lead to a high failure rate among young women.

A number of surgical procedures have been described to establish a neovagina in these patients. Numerous fasciocutaneous flaps have been described for this purpose, based on the external and internal pudendal vessels. The most common design is the modified neurovascular pudendal thigh flap (Singapore flap) (1). This inferiorly based axial pattern flap is based on the internal pudendal artery and vein located at the base of the flap overlying the adductor musculature. In cases of total vaginal reconstruction, bilateral flaps are necessary to effectively line the neovagina. Unfortunately, the Singapore flap often transfers hair-bearing skin, which may be problematic postoperatively.

Both colonic transfers and small-bowel intestinal flaps have been described for this purpose (2). These procedures are commonly used in pediatric patients and gender reassignment surgery. The purported advantages of these techniques include a low risk of postoperative stricture, adequacy of vaginal length, and improved vaginal lubrication during intercourse. Problems with bowel flaps include the need for laparotomy, risk of future adhesive bowel obstruction, and associated abdominal scarring. In addition, the mucosal discharge that may be advantageous during sexual intercourse may cause dissatisfaction because of the constant discharge and persistent perineal soiling.

The use of split-thickness skin grafts to create the neovagina (McIndoe technique) has advantages over other techniques. The donor-site morbidity is relatively low when a suprapubic donor area is used. This provides significant camouflage for the donor scar and allows for a single-sheet graft to be harvested, which lessens the potential for internal scarring. This procedure does require the prolonged use of a vaginal stent, first inserted to mold the skin graft at the time of the initial procedure. The stent must be used for up to 6 months postoperatively in order to prevent the tendency for unfavorable graft contraction. Failure to maintain this space results in severe narrowing and foreshortening of the reconstruction, and a poorly functional reconstruction.

Local complications with the McIndoe procedure or regional flaps are relatively rare. Delayed wound healing is the most common problem but can be lessened by maintaining patients on bed rest for a week following this procedure. This diminishes the risk for graft motion in the early postoperative period, increasing the likelihood of complete graft take. Unusual complications include injury to the surrounding structures (rectum, bladder), which can occur during the initial dissection of the pocket for the neovagina. For this reason, a bowel prep is usually performed so that should an enterotomy be made, a simple repair can be performed without the need for a diverting colostomy. In many circumstances, working in tandem with an experienced gynecologic surgeon is helpful.

Reconstruction of a neovagina in patients with other congenital conditions is often much more demanding. This is usually a result of the multiple prior operations that these patients have undergone. Patients with bladder exstrophy, imperforate anus, and gender dysmorphias often have multiple abdominal incisions and limited abdominal and pelvic soft tissues to use. In addition, creation of a neovagina may require a transabdominal approach to secure the bowel out of the pelvis, which, in most cases, contraindicates the use of skin grafts for reconstruction. Consequently, muscle flaps (with skin grafts) and myocutaneous flaps are typically used. The gracilis flap and the posterior thigh flap are excellent options in these patients because the lower extremities are typically spared from any form of congenital deformity. Coordination of these procedures with a pediatric surgeon and urologist is essential.

Acquired Defects of the Female Perineum

The most common cause of soft-tissue defects in this region is the treatment of gynecologic, urologic, and colorectal malignancies. These wounds may simply be limited to the perineal surface or, at the opposite extreme, may involve resections of the vagina, bladder, and rectum, along with the entire perineal surface. To achieve both the functional goals and primary wound healing, careful planning of these reconstructions must be done. Specific goals for the procedure include restoration of sexual function, maintaining the ability to void, and maintaining fecal continence. If the possibility of fecal and urinary diversion exists, the use of flaps from the anterior abdominal region should be avoided. Experience demonstrates that in these cases, rectus abdominus myocutaneous flaps often lead to wound-healing complications and ventral hernia formation. As with other reconstructive operations, previous radiation therapy to the perineal structures limits the use of local tissues. Providing healthy, well-vascularized tissue to these radiated areas often improves local wound healing and lessens therapeutic delays.

Surface Defects of the Vulva

Skin defects of the female perineum typically result from the resection of in situ or invasive skin malignancies. Most of these tumors are squamous cell carcinomas that can present as either primary tumors or as recurrent lesions. Primary melanoma is a rare circumstance. Given that these tumors are excised with wide margins, large defects of skin and mucosal structures result.

The majority of these defects can be closed with either skin grafts or local flaps (3). Regional muscle flaps or myocutaneous flaps are rarely needed. Given the laxity of the surrounding skin and subcutaneous tissues, smaller defects can usually be closed primarily. For moderate-size defects, local flaps provide an excellent choice for closure and can be designed in a variety of ways. Rhomboid flaps and laterally based advancement flaps

are the most commonly used. The use of local flaps rather than skin grafts allows for early mobilization of the patient without the need for bulky dressings and the risk of graft separation. Donor-site scarring is also reduced.

Skin grafts are typically reserved for use in large defects, including those in areas that were previously irradiated. Split-thickness skin grafts are typically used and are easily harvested from the suprapubic region. Because of the density of hair follicles in the pubic area, healing is rapid and there is minimal discomfort as the patients do not lie on the donor site. Infiltration of the suprapubic area with tumescent fluid prior to harvest creates an even plane for harvesting these grafts as a single sheet (Fig. 72.1). Full-thickness skin grafts are often used for larger defects that typically involve the entire perineal surface and which cannot be closed with a single split-thickness skin grafts. In such cases, the lower abdominal region serves as an excellent donor site. This is limited by the available redundancy of the lower abdominal skin, which allows the donor site to be closed primarily as an abdominoplasty.

Postoperatively, there are limitations on patients who have been treated with skin grafts. To effectively immobilize the grafts, large bolster dressings are placed and secured with permanent sutures. Maintaining patients on strict bed rest for

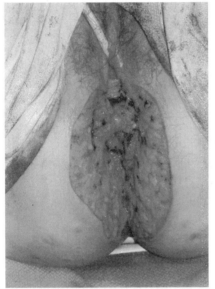

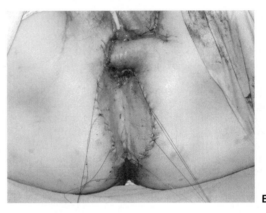

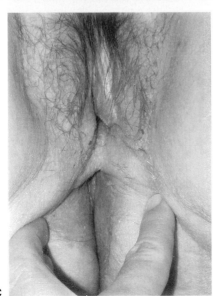

FIGURE 72.1. A: A complex wound of the vagina, rectum, and perineal skin following resection of an advanced squamous cell carcinoma of the perineum. B: Repair using both a local rhomboid flap to separate the rectum from the vagina and a split-thickness skin graft to close the remaining defect. C: Healed wound at 2 months.

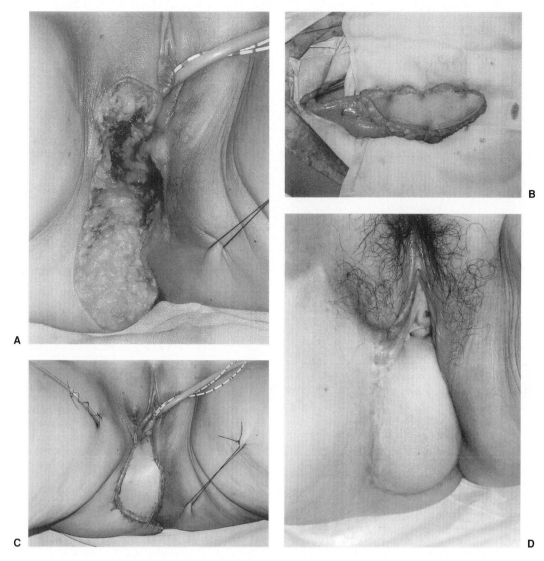

FIGURE 72.2. A 67-year-old woman with recurrent rectal cancer following pelvic irradiation. **A:** Resultant wound following abdominoperineal resection, including the posterior and lateral walls of the vagina. **B:** A vertical rectus abdominus flap prior to transfer to the pelvis. **C:** VRAM skin paddle inset into the defect and **D:** 3-month postoperative result.

periods of up to 1 week is necessary to optimize healing of the grafts. Using a Foley catheter and constipating medications prevents soiling of the bolster dressing. Preventative measures must be taken against deep venous thrombosis. The dressings are removed on postoperative day 7 and local wound care is used to keep the perineum as dry as possible until complete healing occurs.

Acquired Defects of the Vagina

Unlike congenital vaginal defects, acquired defects of the vagina do not lend themselves to the use of skin grafts. A graftable bed is rarely found following ablative procedures. As a result, fasciocutaneous and myocutaneous flaps must be used (4). The decision as to which flaps to use depends on the size of the underlying defect and the presence or absence of previous radiation. In those cases where adjacent organs were removed (rectum, bladder, or both), bulky flaps help prevent the small bowel from descending into the pelvis. Given the number of regional flaps available in this region, free tissue transfers are

rarely needed. Every effort should be made to provide for adequate sexual function; however, there are risks associated with the construction of a neovagina as well as circumstances that preclude the additional operative time. One must be certain, prior to embarking on a complex reconstructive plan, that the patient desires a functional reconstruction. At the extremes of age, or with metastatic or locally advanced tumors, a functional vagina may not be practical and simple wound closure may suffice.

Rectus Abdominus Flap

The rectus abdominus myocutaneous flap remains first choice for partial or total vaginal reconstruction because of the volume of the flap and the generous skin paddle that can be harvested. The skin paddle can be vertically oriented as a vertical rectus abdominis myocutaneous flap (VRAM) or transversely over the lower abdomen (TRAM) (5). Because these resections are performed via a laparotomy incision, the transfer of the flap to the pelvis is simple and in most cases easily reaches the

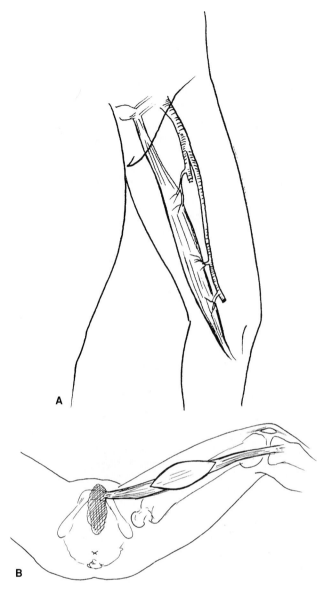

FIGURE 72.3. A: The gracilis muscle has a primary proximal pedicle and several minor pedicles that enter the distal aspect of the muscle. **B:** A myocutaneous flap is designed over the proximal and middle third of the muscle to ensure perfusion to the skin paddle. (From Friedman J, Dinh T, Potochny J. Reconstruction of the perineum. *Semin Surg Oncol.* 2000;19:282, with permission.)

perineal surface. Defects of the anterior or posterior vagina can be closed by insetting the flap along the margins of the wound or, in cases of total vaginal reconstruction, a VRAM can be folded longitudinally and sutured to itself to form an epithelialized cone (Fig. 72.2). The donor site is closed primarily. **Caution should be used when a patient requires both fecal and urinary diversion because in most of these cases, the use of abdominal flaps should be avoided.**

Gracilis Flap and Posterior Thigh Flap

Other flaps have been described for reconstruction of partial or total vaginal defects, including the gracilis muscle and myocutaneous flap, as well as the posterior thigh fasciocutaneous flap. Both transfers are harvested from the thigh region and derive their blood supply from the medial femoral circumflex

and inferior gluteal vessels respectively (Figs. 72.3 and 72.4). Preoperatively, the patient must be examined for the presence of femoral pulses to ensure the patency of these vessels. The posterior thigh flap has the added benefit of being sensate, as it is based on the posterior cutaneous nerve of the thigh, which may be useful in these situations (6). These flaps are particularly useful in cases where a laparotomy is not performed and an isolated perineal approach is used. They avoid the use of the abdomen as a donor site, and may reduce the overall recovery time and donor site morbidity, particularly in obese patients. Certain limitations do exist with these procedures. In general, for total vaginal reconstruction, bilateral flaps are necessary and result in the creation of two donor sites. The skin paddle of the gracilis myocutaneous flap can be unreliable, particularly along the distal third of the muscle. In obese patients, transfer of the muscle and skin paddle to the pelvis may be difficult. In these situations, securing a split-thickness skin graft to each muscle may provide a better option for vaginal lining. The posterior thigh flap provides limited soft-tissue bulk to the pelvis and, in cases where there is a large soft-tissue defect, may prove insufficient for the reconstructive needs of the patient.

FUNCTIONAL RESTORATION OF THE MALE PATIENT

The basic strategies for the male genitalia are similar to those described for female patients. However, the functional and aesthetic goals are quite different because of the specific form and functional requirements unique to the male genital organs. Defects and deformities in these organs result from traumatic injuries or the ablation of malignant processes involving the male genitourinary system and lower gastrointestinal tract. Many tumors, including squamous cell carcinomas of the skin and recurrent malignancies of the anus, require radical excisions of soft tissue. In addition, adjuvant therapy for prostate cancer (external beam or tandem radiation therapy) often produces secondary complications involving the perineal soft tissue such as delayed wound healing and fistulae involving the urethra, bladder, rectum, and perineal skin.

Penile Reconstruction

Efforts to provide functional restoration of the penis require a working knowledge of the physiology of the male phallus (see Chapter 75). Although the overall appearance of the penis is important, form must follow function in order to provide for sufficient outcomes. The essential elements of penile function require the following elements: a phallus of sufficient length to allow for adequate intercourse, appropriate rigidity to provide for penetration, and adequate sensation, both tactile and erogenous, to protect the skin surface and to allow for sexual gratification. All of these requirements must be met to achieve successful functional results.

Defects of the Penile Surface

Surface defects of the penis are common and typically result from traumatic injury or as a complication of circumcision, infection, or excision of squamous cell carcinomas of the penile shaft or glans. When isolated to the skin surface alone, these defects can be treated with skin grafts. Rarely are local flaps or regional transfers necessary. Full-thickness skin grafts or deep split-thickness skin grafts are quite effective in providing durable, expandable skin to this area. Maintaining the grafts in place for at least 1 week is critical to obtaining sufficient take of the grafted skin. Foam dressings that can be sutured in place are useful (Fig. 72.5).

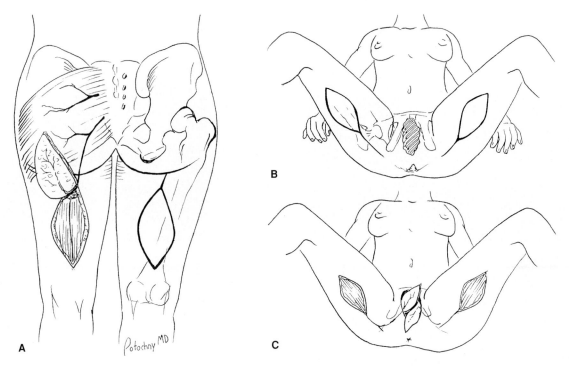

FIGURE 72.4. A: The posterior thigh flap receives its blood supply form the inferior gluteal artery and is designed over the central aspect of the posterior thigh. Bilateral flaps can be raised, tunneled into the perineal defect (**B**), and sutured together to achieve a functional vagina (**C**). (From Friedman J, Dinh T, Potochny J. Reconstruction of the perineum. *Semin Surg Oncol.* 2000;19:282, with permission.)

Secondary deformities of the penis often can be treated in a similar fashion. These problems occur in patients who have significant scarring at the penile base (bladder exstrophy, retraction associated with obesity), which results in positional distortion of the shaft. Contracture release and skin grafting are effective for these problems. Lymphedema of the penile shaft may occur following radiation therapy for carcinoma of the prostate leading to problems of persistent swelling and recurrent infections. Direct excision of the dorsal lymphedematous skin can alleviate this problem. In more severe cases, complete excision of the involved skin and subcutaneous tissue with skin grafting to resurface the entire penile shaft yields good results.

Total Penile Reconstruction

Reconstruction of the entire penis is a much more complex endeavor because of the numerous conditions that must be met to achieve functional and aesthetic results. Consequently, free tissue transfers are often required. Regional flaps often result in a phallus that is insensate or too large to allow for subsequent placement of an inflatable penile prosthesis. Although many free flaps have been described for this purpose (lateral arm flap, fibula osteocutaneous flap), the primary flap of choice is the radial forearm free flap (RFFF) (7). This topic is discussed in detail in Chapter 75.

Scrotal Reconstruction

Most defects of the scrotum are related to either trauma or infection. Although not limited to the scrotal region, Fournier gangrene is an aggressive soft-tissue infection that can lead to significant loss of skin and subcutaneous tissue in the perineal region. This necrotizing infection is most common in patients with attenuated immune systems, including those with diabetes mellitus, poor hygiene, anorectal inflammatory disease, urinary incontinence, and overall debilitated nutritional states. These infections result from mixed aerobic and anaerobic bacteria and require aggressive operative treatment to control. Often multiple debridements are necessary to ensure that all nonviable tissue is removed and a granulation bed suitable for coverage is achieved.

There are two generally accepted methods for scrotal reconstruction and coverage of exposed testes. The most common treatment modality is to simply cover the testicles with a split-thickness skin graft. The testes are typically sutured together in the midline to reduce the surface area of the wound and facilitate closure. Meshed grafts conform to the irregular surfaces of these defects quite well and are favored. Provided there is a well-vascularized recipient bed, graft take is typically 100%. Another technique for coverage of exposed testicles is the use of medial thigh pockets. This involves bilateral subcutaneous elevation of the medial thigh skin and advancing both toward the midline where the two flaps are sutured to each other. The superficial nature of the flaps prevents exposure of the testes to elevated systemic temperatures that can adversely affect spermatogenesis. Clearly, there must be soft tissues of sufficient laxity in the medial thigh for this procedure to be effective. Although this provides effective coverage, the normal contour of the scrotal area is lost and may produce an unusual appearance to this region, which may need to be revised.

Perineal Reconstruction in the Male Patient

Defects in the perineum result from the primary or secondary treatment of rectal or prostate cancers. In the majority of these cases, radiation therapy has either been used as a primary treatment modality or as an adjunct to previous operative extirpation. Consequently, these patients are at high risk for wound-healing complications. This is particularly true in the treatment of acquired fistulas in this region, which can occur following brachytherapy for prostate cancer and commonly occur as a

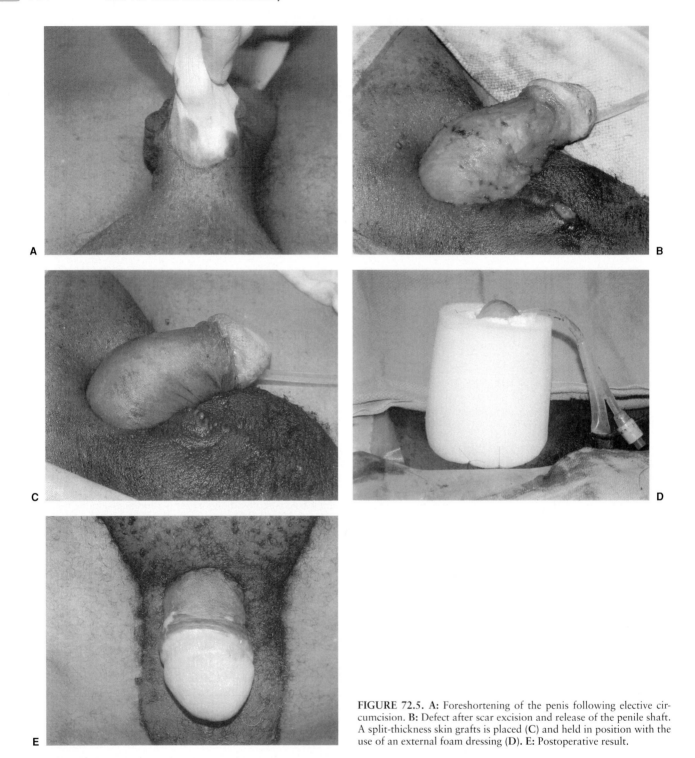

FIGURE 72.5. A: Foreshortening of the penis following elective circumcision. **B:** Defect after scar excision and release of the penile shaft. A split-thickness skin grafts is placed (**C**) and held in position with the use of an external foam dressing (**D**). **E:** Postoperative result.

fistula between the rectum and bladder or as a communication between the prostatic urethra and rectum. Patients typically complain of pneumaturia or of urine leakage from the rectum. Patients who develop local recurrence of rectal cancer are also at high risk for wound-healing problems. Because most of these patients have had previous radiation therapy, providing well-vascularized flaps avoids tension on the closure and is essential to ensuring primary healing of the surgical wound.

In male patients the VRAM flap, gracilis muscle, or myocutaneous flap and the posterior thigh flap remain the workhorse tissue transfers for these defects. Flap selection is based on (a) the amount of soft tissue needed, (b) the adequacy of local blood supply, (c) the presence of surgical scars in the donor region, (d) positioning of the patient during surgery, and (e) the operative approach used (i.e., laparotomy or perineal).

Defects of the Perineum and Pelvic Floor

The majority of patients can be treated using the VRAM flap provided the inferior epigastric pedicle is intact and that no more than one stoma will exit the anterior abdominal wall. This flap is able to fill the pelvis and replace large defects of perineal skin. Thus, the small bowel can be kept out of the pelvis and well-vascularized tissue is provided to facilitate local wound healing. A useful modification of the VRAM flap

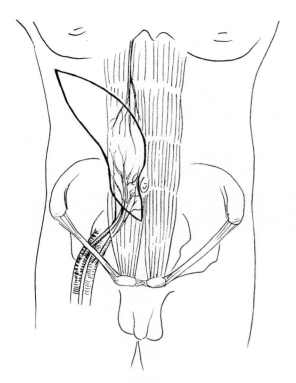

FIGURE 72.6. The extended rectus abdominus myocutaneous flap effectively lengthens the reach of this flap. The skin paddle is based on the periumbilical perforators and extends to the lower costal margin. (From Friedman J, Dinh T, Potochny J. Reconstruction of the perineum. *Semin Surg Oncol.* 2000;19:282, with permission.)

uses an obliquely oriented skin paddle based on the periumbilical perforators (Fig. 72.6). This design lengthens the skin paddle, which greatly increases the reach of the flap into the pelvis. **Because the male pelvis is longer and deeper than that of the female, the additional length provided by this flap ensures sufficient coverage of the wound.** The rectus fascia surrounding the periumbilical perforators is taken while the remaining skin paddle is elevated off the underlying anterior sheath to a point along the costal margin at the anterior axillary line. Donor-site closure is achieved primarily, generally without the need for fascial replacement with prosthetic material.

Should the anterior abdomen be an unsuitable donor area, gracilis myocutaneous flaps are an option. In many cases, unilateral flaps can provide enough soft tissue if the skin paddle is of sufficient volume. **Posterior thigh flaps generally lack the volume necessary to fill large pelvic defects.** In cases where the posterior thigh flap is used, bilateral flaps are generally needed. These procedures, however, are particularly useful in patients who have undergone fecal and urinary diversion. In such cases, a perineal approach can be performed, avoiding the need for laparotomy to gain access to the pelvic wounds. Recovery is rapid and the donor-site scars are quite acceptable.

Acquired Perineal Fistulas

Patients with acquired fistulas in this region are a challenge. As mentioned earlier, the majority of these occur as a result of previous surgery and may be further complicated by the effects of radiation therapy to the surrounding soft tissues. To effectively treat these fistulas, several conditions must be met. First, the fistula tract must be completely excised and the involved structures (rectum, bladder, urethra) must be repaired without tension. This may necessitate the use of interposition skin flaps or mucosal grafts to prevent wound dehiscence and leakage of feces or urine into the wound. **Well-vascularized soft-tissue flaps are interposed to separate the individual repairs from each**

other. This provides greater local blood supply to the area while preventing the surgical repairs from abutting against one another. In most cases, the gracilis muscle flap works very well for these purposes (Fig. 72.7). This is a result of the ease of transfer of this flap to the lower pelvis and the reliability of the muscle, because the medial femoral circumflex vessels are generally outside the local field of radiation.

Special Procedures in the Male Patient

Replantation

Reattachment of the amputated penis is a relatively straightforward procedure provided there has been a sharp, nonavulsive injury to the organ (8). As with other replantation procedures, care of the amputated part is critically important. The organ should be stored in a sterile container and wrapped in a moist, saline-soaked gauze pad. The container is then placed in a plastic bag, or other container, that is filled with ice. As with amputations of other body parts, direct contact should not occur between the amputated part and the ice, otherwise irreversible injury to the penile structures can occur, significantly reducing the possibility of a successful revascularization.

Operative repair begins with debridement of all nonviable soft tissue and dissection of the two dorsal arteries, the dorsal vein, and the two dorsal nerves. The proximal neurovascular structures are then identified. If these vessels are insufficient for microsurgical anastomosis, vein grafts must be considered. A spatulated urethral repair is first performed over a Foley catheter, which provides a stable platform for the remaining repairs. Direct repair of the tunica albuginea of the corporal bodies is then carried out. End-to-end anastomoses are performed for both the dorsal arteries and single dorsal vein. Epineural repairs are performed with 10-0 nylon sutures after suitable nerve endings have been identified and, if necessary, debrided. Vein grafts or nerve grafts are used if there is undue tension on any of the microsurgical repairs. Postoperative care focuses on keeping the amputated part supported with dressings and a scrotal support, avoiding dependent positioning and potential venous hypertension. A Foley catheter is left in place for 2 to 3 weeks to allow healing of the urethral repair and to prevent postoperative stricture formation.

Testicular Autotransplantation

Failure of the testicles to descend into the scrotum predisposes these patients to infertility and increases the risk for testicular malignancies. In most circumstances, the testes can be relocated into the hemiscrotum by using a type of pedicle flap based on testicular perfusion supplied by the vas deferens. There are rare situations in which one or both testes reside high in the abdomen, near the kidney, or within the small-bowel mesentery, which precludes the use of pedicled composite flaps. In these situations, microvascular transfers, or autotransplantation, can be performed to reposition the testes in its appropriate location in the hemiscrotum (9). Although this procedure fails to maintain natural fertility, performing such transfers sustains the hormonal capacity of the testes, avoiding the need for lifelong hormonal replacement. Obviously, the need to perform this procedure is much greater in cases of bilateral cryptorchid testicles than in unilateral cases.

These procedures are ideally performed soon after the diagnosis of high cryptorchid testes is made so as to lessen the negative effects of high intra-abdominal temperatures on the testes. This makes these microsurgical transfers significantly more difficult because of the size of the associated vessels. The autotransplantation procedure allows for transabdominal identification of the testes followed by dissection of the accompanying artery and vein with as long a vascular

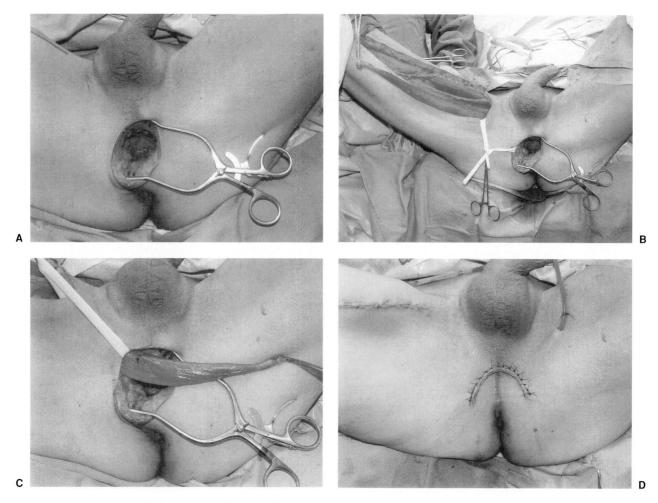

FIGURE 72.7. A 52-year-old male with a recurrent fistula between the rectum and urethra following treatment of prostate cancer with external beam radiation. The fistula tract was excised and both mucosal defects closed primarily (**A**). A gracilis muscle flap was raised (**B**) and transferred to the pelvic defect (**C**) to separate the two repairs and provide greater blood supply to the region. Following wound closure, the fistula did not recur (**D**).

pedicle as possible. Sufficient lengths of vessels can usually be dissected, allowing for primary vascular anastomoses without interposition vein grafts. Recent advances in laparoscopic technique allow harvesting of the testicles without a laparotomy. The laparoscope can also be used to dissect the inferior epigastric vessels off the posterior surface of the rectus abdominus muscle to serve as donor artery and vein for end-to-end microanastomoses. Counter incisions in the inguinal region and base of the hemiscrotum allow the vascular repair and orchidopexy to be performed. Recovery is fairly rapid, although scrotal support is provided for several weeks postoperatively to prevent swelling and for added patient comfort.

Cavernous Nerve Grafting Following Prostatectomy

Radical prostatectomy may require resection of one or both cavernous nerves, which are necessary neural inputs for erectile function. Recently, the concept of interposition sural nerve grafting as a method of maintaining sexual function in these patients has been described. Nerve grafts are performed immediately at the time of the prostatectomy provided that (a) the proximal and distal ends of the cavernous nerves can be identified, (b) the patient has normal preoperative erectile function, and (c) there is no evidence of peripheral neuropathy or a history of radiation therapy. **Although still a controversial**

procedure, some authors have demonstrated a greater rate of spontaneous erectile activity following sural nerve grafting and some patients are able to have unassisted intercourse.

References

1. Wee JT, Joseph VT. A new technique of vaginal reconstruction using neurovascular pudendal-thigh flaps: a preliminary report. *Plast Reconstr Surg.* 1989;83:701.
2. Kim SK, Park JH, Lee KC, et al. Long-term results in patients after rectosigmoid vaginoplasty. *Plast Reconstr Surg.* 2003;112:143.
3. Friedman J, Dinh T, Potochny J. Reconstruction of the perineum. *Semin Surg Oncol.* 2000;19:282.
4. Cordeiro PG, Pusic AL, Disa JJ. A classification system and reconstructive algorithm for acquired vaginal defects. *Plast Reconstr Surg.* 2002;110:1058.
5. Tobin GR, Pursell SH, Day TG Jr. Refinements in vaginal reconstruction using rectus abdominus flaps. *Clin Plast Surg.* 1990;17:705.
6. Hurwitz DJ, Swartz WM, Mathes SJ. The gluteal thigh flap: a reliable, sensate flap for the closure of buttock and perineal wounds. *Plast Reconstr Surg.* 1981;68:521.
7. Chang TS, Hwang WY. Forearm flap in one-stage reconstruction of the penis. *Plast Reconstr Surg.* 1984;74:251.
8. Jordan GH, Gilbert DA. Management of amputation injuries of the male genitalia. *Urol Clin North Am.* 1989;16(2):359.
9. Wacksman J, Billmire DA, Lewis AG, et al. Laparoscopically assisted testicular autotransplantation for management of the intra-abdominal undescended testis. *J Urol.* 1996;152(2 Supple):772.

CHAPTER 73 ■ LYMPHEDEMA

GEORGE H. RUDKIN AND TIMOTHY A. MILLER

Lymphedema is the accumulation of protein-rich interstitial fluid within the skin and subcutaneous tissues that occurs as a result of lymphatic dysfunction. It is estimated that 140 to 200 million cases exist worldwide. Those cases in which the etiology is unknown or that develop as a result of congenital lymphatic dysfunction are termed *primary lymphedema*. All forms of lymphedema that occur as a result of a precipitating cause are referred to as *secondary lymphedema*. **There is no cure for lymphedema; the aim of medical and surgical therapy is to reduce swelling and to prevent complications.**

ETIOLOGY

In primary lymphedema, the disease is thought to be genetically determined, and expression can occur at birth (Milroy disease), puberty (lymphedema praecox), or midlife (lymphedema tarda). In secondary lymphedema, the disease develops as a result of a known inciting event, such as infection or surgical ablation.

However, it is not known why most patients following regional node dissection do not develop lymphedema. A congenital predisposition exists and a spectrum of dysfunction is likely. Patients who are classified as having primary (congenital) lymphedema may, in fact, have a more severe form of lymphatic dysfunction, whereas patients with secondary (acquired) lymphedema develop swelling only after some event further damages already abnormal lymphatics. The capacity for collateral flow and regeneration of damaged lymphatics may vary considerably among patients and may explain whether or not lymphedema develops.

The uncertainties regarding the etiology of primary lymphedema derive from its many unusual, unexplained features: women are afflicted at least three times more often than men and often develop edema around the time of menarche; the left leg is affected more often than the right; and upper extremity involvement is rare.

The most common cause of secondary lymphedema worldwide is direct infestation of lymph nodes by the parasite *Wuchereria bancrofti*. In Western countries, however, damage or removal of regional lymph nodes by surgery, radiation, tumor invasion, or as a result of infection or inflammation are the most common causes of secondary lymphedema. The overall incidence of lymphedema following breast cancer surgery has been reported to be as high as 25%, although severe manifestations are less common. The greatest prevalence of lymphedema occurs among those who undergo extensive axillary surgery followed by axillary radiation. The increasing use of sentinel node biopsy may be diminishing the incidence of this potentially disabling disease (1).

PATHOPHYSIOLOGY

Lymphedema is confined to the subcutaneous compartment; the deep muscle compartments remain uninvolved. Extravasa-

tion of protein-rich fluid occurs when fluid formation exceeds lymphatic transport capacity. The high-protein edema causes shifts in Starling's equilibrium, resulting in the accumulation of more fluid. In time, low oxygen tension, decreased macrophage function, and the presence of increasing amounts of protein-rich fluid give rise to a chronic inflammatory state and consequent fibrosis.

DIAGNOSIS

In the majority of patients, the diagnosis of lymphedema can be made by history and physical examination, excluding alternate causes of edema such as cardiac, renal, hepatic, and venous disease. In true lymphedema, swelling generally begins distally and progresses proximally over months to years. The edema is initially soft and pits easily. It gradually becomes nonpitting as fibrosis develops and the tissue becomes indurated. Skin changes may occur, but ulceration is infrequent. Patients may complain of fatigue or pressure in the extremity, but pain is infrequent. A family history is atypical in lymphedema, but characteristic of lipedema, a lipodystrophy causing symmetric enlargement of the lower extremities, most commonly in females (2).

Imaging techniques may be used in the differential diagnosis and in the assessment of the results of therapy. Lymphoscintigraphy using radiocolloids has been successful in delineating the anatomy of lymph vessels and in evaluating the dynamics of lymph flow. This technique may be useful in planning physiologic forms of surgery. Computed tomography (CT) and magnetic resonance imaging (MRI) are useful to rule out malignancy. Lymphangiography has been largely replaced by these modern techniques.

CLASSIFICATION

Primary lymphedema can be subdivided by age of onset or by lymphangiographic findings. Congenital lymphedema includes all forms of lymphedema present at birth. Milroy disease, a familial sex-linked form of lymphatic aplasia, presents at birth with extremity lymphedema. **The highest incidence of lymphedema, however, occurs during adolescence (lymphedema praecox), accounting for approximately 80% of patients.** The remaining 20% of cases are equally divided between the congenital form and lymphedema tarda, which presents in middle age.

Lymphedema may also be subdivided by lymphangiographic findings. The most common lymphangiographic finding is hypoplasia of the lymphatic vessels. The lymphatics are narrowed and reduced in number. In the hyperplastic pattern (fewer than 10%), the lymphatics are dilated and increased in number owing to obstruction or incompetent valves.

TABLE 73.1

TREATMENT OF LYMPHEDEMA

Medical	Surgical: physiologic	Surgical: excisional
Skin care	Lymphangioplasty	Total skin and subcutaneous excision (Charles procedure)
Elevation	Omental transposition	Buried dermal flap (Thompson procedure)
Compressive garments	Enteromesenteric bridge	Subcutaneous excision beneath flaps (modified Homans procedure)
Pneumatic compression pumps	Lymphovenous anastomoses	
Noninvasive complex lymphedema therapy	Lympholymphatic anastomoses	
Benzopyrenes		
Treatment of infection		

Modified from Rudkin GH, Miller TA. Lymphatic disease: primary lymphedema. In: Ernst CB, Stanley JC, eds. *Current Therapy in Vascular Surgery.* 3rd ed. St. Louis, Mo: Mosby Yearbook; 1995:974 with permission.

MEDICAL MANAGEMENT

The primary treatment for both primary and secondary lymphedema is nonsurgical. Although a variety of therapies are available that may significantly alter the course of disease (Table 73.1), no treatment option is completely and permanently curative. It is imperative that the patient understand the chronicity of the condition as well as the importance of controlling the edema and preventing complications.

Basic skin care is essential in the prevention of infection and may assist in preventing associated skin changes, including dermatitis, hyperkeratosis, and warty verrucosis, as well as breakdown of the epidermis and leakage of lymph fluid (lymphorrhea). Meticulous foot care and daily use of a low-pH, water-based lotion will help to prevent fungal infections of the web spaces. Topical antifungal therapy is recommended for localized fungal infections, but invasive infection may require systemic antifungal therapy. Parasitic infections involving *W. bancrofti* and *Brugia malayi* are initially treated with diethylcarbamazine. Antihistamine and/or anti-inflammatory agents are used to control the allergic reactions to the dying parasite.

Aggressive and prompt treatment of lymphangitis or cellulitis is recommended to prevent development of sepsis. Treatment with a systemic antistaphylococcal and antistreptococcal agent, combined with bed rest and elevation of the affected limb, is suggested. Recurrent lymphangitis or cellulitis occurs in 15% to 25% of patients with lymphedema, and some patients require long-term prophylactic antibiotic therapy.

Diuretics have been used in the treatment of lymphedema, but their effects are short-lived. Benzopyrenes, including coumarin, stimulate macrophage proteolysis and are effective in the treatment of lymphedema of various causes (3). Clinical trials in Europe and Australia have documented improvement in limb volume and skin softness.

Weight reduction and extremity elevation are important simple measures that decrease edema. Patients must elevate the affected extremity at night. This may be accomplished by using a sling for upper extremity edema or elevating the foot of the bed on 4- to 6-inch blocks for edema of the lower extremities. Custom-fitted elastic compressive garments (sleeves or stockings) are often worn during the day to maintain limb volume. The length of the garment should match the extent of disease. A comfortable fit is essential to ensure patient compliance.

Pneumatic compressive machines have been used extensively to treat peripheral lymphedema and are effective if used early in the course of disease, before the development of fibrosclerotic tissue changes. The most advanced pneumatic pumping devices use multicompartmental inflatable sleeves that apply a sequential pattern of compression to the extremity with a pressure gradient, permitting a physiologic distal-to-proximal milking action of the lymphedematous limb. Therapy should be continued at regular intervals, and compressive garments should be worn between treatments. Cardiac failure, active infection, and deep venous thrombosis are contraindications to pump therapy.

Noninvasive complex lymphedema therapy (CLT) consists of manual lymph drainage (massage), compressive bandaging, and physical therapy exercises (4). We have used these treatments in a select group of patients with promising results, but the treatment is time-consuming and labor intensive.

Quantifying the degree of edema is desirable for following the disease and the efficacy of treatment. Although various methods allow assessment of limb volume, including measuring tapes and water displacement, they are cumbersome and prone to error in reproducibility. Having tried several methods, we have found that standardized photography is most helpful in following these patients (5). Photographs are best taken early in the day, to minimize the effect of dependent edema, which typically progresses as the day proceeds.

SURGICAL MANAGEMENT

Surgical intervention should be considered if medical therapy is ineffective in controlling lymphedema or preventing complications. Although numerous surgical procedures for the treatment of lymphedema have been described, none is completely curative. Patients must understand that surgery does not obviate continued medical therapy. **Surgical techniques aim to diminish the size of the affected extremity, with resultant improvement in appearance, function, and prevention of infection.** These procedures may be classified as "excisional" or "physiologic." Physiologic operations attempt to re-establish lymphatic drainage, whereas excisional procedures debulk the limb by removing skin and subcutaneous tissue. Some procedures may have both physiologic and excisional components.

Physiologic Procedures

The concept of reconstructing the lymphatics with microsurgery is an attractive one. Obstructed lymphatics may be drained by surgical anastomosis to either veins or functioning lymphatics. Lymphovenous and lymph node–venous shunts have been performed since the 1960s. In these procedures, a lymphatic vessel or node is anastomosed to a neighboring vein. Lympholymphatic shunts were developed in the 1970s; in these procedures, vein grafts or autologous lymphatic vessels are harvested from a nondiseased extremity and transposed or transplanted to bridge-occluded lymphatics.

Physiologic procedures may be effective for selected patients with localized lymphatic obstruction because of surgery, or cases of primary lymphatic disease demonstrating obstructive patterns. One group has published large studies reporting good results in long-term follow-up (6). In these reports, surgery was found to be most effective when the edema was not advanced or of long-standing duration, or rather before fibrosis developed. It is our experience, however, that patients rarely present to the plastic surgeon before advanced disease is evident. In addition, these techniques are not widely performed in the United States. **Before they can be recommended as a viable alternative to conservative management or excisional surgery, long-term efficacy and anastomotic patency will need to be demonstrated in large studies from more than one center (7).**

Excisional Procedures

Originally described by Charles in 1912, total subcutaneous excision is an extensive procedure that removes virtually all skin, subcutaneous tissue (except in the foot and in the region overlying the calcaneal tendon), and deep fascia, covering the bare muscle with split- or full-thickness skin grafts. Severe secondary skin changes—including ulceration, hyperkeratosis, keloid formation, hyperpigmentation, and a weeping dermatitis—frequently occur, especially if split-thickness grafts are used. This procedure should not be used routinely, but may be an option for patients with severe edema and skin changes (8).

Staged subcutaneous excision beneath flaps was first described by Sistrunk in 1918, and later popularized by Homans. In our opinion, this approach provides the most reasonable surgical compromise as it offers reliable improvement and has a minimum of unfavorable postoperative complications. Improvement is directly related to the amount of skin and subcutaneous tissue removed, as well as the personal care and attitude of each patient. During the operation, as much subcutaneous tissue and skin are removed as possible while attempting to maintain skin flap viability and achieve primary wound healing.

Staged Subcutaneous Excision Beneath Flaps

Absolute bedrest and extremity elevation is instituted 3 days prior to surgery. Edema resolution is often significant, and results in skin laxity, which allows greater amounts of excision. In the current environment of reduced hospital stays, this step is initiated at home, and patients are admitted 24 hours preoperatively. Sequential external pneumatic compression and bladder catheterization are used for those patients with severe edema. A single dose of preoperative antibiotics is administered.

We usually perform this procedure in two stages. A medial resection is performed first, as more tissue can be removed from the medial than from the lateral aspect of both the arm and the leg. If necessary, a lateral procedure is performed 3 months after the initial operation. If bilateral disease is present, the operation may be performed on both involved limbs during the initial procedure, although in cases of massive edema, the prolonged operative time and excessive blood loss mitigates against this approach.

After skin preparation, the leg is exsanguinated and a pneumatic tourniquet is placed as proximally as possible on the affected extremity. A medial incision is made 1-cm posterior to the medial malleolus and extended proximally into the thigh. Anteriorly and posteriorly based flaps of 1.5-cm thickness are elevated to the midsagittal plane in the calf, with less extensive dissection in the thigh and ankle. Subcutaneous tissue beneath the flaps is removed, with care taken to preserve the sural nerve. The deep fascia of the calf is resected, sparing the fascia about the knee and ankle to preserve joint integrity. Redundant skin is resected, and the wound is closed in a single layer with 4-0 nylon over a closed suction drain. The extremity is immobilized in a posterior splint, and the patient is kept at bed rest with the extremity elevated. The drain is typically kept in place for 5 days; sutures are removed on postoperative day 9 and the wound secured by benzoin and tape. The patient is measured for compressive stockings, and extremity dependency is allowed for brief intervals with the extremity tightly wrapped. This regimen is continued for 3 weeks postoperatively. We believe that the use of compression is very important in seroma prevention and in facilitating optimal healing and contour. The lateral procedure is performed 3 months later as indicated. The procedure is essentially the same, with care taken to preserve the superficial peroneal nerve. Figure 73.1 shows the progress of a patient with lymphedema who underwent this procedure.

The arm is prepared as described for the leg. Medial excision is carried out from an incision extending from the distal ulna across the medial epicondyle through the posterior, medial upper arm. Flaps approximately 1-cm thick are elevated to the midsagittal aspect of the forearm and the dissection tapered distally and proximally. The deep fascia is spared. Care is taken to identify and preserve the dorsal sensory branches of the ulnar and radial nerves. If necessary, the tourniquet can be removed to extend the dissection into the axilla. Redundant skin is excised, and the wound is closed over a suction catheter. The postoperative care is similar to that described for the leg.

Results

The senior author has operated on more than 100 patients with lower-extremity lymphedema by staged skin and subcutaneous tissue excisions. Recently, a series of 38 cases was reported with long-term follow-up of between 3 and 17 years (5). Substantial improvement, defined as a significant reduction in extremity size, functional recovery, and reduction in incidence or absence of cellulitis, was seen in at least 75% of patients. With the exception of partial wound separation in one patient and three instances of loss of less than 2 cm of the skin flap, no significant complications were encountered and swelling of the foot was not observed.

However, operative results for postmastectomy lymphedema are much less predictable. In patients with massive swelling, the postoperative improvement is usually significant, and function can often be restored. The results of skin and subcutaneous excision was reported in 14 patients managed over an 11-year period. In 10 patients, the postoperative arm volume was reduced by 250 to 1,200 mL, but four patients noted increased hand swelling postoperatively; arm swelling continued to progress in four other patients despite an initial reduction. **In general, staged skin and subcutaneous tissue**

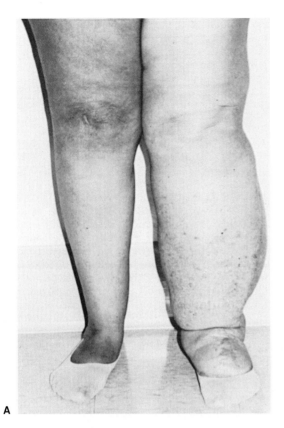
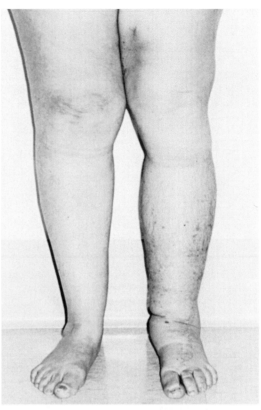

FIGURE 73.1. A: The legs of a 42-year-old woman with lymphedema of 8 years' duration following radical gross dissection. Two dermal flap procedures had been performed 5 years earlier. **B:** The patient's legs 1 year following lateral and medial skin excision and excision of subcutaneous tissue.

excision has not been consistently effective and is not indicated in situations of average postmastectomy lymphedema.

We have found liposuction to be a modestly useful adjunct to excisional procedures in selected cases and most helpful in the thigh. In our experience, the use of this technique alone for the treatment of lymphedema is limited, as the cannula retrieves very little tissue, most likely because of the fibrosclerotic tissue found in chronic lymphedema. One group found the combination of liposuction and compression garments to be effective in the management of postmastectomy lymphedema (9). We have found liposuction to be effective in patients with lipedema (2).

Complications

Recurrent lymphangitis, cellulitis, fibrosis of the subcutaneous tissue, functional impairment, and skin changes have been discussed. Stewart and Treves described the association between postmastectomy lymphedema and lymphangiosarcoma in 1948 (10). The incidence varies between 0.07% and 0.45% (4). This malignant lesion of the lymphatics is almost always associated with chronic lymphedema, most commonly with postmastectomy lymphedema (Stewart-Treves syndrome), but also with filariasis. The lesion has a reddish purple discoloration or nodule and tends to form satellites. It has been confused with Kaposi sarcoma and traumatic ecchymosis. Lymphangiosarcoma generally appears approximately 10 years after the onset of lymphedema and pursues a predictable clinical course with rapid progression and a fatal outcome. The mainstay of therapy has been radical amputation. Average survival is 19 months following initiation of treatment.

CONCLUSION

Lymphedema is a progressive, debilitating, and potentially dangerous condition. The severity of symptoms can vary from mild extremity swelling to serious disabling or life-threatening complications such as recurrent infections and lymphangiosarcoma. Most patients are diagnosed by history and physical examination alone, and may be managed by conservative measures. **Surgical treatment is reserved for cases that are refractory to medical therapy.** Approaches to surgical treatment of lymphedema may be either physiologic or excisional. In our view, the operative procedure that provides the most consistent improvement of lymphedema with the lowest incidence of complications is extensive skin and subcutaneous excision beneath skin flaps. No treatment option is completely and permanently curative of lymphedema. Patients must understand that surgery does not obviate continued medical therapy, and patient cooperation is crucial for successful outcome.

References

1. Golshan M, Martin WJ, Dowlatshahi K. Sentinel lymph node biopsy lowers the rate of lymphedema when compared with standard axillary lymph node dissection. *Am Surg.* 2003;69:209.
2. Rudkin GH, Miller TA. Lipedema: a clinical entity distinct from lymphedema. *Plast Reconstr Surg.* 1994;94:841.
3. Casley-Smith JR, Morgan RG, Piller NB. Treatment of lymphedema of the arms and legs with 5,6-benzo-[alpha]-pyrone. *N Engl J Med.* 1993;329:1158.
4. Boris M, Weindorf S, Lasinski B, et al. Lymphedema reduction by noninvasive complex lymphedema therapy. *Oncology.* 1994;8:95.

5. Miller TA, Wyatt LE, Rudkin GH. Staged skin and subcutaneous excision for lymphedema: a favorable report of long-term results. *Plast Reconstr Surg.* 1998;102:1486.

6. Campisi C, Boccardo F, Zilli A, et al. Peripheral lymphedema: new advances in microsurgical treatment and long-term outcome. *Microsurgery.* 2003;23:522.

7. Gloviczki P. Principles of surgical treatment of chronic lymphoedema. *Int Angiol.* 1999;18:42.

8. Miller TA. Charles procedure for lymphedema: a warning. *Am J Surg.* 1990;139:290.

9. Brorson H, Svensson H. Liposuction combined with controlled compression therapy reduces arm lymphedema more effectively then controlled compression therapy alone. *Plast Reconstr Surg.* 1998;102:1058.

10. Stewart FW, Treves N. Lymphangiosarcoma in postmastectomy lymphedema. *Cancer.* 1948;1:64.

CHAPTER 74 ■ PRESSURE SORES

JOHN D. BAUER, JOHN S. MANCOLL, AND LINDA G. PHILLIPS

Pressure sores are best defined as soft-tissue injuries resulting from unrelieved pressure over a bony prominence. Terms such as *bedsore* or *decubitus ulcer* should be avoided as they suggest all the sores are a result of supine positioning. Although tissue destruction can occur over areas like the sacrum, scalp, shoulders, calves, and heels when a patient is lying down, ischial sores occur in wheelchair-bound patients who are sitting, making "pressure sore" the better term. Relieving the pressure is the key to healing and, more importantly, the key to prevention. Factors such as poor nutrition, incontinence with persistent soilage and moisture, dementia, paralysis, friction, and shear make healing less likely. With so many factors playing a part in pressure sore development, treatment frequently requires input from orthopedic surgery, internal medicine, endocrinology, in-/outpatient nursing, mental health care, and, most importantly, plastic surgery.

The most widely accepted pressure sore staging system was proposed by the National Pressure Sore Advisory Panel Consensus Development Conference, which was held in 1989 (Table 74.1). It divides pressure sores into four groups: stage I with persistent erythema, stage II with dermal injury, stage III with subcutaneous injury, and stage IV with involvement of skin, fat, muscle, and, in the most severe cases, bone. Limitations in this system exist as signs like skin erythema can be present in more than one stage, and dark skin pigmentation can actually obscure the presence of erythema, necessitating other diagnostic signs like increased skin temperature, edema, and induration, to accurately stage the wound. The presence of eschar obscures the severity of the underlying injury, thereby making preoperative staging inaccurate. Furthermore, what is seen on the surface is often merely the *tip of the iceberg*, as confirmed by pressure measurements taken over bony prominences by Le et al. (Fig. 74.1). This system also groups pressure sores with shearing injuries, which can occur in patient transfers, but which have their own characteristics.

EPIDEMIOLOGY

The incidence of pressure sore formation is variable, but the patient populations commonly studied include those in acute care settings, nursing home patients, and paraplegic patients. **In general, approximately 9% of all hospitalized patients develop pressure sores.** The occurrence seen in the acute care setting is as high as 11%. Cited in all studies is the association with other medical problems, including cardiovascular disease (41%), acute neurologic disease (27%), and orthopedic injury (15%). Recently, a large study conducted by Fisher et al. (1) identified key risk factors in acute care pressure sore development using the Braden Scale for Predicting Pressure Sore Risk. These paralleled earlier studies, such as the National Pressure Ulcer Prevalence Survey (1994), and showed age, male gender, impaired sensory perception, moisture, immobility, poor nutrition, and friction/shear as risk factors. With the aging of the population, long-term care has also become a significant focus,

and data from the ongoing National Pressure Ulcer Long Term Care Study suggest that up to 19% of new patients develop a pressure ulcer while in long-term care, and 22% arrive with an existing pressure ulcer. In this study, female gender, age, and cognitive impairment were the key risk factors (2). These data reinforce high rates seen in earlier series, with ranges from 3.5% to 50%.

The incidence in patients with spinal cord injuries varies greatly. Initial reports after World War II recorded pressure sores in up to 85% of patients in the Veteran's Administration's system. Stal et al. cited a 20% incidence in paraplegic patients and a 26% incidence in patients who were quadriplegic (3). A study of large cohort from a statewide Arkansas registry cited significant risk factors in the spinal cord-injured patient, including being underweight, use of pain medications, smoking, suicidal behaviors, history of incarceration, and alcohol and drug use (4).

In terms of pressure sore location, 96% occur below the level of the umbilicus. For the majority of patients, wounds develop in either the supine or seated position. Up to 75% of all pressure sores are located around the pelvic girdle. This is not unexpected, as it mirrors the distribution of pressure in supine and sitting positions (Figs. 74.2 and 74.3).

PATHOPHYSIOLOGY

Compression of soft tissues results in ischemia and, if not relieved, it will progress to necrosis and ulceration, even in well-vascularized areas (Fig. 74.4). In susceptible patients, progression from excessive pressure to irreversible ischemia and tissue necrosis is accelerated by infection, inflammation, edema, and factors that are not yet understood.

Pressure

Landis, in 1930, using a microinjection system, determined that capillary blood pressure in a single capillary ranged from 12 mm Hg on the venous end to 32 mm Hg on the arterial end. **If the external compressive force exceeds capillary bed pressure, capillary perfusion is impaired and ischemia will ensue.** However, this effect is not instantaneous. If it were, we all would suffer from pressure sores. An inverse relationship exists between the amount of pressure and the length of time required to cause ulceration. Early studies demonstrated that pressure of 70 mm Hg applied over 2 hours was sufficient to cause pathologic changes in dogs. Similarly, Daniel et al. demonstrated ischemic changes in a paraplegic pig model (5). They showed that pressure of 500 mm Hg applied for 2 hours, or pressure of 100 mm Hg for 10 hours, was sufficient to cause muscle necrosis. Interestingly, it was not until pressure of 600 mm Hg was applied for 11 hours that ulceration of the skin could be seen. **Not only did these results confirm the relationship between pressure and time, but they also demonstrated that the**

TABLE 74.1

PRESSURE SORE STAGING

Stage	Description
Stage I	Skin intact but reddened for more than 1 hour after relief of pressure
Stage II	Blister or other break in dermis ± infection
Stage III	Subcutaneous destruction into muscle ± infection
Stage IV	Involvement of bone or joint ± infection

initial pathologic changes occurred in the muscle overlying the bone, followed by the more superficial soft tissue, involving the skin last.

Several classic studies investigated pressure and its effects as it relates to location, time, and intensity (Figs. 74.2 and 74.3). In the supine position, the maximal recorded pressures were 40 to 60 mm Hg near the heels, buttock, and sacrum. In the sitting position, pressures were greatest near the ischial tuberosities.

Original dog studies demonstrated an inverse parabolic relationship between the amount of pressure and duration of exposure (Fig. 74.5). Dinsdale confirmed these results in a pig model; perhaps just as importantly, he was also able to demonstrate the absence of injury if pressure could be relieved for as little as 5 minutes, even with pressures as high as 450 mm Hg (6).

Infection

Daniel demonstrated a resistance to ulceration of the skin in his studies in which only pressure and time were altered (7). In the clinical setting, skin involvement occurs with nearly all

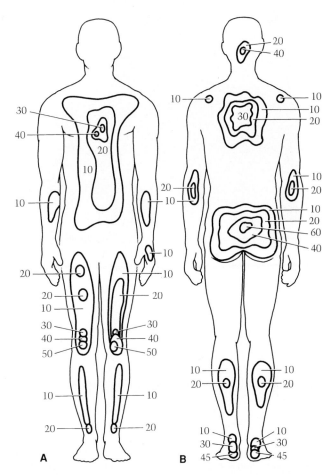

FIGURE 74.2. Distribution of pressures in a normal man. **A:** Prone. **B:** Sitting. (From Lindan O, Greenway RM. Piazza JM. Pressure distribution on the surface of the human body. I. Evaluation in lying and sitting positions using a "bed of springs and nails." *Arch Phys Med Rehabil.* 1965;46:378, with permission.)

pressure sores, suggesting some other relevant factor. As suggested by Nwometh et al. (8), the molecular basis for development of chronic wounds is not clear, although multiple studies now point to an imbalance between matrix metalloproteases (MMPs) and tissue inhibitors of metalloproteases (TIMPs).

It is known that bacterial counts increase in compressed areas. Robson and Krizek quantified the effect of pressure on

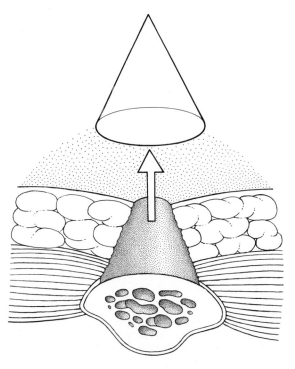

FIGURE 74.1. Cone-shaped pattern of injury resulting from unrelieved pressure. The highest pressure and greatest injury is deep, adjacent to the bone. The cutaneous wound is only the "tip of the iceberg."

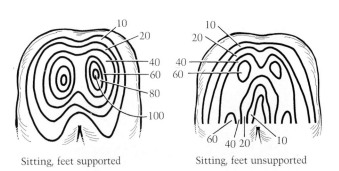

Sitting, feet supported   Sitting, feet unsupported

FIGURE 74.3. Distribution of pressures in a normal man, sitting. (From Lindan O, Greenway RM. Piazza JM. Pressure distribution on the surface of the human body. I. Evaluation in lying and sitting positions using a "bed of springs and nails." *Arch Phys Med Rehabil.* 1965;46:378, with permission.)

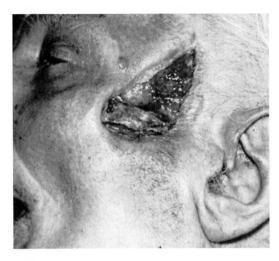

FIGURE 74.4. Pressure sore over the left zygoma in a patient after a cerebrovascular accident.

bacterial count, showing that incisions created in areas of applied pressure and inoculated with known concentrations of organisms allowed for a 100-fold greater bacterial growth than in areas not subjected to pressure. The proposed mechanisms include impaired lymphatic function, ischemia, and impaired immune function.

Inflammation

When tissue is injured, there is a demargination and influx of cells responsible for inflammation. For injuries to heal, a series of events unfolds, including vasoconstriction/vasodilatation, coagulation, influx of proinflammatory cells like neutrophils and macrophages, and, finally, matrix formation/maturation (see Chapter 2). In chronic wounds, there is a breakdown in this sequence, leading to a nonhealing wound. Although this can occur at many levels, intensive investigative efforts have been directed at the balance between a family of proteolytic enzymes known as MMPs, and TIMPs.

In normal wound healing MMPs play an indispensable role in cellular migration by cleaving proteins to clear a path for migrating cells, cleaving intracellular binding proteins, and promoting the release of signaling proteins that promote this migration. Conversely, TIMPs bind to activated proteases to pre-

sumably protect uninvolved matrix and protect cell surface adhesion molecules as the wounds mature. Of specific interest has been the ratio of MMP-1 and MMP-9, to TIMP-1 and TIMP-2. In pressure sores, the ratio of MMP-9:TIMP-1 is higher in chronic pressure sores, and, interestingly, persistently decreases as these wounds heal (9).

Edema

Denervated and compressed skin becomes edematous, which probably plays a significant role in pressure sore formation. As pressure increases, plasma extravasation occurs, leading to edema formation. Further, denervation causes loss of sympathetic tone of the blood vessels, leading to vasodilatation, creating greater engorgement of the vessels, and greater edema. On a molecular level, inflammatory mediators released in response to the trauma of compression can explain edema. The normal homeostasis between prostaglandin F_{2a} (PGF_{2a}) and prostaglandin E_2 (PGE_2) is disrupted in favor of PGE_2, with increased leakage through the cell membranes and increased interstitial fluid accumulation. As interstitial plasma concentrations rise, the concentration of sebum on the skin surface is diluted. Sebum has been shown to be important in the defense against both streptococcal and staphylococcal infections.

PREOPERATIVE CARE

Caring for the pressure sore patient involves more than addressing the wound. Wound healing in chronic wounds requires a systemic strategy, including nutritional assessment and maintenance, control of both systemic and local infection, and pressure and spasm relief. This approach may require input from internal medicine, endocrinology, neurology, urology, nutrition, physical and occupational therapy, and psychiatry, as well as a wound care nurse specialist. Whether the patient is a surgical candidate or not, comprehensive medical care is essential.

Nutrition and Exercise

The nutritional condition of the patient must be evaluated. Normal healing potential exists as long as serum albumin is maintained above 2.0 g/dL. The nutritional literature suggests a requirement of 1.5 to 3.0 g/kg/d of protein to restore lost lean body mass, and 25 to 35 cal/kg of nonprotein calories should be delivered daily. Some evidence suggests that the use of exogenous hormones and resistance exercises may be added to increase both protein synthesis and the anabolic drive. Also important in proper wound healing are vitamins A and C. In addition, zinc is specifically involved with epithelialization and fibroblast proliferation, while calcium is a cofactor for many enzymatic pathways. Ferrous iron and copper are necessary for normal collagen metabolism. Blood levels should be assessed and supplemented as part of the nutritional care. Finally, if oral intake is inadequate, other alimentation, like tube feedings or hyperalimentation, can be delivered.

Infection

Pressure sores may or may not present with local infection. Surgical debridement either at the bedside or operating room is carried out to remove nonviable tissue. A small amount of viable tissue is sent to the microbiology lab for quantitative culture to establish the presence of invasive infection (10^5 organisms per gram of tissue), identify the types of bacteria present, and determine antibiotic sensitivities. Swabbing of the wound is

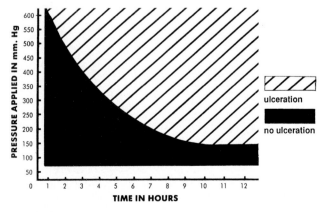

FIGURE 74.5. Inverse relationship between time and pressure in the formation of pressure sores.

discouraged because the specimen may represent only surface contaminants. The use of antibiotics should include topical antimicrobial agents like Dakin solution at 0.025%, silver sulfadiazine, or mafenide acetate, if an eschar exists. Buffered Dakin solution at 0.025% is both bactericidal and nontoxic to cells involved in wound healing. Preoperative systemic antibiotics should cover gram-positive, gram-negative, and anaerobic organisms. The most common organisms cultured from pressure sores are common skin flora *(Staphylococcus, Streptococcus, Corynebacterium)* and enteric organisms *(Proteus, Escherichia coli,* and *Pseudomonas).* Chronic suppressive therapy may be needed to deal with the problem of persistent urinary infections.

Both pulmonary and urinary sources cause seeding and subsequent infection of pressure sores. Indwelling bladder catheters or self-catheterization programs can result in urinary sepsis in one-third of paraplegic patients. If left untreated, urinary infections can be a constant source of bacteremia.

Although all pressure sore patients potentially are at risk for developing pneumonia, acutely ill patients who are bedridden and/or intubated, particularly patients with high spinal cord lesions, are especially susceptible because of poor diaphragmatic function. A program of pulmonary toilet is recommended preoperatively and postoperatively and includes positioning, side-to-side rolling, deep breathing and coughing, chest physical therapy, and bronchodilators.

Relief of Pressure

The initial goal is to avoid any further progression of the sore by relieving the source of pressure, whether the patient is in bed or seated in a wheelchair. Wound healing will not occur in the presence of ischemia or infection.

A simple program of turning the bedridden patient at intervals or intermittently elevating the hips of the patient in a wheelchair will allow for recirculation over bony prominences, and help prevent local ischemia and ulcer formation. As previously stated, Dinsdale demonstrated the ability to counteract the deleterious effects of pressure by relieving it for only 5 minutes every 2 hours (6). In addition, various available mattress and wheelchair padding systems have been designed to relieve pressure, including foam, static flotation, alternating air, low-air-loss pads, and air fluidized beds. The purpose of these systems is to distribute the patient's weight more evenly to minimize pressure in any one area, although the use of these expensive adjuncts does not rule out the need for diligent surveillance.

Spasm

Spasticity is common in patients with spinal cord injuries and is a key contributor in the development of pressure sores, especially as it relates to shear. The incidence varies with the level of injury. The more proximal the lesion, the higher the incidence of spasm: near 100% in the cervical region, 75% in the thoracic region, and 50% in the thoracolumbar region.

Medications available to reduce spasm include Valium, baclofen, and dantrolene. If patients fail to respond to medical therapy, surgical intervention may be required, including peripheral nerve blocks, epidural stimulators, baclofen pumps, and rhizotomy. Rhizotomy, the interruption of spinal roots within the spinal canal, can be surgical or medical, the latter using subarachnoid blocks with phenol (phenol rhizotomy).

Contracture

Bedridden patients, especially those with longstanding denervation and/or altered sensorium, tend to develop joint contractures. They occur because of tightening of both muscles and joint capsules and are common in hip flexors, contributing to the formation of trochanteric, knee, and ankle ulcers. Patients with significant hip and/or knee contractures should have every attempt made to treat the contractures prior to surgery to help prevent recurrence. If physical therapy is unsuccessful at relieving the contractures, tenotomies are performed. In mobile, wheelchair-bound patients, however, releasing the hip contractures can lead to a flail extremity, which may interfere with transfers.

SURGICAL TREATMENT

Debridement

The surgical treatment of pressure sores, like the treatment of any wound, starts with debridement. A dilute solution of methylene blue and hydrogen peroxide can be instilled at the start of the case to help define the cavity and leave a visual guide for excision. After the removal of the necrotic tissue, specimens of viable tissue should be sent for quantitative culture to aid in postoperative systemic and topical antibiotic coverage. Postoperatively, the wound is packed and dressings changed every 6 to 8 hours.

Ostectomy

Removal of the bony prominence is an integral but tricky part of the surgical treatment of pressure sores. Radical ostectomy should be avoided so as to avoid excessive bleeding, skeletal instability, and redistribution of pressure points to adjacent areas. Ischial ulcers best illustrate this as total ischiectomies often result in the formation of a contralateral ischial ulcer. Bilateral ischiectomy has also been proposed, but redistributed pressure has caused perineal ulceration and urethral fistulas. Consequently, removing the minimum amount of bone necessary when debriding ischial pressure ulcers is essential (10).

Pressure Sore Closure

When planning a surgical strategy, the surgeon should consider not only the present surgery, but also the need for subsequent surgical procedures. The choice of closure strategy depends not only on the location, size, and depth of the ulcer, but also on the previous surgeries performed. Primary closure, although tempting, is avoided. These wounds represent an absence of tissue and primary closure leads to tension, a scar over the original bony prominence, and dehiscence. Skin grafting has only a 30% success rate as grafting tends to provide unstable coverage. Musculocutaneous flaps provide blood supply, bulky padding, and are effective in treating infected wounds. Disadvantages include sensitivity to external pressure, functional deformity in ambulatory patients, and lack of bulk in the elderly and in spinal cord patients. Fasciocutaneous flaps offer an adequate blood supply, durable coverage, and minimal potential for a functional deformity, and they more closely reconstruct the normal anatomic arrangement over bony prominences. The disadvantages include limited bulk for the treatment of large ulcers.

Ischial Defects

Ischial pressure sores occur in patients who are in the seated position. These patients tend to have a high recurrence rate, as they almost always return to sitting postoperatively. Conway and Griffith reported on the treatment of 100 ischial pressure sores. Regardless of the type of treatment received (nonoperative or operative), the recurrence rate was 75% to 77%. The advent of improved wheelchair cushions has surely lowered this rate, but recurrence remains a problem.

Figure 74.6 details some of the flap closure strategies. As can be seen with the medially based thigh flap and the gluteus maximus myocutaneous flap, closure can be accomplished with either fasciocutaneous or musculocutaneous flaps. The design should allow coverage of the ulcer but should not prevent the use of other flaps in the future. Additional considerations when designing a flap to close ulcers in this region include the size and depth of the ulcer, quality and pliability of the surrounding skin, presence of previous surgical scars, and the ambulatory status of the patient. The inferior gluteal musculocutaneous flap, based on the inferior gluteal artery, uses only the lower half of the gluteus maximus muscle. This rotation flap does not preclude later use of the posterior thigh flap and is less debilitating in ambulatory patients. In the superiorly based gluteal flap (Fig. 74.7), care is taken to avoid incisions over bony prominences when the patient is in the seated position. The biceps femoris, semimembranosus, and semitendinosus musculocutaneous flaps are said to be effective for ischial ulcers and they can be re-advanced. They are most reliably designed as a V-Y pattern, but do have several disadvantages, including closure is always under tension, the scar is directly over the maximal pressure point, and hip flexion tends to cause dehiscence. The tensor fascia lata (TFL) flap can occasionally be used to close ischial ulcers, although the distal aspect of the TFL flap is usually too thin to offer adequate padding, making the TFL flap, in general, not the best choice. For more complex, deeper, or larger wounds, a combination of flaps may need to be employed.

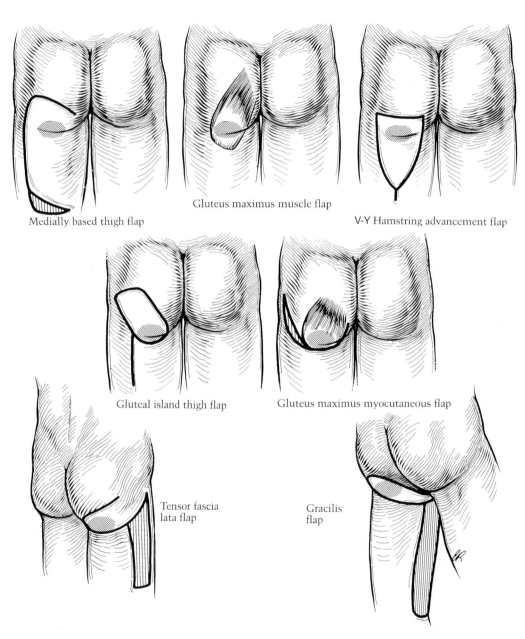

Medially based thigh flap

Gluteus maximus muscle flap

V-Y Hamstring advancement flap

Gluteal island thigh flap

Gluteus maximus myocutaneous flap

Tensor fascia lata flap

Gracilis flap

FIGURE 74.6. Flaps for closure of ischial wounds.

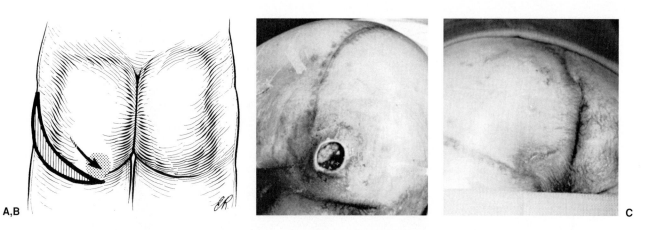

FIGURE 74.7. A: Superiorly based gluteus maximus myocutaneous flap for closure of ischial defect. **B:** Defect. **C:** Late result healed.

Sacral Defects

Sacral pressure sores occur in patients in the supine position. As with ischial defects, musculocutaneous or fasciocutaneous flaps are the mainstays of surgical therapy (Fig. 74.8). One of the first fasciocutaneous flaps was a rotational flap described by Conway and Griffith. In their series of 34 patients, only 16% developed a recurrence. The most commonly described musculocutaneous flaps are based on the gluteus maximus muscle. The gluteal flap can be based superiorly or inferiorly, part or all of the muscle or both muscles may be used, it can be constructed of muscle or muscle and skin, and it may be rotated, advanced, or turned over. Other flaps available include the transverse and vertical lumbosacral flap, based on lumbar-perforating vessels, although these have significantly less bulk and, consequently, are less useful in deeper wounds.

Trochanteric Defects

Trochanteric ulcers develop in patients who lie in the lateral position, especially in those who have significant hip flexion contractures. The most commonly used flap for treatment of this location is the TFL flap (Fig. 74.9). This highly reliable flap is based on the perforating vessels from the tensor fasciae latae muscle, although caution is advised as the distal aspect of the flap has a random blood supply that sometimes necessitates a delay procedure. Sensation from the nerve roots of L1, L2,

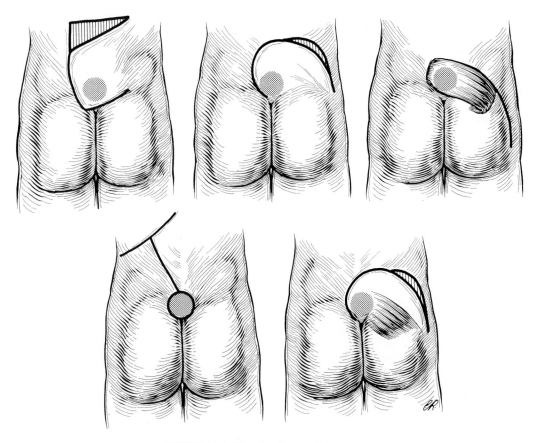

FIGURE 74.8. Flaps for closure of the sacrum.

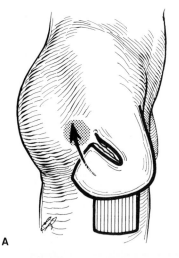

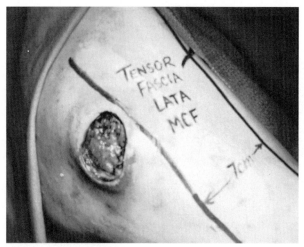

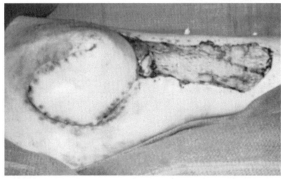

FIGURE 74.9. A: Rotation of tensor fascia lata (TFL) myocutaneous flap. **B:** Defect of trochanter. **C:** TFL flap rotated, donor site skin grafted.

and L3 by the lateral femoral cutaneous nerve makes this a potentially sensate flap in patients with spinal cord injury below L3, representing more than 60% of meningomyelocele patients (11). Rotation of the TFL flap results in a T-shaped junction between the flap and the closed donor site and this area is prone to dehiscence.

Other Considerations

In patients who have multiple pressure sores or who have undergone multiple previous procedures, there may not be any local options remaining. In extreme cases, it may be necessary to consider total thigh flaps in which the femur is removed and the thigh tissue is used to close the wound.

POSTOPERATIVE CARE

Nutrition, medical (for spasm, diabetes, hypertension), psychological, and rehabilitative care continues as required. Careful nursing care is critical to postoperative success. The patients are positioned to avoid pressure on the operative site, with turning every 2 hours, and use of low-air-loss mattresses when available. An absorptive nonocclusive dressing is used in an effort to avoid macerating the wound. The control of urine and stool is important and in the most difficult cases colostomies are required. Drains are placed intraoperatively to remove serous fluid and to aid in apposition of the flaps to the wound bed. Because of probable intraoperative bacteremia, broad-spectrum antibiotic therapy is continued during the perioperative period.

The antibiotics are modified to fit the sensitivity results of intraoperative cultures as these results become available. Patients are kept in the postoperative position, with no pressure allowed on the surgical site for 2 to 3 weeks. It is at this point that most patients have progressed enough to allow weight bearing on the affected site. The process is usually started for 15- to 30-minute intervals and progresses to 2 hours after 6 weeks.

COMPLICATIONS

In addition to the acute complications related to treating pressure sores—hemorrhage, pulmonary and cardiac complications, and infection—a few long-term complications warrant discussion.

Recurrence

The reasons for the high rates of recurrence are multifactorial. The underlying medical problems that contributed to ulcer formation still exist. The presence of spinal cord injury and altered mentation in the elderly persist. The labor-intensive nursing care issues (turning, local wound care, avoidance of urine and fecal contamination) may not have changed from the preoperative setting. Social issues, like the lack of financial resources, inadequate family and/or community support, and the use of drugs and alcohol, may also be present. In short, unless the predisposing factors can be modified (e.g., alter behavior, eliminate spasm, release contractures), there is no reason to provide surgical treatment to an otherwise clean wound (12).

Carcinoma

In 1828, Jean Nicholas Marjolin described a tumor that was present in a chronic wound. However, it was Dupuytren who noted it was a malignancy. **The term *Marjolin ulcer* is used to describe carcinoma arising in a chronic wound.** The most common cell type is squamous cell carcinoma. In contrast to most other tumors of this type, these tumors tend to be aggressive with 2-year survival rates varying from 66% to 80%. Their metastatic rate, as compared to that of Marjolin ulcers arising in burn scars, is significantly higher at 61% versus 34%. The time interval of development is also reduced. The usual time to appearance is 25 years as compared to more than 30 years in burn-related carcinomas, but it can be as short as 2 years. Because of the aggressive nature of the disease, wide surgical excision to clear margins is recommended. Prophylactic lymph node dissection is not recommended, but therapeutic node dissection is indicated in the case of clinically involved nodes. Adjuvant radiation and/or chemotherapy may be indicated in cases of unresectable tumors or if the patient refuses surgery.

NONSURGICAL TREATMENT

The ultimate treatment of pressure ulcers is not necessarily surgical correction. If proper preoperative assessment and preparation are performed, there will usually be a period of time in which the ulcers can be observed. If during this time period the ulcer appears to be healing significantly, continuation of non-operative treatment is indicated. Some patients may never be candidates for surgical correction because of significant medical problems. In these cases, avoidance of unrelieved pressure, control of infection (local and remote), control of incontinence, and improved nutrition may lead to successful ulcer closure, or at least may allow for a stable wound that does not progress.

In some patients, ulcer closure may be accelerated by the use of topical agents other than antibiotics. Robson and Phillips (13) have demonstrated improved healing in ulcers treated with recombinant human platelet-derived growth factor BB and basic fibroblast growth factor. Although the use of growth factors has been shown to improve wound healing, their widespread use has been limited to date. As the cost and accessibility of these agents improves, they may provide an option not available to most patients today. Papaine-urea-derived debridement ointments have been in use since the 1950s and continue to be a valuable tool. Recently, vacuum-assisted closure devices have been used for decreasing the size of these ulcers. Although it shows promise, the presence of liquids like urine and feces, as well as the irregular surface in the area, make application a challenge (14).

In recent years, there has been an explosion of wound-care products available for the nonsurgical treatment of this disease process. As a result, many health care professionals now choose to treat these ulcers by themselves rather than consult a reconstructive surgeon. The practice patterns of health care professionals whose patients require treatment for pressure sores were reviewed and showed that less than 25% of the cases receive consultation by a surgeon (15). The study demonstrated that 82% of the patients' ulcers either had no change or the ulcer actually increased in size during hospitalization. This study underscores the importance of surgical input in the proper care of pressure sores. Even if nonsurgical treatment is chosen, the expertise of the reconstructive surgeon in guiding this form of therapy is critical.

References

1. Fisher AR, Wells G, Harrison MB. Factors associated with pressure ulcers in adults in acute care hospitals. *Adv Skin Wound Care.* 2004;17:80.
2. Horn S D, Bender SA, Bergstrom N, et al. Description of the National Pressure Ulcer Long-Term Care Study. *J Am Geriatr Soc.* 2002;50:1816.
3. Stal S, Serure A, Donovan W, et al. The perioperative management of the patient with pressure sores. *Ann Plast Surg.* 1983;11:347.
4. Krause JS, Vines CL, Farley TL, et al. An exploratory study of pressure ulcers after spinal cord injury: relationship to protective behaviors and risk factors. *Arch Phys Med Rehabil.* 2001;82:107.
5. Daniel RK, Wheatley DC, Priest DL. Pressure sores and paraplegia: an experimental model. *Ann Plast Surg.* 1985;15:41.
6. Dinsdale SM. Decubitus ulcers: role of pressure and friction in causation. *Arch Phys Med Rehabil.* 1974;55:147.
7. Daniel RK, Terzis JK, Cunningham DM. Sensory skin flaps for coverage of pressure sores in paraplegic patients. A preliminary report. *Plast Reconstr Surg.* 1976;58:317.
8. Nwomeh BC, Yager DR, Cohen IK. Physiology of the chronic wound. *Clin Plast Surg.* 1998;25:341.
9. Ladwig GP, Robson MC, Liu R, et al. Ratios of activated matrix metalloproteinase-9 to tissue inhibitor of matrix metalloproteinase-1 in wound fluids are inversely correlated with healing of pressure ulcers. *Wound Repair Regen.* 2002;10:26.
10. Vasconez LO, Schneider WJ, Jurkiewicz MJ. Pressure sores. *Curr Probl Surg.* 1977;14:1.
11. Dibbell DG, McCraw JB, Edstrom LE. Providing useful and protective sensibility to the sitting area in patients with meningomyelocele. *Plast Reconstr Surg.* 1979;64:796.
12. Evans G R, Dufresne CR, Manson PN. Surgical correction of pressure ulcers in an urban center: is it efficacious? *Adv Wound Care* 1994;7:40.
13. Phillips LG, Robson MC. Pathobiology and treatment of pressure ulcerations. In: Jurkiewicz MJ, ed. *Plastic Surgery, Principles and Practice.* St. Louis, Mo: Mosby; 1990: 1223.
14. Greer SE, Duthie E, Cartolano B, et al. Techniques for applying subatmospheric pressure dressing to wounds in difficult regions of anatomy. *J Wound Ostomy Continence Nurs* 1999;26:250.
15. Isenberg JS, Ozuner G, Restifo RJ. The natural history of pressure sores in a community hospital environment. *Ann Plast Surg.* 1995;35:361.

CHAPTER 75 ■ RECONSTRUCTION OF THE PENIS

J. JORIS HAGE

INDICATIONS AND REQUIREMENTS

Reconstruction or de novo construction of the penis may be indicated to treat genital ambiguity, to relieve gender dysphoria in female-to-male transsexuals, or to make up for accidental or (self-) inflicted traumatic loss, oncologic amputation, or infection of the penis.

Genital Ambiguity

Although masculinization can be extreme in newborns presenting with ambiguous genitalia, genetic females recognized in the neonatal period should be raised as girls as it is easier to adapt the genitalia toward the female phenotype (1). Although feminine assignment is probably better than condemning a male patient to a life with an inadequate phallus, it is not necessary to assign the female gender to all such male infants. Three important factors are taken into consideration when deciding on the more appropriate gender for a genetic male newborn with ambiguous genitalia.

First, a urologist and a reconstructive surgeon assess the urogenital anatomy to define the surgical procedures that would be required to construct functional male external genitalia (1,2). Testosterone may be administered to assess the likelihood of penile growth, thus excluding androgen insensitivity and possibly facilitating genital reconstruction (1). Second, the pattern of pubertal change that can be expected at the time of adolescence must be considered. A male role is especially preferable if a male infant has an enzymatic error preventing synthesis of testosterone, because testicular architecture is usually normal. Hence, an endocrinologist evaluates the hormonal status of each patient. Third, a behavioral scientist assesses the social and cultural background of the newborn and the views of the parents on the most appropriate sex for their child. Unbiased sexual orientation is enhanced if the parents show no ambivalence concerning the chosen sex (2).

The above considerations apply only to the newborn. When the diagnosis is initially established in an older child or young adult, all measures should be directed toward restoring the concordance of the phenotype with the sex of rearing (1,3,4). Moreover, there are those in whom no (complete) surgical correction was undertaken even though a proper diagnosis had been made early in life. Complete endocrinologic and urogenital assessment is routine prior to the initiation of reconstructive surgery for such disorders, whether they appear in pediatric, adolescent, or adult cases. Therefore, treatment of genital ambiguity disorders is preferably restricted to multidisciplinary teams capable of well-balanced individualized recommendations for each patient.

Gender Dysphoria

The same principles apply to the treatment of female-to-male transsexuals. Driven by the persistent and unchangeable need to eliminate the difference between the physical reality of the body and gender of the mind, transsexuals seek to adapt their bodies as optimally as possible to the sex they feel they belong to. For the reconstructive surgeon, the key issue prior to considering gender-confirming surgery is to establish beyond reasonable doubt that the transsexual feeling is genuine. The diagnosis of gender dysphoria and the determination of whether sex reassignment surgery is warranted is primarily the task of a behavioral scientist. In addition, appropriate assessment of medical conditions and the effects of the hormonal treatment on liver and other organ systems should be accomplished preoperatively by an endocrinologist. Hence, all specialists involved preferably collaborate closely as members of a gender team (5).

Penile Loss

In male patients with penile loss as a result of amputation or infection, consultation with a psychologist prior to any reconstructive procedures may prevent postoperative disappointment and frustration. In cases where the testes were also lost, the input of an endocrinologist is required and, again, a multidisciplinary approach is preferred.

SURGICAL TECHNIQUES

Reconstruction or construction of the penis should ideally aim at (a) a reproducible one-stage procedure; (b) creation of a competent neourethra to allow urination while standing; (c) return of both tactile and erogenous sensibility in the phallus; (d) sufficient bulk to tolerate the insertion of a prosthetic stiffener; and (e) a result that is aesthetically acceptable to the patient. Additionally, the ideal procedure also requires (f) minimal scarring or disfigurement and (g) no functional loss in the donor area (6).

Correction of Genital Ambiguity

In cases where a decision for male gender assignment has been reached in a child with a small but complete micropenis, several surgical techniques to mobilize the cavernous corpora from the pubic rami, to accentuate the penoscrotal junction, and to reduce the pubic fat may be chosen in order to make the small phallus appear more prominent (2). Gonadal tissue that is inconsistent with the male sex should be removed. Following masculine assignment in a truly intersex patient, genital

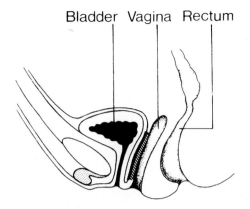
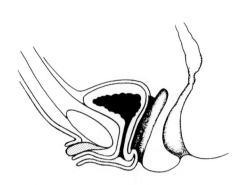

Bladder Vagina Rectum

FIGURE 75.1. In metaidoioplasty, the clitoris is partially released and stretched to become a phallus and the urethra is lengthened to the tip of the phallus using an anterior musculomucosal vaginal flap. (From Hage JJ. Metaidoioplasty—an alternative phalloplasty technique in transsexuals. *Plast Reconstr Surg.* 1996;97:161, with permission.)

correction is similar to that of severe hypospadias. Complete chordectomy is performed to mobilize the cavernous corpora and the urethra is lengthened to bring the perineal urethral orifice to the tip of the glans. Moreover, the ventral aspect of the glans is reconstructed to give it a normal appearance. This can often be accomplished in a single stage with the neourethra being constructed proximally from the midportion of a bifid scrotum meeting a distal rotated vascularized skin flap from the hooded foreskin. If necessary, a thick nonhirsute skin graft can be used to bridge a gap of any length. The prepenile, or "shawl," scrotum that drapes around the base of the penis can be transposed caudally at a later stage and testicular implants may be inserted (1).

Metaidoioplasty

The techniques mentioned above compare to metaidoioplasty, in which a penile substitution with clitoral enlargement and urethral transfer is performed in female-to-male transsexuals (7). The term metaidoioplasty is derived from the Greek, and *meta-* is the prefix denoting the concept of after, or subsequent to; *aidoio* is an archaic combining form relating to the genitals; and *-plasty* is the suffix derived from plastos (formed, shaped) meaning shaping. Indeed, androgen intake may stimulate the growth of the clitoris to the point where this organ can suffice as a phallus. The clitoris is partially released and stretched by resection of the ventral chordae and the urethra is lengthened to reach the tip of this phallus' glans (Fig. 75.1). Although metaidoioplasty is performed according to the principles of hypospadias surgery, the female external genitalia actually has more tissue available for surgical construction of a male phallus than a severe hypospadias patient has available. An overdeveloped clitoris may be distinguished from an underdeveloped penis by the frenulum on the ventral surface of the phallus. In normal males there is only a single midline frenulum, whereas in normal females there are two frenula, each lateral to the midline. Furthermore, in the female clitoris, the so-called chordae holding down the clitoris represent the conjoined continuation of both labial spongiosus corpora toward the glans clitoris rather than solely fibrous strands. The major labia are anterior in position to the scrotum and are "transposed" in relation to the penis (1). The minor labia correspond to the nonfused pendulous urethra and ventral penis covering, whereas the female urethral orifice is comparable to the perineal hypospadias situation.

During the single-stage metaidoioplasty, a caudally based, pedicled musculomucosal flap is raised from the anterior vaginal wall (7,8). The length of this flap is devised in such a way that it will reach beyond the base of the clitoris with a width of about 3 cm. The base of its pedicle envelopes the dorsal half of the perineal urethral orifice. This vaginal flap will serve as the lining of the fixed perineal part of the neourethra. It provides

the urethral angle at the level of the perineal female external orifice with the extra reinforcement needed to prevent fistulation of the urine jet. Subsequently, the vestibular skin between meatus and glans clitoris is incised in a W-like fashion to allow for the release of the clitoral shaft (Fig. 75.2A). Both medial vestibular skin incisions are to be continuous with the parallel incisions on the anterior aspect of the vaginal wall. One lateral upward limb of this W is extended toward the future urethral orifice at the tip of the glans clitoris, while the other limb is extended laterally and upward to include the medial surface of the minor labium. For this, the medial and lateral surfaces of the latter labium are separated and a medially pedicled vestibular-labial skin flap of at least 3 cm width is fashioned. The midline vestibular skin is undermined toward the glans, hence exposing the spongiosus tissue and chordae (Fig. 75.2B). These structures are resected inbetween both crura so as to bare the ventral aspect of both corpora cavernosa. After the phallus is stretched in this way, the vaginal mucosa flap and the vestibular-labial skin flap are rolled on to the catheter and sutured in a watertight fashion (Fig. 75.2C). These flaps are anastomosed in an oblique, or even an interdigital, fashion so as to avoid stricture. To cover and strengthen the neourethra thus created, the medial aspect of the left minor labium is de-epithelialized and sutured to cover the pendulous part of the neourethra in such a way that the labial flap suture line does not overlie the urethral suture line. The lateral surface of the right labium is used to cover the fixed perineal part of the neourethra. Finally, the ventral edge of this labial skin flap is sutured to the dorsal edge of the left labial skin flap (Fig. 75.2D). In most patients the metaidoioplasty is combined with the construction of a bifid scrotum in which testicular prostheses are implanted, hence effecting the dorsal transposition of the major labia by bilateral V-Y advancement.

This technique allows the base of the clitoris to be anteriorly advanced for approximately 3 cm (7,8). If provided with a sufficiently lengthened urethra the clitoris-penoid will act as a normal and complete penis, albeit a small one hardly capable of sexual penetration. In cases where the clitoris seems to be large enough to provide a phallus that will satisfy the patient, this one-stage procedure is the method of choice.

Phalloplasty

Alternatively, efforts may also be made to construct a phallus de novo. The relevant differences between the female and male urogenital anatomy represent the surgical goals for phalloplasty in female-to-male transsexuals (Fig. 75.3). The internal genitalia are superfluous but the urethra requires lengthening, and some sort of phallus with a urethra has to be added. Because the male scrotum has abundant skin as compared to the female major labia, the labial skin requires augmentation and

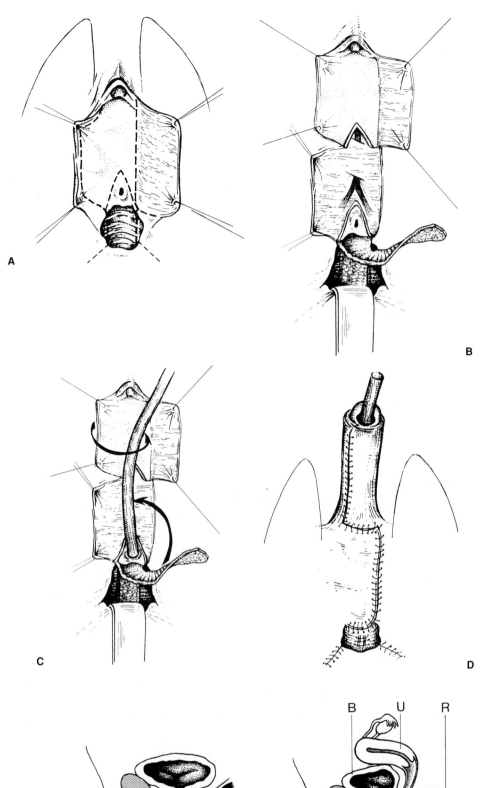

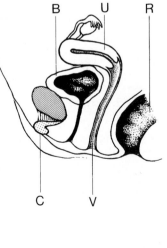

FIGURE 75.2. A: To allow for the release of the clitoral shaft and to secure neourethral lining and cover, the vestibular skin between meatus and glans clitoris is incised in a W-like fashion. **B:** The midline vestibular skin is undermined toward the glans thereby exposing the spongiosus tissue and chordae. These structures are resected to bare the ventral aspect of both cavernous corpora. **C:** After the phallus is stretched, the vaginal mucosa and vestibular skin flaps are rolled onto the catheter and sutured in a watertight fashion. Both flaps are anastomosed in a beveled fashion to prevent strictures. **D:** To strengthen the neourethra thus created, the medial aspect of the left minor labium is de-epithelialized and sutured to cover the pendulous part of the neourethra. The lateral surface of the right minor labium is used to cover the perineal fixed part of the neourethra. (From Hage JJ. Metaidoioplasty—an alternative phalloplasty technique in transsexuals. *Plast Reconstr Surg.* 1996;97:161, with permission.)

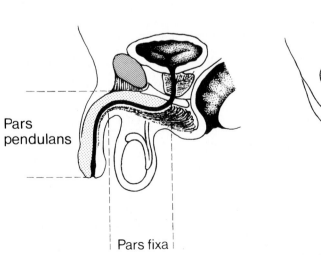

FIGURE 75.3. The relevant differences between female and male representing the surgical goals for phalloplasty in transsexual patients, involve the superfluous female internal genitalia like the vagina (*V*) and uterus and ovaries (*U*). Conversely, the female body is short of erectile tissues (*C*), testes, and sufficient scrotal skin. Furthermore, in female-to-male surgery, the urethra should be lengthened (*B*, bladder and urethra; *R*, rectum).

the insertion of testicular prostheses. Female erectile tissues are much less developed than their male counterparts and they are ideally replaced by an implant in female-to-male transsexuals. Phalloplasty in female-to-male transsexuals can seldom be achieved in one stage because of the need to create a competent neourethra allowing a urine stream to break cleanly from the tip of the newly constructed phallus (6). Urethral construction in a properly situated phallus involves fitting the phallus with the pendular part of the urinary conduit, and also advancing the original female urinary orifice to a more anterior position. Advancement up to the base of the clitoris may be accomplished by construction of the perineal part of the neourethra using a flap raised from the anterior vaginal wall (6,9). Construction of this fixed part is performed separately from phalloplasty, but may be combined with the hysterectomy. Other surgeons construct this pars fixa using an extra-long urethral part of the flap used for phalloplasty or, even, free grafts (10).

A variety of techniques have been used for the actual phalloplasty, and most are also applicable in men who have sustained loss of their penis. In these latter patients, the loss is often partial, necessitating the reconstruction of the extracorporal, or pendulous, part of the penis only.

The development of techniques for phalloplasty has paralleled the evolution of plastic surgery (11). Following randomly vascularized skin flaps, axial skin flaps depending on one or more well-defined vascular pedicles were recognized and used for phalloplasty. Subsequently, myocutaneous pedicled flaps were introduced. Use of these flaps has some advantages but obvious scarring of the donor site is inevitable and, as in most pedicled skin flaps, no sensibility is obtained in these myocutaneous flaps. Nevertheless, phalloplasty techniques currently applied still include the superficial inferior epigastric skin flap, the extended groin skin flap, the rectus abdominis myocutaneous flap, and the tensor fascia lata myocutaneous flap (11). Of these pedicled flaps, the extended groin flap has the fewest drawbacks and has the least donor site disfigurement (3). Because no sensibility in the phallus is to be expected, however, no stiffeners can be used in any pedicled flap. Consequently, I regard these to be techniques with few indications for phalloplasty.

Although the ideal requirements of phalloplasty have not all been met by any single technique, microsurgical free flap techniques lead to superior functional and aesthetic results. To construct the pendulous or phallic part of the neourethra, the technique of a roll-in-a-roll is frequently used (6,10). Alternatively, the neourethra may be preconstructed by burial of a full-thickness skin graft in the flap to be used for the phalloplasty at a later stage (12,13). Using free flaps, it is possible to provide the phallus with protective sensibility by coapting one of the dorsal clitoral or inguinal nerves to a cutaneous nerve in the flap (6). Because no erogenous phallic sensibility is to be expected in the neophallus, the second dorsal clitoral nerve should be left unharmed. Phallic sensibility is a condition sine qua non for the use of implants or transplants and, hence, rigidity techniques should only be performed after free flap phalloplasty. Because a constant rigid phallus may serve as a source of embarrassment to the patient, inflatable hydraulic prostheses are preferred (6,14). Because such prostheses demonstrate mechanical failure, however, some authorities have their patients use external devices for erection, whereas others fully rely on edema, scar fibrosis, or congestion to give sufficient rigidity. Apart from the need to give the perineum a scrotumlike appearance, aesthetic considerations require the construction of a glanslike tip of the neophallus. The Norfolk technique of coronal ridge and sulcus construction leads to superior results when a circumcised appearance is desired (6). Triangular flaps at the distal end of the flap give the phallus a conic glans and a sagittally slitted aspect of the urethral orifice and prevent meatal stricture (Fig. 75.4). As surgical techniques further develop, combinations of pedicled and free flaps, or even of two

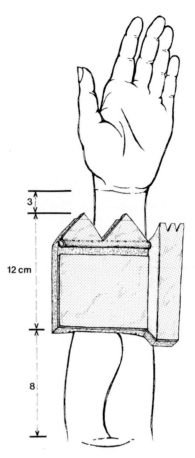

FIGURE 75.4. Design of a forearm free flap allowing the construction of the phallic part of the neourethra by the tube-within-a-tube roll technique. The 2.5-cm narrow ulnar skin strip is tubed outside-in to become the neourethra. Next to this strip, the flap is de-epithelialized over a width of 1 cm. This allows for the wider radial skin flap to be tubed and sutured in a watertight fashion over the urethral part to become the outer aspect of the phallus. Proximally, the urethral skin flap is extended 1 cm beyond the outer radial flap to reinforce the anastomosis between this phallic part of the neourethra and its fixed perineal part. Triangular flaps at the distal end of the flap give the phallus a conic glans and a sagittally slitted aspect of the urethral orifice and prevent meatal stricture. A distally based circumferential skin flap is dissected to be sutured to its own base in order to form the coronal ridge. Its donor site is covered with a split-thickness skin graft to mimic the coronal sulcus. A, artery; N, nerve; V, vein. (From Hage JJ, de Graaf FH. Addressing the ideal requirements by free flap phalloplasty: some reflections on refinements of technique. *Microsurgery.* 1993;14:592, with permission.)

free flaps, are applied (15). Such sophisticated methods do not always lead to better results. Microsurgical techniques further allow the surgeon to choose the flap's donor site from all over the body. As such, the choice includes the most frequently used radial forearm flap (10), the ulnar forearm flap (4), the lateral upper arm flap (12), and the fibula flap (13). The donor site may be chosen in such a way as to prevent obvious scarring. Still, laborious techniques such as pretransfer tissue expansion and posttransfer correction of the donor site may be indicated. Consequently, the quest for other free flap donor sites to be used for phalloplasty continues.

COMMENTS

In cases of severe micropenis or genital ambiguity the main question for the reconstructive surgeon concerns what the fate of the presented organ will be—can it be made any bigger or should gender reassignment be contemplated (1,2). A useful objective criterion for function is the ability to void standing up through an opened fly. It is surprising how short a penis can be used to accomplish this task, especially if a boy is given adequate instruction and trousers with adequate openings (2). The same applies for male amputees and for female-to-male transsexuals who had a metaidoioplasty: a very small penis is compatible with the normal male role. Thus the prospect of a very small penis should not, on its own, be an indication for assignment to the female gender or phalloplasty (2).

Although a small phallus may perform normal urination, it is more difficult to get away with an abnormal appearance. Little boys are very conscious of their genitalia and only a few men with a micropenis will feel confident to change clothes or shower in public. No operation has yet been devised to predictably make the corpora of the truly small penis longer, but the techniques for phalloplasty used for female-to-male gender confirmation can be applied to male adults. The disadvantage in infants is that the constructed phallus may not grow (3,4). Now that neophailic sensibility and possible rigidity may be secured, these techniques may be appropriate for the adult male patient with a small but sexually sensitive penis or penile stump. Still, the plethora of techniques for penile construction suggests that none is ideal and neophalloplasty remains one of the most challenging procedures in reconstructive surgery.

References

1. Donahoe PK, Schnitzer JJ. Evaluation of the infant who has ambiguous genitalia, and principles of operative management. *Semin Pediatr Surg.* 1996;5:30.

2. Woodhouse CRJ. Problems of intersex, gender identity and micropenis. In: Woodhouse CRJ, ed. *Long-Term Pediatric Urology.* London: Blackwell; 1991:176.

3. Perovic S. Phalloplasty in children and adolescents using the extended pedicle island groin flap. *J Urol.* 1995;154:848.

4. Gilbert DA, Jordan GH, Schlossberg SM, et al. Forearm free flap for pediatric phallic reconstruction. In: Ehrlich RM, Alter GJ, eds. *Reconstructive and Plastic Surgery of the External Genitalia—Adult and Pediatric.* Philadelphia: Saunders; 1999: 327.

5. Meyer WM III, Bockting WO, Cohen-Kettenis P, et al. The Harry Benjamin International Gender Dysphoria Association's standards of care for gender identity disorders, sixth version. *J Psychol Hum Sexual.* 2001; 13:1.

6. Hage JJ, de Graaf FH. Addressing the ideal requirements by free flap phalloplasty: some reflections on refinements of technique. *Microsurgery.* 1993;14:592.

7. Hage JJ. Metaidoioplasty—an alternative phalloplasty technique in transsexuals. *Plast Reconstr Surg.* 1996;97:161.

8. Perovic SV, Djordjevic ML. Metaidioplasty: a variant of phalloplasty in female transsexuals. *BJU Int.* 2003;92:981.

9. Chesson RR, Gilbert DA, Jordan GH, et al. The role of colpocleisis with urethral lengthening in transsexual phalloplasty. *Am J Obstet Gynecol.* 1996;175:1443.

10. Gottlieb LJ, Levine LA. A new design for the radial forearm free-flap phallic reconstruction. *Plast Reconstr Surg.* 1993;92:276.

11. Hage JJ, Bloem JJAM, Suliman HM. Review of the literature on techniques for phalloplasty with emphasis on the applicability in female-to-male transsexuals. *J Urol.* 1993;150:1093.

12. Khouri RK, Young VL, Casoli VM. Long-term results of total penile reconstruction with a prefabricated lateral arm free flap. *J Urol.* 1998;160: 383.

13. Hage JJ, Winters HAH, van Lieshout J. Fibula free flap phalloplasty: modifications and recommendations. *Microsurgery.* 1996;17:358.

14. Hoebeke P, de Cuypere G, Ceulemans P, et al. Obtaining rigidity in total phalloplasty: experience with 35 patients. *J Urol.* 2003;169:221.

15. Laub DR, Laub DR Jr, Hentz RV, et al. The post-modern phalloplasty: forearm flap urethroplasty with superficial external pudendal artery-abdominal tube pedicle flap. In: Ehrlich RM, Alter GJ, eds. *Reconstructive and Plastic Surgery of the External Genitalia—Adult and Pediatric.* Philadelphia: Saunders; 1999:335.

CHAPTER 76 ■ PLASTIC SURGEONS AND THE DEVELOPMENT OF HAND SURGERY

J. WILLIAM LITTLER

Our primitive pentadactylate hand is a structure with finely articulated cantilever digits radiating from a fixed semicircular carpal base, arranged and endowed for prehension by precision movement, strength, and sensibility—so perfect in design, that little change or specialization (unlike the foot) was needed for compliance and adaptability to the creativity so essential in human cultural development. Its form embodies not only the physical characteristics of geometry repeated in nature, but with its movement and tactility, a spatial stereognostic sense as well.

The hand can be rugged and its palmar coniferous skin durable, yet its vulnerability to diverse intrinsic or acquired disorders often requires the highest and most ingenious surgical skill for correction. Specialty attention is essential, and it is here that plastic surgeons have served well the structural, functional, and aesthetic requirements of this guided instrument of instruments. Basic principles of tissue care set forth by John Hilton in his lectures on "Rest and Pain" (1863) have withstood the test of time (1). Hilton, a distinguished anatomist and surgeon, stated that "where possible, a guiding principle of wound treatment is immobilization. This perceptive work was considered so important that nearly a century later Frederic Wood-Jones declared, "... (it) should be read by every medical student during his medical career (2)."

ANATOMIC UNDERSTANDING AND ITS ILLUSTRATION

The mastery of hand anatomy and function is the absolute basis of diagnosis and treatment. As understanding evolved, the importance of illustration for clarification and dissemination of that knowledge also developed.

Sir Charles Bell (1774–1842), the hand's most articulate advocate, was a Scot from Edinburgh and later London. His (4th) Bridgewater Treatise, *The Hand—Its Mechanism and Endowments as Evincing Design* (1834), is dedicated to a philosophic and predarwinian comparative anatomic survey that expresses the hand as an agent of ingenuity with reliance on guidance for adaptation as its principal characteristic (3).

Duchenne's exhaustive *Physiology of Motion* (1867) remains fundamental and includes a superior fundamental presentation of the hand's intrinsic musculature, selectively illustrated by engraving (4).

The fine art of anatomic illustration began with the Renaissance master, Leonardo da Vinci (1452–1519). His dissections and dissertations on the human body, astute observations, and remarkably accurate drawings in all probability inspired the young Belgian anatomist Andreas Versalius (1514–1564), whose dissections in Padua were published as *De Corporis Humani Fabrica* in 1543, when he was 29 years of age. They were dramatically illustrated by his countryman Jan Van Cal-

car, who was a student of Titian. This treatise broke the millennial Galenic tradition. *Praktische Anatomie* (1935) by T. von Lanz and W. Wachsmuth of Wurzburg was one of the most thorough and elegant anatomic presentations of the upper limb in the 20th century.

M.F. Landsmeer of Leydon (5) made an exhaustive analysis of the dynamic aspects of retinacular components serving the finger extensor system (1955), which aided surgical correction of finger deformities and malformations. Artistic illustration of structural and functional concepts are indispensable, as textual descriptions alone become obscure if not incomprehensible. **Of all anatomic dissertations related to the hand, however, a single volume, *The Principles of Anatomy as Seen in the Hand* (first edition 1920) by Frederic Wood-Jones holds unique status (2). It is still unsurpassed for lucidity of text and illustrations and is most rewarding as a foundation for residents and fellows of hand surgery programs.**

In 1981, anatomic studies stimulated by evolving surgical procedures incited fresh dissections by Robert Beasley and his colleagues (6). These are informative, special for their clarity and accuracy, and ideal for surgical training because of their rendering in lifelike color by master anatomic illustrator Leon Dorn.

EVOLUTION OF HAND SPECIALIZATION

At the turn of the 19th century, major advances were being made in general surgery but only limited attention was paid to the disabled hand. Principles of care were lacking; surgical intervention was unpredictable and often complicated by infection. Allen Kanavel of Chicago (1912) clarified the digital synovial tendon sheaths and palmar spaces with descriptions of nondisabling incisions for the draining of infections. He also exemplified the research-oriented surgeon by contributing to the clinical care of other hand disorders beyond infections.

Progress was occurring elsewhere, notably in Germany, where special attention was given to amputated thumbs. Carl Nicoladone (1849–1903) of Vienna and Gratz, but of Italian ancestry, was a pioneer who focused on the thumb (1891) and development of hand surgery. He applied the Tagliacozzi (1598)-type pedicle flap for thumb coverage, originating osteoplastic thumb reconstruction, as it is known today. This talented surgeon not only did tendon transfers, but he used the pedicle flap concept of Tagliacozzi for the transfer of a second toe for thumb reconstruction in three cases. However, keeping the hand and foot attached during transfer was fraught with difficulties.

In France, an interest in thumb reconstruction had been kindled. Ipsilateral finger transfer for thumb reconstruction was favored by Guermonprez (1887) and later championed

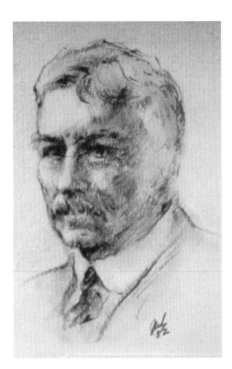

FIGURE 76.1. George H. Monks (1853–1933). An American pioneer of unprecedented ability in the early development of plastic surgery. (Illustration by J. William Littler.)

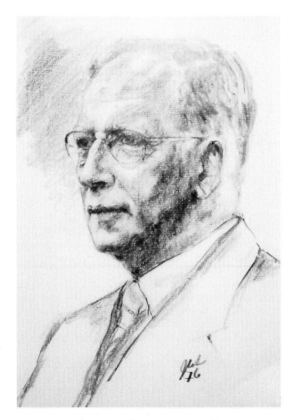

FIGURE 76.2. Sterling Bunnell (1882–1957), whose vast experience and presence in the Army General Hospital Hand Centers, and whose 1944 edition of *Surgery of the Hand* during World War II were critical to the development and establishment of hand surgery as a major specialty. (Illustration by J. William Littler.)

by Marc Iselin (1937) and Jean Gosset (1949). Gosset was one of the first to use the neurovascular pedicle technique for index finger transposition.

According to Goldwyn (7), a glimpse of the future came at the turn of the 20th century from a report by George Monks of Boston (Fig. 76.1). It concerned the isolation of a composite tissue island from the forehead on a single superficial temporal arteriovenous pedicle, passed subcutaneously and used to resurface a lower eyelid. The elegance of the procedure complimented Monks, its brilliant innovator, who was one of America's first plastic surgeons.

About 1897, John Murphy of Chicago turned his interest to vessel anastomosing and to the critical problem of severed nerves and tendons in the hand and wrists. Murphy's work was followed by that of Guthrie whose text, *Blood Vessel Surgery and Applications*, was published in 1912. This work had attracted Alexis Carrel to Chicago and he continued the study of vascular repairs for which he was awarded a Nobel Prize in 1929.

The Chicago hand group continued to provide leadership. Sumner Koch who had gained both interest and experience in World War I, was joined by the research-oriented Michael Mason and Harvey Allen. They laid out the scientific basis for successful tendon repairs. At the same time, in England, Sir Herbert Seddon was establishing the scientific basis for nerve repairs and grafting.

THE WORLD WAR II ERA

Concentrated effort always accelerates medical progress and most often occurs during wars. This has been especially true for the repair of hands. World War II was a medically historic event with improved transport, free use of blood transfusions, and other advances resulting in the survival of great numbers of battle casualties who became healthy but physically handicapped, especially from upper limb injuries. Surgery of the hand moved dramatically from wound closure and the drainage of infection to reparative surgery with ever-increasing momentum

and recognition of its importance. The first book in English dealing principally with the repairs of hands was *The Hand, Its Diseases and Disabilities* (1942) by Condict Cutler of New York. Dr. Sterling Bunnell (Fig. 76.2) followed this with his monumental book, *Surgery of the Hand* (1944) (8). He served as civilian consultant to the Secretary of War (now Department of Defense) with the directive to "guide, integrate, and develop the special field of hand surgery."

Perhaps the greatest credit for the surge of improvement in the care of injured hands during World Was II should go to Surgeon General Norman Kirk, an orthopedist by training and a wise and open-minded chief. General Kirk's directive for dealing with serious hand injuries reflects great insight. First, he stated that hand injuries could not be given adequate care in a battle zone and therefore should be evacuated back to the "Zone of Interior," meaning the United States proper. Second, he stated that care of this small and complex part required regional specialization, one surgeon mastering and integrating into treatment the appropriate aspects of traditional plastic, orthopedic, and neurologic surgery. **Third, centers for hand surgery should be organized, but not as separate services, and because soft-tissue management was the greatest determinate of treatment outcome, the centers should be developed within existing Plastic Surgical Services of General Hospitals, and where needed, he would assign additional orthopedic or neurologic surgeons to augment the plastic surgical staffs.**

By the end of World War II, nine hand centers had been established in the military hospitals. The first was at Cushing General Hospital near Boston, where I served (Fig. 76.3), which became the model for developing others. The regional reorganization allowed a concentration of interest, crossing traditional lines for discovery, and giving relevance to significant background work that was lying dormant or previously had been

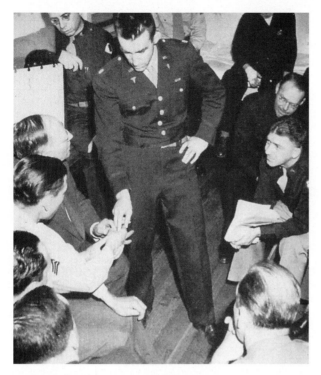

FIGURE 76.3. With Dr. Bunnell (seated at my right hand) discussing an ulnar nerve problem with hand surgery staff at the Cushing General Hospital, 1946.

passed over casually. There developed a cadre of new regional specialists—the hand surgeon. Despite the jealous clinging to territorial boundaries, the concept of regional specialization established in World War II for hands is the organizational pattern of most surgical specialties today.

Because of space constraints, only a few of the many achievements of the World War II are mentioned here.

Isolation and Transfer of Single Functional Units

The poor prognosis and unpredictable regeneration following nerve repairs focused increased attention on elective transfer of intact muscle–tendon units for paralytic deficits, which were found to be useful despite sensory impairments. Loss of thumb opposition attracted particular attention. Ideas were revived, developed, and refined. E. Huber of Germany and J. Nicolaysen of Norway concurrently (1921) had introduced radial transposition of the abductor digiti quinti muscle, isolated on intact neurovascular pedicles, to the thenar area to restore thumb opposition.

This concept of a muscle isolated on its neurovascular pedicle for transfer was precursory to the development of today's many arterialized (axial) cutaneous and myocutaneous composite tissue flaps. Brash's publication in England of *Neurovascular Hila of Limb Muscles* (1945) was timely, and provided much of the basic support for microvascular free tissue transfers done today as part of many reconstructive operations.

Thumb Reconstructions

Recognition by Colonel Radford Tanzer and others of the special problems of thumb loss led to a perusal of many papers on the subject. The results of past efforts were not encouraging, either functionally or aesthetically. This, in itself, stimulated greater determination for the development of more re-

fined methods during and after World War II, culminating in finger transposition on intact neurovascular pedicles. This allowed proper length and mobility for strategic positioning, while incisional design accuracy for both donor and recipient sites resulted in adequate interdigital commissures. Development of the neurovascular pedicle finger transposition procedure for thumb reconstruction in America was coincidental to that of Jean Gosset in France and Otto Hilgenfeldt in Germany.

Axial-Based Flaps

Shaw, of the Jerome Webster plastic surgical program, and Payne published their vanguard paper, *One Stage Tubed Abdominal Flaps*(1946). They used the superficial inferior epigastric artery and vein for a central vascular circuit. This reliable and versatile "axial" flap displayed clarity of concept and simplicity of application to qualify it as a "milestone" in the progress of reconstructive surgery. The concept later was of prime importance in development of free composite tissue transfers by microvascular direct anastomosis.

THE POST-WORLD WAR II ERA

The surgical experiences of World War II produced a sizable cadre of hand surgeons who eventually became available for civilian service. Hand surgery had emerged and the potentials and advantages of regional specialization had been established. After the war, this group of military hand surgeons founded the American Society for Surgery of the Hand (ASSH) (1945) with Dr. Bunnell as its first president. Of the 35 founding members of the ASSH, 14 were general surgeons, 13 were plastic surgeons, and 8 were orthopedic surgeons. For more than 50 years the ASSH has provided a prime forum for the specialty and has been notable for its continued educational activities.

In 1970, a second American national organization for surgery of the hand, the American Association for Surgery of the Hand, was organized in response to an exploding interest. The prime movers in the formation of this organization also had plastic surgery backgrounds.

Professional societies for surgery of the hand are now thriving in most countries today, and recognition is given to the indefatigable French plastic surgeon Raoul Tubiana (Fig. 76.4), who has given direction and help to many of these societies. His editing and bringing to reality the five-volume magnum opus, *The Hand* (1995) (9), reflects an incomparable dedication and contribution to the specialty.

With only a short reprieve from World War II, the Korean War broke out (1950) and the lessons learned from World War II were applied on an appropriately smaller scale, with the reconstructive center at Valley Forge General Hospital being the primary hand surgery center. I was privileged to serve as civilian consultant for these efforts, as Dr. Bunnell had done in World War II.

The postwar era was also a period of development of in-depth, high-quality graduate teaching courses. It was the time when Robert Chase, working with plastic surgeon William White of Pittsburgh (1960), developed the epic film "Functional Anatomy of the Forearm and Hand," which has served such a multitude of students and surgeons as to attain classic status. Of the graduate continuing education programs that developed, notable courses were those on the hand, which were given at New York University by Dr. Robert Beasley and in Pittsburgh by Dr. William White, both having general and plastic surgery backgrounds.

The postwar era was also a time of renewed interest and efforts to apply basic science to surgery, most notably to tendon

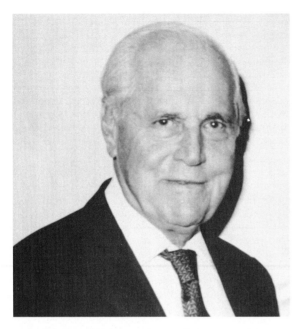

FIGURE 76.4. Raoul Tubiana (1917–), whose tenacity over 25 years has given hand surgeons five volumes of comprehensive subject matter comparable to the earlier great work of Duke-Elder on the eye.

surgery. The discouraging tenets of flexor tendon repairs finally gave way to the recognition that tendons have intrathecal healing capabilities. More important were the technical refinements made. Verdan of Switzerland at a Plastic Surgical Meeting in 1958 reported disregard for the traditional "no-man's land" and unprecedented success for primary repair of severed digital flexor tendons. These results were confirmed by Kleinert and reported at the ASSH in 1967 (10), with results so good as to be doubted by some at the time. Progressively flexor tendon grafting gave way to primary repairs, and one's success with flexor tendon grafting as the measure of competence as a hand surgeon was swept away.

In a similar manner, more sophisticated research was applied to the problems of small-vessel repair and better nerve junctures. Because the Tagliacozzi method of tissue transfers is restricted by their pedicle attachments to the donor site, freedom from this restraint had been a primary goal for decades. A new era was heralded when Jacobson (1960) demonstrated successful small-vessel anastomosis using magnification with refined instruments and supersmall sutures. Successful repair of digital vessels in a thumb by Kleinert in 1963 (11) was a landmark event, leading to the regular reunion of completely severed digits. It was exhilarating to discover that composite tissues could be reliably transferred by direct vessel anastomosis, unrestrained by pedicle attachments. In 1979, plastic surgeon Buncke of San Francisco did the first free transfer of a primate toe to thumb (12). Plastic surgeons O'Brien and Morrison in Australia, John Cobett in the United Kingdom, Viktor Meyer in Switzerland, and others set new standards for microsurgical skills.

It is obligatory for the hand surgeon to know and to use the basic elements of muscle physiology in the restoration of functional losses secondary to paralysis. The basic principles were well established in World War II. In 1979, Robert Beasley presented to the American Association of Plastic Surgeons a uniquely successful plan for restoring hand function for C5–C6 spinal cord injured. His procedure optimally uses the remaining four functioning muscles distal to the elbow for an unequaled efficient and biomechanically sound reconstruction for this severe impairment.

Manktelow, a plastic surgeon in Toronto, with McKee have presented impressive examples of the value of free muscle transfers by direct vessel anastomosis and nerve repairs (13).

CONGENITAL MISHAPS

Few matters dismay the surgeon and family more than realization of surgical limitations in what can be done for the child with a developmental defect, and no greater elation is experienced than by a meaningful correction. Again, there have been many contributors to this, but two plastic surgeons deserve special recognition for leadership in this field: Joseph Upton of Boston and Dieter Buck-Gromko of Hamburg.

Also, with the ever-increasing awareness of the significance of disfigurement to one's psychological composure and socio-economic well being, the potential help from modern prostheses, alone or in conjunction with surgical reconstructions, has come to be recognized. Extremely high quality is essential and much credit goes to Genevieve deBese of New York, whose unrelenting pursuit of excellence has set standards for hand prostheses.

REFLECTIONS

The importance of the hand to the well-being of every individual is self-evident and the hand's variable afflictions offer an unlimited opportunity, through originality of thought and ingenuity, for correction by surgical reconstruction. Proficiency in the assessment of what parts can be saved within the injured hand and how they can best be redistributed for maximal usefulness fall within the traditional concepts of plastic surgeons and is a salient attribute of all experienced hand surgeons of all primary backgrounds.

It is equally evident that the high quality of care increasingly available today is the product of innumerable contributors but could never have been achieved without regional specialization. The hand surgeons were leaders in what has become the modern organization of essentially all surgical specialties.

From this brief overview of the evolution of reparative hand surgery to the standards now achieved, plastic surgeons can appreciate and justly take pride in the prime and often pivotal role their forerunners and colleagues have played.

Manus Mani, Homo Hominis

References

1. Hilton J. *Rest and Pain*. London: Royal College of Surgeons; 1863.
2. Wood-Jones F. *The Principles of Anatomy as Seen in the Hand*. Philadelphia: Blakeson and Son; 1920.
3. Bell C. *The Hand—Its Mechanisms and Vital Endowments as Evidencing Design*. London: William Pickering; 1834.
4. Duchenne GB. *Physiology of Motion*. Paris: Bailliene; 1867. Translated to English by Kaplan E, translator. Philadelphia: Lippincott; 1959.
5. Landsmeer JM. Anatomical and functional investigation of the articulations of human fingers. *Acta Anat Suppl*. 1955;24:2511.
6. Beasley RW, et al. Surgical anatomy of the hand. In: *Hand Injuries*. Philadelphia: WB Saunders; 1981.
7. Goldwyn R, Monks GH.*J Plast Reconstr Surg*. 1971;48:478.
8. Bunnell S. *Surgery of the Hand*. Philadelphia: Lippincott; 1944.
9. Tubiana R. *The Hand*. Philadelphia: WB Saunders; 1995.
10. Kleinert H, et al. Primary repair of lacerated flexor tendons in no-man's land. *J Bone* Joint Surg. 1967;49A:577.
11. Kleinert H, et al. Small vessel anastomosis for the salvage of the severely injured extremity. *J Bone Joint Surg*. 1963;49A:788.
12. Buncke H, et al. Nicoladoni procedure in rhesus monkey or hallux hand transplantation utilizing microminiature vascular anastomosis. *Plast Reconstr Surg*. 1979;63:607.
13. Manktelow R, Mckee N. Free muscle transplantation to provide finger flexion. *J Hand Surg*. 1978;3:416.

CHAPTER 77 ■ PRINCIPLES OF UPPER LIMB SURGERY

BENJAMIN CHANG

PREOPERATIVE PRINCIPLES

History

In no area of medicine is obtaining an accurate history before initiating treatment more important than in upper limb surgery. The patient's age, hand dominance, occupation, and history of prior upper-extremity problems are obtained. The date, time, mechanism, and circumstances (e.g., work related, contaminated) of injury are elicited. Information about the position of the limb during the injury (e.g., fall on outstretched hand, hand open or grasping) and prior treatments may also be useful. For chronic or nontraumatic problems, it is essential to list details of the onset and course, and to prioritize the patient's complaints in the order of importance to the patient. A clear, prioritized list of complaints facilitates the physician's orderly follow-up on each problem at every visit so that progress or lack of progress can be systematically documented. Once the chief complaints are delineated, their effect on the patient's functional ability in his or her occupation and activities of daily living can be evaluated.

Pertinent past medical history, including anesthetic experiences, bleeding disorders, prior operations, current medications, allergies, and tetanus immunization status, are recorded.

Physical Examination

Together with a thorough history, the physical examination is the only diagnostic test needed in the vast majority of problems seen by the hand surgeon. A precise knowledge of the anatomy of the upper limb and its variations are essential for accurate diagnosis. The entire upper limb should be exposed and examined systematically: circulation, sensibility, soft tissues, bones, joints, and active muscle functions.* Of course, the examination should be tailored to each patient's problem as guided by symptoms and history; not every test needs to be performed on every patient.

Circulation can be evaluated by observing the color of the skin and nail beds, checking the temperature of the skin and the timing of capillary refill after blanching the skin with light pressure. Findings are interpreted by comparing them with those of normal parts. **Arterial insufficiency produces a pale, cool limb with prolonged capillary refill and loss of tissue turgor. Venous insufficiency will result in a purple, congested extrem-**

ity with faster-than-normal capillary refill. These clinical parameters can be combined with pulse oximetry and Doppler examination if needed, but conclusions must be based on the composite of findings, as no single test is infallible. Testing for viability with needle puncture is condemned. A digit with no arterial inflow for several hours can still "bleed" when pricked. This test serves only to provide avenues for infection. Brachial, radial, and ulnar pulses are palpated. Performing the Allen test (2) is useful to determine patency of both ulnar and radial arteries. The patient should raise and clench the fist to exsanguinate the hand while the physician compresses both radial and ulnar arteries at the wrist. As the patient opens the hand, the examiner releases pressure on the radial artery and observes the capillary refill across the hand. The test is repeated, releasing pressure on the ulnar artery, and filling from the ulnar side is observed. Incomplete refill across the hand may occur in 10% to 15% of patients, and may indicate an incomplete superficial palmar arterial arch or occlusion of the radial or ulnar arteries.

Sensibility is essential to hand function and is tested if there is any question of nerve damage from a direct injury, compression, or degenerative process. **Denervated skin is dry and becomes smooth as it loses papillary skin ridges. Also, it does not wrinkle with immersion in water.** These observations can be useful in examining children who are too young to cooperate and for identifying malingerers. The most useful screening test in the case of acute injury is to check light-touch perception by comparing it with that of an uninjured part. Using a soft cotton-tipped applicator stick alleviates anxiety, especially in children. Static and moving two-point discrimination (2PD) measure innervation density and can be performed with a bent paperclip or blunt caliper to quantitate the level of sensibility. Moving 2PD is a more sensitive indicator of the levels of sensibility needed for hand function. Abnormal measurements (>6 mm static and >3 mm moving 2PD at the fingertips) indicate axonal impairment (3). Two-point discrimination has the advantage of being somewhat quantitative, which allows for comparisons over time and between patients. Even more sensitive than 2PD is vibration sensibility (tuning fork) and pressure thresholds (Semmes-Weinstein monofilament testing). Although some variations and overlap exist in the sensory innervation of the upper limb, there are three autonomous areas on the hand, each of which is innervated by only one of three major nerves. The autonomous zone for the median nerve is the index fingertip, for the ulnar nerve it is the small finger's tip, and for the radial nerve it is the dorsal side of the first web space.

Soft-tissue coverage should be restored before reconstruction of deeper structures is undertaken. Thick scars along the route of tendon transfers or across joints will limit mobility. During open wound examination, any skin deficits or devitalized areas are noted and recorded on a sketch, but deep probing is not performed in the emergency room without appropriate anesthesia, lighting, and instruments.

---

*For a complete description of the physical examination, the reader is referred to an excellent handbook, *The Hand: Examination and Diagnosis*, published by the American Society for Surgery of the Hand, 3025 South Parker Road, Suite 65, Aurora, CO, 80232.

741

Bone injuries are considered if gentle palpation reveals localized skeletal tenderness. **A fracture is suspected when sharp pain is accompanied by deformity, abnormal mobility, progressive swelling, and/or prominent ecchymosis.** Radiographs of good quality and a minimum of posteroanterior (PA), lateral, and oblique views are essential. Specialized views may be required to rule out fractures of a specific bone (e.g., scaphoid or hook of the hamate). A fracture should be described according to location, type, and deformity. The *location* is specified by the name of the bone and the portion involved (base, midshaft, neck, intra-articular, etc.). The *type* of fracture is described according to the pattern (transverse, oblique, spiral, comminuted, undisplaced) and whether a communicating skin wound (open or closed) is present. Describe the *deformity* according to the displacement (dorsal, volar, radial, ulnar) and angulation. By tradition, angulation is named for the direction of the apex and rotation for the distal segment in relation to the proximal one. Rotational malalignment in the fingers can best be observed by having the patient slowly bring all the fingers from a fully extended position into flexion. Any scissoring (crossing of fingers) usually indicates a rotational malalignment. For example: "The patient has a right fifth metacarpal neck fracture that is closed and comminuted with 3-mm volar displacement and 45 degrees of dorsal angulation, but no rotational malalignment."

Joints are examined for tenderness, active and passive range of motion, stability, and deformity. Abnormal physical findings necessitate radiographic examination. A "chip" fracture may indicate a ligamentous avulsion injury. Stress radiographs may be required in diagnosing ligamentous injuries, and should be performed after injecting local anesthetic to prevent pain and guarding.

Muscle function depends on skeletal stability, functioning joints, and intact motor nerves and muscle–tendon units. Each unit for which there is reason to suspect injury should be tested, first without resistance to assess active range of motion, and then with resistance to assess strength. **Pain or weakness against resistance suggests a partial tendon laceration.** Dynamometers that measure grip and pinch forces are of little use with acute injuries, but are essential for evaluating and following chronic problems. The absolute numbers are less important than comparison with those of the unaffected side. Some information may be gained by observing the resting posture of the hand. In the supine position, the resting hand should have the fingers in a partially flexed position, falling into a smooth cascade of progressively more flexion from the index to the small finger. A complete tendon laceration will cause the injured digit to fall out of line at rest. The tenodesis effect from passive wrist flexion/extension can also help evaluate suspected tendon injuries, even if the patient is under anesthesia. Wrist flexion increases tension on the digital extensor tendons causing passive digital extension. A digit with a transected extensor tendon will fail to extend when the wrist is passively flexed. This tenodesis effect can also be used to test the flexor tendons, observing the digital cascade, as the wrist is hyperextended. However, a partially severed tendon cannot be diagnosed or excluded by any of these manipulations. Wound exploration is often the only means to establish the presence of partially severed tendons with certainty.

Acute Injury

The first priority is to rule out injuries to other parts of the body. **To minimize patient discomfort, as much information as possible is obtained from observation rather than manipulation. Proceeding from distal to proximal, every structure in the zone of injury is systematically tested.** The entire examination need not be performed in the emergency room. There are two important questions to be answered in the emergency room. First, are any parts threatened by ischemia? Second, does this injury need to be treated in the operating room? If the answer to either question is yes, extensive exploration of wounds should be deferred to the operating room. Often, the basic information is gained by examining the areas distal to the wound, including circulation, sensibility, and muscle/tendon integrity. The physical findings and appropriate radiographs guide exploration.

It is helpful to triage injuries into three categories according to severity and urgency: (a) severe injuries that require immediate treatment; (b) severe injuries that require early treatment; and (c) less-severe injuries. Severe injuries that require immediate treatment include life-threatening situations and injuries that have resulted in ischemia and threaten survival of the parts. **There are only two life-threatening upper limb problems: exsanguinating hemorrhage and necrotizing infection** (see Chap. 85). *Hemorrhage* in the absence of a coagulopathy can be controlled by elevation and direct pressure on the bleeding point. Makeshift tourniquets should not be used because they can apply dangerously high pressures, causing permanent damage to underlying muscles and nerves. Clamping of "bleeders" in the emergency room is strongly discouraged because of the risk of injury to adjacent nerves.

Tetanus prophylaxis should be considered for every patient with a wound. For clean wounds, tetanus toxoid should be administered if the patient has not been immunized within 10 years or has had fewer than the usual series of immunization doses. For highly contaminated or extensive wounds, tetanus toxoid usually should be administered, and if the patient has not been immunized within 5 years, tetanus immune globulin is recommended.

Injuries that result in *ischemia* include amputations, vascular injuries, crush injuries, and electrical injuries. Muscle is the tissue most vulnerable to hypoxia and must be reperfused within about 6 hours if it is to survive. Hypothermia is our only means of prolonging this time limit, as it lowers the metabolic rate of the tissues. Ischemic parts not amputated should be kept cool with ice, but taking care not to freeze them. One should suspect a *compartment syndrome* if the patient complains of progressive pain disproportionate to the injury, if a muscle compartment feels tense on palpation, and especially if passive muscle stretching dramatically increases pain.

High-pressure injection injuries can cause progressive tissue damage. These injuries vary in severity depending on the toxicity and volume of the injected agent. The history is the key to diagnosis, as the toxic agent may be forced through a tiny, innocuous-appearing wound. Often, injection is at a fingertip with dissection of the material along the tendon sheaths all the way into the forearm. Left untreated, there will be progressive inflammation and destruction of the surrounding tissues and often this is inevitable despite early recognition and immediate operative debridement.

Severe injuries that require early surgical repair include those of flexor tendons, open fractures, and joint injuries. If the skin wound is not extensive, it can be irrigated and closed in the emergency room, except for human bites, with delayed primary repair performed within a week. Extensor tendon and nerve injuries can be handled in a similar fashion except that definitive repair can be delayed for a longer period with the exception of independent units such as the extensor pollicis longus (EPL), which will contract and shorten rapidly. Severe injuries that require early treatment, not necessarily surgical, include frostbite, most chemical and thermal burns, and electrical injuries for which specific treatment is discussed in other chapters. The quality of the initial care for injuries is the most important single determinant of the final degree of recovery.

RECONSTRUCTIVE PRIORITIES IN THE UPPER LIMB

1. Restore *circulation*
2. Obtain good *soft-tissue coverage*
3. Align and stabilize the *skeleton*
4. Restore *nerve function*
5. Mobilize *joints*
6. Restore *tendon function*

Reconstructive Cases

Planning of surgical reconstruction should begin with the initial treatment, even though the reconstruction may take operations over many months to complete. The first step is to identify all of the injured structures by history, physical examination, and operative exploration. Once the deficits are understood, they should be prioritized if there is no potential for full recovery. Often, mechanical design must be simplified to a lower order of function. **It is generally better to have a few things work well than many that work poorly.** The following order of reconstructive priorities serves as a general guide based on prerequisites; each step in the sequence depends on successful completion of the preceding steps (Table 77.1). Restoring adequate *circulation* is the first priority. Inadequate perfusion will impair wound healing, predispose to infection, and result in a cold intolerance. The next priority is good *soft-tissue coverage*, which might require replacement with skin graft, local flap, or distant tissue transfer. Delayed primary closure is indicated for badly contaminated wounds. Without adequate circulation and soft-tissue coverage, repair of underlying structures is futile. Even if they heal, it will be with excessive scar and adhesions. The third priority is to align and *stabilize the skeleton*. Fractures and dislocations should be reduced and stabilized. The fourth priority is to restore *nerve function* by repair or nerve grafting. The fifth priority is to *mobilize joints* that may have become stiffened as a result of chronic edema, inflammation, and disuse. Severely stiffened joints may require surgical release. The last priority is to restore *tendon function* by repair, grafting, tendon transfer, or tenolysis. It is important that passive range of motion of joints crossed by a tendon be maximized before that tendon is reconstructed.

The priorities listed above should be incorporated into a master plan, not necessarily separate operations. Replantation is an example of combining all of the steps into one operation. Several staged operations may be needed if the postoperative regimen for one part of the operation is different from that of another part. For example, osteotomy for malunion should not be done at the same time as tenolysis because the first requires immobilization and the second necessitates prompt mobilization. Once the deficits are identified and prioritized, steps with compatible postoperative regimens are combined as far as feasible. Each stage should be deferred until the tissues are soft, edema is resolved, and the joints are supple. This approach of identifying and prioritizing deficits, then grouping them into staged operations, can also be applied to nontraumatic reconstructive problems.

OPERATIVE PRINCIPLES

Anesthesia

Surgery on the upper limb can be performed with a variety of anesthetic techniques: general, regional, or local infiltration. Use of local infiltration anesthesia is limited to small lesions or to supplement a regional nerve block. General anesthesia is usually indicated for children, for uncooperative patients, when multiple operative fields are required, and for long procedures.

The upper limb lends itself well to regional block anesthetics, which can be combined with judicious sedation if required for anxiety. The chief disadvantages of regional blocks are the time interval for its full effectiveness, the risk of incomplete anesthesia, and the limited tourniquet time. For a detailed review of local anesthetic agents, see Chapter 11. The most commonly employed regional anesthetic blocks are brachial plexus blocks, intravenous regional (Bier) blocks, median and ulnar wrist blocks, and digital blocks.

Either interscalene or supraclavicular brachial plexus blocks can give deep and superb anesthesia of the entire upper limb and allow long tourniquet times but require great skill to administer, are not always complete, and carry a significant risk of pneumothorax or other complication. Blocks of the median or ulnar nerves, or both, at the wrist are safe, easy to perform, hurt less than palmar or digital blocks, and are useful for both emergency and elective operations. Anesthetic injections should be adjacent to and not into the nerves.

Intravenous regional anesthesia (Bier block) anesthetizes the whole arm distal to the tourniquet. Thus for some purposes, it fills the gap between brachial plexus blocks and wrist blocks. The Bier block is conceptually simple: exsanguinate the arm and fill the veins with a local anesthetic. The details of administration can be found in all anesthesiology texts. The main advantage of the Bier block is that it is easy to perform and reliable in giving a good anesthetic block. Its main disadvantages are tourniquet pain, which limits operative time; compromised visibility for precision dissections as the anesthetic flows into the line of dissection with every cut; and loss of anesthesia immediately when the tourniquet is deflated. Its risks are essentially that of tourniquet failure, which could allow a toxic dose of the anesthetic to be sent as a bolus into the body. Thus, although simple, this technique should be used only when equipment for resuscitation is readily available.

At the wrist, the *median nerve* is located medial to the flexor carpi radialis (FCR) and directly deep to the palmaris longus (PL) tendon when present. A good block can be expected by simply injecting the anesthetic solution into the carpal tunnel without eliciting paresthesia (Fig. 77.1). Anesthetic is also injected into the subcutaneous tissues between the PL and the FCR tendons to block the palmar cutaneous branch of the median nerve.

At the wrist, the *ulnar nerve* is situated against the lateral side of the flexor carpi ulnaris (FCU) and directly deep to the ulnar artery. To block it, 5 mL of anesthetic is injected deep to the ulnar artery from the side of the wrist, just deep to the FCU tendon (Fig. 77.2). The dorsal branch of the ulnar nerve can be blocked in the subcutaneous tissues alongside and just distal to the ulnar styloid.

The superficial division of the *radial nerve* emerges from beneath the brachioradialis muscle in the midforearm and usually divides into several branches proximal to the radial styloid. Block the branches by injecting 4 to 5 mL of anesthetic solution subcutaneously over the radius or the midforearm, where it often can be felt to roll under a palpating fingertip (Fig. 77.3).

Except for the thumb, which has a good dorsal blood supply, *digital nerve* block should be in the distal palm, where there is good collateral circulation, rather than in the base of the finger. Epinephrine is not recommended for any digital nerve block. A dorsal approach through the interdigital web or a volar injection just distal to the distal palmar crease can be used (Figs. 77.4 and 77.5). To get complete dorsal anesthesia over the proximal and middle phalanges, a subcutaneous injection

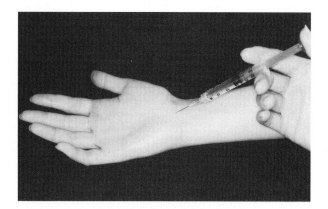

FIGURE 77.1. Median nerve block.

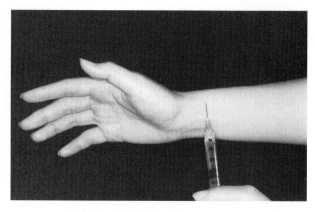

FIGURE 77.3. Radial nerve block.

over the base of the proximal phalanx is required. A circumferential "ring block" at the base of a finger is unnecessary and is dangerous.

Tourniquets

A bloodless field maintained by a pneumatic tourniquet has become a standard and indispensable instrument for upper limb surgery. The current method of exsanguinating the arm with a flat rubber bandage can be traced back to Esmarch in 1873, and Cushing is credited with introducing the pneumatic tourniquet in 1904, although it was intended for use in craniotomies (1). The main factors of tourniquet safety are pressure and its area of distribution. The pressure must exceed systolic pressure by about 100 mm Hg to maintain a bloodless field, but excessive pressure can cause direct injury to tissues under the tourniquet, especially the nerves. Pneumatic tourniquets should have accurately calibrated pressure gauges. The duration of tourniquet application should be limited to about 1.5 to 2 hours. For a longer operation, the tourniquet should be deflated and the arm reperfused for 12 to 15 minutes per hour of ischemia to clear the acidosis (4). When the tourniquet is no longer needed, maximally elevate the arm and completely remove the cuff and padding to prevent them from acting as a venous tourniquet. In general, it is safer to release the tourniquet before skin closure and to check hemostasis.

Exsanguination of the arm with an Esmarch bandage before tourniquet inflation is contraindicated in the presence of infection or malignant tumors. Instead, the limb should be elevated for several minutes for gravity to drain it of blood before the tourniquet is inflated.

When the operation is limited to a finger, a digital tourniquet can be used but with care that it not be too tight and that its pressure is widely distributed, as with a flat Penrose drain. Rubber bands and cut off pieces of latex glove rolled down on the finger are hazardous because an unknown pressure is applied over a small area.

Magnification

Good visualization is essential for atraumatic surgical technique. Loupes with ×2.5 to ×3.5 magnification are ideal for most upper extremity surgery. The binocular operating microscope is preferable for repair of small vessels and for some nerve surgery.

Elective Incisions and Wound Extensions

All incisions heal with a scar, and all scars contract. **To avoid contracture, incisions must not cross skin flexion creases at joints.** Stated another way, they should be along lines that undergo no change in length with movements of the part. There is much more latitude for dorsal skin incisions. The elastic and loosely attached skin can substantially compensate for scar shortening, avoiding restriction of motion.

The two most useful incisions in the finger that satisfy the above principles are the midaxial and the Bruner, or zigzag, incisions. The midaxial incision gives access to both volar and dorsal structures but may require very extensive undermining. The Bruner incision is only for the palmar surfaces and crosses

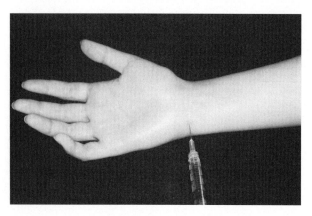

FIGURE 77.2. Ulnar nerve block.

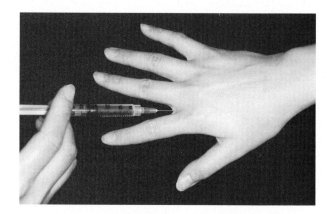

FIGURE 77.4. Digital nerve block.

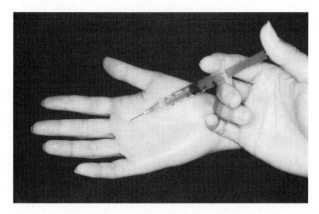

FIGURE 77.5. Digital nerve block.

the volar skin between flexion creases in a zigzag fashion, which creates a series of short, broadly based, opposing flaps.

Wound Closure

Incisions and wounds of the hand can generally be closed with a single layer of interrupted sutures. Vertical mattress sutures are needed if the skin edges tend to invert. Lacerated wounds that cross flexion creases need reorientation by Z-plasties. Wound closure for children with 5-0 or 6-0 plain gut avoids the trauma to patient, family, and surgeon of suture removal. Except in areas of unavoidable tension, such as posterior to the elbow, sutures are removed after 7 to 10 days to minimize suture marks. On the forearm and upper arm, elective incisions can be closed with a continuous intradermal monofilament suture.

POSTOPERATIVE PRINCIPLES

Dressing

A well-applied dressing is an integral part of the operation in hand surgery and requires the same attention to details as the operation itself. It should conform to the limb to provide support but without compression, which can act as a venous tourniquet to promote edema. The basic hand dressing consists of three layers. The first layer is flat, with slightly moist gauze applied directly to the wounds. The second layer is fluffed gauze placed between the fingers to prevent skin maceration and to cover potential pressure points, such as the ulnar head. The third layer is a 2- or 3-inch roll gauze applied circumferentially to hold the other layers in place but with diminishing pressure from distal to proximal to promote venous return. The original dressing placed in the operating room is left on until suture removal unless there is a specific indication to remove it sooner. Any patient who complains of an unexpected degree of pain after surgery should have the dressing split down to the skin to ensure that the dressing is not too tight. As swelling correlates with pain, this will give great relief to the majority of such patients.

Immobilization

Effective immobilization favors wound healing and is essential for the healing of many structures, such as bones and skin grafts. However, because prolonged immobilization can lead to stiffness of the small joints, immobilization should be main-tained where essential for the minimal amount of time needed while continued movement of other parts is encouraged.

Protective Position

When immobilization is essential, it should be in the "protective" or "safe position." This keeps ligaments under maximum stretch to prevent their shortening and subsequent restriction of joint mobility.

There are just three essential elements of the protective position: interphalangeal (IP) joint extension, metacarpophalangeal (MCP) joint flexion, and palmar abduction of the thumb. Maintaining the interphalangeal joint in extension prevents shortening of the volar plate and flexor tendon sheath. Because of the camlike shape of the metacarpal heads, collateral ligaments of metacarpophalangeal joint are maximally stretched when the joint is in full flexion. Therefore, keeping the MCP joints in flexion prevents shortening of their collateral ligaments and loss of joint mobility during immobilization. Holding the wrist in slight extension takes advantage of the tenodesis effect to make it easier to keep the MCP joints in flexion. Finally, palmar abduction of the thumb simply keeps the soft tissues of the first web space stretched to prevent an adduction contracture.

Either a splint or a cast can be used to immobilize the hand. A splint is easier to remove and allows for some expansion to accommodate swelling but a cast can be molded to apply selective pressure to a wound or graft without circumferential constriction. For children, an above-elbow cast is the only reliable dressing. The cast and padding should be split if the patient complains of excessive tightness, progressive pain, or numbness in the digits.

Elevation

An accidentally or surgically injured limb should be continuously elevated until effective pumping activity is again functioning to propel venous blood and lymph back to the body. The heart is the point of reference for elevation. While walking, the patient should hold the hand over the contralateral shoulder or even rest it on the head. Slings tend to promote edema by holding the hand at the level of the umbilicus, which is lower than the heart. In the sitting position one should prop the elbow on a table with the hand upright and at night one should rest the hand on pillows or on the chest.

References

1. Green DP. General principles. In: Green DP, ed. *Green's Operative Hand Surgery.* 5th ed. New York: Churchill Livingstone; 2005.
2. Levinsohn DG, Gordon L, Sessler DI. The Allen's test: analysis of four methods. *J Hand Surg.* 1991;16A:279.
3. Louis DS, Greene TL, Jacobson KE. Evaluation of normal values for stationary and moving two-point discrimination in the hand. *J Hand Surg.* 1984;9(4):552.
4. Wilgis EF, et al. Observations on the effects of tourniquet ischemia. *J Bone Joint Surg AM.* 1971;53(7):1343.

Suggested Readings

American Society for Surgery of the Hand. *The Hand: Examination and Diagnosis.* 3rd ed. New York: Churchill Livingstone; 1990.
Beasley RW. *Beasley's Surgery of the Hand.* New York: Thieme; 2003.
Green DP, ed. *Green's Operative Hand Surgery.* 5th ed. New York: Churchill Livingstone; 2005.
Smith P. *Lister's The Hand: Diagnosis and Indications.* 4th ed. New York: Churchill Livingstone; 2002.

CHAPTER 78 ■ RADIOLOGIC IMAGING OF THE HAND AND WRIST

CORNELIA N. GOLIMBU

The first x-ray image obtained was of a hand. Since then advancements have produced revolutionary changes in the way anatomy and pathology of the human body are imaged: Magnification radiography, arthrography, angiography, nuclear medicine, ultrasound, computed tomography (CT), and magnetic resonance imaging (MRI) all contribute in specific ways to detection and characterization of bone, joint, and soft-tissue abnormalities.

RADIOGRAPHS

With the exception of those cases in which it becomes very obvious that the abnormality is limited to the skin and to the superficial soft-tissue layers (burns, skin disorders, superficial lacerations), almost all patients with hand and wrist problems should have roentgenograms obtained.

The most important initial step for radiographic examination of the hand and wrist is to establish where and what is the most likely abnormality. It is obvious that a crush injury to a single distal phalanx can be fully seen simply by obtaining a finger view in frontal and lateral projection. Hand views are necessary when the injury involves the base of fingers or metacarpals, and should include oblique views, as overlapping limits lateral visualization. Acute or chronic trauma to the carpal complex is screened by the three standard radiographic positions of the wrist (posteroanterior, oblique, and lateral). In specific situations additional views can be obtained, such as for the scaphoid, carpal tunnel, or hamate hook. When intermittent abnormal alignment is suspected, special stress views may be needed to diagnose a dynamic instability. Also, stress views may be needed to evaluate digital ligamentous injuries. Studies for suspected foreign bodies may be helpful only when radiopaque materials are retained in the tissues; wood splinters are usually nondetectable by radiographs.

Radiologic imaging will aid diagnosis and illustrate the extent of involvement of arthritis. Comparable views of both hands generally are needed to establish the full extent of the disease, for which the symmetry of the lesions is often a strong diagnostic feature, especially with inflammatory types of arthritis.

Degenerative Arthritis

The common osteoarthritis usually associated with increasing age and traumatic arthritis are the two types of degenerative arthritis. They are indistinguishable radiographically, and even histologically, and the designation of traumatic arthritis depends entirely on the history of direct trauma to the in-

volved part, such as an intra-articular fracture, to which initiation of the degenerative process can reasonably be attributed. The basic radiographic findings of degenerative arthritis are:

1. Narrowing of the joint space normally occupied by articular cartilages
2. Subchondral bone sclerosis
3. Osteophyte formation along articular margins

Inflammatory Arthritis

The most frequent forms of inflammatory arthritis are the common rheumatoid arthritis (RA), the less common psoriatic arthritis, and the rare form associated with lupus erythematosus disorders. The classic radiographic signs of RA are:

1. Symmetry of involvement/both hands, progressive from intercarpal joints to metacarpophalangeal (MCP) and proximal interphalangeal (PIP) joints
2. Narrowing of the joint spaces
3. Erosion of articular cortex
4. Malalignment (ulnar deviation of fingers)
5. Soft-tissue swelling centered on the joints
6. Periarticular osteoporosis

The classic radiographic findings of psoriatic arthritis are:

1. Distal to proximal progressive involvement of interphalangeal joints
2. Periosteal new bone deposition in paraarticular location
3. Erosions of articular cortex with "pencil-in-cup" deformity
4. Lack of osteoporosis

The typical radiographic findings of arthritis associated with lupus erythematosus are:

1. Dominant malalignment deformities
2. Absence of articular cortex erosions
3. Profound, generalized osteoporosis (more than juxta-articular)

Metabolic Arthritis

Gout and pseudogout are the most frequently encountered forms of metabolic arthritis. Typical radiographic presentations of gout include:

1. Bone erosions with "overhanging margins" in juxta- or intra-articular locations
2. Preservation of joint space
3. Soft-tissue masses representing the tophi

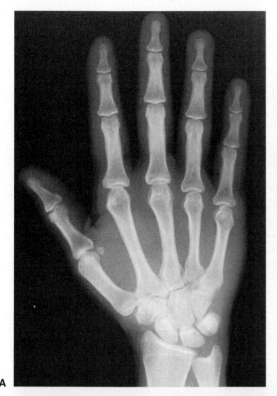

A

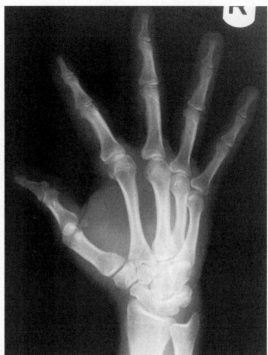

B

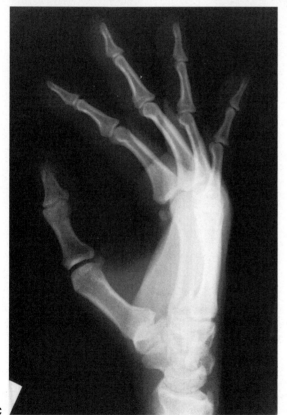

C

FIGURE 78.1. Standard radiographic views of the hand.
A: Posteroanterior frontal view. B: Posteroanterior oblique
view. C: Lateral view.

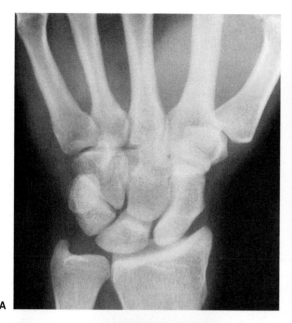 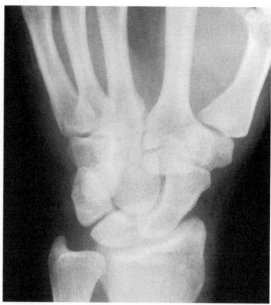

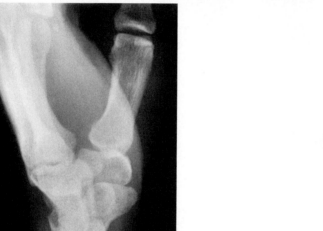

FIGURE 78.2. Standard radiographs of the wrist. **A:** Posteroanterior frontal view. **B:** Posteroanterior oblique view. **C:** Lateral view.

Pseudogout is characterized by:

1. Calcifications in the hyaline cartilage covering the carpal bones or ulnar head
2. Narrowing of the intercarpal and MCP joint spaces
3. Collapse of the lunate
4. Calcium pyrophosphate crystals detected in the synovial fluid analyzed in polarized light microscopy

STANDARD RADIOGRAPHS

The complexity of the bone and joint anatomy of the hand and wrist necessitates a multitude of positions for visualization of all the bone surfaces in profile views, in relaxed or stressed position, and in supination or pronation. This chapter succinctly presents the projections most commonly used in the diagnosis of hand and wrist abnormalities. Detailed textbooks dedicated to this topic can be consulted for additional information.*

Hand Views

Roentgenograms of the hand taken as part of the routine radiologic investigation should consist of frontal and oblique, posteroanterior (PA) views. The *frontal view* outlines the carpal bones, the carpometacarpal and metacarpophalangeal joints, and the phalanges (Fig. 78.1A). The thumb is seen in oblique or almost lateral view. The *oblique view* (Fig. 78.1B) is impor-

---

* A recommended comprehensive text is Gilula LA, Yiu Y. *Imaging of the Wrist and Hand.* Philadelphia: WB Saunders; 1996.

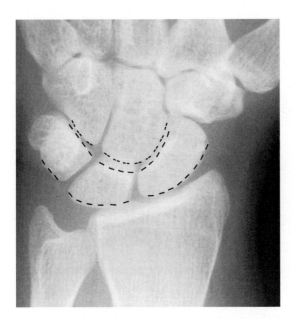

FIGURE 78.3. Carpal alignment in frontal view. The contour of the proximal and the distal surfaces of the first carpal row describes two arches that should be parallel to each other. The proximal surface of the capitate and hamate represents the third arch, concentric with the first two.

tant for profile visualization of the metacarpophalangeal joints and for perception of depth localization of any abnormality seen in the frontal views.

Occasionally, a *lateral view* is needed when alignment of the interphalangeal joints is in question. For this purpose the lateral projection of the hand should be obtained with the fingers in a progressive degree of flexion; in such a position, each middle and distal phalanx is projected separately (Fig. 78.1C). In this view, the thumb is projected in a frontal position.

Finger Views

Finger radiographs are obtained in lateral and posteroanterior views when the abnormalities are likely to be limited to the

distal and middle phalanges of one or more fingers. Such a small field of view is advantageous because it allows tailoring of the exposure factors fit for thin tissue parts, consequently producing films of ideal radiographic density for the small segments in question. Moreover, the hand and wrist are spared the radiation exposure by being purposely omitted.

Wrist Views

The minimum accepted views necessary for roentgenographic study of the wrist include three projections: posteroanterior, lateral, and oblique (1). The normal *posteroanterior frontal view* outlines the contour of the distal radius and ulna, and the carpal bones and their articulations with the metacarpals. The intercarpal articulations are seen as uniform spaces of 1 to 2 mm; only the scapholunate space may be slightly larger. The ulnar styloid is profiled on the medial side of the ulnar head (Fig. 78.2A). In the frontal projection of the wrist, the joint between trapezium and trapezoid is not well visualized. This anatomic area is better visualized in the *posteroanterior oblique projection* (Fig. 78.2B). In this view the trapezium is not overlapped by the trapezoid; the articulation of these two carpals with the surrounding bones is projected clearly. The dorsal surface of the triquetrum is seen almost in profile in this position and its dorsal cortex is not overlapped by any other carpal structures. A true *lateral projection* is essential in determining the position of the lunate in relation to the long axis of the radius and capitate (Fig. 78.2C). The lateral view must be obtained in a neutral position of the forearm (90-degree abduction of the shoulder, 90-degree flexion of the elbow), without pronation or supination, so as to allow exact measurements of the relative length of the radius and ulna (for ulnar variance) or the angle described by the axis of the scaphoid, lunate, and capitate. An easy way to determine the correctness of positioning in the lateral view is to check the overlap of the scaphoid and pisiform. The pisiform's anterior margin should project halfway between the anterior margin of the scaphoid and the lunate (Fig. 78.2C). The anterior and posterior poles of the lunate should be in symmetric position in a normal wrist; the long axis of the scaphoid describes a 120- to 150-degree angle with the long axis of the wrist.

The proximal and distal surfaces of the first carpal row (scaphoid, lunate, triquetrum) and the proximal surface of the

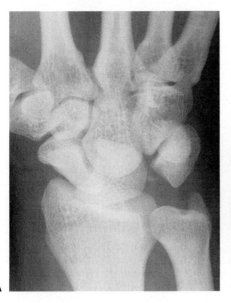

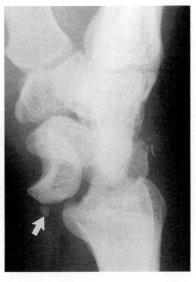

A   B

FIGURE 78.4. Anterior lunate dislocation. A: Posteroanterior view: The lunate is tilted and no longer articulates with the adjacent carpal bones. B: Lateral view: The lunate is dislocated and rotated 90 degrees in a palmar direction. A small fragment of bone represents an avulsion fracture of the intercarpal ligaments insertion site (*arrow*).

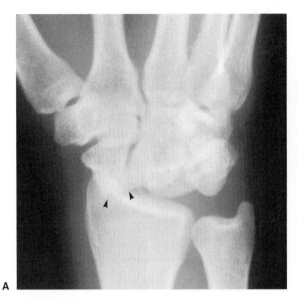

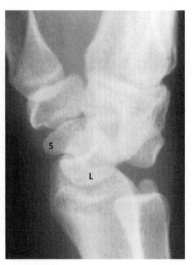

FIGURE 78.5. Transcaphoid posterior perilunate dislocation. **A:** Posteroanterior view: Scaphoid is fractured at the waist (*arrowheads*). Midcarpal joint space is not seen. **B:** Lateral view: Distal carpal row is dislocated posteriorly in relation to the lunate (*L*). The scaphoid (*S*) fracture is obscured by the slight palmar tilt of the lunate.

capitate and hamate describe the configuration of three parallel arches (Fig. 78.3). Interruption of these arches represents an abnormality such as fracture of carpals, dislocation of lunate, or complex injuries, such as transcaphoid perilunate dislocation (Figs. 78.4 and 78.5).

The *scaphoid projection* (PA with maximum ulnar deviation of the wrist) is necessary for all patients who have pain in the radial side of the wrist following trauma. In this view, the scaphoid appears elongated, allowing visualization of the cortex and trabeculae of its waist (Fig. 78.6). In many instances it is the only view in which a nondisplaced fracture of the scaphoid becomes visible.

When the clinical history and localized tenderness indicate possible injury to the hook of the hamate, additional views are indicated in the search for a fracture. The *oblique view of the hamate* projects the hook in profile, thus often making possible the detection of subtle, nondisplaced fractures (Fig. 78.7). A *carpal tunnel view* is obtained by directing the central x-ray beam tangential to the floor of the carpal tunnel and, because its bony medial wall is formed by the hook of the hamate, fracture there may be demonstrated. The more proximally situated pisiform also is well visualized in this view. Sagittally oriented fractures of the pisiform may be seen only in this view

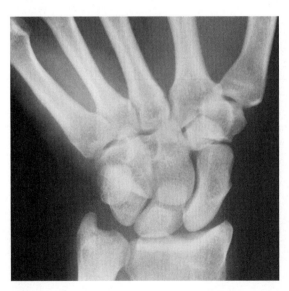

FIGURE 78.6. Scaphoid view. The ulnar tilt of the hand allows better visualization of the scaphoid with better detail of the cortical surface and bone trabeculae at its waist.

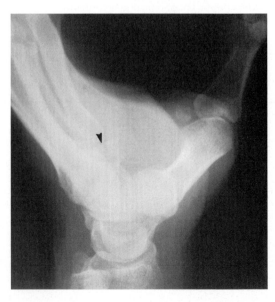

FIGURE 78.7. Oblique views for hamate hook. At the base of the hamulus, a lucent line suggests a fracture (*arrowhead*). A CT scan will consistently identify the fracture if more information is necessary to make the diagnosis. See Fig. 78.17.

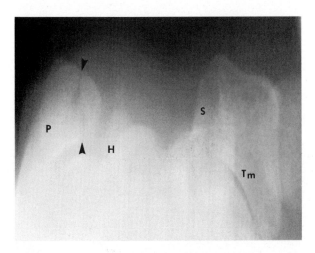

FIGURE 78.8. Carpal tunnel view. Sagittally oriented fracture of the pisiform is seen (*arrowheads*). Trapezium (*Tm*) and distal pole of the scaphoid (*S*) make the lateral wall of the carpal tunnel. The medial wall is made of the pisiform (*P*) and hook of the hamate (*H*).

(Fig. 78.8). The carpal tunnel view allows for a profile view of the scaphoid tubercle.

DYNAMIC STUDY

If fractures and dislocations have been excluded by normal radiographs, one must consider that persistent pain and focal swelling of a wrist following acute trauma may be a result of ligament disruption. When untreated, such injuries may allow abnormal motion between the carpal bones, which can subsequently lead to degenerative disease of the wrist.

For the hand surgeon treating the patient with ligament injuries, it is important to know (a) the precise location of the injury, (b) the character of the lesion (sprain, complete tear, bony avulsion), (c) the significance of this injury to joint stability, and (d) if any instability is present (1). In the search of these answers, the diagnostic test employed is a dynamic study. The motion can be active, performed by the patient (instability series), or passive, performed by an examiner (stress views).

Motion Views (Instability Series)

The wrist is positioned in the extremes of its physiologic range of motion. These *motion views* are posteroanterior views in maximum radial and ulnar deviation, clenched-fist PA and anteroposterior (AP) views, and lateral views with radial and ulnar tilt, as well as maximum flexion and extension. Collectively, these are referred to as an *instability series*. When abnormal joint openings are demonstrated, a ligamentous tear with dynamic instability is documented. For example, scapholunate dissociation resulting in an abnormally large gap between these two bones may be clearly seen in the clenched-fist AP (supinated) view and not even suggested by routine radiographs (Fig. 78.9).

Stress Views of the Wrist and Digits

Stress views are radiographs obtained while passive stress is applied. The stress applied to the wrist may be physiologic

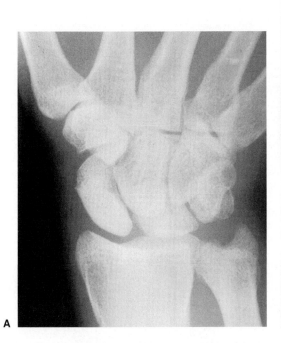
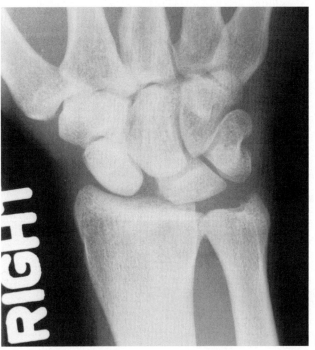

FIGURE 78.9. Scapholunate dissociation (rotatory subluxation) of the scaphoid. **A:** Posteroanterior view with ulnar deviation: The scapholunate space is slightly larger than the other intercarpal joints, but not definitely abnormal. **B:** Anteroposterior (supinated) view with clenched fist: The stress on the carpal bones produced by the tightly clenched fist shows scapholunate dissociation caused by rotatory subluxation of the scaphoid. The ring sign representing projection of the distal pole on the rest of the scaphoid can be seen.

(radial-ulnar deviation in frontal view or flexion–extension in lateral view) or nonphysiologic (radial and ulnar transposition; passive pronation and supination). The most commonly helpful views are passive ulnar deviation and radial transposition, which may show instability in the scaphotrapezial and scapholunate joints, respectively. In lateral views, dorsally directed stress may unmask subtle midcarpal joint instability, seen as dorsal translation of the capitate in relation to the lunate.

Among the most useful stress studies are those of the metacarpophalangeal joint of the thumb. Reliability of observations is enhanced by injection of a local anesthetic into the MCP joint. This not only prevents pain, but also prevents splinting from thenar muscle spasm, which may give a false impression of stability. Frontal views are obtained with ulnar and radial stress with comparison views of the normal thumb. Small tears of the radial or ulnar collateral ligaments are reflected in stress views as 15 to 20 degrees greater angulation of the abnormal joint compared with the normal side. Greater differences in angulation, especially subluxation of the phalanx on the metacarpal head, occur with a complete collateral ligament disruption.

VIDEOFLUOROSCOPY

Fluoroscopic observation of motion of the hand and wrist can be recorded on videotape. Because the time of examination is short, irradiation to the hand is minimal, and the opportunity for repeated viewing of the videotapes results in more accurate conclusions about the movement of each carpal bone and degree of opening of individual joint spaces. This is the best method to study the cause of a painful click and intermittent or "dynamic" scapholunate instability in which the abnormality may be only an instantaneous change in position of the carpal bones.

Examination begins with a PA view of the wrist while the patient actively moves the hand in maximum ulnar and then radial tilts. This is first done with an open hand and then repeated with a closed fist. The compressive pressure produced by clenching of the wrist may enlarge the space between the scaphoid and the lunate to a degree indicative of scapholunate dissociation. Generally, for comparison, the asymptomatic wrist should also be studied while the same maneuvers are performed as on the abnormal side. Laxity of joints varies considerably from person to person and during the lifetime of each individual. Therefore, the asymptomatic side serves as a "control" of normal joint laxity for each patient. Only very substantial differences of joint opening between the normal and the painful side warrant diagnosis of scapholunate dissociation. The term *rotatory subluxation* of the scaphoid refers to a scapholunate dissociation characterized by palmar tilt of the scaphoid's distal pole seen on lateral views and, again, by enlargement of the scapholunate joint space observed on frontal views.

In lateral projection, each wrist is studied while the patient performs active flexion, extension, followed by ulnar and radial tilt. The lateral view is most informative for alignment in the central axis of the wrist (radius-lunate-capitate). Subtle instability of the carpal bones (dorsal intercalated segment instability [DISI] or volar intercalated segment instability [VISI]) can be detected during these movements. Subluxation of the distal radioulnar joint is not easily documented by fluoroscopy of wrist motion (see Computed Tomography below).

ARTHROGRAPHY

Introduction of iodinated contrast material into the synovial spaces of the wrist and carpometacarpal joints has been devised to aid in diagnosis of injuries to the triangular fibrocar-

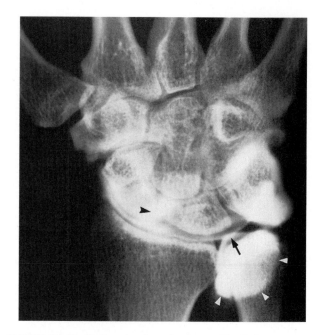

FIGURE 78.10. Abnormal wrist arthrogram with all three compartments filled from a single injection. Iodinated contrast material introduced in the radiocarpal joint enters through a tear in the triangular fibrocartilage (*arrow*) into the distal radioulnar joint space (*white arrowheads*). Also, presence of contrast material in the midcarpal joints (*black arrowhead*) indicates a tear in the scapholunate ligament.

tilage complex (TFCC), intercarpal ligaments, and/or capsular tears around these joints. Contrast material injected into the radiocarpal joint can traverse torn intercarpal ligaments (scapholunate, lunotriquetral ligaments) and can be seen to accumulate in the midcarpal compartment. Similarly, it can enter the distal radioulnar joint through a gap in the TFCC (Fig. 78.10). When such communications are not seen but are still clinically suspected, separate injections of the midcarpal joint space or distal radioulnar joint may detect unidirectional abnormal flow of contrast medium through tears of ligaments or the triangular fibrocartilage complex (triple-compartment arthrogram) (2). Recent technical advances, such as digital subtraction radiography, have made triple-compartment arthrography more reliable, but its usefulness is diminishing as other means of imaging develop. Arthrography produces a disturbingly high number of false-positive results. The mere flow of contrast from one compartment to the next does not prove that the abnormality of morphology is clinically significant (3,4). For example, a small perforation in the center of the TFCC is present in approximately 50% of all individuals 40 years of age or older (5), most of whom are completely asymptomatic. Arthrography has been replaced by MRI, which is noninvasive and provides much more precise information about synovial cavities, ligaments, and other soft-tissue structures.

BONE SCINTIGRAPHY

Radionuclide imaging is useful, but the scans must be interpreted with careful clinical correlation and in conjunction with radiographs. Bone scintigraphy is based on two basic processes: the physical properties of technetium 99m and the metabolic rate of bone absorption of phosphate compounds. The

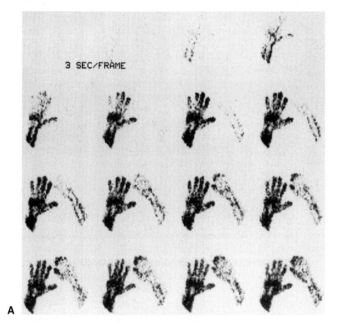

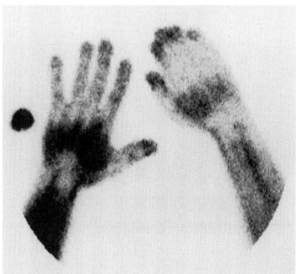

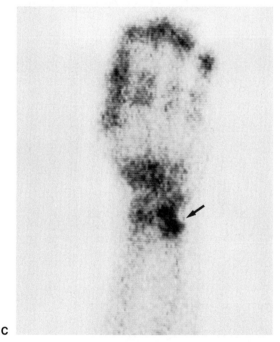

FIGURE 78.11. Three-phase technetium 99m bone scan in reflex sympathetic dystrophy (RSD). **A:** First phase: Blood flow is diminished on the abnormal side. **B:** Second phase: Decreased activity in the abnormal hand is consistent with ischemia. **C:** Delayed phase shows moderate increase in the uptake of multiple joints consistent with RSD. Focal intense activity in the ulnar head (*arrow*), site of minor bone injury that triggered the disorder.

radioisotope scan is an excellent, sensitive, and relatively inexpensive screening method for many disorders, but is limited by its lack of specificity.

Diphosphonate compounds normally cross from the blood to bone, where they are deposited in proportionally larger amount on those segments of the skeleton where metabolic rate of bone turnover is greater or where active deposition represents a repair process (callus, reactive bone sclerosis, etc.). Using diphosphonate compounds bound to a radioisotope such as technetium 99m, we can follow the activity of the radioactive tracer to detect zones of active metabolic turnover. The physical properties of technetium 99m make it an ideal clinical tracer: It is readily available, has a short half-life (6 hours), and emits γ photons with monoenergetic disintegration energy at 140 keV, which can be detected by sodium iodide scintillation crystal. The Anger γ scintillation camera detects these photons, and by usage of collimators and electronic processing, this information is visually displayed as anatomic structures with diverse levels of isotope activity.

For the study, technetium 99m bound to methydiphosphonate is injected intravenously. In a few seconds it reaches the hand through arterial blood flow, diffuses in the capillaries, and returns via the draining veins into the general circulation. In about 5 minutes, it is uniformly mixed in the entire blood pool. Gradually, the technetium bound to diphosphonate is excreted by the kidneys. About 3 to 4 hours after injection, 30% to 40% of the technetium is deposited in the bones, 10% to 15% is diffusely dispersed in other tissues, and 5% is still in the blood, while 35% of the administered dose has been excreted into the urine (1).

The study is conducted in three phases.

1. *Phase 1: radionuclide angiogram.* Following a bolus intravenous injection of tracer, radioactivity is detected

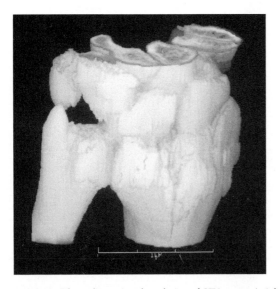

FIGURE 78.12. Three-dimensional rendering of CT images. Axial images were reformatted to represent the wrist seen from the dorsal side. Comminuted, impacted fractures are seen in the distal radius and ulna.

at its first pass in the ulnar and radial arteries. Venous drainage of the isotope can be seen 10 to 20 seconds later.

2. *Phase 2: blood pool phase.* At 5 to 8 minutes after injection, an equilibrium is reached in the distribution of the isotope in the entire blood pool. Areas of increased metabolic activity represent hyperemic zones in the tissues.

3. *Phase 3: metabolic images or delayed phase.* Images obtained at 3 to 4 hours after injection reflect the activity of the technetium bound to diphosphonate deposited in the bone. Foci of abnormally high uptake of isotope seen in the delayed images represent areas of increased absorption of the phosphate compounds bound to the technetium.

The early phases of a bone scan can be used as a crude angiogram, useful to differentiate fast-flowing blood seen in arteriovenous malformations from the slow flow of hemangiomas. In most arteriovenous malformations, a large dominant feeding artery can be detected in the earliest images of radionuclide angiogram. The flow of isotope toward and into the malformations is rapid, and it reaches the hand much faster than the opposite normal side. In hemangioma, the activity of the tracer

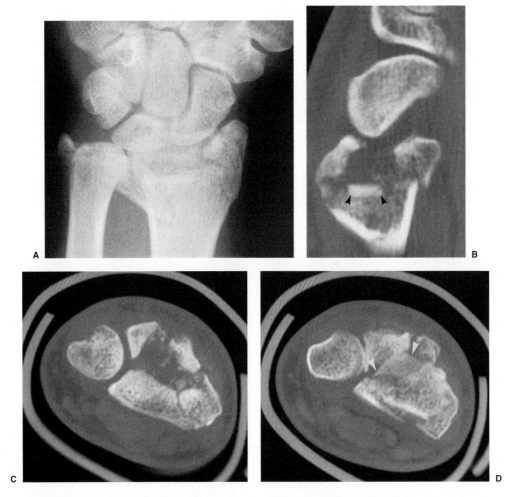

FIGURE 78.13. "Die-punch" fracture of distal radius. **A:** Posteroanterior view of the wrist shows comminuted intra-articular fracture of the distal radius. **B:** Sagittal CT image: A fragment of articular cortex is displaced proximally, impacted in the spongy bone of the metaphysis (*arrowheads*). **C:** Axial CT image in the distal surface of the radius shows the degree of comminution and the central gap left by the displacement of the articular fragment. **D:** Axial CT image 6 mm proximal to C shows the missing articular cortex fragment (*arrowheads*) trapped between the metaphyseal fragments.

is most intense in the second phase of the bone scan, when the entire blood pool is uniformly radioactive (capillary phase). The radionuclide angiogram is useful in assessing the arterial blood flow in patients with acute thrombosis, frostbite, or recent surgery for limb reattachment. Pins, orthopedic hardware, bulky dressings, and skin abnormalities seen in these patients often make MRI or conventional angiography impractical. The first phase of a bone scan can be a practical substitute.

The third phase is the most important part of the bone scan for detection of osseous lesions. Delayed images with focally abnormal increased uptake of tracer activity will be seen at fracture sites in their acute phase, during healing when calcified callus is being formed, or even much later as high metabolic activity of the remodeling of the fracture site continues for months after the injury. Technetium bone scan is so sensitive that a negative examination practically excludes any significant osseous abnormality. Thus, the radioisotope bone scan is a good screening modality to exclude bone pathology. The problem with the bone scan is its lack of specificity: Focal uptake may appear the same from fractures, avascular necrosis of bone, erosive arthritis, infection, osteoid osteoma, bone tumors, and so forth.

Diffuse, generalized, increased uptake may be a sign of rheumatoid arthritis, septic joint, acute disuse osteoporosis, or other generalized diseases. In reflex sympathetic dystrophy (RSD), a characteristic pattern of abnormalities has been described in the bone scan (1). It consists of diffuse increased activity in all joints of the hand, from radiocarpal to interphalangeal articulations. Less specific for RSD is the asymmetric activity seen in the first and second phase of the bone scan, a manifestation of disturbed blood perfusion to the affected hand (Fig. 78.11). Although these are frequent findings with RSD, as with many other tests, when used alone they are not pathognomonic of the disorder (6).

ULTRASOUND

Ultrasound (US) is an imaging modality that is extremely suitable for detection of fluid collections. It can also visualize superficially located tendons of the extremities in different positions. As such it would appear to be the modality of choice for imaging ganglion cysts of the wrist and hand (7). However, two drawbacks diminish significantly the usefulness of ultrasound: US does not visualize the bone structures and it is extremely operator dependent. Only radiologists trained specifically and experienced in the subtle variations of ultrasonography of the musculoskeletal structures can make consistently accurate diagnosis and more specifically so in the hand and wrist where the anatomy is complex. A ganglion cyst appears in ultrasound images as a discrete hypoechoic mass. Cysts located deep between the tendons or those related to pathology of adjacent synovium or intercarpal ligaments are better demonstrated by MRI, which detects all soft-tissue and bone structures and thus gives a more thorough understanding of related pathology. For these reasons ultrasound studies of the hand and wrist are infrequently performed.

COMPUTED TOMOGRAPHY

CT of the hand and wrist is the modality of choice for imaging the abnormalities of cortical bone. It can obtain primary images in all planes, with sections as thin as 0.5 to 1 mm (8). For example, small avulsion fractures that may be obscured in routine radiographs by complex overlapping of carpal bone are easily detected in CT images. Another advantage of CT is the ability to obtain from multiple axial images a three-dimensional rendering of the anatomy viewed from different

angles (Fig. 78.12). This provides a direct three-dimensional visual representation of the relationship between the bone structures, especially useful in complex fractures or dislocations.

Distal Radial Fractures

The vast majority of fractures in the distal radius and ulna are readily detected from plain films. However, details of comminuted fractures that intersect complex articular surfaces can be better visualized by CT images. Specifically, the burst fractures that involve the distal radioulnar joint are seen at best advantage in the axial CT images. Displacement of fragments that can cause permanent incongruity of the distal radioulnar joint can be detected initially by CT scan or the correctness of their reduction verified.

Die-punch fractures of the distal radius present difficulty in reduction and stabilization. Planning appropriate treatment requires precise knowledge of the extent of comminution, the size of fragments, and the degree of their displacement into the metaphysis. This information can be readily obtained from CT images (Fig. 78.13). The axial slices evaluate the size and position of the displaced fragment as well as distal radioulnar joint congruency. Sagittal and coronal images show the exact position of the displaced cortical fragment of the radius embedded in the cancellous bone of the metaphysis.

Distal Radioulnar Joint Injuries

Distal radioulnar joint (DRUJ) alignment is difficult to assess from plain films or even from videodynamic studies. Axial CT images obtained at the level of the sigmoid notch of the radius directly demonstrate the position of the ulnar head in relation to the radius. Subtle subluxations are more readily diagnosed if these axial images are obtained in three positions: neutral, pronation, and supination, each time simultaneously imaging both wrists. Only three to four sections exactly centered on the distal radioulnar joint are necessary for each position. Such

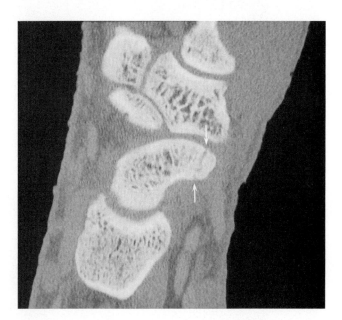

FIGURE 78.14. Oblique sagittal CT image in the long axis of the scaphoid. Hairline, nondisplaced fracture of the scaphoid (*arrows*).

an examination is expeditious and practical, and provides precise information on the degree of dislocation, subluxation, and the position in which such alignment abnormalities are most pronounced (8).

Scaphoid Fractures

Nondisplaced *fractures of the scaphoid* are notoriously difficult to detect by plain films obtained early after injury. When initial films of patients with clinically suspected scaphoid fractures appear to be normal, the most frequent therapeutic attitude is to immobilize the wrist as if an undisplaced fracture had

been demonstrated and to repeat radiographs in 7 to 10 days. With a fracture, resorption of bone at the fracture margins will generally make it detectable in the follow-up radiographs. For high-performance athletes and others for whom an immediate diagnosis is of practical necessity, CT can be employed for early detection of scaphoid fractures (Fig. 78.14).

Computed tomography of the scaphoid should include sagittal views obtained in the long axis of this bone (8). Such images (1- to 2-mm thick slices) will depict the contour of the cortex from the distal to the proximal pole and detect any sagittal angulation between fracture fragments. Displacement of more than 1 mm between fragments and any palmar angulation of the distal pole detected by CT are of great

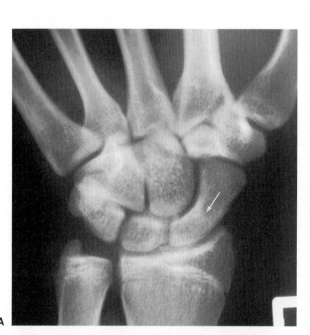

A

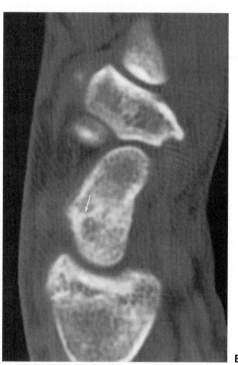

B

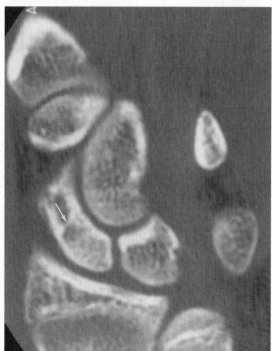

C

FIGURE 78.15. Healing scaphoid fracture. **A:** Scaphoid view at 4 months follow-up, treated with a cast. Healing of the fracture (*arrow*) is difficult to assess. Oblique sagittal CT image (**B**) and coronal CT image (**C**) both demonstrate that fracture gap is obliterated by callus, an indication of normal healing (*arrow*).

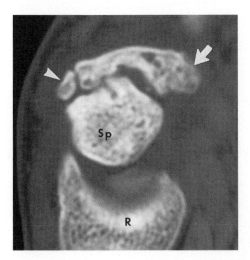

FIGURE 78.16. Nonunion of scaphoid fracture. Oblique sagittal CT image: Distal fragment is tilted in a horizontal position (*arrow*); the small comminuted fragment on the dorsal side contributes to the "humpback" deformity of the scaphoid (*arrowhead*). The fracture surfaces are sclerotic, and the gap between them is irregular. *R*, radius; *Sp*, scaphoid proximal fragment.

clinical significance. Also, CT can demonstrate the early healing stage of callous formation, seen in the CT images as blurring or complete obliteration of the fracture line in the bone marrow (Fig. 78.15). Cortical bone healing lags several weeks behind healing of the cancellous bone. Of course, complications of scaphoid fractures, such as nonunion or avascular necrosis of bone (AVN), are also seen in the CT images.

Nonunion of a scaphoid fracture is characterized by enlargement of the gap between fragments and sclerosis of the fracture surface (Fig. 78.16). Sagittal CT images obtained in flexion and extension can demonstrate directly motion between the fracture fragments, thus permitting differentiation between fibrous callus and true nonunion. In late stages of nonunion, changes consistent with posttraumatic arthrosis,

such as eburnation of adjacent spongy bone, cystic erosion of bone surface, and marginal osteophytes, develop at the fracture site.

Avascular necrosis of bone in the early stage is more readily demonstrated by MRI than by CT; however, subtle changes in density in the trabecular bone can be detected by CT. Care should be exercised in making an early diagnosis of avascular necrosis. During the normal healing of a fracture there is diminished blood supply to the proximal pole of the scaphoid, which consequently is less affected by the natural osteoporosis of disuse seen in all other segments of the carpus. In the first weeks after immobilization, mild, proximal pole high density may be only a transitory phase of the healing process rather than a sign of avascular necrosis of bone. Demonstration of the deposition of calcified callus at the fracture site is a strong indication that normal healing is occurring and supersedes the transitory phase of retained normal density of the proximal fragment of the scaphoid for healing assessment.

Hamate Fractures

Hamate hook fractures cannot always be seen on special oblique or carpal tunnel views but are easily detected in axial CT images (Fig. 78.17). Sagittal views can be used to determine any angulation or displacement of the hook fragment in a craniocaudad direction. Computed tomographic images are also useful in evaluation of those fractures of the body of the hamate that intersect and displace part of the carpometacarpal joint surfaces (Fig. 78.18).

Congenital Anomalies

Congenital abnormalities of the hand and wrist may have complex involvement of the bones, which necessitates clarification by a multisectional imaging modality such as CT. Especially useful to planning of surgery is the three-dimensional rendering of the deformed bones.

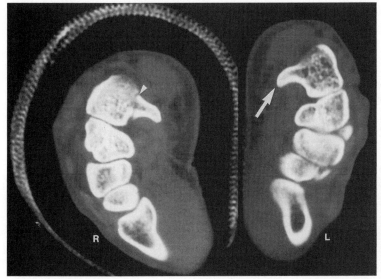
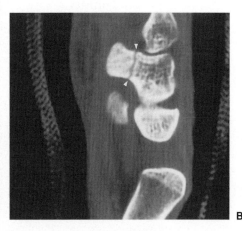

FIGURE 78.17. Fracture of hamate hook. **A:** Axial CT image of both wrists: left hook is normal (*arrow*); the right one has a fracture through its base (*arrowhead*). **B:** Sagittal CT image: nondisplaced fracture through the base of hamate hook (*arrowheads*). See fig 78.7.

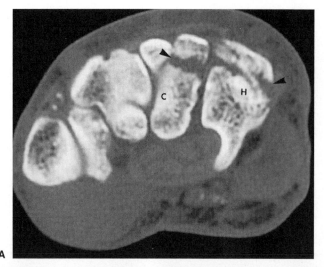

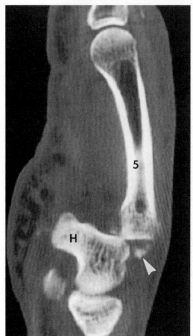

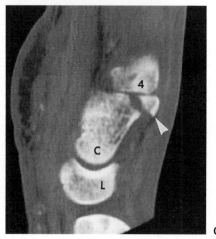

FIGURE 78.18. Fracture-dislocation of the carpometacarpal joints. **A:** Axial CT image: fractures (*arrowheads*) in the dorsal part of the capitate (*C*) and body of the hamate (*H*). **B:** Sagittal image through the hamate: dorsal dislocation of the fifth (*5*) metacarpal together with a small fragment (*arrowhead*) detached from the dorsal margin of the hamate (*H*). **C:** Sagittal CT image through capitate (*C*) and lunate (*L*). The base of fourth metacarpal (*4*) is displaced dorsally, together with a fragment of capitate (*arrowhead*).

Tumors

Tumors of all the anatomic structures of the hand and wrist are generally best elucidated by MRI. The role of CT is limited to characterization of matrix calcification and cortical bone involvement, giving little more information than routine roentgenograms. The important soft tissue extent of any tumor is the domain of MRI rather than CT. An exception is osteoid osteoma, for which the detection of the nidus, the reactive bone sclerosis around it, and the thickening of the cortex adjacent to the nidus are superbly portrayed in the CT images (Fig. 78.19).

Degenerative Disorders

Cystic erosions of carpal bones that communicate with joint spaces are occasionally seen in posttraumatic arthritis or other chronic arthritides of the wrist, including pseudogout. Even though their existence is suspected from the plain films, it is only in CT images obtained in multiple planes that the exact location of any cortical interruptions can be visualized (Fig. 78.20). Differentiation can be best made between cystic bone marrow abnormalities seen in generalized diseases (sarcoidosis, amyloidosis, etc.) and local diseases related to synovial pathology, leading to erosions or fissures of the cortical bone and cystic lesions in the immediately adjacent spongy bone (posttraumatic arthritis, pseudogout).

Technical Limitations of Computed Tomography

Metallic artifacts generated by orthopedic fixation devices such as plates and screws degrade CT images each time the path of the x-ray beam encounters the extreme density of a metal piece. When the metal is large and unavoidable by any change in the orientation of the CT slices, the CT images may be so degraded by artifacts as to become useless. However, by careful inspection of routine radiographs, a compromise can be reached in many cases: The hand and wrist can be placed in the gantry

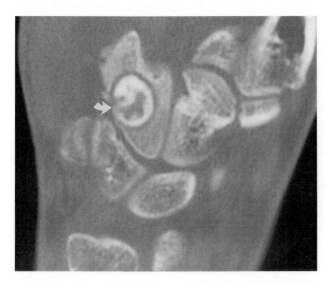

FIGURE 78.19. Osteoid osteoma. Coronal CT image: Ring of sclerosis (*arrow*) surrounds the nidus of an osteoid osteoma in the hamate.

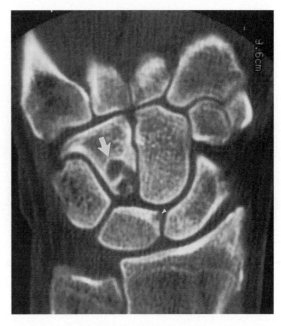

FIGURE 78.20. Carpal cystic erosions. Coronal CT image shows a cystic erosion of proximal pole of the hamate with fragmentation of the articular cortex (*arrow*). A small erosion is also seen in the lunate (*arrowhead*).

in such a position as to obtain at least several slices that do not pass through the metal pieces. These would not contain artifacts and can be of diagnostic value. An example of such a situation is the CT obtained for follow-up of scaphoid fractures treated with Herbert screw fixation. Care is taken to position the hand so as to align the screw with the exact plane of the oblique sagittal slices. Consequently, only two or three slices will contain artifacts; all the others have the necessary resolution for detection of calcified callus obliterating the fracture gap (Fig. 78.21).

MAGNETIC RESONANCE IMAGING

A true revolution of musculoskeletal radiology took place with the advent of MRI. Structures previously invisible by radiologic means became clearly depicted by this new multisectional imaging modality, which does not deliver any radiation to the patient. Imaging the tendons, ligaments, vessels, and nerves in addition to the bone and joint structures is now possible. Knowledge of nature and exact location of pathology is accomplished better by MRI than by any other imaging modality (9).

Magnetic resonance imaging is based on the spinning properties of the hydrogen atom nucleus (a single proton). In the strong magnetic field inside the scanner, these protons line up their spinning vector in a parallel or antiparallel direction. When a radiofrequency (RF) pulse is applied, these protons flip their angle of rotation (are excited); when the RF pulse is interrupted, they return to a resting state (relax) at different rates, depending on their bonding environment (molecules

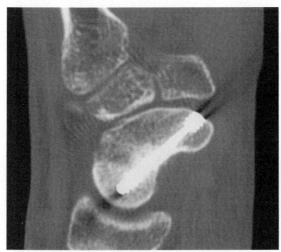

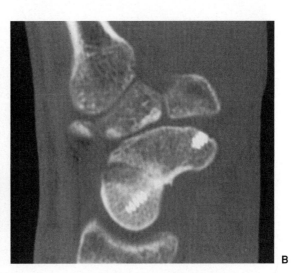

A

B

FIGURE 78.21. Scaphoid fracture treated with Herbert screw. **A:** Sagittal CT image aligned with the screw contains artifacts from the metallic density. **B:** Adjacent slice carefully planned to reduce the metallic artifact shows some fracture healing, mostly on the palmar side.

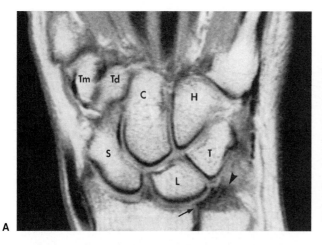

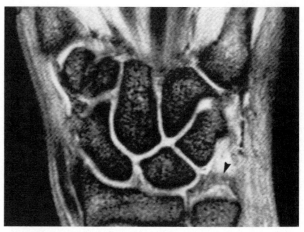

FIGURE 78.22. Coronal MRI of normal wrist. **A:** Coronal proton density-weighted image of the wrist shows the carpal bones: scaphoid (*S*), lunate (*L*), and triquetrum (*T*) form the proximal carpal row; trapezium (*Tm*), capitate (*C*), trapezoid (*Td*), and hamate (*H*) form the distal carpal row. The articular cartilage of distal radius is continuing medially to form the surface of the distal radioulnar joint (*arrow*). The bone marrow signal is uniformly high, giving a light-gray appearance of the carpal bones. The fibrocartilage of the wrist appears as a triangular low signal structure (*black arrowhead*). **B:** Coronal T2*-weighted image obtained at same level as (A) demonstrates the high signal—manifested as a white line—representing summation of the articular fluid and the superficial layer of hyaline cartilage covering the carpal bones. The bone marrow is uniformly low in signal. The triangular fibrocartilage is seen as a low-signal structure against the background of the high signal of the articular fluid (*black arrowhead*).

of fat, water, etc.). Capturing the radiofrequency generated by these protons returning to their relaxed state of spinning is done by "resonating" their RF with that of a receiving coil, which is extremely sensitive to infinitely small variations of the RF signal intensity. These variations are processed by a computer, which calculates through the Fourier transform formula the intensity of signal in each pixel of the tissue slice in which the protons are relaxing. These pixels are presented in a digital image, with shades of gray proportional to the RF signal intensity of the protons in that volume of tissue. Thus it becomes

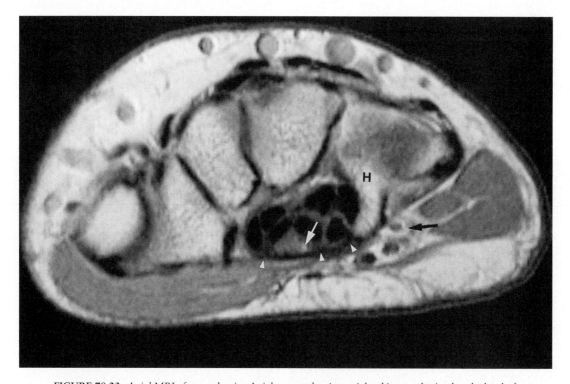

FIGURE 78.23. Axial MRI of normal wrist. Axial proton density-weighted image obtained at the level of the hamate hook (*H*) shows the carpal tunnel and the transverse carpal ligament (*arrowheads*) underneath which the median nerve is illustrated with a median artery within it (*white arrow*). On the medial side of the wrist, next to the hook of the hamate, the ulnar artery and ulnar nerve are identified (*black arrow*). The black oval-shaped structures in the carpal tunnel represent cross-sections of the flexor tendons, separated by a gray layer of synovial sheaths.

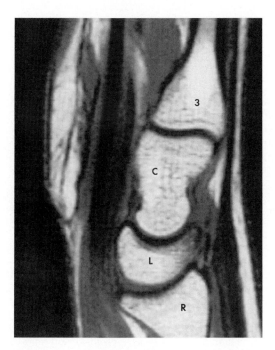

FIGURE 78.24. Sagittal MRI of normal wrist. Sagittal T1-weighted image obtained in the center of the wrist demonstrates the longitudinal alignment of the radius (*R*), lunate (*L*), capitate (*C*), and third metacarpal (*3*). The lunate has no tilt of the palmar or dorsal poles.

possible to differentiate tissues based on the rate of relaxation of the protons they contain.

Technique

Satisfactory-quality MRI of the hand and wrist necessitates medium- or high-field scanners (1.0 to 1.5 Tesla units), use of dedicated surface coils capable of producing images with a field of view of 100 mm or less, and meticulous attention to the scanning parameters. The most common sequences of RF pulse excitation are spin-echo T1- and T2-weighted images. Each manufacturer of magnetic resonance scanners has devised pulse sequences aimed at showing at best advantage zones of higher water content (tumors, inflammation, cysts, articular fluid). The common denominator of such sequences is T2*-weighted; however, each type of magnetic resonance scanner would have a particular name for these images (abbreviated in groups of letters: FLASH, FISP, STIR, etc). In this chapter, illustrations of T2*-weighted images are selected from the FLASH protocol. In all these sequences the bone cortex, ligaments, tendons, and fibrocartilage appear as signal void structures (black in the image). Proton density is a variant of T1-weighted image the sequences with suppression of signal from fat have the advantage of making any zone of edema or intra-articular fluid more conspicuous.

In T1-weighted images, the marrow and subcutaneous fat have high signal (white or light-gray shade in the image). The articular fluid, synovial cyst, or any other dominant water zone is showing an intermediate signal (medium-gray in the image). Muscles also are seen as intermediate signal intensity structures and are at times difficult to distinguish from collections of fluid.

T2-weighted images show the fat in the bone marrow and subcutaneous layer as a low-intermediate signal tissue (dark gray in the image). Contrary to T1-weighted images, in T2-weighted images, the fluid in the joint, cystic structures, and zones of edema exhibit high signal intensity (white in the image).

T2*-weighted images (FLASH) and fat-suppressed T2-weighted images are characterized by a marked contrast between zones of fluid (white in the image) and bone or fibrocartilage that have low or absent signal (black). This striking difference in signal resembles an arthrographic effect and is especially useful in the evaluation of the TFCC.

A complete wrist or hand examination usually consists of coronal T1-weighted coronal FLASH, sagittal T1-, and axial T2-weighted images, but tailoring of the examination to suit the clinical problem is necessary. For example, in Kienböck

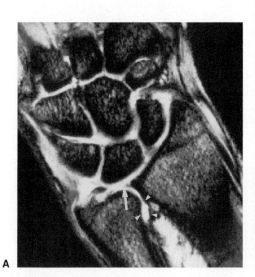

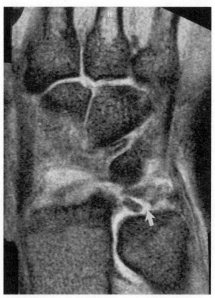

FIGURE 78.25. Acute traumatic tear of the triangular fibrocartilage of the wrist. **A:** Coronal T2*-weighted image: gap in the fibrocartilage avulsed from the radius (*arrow*) and prominent fluid in the distal radioulnar joint (*arrowheads*). **B:** Another patient with TFCC avulsed from the ulna with gap marked by arrow.

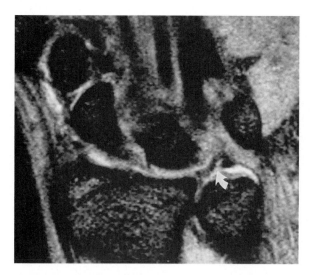

FIGURE 78.26. Flap tear of the triangular fibrocartilage. Coronal T2*-weighted image shows a horizontal tear detaching a flap of the TFCC (*arrow*).

disease, sagittal FLASH images show with better advantage the surrounding synovitis and highlight any fragmentation with displacement of lunate parts.

Gadolinium administered intravenously is used to detect small vascular masses (glomus tumor, etc.) and to determine the differential of blood perfusion between normal tissues and tumoral or inflammatory lesions. Gadolinium is also used to enhance the signal in the lumen of the vessels during magnetic resonance angiography (MRA).

Magnetic resonance angiography is performed by rapid acquisition of axial slices in a "slab of tissue" configuration, each sequence repeated at 30 seconds. The electronic processed data are displayed as a three-dimensional representation of the vessels seen from different vantage points. The precise timing of the scanning in relation to the bolus of gadolinium injection enables one to visualize separately the arteries or the veins. In cases in which no contrast is used, this is accomplished by modifying the scanning parameters related to the velocity of blood flow.

Normal Magnetic Resonance Imaging Demonstrated Anatomy

Coronal images obtained in the center of the wrist and hand show the distal radius and ulna, the carpals and metacarpals in their longitudinal orientation, and their articulations (Fig. 78.22). The triangular fibrocartilage complex is seen as a signal-void band stretching from the medial margin of the radius across the ulnar head to where it is attached at the base of the ulna styloid. The marrow has characteristic light signal with the bone trabeculae seen as a fine lattice of intersecting thin black lines. *Coronal T2-weighted* images outline the articular surface of the TFCC and intercarpal ligaments.

Axial images are necessary for study of the carpal tunnel. The bone walls, the palmar aponeurosis, the median nerve, and other soft-tissue structures located in the tunnel are clearly visualized (Fig. 78.23). The individual compartments of the extensor tendons will be seen on cross section, on the dorsal side of the wrist. *Sagittal T1-weighted images* are essential for evaluation of the alignment in the central axis of the wrist and hand: radius–lunate–capitate–third metacarpal (Fig. 78.24).

Common Pathologic Disorders Detectable by Magnetic Resonance Imaging

Triangular Fibrocartilage Tears

Lesions of the TFCC are divided in two groups: acute tear secondary to trauma and chronic degeneration. The acute tears are seen in the magnetic resonance images as interruption of the low-signal void representing the TFCC (Fig. 78.25). Fluid from the synovial spaces of the medial side of the wrist enters through the gap of the tear, seen in FLASH images as a white zone in the normally black cartilage band (10). Most acute tears seen in young individuals are from the ulnar attachment. Partial tears may split the TFCC horizontally, leaving a flap of fibrocartilage free to displace toward the ulnar head (Fig. 78.26).

Degenerative disease of cartilage, a ubiquitous process histologically demonstrable in the middle-age population, is often observed in the TFCC beginning in the fourth decade. By age 60 years, more than 50% of the population has fissures and perforations in the TFCC (5,10). These abnormalities translate in MRI as thinning of the TFCC, irregular frayed surfaces, fenestration, or large gaps containing fluid. Such appearance of TFCC seen in MRI may be asymptomatic and represent the "normal for age." This is why images of the magnetic resonance study must be interpreted only with clinical correlation to avoid false-positive interpretations (5).

Thumb Ulnar Collateral Ligament Tears

Chronic (gamekeeper's thumb) or acute disruption of the ulnar collateral ligament (UCL) of the thumb's metacarpophalangeal joint (ski-pole injury) is easily diagnosed by MRI. Occasionally the distal end of the ruptured UCL will be displaced outside the adductor aponeurosis (Stener lesion). With acute injury, the

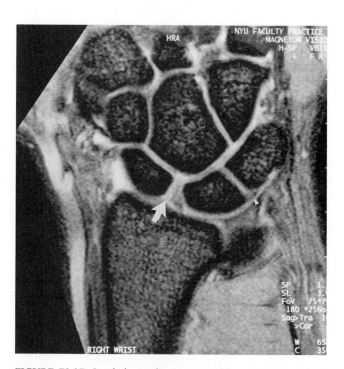

FIGURE 78.27. Scapholunate ligament tear. Coronal T2*-weighted image shows wide space between scaphoid and the lunate. The scaphoid attachment of the ligament is interrupted (*arrow*). The normal lunotriquetral ligament is represented by a slender black line on the proximal margin of the joint (*arrowhead*).

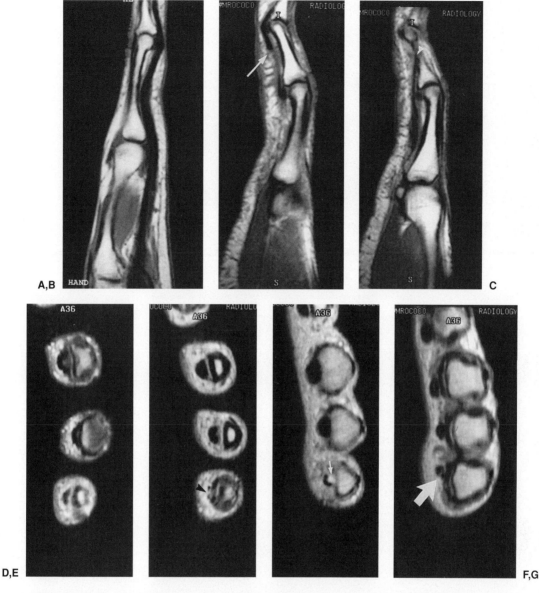

FIGURE 78.28. Ruptured flexor profundus tendon of the fifth digit. **A:** Sagittal T1-weighted image of the fourth digit presented as reference demonstrates the longitudinal direction of a continuous flexor tendon from distal phalanx across the metacarpophalangeal joint. **B:** Sagittal T1-weighted image of the fifth digit: Only the distal portion of flexor digitorum profundus (FDP) is demonstrated with an abrupt discontinuity at the site of rupture (*arrow*). **C:** The normal flexor digitorum superficialis (FDS) tendon is visualized as a thin band attaching on the middle phalanx (*arrowhead*). **D to G:** Axial images of third, fourth, and fifth digits demonstrate a normal appearance of the FDP at the level of the distal phalangeal base in (**D**) and the empty sleeve of the flexor tendons at the site of tear (see *arrowhead* in **E**). The two black dots on the palmar surface of the middle phalanx represent the two insertion slips of the FDS. The space between them should be occupied by the normal flexor profundus tendon, which is retracted proximally and is therefore absent at this level. Compare with the normal appearance of third and fourth digits. **F:** The empty sleeve of the flexor digitorum profundus is represented by white zone (fluid in the sleeve) (*arrow*). **G:** At the level of the metacarpal head there is normal appearance of both FDS and FDP tendons (*arrow*). (Courtesy of Dr. E. Lubat.)

T2-weighted images show adjacent edema and hemorrhage as diffuse zones of increased signal surrounding the torn UCL. Bone bruises in the metacarpal head show increased/decreased signal intensity in the T2-/T1-weighted images, respectively.

Intercarpal Ligament Tears

Scapholunate and lunotriquetral ligament tears are diagnosed by MRI when the low-signal band of the ligament being evaluated is interrupted. Often the instability of the joint will be evident from an abnormally large space between opposing articular surfaces (Fig. 78.27).

Digital Tendon Lesions

In most cases, complete *tears of finger tendons* can be diagnosed by clinical examination. Standard radiographs may show a flake of bone detached from the insertion site of the tendon. Demonstration of the quantity of fibrous tissue in the digital fibro-osseous tunnel and knowledge of the exact location of

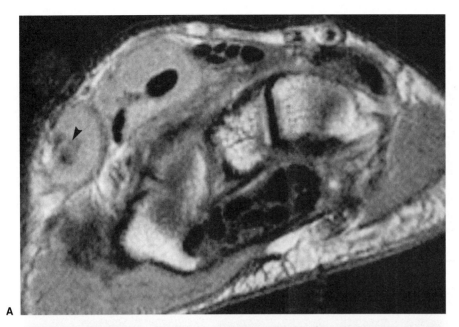

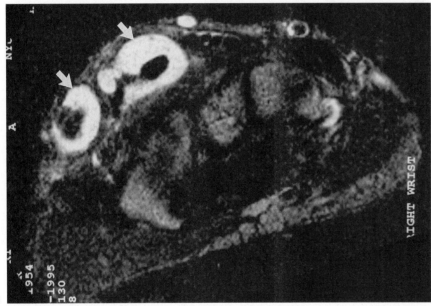

FIGURE 78.29. Partial extensor tendon tear and tenosynovitis. **A:** Axial proton density image shows fluid in the second and third extensor compartments. The abductor pollicis longus tendon has abnormal contour and abnormally high signal consistent with a partial tear (*arrowhead*). **B:** T2-weighted axial image at the same level with (**A**) shows with sharper contrast the fluid accumulated in the tendon sheaths of the second and third extensor compartment (*arrows*).

the end of the retracted proximal segment of the tendon can be helpful in planning surgery. This information can be obtained precisely from sagittal and axial magnetic resonance images (Fig. 78.28).

Tendonitis and Tenosynovitis

Tenosynovitis or *chronic partial tears* longitudinally oriented in tendons are characterized in the axial T2-weighted images by central zones of high signal within the tendon, distention of sleeve by fluid, and thickening of the synovium, which becomes visible as a cuff around the tendon (Fig. 78.29).

Carpal Tunnel Syndrome

Carpal tunnel syndrome (CTS) is essentially a clinical diagnosis from its characteristic signs of nerve compression, and generally can be confirmed by electrodiagnostic studies. Thus, MRI is rarely needed or performed for this condition. The MRI findings of carpal tunnel syndrome include anterior bowing of

the transverse carpal ligament and edema of the median nerve just proximal to its entrance in the carpal tunnel, seen in axial MRI as increased diameter and higher signal intensity of the nerve. As CTS is a nerve compression caused by tenosynovitis, thickening of the synovium investing the digital flexor tendons may be seen on MRI as intermediate signal layers separating individual tendons.

As CTS that is successfully relieved by surgical decompression does not recur, MRI may be strongly indicated for a patient who presents with recurrent symptoms of median nerve compression. Often MRI will reveal discrete masses or other space-occupying lesions, such as ganglion cysts in the carpal tunnel, accounting for the recurrence of nerve compression symptoms.

Avascular Necrosis of Carpal Bones

AVN of the proximal fragment of a fractured scaphoid and idiopathic osteonecrosis of the lunate (Kienböck disease) are two frequently encountered and serious wrist problems about

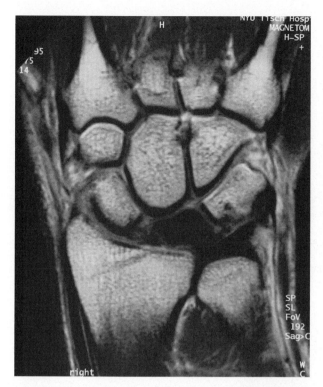

FIGURE 78.30. Kienböck disease. Coronal T1-weighted image shows abnormal low signal in the bone marrow of the lunate consistent with avascular necrosis of bone.

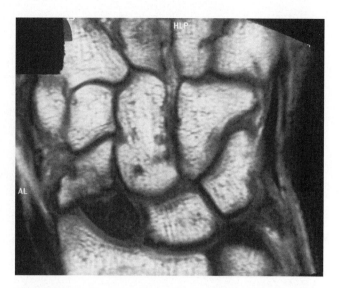

FIGURE 78.32. Avascular necrosis of proximal fragment of fractured scaphoid. Coronal T1-weighted image shows fracture through the waist of the scaphoid and low signal in the bone marrow of the proximal fragment consistent with AVN.

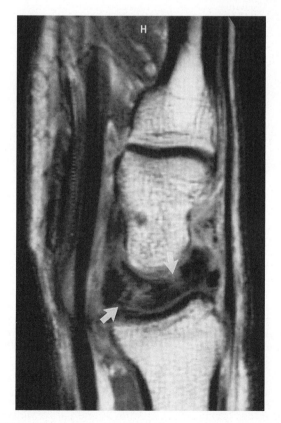

FIGURE 78.31. Advanced Kienböck disease with collapse and fragmentation. Sagittal T1-weighted image shows the fragmentation of the lunate (*arrows*) through the zone of aseptic necrosis manifested as low signal in the bone marrow.

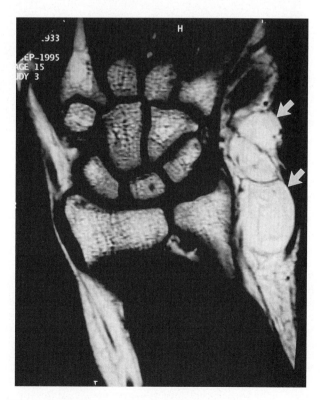

FIGURE 78.33. Lipoma. Coronal T1-weighted image shows a fat-containing mass on the ulnar side of the wrist (*arrows*).

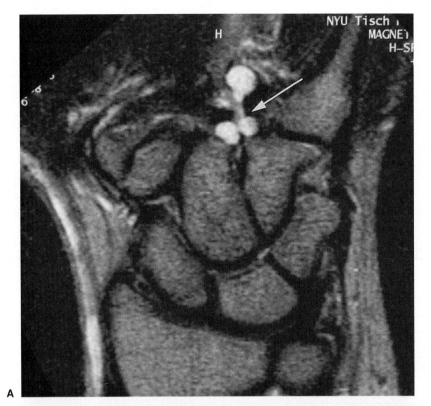

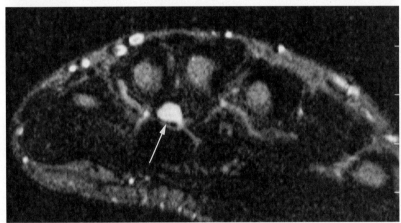

FIGURE 78.34. Ganglion cyst. **A:** Coronal T2-weighted image shows the multiloculated ganglion cyst located in the palmar surface, near the joints between the capitate, hamate, and metacarpal basis (*arrow*). **B:** Axial T2-weighted image shows the deep location of the ganglion cyst (*arrow*).

which precise information is needed. A rare similar spontaneous disorder, Preiser disease, occurs to the scaphoid.

Magnetic resonance imaging is able to detect the earliest changes in the bone marrow, thus allowing a specific diagnosis even at a time when all radiographs are normal. The most accepted theory of etiology of Kienböck disease is that initially forces transmitted axially from the forearm converge on the convex surface of the lunate to produce microfractures. A short ulna (negative variance) may be a predisposing factor (see Wrist Views above). This stage can be regarded as the precursor of AVN and is manifested on MRI as lines of low signal traversing the bone marrow horizontally and parallel to the proximal surface of the lunate (9). If the process continues zones of bone marrow become necrotic, appearing in MRI as low-signal areas in T1-weighted images. When most of the bone marrow of the lunate becomes necrotic, subtle increase in the bone density appears in radiographs. At this time, the entire lunate appears low in signal (Fig. 78.30). Fissures of the cortex and collapse of the lunate indicate advanced

and irreversible Kienböck disease (Fig. 78.31). MRI can detect Kienböck disease at a very early stage, hopefully at a time when treatment can arrest the process. MRI is also helpful in early detection of *AVN in the proximal fragment of a fractured scaphoid.* Observing zones of abnormal signal in most of the bone marrow and lack of enhancement following intravenous administration of gadolinium are indications of AVN. Such findings at 3 months following injury are a strong indication that healing is not occurring with conservative treatment (Fig. 78.32).

Tumors

Tumors of either bone or soft tissues are well visualized in magnetic resonance images. The precise location of the tumor, its extent, and its relationship with adjacent muscles, bones, and neurovascular bundles also can be determined, a significant help in the planning of tumor excision (11). In many instances, the histology of the masses can be reliably concluded: Lipomas

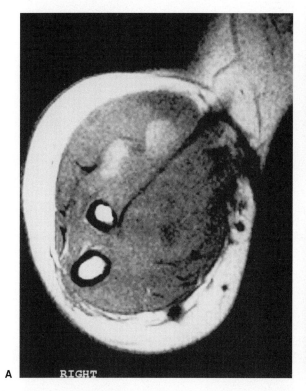
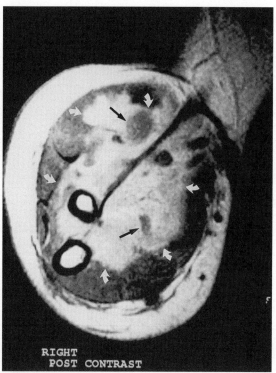

FIGURE 78.35. Synovial sarcoma of the forearm. **A, B**: Axial T1-weighted images before (**A**) and after (**B**) intravenous administration of gadolinium show an aggressive infiltrating mass in the forearm with high vascularity. The margins are better defined (*white arrows*) and necrotic parts of the tumor appear more conspicuous after contrast enhancement (*black arrows*).

have homogeneous fatty content seen in T1-weighted images as a bright signal (Fig. 78.33). Cystic collections of fluid such as those seen in ganglion cysts are characterized in T2-weighted images by a homogeneous bright signal with no internal structure (Fig. 78.34).

Malignant soft-tissue tumors often appear in MRI as infiltrative masses with ill-defined margins. Gadolinium administered intravenously enhances the hypervascular parts of these tumors, making more conspicuous the extent of the lesion and any central zone of necrosis (Fig. 78.35). Such information is essential for planning of biopsy and treatment.

Hemangiomas or arteriovenous malformations give characteristic magnetic resonance images of a mixture of vascular elements on the background of fat and serpiginous, dilated vascular channels feeding or draining the masses.

Retained Foreign Bodies

Suspected and symptomatic *foreign bodies* that are not radiopaque cannot be seen in radiographs, although occasionally CT may detect them. MRI is a much more sensitive modality of detecting nonmetallic foreign bodies and can provide precise information regarding their exact position and relation to adjacent anatomic structures, such as nerves, vessels, tendons, and their synovial sleeves.

Magnetic Resonance Angiography

MRA is extremely useful in studying the abnormal vascular channels related to arteriovenous malformations. It is also reliable in diagnosis of thrombosis of an ulnar or radial artery.

In Raynaud disease or other nontraumatic ischemic processes (e.g., Buerger disease), MRA can be used as an objective determination of the response to different therapy protocols: Its being noninvasive and the short time necessary for scanning (<1 minute for each arterial and venous phase) make it an excellent method for sequential follow-ups (Fig. 78.36). It is now predictable that selective angiography, performed with catheters introduced through the femoral artery, will become a rarity, limited to those instances when the diagnostic imaging of the vascular system is being combined with endovascular treatment of occlusion or, conversely, for embolization of hypervascular masses.

Contraindications for Magnetic Resonance Imaging

Patients who have cardiac pacemakers, surgical clips in the cerebral arteries, or fragments of metal embedded in the globe of the eye should not be admitted in the room of the powerful magnetic fields of an MRI scanner. Ferromagnetic fragments may change position in the body when they align with the direction of the high-strength magnetic field permanently present in and near the scanner. The torque force generated when such metallic fragments move is strong enough to lacerate adjacent tissues, with subsequent serious or even fatal consequences. Patients who need MRI should be screened by clinical history, and in cases of persons previously involved in metal tool working, screening with radiographs can be considered for the area suspected of containing retained ferromagnetic metal fragments.

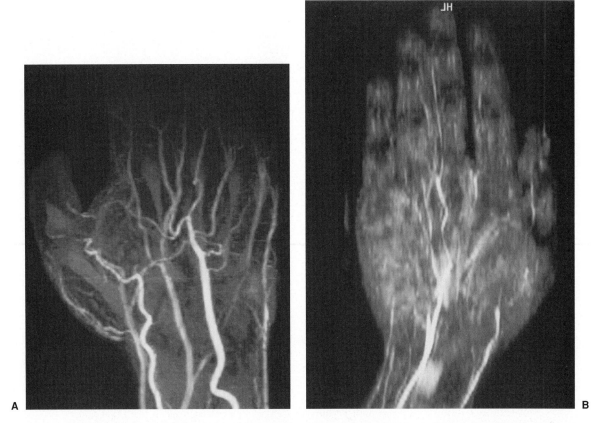

FIGURE 78.36. Magnetic resonance angiogram. **A:** Normal flow through the arterial branches of radial and ulnar arteries. **B:** Severe attenuation of the digital branches is consistent with vasospastic disease.

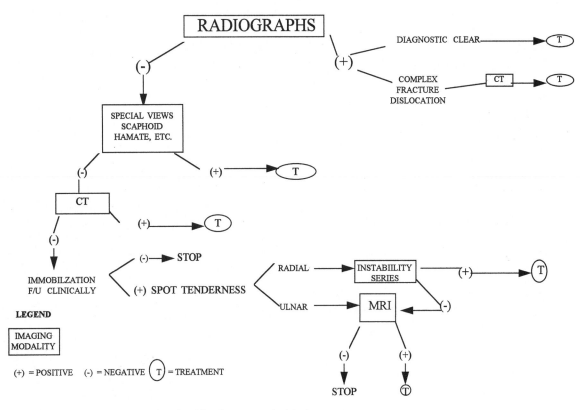

FIGURE 78.37. Imaging algorithm for acute wrist injuries.

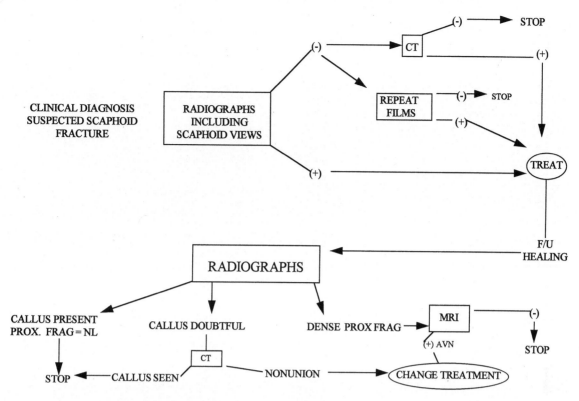

FIGURE 78.38. Imaging algorithm of acute scaphoid trauma.

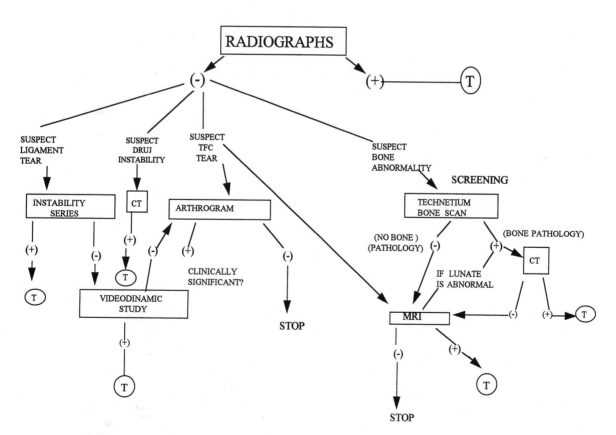

FIGURE 78.39. Imaging algorithm for chronic wrist pain.

IMAGING ALGORITHMS FOR HAND AND WRIST PATHOLOGY

In concluding this chapter, I present several algorithms of radiologic investigation of common clinical problems encountered in hand and wrist. They should not be regarded as constraining rules of work-up, but rather as suggested pathways that lead to a high degree of accuracy in diagnosis (Figs. 78.37 to 78.39).

References

1. Gilula LA, Yiu Y. *Imaging of the Wrist and Hand.* Philadelphia: Saunders; 1996.
2. Levinsohn EM, Rosen ID, Palmer AK. Wrist arthrography: Value of the three compartment injection method. *Radiology.* 1991;179:231.
3. Manaster BJ. The clinical efficacy of triple injection wrist arthrography. *Radiology.* 1991;178:267.
4. Yin YM, Evanoff B, Gilula LA, et al. Evaluation of selective wrist arthrography of contralateral asymptomatic wrists for symmetric ligamentous defects. *AJR Am J Roentgenol.* 1996;166:1067.
5. Metz VM, Schratter M, Dock WI, et al. Age-associated changes of the triangular fibrocartilage of the wrist: Evaluation of the diagnostic performance of MR-imaging. *Radiology.* 1992;184:217.
6. O'Donoghue JP, Powe JE, Mattar AG, et al. Three-phase bone scintigraphy: Asymmetric patterns in the upper extremities of asymptomatic normals and reflex sympathetic dystrophy patients. *Clin Nucl Med.* 1993;18:829.
7. Van Holsbeeck M, Introcaso JH. Sonography of the elbow, wrist and hand. In: Van Holsbeeck M, Introcaso JH, eds. *Musculoskeletal Ultrasound.* St. Louis: Mosby–Year Book; 1991:285.
8. Golimbu C. The wrist. In: Firooznia H, Golimbu C, Rafii M, et al., eds. *MRI and CT of the Musculoskeletal System.* St. Louis: Mosby–Year Book; 1992:615.
9. Golimbu C, Firooznia H, Rafii M. Avascular necrosis of carpal bones. *MRI Clin North Am.* 1995;3:281.
10. Totterman SMS, Miller RJ. MR imaging of the triangular fibrocartilage complex. *MRI Clin North Am.* 1995;3:213.
11. Binkovitz LA, Berguist TH, McLeod RA. Masses of the hand and wrist: Detection and characterization with MR imaging. *AJR Am J Roengenol.* 1990;154:323.

CHAPTER 79 ■ SOFT-TISSUE RECONSTRUCTION OF THE HAND

JOHN TYMCHAK

The objective in the management of soft-tissue injuries of the hand is to achieve primary wound healing. Primary wound healing minimizes the inflammatory reaction, scar formation, and joint stiffening. Surgical approaches include primary closure, skin grafts, flaps, and free tissue transfers. The choice of treatment is based on the mechanism of injury, the size of the defect, location and status of the wound, and injuries to other parts of the hand, as well as the patient's age, sex, general health, and occupation.

The principles pertaining to the timing of soft-tissue replacement are the same as elsewhere in the body. Soft-tissue replacement is performed as early as feasible but not necessarily at the time of injury. Initial treatment may consist of wound debridement alone. Tissues of uncertain viability are retained and inspected for viability at a second procedure. Once loss is certain, the tissue is excised, discarded, and replaced before an inflammatory reaction or infection complicates the wound.

In selecting donor sites for soft-tissue reconstruction, the hand itself is superior to other sites for several reasons: the tissue match is the best, recovery of sensibility is superior, and care is facilitated because the wounds are in a single region. When distant donor sites are chosen, the results achieved for the injured hand must justify the disfigurement and potential problems at the donor site.

SKIN GRAFTS

The dorsal and volar surfaces of the hand have different requirements when considering the replacement of skin. Dorsal skin is thin and loose enough so as not to restrict flexion, yet it must protect tendons and joints. Volar skin must be thicker and tougher, while still allowing motion, and requires sensibility. The glabrous volar hand skin is characterized by the absence of pilosebaceous structures and the presence of specialized encapsulated nerve endings. Consequently, volar skin cannot be replaced by ordinary grafts as only glabrous skin can provide the special dermal neural mechanoreceptors.

Full-thickness grafts are used primarily for small defects. Advantages of full-thickness grafts include a thicker, protected tissue covering, establishment of better sensibility, and less contraction than split-thickness grafts. Graft donor sites for harvesting of glabrous skin include the hypothenar eminence of the hand, and the non–weight-bearing region of the instep of the foot. Grafts harvested from the hypothenar eminence provide a location within the same operative field and a donor site that can be primarily closed. Additional donor sites for full-thickness skin graft harvesting include the volar wrist, and the hairless inguinal fold region.

Split-thickness skin grafts are used for closure of major skin defects. Most wounds are best covered by grafts approximately 0.015-inch thick in adults, and thinner in children. Grafts thicker than 0.018 inches are seldom indicated because of donor-site morbidity. If thick skin is necessary, a full-thickness graft should be used. Furthermore, the thicker the graft, the more hair follicles are transferred. Thus care should be taken to select a relatively hairless area as a donor site for the hand.

FLAPS

Flap tissue is attached temporarily or permanently to its donor site by a pedicle through which vascularization is maintained. Beasley (1) cites three indications of flaps coverage: (a) the wound is unsuitable for revascularization of a skin graft; (b) there is need for subcutaneous tissue replacement as well as skin; and (c) protection is required of an exposed vital structure, such as nerve or joint. Flap donor sites can be divided into local, regional, and distant.

Local Flaps

Bilateral V-Y Advancement Flaps

In 1947, Kutler (2) described the use of bilateral V-Y advancement flaps for coverage of fingertip injuries (Fig. 79.1). These flaps are ideally suited for transverse or slightly volar amputations at the midnail level. Bilateral V-Y advancements flaps are cut from the sides of the injured finger and advanced over the tip by dividing the fibrous septa. Unless vertical septa are severed, almost no distal advancement of the flap is possible. Care must be taken to avoid injury to the lateral pulp tissues in which the terminal elements of the neurovascular bundles pass into the mobilized flaps. Disadvantages of bilateral V-Y advancement include the limited mobility of these flaps, and placement of a scar directly on the fingertip.

Volar V-Y Advancement Flaps

Another surgical approach for transverse midnail or dorsally directed fingertip amputations is the volar V-Y advancement flap (Fig. 79.2) as described by Atasoy (3). A single V-shaped volar flap is cut on the remaining distal phalanx with the tip of the flap at the distal interphalangeal (DIP) joint crease. After division of the fibrous septa from the underlying distal phalanx, the flap is advanced and the donor defect closed. As with all flaps, a tension-free closure is mandatory. The use of V-Y advancement flaps to repair inappropriately large defects can stretch the innervating nerves with resultant dysesthesia.

Volar Neurovascular Advancement Flap (Moberg Flap)

The entire volar surface of an injured digit can be advanced distally as a neurovascular flap to reconstruct an amputated

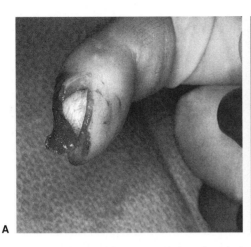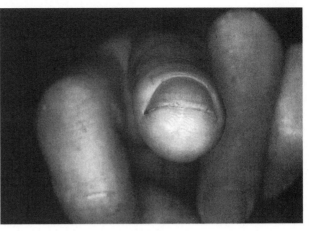

FIGURE 79.1. **A:** Kutler bilateral V-Y advancement flaps elevated on subcutaneous tissue pedicles. **B:** Postoperative result. (Courtesy of Dr. Robert W. Beasley.)

fingertip. This technique was first described by Moberg (4) in 1964 for thumb tip reconstruction. **Although this procedure has been described for all digits of the hand, the Moberg flap is best suited for transverse thumb tip amputations.** Two parallel incisions to create the flap are made just dorsal to the neurovascular bundles of the thumb. The flap is elevated from the flexor tendon sheath with the neurovascular bundles included in the flap. The base of the flap is usually placed at the metacarpophalangeal joint flexion crease and the flap advanced to cover the tip defect. Additional flap advancement may be achieved by excision of burrow triangles at the flap base, or by conversion to an island flap with skin grafting of the secondary defect. **Use of a volar neurovascular advancement flap for digits other than the thumb, may lead to dorsal skin necrosis.** The dorsal skin of the thumb however, is protected against necrosis by dorsal arterial branches from the radial artery.

Cross-Finger Flap

A flap of dorsal skin and subcutaneous tissue from the middle phalanx of an adjacent finger (Fig. 79.3) was first described by Gurdin and Pangman(5) in 1950. **The standard cross-finger flap is best performed for cases of volar fingertip pulp amputation.** The flap is designed over the dorsal surface of the middle phalanx of an adjoining digit and elevated superficial to the extensor peritenon. After turning the flap over like the page of a book, the injured finger is flexed and the flap sutured over the volar tip defect. The donor site is skin grafted and the digits immobilized. Because adipose tissue is absent, revascularization is rapid and the pedicle may be divided on the eighth or ninth postoperative day. This short period of attachment lessens the risks of postoperative joint stiffness. Complications associated with the use of cross-finger flaps include donor-site depression, skin graft hyperpigmentation, digital stiffness, and cold intolerance.

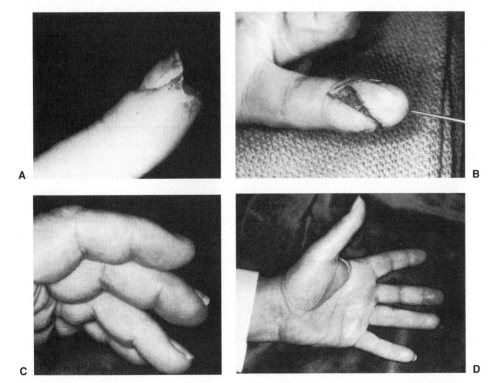

FIGURE 79.2. **A:** Traumatic amputation of the middle fingertip. **B:** Mobilization and advancement of volar V-Y advancement flap. **C** and **D:** Postoperative results. (Courtesy of Dr. Robert W. Beasley.)

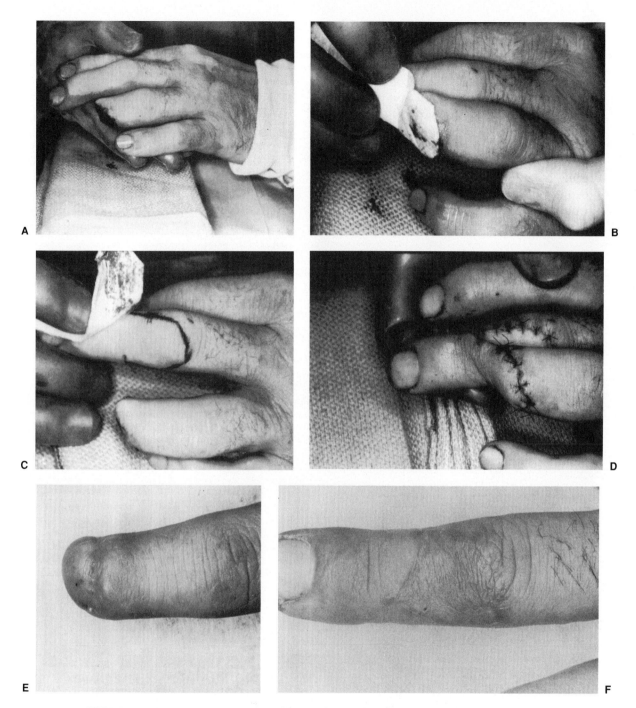

FIGURE 79.3. A: Traumatic amputation of the ring finger to be closed with a distally based cross-finger flap. **B:** Pattern material is applied to defect. **C:** Design of the flap based on the applied pattern. **D:** Flap transfer with skin grafting of the flap donor site. **E and F:** Postoperative results. (Courtesy of Dr. Robert W. Beasley.)

Reversed Cross-Finger Flap

A modification of the standard cross-finger flap is the reversed cross-finger flap. This flap can be used for soft-tissue coverage of dorsal digital injuries. A standard cross-finger flap is designed and de-epithelialized. The flap is then elevated in a routine fashion and turned 180 degrees upside down to cover a dorsal defect on an adjacent finger. The donor defect and undersurface of the flap are then skin grafted.

Flag Flap

Cross-finger flaps can be based proximally, laterally, or distally with length-to-width ratios of 2:1. Distally based pedicles are necessary when cross-finger flaps are used to close distal finger amputations. Cross-finger flaps are ideally designed as axial flaps based on the dorsal branches of the digital vessels (Fig. 79.4), allowing for a very narrow pedicle and thus a mobile flap. Because of their configuration, these flaps are referred to as flag flaps.

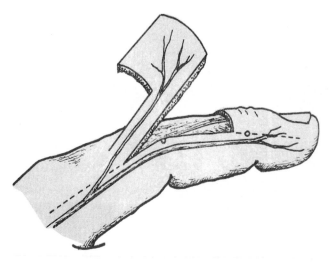

FIGURE 79.4. An axial-based "flag flap" named for its configuration. The designed narrow pedicle allows for great mobility of the flap. (Courtesy of Dr. Robert W. Beasley.)

Volar Cross-Finger Flap

To close a distal thumb amputation site, a cross-finger flap from the dorsal surface of the index finger can be used, however the results often mutilate the donor site. To overcome this problem and to provide better subcutaneous padding, an alternate method of reconstruction is the volar cross-finger flap (Fig. 79.5). Although this flap is best when the amputation is through the terminal phalanx of the thumb, it can also be used for amputations through the distal end of the proximal phalanx. The flap is constructed from the volar surface of the middle or proximal phalanx of the middle finger. Immobilization during the period of attachment is thus possible in a comfortable, protective position.

The volar cross-finger flap requires care in planning and attention to details. The flap is designed with the amount of donor tissue needed but with margins carried to the functional

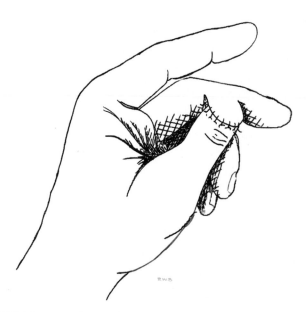

FIGURE 79.5. Closure of a distal thumb amputation with a volar cross-finger flap from the middle finger. (Courtesy of Dr. Robert W. Beasley.)

lines to avoid contracture development. In planning dorsal and volar cross-finger flaps, there are fundamental anatomic differences that must be considered (Fig. 79.6). **The blood supply to the volar tissue is essentially vertical with only short horizontal patterns.** Consequently, the size of volar flaps that can be elevated without necrosis is limited. In contrast, dorsal tissue has a longitudinally oriented vascular network, which permits larger flaps. The pedicle of the volar cross-finger flaps, in contradistinction to that of the dorsal cross-finger flap, must not be dissected free of the digital neurovascular pedicle near its base as there is no longitudinal vascular network. Subsequently, when the pedicle is divided, care must be taken not to injure the neurovascular bundles.

Innervated Cross-Finger Flap

In 1983, Cohen and Cronin (6) described the innervated cross-finger flap. This flap incorporates the dorsal sensory branch of the proper digital nerve into a flap of skin elevated from the dorsum of the middle phalanx of an adjacent finger. By dividing this branch at its origin from the digital nerve on the uninjured digit, a neurorrhaphy can be performed to the divided digital nerve. The donor site is then skin grafted.

Thenar Flap

The concept of a flap elevated from over the thenar eminence was first described by Gatewood (7) in 1926 (Fig. 79.7). Subsequent authors have described various modifications. **The thenar flap must not be confused with a palmar flap, which has associated unacceptable complications.** Complications associated with palmar flaps include fixed flexion contractures of the proximal interphalangeal (PIP) joint of the recipient finger and persistent tenderness of the flap donor site scar on the palm. The thenar flap, however, is an excellent technique for reconstruction of major distal phalangeal amputations. The tissue match is exact, there is sufficient subcutaneous tissue to restore the lost pulp, and the donor site is inconspicuous during most activities. The serious complications associated with palmar flaps can be avoided with thenar flaps if the guidelines set forth by Beasley (1) are followed: (a) the metacarpophalangeal joint of the recipient finger is fully flexed in a protective position, minimizing proximal interphalangeal joint flexion. Flexing of the distal interphalangeal joint when present, further improves the position of immobilization, (b) the thumb is placed in full palmar abduction or opposition, (c) the thenar flap is designed with a proximally based pedicle, high on the thenar eminence so its lateral margin is at the metacarpophalangeal skin crease, and (d) the pedicle of the flap is severed after 10 to 14 days (1).

If simple wound closure of a fingertip amputation is desired, the width of the flap should equal the diameter of the finger. However, the fingertip will then have a flat appearance. To restore the roundness of a normal fingertip, the width of the flap must be 1.5 times the diameter of the digit, as the tip is a half-circle (Fig. 79.8). The flap donor site may be closed primarily or may require placement of a skin graft.

Following division of the thenar flap pedicle after 10 to 14 days, active exercises are begun to remobilize the hand. Age is not a contraindication to the use of thenar flaps. Thenar flaps have been used with equal success with patients from 1 to 76 years of age. A review of 150 thenar flaps involving all age groups revealed not one incident of joint restriction or other serious complication (8).

Neurovascular Island Flaps

The neurovascular island flap for loss of thumb pulp was well described by Littler (9) in 1960. Sensate, vascularized tissue from the ulnar side of the ring or long finger is transferred to the thumb in a single stage (Fig. 79.9). The neurovascular bundle is

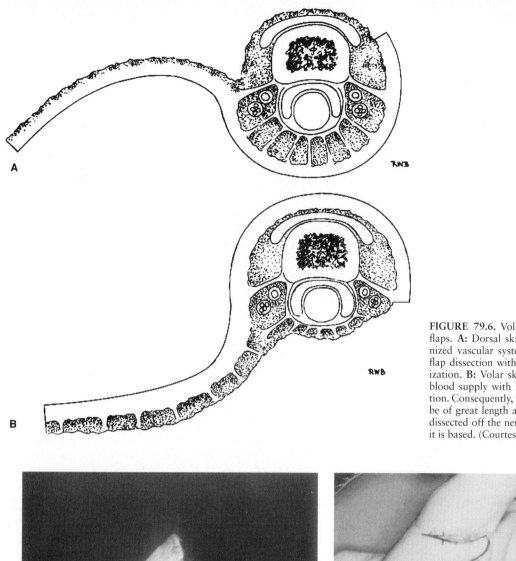

FIGURE 79.6. Volar versus dorsal cross-finger flaps. **A:** Dorsal skin has a longitudinally organized vascular system that allows for extensive flap dissection without potential for devascularization. **B:** Volar skin has an essentially vertical blood supply with limited longitudinal distribution. Consequently, volar cross-finger flaps cannot be of great length and their pedicle must not be dissected off the neurovascular bundle on which it is based. (Courtesy of Dr. Robert W. Beasley.)

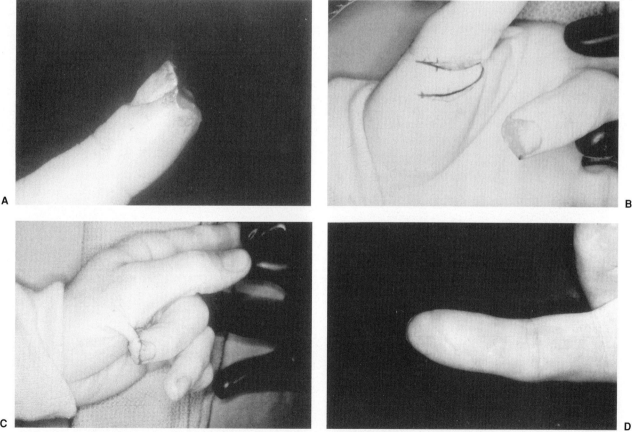

FIGURE 79.7. Thenar flap. **A:** Traumatic amputation of the middle fingertip. **B:** Design of the flap high on the thenar eminence. **C:** Flap inset into soft-tissue defect with maximal metacarpophalangeal flexion and minimal proximal interphalangeal joint flexion. **D:** Postoperative result. (Courtesy of Dr. Robert W. Beasley.)

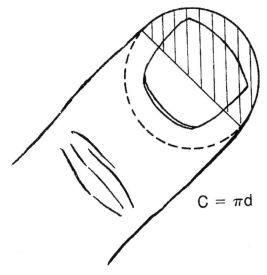

FIGURE 79.8. A normal round fingertip is essentially half a circle when viewed dorsally. Consequently, restoration of this contour requires the flap to be 1.5 times the finger's diameter. (Courtesy of Dr. Robert W. Beasley.)

$$C = \pi d$$

dissected from the level of the palmar arch. The proper digital nerve must be split from its adjacent digit counterpart along the course of the common digital nerve with the dissection carried proximal enough to effect the transfer to the thumb. Because the distal nerve must be divided, sensory loss is experienced in the donor finger. The soft tissue on the donor finger is then skin grafted. It is important in designing and performing the

neurovascular island flaps that the digital nerve not be placed on tension, for this may result in altered sensation.

Radial and Ulnar Artery Forearm Flaps

One flap that can be used to cover defects on the dorsum of the hand or palm is the distally based radial forearm flap. This flap is based distally on the radial artery and its accompanying venae comitantes. The multiple anastomoses between these veins permit reversal of flow in the venae comitantes without valvular obstruction. Retrograde flow is provided by the ulnar artery, providing that the palmar arterial arches are intact. The radial forearm flap may provide up to 8 × 10 cm of thin, hairless skin, which can be used to resurface the dorsum of the hand or palm. The major objection to use of this flap is the associated disfigurement of the skin-grafted donor site. A forearm flap based on the ulnar arterial system can also be designed. However, because the ulnar artery is the hand's dominant arterial system, this flap is less desirable.

Distant Flaps

Distant flaps come from body parts outside of the injured upper extremity. They can be divided into three types: (a) axial (flaps that have a specific vascular pedicle), (b) random (flaps that lack a specific vascular pedicle), and (c) free flaps.

Axial Flaps

The abdomen is a favorite donor site of large, distant, axial flaps for hand resurfacing (Fig. 79.10). The two best abdominal flaps—the superficial inferior epigastric artery flap and the superficial circumflex iliac artery (groin) flap—are based on

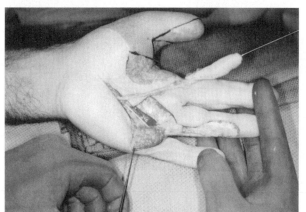

A

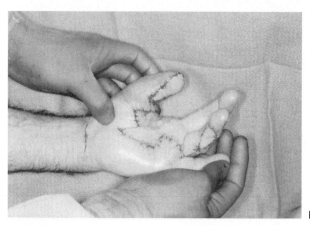

B

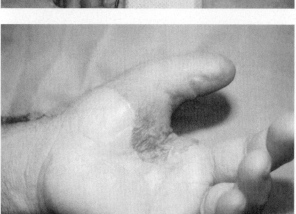

C

FIGURE 79.9. A: Neurovascular island flap harvested from ulnar border of the ring finger for thumb resurfacing. **B:** Inset of the flap on the thumb with skin grafting of the flap donor site. **C:** Postoperative result. (Courtesy of Dr. Robert W. Beasley.)

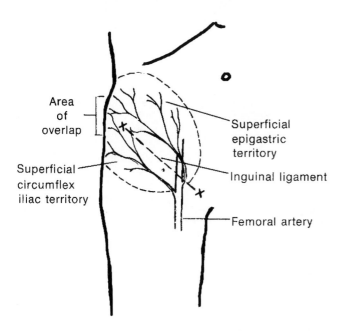

FIGURE 79.10. Axial blood supply for the superficial inferior epigastric artery flap and the superficial circumflex iliac artery (groin) flap. Laterally, the vessels communicate with branches of the lateral thoracic artery system. (Courtesy of Dr. Robert W. Beasley.)

branches of the femoral artery. The two systems communicate with each other and with the lateral thoracic artery system descending from the axilla.

Superficial Inferior Epigastric Artery Flap. Shaw and Payne (10) described a tubed abdominal axial flap based on the superficial inferior epigastric artery (Fig. 79.11), which is useful and reliable for coverage of hand wounds and is usually situated on the side contralateral to the injury. In the adult, the donor site can be closed directly for flaps up to 12 cm wide. Furthermore, the end of the flap has minimal hair and the donor scar does not extend onto the chest. The contralateral location of the flap usually allows the injured extremity to lie comfortably across the lower body, producing minimal elbow or shoulder pain.

Superficial Circumflex Iliac Artery (Groin) Flap. The groin flap is an axial flap based on the superficial circumflex iliac artery system (11) (Fig. 79.12). These flaps can be long, and donor sites as wide as 15 cm can be closed directly. It is usually necessary to elevate the flap from the same side as the injured hand unless one raises a flap that is greatly in excess of the length needed in order to have a long and mobile pedicle. This ipsilateral arrangement leaves a "dangling" elbow, which makes immobilization very difficult as compared with a flap from the contralateral abdomen. In addition, the shoulder usually must be externally rotated, often to a degree that produces discomfort. The chief advantage of the groin flap is minimal hair transfer.

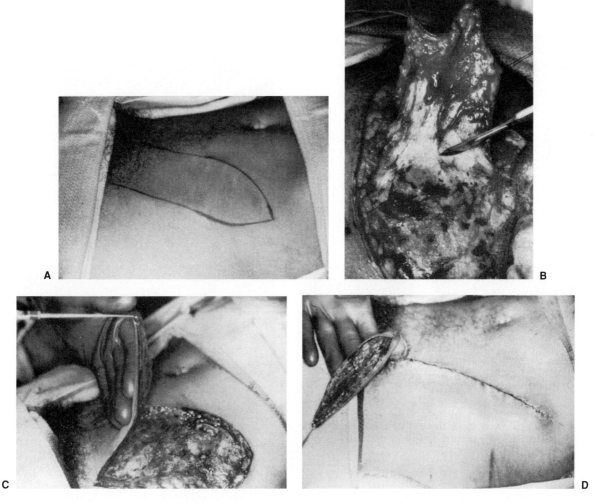

FIGURE 79.11. Superficial inferior epigastric flap. A: Flap design based on the superficial inferior epigastric artery system. B and C: Flap elevation. D and

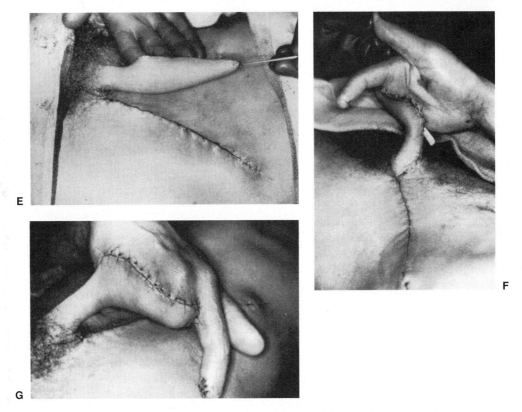

FIGURE 79.11. (*Continued*) E: Rotation and tubing of the elevated flap. F and G: Flap inset for soft-tissue reconstruction of the traumatic defect. (Courtesy of Dr. Robert W. Beasley.)

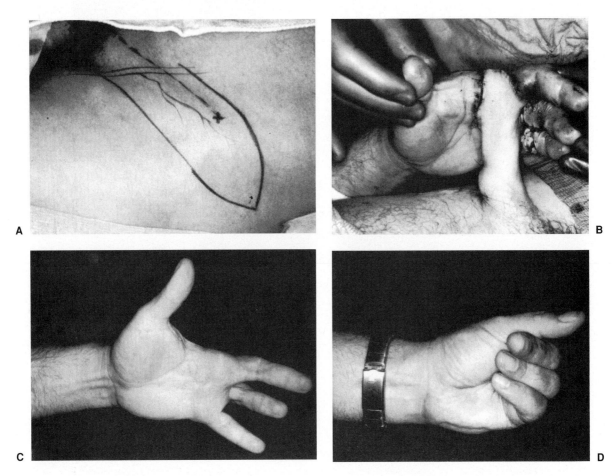

FIGURE 79.12. Groin flap. A: Flap design based on the superficial circumflex iliac artery system. B: Flap elevation and insetting into soft-tissue defect. C and D: Postoperative result. (Courtesy of Dr. Robert W. Beasley.)

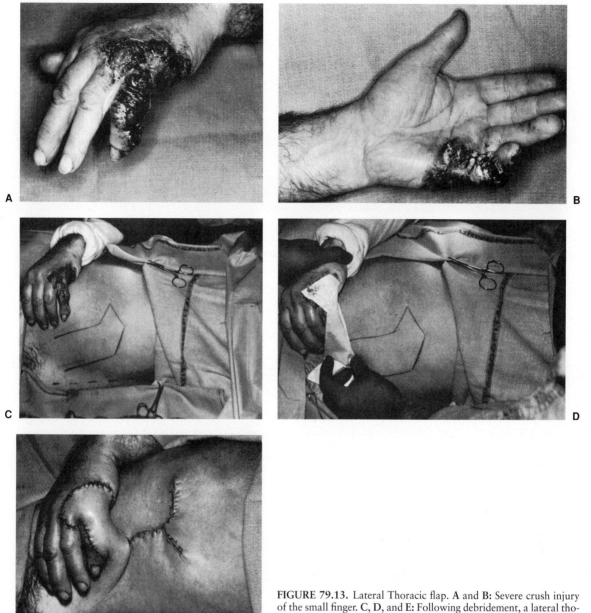

FIGURE 79.13. Lateral Thoracic flap. **A** and **B**: Severe crush injury of the small finger. **C, D,** and **E**: Following debridement, a lateral thoracic artery flap was designed and inset for soft-tissue reconstruction. (Courtesy of Dr. Robert W. Beasley.)

Lateral Thoracic Artery Flap. The lateral thoracic artery flap is a superiorly based axial flap (Fig. 79.13). The artery passes downward from the axilla toward the anterior superior iliac crest, parallel to the anterior border of the latissimus dorsi muscle. The flap is relatively thin with skin that is usually hairless, soft, and pliable. However, there can be substantial disfigurement of the donor site. The lateral thoracic artery flap is used mainly for patients who must remain ambulatory and are willing to accept the resulting scars. In designing the flap, the contralateral side is used, fixation is easy to maintain, and the position is well tolerated.

Random Flaps

The abdomen and contralateral arm can also provide random-circulation distant flaps. Random flaps can be elevated from any part of the abdomen and be based either inferiorly or superiorly. With the abdominal flaps, the length-to-width ratio is generally restricted to about 1.5:1.

The medial surface of the contralateral arm is also a good donor site for a random flap. Although it is a random flap, the excellent vascularity of the area permits length-to-width ratios of 2:1 if tension is avoided. The tissue match is better than that of the abdomen, and positioning is tolerable. Great care must be taken in the design and insetting of cross-arm flaps to prevent kinking of the pedicle or difficulty in fitting the flap to the defect.

Free Flaps

Free tissue transfer provides wound coverage and potential transfer of bone, nerve, and tendons. Each free flap donor site has its own advantages and disadvantages. A commonly used free tissue transfer for hand reconstruction is the fasciocutaneous lateral arm flap, which is supplied by the posterior radial collateral artery, a branch of the profundi brachial artery (12) (Fig. 79.14). This flap may be raised so as to include vascularized triceps tendon and a segment of humerus bone. In addition, the flap can be innervated by use of the associated

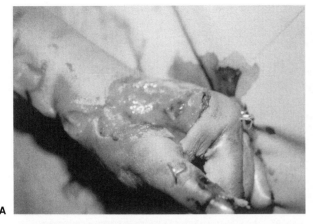

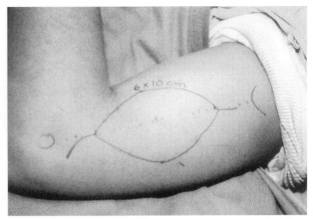

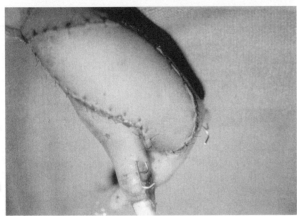

FIGURE 79.14. Lateral arm flap. **A:** Soft-tissue defect following debridement and stabilization of right hand metacarpal fractures. **B:** Design of a lateral arm flap supplied by the posterior radial collateral artery. **C:** Lateral arm free flap transfer completed.

lateral cutaneous nerve of the arm. A disadvantage of the lateral arm flap is that the flap donor site is limited to 6 cm in width so that a primary closure can be achieved. Larger defects require skin grafting.

The temporoparietal fascia free flap is another useful flap in hand reconstruction. Harvested from the temporoparietal area of the skull, this flap provides for thin, supple, soft-tissue coverage and is suitable for secondary tendon and nerve reconstructions. The donor site is closed primarily and the flap is skin grafted after insetting. Other free flaps for hand reconstruction are the scapular flap, groin flap, and dorsalis pedis flap. In instances where muscle coverage is desired, the latissimus, serratus anterior, and rectus abdominus muscles can be used.

References

1. Beasley RW. *Beasley's Surgery of the Hand*. New York: Thieme; 2003.
2. Kutler W. A new method for finger tip amputation. *JAMA*. 1947;133:29.
3. Atasoy E, Loakimidis E, Kasdan ML, et al. Reconstruction of the amputated fingertip with a triangular volar flap. A new surgical procedure. *J Bone Joint Surg*. 1970;52A:921.
4. Moberg E. Aspects for sensation in reconstructive surgery of the upper extremity. *J Bone Joint Surg*. 1964;46A:817.
5. Gurdin M, Pangman WI. The repair of surface defects of fingers by transdigital flaps. *Plast Reconstr Surg*. 1950;5:368.
6. Cohen BE, Cronin ED. An innervated crossfinger flap for fingertip reconstruction. *Plast Reconstr Surg*. 1983;72:688.
7. Gatewood: A plastic repair of finger defects without hospitalization. *JAMA*. 1926;87:1479.
8. Melone CP, Beasley RW, Carstens JH. The thenar flap: An analysis of its use in 150 cases. *J Hand Surg*. 1982;7:291.
9. Littler JW. Neurovascular skin island transfer in reconstructive hand surgery. In: *Transactions of the Second Congress of the International Society of Plastic Surgeons*. London: Livingstone; 1960.
10. Shaw DT, Payne RL. One-stage tubed abdominal flaps. *Surg Gynecol Obstet*. 1946;83:205.
11. McGregor IA, Jackson IT. The groin flap. *Br J Plast Surg*. 1972;25:3.
12. Katsaroj J, Tan E, et al. The use of the lateral arm flap in upper limb surgery. *J Hand Surg*. 1991;16A:598.

CHAPTER 80 ■ FRACTURES AND LIGAMENTOUS INJURIES OF THE WRIST

HANNAN MULLETT AND MICHAEL HAUSMAN

The wrist is the most complex joint in the body, acting as a structural and functional link between the hand and the forearm. It has no representative analog or machine model. It allows precise placement of the hand for activities beyond the eye's resolution, such as microvascular surgery, while providing stability for lifting multiples of the body's own weight. Although robust, the wrist is vulnerable to injury, and wrist pain and stiffness are common clinical problems.

ANATOMY

The wrist functionally consists of the eight carpal bones but functionally includes the distal radius, ulna, and bases of the metacarpals. For descriptive purposes the carpal bones are divided into the proximal and distal rows, each composed of four bones. This divides the wrist into radiocarpal and midcarpal joints. The ulnocarpal joint consists of the theoretical articulation between the distal ulna and the lunate and triquetrum and the interposed triangular fibrocartilage complex (TFCC). In the normal wrist, the ulnar head is extra-articular, excluded from the wrist by the unfenestrated, intact TFCC. The distal row includes of the trapezium, trapezoid, capitate, and hamate, which are bound together by strong interosseous ligaments and act as a single unit. The proximal row is comprised of the scaphoid, lunate, and triquetrum, and acts as a link between the relatively rigid distal row and the radioulnar articulations. The pisiform is not an active element, but rather a sesamoid bone in the flexor carpi ulnaris (FCU) tendon. There are no muscular attachments to the proximal carpal row; it is stabilized only by ligaments. The proximal row is subjected to compression and shearing load as the wrist is loaded. Sixty percent of the ratio of the joint axial load distributed across the proximal carpal row is borne by the radioscaphoid joint and 40% is borne by the radiolunate joint.

Intrinsic and extrinsic ligaments provide stability to the carpus (Fig. 80.1). The two most important ligaments—the scapholunate and lunotriquetral—are divided into dorsal, proximal, and palmar regions. The thickest and strongest region of the scapholunate ligament is located dorsally and is composed of dense transversely oriented collagen. The central region is composed of fibrocartilage, and the palmar region has thin obliquely oriented collagen fibers. In contrast the palmar fibers of the lunate-triquetrum ligament are strongest.

KINEMATICS

Sixty percent of flexion occurs at the midcarpal joint and 40% occurs at the radiocarpal joint. The reverse is true of wrist extension where the majority occurs at the radiocarpal joint (60%) and the remainder at the midcarpal joint. Wrist extension is accompanied by a degree of radial deviation and

wrist flexion by ulnar deviation. During radial deviation the radial column shortens (scaphoid flexion) and the ulna column lengthens (triquetrum slides proximally on the hamate). In ulnar deviation, the radial column lengthens (scaphoid extends) and the ulna column shortens (triquetrum slides distally on the hamate).

There are several conceptual models to describe wrist biomechanics (Fig. 80.2). The columnar model was introduced by Navarro and suggests the carpus is composed of three vertical columns each with a separate function: the central (flexion–extension), lateral (mobile), and medial (rotational) columns (1).

Talesisnik modified this theory adding the trapezium and trapezoid to the central column and eliminating the pisiform from the medial column (2).

Lichtman described the "oval ring" concept, which suggested that the proximal and distal rows of carpals are joined by two physiological links to form a ring (3). One is a mobile radial link at the scaphotrapezial joint, and the other is rotational at the triquetral–hamate articulation. The two links appear to allow the motion needed between proximal and distal carpal rows as well as medial–lateral deviations. Carpal instability is classified according to which of the links has been disrupted.

CARPAL INSTABILITY

Carpal instability occurs when there is an injury to the carpal bones or extrinsic or intrinsic ligaments that affect the normal carpal alignment and kinematics (4). There are a number of different classifications of carpal instability, which evolved as our understanding of wrist mechanics improved. Carpal instability dissociation (CID) describes carpal malalignment resulting from fractures or ligamentous disruptions within either the proximal or distal carpal rows. Common examples include injuries to the scapholunate or lunate-triquetrum interosseous ligaments resulting in patterns of dorsal or volar collapse, respectively (Fig. 80.3). Carpal instability nondissociative (CIND) relates to instability between carpal rows, and can be caused by ligament injury, or bony fracture, or both. Carpal instability complex (CIC) results from a combination of CID and CIND (e.g., metacarpal instabilities or perilunate dislocations and fracture/dislocations). Another category of carpal instability—adaptive—results from extrinsic factors such as a distal radial fracture, which may lead to loss of palmar tilt, radial height, and ulnar inclination. Another classification is based on the appearance of the lunate on the lateral radiograph (5). In dorsal intercalated segment instability (DISI), the lunate is angulated dorsally and the capitate is displaced dorsal to the radiometacarpal axis. In volar intercalated segment instability (VISI), the lunate angulates in a palmar direction, which causes the capitate to become displaced palmer to the radiometacarpal axis. A more recent classification incorporates the following six

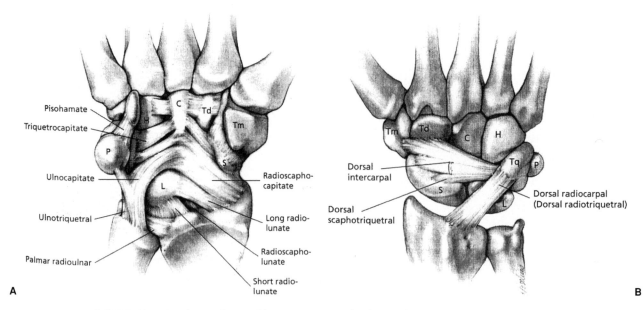

FIGURE 80.1. A: Palmar radiocarpal ligaments. **B:** Dorsal radiocarpal ligaments.

important parameters: (a) tonicity, (b) constancy, (c) etiology, (d) location, (e) direction, and (f) pattern.

The most commonly encountered carpal instability problems are scapholunate dissociation, scaphoid nonunion causing carpal instability, carpal instability secondary to radial fracture malunion, lunotriquetral dissociation, and midcarpal instability.

Scapholunate Instability

Scapholunate instability ranges from mild nondissociative instability to complex perilunate dislocations. Mild scapholunate ligament injury may present as a dorsal ganglion or "dorsal capsule syndrome." This is the first stage of progressive perilunate instability for which Mayfield has described the following four stages (Fig. 80.4) (6):

Stage I: Scapholunate instability results from tearing of the scapholunate and volar radioscaphoid ligaments.

Stage II: The midcarpal joint capsule ruptures dorsally, allowing the capitate to dislocate dorsally over the lunate.

Stage III: The triquetrum separates from the lunate as a result of tearing of the radial–lunate–triquetral ligaments.

Stage IV: The lunate is dislocated into the carpal tunnel, while the rest of the carpus remains in line with the radius.

Radiographic Examination

Scapholunate dissociation may be static or dynamic. In the case of the former, wrist radiographs are always abnormal, demonstrating a widened scapholunate space known as a Terry-Thomas sign (Fig. 80.5). A gap greater than 5 mm is clearly diagnostic of scapholunate dissociation. The "scaphoid ring" sign occurs when the scaphoid is flexed and the shadow of the distal pole is projected through the scaphoid waist on the anteroposterior (AP) view (Fig. 78.9). In the case of dynamic scapholunate dissociation, standard radiographs are normal. The diagnosis is based on clinical examination and specialized radiographic studies such as stress views, but videodynamic radiography is the best test.

Treatment of Scapholunate Instability

Appropriate management of acute injuries helps to avoid long-term sequelae such as posttraumatic arthritis. Controlling the position of the scaphoid and lunate by closed means is not recommended. Open reduction and primary repair of the scapholunate ligament is advocated by some, but is prone to recurrent diastasis of the scapholunate joint. The restored intercarpal relationship is maintained by Kirschner wire (K-wire) fixation, which neutralizes rotational forces. Interosseous sutures are passed and secured using either bone tunnels or suture anchors. This procedure is frequently combined with a dorsal capsulodesis to support the weakened scapholunate intercarpal ligament (SLIL). More recently the arthroscopic treatment of acute scapholunate dissociation has been described.

The term *chronic scapholunate dissociation* is somewhat arbitrary, but generally refers to a period of greater than 3 or 4 weeks after the initial injury. Treatment options at this stage depend on the severity of symptoms, demand of the patient, and presence or absence of scapholunate advanced collapse (SLAC) changes. Patients with mild symptoms may be treated conservatively using activity modification, anti-inflammatory medication, and intermittent splinting. In early stages without degenerative changes, arthroscopic debridement of the SLIL may be of benefit.

Definitive surgical procedures are generally either soft-tissue procedures designed to correct the alignment of the scaphoid or intercarpal fusions that can be limited or involve total wrist fusion. Numerous techniques exist that attempt to stabilize the scaphoid using either late ligamentous repair, tendon grafting, or capsulodesis. However, none of these procedures is reliable for long-term pain relief and maintenance of the anatomical position of the scaphoid. Limited intercarpal fusion is the technique of choice. Although it would seem logical that a scapholunate fusion is the most anatomic procedure, the rate of successful fusion is unacceptable. Either scaphotrapezio-trapezoid or scaphocapitate fusion is a reliable technique to prevent the progression of degenerative changes in patients with minimal or no degenerative changes. **In the presence of arthritis involving the radioscaphoid joint, with or without involvement of the capitolunate joint, either a four-corner fusion (capitate–lunate–hamate–triquetrum) with scaphoid excision or a proximal row carpectomy is recommended.** Rosenwasser et al. (7) described a technique of controlling the alignment

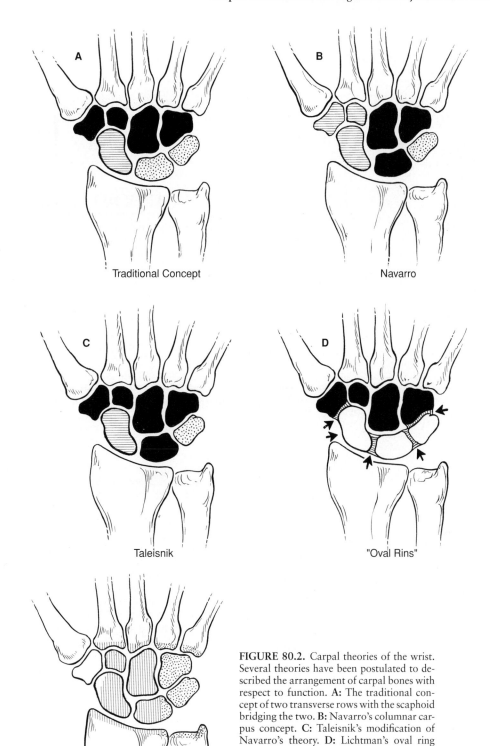

FIGURE 80.2. Carpal theories of the wrist. Several theories have been postulated to described the arrangement of carpal bones with respect to function. **A:** The traditional concept of two transverse rows with the scaphoid bridging the two. **B:** Navarro's columnar carpus concept. **C:** Taleisnik's modification of Navarro's theory. **D:** Lichtman's oval ring concept. **E:** Weber's view of the carpus is that of two longitudinal columns. The control column (*stippled*) occupies the ulnar portion of the wrist, emphasizing the importance of the helicoid configuration of the triquetrohamate joint. The force-bearing column (*striped*) is on the radial side.

of scapholunate articulation by means of a Herbert screw (Zimmer, Inc., Warsaw, IN). This prevents scapholunate diastasis while permitting rotation. They report satisfactory maintenance of the restored scapholunate articulation with good range of wrist motion in a series of 21 patients at a mean of 32 months.

Lunotriquetral Instability

Lunotriquetral dissociation results from posttraumatic incompetence of the strong palmar portion of the lunotriquetral ligament. The mechanism of injury is a fall on an extended, outstretched hand. Symptoms are ulna-sided wrist pain, stiffness,

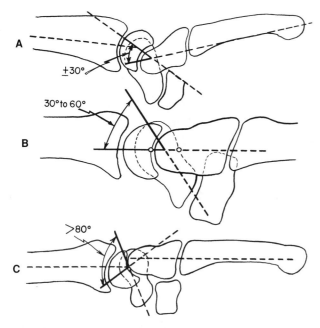

FIGURE 80.3. **A:** Abnormal volar flexion of the lunate and scaphoid with ± 30 degrees volar tilt, diagnostic of a volar intercalated segment instability (VISI) deformity. **B:** Normal carpal alignment with lunate and capitate colinear and scaphoid angled 45 degrees (normal: 30 to 60 degrees, ± 15 degrees) to the sagittal plane of the forearm. **C:** Abnormal dorsiflexion of the lunate with a vertical scaphoid; scapholunate angle 80 degrees (normal: 45 to 60 degrees), typical dorsal intercalated segment instability (DISI) deformity (Chapter 78). (From Cooney WP, Linscheid RL, Dobyns JH. Fractures and dislocations of the wrist. In: Rockwood CA, Green DP, Bucholz RW, et al., eds. *Fractures in Adults.* 4th ed. Philadelphia: Lippincott-Raven; 1996:762, with permission.)

and weakness. Physical examination reveals focal tenderness, limited range of motion, and reduced grip strength. A definitive radiologic diagnosis is difficult to secure. Plain radiographs may be negative, although a VISI deformity may be seen in chronic cases. Magnetic resonance imaging (MRI) is a poor modality for identifying lunotriquetral ligament injury but might exclude other causes of ulna wrist pain, such as TFCC pathology. The diagnostic gold standard at present is wrist arthroscopy.

Treatment depends on the severity of symptoms and the presence of degenerative changes. If conservative treatment fails, the goals of surgical reconstruction are similar to other types of carpal instability—the restoration of stable carpal alignment and pain-free function. Lunotriquetral arthrodesis and ligament reconstruction are treatment alternatives. A significant nonunion rate has been reported for lunotriquetral arthrodesis, and the overall success for either treatment is probably improved by combining arthrodesis or ligament reconstruction with an ulnar-shortening osteotomy.

Adaptive Instability

Adaptive instability results from an osseous deformity affecting the normal carpal alignment most commonly seen following malunion of the distal radius. The secondary effect on carpal alignment frequently occurs at the midcarpal joint as the lunate rotates dorsally and the axis of the capitate aligns dorsal to that of the radius along the inclined surface of the distal radius. Dorsal angulation greater than 20 degrees has been reported to result in symptoms and a DISI pattern.

CARPAL FRACTURES

Carpal bone fractures account for 18% of hand fractures, and the bones in the proximal row are the most frequently fractured. **The scaphoid is by far the most common carpal bone fractured, representing 79% of fractures in the carpal group and 10% of all hand fractures.** Triquetral fractures are the second most common, accounting for 14% of wrist injuries. The incidence of isolated fractures of any of the remaining carpal bones is on the order of 1%.

SCAPHOID FRACTURES

Scaphoid fractures represent the most common carpal fracture, with an annual estimated incidence of 38 fractures per 100,000 men. Fractures of the scaphoid most frequently occur in young adult males and usually involve the waist of the scaphoid. The usual mechanism of injury is falling on the outstretched hand, causing axial loading in dorsiflexion. This causes the distal aspect of the scaphoid to impact on the dorsal rim of the radius, creating a fracture through the waist.

Correct diagnosis and treatment of scaphoid fractures is particularly important because of the vital role of this bone in wrist motion.

Bone healing may be problematic, particularly with proximal pole fractures, as the vascular supply is by retrograde intraosseous blood flow from distal dorsal vessels.

Diagnosis

The clinical findings are swelling, snuffbox tenderness, and a positive axial compression test. Fullness in the snuffbox indicates a wrist effusion. Mandatory radiographs include a scaphoid view in ulnar deviation, 20 degrees of dorsiflexion, and 20 degrees of supination from the posteroanterior (PA) view. **On initial radiographs, 2% to 3% of fractures are "occult," and if a fracture is suspected after repeated physical examinations, high-quality radiographs should be repeated after a 10- to 14-day interval.** The true lateral view should be carefully examined for an associated ligamentous injury demonstrated by abnormal posture of the lunate. A negative three-phase bone scan 48 or more hours after injury rules out any fracture, but unlike an MRI scan, gives no imaging of ligamentous structures (see Chapter 78). Positioning of the long axis of the scaphoid parallel to the plane of the scanner improves imaging and accuracy, and this nonstandard position should be coordinated with the radiologist. A sagittal cut parallel to the long axis of the scaphoid is the best way to demonstrate the fracture and any associated deformity. High-resolution computed tomography (CT) is best to assess displacement and angulation, which is frequently greater than suspected, and may, therefore, be an indication for surgery (Fig. 80.6).

Classification

There are two commonly used scaphoid fracture classifications—Herbert and Russe. Herbert (Fig. 80.7) classifies stable fractures as type A (incomplete fracture through the waist or fracture of the tubercle), and unstable fractures as type B (e.g., distal oblique fracture, displaced fracture through the waist, proximal pole fracture, transcaphoid perilunate fracture dislocation) (8).

Russe classified scaphoid fractures into three types according to the relationship of the fracture to the long axis of the

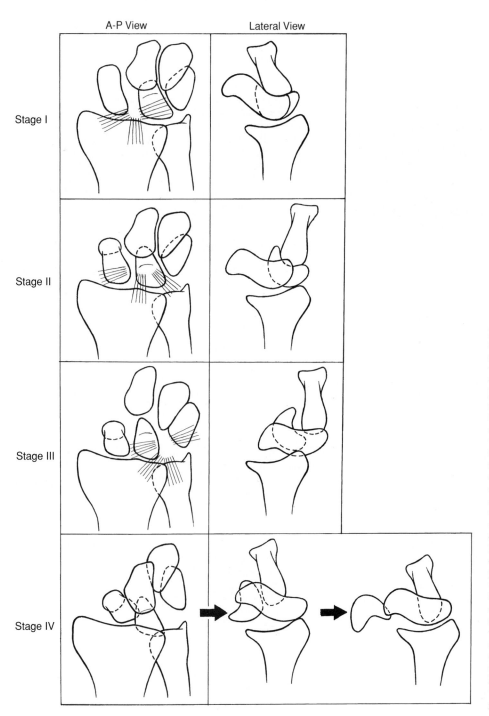

FIGURE 80.4. Progressive perilunate instability. Mayfield based his observations on cadaveric wrists that were subjected to extension, ulnar deviation, and intercarpal supination. Four stages of ligamental injuries with resulting carpal malalignment were noted, which eventually led to lunate dislocations. In stage I, the scapholunate ligament is disrupted, leading to scapholunate dissociation. In stage II, the midcarpal capsule is also disrupted at the capitolunate joint, allowing the capitate to dislocate dorsally. In stage III, an avulsion fracture of the triquetrum or lunotriquetral ligament disruption occurs, causing separation of the two carpal bones. The lunate and radius are still collinear, whereas the remaining carpus tends to separate from the lunate (usually dorsally), thus producing perilunate dislocations. In stage IV, the dorsal radiocarpal ligament is severed, allowing the lunate to displace volarly while the rest of the carpus remains aligned to the radius. The volar radiolunate ligament usually remains intact, acting as a tether upon which the lunate can rotate. This produces the "spilled teacup" sign on lateral radiographs (*Lateral B*).

scaphoid. Horizontal oblique and transverse fractures are stable, whereas vertical oblique fractures are unstable (9).

Treatment

Stable Undisplaced Fracture

This is the most favorable situation. The union rate exceeds 95% in undisplaced stable scaphoid waist fractures that are diagnosed soon after injury and casted until fracture union. Undisplaced fractures of the proximal pole have a lower union rate of approximately 70%.

The standard treatment for stable undisplaced fractures is a short-arm cast until union is radiographically demonstrated, an average of 3 to 6 months. If the patient is noncompliant, a long-arm cast is advisable. A neutral position is best as radial deviation–palmar flexion reduces the fracture but causes collapse, whereas ulna deviation reduces angulation but distracts the fracture. It is usual to include the thumb in the cast, although this requirement has not been proven to affect union rates. If union is in doubt, fracture healing is monitored with serial radiographs or CT scans. Given the long period of immobilization required and advances in minimally invasive operative techniques, internal fixation is increasingly seen as a preferable alternative to conservative treatment.

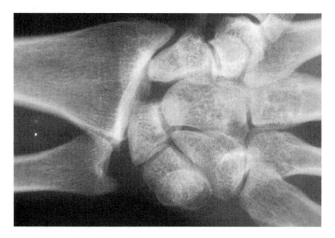

FIGURE 80.5. Wrist radiograph demonstrating a widened scapholunate space known as a Terry-Thomas sign (after British film actor).

Operative Fixation of Acute Scaphoid Fractures

There are clear advantages to early operative treatment of acute displaced scaphoid fractures. Technologic advances provide improved imaging and minimally invasive techniques that make operative intervention attractive, and obviate long periods of cast immobilization, resulting in joint stiffness and muscle weakness. Early anatomic reduction reduces the incidence of delayed, union, nonunion, or malunion.

Open Technique

Enhanced fixation techniques, better instrumentation and the ready availability of high-quality operative fluoroscopy have fueled the trend toward early surgical treatment of acute scaphoid fractures.

The volar (Russe) approach is cited as protective of blood supply and is useful when a bone graft is used to correct angular deformity. However it may require partial resection of the trapezium to access the center of the scaphotrapezial articular surface. The dorsal approach provides easier exposure and central screw placement is facilitated. Inspection of the capitate facet on the medial border of the scaphoid allows confirmation of reduction. It is essential to protect the dorsal ridge vessels and scapholunate ligaments.

Percutaneous and Arthroscopic Techniques

There is also a trend toward acute fracture fixation using percutaneous screw fixation to shorten immobilization. Inoue and Shionoya reported 40 patients with acute scaphoid fractures who were treated using a limited-access technique (10). The average time to union of all Herbert type B fractures treated with this technique was 6.5 weeks, with a much earlier return to manual work when compared with conservative management.

Slade et al. reported a technique using a percutaneous dorsal approach and a combination of arthroscopy and fluoroscopy to ensure anatomic reduction and accurate implant placement (11) (Fig. 80.8). They felt that arthroscopy had the advantage of detection of concurrent ligament injuries in addition to less soft tissue trauma.

Scaphoid Nonunion

Nonunion of scaphoid fractures has traditionally been considered as a complication of displaced fractures but can result from undiagnosed or undertreated nondisplaced scaphoid fractures. Progressive collapse and deformity usually occur at the fracture site, leading to subluxation of the midcarpal joint and dorsal rotation of the lunate. The natural history of nonunion is late radioscaphoid degenerative changes, followed by pan carpal arthritis. Lichtman has proposed a useful classification system (Table 80.1).

Treatment of Nonunion with No Degenerative Changes

The natural history of scaphoid nonunion is such that re-establishment of normal carpal alignment and stability should be attempted even if the patient is asymptomatic. The selected treatment depends on the location of the fracture and the quality of bone stock. Sagittal CT scans greatly aid the making of an accurate assessment. MRI provides the most reliable method to evaluate the vascularity of the proximal pole. The presence of avascular necrosis does not preclude healing. Scaphoid waist nonunion with good vascularity of the proximal pole may be approached using a volar approach. A minimally invasive technique using a cannulated screw inserted through a dorsal approach is optimal for selected cases. A "humpback" deformity may be addressed by using a volar bone graft. If the proximal pole is avascular, or if there have been previous unsuccessful surgical efforts to obtain fracture healing, a vascularized bone graft should be considered. A high success rate has been

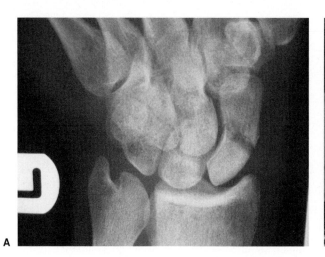

A

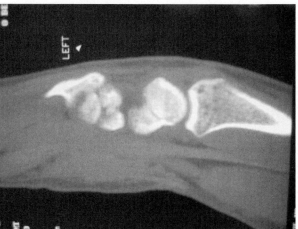

B

FIGURE 80.6. A and B: Scaphoid fracture diagnosed by CT scan after plain radiographs failed to indicate a fracture.

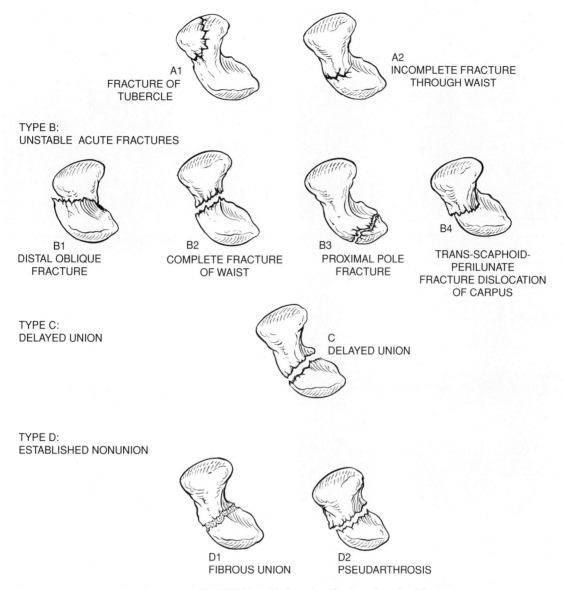

FRACTURE OF
TUBERCLE A1

A2 INCOMPLETE FRACTURE
THROUGH WAIST

TYPE B:
UNSTABLE ACUTE FRACTURES

B1
DISTAL OBLIQUE
FRACTURE

B2
COMPLETE FRACTURE
OF WAIST

B3
PROXIMAL POLE
FRACTURE

B4
TRANS-SCAPHOID-
PERILUNATE
FRACTURE DISLOCATION
OF CARPUS

TYPE C:
DELAYED UNION

C DELAYED UNION

TYPE D:
ESTABLISHED NONUNION

D1
FIBROUS UNION

D2
PSEUDARTHROSIS

FIGURE 80.7. Herbert classification of scaphoid fractures.

reported using a vascularized distal dorsal radius graft based on the 1,2 intercompartmental supraretinacular artery (12). An alternative donor site is the volar pronator-based graft.

Scaphoid Nonunion Advanced Collapse Wrist

The treatment of the scaphoid nonunion advanced collapse (SNAC) wrist depends on the stage of disease and the symptoms and requirements of the patient. In selected cases, attempts to salvage the scaphoid are probably warranted, as symptoms do not always correlate with radiographic appearance. Salvage procedures involve either scaphoid excision and intercarpal fusion or proximal row carpectomy. A medial column or four–corner fusion (capitate–lunate–triquetrum–hamate) is a reliable procedure, and the use of specifically designed fusion plates has reduced the period of immobilization required postoperatively. Good results have also been reported with proximal row carpectomy. This is most useful when arthritic changes are confined to the radioscaphoid articulation. Degenerative changes of the proximal capitate or lunate fossa of the radius are relative contraindications to the procedure, although the procedure might succeed if changes are minimal. In the case

of advanced degenerative arthritis, the treatment of choice is a wrist arthrodesis.

Other Carpal Fractures

The other carpal bones account for the 21% of carpal fractures or 1.1% of all fractures. Apart from fractures of the lunate associated with Kienböck disease, the triquetrum is most commonly fractured. Fractures may occur in isolation as either an impaction or avulsion injury, such as a hamate hook fracture (direct impact) or a dorsal chip fracture of the triquetrum. They may also represent part of a more complex injury pattern such as a perilunate fracture dislocation.

Lunate

Fractures of the lunate are rare except in association with Kienböck disease. Teisen and Hjarbaek classified fresh lunate fractures into the following five groups: group 1, palmar pole; group 2, marginal chip fracture; group 3, dorsal pole; group 4, sagittal fracture; and group 5, transverse fracture (13). In a long-term follow-up study of 11 patients they found no patients

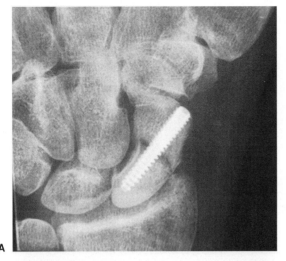

A

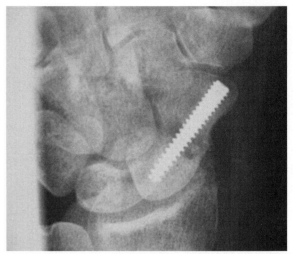

B

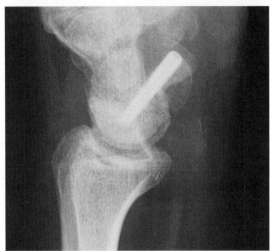

C

FIGURE 80.8. Internal fixation of scaphoid waist fracture by percutaneous headless cannulated screw as seen in (**A**) AP, (**B**) oblique, and (**C**) lateral views.

had pain, muscle atrophy, or reduced grip strength. The majority of lunate fractures occur in association with Kienböck disease. Although this condition was described in 1910 by Kienböck, an Austrian radiologist, there remains no consensus as to the etiology of this condition. Possible causes include heavy use or trauma. It is usually diagnosed between the ages of 15 and 40 years. Symptoms typically include progressive wrist pain, which may radiate proximally to the forearm, with associated loss of motion and grip weakness. There are recognized radiologic changes that correlate with the progression of the condition. The Stahl classification system, modified by Licht-

man and subsequent authors, is useful in guiding treatment (14) (Fig. 80.9).

Stage I: There are no visible changes on plain radiographs but bone scans and MRI studies will be positive.

Stage II: Plain radiographs demonstrate lunate sclerosis without collapse.

Stage IIIA: Sclerosis with fragmentation or collapse of the lunate, or both.

Stage IIIB: Stage IIIA changes combined with fixed rotation of the scaphoid.

Stage IV: There are established degenerative changes at the radiocarpal or midcarpal level, including subchondral cyst formation, sclerosis, and articular cartilage narrowing.

Patients with stage I disease may benefit from immobilization and activity modification. There is insufficient evidence to recommend surgical intervention in this group. Treatment of stage II disease is generally directed at decreasing the axial load on the lunate by means of radial shortening, ulnar lengthening, or capitate shortening. Some success has occurred using reverse flow pedicle radius vascularized bone grafts. The salvage procedures for advanced disease (stages IIIB and IV) include proximal row carpectomy and total wrist fusion.

Hamate

Fracture of the hook of the hamate often results from a fall on the outstretched hand, although it may be seen in golfers and racket sport players who frequently do not recall a specific

TABLE 80.1

TYPES OF SCAPHOID NONUNION

1. Simple	No displacement
	No degenerative change
2. Unstable	Displacement >1 mm
	Scapholunate angle >70 degrees
3. Early arthritic	Radioscaphoid arthritis present
4. SNAC wrist	Radioscaphoid and midcarpal arthritis
5. SNAC plus	Arthritis throughout wrist

Abbreviation: SNAC, scaphoid nonunion advanced collapse.

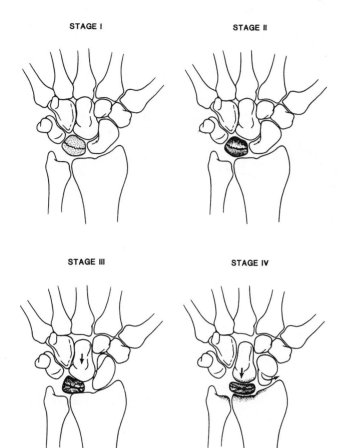

STAGE I

STAGE II

STAGE III

STAGE IV

FIGURE 80.9. Staging of Kienböck disease (after Lichtman). *Stage I:* Routine radiographs (PA, lateral) are normal, but CT may show a linear fracture, usually transverse through the body of the lunate. MRI will confirm avascular changes. *Stage II:* Bone density increase (sclerosis) and a fracture line are usually evident on the PA radiograph. PA and lateral tomograms demonstrate sclerosis, cystic changes, and often a clear fracture. There is no collapse deformity. *Stage IIIa* (not pictured): Advanced bone density changes are present with fragmentation, cystic resorption, and collapse. The diagnosis is evident from PA x-ray tomograms (PA, lateral), which demonstrate the degree of lunate infraction and the amount of fracture displacement. Proximal migration of the capitate is present. *Stage IIIb* (not pictured): There is additional mild to moderate rotary malalignment of the scaphoid. *Stage IV:* Perilunate arthritic changes are present with complete collapse and fragmentation of the lunate. Carpal instability is evident with scaphoid malalignment and capitate displacement into the lunate space. (From Cooney WP, Linscheid RL, Dobyns JH. Fractures and dislocations of the wrist. In: Rockwood CA, Green DP, Bucholz RW, et al., eds. *Fractures in Adults*. 4th ed. Philadelphia: Lippincott-Raven; 1996:843, with permission.)

traumatic incident. They present with pain distal and radial to the pisiform, which may be aggravated by grasping as the flexor tendons to the ring and small fingers pull against the hook of the hamate as they exit the carpal tunnel. Standard radiographs rarely reveal this fracture, although it may be seen on a carpal tunnel view. A hamate hook lateral radiographic view (30 degrees, palmar-tilted lateral wrist projection) with the thumb in palmar abduction is advocated. The most reliable diagnostic study is a high-resolution CT scan. Delayed

diagnosis is the norm with this injury and the fracture has frequently progressed to a state of nonunion. The definitive treatment of established nonunion of the hamate is subperiosteal excision with careful preservation of the motor branch of the ulnar nerve.

Trapezium

These are the second most common nonscaphoid carpal fractures. It is a rare, isolated injury, and is usually associated with other injuries, such as distal radial fractures or fracture of the first metacarpal. They are usually identified on plain radiographs, including oblique and carpal tunnel views. The Robert view (hyperpronated AP view) and the Bett view (elbow raised from cassette, 25 degrees pronation and thumb abducted) are useful. Nondisplaced fractures may be treated by cast immobilization. Unstable fractures and those with intra-articular incongruity are treated by reduction and fixation. Nonunion of the palmar ridge occurs often and may be treated by excision.

Capitate

Capitate fractures are uncommon but may occur in conjunction with major injuries, such as perilunate dislocation. Scapholunate syndrome involving capitate and scaphoid waist fractures has been described. Accurate diagnosis usually requires a high-resolution CT scan. If the diagnosis is secured acutely, union may result from immobilization. Anatomic reduction is required for restoration of carpal kinematics. The use of a headless cannulated screw is helpful. Even with optimal treatment some posttraumatic carpal arthrosis may be found with long-term follow-up. Nonunion may be treated by bone grafting and internal fixation.

References

1. Navarro A. *Anales de Instituto de Clinica Quirurgica y Cirugia Experimental*. Montevideo: Imprenta Artistica de Dornaleche Hnos; 1935.
2. Taleisnik J. Post-traumatic carpal instability. *Clin Orthop*. 1980;73–82.
3. Lichtman DM, Schneider JR, Swafford AR, et al. Ulnar midcarpal instability—Clinical and laboratory analysis. *J Hand Surg [Am]*. 1981;6:515–523.
4. The Anatomy and Biomechanics Committee of the International Federation of Societies for Surgery of the Hand. Definition of carpal instability. *J Hand Surg [Am]*. 1999;24:866–867.
5. Linscheid RL, Dobyns JH, Beabout JW, et al. Traumatic instability of the wrist. Diagnosis, classification, and pathomechanics. *J Bone Joint Surg [Am]*. 1972;54:1612–1632.
6. Mayfield JK. Wrist ligamentous anatomy and pathogenesis of carpal instability. *Orthop Clin North Am*. 1984;15:209–216.
7. Rosenwasser MP, Strauch RJ, Miyasaka KC. The RASL procedure: Reduction and association of the scaphoid and lunate using the Herbert screw. *Techniques in Hand and Upper Extremity Surgery* . 1997;1(4):263–272.
8. Herbert TJ. Scaphoid fractures and carpal instability. *Proc R Soc Med*. 1974;67:1080.
9. Russe O. Fractures of the carpal navicular: Diagnosis, non-operative treatment, and operative treatment. *J Bone Joint Surg*. 1960;42A:759–768.
10. Inoue G. Capitate-hamate fusion for Kienböck's disease. Good results in 8 cases followed for 3 years. *Acta Orthop Scand*. 1992;63:560–562.
11. Slade JF III, Grauer JN, Mahoney JD. Arthroscopic reduction and percutaneous fixation of scaphoid fractures with a novel dorsal technique. *Orthop Clin North Am*. 2001;32:247–261.
12. Zaidemberg C, Siebert JW, Angrigiani C. A new vascularized bone graft for scaphoid nonunion. *J Hand Surg [Am]*. 1991;16:474–478.
13. Teisen H, Hjarbaek J. Classification of fresh fractures of the lunate. *J Hand Surg [Br]*. 1988;13:458–462.
14. Allan CH, Joshi A, Lichtman DM. Kienböck's disease: Diagnosis and treatment. *J Am Acad Orthop Surg*. 2001;9:128–136.

CHAPTER 81 ■ FRACTURES, DISLOCATIONS, AND LIGAMENTOUS INJURIES OF THE HAND

DAVID W. FRIEDMAN, AMY KELLS, AND ALBERTO AVILES

Injuries to the phalanges and metacarpals are common and can result in acute morbidity and long-term disability. Evaluation of all hand injuries begins with gross inspection for apparent deformities, including areas of edema and ecchymosis, and a neurovascular examination. The examination is performed systematically and proceeds from relatively uninjured areas to those areas of suspected injury, so as to gain the cooperation and trust of the patient by minimizing discomfort. **The neurovascular status and the degree of concomitant soft-tissue injury are assessed; they determine the mode of treatment and the ultimate outcome.** If a fracture or dislocation is suspected, obtain radiographs. A minimum of three views is required to accurately diagnose the presence and pattern of fractures. The precise areas of suspected injury are conveyed to the radiologist to allow for a more critical assessment of these specific areas. Open fractures and fractures associated with lacerations often involve soft-tissue injuries, which are discussed in Chapter 79.

Early motion is absolutely essential if the patient is to regain normal function. Because long-term stiffness and disability from either tendon or joint capsular scarring will occur if the fingers are immobilized for more than 4 weeks, **sufficient stabilization of fractures must be achieved to allow for motion at no later than 4 weeks whenever possible.** Moreover, any treatment must also minimize the surgical trauma to the surrounding tissues, as the condition of the soft-tissue envelope will ultimately determine outcome. **A delicate balance must be achieved between accurate stable fixation and surgically created soft-tissue disruption** (Fig. 81.1).

DISTAL PHALANX

Distal phalanx fractures are classified by location: tuft, shaft, or base. Tuft fractures are among the most common hand fractures and most can be treated in a closed fashion with splinting of the distal interphalangeal (DIP) joint, while encouraging motion at the proximal interphalangeal (PIP) joint. Prior to immobilization, the soft tissues are evaluated as the crushing force can often be associated with a significant nail bed injury. A breach in the nail plate is an indication for its removal and suture repair of any underlying nail bed laceration. Irrigation and accurate (open) reduction of the fracture can be accomplished at that time, with the matrix repair acting as an internal splint. Motion at the DIP joint can be started after 3 to 4 weeks of immobilization with protective splinting as required until discomfort has resolved.

Nondisplaced shaft fractures can be treated with splinting of the DIP joint for 3 to 4 weeks with gentle, progressive motion instituted after that time. Displaced shaft fractures may require Kirschner (K) wire fixation as soft-tissue disruption often adds to fracture instability. A single axial K-wire transfixing the DIP

joint in extension is usually sufficient and should remain for 4 weeks.

Avulsion of the extensor tendon is often associated with a bony articular fragment. These injuries are classified by the size of the avulsed bony fragment and most can be treated nonoperatively with extension splinting for 8 weeks. **However, if more than one-third to one-half of the articular surface is displaced, and/or if there is volar subluxation of the distal phalanx, operative treatment is indicated.** The most suitable approach is K-wire stabilization, performed closed or open, with correction of any subluxation and transarticular fixation of the DIP joint in extension. With large fragments, fixation of the avulsed segment can be accomplished with either interfragmentary wiring, Kirschner pinning, or screw fixation. Patients should anticipate some degree of extensor lag (incomplete extension) following treatment, and can expect approximately 50% of the preoperative lag to be corrected (1).

A dorsally directed axial load can create a dorsal fracture dislocation with resultant impaction fracture at the volar base of the distal phalanx. These fractures are analogous to the pilon fracture of the PIP joint and can be difficult to treat because of the degree of comminution. Closed reduction with percutaneous pinning, if necessary, plus extension block splinting is the most effective treatment. Open reduction with internal fixation can be difficult to achieve and should be a last resort. DIP volar plate arthroplasty has been described as an alternate option for highly comminuted volar base fractures or chronic dorsal dislocations of the distal phalanx (2).

MIDDLE AND PROXIMAL PHALANX

Condylar Fractures

Because fractures of the middle and proximal phalanx have similar properties, they are discussed together. Torsion- and valgus-directed forces at the DIP and PIP joints can lead to condylar fractures of either the middle or proximal phalanx. These injuries are often misdiagnosed as a "sprain" and often lose their reduction in the early postinjury period. As these fractures are intra-articular, appropriate management is crucial to maximize interphalangeal joint mobility and overall hand function. The goal of any operative treatment should be to accurately re-establish joint congruity.

Condylar injuries are broadly classified into either unicondylar or bicondylar fracture patterns. Completely nondisplaced fractures can be treated closed with extension splinting. Any displacement, either initially, or that which is identified during close follow-up, must be treated to achieve

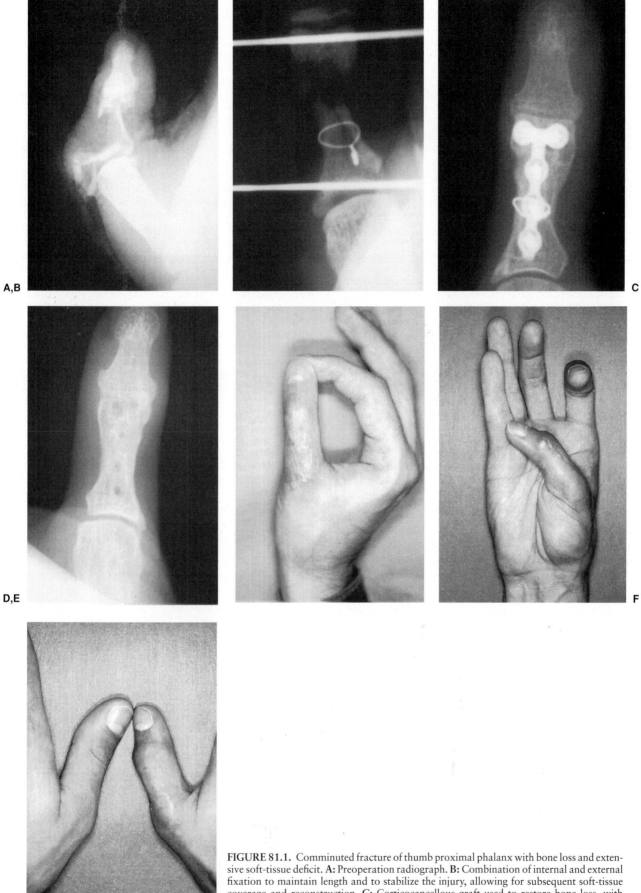

FIGURE 81.1. Comminuted fracture of thumb proximal phalanx with bone loss and extensive soft-tissue deficit. **A:** Preoperation radiograph. **B:** Combination of internal and external fixation to maintain length and to stabilize the injury, allowing for subsequent soft-tissue coverage and reconstruction. **C:** Corticocancellous graft used to restore bone loss, with dorsal plate fixation. **D:** Subsequent removal of hardware and tenolysis to restore mobility. **E** to **G:** Final result.

accurate reduction and fixation. Percutaneous fixation should include at least two K-wires as these fractures are subject to significant deforming forces from the attached collateral ligaments. Stable fixation should allow for early motion at the PIP joint or the outcome may well be a stiff and painful finger.

Condylar fractures that are not amenable to closed treatment require an open technique to achieve precise reduction. Unicondylar injuries can be approached using a midaxial incision, and fixation is achieved with 1.0- to 1.2-mm screws, K-wires, or a combination of both. **Care must be taken in maintaining the collateral ligament attachment to the displaced fragment, as much of the condylar blood supply is derived from this structure.** Rigid fixation should be achieved, if possible, to permit early interphalangeal (IP) joint motion or a poor outcome will likely result despite the creation of a perfectly congruent articular surface.

Bicondylar fractures are inherently too unstable to permit closed treatment and require open reduction and internal fixation. The operative planning must include exposure of both condyles and can be achieved using a dorsal skin incision. Parallel incisions between the central slip and lateral bands will allow for joint exposure while carefully preserving the central slip attachment at the base of the uninvolved middle phalanx. If the intercondylar and shaft fracture patterns are short and oblique, the joint surface may be re-established with interfragmentary lag screws. A transverse fracture pattern at the condylar–shaft interface may require an oblique K-wire or a small 1.3-mm T plate to align and fix the condyles to the shaft. Alternatively, these fractures can be treated with minicondylar blade plates. Familiarity with use of these plates is essential as precise application is requisite to a favorable outcome. Complications, including joint stiffness, tendon adhesions, and infections, occur more frequently than when K-wire stabilization is used, and should be anticipated and discussed with the patient preoperatively.

Shaft Fractures

Shaft fractures of the middle and proximal phalanx require operative treatment when rotational deformity is present or the fracture pattern is deemed unstable. Finger rotation is best evaluated clinically during flexion and extension while observing the posture and directional plane of the dorsal aspect of the distal phalanges and nail plates, with careful comparison to the normal contralateral hand. Any overlapping of the digits with such maneuvers constitutes a deformity requiring surgical intervention. If the clinical appearance and positioning of the digits is adequate, then the fracture pattern must be addressed.

Nondisplaced fractures in a digit can be buddy taped to an adjacent uninjured digit; however, the potentially unstable spiral or oblique fracture patterns require splinting. Displaced transverse fractures are usually stable when reduced and can be treated with immobilization. The hand is placed in the "intrinsic plus" position, maintaining the metacarpophalangeal (MCP) joints in flexion and the IP joints in extension, with the adjacent digits included in a well-molded cast. Displaced spiral and short oblique fractures tend to be unstable and often lose reduction with casting alone. The loss of reduction with these fractures is particularly problematic as a few millimeters of shortening or malrotation cannot be tolerated. Careful and close follow-up evaluation, with frequent radiographic documentation is essential.

The fracture pattern often determines the operative technique used. Transverse fractures that require operative reduction and fixation are most amenable to percutaneous crossed K-wire fixation (Fig. 81.2). To achieve maximal rotational stability, when feasible, wires should be bicortical and should not both cross at the fracture site. Fixation requires enough stability to allow for PIP motion to begin no later than at 4 weeks. Short oblique fractures can be treated with K-wire fixation as well; however, long spiral oblique fractures are best managed with precise interfragmentary screw fixation for improved rotational stability that allows early mobilization (Fig. 81.3). To achieve ideal stable fixation, the length of the fracture should be approximately three times the width of the shaft. Compression screws are placed via a midaxial approach to avoid tendon entrapment, and, if possible, all screw heads should be carefully countersunk. The use of three screws is equivalent to the biomechanical stability of plating (3).

Although offering maximal stability, plating of phalangeal shaft fractures has limited use because of the extensive dissection required, which often results in stiffness, necessitating eventual plate removal and concomitant tenolysis. Use of plates should be limited to severely comminuted fractures, open fractures, or fractures with significant bone loss. A dorsal approach with splitting of the extensor mechanism is used for dorsal plating, whereas a midaxial approach with excision of one sagittal band can be used for lateral plate application. Regardless of plate or approach, patients must begin immediate protected motion in an effort to avoid stiffness and a resultant poor outcome.

Most important, the operative approach is often dictated by the associated soft-tissue injury in addition to the fracture pattern. Open fractures with significant soft-tissue injury are best treated with external fixation. Fixators should be positioned midaxially when possible, using an open approach with small incisions to avoid injury to the nearby neurovascular bundles. External fixation can either be used as the first stage in a multistage operative plan or as a definitive treatment.

Base Fractures

Fractures of the base of the middle and proximal phalanx are described as either extra- or intra-articular. Extra-articular fractures can be managed by closed reduction and casting with the MCP joints positioned in approximately 70 degrees of flexion and the PIP joints in neutral. These fractures must be carefully evaluated for any rotational deformity, which if present, will necessitate correction and some form of fixation. A dorsal approach with excision of the sagittal band over the fracture site gives adequate exposure for precise open reduction and fixation. Open treatment is often associated with tendon adhesions, and, thus, fixation should be sufficiently stable to allow for early motion in an effort to avoid this complication.

Intra-articular fractures of the base of the phalanx can also be managed with closed treatment if nondisplaced. However, the inherently unstable oblique fracture pattern will need percutaneous fixation, even if nondisplaced. Displaced fractures require open reduction and internal fixation to re-establish joint congruity. The approach to these fractures is similar to that described for extra-articular fractures with the addition of a capsulotomy. Cortical screws and/or K-wires may be used for internal fixation, with external fixation being occasionally required for more complex fracture patterns (Fig. 81.4).

FINGER METACARPALS

Head Fractures

Metacarpal head fractures are uncommon and can be associated with collateral ligament injuries such as that commonly seen in the thumb. Radiographs should include specialized Brewerton views, which are obtained by maintaining the wrist

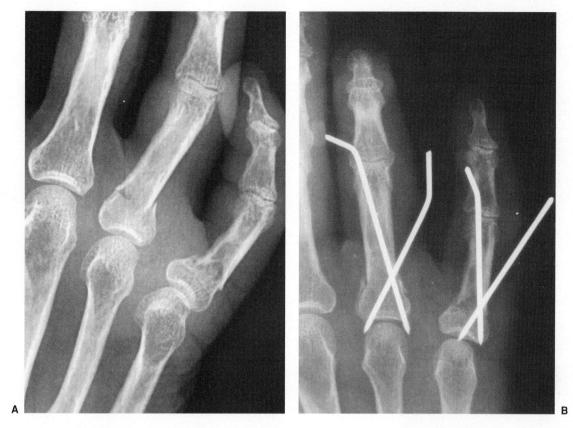

FIGURE 81.2. Displaced transverse fractures at the base of the ring and small finger proximal phalanges with rotational deformity. **A:** Preoperation radiograph. **B:** Closed reduction and percutaneous 0.045 K-wire fixation.

in neutral and at 45 degrees to the tabletop, and the dorsum of the phalanges flat on the cassette with the MCP joints flexed 45 to 65 degrees. Intra-articular fractures should be treated with open reduction and internal fixation if there is >1 mm displacement of the fragments, or if more than 20% of the joint surface is involved. As with all intra-articular fractures,

precise fragment reduction to create a congruent MCP joint is essential to achieve optimal results. Computed tomography (CT) evaluation can accurately define fragment alignment and can aid in treatment planning. If operative intervention is required, the modality is dictated by the fracture pattern with unilateral sagittal band division used for exposure. Small

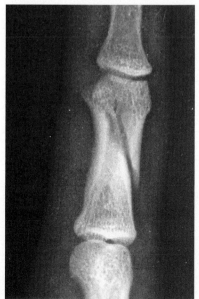
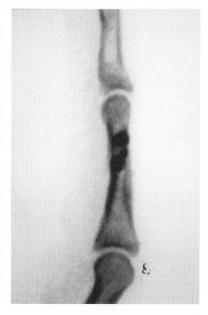
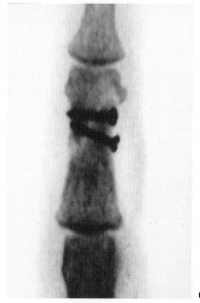

FIGURE 81.3. Long spiral oblique fracture of the middle phalanx. **A:** Preoperation radiograph. **B and C:** Lateral and posteroanterior views of interfragmentary screw fixation.

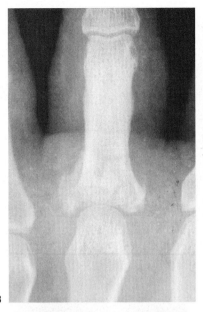
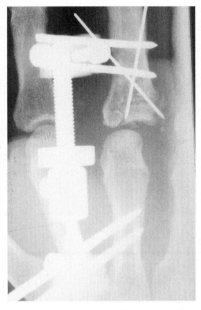
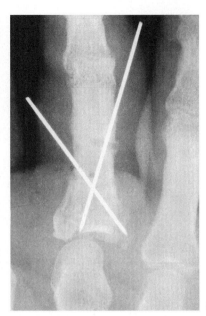

A,B

C

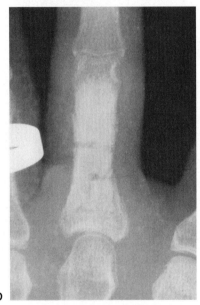

D

FIGURE 81.4. Intra-articular, comminuted, and impacted fracture of the proximal phalangeal base. A: Preoperation radiograph. B: External fixation device placed to neutralize
MCP joint, bony fragments disimpacted and stabilized with bone grafting, and 0.045 K-
wires. C: Early removal of external fixation device, allowing digital motion with K-wires
still in place. D: Final result after hardware removal and bony contour restored.

cortical screws can be used and should be buried and placed
outside the MCP joint articular surface. Small joint arthroscopically assisted reduction and fixation is often possible and has
the added benefit of limiting surgical trauma. Following reduction, K-wires can be used alone or in combination with interosseous wires. The goals of fixation should be to adequately
stabilize the fracture and allow for early mobilization to limit
adhesions of not only the extensor tendons, but of the MCP
joint as well.

Neck Fractures

Neck fractures can occur with any digit but are most common
in the little finger. A fracture of the fifth metacarpal neck is
known as boxer's fracture because these injuries are often associated with a blow delivered during an altercation. Prior to
appropriate fixation, patients with skin breaks, regardless of
size, must be treated as if they have a contaminated joint, and
the MCP joint carefully inspected and irrigated. If these frac-

tures are determined to be closed, they can often be treated
by closed reduction and carefully fitted cast immobilization.
The amount of acceptable angulation for these fractures varies
within the literature and between the metacarpals. The index
and middle metacarpals can generally tolerate 20 to 30 degrees of angulation; however, in the ring and little fingers,
50 to 70 degrees of angulation can be considered acceptable
in some individuals. Increasing fracture angulation may be
associated with a prominent metacarpal head in the palm,
which is often problematic for laborers and athletes. Treatment,
therefore, must be appropriately tailored to each individual
patient.

Fractures with an unacceptable reduction can be treated
with an open procedure and plate fixation using either a lateral or dorsal approach. Simple longitudinal K-wire placement, supplemented with a well-molded plaster cast to control
rotation, often suffices, and limits surgically created trauma
(Fig. 81.5). Newer percutaneous intramedullary nails introduced into the metaphyseal base of the metacarpal can also be
used. K-wire fixation can be effective particularly with border

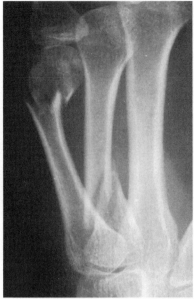
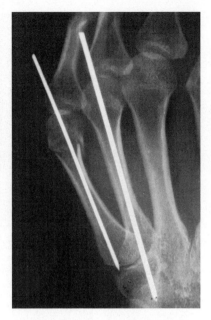
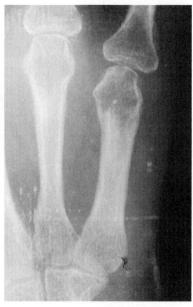

A,B   **C**

FIGURE 81.5. Displaced metacarpal neck fracture of the small finger and displaced extra-articular oblique metacarpal base fracture of the ring finger. **A:** Preoperation radiograph. **B:** Closed reduction and percutaneously placed, longitudinal 0.062 K-wire stabilization. **C:** Long-term results demonstrating accurate alignment and fracture healing.

metacarpals by the placement of transverse wires proximal and distal to the fracture site supplemented with a single longitudinal wire.

Shaft Fractures

The treatment of metacarpal shaft fractures is dictated by fracture pattern, position of the involved metacarpal, and by the number of metacarpals injured. Metacarpal shaft fractures generally have an apex dorsal angulation as a result of the deforming forces of the attached interosseous muscles. Closed reduction can often be achieved with distraction and direct pressure on the fracture apex. The amount of acceptable angulation following reduction varies with the involved digit. The ring and small finger metacarpals can tolerate 40 degrees of angulation because of motion provided by the carpometacarpal (CMC) joint. However, only approximately 15 degrees of angulation is acceptable at the index and middle metacarpals. The length of acceptable shortening is only approximately 5 mm because of the carefully balanced extensor mechanism; however, any degree of rotation that results in finger overlap must be corrected.

Although transverse fracture patterns are the most amenable to closed treatment, multiple transverse shaft fractures are an indication for internal fixation to allow for early motion (Fig. 81.6). Stabilization can most often be achieved with percutaneous intramedullary nails or K-wires. Oblique fractures are often unstable even after adequate reduction and thus require operative treatment. Short oblique fractures may be treated with intramedullary nails or crossed K-wires with placement of an additional longitudinal wire after reduction. In addition, perpendicular K-wires traversing the adjacent uninjured metacarpal can also be used to stabilize fractures of the border digits. Short oblique fractures that require open reduction should be approached dorsally with the incision centered along the injured metacarpal or in the intermetacarpal space when multiple adjacent fractures are present; 2.0- or 2.4-mm dorsal plates should be used for fixation (Fig. 81.7).

Long oblique fractures are more difficult to reduce and often require open reduction and internal fixation. A dorsal approach with plate fixation as described for short oblique fractures can be used with the addition of supplementary compression screws. Screw fixation alone can be adequate for long oblique fractures if the length of the fracture line is twice the diameter of the bone. Fractures associated with significant soft-tissue damage should be treated with external fixation, while coverage is expeditiously established.

Base Fractures

Metacarpal base fractures are considered high-energy injuries. These injuries are divided into extra- or intra-articular fractures. If the carpus is involved, CT evaluation is often needed to accurately rule out fractures or dislocations. Extra-articular base fractures can be treated with closed reduction if treated before significant edema develops. A distraction maneuver with force directed over the displaced apex is usually successful in gaining reduction. Degrees of acceptable angulation and shortening vary with the involved digits. The ring and little finger metacarpals can tolerate 10 to 15 degrees of angulation and up to 2-mm of shortening, as there is compensatory motion at their corresponding CMC joints. The index and long fingers, however, are only able to tolerate 5 degrees of angulation. If reduction cannot be maintained in these extra-articular fractures, closed or open reduction with K-wire fixation or dorsal plate application is required (Fig. 81.5).

Intra-articular metacarpal base fractures result from high-energy axial loads that cause T- or Y-shaped injuries comparable to the Bennett or Rolando fracture seen in the thumb. These fracture patterns often occur in the fifth metacarpal and are often referred to as either a "baby" or "reverse" Bennett- or Rolando-type fracture. Generally, these fractures require open reduction and internal fixation with K-wires or a mini T or Y plate. Avulsion fractures of the metacarpals are usually associated with forced palmar flexion of the wrist and can be treated closed by placing the wrist in extension as long as less than 20% of the articular surface is involved. Avulsion fractures with more than 20% joint involvement will require open

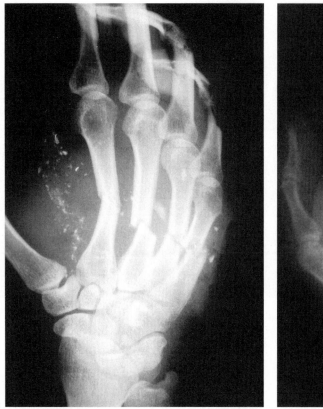
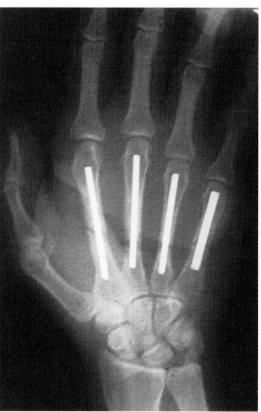

FIGURE 81.6. Multiple transverse metacarpal shaft fractures after gunshot wound with significant soft-tissue loss. **A:** Preoperation radiograph. **B:** Intramedullary rod placement for stabilization.

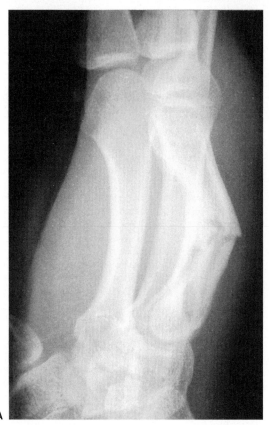
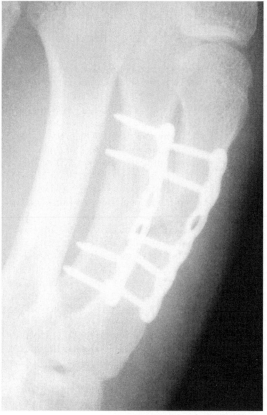

FIGURE 81.7. Transverse midshaft fractures of fourth and fifth metacarpals with dorsal angulation. **A:** Preoperation radiograph. **B:** Reduction and placement of 2-mm plates for rigid fixation, allowing early motion.

reduction and internal fixation, remembering that these patients must be carefully evaluated for associated carpal injuries.

THUMB FRACTURES

Distal and Proximal Phalanx

Fractures of the thumb phalanges are less common and tend to result from a direct blow. Distal phalanx fractures can be divided into either tuft-, transverse-, or longitudinal-type fractures. Treatment is based on both location and fracture pattern. Tuft fractures, as in the other digits, are treated with appropriate attention to injuries of the nail bed and surrounding soft tissues as described earlier. Transverse fractures, however, differ from those seen in the other fingers because of the strong pull of the flexor pollicis longus (FPL) tendon. The pull from the FPL causes displacement of these fractures, rendering them unstable. Reduction and fixation using percutaneous K-wires that cross the IP joint are required for stabilization. Longitudinal fractures are rare and frequently require open reduction and internal fixation. Nondisplaced transverse and longitudinal fractures can be treated with cast immobilization or protective splinting.

Mallet injuries of the thumb, as with other digits, are treated in a similar manner. If no volar subluxation of the distal phalanx is present, these injuries are treated with dorsal extension splinting for 6 to 8 weeks. Volar subluxation or significant (greater than 33%) involvement of the joint surface requires operative treatment with reduction and K-wire fixation, or open reduction with interosseous wiring or screw fixation if fragment size permits.

Thumb Metacarpal Fractures

Thumb metacarpal fractures are divided into shaft and base fractures with base fractures further classified into either extra- or intra-articular. Shaft fractures are usually the result of direct trauma and are much less common than metacarpal base fractures. These injuries are treated by their radiographic pattern with unstable fractures requiring operative reduction and fixation with percutaneous K-wires. **Metacarpal base fractures are much more common than shaft fractures, and the intra-articular types are described as either Bennett- or Rolando-type fractures.**

Unlike shaft fractures that are usually the result of a direct blow, base fractures occur from an axial load through the metacarpal shaft. Extra-articular (epibasilar) fractures are most commonly transverse or oblique in nature and can be treated with casting if stable. Following closed reduction, these fractures are immobilized for 4 weeks in a thumb spica cast. Mobility of the adjacent CMC joint allows for up to 30 degrees of acceptable angulation at the fracture site. If these fractures prove to be unstable with eventual loss of reduction, operative reduction and percutaneous K-wire fixation is recommended.

The pattern of intra-articular base fractures reflects the contributions of the complex and extensive ligamentous structures at the CMC joint, most notably of the volar oblique ligament. In the Bennett-type fracture, which consists of an intra-articular fracture through the volar–ulnar aspect of the metacarpal base, the fracture fragment is held in anatomic position by the volar oblique ligament. The remainder of the metacarpal is displaced dorsally and radially by the strong pull of the abductor pollicis longus. Thus, treatment is aimed to restore articular congruity by reduction of the dorsally displaced metacarpal. If reduction of the metacarpal shaft to the Bennett fragment can be accom-

plished satisfactorily with a 1-mm or less articular step-off, closed reduction with percutaneous pinning is an acceptable treatment option. With this technique, closed reduction of the metacarpal base to the Bennett fragment is accomplished with longitudinal traction, pressure at the thumb metacarpal base, and pronation. A transarticular K-wire is then passed from the metacarpal to the trapezium or second metacarpal for stabilization (Fig. 81.8). If unacceptable reduction is obtained with the closed technique, open reduction is performed. Open fixation can then be obtained with K-wires, screws, or plate fixation, with stabilization of the metacarpal–trapezial joint if needed. Regardless of the technique used, the thumb is immobilized for 4 weeks in a well-fitted thumb spica cast.

The Rolando-type fracture is a high-energy fracture that is made up of at least three fragments, with all comminuted base fractures commonly placed in this category. The classic Rolando fracture, as described in 1910, is a T- or Y-shaped metacarpal base fracture composed of three fragments. These fractures are difficult to treat as they require restoration of both the articular surface as well as the length of the metacarpal. Open reduction with internal fixation using or condylar blade T or Y plate, multiple K-wires, or interosseous wiring is the treatment of choice for these complex fractures (Fig. 81.9). External fixation remains an option with highly comminuted fractures.

JOINT DISLOCATIONS AND LIGAMENTOUS INJURIES

Dislocations and injuries to the ligaments of the hand can occur from hyperextension, hyperflexion, lateral deviation, torsion, or impaction. These stress forces lead to subluxation or dislocation that can occur with or without associated fractures. Many of these injuries are primarily from impaction forces that result in fractures that were discussed previously. The following sections focus on the treatment of dislocations and their associated ligamentous and soft-tissue injuries. Various tissues stabilize the joints of the hand, including the collateral ligaments, volar plates, capsular attachments, and numerous tendon insertions. Disruption of any or all of these structures will often require operative repair because of joint instability, or irreducible dislocation secondary to soft-tissue interposition.

Distal Interphalangeal Joint Injuries

Commonly encountered dorsal dislocations of the DIP joint are often open and must be treated as a contaminated joint. Patients are treated with antibiotics, copious irrigation of the joint, and accurate reduction and stabilization. Closed dislocations can be reduced using longitudinal traction, with the distal phalanx held in slight flexion. Irreducible dislocations tend to be held by intervening soft tissue, most commonly the volar plate or flexor tendon, which becomes entrapped by the condyle of the middle phalanx. The DIP joint is splinted in slight flexion for 2 to 3 weeks following reduction, but with protected motion begun after 1 week. Although less common, volar dislocations of the DIP joint can occur and are treated with closed reduction and extension block splinting for 6 to 8 weeks. Inability to reduce volar dislocations is usually secondary to partial entrapment of the extensor tendon within the DIP joint and requires open reduction.

Hyperextension injuries that do not cause joint dislocation can result in flexor digitorum profundus (FDP) tendon avulsion, commonly referred to as a "jersey" finger, the result of the injured digit being caught in a football "jersey," resulting in hyperextension and tendon avulsion. These injuries occur

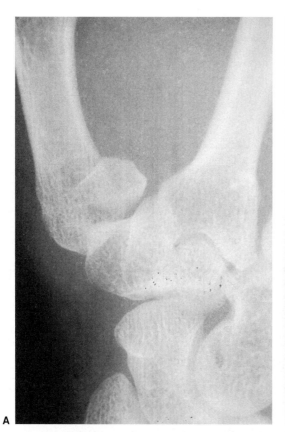
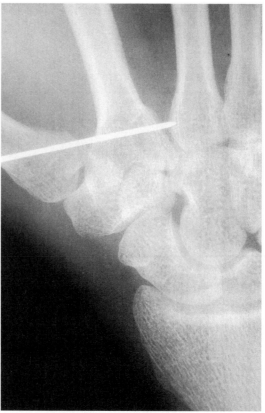

FIGURE 81.8. Bennett fracture: avulsion of volar–ulnar fragment with displacement of metacarpal shaft. **A:** Preoperation radiograph. **B:** Single 0.062 K-wire transfixed to index metacarpal to stabilize thumb metacarpal shaft and maintain reduction to Bennett fragment.

most commonly in the ring finger and can be associated with vincula or bony fragment avulsion. The FDP tendon can retract into the palm with complete rupture of the vincula or can be held at the level of the PIP joint if the vincula remain intact. Both types of avulsions should be treated with anatomic reattachment of the FDP tendon with a heavy, nonabsorbable, pullout suture tied over a dorsally placed button. FDP avulsions with an attached bony fragment tend not to retract beyond the distal extent of the A-4 pulley because of catching of the associated fragment on the distal edge of the pulley system. These injuries can be treated by fixation of the avulsed bony fragment if sufficiently large. FDP avulsions associated with an intact vincula are the most common type of injury and have a better prognosis than those with complete separation of the vincula, as the blood supply to the tendon is not disrupted.

Proximal Interphalangeal Joint Dorsal Dislocations

The PIP joint, like the DIP joint, is a bicondylar hinge joint with minimal motion permitted in more than one plane. In addition to strong capsular ligaments, the proper and accessory collateral ligaments are the primary joint and volar plate stabilizers, respectively. Stress forces on the PIP joint can lead to failure of these structures, leading to painful ligamentous injury and joint instability, as well as incomplete or complete dislocation. Dorsal dislocation of the PIP results from hyperextension, which disrupts the volar plate attachment to the base of the middle phalanx. **These dislocations are not only the most common type of PIP dislocation, but also represent the most common injury to the joints of the hand (4).** Hyperextension

injuries of the PIP can be seen as part of a spectrum of increasing pathology ranging from subluxation to dislocation, and ultimately, fracture dislocation. Subluxation or simple hyperextension results in isolated volar plate injury and can be treated with buddy taping and early range of motion, after 7 to 10 days of immobilization in slight flexion. Failure of the volar plate along with a longitudinal split in the collateral ligaments from hyperextension and torsion can result in dorsal dislocation with or without an associated fracture. Pure dorsal dislocations must be reduced and assessed for stability. Although reduction can usually be achieved by digital block and longitudinal traction, the volar plate occasionally blocks attempts at reduction. If difficulty is encountered with simple traction during reduction, the injury pattern should be reproduced with hyperextension and pressure applied to the base of the middle phalanx in an attempt to achieve reduction. After reduction, joint stability is evaluated and radiographs should be obtained to confirm joint congruity, assess reduction, and search for occult fractures. If stable, dorsal dislocations can be treated with buddy taping and early active motion after a brief period of immobilization. If the joint is found to be unstable, an extension block splint is used, with the PIP blocked at 10 degrees short of instability, but to no more than 20 degrees. Motion is progressively increased by 10 degrees of extension on a weekly basis.

Fracture dislocations can be classified as stable or unstable. Fractures that involve less than 30% of the joint surface are considered stable and can be treated with reduction and extension block splinting. The unstable fracture dislocation pattern, those involving greater than 30% of the joint surface, or those exhibiting subluxation, can be difficult to treat and almost always results in residual PIP stiffness. Dynamic traction can allow reduction and fracture stabilization as well as permit

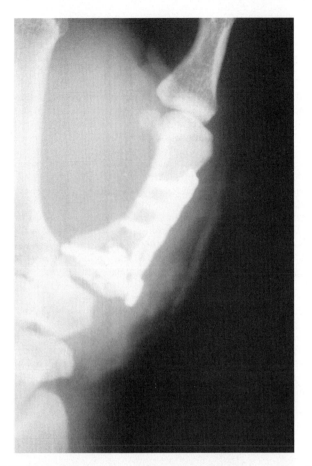

FIGURE 81.9. Reduction and rigid fixation of highly comminuted Rolando fracture using a contoured Y-plate.

early motion with an acceptable outcome. Transarticular K-wire fixation of the joint in less than 30 degrees of flexion is an alternative option to achieve and maintain reduction and joint congruity in these unstable fractures. Patients treated by this method should have early pin removal and protected range of motion instituted by 3 weeks. External fixation, either static or dynamic, is another modality for treatment of these complex fracture patterns. This includes the use of the newer "compass hinge" devices that maintain fracture reduction while allowing controlled passive and active motion (Fig. 81.10). Open reduction and internal fixation can be used if the fracture fragments are sufficiently large, but should be reserved for irreducible fractures or dislocations as this is associated with a greater than 50% complication rate, including joint stiffness, infection, instability, and early arthritis. Volar plate arthroplasty has been proposed as an acute treatment option for these fractures (5). However, recurrent dislocation has been reported as the most common complication with this procedure, particularly when more than 50% of the joint surface has been displaced. Osteochondral hamate grafts can be used as a salvage procedure to restore the volar bony restraint of the middle phalangeal base (6).

Proximal Interphalangeal Joint Volar Dislocations

Volar dislocations of the PIP joint are much less common than dorsal dislocations and are usually associated with a central slip injury and avulsion fracture. Volar dislocations can also occur in combination with torsion, which can lead to capsular disruption, resulting in the proximal phalangeal condyle becoming trapped between the central slip and the lateral band. Simple volar dislocations can be reduced with longitudinal traction and, although there may be disruption of the central slip,

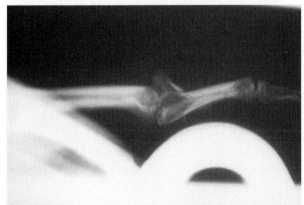

A

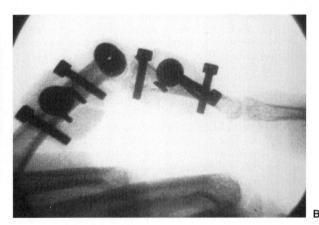

B

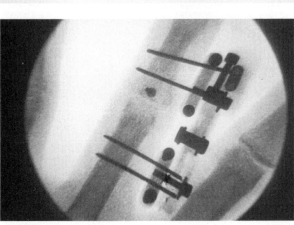

C

FIGURE 81.10. Comminuted, impacted "pilon" fracture at base of proximal phalanx. A: Preoperation radiograph. B and C: Reduction and screw fixation with placement of compass hinge dynamic external fixator to maintain reduction and allow early mobilization.

can be treated nonsurgically with extension splinting of the PIP joint for 6 weeks while allowing DIP motion. However, if joint instability is noted, early operative repair is indicated. Volar dislocations associated with torsional forces often require open reduction, as the proximal phalangeal condyle tears the interval between the central slip and the lateral band, ultimately becoming entrapped. Thus, if closed reduction with traction is unsuccessful, reduction with the PIP and DIP joints flexed can be attempted; however, surgical intervention is necessary if this maneuver fails. At the time of open joint reduction the central tendon can be assessed and, if intact, motion can be instituted after a brief period of 2 to 3 weeks of immobilization. If associated with a minimally displaced (less than 1 mm) avulsion fracture, these volar dislocations can be treated in a similar way to simple dislocation. Avulsion fractures with more than 1 mm of displacement should be treated with precise reduction and internal fixation. K-wire fixation or open reduction with screw fixation can be used for larger fragments.

Proximal Interphalangeal Joint Collateral Ligament Injuries

Collateral ligament injuries can occur with or without dislocations. Most of these injuries can be treated with buddy taping the injured digit to an adjacent uninjured digit after a brief 7- to 10-day period of immobilization. **Complete rupture of the radial collateral ligament of the index finger, however, should be repaired using a midaxial incision and a suture anchor or pullout suture, because of the substantial forces generated during pinch.** Collateral ligament injuries in association with volar plate disruption often occur with lateral dislocations. These injuries are treated with closed reduction and a short period of static splinting followed by protected motion and buddy taping. Operative intervention is indicated for irreducible dislocations or those associated with displaced fractures or fractures involving more than 25% of the joint surface. Purely ligamentous injuries can be repaired as above following open reduction, while those associated with fractures are repaired by bony stabilization alone with K-wires, screws, or suture anchors.

Metacarpophalangeal Joint Injuries

Ligamentous injury to the MCP joint can occur with either subluxation of the joint or pure dislocation. Lateral subluxation can result in collateral ligament disruption. These injuries are uncommon, but if they result in joint instability, or occur in the index radial position, require operative repair. Stability can be assessed by examining proximal phalanx deviation with the MCP held in 30 degrees of flexion. If stable, the injured digit can be buddy taped to an adjacent digit for 6 weeks. Deviation of greater than 20 degrees, or an avulsion fracture with greater than 2 mm displacement, are indications for operative repair (7). Similar to that described for PIP collateral ligament injuries, a midaxial approach using suture anchors or K-wire fixation can be used for repair. MCP dislocations are usually dorsal or ulnar, and often result in a volar plate injury that can be associated with metacarpal head fractures. Reduction of most dislocations can be achieved with wrist flexion and pressure on the dorsal aspect of the base of the proximal phalanx. Following reduction these injuries are treated with an extension block splint to allow the volar plate to heal. Inability to reduce an MCP dislocation is likely secondary to volar plate entrapment and should be treated with open reduction via a dorsal approach, freeing the entrapped volar plate. Once reduced, MCP dislocations associated with metacarpal head fractures are treated as previously described.

Thumb Joint Injuries

Ligamentous injuries of the thumb are common and typically involve the ulnar collateral ligament (UCL) of the MCP joint. When forced radial deviation occurs on an outstretched hand while the thumb is adducted, disruption of the ulnar collateral ligament at its distal insertion site occurs. This can occur as a purely ligamentous disruption or include a bony fragment at the proximal phalangeal point of attachment. Diagnosis of UCL injuries is usually by clinical examination. Plain radiographs may demonstrate volar subluxation of the proximal phalanx relative to the metacarpal with complete collateral ligament ruptures. Magnetic resonance imaging (MRI) may occasionally be helpful in identifying a Stener lesion (see below), which is pathognomonic for complete ligamentous disruption. Partial tears can also be differentiated from complete tears by stress testing under local anesthetic block, with or without radiographs, with the finding of an end point in partial tears (Fig. 81.11). Partial tears can be treated with immobilization for 6 weeks. Although there is controversy regarding treatment of complete UCL tears, most clinicians, including the authors, agree that the most favorable outcome is with operative repair.

UCL injuries often result in entrapment of the avulsed distal end by the leading proximal edge of the adductor aponeurosis (Stener lesion), which, unless released, will lead to nonhealing of the ligament and instability. Operative repair of UCL injuries is through a sinusoidal incision centered over the ulnar aspect of the MCP joint, with the more distal limb being

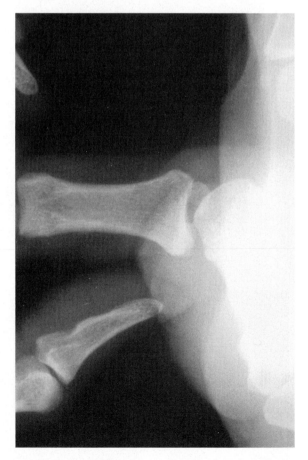

FIGURE 81.11. Stress view of thumb MCP joint after anesthetic block, indicative of complete ulnar collateral ligament tear demonstrating subluxation and >75 degrees of laxity.

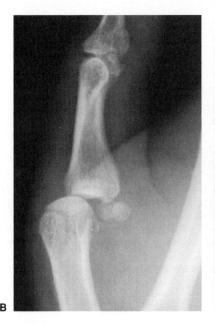
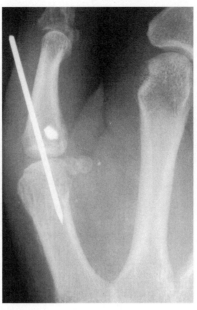
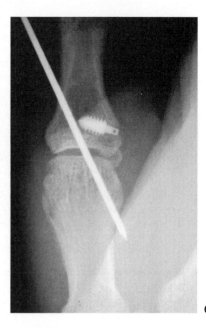

A,B
C

FIGURE 81.12. Volar subluxation of proximal phalanx indicative of complete ulnar collateral ligament tear. **A:** Preoperation radiograph. **B** and **C:** Ulnar collateral ligament reinsertion using bone anchor and transarticular MCP joint K-wire fixation for stabilization.

more volar. Repair of the torn UCL can be achieved with direct suture repair, suture anchor, pullout suture, or bony fixation if associated with an avulsion fracture (Fig. 81.12). Delayed repair of UCL injuries more than 3 weeks after injury may require the use of a tendon graft. Injuries to the radial collateral ligament of the thumb are much less common than UCL injuries. A Stener lesion homolog is not present with these injuries because of the broadness of the abductor aponeurosis. However, guidelines for management of these injuries follow those for

the ulnar side, with identification of no end point on stress testing indicative of complete tears. Injuries with >30 degrees of laxity but with an end point relative to the contralateral thumb, are treated as a partial tear with thumb spica immobilization. Complete tears can be treated with immobilization or operative repair, but in patients whom the injury occurs in the dominant hand or who require bilateral manual dexterity, open repair will yield more reliable results, and is the treatment of choice (Fig. 81.13). Fifty percent of radial collateral ligament

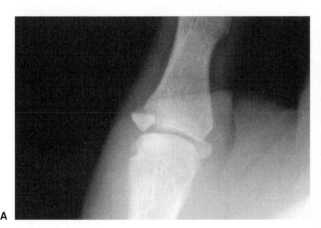

A

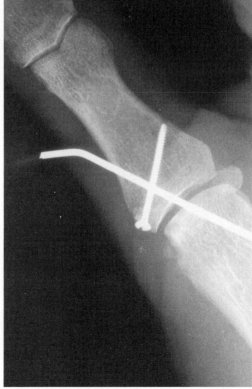

B

FIGURE 81.13. Radial collateral ligament injury of thumb MCP joint with bony avulsion. **A:** Preoperation radiograph. **B:** Reduction of bone fragment and attached collateral ligament using a single lag screw and MCP stabilization using 0.062 K-wire.

tears will be midsubstance, as opposed to UCL tears, which, as previously mentioned, usually occur at their distal insertion site.

In addition to collateral ligament injuries, dislocations of the joints of the thumb can occur and are often associated with volar plate disruption. IP dislocations of the thumb are relatively uncommon and are usually dorsal in direction. Closed reduction and immobilization with the joint in 20 degrees of flexion is the treatment of choice. Inability to reduce an IP dislocation is likely a result of entrapment of the volar plate and therefore requires open reduction. MCP dislocations usually occur dorsally and are associated with volar plate disruptions as well as collateral ligament and capsular tears. The majority of dorsal dislocations can be reduced by closed reduction and should be treated with 4 to 6 weeks of immobilization in 20 degrees of flexion. Joint stability assessment by stressing the collateral ligaments should be performed, as well as stability testing with hyperextension to assess the continuity of the volar plate. Instability in any direction should be addressed with operative repair. Irreducible dorsal dislocations, as well as most volar dislocations, will require open reduction and appropriate ligamentous or capsular repair. Radiographs that show significant hyperextension of the MCP joint are often associated with irreducible dislocations. Repeated, forceful attempts at reduction of thumb MCP dislocations should be avoided as this indicates entrapment of the volar plate, sesamoids, or flexor pollicis longus tendon. If the sesamoids (and associated volar plate) are noted to be within the MCP joint, open reduction is required. A dorsal or volar approach may be used for open reduction of irreducible MCP joint dislocations, although a dorsal approach is preferred. Following open reduction, the thumb is immobilized for 2 weeks in a thumb spica cast with the MCP joint in 20 degrees of flexion. A removable splint is then fashioned to allow for protected early motion of the MCP and IP joints for an additional 2 to 4 weeks.

Purely ligamentous injuries at the base of the thumb in association with first CMC dislocation are extremely rare, as the Rolando and Bennett fracture patterns are much more common. Disruption of the volar oblique ligament occurs with dorsal dislocation of the first CMC joint. These dislocations tend to easily reduce but are inherently unstable and usually require ligament reconstruction. If stable, immobilization for 6 weeks in a thumb spica cast is required.

CONCLUSION

Attention to the soft tissues of the hand is critical if one is to achieve a satisfactory outcome, particularly with more complex injuries and those involving the joint spaces. Generally speaking, the least-invasive form of fixation will serve the patient best and minimize surgical trauma. A careful balance must be reached between achieving stable, rigid fixation, minimizing soft-tissue trauma, and allowing for early, active motion.

References

1. Foucher G, Binhamer P, Cange S, et al. Long-term results of splintage for mallet finger. *Int Orthop*. 1996;20(3):129–131.
2. Rettig ME, Dassa G, Raskin KB. Volar plate arthroplasty of the distal interphalangeal joint. *J Hand Surg [Am]*. 2001;23(5):940–944.
3. Hastings H. Unstable metacarpal and phalangeal fracture treatment with screws and plates. *Clin Orthop*. 1987;214:37–52.
4. Glickel SZ, Barron OA. Proximal interphalangeal joint fracture dislocations. *Hand Clin*. 2000;16(3):333–344.
5. Eaton RG, Malerich MU. Volar plate arthroplasty of the proximal interphalangeal joint. A review of ten years' experience. *J Hand Surg [Am]*. 1980;5(3):260–268.
6. Williams RMM, Kiefhaber TR, Sommerkamp TG, et al. Treatment of unstable dorsal proximal interphalangeal fracture/dislocations using a hemihamate autograft. *J Hand Surg [Am]*. 2003;28(5):856–865.
7. Delaere OP, Suttor PM, Degolla R, et al. Early surgical treatment for collateral ligament rupture of metacarpophalangeal joints of the fingers. *J Hand Surg [Am]*. 2003;28(2):309–315.

CHAPTER 82 ■ TENDON HEALING AND FLEXOR TENDON SURGERY

PAUL ZIDEL

Successful flexor tendon surgery remains a great surgical challenge. Many biologic factors remain beyond our control. Nevertheless, an accurate diagnosis and knowledge of the biology of wound healing, coupled with meticulous surgical technique and postoperative care, are the controllable factors that optimize results.

HISTORY

Kleinert among others reviewed the history of flexor tendon surgery. Galen, who lived in the 2nd century AD and was a surgeon to the gladiators, believed that a tendon was a combination of nerve and ligament, as the nerve entered a muscle and ended in a white cord. Avicenna, a Persian physician who lived 800 years later, was the first to recommend repair of this structure. However, it was not until 1752, when Albrecht von Haller, a Swiss investigator, concluded that this tendinous structure was insensitive to pain, that repair began to be accepted. Poor results led to controversy and experimentation. In 1916, Mayer described the blood supply and avascular zone of tendons. Bunnell used the term "no man's land" to describe the consistently unfavorable zone of repair in the fingers. Mason developed a clinical guide differentiating between primary and secondary tendon suture repairs and strengthening with stress. In 1959, Verdan described the zones of flexor tendon repairs in the hand. In 1967, Kleinert reported his remarkably high percentage of good results in zone two, the "no man's land" of Bunnell. Potenza studied tendon healing based on extrinsic fibroblastic invasion and proliferation with adhesion formation. Lundborg, believing tendons had the intrinsic requirements to heal, explored intrinsic tendon healing based on synovial fluid nutrition. Strickland, Manske, Gelberman, and others have studied the delicate balance between healing and motion with regard to such factors as the role of growth factors and fibronectin, the ratio of extrinsic to intrinsic healing, tendon suture techniques and the strength of repairs, and the effects of early active postoperative motion on outcome. Nevertheless, many questions remain unsettled.

TENDON ANATOMY

In a complex functional system, muscle fibers extend from their osseous origin and taper into long, narrow, glistening white structures called tendons. Tendons have no inherent contractile properties, but are the important link between muscle and bone, causing motion of the intercalated joint.

Tendons are composed of dense, metabolically active connective tissue, the collagen bundles of which are oriented in regular, spiraling patterns. This arrangement of fibers provides a maximal vector of tissue force parallel to the longitudinal muscle fibers. Tendons are exceptionally strong for transmitting forces, yet are designed to glide easily. Microscopic analysis of the tendon reveals it to be composed of very few tendon cells (*tenocytes*) and even fewer synovial cells and fibroblasts. There is an abundance of intercellular tissue matrix, mainly type I collagen with small amounts of types III and IV collagen and elastin. The *endotenon* encloses tendon bundles and is continuous with the perimysium proximally and the periosteum distally. If the tendon is within a synovial sheath, the outer layer of the tendon is called the *epitenon*, which is vascular and cellular, although the intrasynovial tendon has avascular watershed areas or zones. Early observation of the relative lack of cells and the avascular zones led to the erroneous conclusion that tendons did not have within them the intrinsic capability for repair and needed extrinsic adhesions for healing. Both endotenon and epitenon cells can bridge the tendon gap. If the tendon is outside the sheath (extrasynovial), then the outer, loose, circumferential areolar adventitial layer is called the *paratenon*, through which blood vessels run longitudinally.

Tendons vary both in size and shape from one to another as well as within an individual tendon. The flexor tendons of the wrist, flexor carpi radialis (FCR) and flexor carpi ulnaris (FCU), are strong and thick, while the flexor pollicis longus (FPL) has a distal muscle belly. **The flexor tendons of the fingers are arranged into three layers as they approach the carpal tunnel from the distal wrist.** The flexor digitorum superficialis (FDS) tendons to the middle and ring fingers are most superficial; deeper are the superficialis tendons of the index and small fingers. The deepest layer is composed of the FPL and the four flexor digitorum profundi (FDP) tendons to the index, middle, ring, and small fingers, which are derived from a common muscle belly. The greatest variability is seen in the FDS to the small finger with deficiency or absence. There is often a tendon slip from the FDP of the index to the FPL, which may require excision to prevent postsurgical complications.

At the base of the fingers, the superficialis tendons divide, allowing the deeper profundi tendons to pass through them to become volar or superficial to the FDS (Fig. 82.1). Each of the two slips of the penetrated FDS cross under the FDP, rotate 180 degrees, and rejoin at the Camper chiasm, and insert on the middle phalanx as the prime flexor of the proximal interphalangeal (PIP) joint.

The lumbrical muscles originate from the substance of the profundi tendons in the hand, passing palmar to the metacarpophalangeal (MCP) joint and then dorsal to the interphalangeal (IP) joints, inserting into the extensor mechanism at the level of the proximal phalanx. **Lumbrical muscle contraction thereby produces flexion at the MCP with simultaneous extension at the IP joints.**

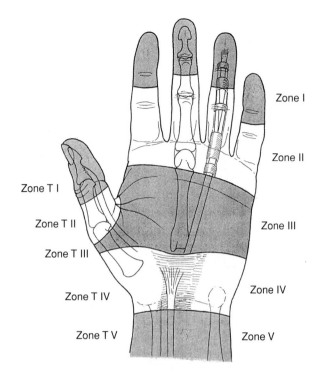

FIGURE 82.1. The vincular mesentery system. (Reproduced by permission of The Foundation for Hand Research, Inc.)

Clinical Tendon Zones

Verdan described five flexor tendon zones in the hand based on anatomic factors influencing the prognosis of repairs (Fig. 82.2). Zone I lies distal to the insertion of the FDS and contains only the profundus. Zone II begins at the proximal portion of the flexor tendon sheath A1 pulley and extends to the FDS insertion; it corresponds to Bunnell's "no man's land." Zone III is between the distal palmar crease distally and the distal margin of the carpal tunnel proximally. Zone IV is within the carpal tunnel, where the median nerve and nine flexor tendons are in intimate relation. Injury there almost always includes the median nerve and, being amid fixed fibrous structures, it is in a difficult zone for successful repairs. Zone V is proximal to the carpal tunnel in the distal forearm. In the thumb, Zone T I is distal to the IP joint. Zone T II is over the proximal phalanx

from the A1 pulley to the IP joint. Zone T III is in the thenar eminence. Zones T IV and T V are the same as for fingers.

Digital Fibro-osseous Sheath

The fibro-osseous sheath is a synovial-lined canal that originates from the periosteum and encloses the flexor tendons in the digits. The sheath is a multilayered double-walled covering. The synovial lubricating fluid is rich in hyaluronate and protein, which contributes to the nutrition of the tendon through imbibition as well as providing lubrication for gliding. It extends from the distal palmar crease to just beyond the distal interphalangeal (DIP) joint. Doyle and Blythe described the pulley system in detail, as there are thickenings of the sheath that act as a biomechanically essential restraining pulley system to keep the tendons tight to the bones regardless of the position of the fingers or wrist. The pulley system maintains a constant moment arm of force and prevents bowstringing. The average excursion is 1.5 mm per 10 degrees of flexion. There are five annular (A) pulleys and three thinner, collapsible crisscross cruciate (C) pulleys (Fig. 82.3). The thumb has two annular pulleys (at the proximal and distal phalanx) and an oblique pulley between them that is important and needs to be preserved. There is also a palmar aponeurosis pulley from the palmar fascia proximal to the A-1 pulley in the palm. The A-1 pulley is the most common site for stenosing tenosynovitis to occur, resulting in a trigger finger. The essential A-2 pulley is found at the proximal portion of the proximal phalanx, and the other essential A-4 pulley is at the middle portion of the middle phalanx. **These are the two pulleys that should be preserved to prevent flexor tendon bowstringing.**

TENDON HEALING

It is now established that tendons have intrinsic healing capability provided that adequate blood supply and nutrition are present. Within the tendon sheath, the blood supply runs through the "mesotenon" to form a vascular mesentery called a vincula (Fig. 82.1). There are two vincula to each FDS and FDP. Their origin is the digital vessels, which join in a four-step ladderlike plexus. Between the vinculum are relative avascular watershed zones. Retraction of a disrupted flexor tendon may avulse its vincular blood supply. Synovial fluid, as well as extracellular tissue fluid, has also been shown to contribute to tendon nutrition. This filtrate of plasma, similar to joint fluid and rich in hyaluronate and protein, bathes the tendons within

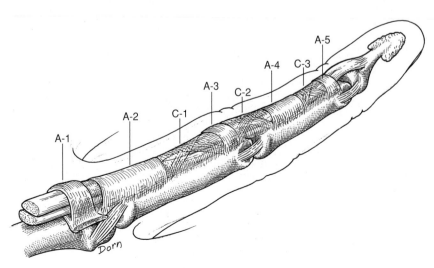

FIGURE 82.2. Zones of the hand. Note the relationship to underlying structures.

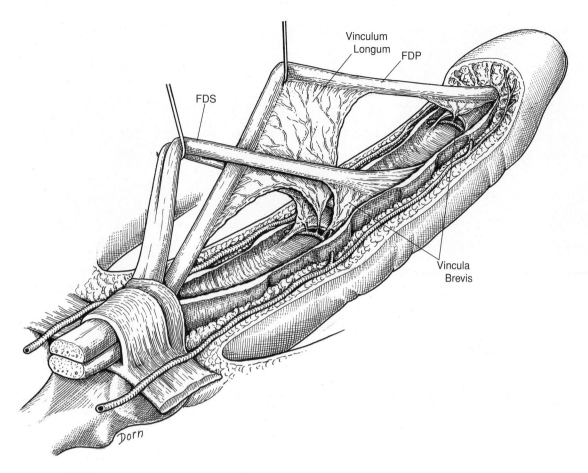

FIGURE 82.3. Flexor tendon sheath pulley system.

the digital tendon sheath to preserve vitality and contribute to repair. Repair of the tendon sheath when feasible has been advocated to not only aid in healing, but to preserve gliding and prevent catching of the tendon. Extrasynovial tendons receive their blood supply via randomly arranged small vessels from the peritendinous soft tissue and this vascular supply may also be diminished by injury.

Severed tendons become united or cemented together by macromolecules of collagen commonly known as scar. The healing process is divided into three overlapping phases. The first is the exudative or inflammatory phase, which is initiated immediately after injury. All cut surfaces, whether tendons or other structures, are flooded with exudate and debriding macrophages. This gives way on about the fifth day to the second phase of fibroplasia, or the proliferative phase, during which macromolecules of collagen are extruded at random into the exudate from fibroblast migration. This "common wound," described by Littler and Peacock, has the elements of healing distributed over all injured surfaces. The third remodeling phase of wound healing begins 3 to 6 weeks after injury and is one of differentiation and maturation of the common scar and last for months.

Adhesions, which are byproducts of fibroplastic proliferation and collagen formation from extrinsic cellular activity, need to be minimized for gliding to occur. As all parts of a wound are initially cemented together equally, tendons that adhere to mobile soft tissue will move with those tissues. When healing firmly unites the repaired tendon to fixed structures, favorable remodeling is precluded. Thus, the functional recovery of a repaired tendon is substantially determined by the mobility or rigidity of those tissues in contact with the site of tendon repair. **The strength and size of a tendon repair and its**

vascularity can be increased with exercise and motion and diminished with immobilization. Appropriately stressed tendons heal faster, have fewer adhesions, better excursion, and increase tensile strength faster than unstressed tendons. Repair strength decreases (10% to 50%) between days 5 and 21, although it might not decrease significantly in appropriately stressed repairs. Hence, appropriate early active mobilization can improve results. The exact balance between intrinsic and extrinsic healing and subsequent strength and motion is still being studied.

DIAGNOSIS OF FLEXOR TENDON INJURIES

A careful history allows an appreciation of the mechanism of injury and guides the subsequent examination. It is assumed that every structure in the area of injury has been damaged and each should be methodically evaluated. The location and size of the wound often define the extent of the injury. Noting the disruption of the normal flexion cascade posture of the resting fingers by a single extended finger, in conjunction with an appropriately located wound, makes the diagnosis of a finger flexor tendon injury virtually certain (Fig. 82.4). Asking the patient if pulsating blood flow occurred following a digital laceration with impaired sensation will aid in the diagnosis of a concomitant neurovascular injury. The flexor tendons move proximally as the finger is flexed. If the finger is examined in extension but was injured while flexed, the cut tendon will be found more distal than the skin wound (Fig. 82.5).

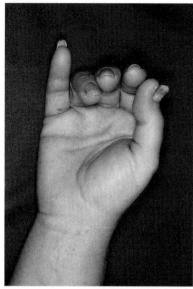
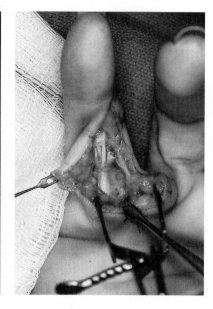
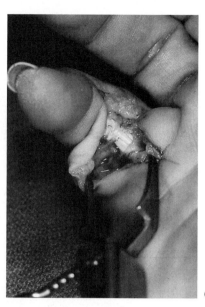

FIGURE 82.4. A: Note the small laceration at the base of the small finger proximal phalanx and the posture of the fingers. **B:** Note the complete profundus tendon laceration with the proximal tendon edge out of the Camper chiasm. **C:** The repair is under the A-4 pulley.

Profundus and superficialis tendons are tested individually. **Isolated superficialis function is tested by preventing profundus action by holding the distal interphalangeal finger joints fully extended for all fingers except the one being tested.** With a common muscle belly supplying all four of the flexor digitorum profundi, blocking DIP joint flexion nullifies FDP flexion of the finger being examined. If strong PIP joint flexion is observed, it can only be the result of an intact, functionally independent FDS. **Full, active flexion of the DIP joint can only result from an intact FDP.**

In the absence of an open wound, failure of digital flexion may be a result of either tendon rupture or nerve palsy. Often the differentiation can be made by placing pressure on the flexor muscle mass in the patient's forearm and observing for passive digital flexion, which will occur if the tendon is intact or with a tenodesis maneuver. Specific muscle electrical stimulation is also useful in clarifying the differential diagnosis of nerve versus tendon injuries.

Partial flexor tendon severance is suspected when there is a corresponding wound with weakness of tendon pull, limited motion, and/or pain produced by the effort. These are often treated conservatively with early mobilization. If rupture occurs, prompt repair is indicated.

Tendon ruptures may occur at the insertion on the bone or musculotendinous junction, or occasionally at a diseased tendon's midsubstance in conditions such as rheumatoid arthritis, fractures, gout, infection, steroid injection, or just "spontaneous" rupture.

Tendon avulsion injuries, usually of the FDP and most frequently of the ring finger, result from forced extension while the profundus is being maximally contracted. It may have an associated bony avulsion fracture fragment seen on radiographs and may even retract into the palm. Prompt repair usually has a good prognosis in contrast to secondary repairs.

SURGICAL RECONSTRUCTION OF FLEXOR TENDON CONTINUITY

The repair of flexor tendons can be classified as primary, delayed primary, or secondary (early and late). "Primary" indicates repair is performed within 24 hours after injury. Contraindications to primary repair are high-grade contaminations, such as human bites and infection. "Delayed primary" repair is done from 1 to 14 days after injury while the wound can still be pulled open without an incision. A child may have a little more leeway in terms of timing to repair, but presents compliance obstacles. "Early secondary" repairs are performed between 2 and 5 weeks. "Late secondary" repairs are performed

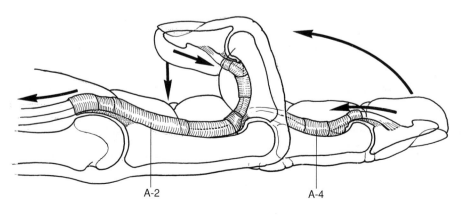

FIGURE 82.5. Note that the position of the tendon relative to the skin creases is dependent on the posture of the finger. The fingertip moves toward the palm with the tendon force vectors both distal (at DIP) and proximal (at MCP). If the flexor tendons are severed while the finger is fully extended, the level of skin wounding and tendon severance will be the same. If injury occurs with the finger flexed, the tendon division will be distal to the skin wound.

5 weeks or more after injury and may require tendon substitution procedures rather than a direct repair. This may be a primary tendon graft, a two-stage procedure, a tendon transfer, free vascularized tendon transfer, or a salvage procedure, such as tenodesis (static or dynamic), capsulodesis, or arthrodesis.

Repair of flexor tendons should be carried out only under ideal conditions. A failure of primary repair will always compromise the ultimate recovery. Creation of a clean, uncontaminated wound is mandatory. The wound is debrided under adequate anesthesia—regional or general—and with absolute visualization of structures to prevent iatrogenic injuries. A tourniquet is inflated 100 to 150 mm Hg greater than systolic blood pressure after exsanguination with an Esmarch elastic bandage to ensure a bloodless field. Extending the traumatic laceration to allow for adequate exposure requires a thoughtful respect for the lines of skin tension. These extensions may be either proximal or distal or both, in a zigzag or, preferably, a nondominant-side midaxial location, whenever possible. Basic principles include atraumatic technique, which minimizes the handling of the tendon to lessen scar and adhesion formation. Windowing of the intact flexor tendon sheath for tendon retrieval and repair should be performed between the annular pulleys of the sheath. Repair of the sheath, if possible, may help as a barrier against development of fixed adhesions and preserve essential biomechanics. Lister uses an L-shaped funnel incision at the cruciate pulleys for the window from which to retrieve the cut tendon ends.

The flexor tendons may require retrieval if they retract away from the initial injury site. Multiple maneuvers using catheters, tendon retrievers, and even endoscopy and other instruments allow for tendon retrieval, preferably under direct vision and as atraumatically as possible. Using a metal probe with eyelet sutured proximally with a slipknot to the cut tendon end and bring it distal, using a thin sheet of silicone background material folded like a funnel to ease the tendon under pulleys. Other techniques include circumferential suturing of the proximal tendon to a cut, beveled small feeding tube or commercially available tendon retrieval kits are frequently used.

The tendon ends need to be coapted without undo tension. Tension can be alleviated during the repair with a tendon approximator or by a "blocking technique" whereby a small needle is passed through the sheath and tendon proximal to the repair. Many suture techniques for flexor tendon repairs have been advocated, including the Bunnell, modified Kessler-Kirchmayr and Tajima, Tsuge, augmented Becker, modified Pennington, Pulvertaft, looped repairs of Lee, Lim, and Tsai, locked cruciate, and Sandow's single cross-grasp four-strand tenorrhaphy (Fig. 82.6). The significance of the number of sutures crossing the repair site or "core" sutures, the difference between locking, looping, and grasping sutures, and strength versus gap and resistance to gliding have been studied. **Present recommendations include a running circumferential or epitenon suture in addition to the core sutures (Fig. 82.7).** Strickland advocates four strands of core sutures. A 3-0 or 4-0 synthetic, nonabsorbable braided polyester or polyfilament material is used, placed dorsal. The running circumferential suture of 6-0 Prolene can be simple, locking, or inverting mattress, or a crisscross locking stitch, Silfverskiöld, or other variation, depending on the circumstances. The running circumferential suture greatly increases the strength of repair. The tendon should be free of entrapped soft tissue and should be seen to be freely gliding.

If other injuries are noted, these are repaired in a logical manner; that is, volar plate first, neurovascular bundles last. The repair of partial tendon lacerations has been controversial. If less than 25% of tendon substance has been injured, repair may not be needed. Usually a single suture repair of laceration

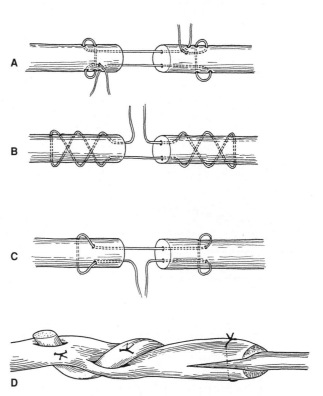

FIGURE 82.6. A: Kessler suture, **(B)** Bunnell suture, **(C)** modified Kessler suture, and **(D)** Pulvertaft (weave suture results in a very strong juncture, but is not suitable for use within the flexor tendon sheath because of its bulk).

is performed for a smoother surface. A dorsal extension blocking splint is applied for protection during the initial phases of healing.

Author's Preferred Method of Tendon Repair

If the tendon ends are in close, tension-free approximation, then the back wall is repaired using a 6-0 epitenon suture of at least 2 mm in a simple locking or Silfverskiöld technique. Next, two to four, double-loop, locked, longitudinal core sutures are placed dorsally and as peripheral as possible (Arthrex looped FiberWire when available, otherwise Supramid). If the ends of the tendons are significantly separated, the core sutures are placed in one tendon first without the epitenon and the tendon is retrieved. The running circumferential epitenon suture is finished in the Silfverskiöld Chinese finger-trap manner. **The repair is examined so as to be free from trapped tissue and able to glide under the pulleys.**

POSTOPERATIVE THERAPY

Many factors are involved in postoperative therapy considerations, including age, extent of injury, number of tendons involved, location, concomitant injuries, swelling, motivation and number of core sutures. **There has been a steady trend toward early controlled active motion following tendon repair.** This appears to facilitate strengthening of the repair, provided it does not exceed the critical rupture force. Many factors are involved in the calculation of bursting strength such as edema formation and bulk of repair, making the friction coefficient difficult to calculate. The

A
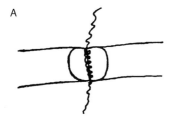

B
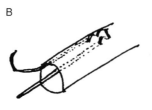

C
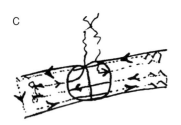

D
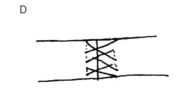

FIGURE 82.7. Author's preferred method for tendon repair: **A:** The back wall is sutured first with Silfverskiöld or cross-locking 6-0. **B:** 3-0 or 4-0, looped if available. Arthrex or supramid, is first placed from the inside and then brought back along the periphery. **C:** 4-core sutures (or 8 if looped) locking are placed and tied in the center. **D:** Silfverskiöld finishes repair.

presently estimated average tensile strength needed for passive motion without resistance on a normal flexor tendon is 500 g; light grip is 1,500 g; and strong grip is 5,000 g. There are several postoperative therapy splinting protocols, including the Duran and the Kleinert rubber-band traction, the Brooke Army palmar-bar modification, the Mayo Clinic synergistic wrist splint, Evan's short arc motion, and the Strickland hinged wrist splint and active tenodesis. The relationship of tendon excursion with respect to tendon and joint motion and finger position helped determine aspects of these protocols. Wehbe and Hunter et al. showed the three finger positions for maximal differential gliding of FDP to FDS to minimize adhesions. Increasing wrist motion with tenodesis is also considered. However, standard protocols employ a dorsal shell with the wrist, MCPs, and IPs flexed. Active extension (to prevent PIP contracture) and passive flexion are encouraged after the first postoperative day, when bleeding should not be provoked. After 2 to 3 weeks, "place and hold no power" can be initiated along with protected passive motion to maintain joint mobility and avoid contractures especially the PIP joint. Differential gliding of the uninjured tendons can also start at that time with wrist tenodesis and "suitcase" power fist. Isolated active tendon differential gliding of the injured tendon begins by at least 4 to 6 weeks and active, assisted, complete fist and passive range of motion. Protective splinting may continue with progressive resistance exercises for up to 8 weeks total, with gradually increased active resistance-strengthening exercises up to 12 weeks.

To evaluate results, Boyes' method of "fingertip to distal palmar crease" can be used. To standardize and compare results, the Strickland classification based on total active motion (TAM) can be used. The formula is

Strickland's Adjusted System:

(PIP + DIP) flexion − extension deficit × 100/175

degrees = %normal

Excellent	75–100%
Good	50–74
Fair	25–49
Poor	<25

or

American Society for Surgery of the Hand System:

(MP + PIP + DIP) flexion − extension LAG = TAM

COMPLICATIONS OF TENDON REPAIR AND THEIR MANAGEMENT

The ideal end result of tendon repair is full recovery of unrestricted, pain-free motion and strength. For many reasons, whether by the nature of the injury or other factors, this may not be achieved. **When full active motion is restricted following tendon repair, the surgeon must determine if the decreased motion is secondary to a disruption of the repair, a joint problem, contracture, tendon adhesion, or other problem.** If separation of the repaired tendon is promptly recognized and repaired again, the results are not necessarily compromised and are much more favorable than if a late secondary repair is attempted.

Other complications include the "quadriga effect" from excessive FDP tendon shortening, with a flexion deformity of the repaired finger causing incomplete flexion of the other fingers. Excessive tendon length, as may occur with a graft, can result in a "lumbrical-plus finger" as the lumbrical's origin is too proximal and thus too tight. A "superficialis finger" may be indicated when DIP motion is not achievable, especially as it accounts for only approximately 15% of the arc of flexion. When tendons cannot be repaired adequately, function may best be optimized with salvage procedures such as tenodesis, arthrodesis, or rarely amputation.

Tenolysis

Tenolysis is considered when tendon adhesions limit motion. The flexor tendon is intact and exerting its force but unable to pull through. **This restriction of motion, caused by tendon adhesions, is diagnosed when the passive motion is much greater than the active range of motion.** Generally, surgical tenolysis is not considered until the patient is at least 3 to 6 months posttendon repair with no improvement for the prior 1 to 2 months. Immediate motion exercises and therapy are needed following tenolysis. A major complication of tenolysis is tendon rupture. The patient should also be made aware that rupture may occur intraoperatively, as well as be prepared for tendon grafting or silicone rod placement or overall worsening of the situation.

Tendon Grafts

Tendon grafts are used to achieve a functional result, usually in the face of a biologically unfavorable zone II injury with crush or scarring. The concept of a tendon graft or tendon transfer is to traverse through the zone of injury with a relatively normal tendon surface, minimizing adhesion formation and transferring the site of repairs from biologically unfavorable for gliding to more favorable ones. The proximal juncture repair is usually done in the uninjured palm or forearm with a Pulvertaft weave (Fig. 82.6) and the distal repair at the distal phalanx. Tendon grafts can be performed as a single operation, or possibly with an "active tendon graft," but usually a two-stage reconstruction is used. The decision can be based on preoperative factors after a trial of therapy to optimize the tissue. The Boyes classification for tendon grafting helps guide the procedure of choice, yet the final decision is confirmed only at the time of surgery, based on the status of the tissue. The first stage is removal of tendon remnants and scar with implantation of a pliable silicone rod to preserve the space and for "sheath induction" of the tissue bed. The rod is fixed distally to the FDP stump or screwed securely to the distal phalanx and left free proximally between the FDS and the FDP in the forearm. This is combined with essential A-2 and A-4 pulley reconstruction over the rod if needed. Also, excision of scarred lumbricals to prevent a lumbrical-plus (PIP hyperextension) finger, joint ligament release, and capsulotomies may need to be done at this stage. The second stage is removal of the silicone rod, usually 3 months later, and replacement with an autogenous tendon graft without opening or creating raw surfaces in the unfavorable zone of injury. There exist variations of the two-stage procedure, such as the FDS being first sutured and advanced after healing to replace the FDP. Tendon-grafting procedures for the FDP in the presence of an intact FDS remain controversial and need to be individualized. The two-stage tendon graft may improve function dramatically but also is fraught with complications. Other variations include the Paneva-Holevich two-stage tendon reconstruction.

CONCLUSION

Flexor tendon repairs remain a basic and challenging task.

Suggested Readings

Barrie KA, Wolfe SW. The relationship of suture design to biomechanical strength of flexor tendon repairs. *J Hand Surg.* 2001;6(1):89.

Beasley RW. *Beasley's Surgery of the Hand.* Thieme Medical, New York: Stuttgart, 2003.

Boyer MI. In: Green D P, ed. *Green's Operative Hand Surgery.* 5th ed. Vol. 1. Philadelphia: Elsevier; 2005: 219.

Hunter JM, Mackin EJ, Callahan AD, eds. *Tendon Injuries. Rehabilitation of the Hand and Upper Extremity.* 5th ed. St. Louis: Mosby; 2002.

Kleinert HE. Primary repair of flexor tendons in "no man's land." *J Bone Joint Surg.* 1967;49A:577.

Kleinert HE, Spokevivius S, Papas NH. History of flexor tendon repair. *J Hand Surg.* 1995;20A:S46.

Lister GD. Incision and closure of the flexor tendon sheath during primary tendon repair. *Hand.* 1983;15:127.

Littler JW. Principles of reconstructive surgery of the hand. *Am J Surg.* 1956;92:88.

Manske PR. Flexor tendon healing. *J Hand Surg.* 1988;13B:237.

Strickland J W Flexor tendon injuries. I. Foundations of treatment. *J Am Acad Orthop Surg.* 1995;3:44.

Strickland JW, Schneider LH, McCarroll HR. Tendons. In: Manske PR, ed. *Hand Surgery Update.* Englewood, CO: American Society for Surgery of the Hand; 1994: 13–1.

Taras JS, Schneider LH. *Atlas of the Hand Clinics—Flexor Tendon Repair.* Vol. 1. Philadelphia: Saunders; 1996.

CHAPTER 83 ■ REPAIR OF THE EXTENSOR TENDON SYSTEM

STEVEN J. BATES AND JAMES CHANG

The complex extensor system is covered by thin, pliable dorsal skin, leaving the tendons susceptible to trauma and exposure. Contrary to popular belief, these injuries may be more difficult to treat than those of the flexor tendon system. Because of the complex anatomy of the extensor system, minimal discrepancies in tendon length and tension can lead to significant functional deficits following tendon injury and repair. An understanding and respect for the complexity of extensor tendon anatomy and function will ultimately lead to favorable outcomes for most injuries.

This chapter reviews the anatomy, treatment, and rehabilitation of acute injuries by zones. Several specific extensor tendon problems that are commonly encountered by plastic surgeons are highlighted.

ANATOMY

The radial nerve innervates the extensor muscles of the wrist, thumb, and fingers. Direct branches from the radial nerve innervate the brachioradialis and the extensor carpi radialis brevis and longus muscles. The remainder of the extensor muscles are innervated by the posterior interosseus nerve, a branch of the radial nerve. The extensor tendons are covered by a thin layer of paratenon through which they receive nutrition. At the level of the wrist, the tendons are covered by a synovial lined sheath, the extensor retinaculum. The retinaculum is composed of both vertical and horizontal fibers that separate the tendons into six distinct anatomic compartments (Fig. 83.1). At this level, one may palpate the Lister tubercle, a dorsal bony prominence of the radius around which the extensor pollicis longus, in the third compartment, courses radially as it travels toward the thumb.

Distal to the extensor retinaculum, the tendons to the index, middle, ring, and small fingers are often connected by juncturae tendineae at the level of the metacarpals. There is a consistent connection from the ring finger to both the middle and small fingers and a variable connection between the index and middle fingers. Both the index finger and small finger have separate extensor tendons in addition to slips from the extensor digitorum communis tendon. **These individual extensors always lie ulnar to the communis slip and can often be employed as a "spare part" for tendon transfers to other fingers.** It is important to note that the communis tendon to the small finger may be absent up to 80% of the time. When this is the case, there is replacement by a substantial juncturae tendinum from the ring finger.

At the level of the metacarpophalangeal (MCP) joint, the common extensor tendon is stabilized over the dorsum of the MCP joint by the sagittal bands that prevent ulnar or radial subluxation of the tendon during flexion and extension. Distal to this level, the extensor mechanism forms a broad, flat hood over the proximal phalanx with both oblique and transverse fibers (Fig. 83.2). It is at this level that the extensor mechanism receives tendinous contributions from the intrinsic muscles of the hand through the lateral bands. The lumbrical muscles pass volar to the MCP joint and then dorsal to the proximal interphalangeal (PIP) joint through the lateral bands allowing for simultaneous flexion of the MCP and extension of the PIP joint. At the level of the PIP joint, the extensor tendon becomes the central slip and attaches to the dorsal base of the middle phalanx along with oblique fibers from the lateral bands to allow for extension of the PIP joint. Distally, the lateral bands join to insert into the base of the distal phalanx for distal interphalangeal (DIP) joint extension. The triangular ligament stabilizes the lateral bands dorsally over the middle phalanx, thereby preventing volar subluxation and the boutonnière deformity. At the same level, the transverse retinacular ligament stabilizes the terminal lateral bands volarly, thereby preventing dorsal subluxation and the swan neck deformity.

ANATOMIC PEARLS

Once the hand surgeon becomes familiar with the extensor tendons, certain anatomic pearls that have direct surgical implications are appreciated. The first dorsal compartment, commonly released for de Quervain tenosynovitis, is likely to have subcompartments that require separate release to adequately relieve tightness of the abductor pollicis longus (APL) and extensor pollicis brevis (EPB) tendons. The APL usually has several slips, and these may be used for tendon rerouting or interposition. In the third extensor compartment, the extensor pollicis longus (EPL) tendon glides freely without junctural connections to the other extensors. **A complete laceration of the EPL results in retraction of the proximal end, preventing easy repair.** Many surgeons have searched wounds in vain in the emergency room for this elusive tendon! Unlike the EPL, the extensor digitorum communis (EDC) tendons are prevented from retraction by the juncturae tendineae. If the extensor indicis proprius (EIP) or extensor digiti minimi (EDM) tendons are used for tendon transfer, it is helpful to remember that these accessory tendons lie ulnar to the EDC tendons at the level of the MCP joint. Lastly, another trick to identify the EIP tendon is to look for the tendon having the most distal muscle belly in the floor of the fourth extensor compartment.

TENDON ZONES OF INJURY

Like the flexor tendon system, injuries to the extensor tendons are classified by anatomic zones. Unlike the five zones in the flexor tendon system, there are nine zones of extensor tendon injury that help divide specific treatment and therapy (Fig. 83.3). The nine zones are as follows:

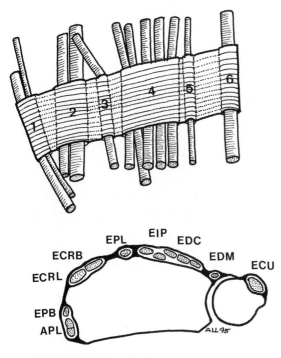

FIGURE 83.1. Dorsal wrist compartments.

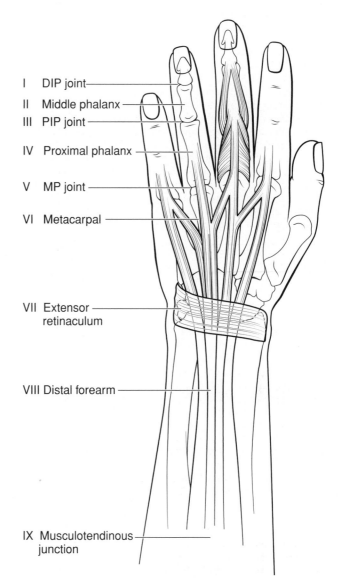

I   DIP joint
II Middle phalanx
III PIP joint
IV Proximal phalanx
V   MP joint
VI Metacarpal
VII Extensor retinaculum
VIII Distal forearm
IX Musculotendinous junction

FIGURE 83.3. Extensor tendon zones of injury.

Zone I injuries are located at the terminal extensor slip, at the level of the distal phalanx and distal interphalangeal joint.

Zone II spans the area of the lateral bands over the middle phalanx of the fingers or the proximal phalanx of the thumb.

Zone III spans the proximal interphalangeal joint of the fingers corresponding to insertion of the central slip. Injuries in this area that disrupt the central slip attachment can lead to boutonnière deformities.

Zone IV spans the area overlying the proximal phalanx of the finger.

Zone V includes injuries over and around the metacarpophalangeal joints of the fingers. There is often joint involvement at this level, and the sagittal bands may be damaged causing subluxation of the tendon.

Zone VI spans the area overlying the metacarpals in the hand. In this zone, the junctura tendineae may be involved.

Zone VII is directly over the extensor retinaculum, which may protect the tendons from injury.

Zone VIII spans the area between the extensor retinaculum and the musculotendinous junction.

Zone IX is the most proximal zone and is in the region of the musculotendinous junctions and muscle bellies, in the forearm.

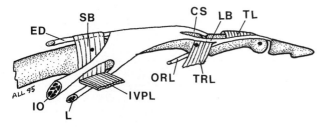

FIGURE 83.2. Anatomy of the extensor apparatus of the finger.

ACUTE TENDON INJURIES

Treatment of Zone I Injuries

Injuries to the distal end of the extensor tendon mechanism in zone I are also known as mallet finger injuries. These injuries consist of disruption of the terminal slip of the extensor tendon mechanism from the base of the distal phalanx. Patients often present with a history of hyperflexion of the joint. The DIP joint is flexed at rest and there is an inability to actively extend the distal phalanx.

Doyle and others have classified mallet finger injuries into four distinct types. Type I injuries are closed injuries with attenuation or disruption within the substance of the extensor tendon. These may be associated with a small bone fragment (<20% of the articular surface) attached to the tendon. Type II injuries are open injuries that occur after direct laceration of the distal extensor tendon insertion. Type III injuries are also open injuries but occur after abrasion or avulsion of the soft tissues overlying the extensor tendon at its distal insertion. Type IV injuries involve the distal phalangeal bone and are subclassified into three groups: (a) transphyseal fractures in children;

(b) hyperflexion injuries involving 20% to 50% of the articular surface; and (c) hyperextension injuries that usually involve 50% of the articular surface, with associated volar subluxation of the distal phalanx.

Treatment for types I, IVa, and IVb injuries consists of splinting the finger in hyperextension. We favor custom-fitted plastic splints rather than poorly fitting prefabricated splints. **Successful treatment of these closed injuries requires strict adherence to the splinting protocol for as long as 8 weeks.** Type II injuries require direct repair of the skin laceration, usually with 4-0 or 5-0 nylon suture. Deep passage with the sutures will allow for simultaneous tendon and skin approximation (tenodermodesis). Because of the proximity to the DIP joint in these injuries, appropriate steps should be taken if joint involvement is suspected. Patients are splinted as with closed injuries with the exception of suture removal at 12 to 14 days after repair. Type III mallet injuries require soft-tissue coverage of exposed tendon. Reconstruction of these injuries is often facilitated by Kirschner wire pinning across the DIP joint to hold the joint in extension. A local flap, such as the reverse cross-finger flap or homodigital island flap, can be used for coverage of exposed tendon and joint.

Type IVc injuries require reduction of the distal phalanx and the large articular fracture piece, which is often pulled 90 degrees to the normal joint axis by the extensor mechanism. There may be collateral ligament rupture leading to volar subluxation of the distal phalanx. Subluxation may appear immediately or may present later in fractures that have been inadequately reduced. For those fractures seen early, closed reduction with percutaneous pinning can be successful. However, it is often necessary to proceed with open treatment so as to obtain adequate reduction and maintenance of the articular surfaces. The distal phalanx is first pinned into reduction with a transarticular wire. Once the joint is stabilized, the dorsal fracture fragment must be rotated back into position. The fragment is then held in place with a 0.028-inch Kirschner wire or a small fragment screw. If the fragment cannot be adequately reduced, it may be debrided. The edge of the extensor tendon is then advanced onto the distal phalanx and affixed with a suture anchor or tie-over button, taking care to avoid disruption of the nail germinal matrix.

Splinting remains the hallmark of treatment for most mallet finger injuries, especially closed injuries without subluxation of the distal phalanx. The mallet finger splint is best customized. To increase patient compliance and avoid the complication of tissue maceration and necrosis, the splint must be properly fitted. The DIP joint should be placed into slight hyperextension. **The PIP joint is left free, and immediate range-of-motion exercising of this and all other joints is continued.** All patients should be continuously splinted for 6 to 8 weeks. If at any time the patient removes the splint, the volar surface of the finger should be rested against a rigid surface to ensure continuous extension. After 6 to 8 weeks, the splint is removed. If there is no extensor lag, the patient is progressed to night splinting for an additional 2 weeks, after which the splint is discontinued. If extensor lag remains, the patient is again splinted for another 6 weeks or until the extensor lag has resolved. The patient may then need controlled active flexion exercises to regain DIP flexion.

Treatment of Zone II Injuries

Zone II injuries, which occur at the level of the middle phalanx of the fingers or proximal phalanx of the thumb, are likely the result of a direct laceration to the tendon. Lacerations involving <50% of the tendon substance can be treated conservatively, adhering to usual wound-care protocols. For partial tendon lacerations, the DIP is splinted in extension for 14 days until sutures are removed, at which time active and gentle passive range-of-motion exercising is begun at the DIP joint.

Lacerations involving >50% of the tendon should be repaired primarily with a fine running suture that approximates the tendon ends. Inadvertent bunching or shortening of the tendon will lead to incomplete DIP flexion after healing. For complete tendon lacerations requiring repair, splinting protocols are similar to those for zone I mallet finger injuries.

Treatment of Zone III Injuries

Zone III injuries, which occur over the PIP joints, consist of disruption of the central slip from the base of the middle phalanx. **If untreated, these injuries can give rise to the characteristic boutonnière deformity in which the PIP becomes flexed and the DIP becomes hyperextended as a result of volar migration of the lateral bands.** These injuries may be the result of direct tendon laceration or of closed avulsion of the tendon occurring after hyperflexion or volar dislocation of the PIP joint. The injury might not be immediately evident and can present as late as 3 weeks after trauma. A boutonnière lesion is tested by placing the finger in 90 degrees of flexion at the PIP joint and then testing the ability to actively extend the PIP joint against resistance. The ability to extend against resistance is an indication of central slip continuity.

Closed central slip injuries usually represent avulsion of the central slip from its attachment. These may be treated with splinting, which keeps the PIP joint in extension while allowing for flexion and extension of the DIP joint. A closed central slip injury should be treated operatively when radiographs reveal that a small fragment of bone has been avulsed from the middle phalanx and there is volar subluxation of the joint. These injuries are treated with a dorsal approach and anatomic reduction and fixation of the fracture fragment. If the bone fragment is too small, then micro bone anchors placed into the dorsal base of the middle phalanx can be used.

Because of the importance of PIP joint extension, lacerations of the central slip should be primarily repaired. Again, care should be taken to avoid any length discrepancy in the tendon after repair. In both closed injuries and postprocedure repaired central slip injuries, the finger is placed into a splint with the PIP joint extended and the DIP joint left free. At 3 weeks, the patient is placed into a spring-loaded splint, which allows for active PIP flexion and passive extension. The splint is worn at all times up to 8 weeks after a closed injury or an open repair. Night splinting and active and passive range-of-motion exercises are instituted between 8 and 11 weeks after the operation.

Treatment of Zone IV Injuries

The extensor tendon is very broad in this zone—it lies over the proximal phalanx of the fingers—and injuries are often partial lacerations. As with zone III injuries, those injuries of <50% may be treated conservatively with range-of-motion exercises beginning after the skin laceration has healed. For more substantial injuries, the tendon is meticulously repaired with figure-of-eight sutures.

Early, controlled, active range-of-motion protocols may be carefully instituted to reduce the need for secondary tenolysis.

Treatment of Zone V Injuries

Human bite wounds commonly occur in zone V, which is over the MCP joints. This is generally the result of striking someone in the mouth with a clenched fist. These open wounds are often associated with partial tendon lacerations. The MCP joint should be explored in all cases as joint involvement is common. After exploration and irrigation of the wound, lacerations may be left unrepaired in these contaminated wounds as the proximal tendon does not to retract at this level. Patients should receive appropriate antibiotic prophylaxis pending wound culture results. A splinting regimen is then instituted.

Lacerations are often partial in zone V and should be repaired when >50%. The sagittal bands should be inspected for involvement. **Failure to repair a sagittal band laceration will lead to subluxation of the tendon over the MCP joint and loss of effective joint excursion (see Sagittal Band Injuries below).**

Treatment of Zone VI Injuries

The extensor tendons in Zone VI, which lies over the metacarpal bones, have a more cordlike structure that is similar to that of the flexor tendons. Consequently, injuries in this area often result from lacerations and are less likely the result of spontaneous rupture. The tendon ends are stout enough to hold core sutures and epitenon sutures. The greater strength of repair will allow early range of motion. Because of the juncturae tendineae, tendon ends rarely retract, allowing easier retrieval. However, if the tendon ends are not approximated correctly, then the abnormal tension in one finger may affect the flexion–extension arc of the other fingers via these same juncturae.

Treatment of Zone VII Injuries

Injuries within zone VII involve the extensor retinaculum. At this level, multiple tendons are often involved, making repair more tedious and time-consuming. Once the tendon ends are approximated, the retinaculum directly overlying the repair should be released to avoid postoperation adhesion formation. A portion of the distal or proximal retinaculum should be preserved so as to prevent tendon bowstringing. Fractures of the distal radius may cause rupture of the extensor tendons in zone VII, and these injuries should be ruled out when evaluating such fractures.

Treatment of Zone VIII Injuries

These injuries proximal to the extensor retinaculum are treated similarly to zone VII injuries. At the level of the musculotendinous junction, the tendon fibers should be isolated and repaired with a core suture or figure-of-eight suture. Careful identification of the proximal and distal ends should be performed so that correct reconnections can be made.

Treatment of Zone IX Injuries

These injuries occur through the extensor muscle substance with denervation of the muscle distal to the laceration. **For this reason, return of function after primary repair may be limited.** The muscle fascia should be directly approximated with figure-of-eight sutures to ensure a strong repair.

Following tendon repair in zones VI through IX, patients are placed in a static volar splint with the wrist in 30 degrees of extension, the MCP joints in 0 to 15 degrees of flexion, and the interphalangeal (IP) joints in full extension. Wrist extension provides the majority of "unloading" of tension across the repair. The splint is worn at all times and no active or passive motion is allowed at the fingers. While wearing the splint, the patient may start passive MCP hyperextension exercises. Between 3 and 6 weeks, the patient is placed into a dynamic splint with the wrist in 30 degrees extension, the MCP is in

increasing flexion, and the IP joints are held in full dynamic extension by the splint. Guarded active flexion is begun at the IP joints, using a volar guard to block the amount of flexion allowed. The static splint should be worn at night. Between 6 and 8 weeks, the patient may begin exercises, consisting of active digital flexion with the wrist in extension and active finger extension, out of the splint. Wrist flexion and extension are also begun with the fingers in a relaxed, extended posture. At 8 to 12 weeks postrepair, the patient is slowly weaned from the splints. Full range of motion is allowed with the avoidance of simultaneous finger and wrist flexion. The patient should also start light grip-strength activities. At 12 weeks postoperative, the patient is allowed to flex both the fingers and the wrist. These protocols may be advanced more quickly in the compliant patient.

COMMON EXTENSOR TENDON RECONSTRUCTIVE PROBLEMS

The extensor tendon mechanism represents a complex balance between extrinsic and intrinsic tendons and ligamentous support. Disruption of any one of these contributions may lead to instability and loss of function. Chronic imbalance in the extensor tendon system leads to characteristic deformities that are challenging reconstructive problems. **When evaluating a patient for possible reconstruction, it is important to differentiate between *intrinsic* and *extrinsic* tightness within the extensor system.** Normally, the intrinsic muscles are tightened with MCP joint extension and unloaded with MCP joint flexion. In the case of intrinsic tightness, there is less passive flexion of the PIP joint when the MCP joint is held extended than when the MCP joint is flexed. With extrinsic tendon tightness, the opposite is observed. The extrinsic extensor tendon limits the ability of the finger to achieve combined flexion of the MCP joint and the PIP joint. Hence, there is less passive flexion of the PIP joint when the MCP joint is held flexed than when the MCP joint is extended. Proper diagnosis of intrinsic versus extrinsic tightness will help to guide the surgeon toward correct treatment of these complex clinical problems.

Sagittal Band Injuries

As the extrinsic extensor tendon passes over the metacarpal head it is stabilized in a central position by the sagittal bands. The fibers of these bands arise from the extensor tendons, pass around the metacarpal head on the radial and ulnar sides, and insert into the volar plate. With MCP joint flexion and extension, the sagittal bands ensure centralization of the extensor tendon over the apex of the metacarpal head as the tendon glides over the joint. With laceration or rupture of one of the sagittal bands, the extensor tendon slips off the apex of the metacarpal head, losing its central position and mechanical advantage.

Lacerations in zone V can involve the sagittal bands, and these injuries should be recognized and corrected at the time of primary tendon repair. **Closed sagittal band injuries are often seen in patients with rheumatoid arthritis.** These injuries occur spontaneously during power-grip activities. **Because power grip is stronger in the ulnar half of the hand, spontaneous rupture occurs on the radial side, causing ulnar subluxation of the extensor tendons. The middle finger is most often involved.**

Patients with sagittal band injuries often present with pain and swelling over the MCP joint and describe "snapping" and "locking" with active extension of the affected finger. There is an inability to fully extend the affected finger, but normal MCP joint flexion is preserved. It is important to differentiate sagittal band rupture from other problems around the MCP joint.

Radiographs will reveal if arthritic changes have caused MCP joint subluxation. While examining the hand, the palmar surface should be inspected to rule out trigger finger as the cause of "snapping" and "locking." The affected finger should then be passively extended to zero degrees. If there is a proximal tendon disruption, the patient will be unable to maintain the finger in full MCP joint extension. If radial nerve palsy is present, no degree of active extension will be possible. In contrast, if the sagittal band was, indeed, ruptured, passive extension returns the extensor tendon to the apex of the metacarpal head, and the patient is able to actively maintain this position.

When diagnosed within the first 2 to 3 weeks after injury, sagittal band ruptures may be treated conservatively. The fibers of the affected band have not contracted, and often splinting of the MCP joint into full extension will allow for healing. The PIP joint should be left free to allow for active motion. The MCP joint is continuously splinted for 3 weeks. After 3 weeks, the splint is removed several times a day to allow for active MCP joint flexion and passive extension.

Any open injury to zone V warrants inspection of both sagittal bands, and lacerations should be repaired. Suture of the sagittal bands must be meticulous so as to restore correct length and to prevent imbalance. The sagittal band fibers are thin and friable. If diagnosis is delayed, the fibers often contract, making direct suture impossible.

Late repair of the sagittal band may be accomplished by using tendon tissue around the region of the extensor hood/sagittal band defect. For this purpose, one may use a juncturae tendinum or a proximally or distally based portion of the extensor tendon itself. These are either sutured to the remaining extensor hood, or are passed around the lumbrical tendon. Tension is set to ensure centralization with both flexion and extension of the finger. Postoperative care is similar to nonoperative splinting. The MCP is placed into full extension and the PIP is left free. Active PIP motion is begun at 1 week. MCP joint active flexion and passive extension are begun at 3 weeks.

Swan Neck Deformity

The swan neck deformity is characterized by DIP joint flexion and PIP joint hyperextension. The imbalance in this deformity is usually caused by intrinsic muscle tightness as the lateral bands sublux dorsal to the axis of PIP joint rotation (Fig. 83.4). The associated ligamentous abnormalities include tightening of the triangular ligament and laxity of the transverse retinacular ligament. Chronic mallet finger deformities and congenital or traumatic volar plate laxity of the PIP joint can also lead to the swan neck deformity. Patients may have a dynamic deformity that manifests during attempted maximum extension or a

fixed deformity with underlying contracture and joint changes. **Swan neck deformities usually do not respond to conservative measures such as splinting trials or exercises.** These therapy regimens may improve underlying joint contractures, but extensor tendon imbalance is refractory to such treatment.

Operative management of swan neck deformity is reserved for those patients with a dynamic imbalance but normal underlying joint architecture. Patients with severe contracture or PIP joint arthritis are best managed by arthrodesis. If the imbalance is secondary to a mallet deformity, then correction of that deformity at the DIP joint will often restore normal length–tension relationships around the PIP joint.

Patients with PIP volar plate laxity may be treated by either of two "tenodesis" procedures. The common principle behind these two procedures is the use of tendon grafts or tendon rerouting to check-rein the PIP joint and prevent hyperextension. The spiral oblique retinacular ligament (SORL) reconstruction described by Thompson uses a free tendon graft for tenodesis. In this procedure, the free tendon graft (usually palmaris longus) is passed through the base of the distal phalanx in a dorsal-to-volar direction. It is then routed along the side of the finger through the subcutaneous tissue deep to the neurovascular bundle. The graft spirals volar and obliquely across the PIP joint to the opposite side of the finger where it is then routed through the base of the proximal phalanx in a transverse fashion. The graft is pulled through the finger from the proximal direction until tension is set with the PIP joint in 20 degrees of flexion and the DIP joint neutral. The tendon ends are then anchored to the periosteum.

In the superficialis tenodesis technique described by Littler, a slip of the flexor digitorum superficialis (FDS) is used for tenodesis at the PIP joint. This method is often preferred when correcting multiple fingers or when a particularly stout repair is required. A volar zigzag incision is made and the FDS is isolated between the A2 and A4 pulleys. One slip is transected proximally, leaving a distally based slip of tendon. The proximal end is passed through the proximal phalanx in a volar-to-dorsal direction and secured by the tie-over button technique. Tension is set with the PIP joint in 20 degrees of flexion and the joint is secured with a K-wire.

Postoperative care is the same for both techniques and consists of continuous splinting for 4 weeks, after which patients are placed into a dorsal blocking splint that maintains the PIP joint flexed at 20 degrees and the DIP joint neutral. Active joint flexion and extension exercises are begun with the splint preventing extension beyond 20 degrees. At 10 weeks postoperative, the splint is adjusted to allow the PIP joint to straighten another 10 degrees. Because the goal is to prevent PIP joint hyperextension, the joint is limited from obtaining full extension. A final 10-degree extensor lag is ideal.

Boutonnière Deformity

The boutonnière deformity refers to DIP joint hyperextension and PIP joint flexion. The mechanism leading to this deformity is usually disruption of the central slip from the base of the middle phalanx secondary to trauma or attenuation from underlying arthritis. The disruption causes subluxation of the lateral bands volar to the axis of PIP joint rotation (Fig. 83.5). The ligamentous abnormalities are opposite to those seen in the swan neck deformity and consist of transverse retinacular ligament contraction and triangular ligament laxity. Initially, patients have full active flexion and passive extension of the IP joints. As the time from initial injury increases, the lateral bands begin to displace volar to the PIP joint axis and become shortened and fixed in this position. The patient is then unable to passively extend the PIP joint. Joint contractures and arthritic changes of the PIP joint can follow.

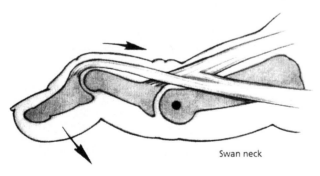

Swan neck

FIGURE 83.4. Swan neck deformity of digit with flexion of the distal interphalangeal joint and hyperextension of the PIP joint. Note the course of the lateral bands dorsal to the PIP joint axis of rotation.

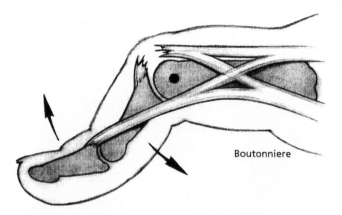

FIGURE 83.5. Boutonnière deformity of digit with hyperextension of the distal interphalangeal joint and flexion of the PIP. Note rupture of the central slip and the course of the lateral bands volar to the PIP joint axis of rotation.

Initial treatment of the boutonnière deformity consists of conservative management with static extension splinting of the PIP joint and active motion at the DIP joint. **When diagnosed early, the boutonnière deformity will almost always respond to conservative management.** In late cases, fixed deformities should also be treated with splinting and exercise prior to any surgical release. Serial splinting of the PIP joint into greater degrees of extension can gradually alleviate any flexion contracture of the PIP joint.

Surgical correction of the boutonnière deformity is extremely difficult and should be reserved for those patients who do not respond to splinting. A number of procedures have been advocated, all of which attempt to divert the increased tone at the DIP joint toward the PIP joint. In the Fowler procedure, the extensor mechanism is approached through a dorsal incision over the PIP joint. The extensor mechanism is incompletely divided in a transverse direction at the junction of the middle and proximal thirds of the middle phalanx. Care is taken to preserve the oblique retinacular ligaments and to avoid complete division of the extensor mechanism. The release allows the lateral bands to slide proximally, thereby increasing tone over the PIP joint, bringing the joint back into extension. At the same time, tone is relaxed across the DIP joint, allowing this joint to move into greater flexion. Postoperatively, the PIP joint is splinted into full extension, leaving the DIP joint free for immediate range-of-motion exercises. After several weeks, the patient is advanced to dynamic splinting protocols.

In a similar procedure, Littler recommended division of the lateral bands as described above. However, the lateral bands are shifted dorsally and sutured to the central tendon, transforming these bands into active extensors of the PIP joint. The PIP joint is then immobilized in full extension with a K-wire. The oblique retinacular ligament remains intact to control the DIP and acts to passively extend this joint when the PIP joint is extended. This procedure is recommended when the lateral bands are shortened and adherent to the underlying capsule, preventing their ability to slide proximally after distal division. After several weeks, the splint and K-wire are removed, and dynamic splinting protocols are instituted.

A large central tendon deficit over the PIP joint will preclude both aforementioned procedures. In this situation, the lateral bands may be centralized dorsally, or, alternatively, a tendon graft may be used to bridge the gap in the central slip. With either method, the lateral band or the tendon graft is anchored to the base of the middle phalanx to recreate the central slip insertion and to redirect the force to the middle phalanx. The PIP joint is then immobilized with a K-wire.

Extensor Tendon Rupture

Spontaneous rupture of extensor tendons is commonly seen in rheumatoid arthritis and osteoarthritis (Fig. 83.6). Rupture is often caused by attrition of the tendon substance after prolonged abrasion against bony surfaces or by inflammatory processes such as tenosynovitis. Patients present with an extensor lag and an inability to actively extend a finger. Often there is no history of trauma or excessive force placed on the tendon. In the case of rheumatoid arthritis, the tendons rupture in an ulnar-to-radial fashion, starting with the EDC and EDM of the little finger and progressing sequentially toward the index finger. As discussed previously, fractures of the distal radius can also cause extensor tendon rupture, with the EPL most often affected. With early diagnosis, primary tendon suture or short tendon grafts may be used for repair. However, tendon transfers may be necessary in the setting of multiple tendon ruptures or delayed diagnosis with retracted extensor muscles.

Rupture of the EPL is usually treated by EIP or palmaris longus (PL) transfer. Rupture of the APL or the EDC may also be treated with transfer of the EIP tendon. An alternative transfer for EDC rupture involves a side-to-side tenodesis of the adjacent intact communis tendon. Rupture of the extensor carpi radialis longus (ECRL) or extensor carpi radialis brevis (ECRB) is best treated by transfer of the pronator teres (PT) tendon.

Dorsal Hand Degloving Injuries

The thin, pliable skin of the dorsal hand makes this area susceptible to traumatic degloving injuries with exposure and/or damage of the extensor tendons. Principles of management include thorough debridement of all nonviable tissues, definitive repair of fractures, coverage with durable tissue, and tendon reconstruction. In the setting of tendon exposure or injury, skin grafting often is not a viable option because of likely adhesion formation. Because of proximity and ease of harvest, the ipsilateral reverse radial forearm fasciocutaneous or fascia-only flap is the "workhorse" flap for these injuries (Fig. 83.7A). An Allen test should be performed prior to flap elevation to ensure patency of the palmar arch. Another useful regional flap is the posterior interosseous artery flap; the "lifeboat" distant flap is the pedicled groin flap. When local, regional, or distant flaps are unavailable, free-tissue transfer can be considered. Free flaps should be thin and pliable over the dorsal surface of the hand. The contralateral radial forearm flap, anterolateral thigh flap, temporoparietal fascia flap, and lateral arm flap are possible options. With segmental tendon losses, staged tendon

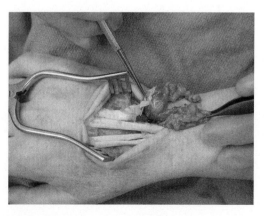

FIGURE 83.6. Spontaneous tendon rupture. This patient was found to have ruptures of the ring and small finger EDC tendons from dorsal tenosynovitis.

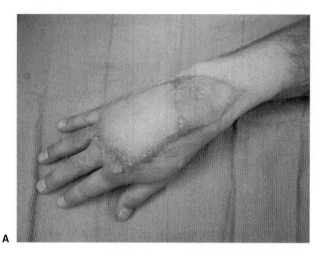
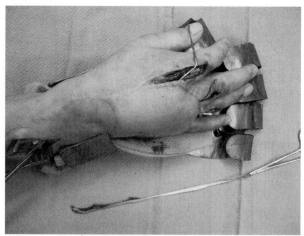

FIGURE 83.7. Reversed radial forearm flap. **A:** This patient has undergone wound coverage of the dorsum of the hand with a reversed radial forearm fasciocutaneous flap. **B:** Staged tendon reconstruction with toe extensor grafts after silastic tendon implant removal.

reconstruction can be performed with silastic rods placed at the time of flap coverage. The second stage can be performed after the flap has healed and maximal passive flexion and extension are achieved. This stage consists of silastic rod removal and placement of free autologous tendon grafts from the palmaris, plantaris, or toe extensors to bridge defects between proximal motors and distal tendons (Fig. 83.7B).

Suggested Readings

Burton RI, Melchior JA. Extensor tendons—late reconstruction. In: Green DP, ed. *Operative Hand Surgery*. 4th ed. New York: Churchill-Livingstone; 1999: 1988–2021.

Doyle JR. Extensor tendons—acute injuries. In: Green DP, ed. *Operative Hand Surgery*. 4th ed. New York: Churchill-Livingstone; 1999: 1950–1987.

Fowler SB. The management of tendon injuries. *J Bone Joint Surg Am.* 1959;41A:579–580.

Hentz VR. Tendons and muscles. In: Hentz VR, Chase RA, eds. *Hand Surgery, A Clinical Atlas.* Philadelphia; WB Saunders; 2001:320–506.

Littler JW. The finger extensor mechanism. *Surg Clin North Am.* 1967;47:415–432.

Littler JW. The digital extensor-flexor system. In: Converse JM, ed. *Reconstructive Plastic Surgery.* Vol. 6. Philadelphia: WB Saunders; 1977: 3166–3183.

Littler JW, Eaton RG. Redistribution of forces in correction of boutonnière deformity. *J Bone Joint Surg.* 1967;49A:1267–1274.

Lluch AL. Repair of the extensor tendon system. In: Aston SJ, Beasley RW, Thorne CH, eds. *Grabb and Smith's Plastic Surgery.* 5th ed. New York: Lippincott-Raven; 1997: 883–888.

Nichols HM. Repair of extensor tendon insertions in the fingers. *J Bone Joint Surg Am.* 1951;33A:836–841.

Thompson JS, Littler JW, Upton, J. The spiral oblique retinacular ligament. SORL. *J Hand Surg Am.* 1978;3:482–487.

Trumble TE. Extensor tendon injuries. In: Trumble TE, ed. *Principles of Hand Surgery and Therapy.* Philadelphia: WB Saunders; 2000: 263–278.

CHAPTER 84 ■ INFECTIONS OF THE UPPER LIMB

JAMES J. CHAO AND BLAKE A. MORRISON

Infections in the hand and upper extremity are common, accounting for as many as 35% of patients admitted to hand surgery services. The majority of hand infections are the result of minor trauma for which appropriate treatment was neglected or delayed. Occasionally, patients will attempt to drain an infection, using a less-than-ideal aseptic technique, only to present with a substantial infection later. **Prompt evaluation and proper treatment of hand infections can mean the difference between an excellent outcome and permanent disability.**

Antibiotics are the only treatment necessary in cases of uncomplicated cellulitis. However, for more evolved infections with localized collections of purulence, surgical drainage remains the cornerstone of the treatment plan with antibiotics as a necessary adjunct.

This chapter discusses the most frequently encountered hand infections and their typical presentations, although the clinician should also be aware of rare infectious agents ("zebras"). "Zebras" should be considered more carefully when a patient's clinical course fails to follow the expected trajectory. This chapter offers a foundation of acceptable practices, as well as suggestions regarding surgical pitfalls. Any surgeon who accepts the responsibility for draining a hand infection must undertake comprehensive management responsibility, including preoperative planning, surgical approach, postoperative care, and, most importantly, rehabilitation.

GENERAL PRINCIPLES

Evaluation

Evaluation of the patient begins with a thorough history, which may reveal the source of inoculation or factors that predispose to infection. Previous injury to the site is a critical element of the history, which includes bites, splinters, needle sticks, and previous attempts at treatment by other physicians or the patient. The examiner should determine hand dominance and occupation, which may increase exposure to certain infectious agents. In addition, history of systemic disease, such as diabetes and immunocompromised states, should be ascertained, as well as tetanus status and the presence of other sources of infection.

Symptoms should be explored in detail, including timing of events. Pain, loss of function, drainage, fever, or chills all suggest infection. A throbbing pain that causes loss of sleep almost invariably heralds pus accumulation in a confined space.

The physical examination should include exposing the entire upper extremity involved. This allows examination for lymphadenopathy and signs of lymphangitis. A systematic approach to the physical examination helps avoid missing important signs.

Radiographs of the affected part are generally obtained to document retained foreign bodies, rule out osteomyelitis or gas in the soft tissues, and to serve as a baseline for future comparison. Imaging and laboratory studies may be enlightening in specific circumstances, but the vast majority of hand infections are diagnosed on purely clinical diagnoses.

Operative Principles

Specific incisions for various indications are covered in the sections to follow, but a few general concepts apply to all. The placement of incisions must follow accepted principles of hand surgery. An incision should never cross a flexion crease at a right angle so as to avoid the development of flexion contracture. Anatomic locations of critical structures must be noted to avoid iatrogenic injuries. Incisions may have to be lengthened and should be planned accordingly by making potential extensions with a marking pen so as to avoid inappropriate choices.

Tourniquet control is helpful in infection cases, as the inflammation accompanying an infection can lead to profuse bleeding that obscures the operative field. For minor procedures such as drainage of a felon, a simple finger tourniquet may be fashioned from a Penrose drain or section of sterile glove wrapped from distal to proximal and secured with a hemostat. In more involved cases, a standard pneumatic tourniquet is placed; but to prevent proximal migration of accumulated pus, use Esmarch bandaging with caution. An alternative for venous exsanguination of the upper extremities is elevation of the arm with digital pressure on the brachial artery for 2 minutes prior to tourniquet insufflation.

Rest, Heat, and Elevation

Rest, heat, and elevation are important adjuncts to surgical treatment of hand infections. Immobilization of the affected extremity limits the opening of tissue planes, restricting the spread of infection. Splinting should always be in a position of function to reduce the stiffness that will have to be overcome in subsequent hand therapy.

Application of heat increases the delivery of inflammatory cells to the affected area by local vasodilatation, and also improves patient comfort. Moist heat is more effective than dry heat, and can be combined with sink hydrotherapy on an inpatient or outpatient basis. Warm soaks reach maximum vasodilatory effect in approximately 10 minutes. Consequently, short but frequent soaks are preferred over continuous immersion. For more severe infections for which soaks are inadvisable, the affected part can be wrapped in moist hot towels, and then covered with plastic wrap to create a vapor barrier, with a dry towel to insulate.

Elevation helps to reduce edema by improving venous and lymphatic return to the heart. The goal of elevation is to keep the hand above the level of the heart so that dependant drainage can occur. Thus simple arm slings provide poor therapeutic support. Patients should be counseled to rest with the extremity above their chest, or on pillows while sitting. Commercially available supports, such as the foam block arm elevation pillow, are excellent at maintaining effective elevation.

Inpatient Care

Many patients will present with infections that meet the criteria for inpatient hospitalization. The need for intravenous antibiotics is the most common justification for admission to the hospital, but admission to the hospital allows many treatment options that are simply impractical on an outpatient basis. Some patients may require continuous or intermittent wound irrigation. Another obvious indication is the need for frequent dressing changes. Although home health care may be available in some areas, it may not be feasible. Dressing changes by nursing staff serve to educate the patient on appropriate technique and relieve anxiety over potentially painful wound care. The patient can then continue dressing changes reliably as an outpatient.

For patients with substantial infections for which extensive debridement and complex reconstruction are required, inpatient care is mandatory. The care of such patients is divided into three phases. Phase I consists of rapid infection control and staged debridement. The surgeon should not feel compelled to address every component of a complex case at the initial setting. Devitalized tissue is excised, the patient is splinted, and a planned "second look" exploration in 24 to 48 hours is scheduled. This approach may reduce the total defect that requires eventual reconstruction. Phase II consists of salvage of vital structures and soft-tissue coverage. Once the infection is cleared, it is important to identify structures that require reconstruction later, repair the ones that are amenable to delayed primary repair, and obtain soft-tissue coverage. Edema control in the hand is very difficult to obtain with open wounds present. The presence of edema makes the goals of occupational therapy and useful motion almost impossible. Reconstructive surgery (phase III) is performed once stable soft-tissue coverage is possible and additional time allows for thorough discussion of all available reconstructive options.

Occupational therapy services are invaluable for initiating early hand therapy during the patient's stay in the hospital. Occupational therapists or cast technicians can fabricate custom thermoplastic splints that can be removed for daily wound care.

ANTIMICROBIAL THERAPY

Antibiotics are indispensable adjuncts to surgical management of hand infections. Cultures are obtained prior to initiation of antibiotics. However, initial antibiotic therapy is always empirical, based on the likelihood of pathogen for a given presentation. Because the vast majority of acute bacterial infections in the hand are caused by *Staphylococcus* or *Streptococcus* species, therapy is usually directed at these common, gram-positive organisms. However, specific elements of the history, particularly mechanism of injury, may suggest alternative antibiotic choices. For example, cat bites require coverage for *Pasteurella multocida*.

Unfortunately, patterns of emerging antimicrobial resistance complicate the selection of antibiotics. In particular, the increasing prevalence of community-acquired methicillin-resistant *Staphylococcus aureus* (MRSA) may render first-generation cephalosporins and synthetic penicillins ineffective as choices for empiric treatment of hand infections. The clinician should observe patterns of resistance in their area of practice and adjust antibiotic choices accordingly.

Table 84.1 presents suggestions for empiric treatment of hand infections. Therapy should be tailored to the clinical scenario and guided by culture results. Like all pharmaceuticals, antibiotics have finite therapeutic windows, and selection of particular drugs (e.g., gentamicin, vancomycin) may necessitate serum level determinations to adjust dosages and limit risk of iatrogenic injury. Alternative antibiotics for treating MRSA are suggested, and should be used when regional resistance patterns warrant such coverage (Table 84.1).

ACUTE PROCESSES

Cellulitis

Virtually all hand infections begin as cellulitis, a superficial process that presents with pain, swelling, and erythema. Lymphadenopathy may occasionally occur. The vast majority of cases will respond to oral antibiotics, rest, warm soaks, and elevation. Because gram-positive organisms are typically the responsible agents, a first-generation cephalosporin or penicillin is appropriate. First-line agents should be adjusted when MRSA is prevalent.

Lymphangitis is diagnosed when cellulitis is accompanied by erythematous streaks up the arm. Consideration for inpatient treatment with intravenous antibiotics should be made for this complication, particularly in the diabetic or otherwise immunocompromised patient.

Paronychia

A paronychia is an infection of the soft tissues surrounding the fingernail and is the most common infection in the hand (Fig. 84.1). This typically results from inoculation of bacteria between the nail and surrounding structures, often as a consequence of relatively minor trauma such as nail biting, poor manicuring, or a small puncture wound. *S. aureus* is the most common isolate, but anaerobes are frequently present and usually attributed to contamination of the wound with oral secretions (2).

If a paronychia is diagnosed at an early stage, before a discreet abscess cavity has formed, oral antibiotics, warm soaks, rest, and elevation may be sufficient treatment. For an abscess localized to one lateral nail fold, the fold can be elevated bluntly using a small hemostat or Freer elevator. Alternatively, a no. 11 blade can be used, paying careful attention to direct the point away from the nail bed. This can often be done without anesthesia through the insensate distended epithelium where the abscess is pointing. A small portion of gauze is placed under the elevated nail fold, and sink hydrotherapy is begun in 48 hours.

An infection that involves the proximal nail and one lateral fold is known as an eponychia. When an abscess dissects under the nail sulcus to the opposite lateral fold, it is known as a "runaround" abscess. A confined collection of pus can place pressure on the germinal matrix, resulting in a nail deformity if left untreated. Failing conservative management, surgical debridement and drainage of this condition is warranted. Two incisions are made at the edges of the nail fold, the proximal nail is excised, and the fold is elevated and packed with gauze (Fig. 84.2). Only the loose portion of the nail plate needs to be removed. Rarely, the pus collection will elevate the entire nail plate, necessitating removal of the entire nail. Improved results have been reported by some authors with limited removal of the nail plate, sparing the incisions in the nail fold (3).

TABLE 84.1

ANTIBIOTIC CHOICES FOR HAND INFECTION TREATMENT

DIAGNOSIS	ORGANISM	ANTIBIOTICS OF CHOICE	DURATION	SURGICAL TREATMENT
Cellulitis (nondiabetic)	Group A *Streptococcus* (occasionally group B, C, or G), *Staphylococcus aureus*[a]	Mild: cephalexin, erythromycin, AM/CL, azithromycin, clarithromycin, dicloxacillin; Severe: cefazolin, nafcillin, oxacillin, penicillin G	5–7 days	No surgical treatment, but may benefit from splinting
Cellulitis (diabetic)	Group A *Streptococcus*, *Staphylococcus*, Gram-negative organisms	Mild: AM/CL, second- or third-generation cephalosporin; Severe: IMP, meropenem, AM/SB, PIP/TZ	7–10 days	
Paronychia Nail biting, etc.	*Staphylococcus*	Clindamycin 300 mg p.o. q.i.d.; Erythromycin 500 mg p.o. q.i.d.	5–7 days 10 days	Drain when fluctuant
Oral contact Dishwashing	HSV (Whitlow) *Candida*	Acyclovir 400 p.o. t.i.d.; Clotrimazole (topically)	t.i.d.–q.i.d. × 7–14 days	
Felon	*Staphylococcus*, *Streptococcus*, polymicrobial	See drugs for cellulitis	7–10 days	Surgical drainage
Herpetic whitlow	HSV	None (most patients); Acyclovir (HIV+)	10 days	Contraindicated unless secondarily infected
Palmar space abscesses, flexor tenosynovitis	*Staphylococcus*, *Streptococcus*, polymicrobial	IMP, meropenem, AM/SB, PIP/TZ	10–14 days	Surgical drainage, hospital admit, consider second look
Bites Human	*Streptococcus viridans*, *S. epidermidis*, *S. aureus*[a], *Eikenella*, *Bacteroides*, *Corynebacterium*	Early: AM/CL; Infected: AN/SB, cefoxitin, or PIP/TZ; Clindamycin+ fluoroquinolone or TMP/SMX if penicillin allergic		Irrigate, debride, do not close
Dog	*Pasteurella multocida*, *E. aureus*, *Bacteroides*	AM/CL[b]	Clindamycin+ fluoroquinolone (adults) or clindamycin+ TMP/SMX (children)	Most can be closed loosely after sharp debridement
Cat	*Pasteurella*, *S. aureus*[a]	AM/CL[c]	Cefuroxime or doxycycline	Closure almost never indicated

[a] Consider substituting *S. aureus* coverage when MRSA is prevalent in the community. Oral agent choices include TMP/SMX, clindamycin, tetracycline, minocycline, doxycycline, rifampin, and linezolid. Intravenous agents include vancomycin, gentamicin, and daptomycin.
[b] Few dog bites ≅50% become infected. Consider rabies exposure.
[c] Most cat bites (80%) become infected. Consider rabies exposure.
Abbreviations: AM/CL, amoxicillin + clavulanate; AN/SB, ampicillin + sulbactam; HSV, herpes simplex virus; IMP, imipenem + cilastatin; PIP/TZ, piperacillin + tazobactam; TMP/SMX, trimethoprim + sulfamethoxazole.

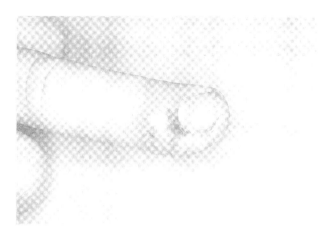

FIGURE 84.1. An advanced paronychia with purulence requiring drainage to avoid expansion beneath the fingernail plate. (Courtesy of Robert W. Beasley, MD.)

Felon

A felon is an abscess of the distal pulp of the thumb or finger (Fig. 84.3). Because of the unique anatomy of the pulp, with 15 to 20 longitudinal septa anchoring the skin to the distal phalanx, the pulp is divided into multiple small closed compartments. Abscess formation within these small closed compartments results in rapid development of swelling and throbbing pain. The pain is usually worsened by dependency, and may keep the patient from sleeping at night. Delayed presentation or inadequate treatment may lead to necrosis of the entire pulp, or extension of the infection into the flexor tendon sheath, distal interphalangeal joint, or the distal phalanx.

Felons typically present after a history of a puncture wound, thus radiographs should be examined carefully for evidence of retained foreign body. Tetanus status must be assured. The most common pathogen involved is *S. aureus*, but gram-negative infections also occur, particularly in the immunocompromised patient (4). Early felons may resolve with oral antibiotics, warm soaks, rest, and elevation; however, any sign of fluctuance requires surgical drainage.

A variety of incisions have been described for the drainage of felons. The chosen incision should adhere to the following basic principles: (a) Avoid iatrogenic injury to neurovascular structures, (b) leave an acceptable scar, (c) avoid the flexor tendon sheath, and (d) drain all fluid collections adequately. If the abscess is pointing, the preferred approach is a longitudinal volar incision through the tip of the abscess. If no draining sinus tract or pointing is apparent, the incision is made through the point of maximum tenderness or fluctuation. Alternatively, a longitudinal incision is made just dorsal to the midlateral line, and may be extended around the tip of the finger in a "hockey stick" fashion for extensive felons (Fig. 84.4). Particular care is made to stay dorsal to the neurovascular bundle. All incisions are kept distal to the distal interphalangeal (DIP) flexion crease.

The abscess cavity is packed loosely with gauze, which is removed after 48 hours and sink hydrotherapy begun. Splinting and elevation are valuable adjuncts.

Herpetic Whitlow

Herpes simplex virus infection of the hand may occur as a primary or recurrent infection and is known as herpetic whitlow (Fig. 84.5). This process tends to occur in children, adolescents with genital herpes infections, and health care workers with frequent exposure to oral secretions (e.g., dentists, surgeons, anesthesiologists, and nurses) (5). Herpetic whitlow is easily mistaken for a bacterial paronychia or felon. The correct diagnosis is critical, because incision and drainage of herpetic whitlow is generally contraindicated (5).

The distinction is made primarily from the history. Herpetic whitlow usually presents with a prodromal phase of 24 to 72 hours of burning pain *prior* to the development of skin changes. This is followed by erythema and swelling, then the formation of clear vesicles. The vesicles may coalesce, often around the nail fold. The fluid within may become turbid, but not frankly purulent without bacterial superinfection. The pulp of the affected digit is not tense as in a felon.

This process occurs over approximately 2 weeks and then resolves over the next 7 to 10 days. The diagnosis may be confirmed by viral culture or Tzanck smear, which is quick and relatively inexpensive, albeit less sensitive than viral culture. Treatment is conservative and includes rest, elevation, and anti-inflammatory agents. Recurrence affects approximately 20% of patients, but is typically less severe than the primary attack. Acyclovir may be used in severe cases, or in the immunocompromised patient at risk for a life-threatening viremia.

All physicians who treat hand infections should keep herpetic whitlow in the differential diagnosis when evaluating a painful digit with skin changes as described above. **Incision and drainage of a whitlow will invariably lead to a worse outcome than conservative management.** Drainage should be limited to those cases with secondary bacterial infection and well-defined fluctuant fluid collections (6).

Palmar Space Infections

The hand contains several potential spaces that become clinically relevant when they become infected and harbor localized collections of pus. These include the thenar space, the midpalmar or subtendinous space, the hypothenar space, the dorsal subaponeurotic space, and the web spaces. Of these, the thenar and midpalmar spaces are clinically the most important.

A penetrating injury such as a splinter is often the inciting event in a palmar space infection, and *S. aureus* is the most common pathogen. Antibiotics, rest, heat, and elevation may prove adequate for early, limited cases, but the majority will present with substantial infections that require operative drainage. The key to success in treatment is adequate drainage while avoiding iatrogenic injury to important neurovascular structures. Incisions must be chosen to avoid subsequent scar contractures.

Several approaches have been described for the various spaces. For infections in the midpalmar space, we prefer a gently curved longitudinal incision in the palm (Fig. 84.6A). Care is taken to avoid injury to the superficial palmar arch and digital vessels once the dissection proceeds deep to the palmar fascia. The wound is packed open and daily dressing changes started on postoperation day one. Alternatively, the wound can be closed loosely over an irrigation catheter in the proximal wound and a small Penrose drain in the distal wound. For thenar space infections, we prefer combined dorsal and volar incisions. A slightly curved longitudinal incision is made in the dorsum of the first web space (Fig. 84.6B). Dissection between the first dorsal interosseous muscle and adductor pollicis usually reveals a collection of pus. A separate incision is made on the thenar eminence, parallel to the thenar crease. Great care is taken to avoid injuring the palmar cutaneous branch of the median nerve in the proximal subcutaneous portion of the incision, and the motor branch of the median nerve, which is located at the point where a flexed middle finger touches the palm. Postoperative care includes splinting and dressing changes or catheter irrigation as above.

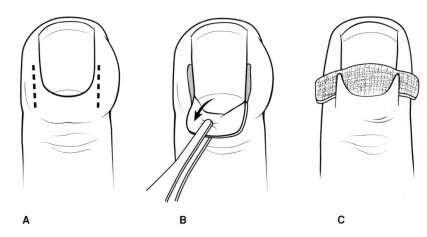

A   **B**   **C**

FIGURE 84.2. **A** to **C:** Incisions and procedure for elevating the eponychial fold with excision of the proximal third of the nail. A gauze pack prevents premature early closure of the cavity.

When draining any closed space infection, the hand surgeon should be aware of the possibility of a *collar button* abscess, also known as a collar stud abscess. This occurs when an abscess spreads between distinct tissue layers through a small sinus tract, leading to an hourglass configuration. A high index of suspicion and thorough exploration will avoid the mistake of draining the superficial component only, leaving the bulk of the process surgically untreated.

Pyogenic (Suppurative) Flexor Tenosynovitis

Although flexor tenosynovitis is not the life-threatening condition it was it the preantibiotic era, this purulent infection of the tendon sheath is still among the most serious hand infections encountered. **Left untreated, this infection can lead to destruction of the gliding surfaces in the sheath, necrosis of tendons, osteomyelitis, and even amputation.** The ring, middle, and index fingers are most commonly affected, and *S. aureus* is the most common isolate. Although a history of penetrating injury is typical, a few cases are a result of hematogenous spread, usually caused by gonococcus.

Kanavel described the four cardinal signs of flexor tenosynovitis that bear his name: *(a) fusiform swelling of the finger, (b) partially flexed posture of the digit, (c) tenderness over the entire flexor tendon sheath, and (d) disproportionate pain on passive extension* (8). The latter sign is the most constant and typically the first present in early cases.

Early cases of flexor tenosynovitis (i.e., less than 48 hours into the process) may respond to conservative management, in-

cluding intravenous antibiotics, rest, heat, and elevation. Failure to respond within 24 to 48 hours warrants immediate operative intervention. In our experience, the overwhelming majority of cases present as advanced processes, when surgical management is mandatory.

Less severe cases of flexor tenosynovitis may be treated with a limited incision and catheter irrigation technique. A transverse or oblique incision is made just distal to the distal flexion crease. A similar incision is made in the palm over the proximal edge of the A-1 pulley (Fig. 84.7). The sheath is copiously irrigated with sterile normal saline and an irrigation catheter

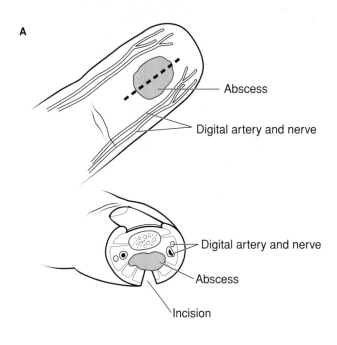

A

Abscess

Digital artery and nerve

Digital artery and nerve

Abscess

Incision

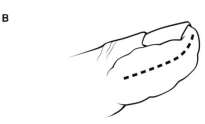

B

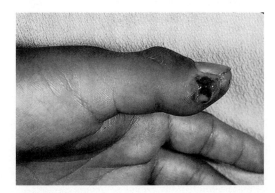

FIGURE 84.3. A felon that was neglected and drained spontaneously. (Reproduced from Doyle JR. *Orthopaedic Surgery Essentials: Hand and Wrist*. Philadelphia: Lippincott Williams & Wilkins; 2006:8 with permission.)

FIGURE 84.4. Drainage of a felon. **A:** Longitudinal incision is made over the point of maximum fluctuance. **B:** Hockey stick or J incision should be reserved for severe abscess.

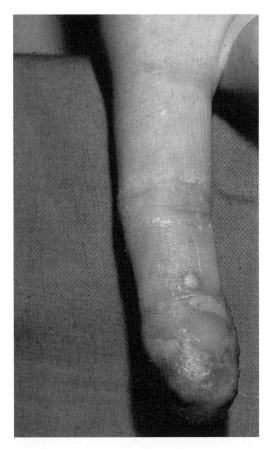

FIGURE 84.5. Herpetic whitlow of the index finger. (Image provided by Stedman's.)

sutured in place proximally with a small Penrose drain sutured distally to allow outflow. The extremity is splinted and irrigation can be performed in a continuous or intermittent manner. Inpatient treatment and intravenous antibiotics are standard of care. For severe cases, the previously described incisions are extended in a Bruner-type, zigzag fashion over the entire course of the flexor sheath. The wound is packed open, and is loosely approximated when the infection has subsided. Early and aggressive hand therapy is indicated for all cases.

Bite Wounds

Human Bites

Human bite wounds to the hand are potentially serious injuries because of the virulence of the organisms comprising the human oral flora. The most common mechanism is striking a tooth with a clenched fist, hence the nickname "fight bite." The patient may present in a delayed fashion or withhold details of the altercation, thus a high index of suspicion should be maintained for what may be a very unimpressive external wound. The wound is most commonly over the metacarpophalangeal joints, putting the extensor mechanism and joint surfaces at risk of injury. The relationship of the various tissue layers varies from flexion to extension, thus the hand must be examined with the fingers fully flexed, reproducing the position at the point of impact (Fig. 84.8). Radiographs are mandatory, and may reveal a tooth fragment, fracture of the metacarpal head, or air in the joint.

All human bites to this region should be explored (9). The joint space should be irrigated and wound edges debrided. Human bite wounds should not be closed primarily, but in selected cases, large wounds may undergo secondary closure after 7 to 10 days of dressing changes and antibiotics. The extremity is elevated, splinted in a position of function, and hand therapy initiated within 48 to 72 hours. Although *S. aureus* and *Streptococcus viridans* are the most common pathogens, antibiotic coverage must include anaerobes commonly found in human saliva, including *Bacteroides* sp. and *Eikenella corrodens*.

Animal Bites

Domestic dogs are responsible for the vast majority of animal bites (10). Although these wounds tend to become infected less often than human or cat bites, the powerful jaws of a dog can inflict substantial crush injuries in addition to puncture wounds and lacerations. Cat bites are usually small puncture wounds because cat teeth are long and sharp. The tetanus status of the patient must be assured and the possibility of rabies explored and treated appropriately.

All animal bites should be thoroughly irrigated and joints explored when potentially violated or as indicated by radiographs. The majority of acute dog bite wounds may be loosely approximated after debriding the edges sharply. Cat bites rarely require closing, but may be if needed. Substantial bite injuries may benefit from splinting, elevation, and hand therapy. Cat bites have a tendency to close quickly, trapping bacteria and subsequently producing the late sequelae of a closed space abscess.

Antibiotic coverage for animal bites should cover the mixed flora found in animal saliva. This includes the gram-positive *Staphylococcus* and *Streptococcus* spp., anaerobes such as *Bacteroides* sp., and *Pasteurella multocida*, a small, gram-negative coccus.

Cat bites may also cause cat-scratch fever. The patient presents with a small pustule with surrounding edema at the site of a cat bite and painful lymphadenopathy. Treatment is symptomatic, with anti-inflammatory agents for pain, and antibiotics for the primary infection when present. The pain usually resolves within 2 weeks, although the lymphadenopathy may last 6 weeks or, occasionally, years.

Septic Arthritis

Infection of a joint space in the hand can lead to rapid destruction of the articular surfaces with devastating consequences for the function of the digit. The articular cartilage is avascular, thus particularly prone to such damage. Joint infections most commonly occur as the result of penetrating trauma, but may also be caused by local extension of an adjacent infection, such as flexor tenosynovitis. Septic arthritis may also occur from hematogenous seeding. In children, an infected joint should prompt a search for infection elsewhere, with *Streptococcus* sp., *Staphylococcus* sp., and *Haemophilus influenzae* the most important pathogens to cover. In adults with no history of trauma, gonococcus must be suspected.

The septic joint will present swollen, warm, and tender, with marked pain on passive motion. The patient will tend to hold the joint in the position that maximizes joint space volume; that is, full extension in the metacarpophalangeal joints and 30 degrees flexion in the interphalangeal joints. The joint may be aspirated to confirm the diagnosis.

All septic joints must be explored. The joint space is copiously irrigated and debrided. The joint may be packed open, and dressing changes performed until the wound closes by secondary intention. Alternatively, the joint is closed over an

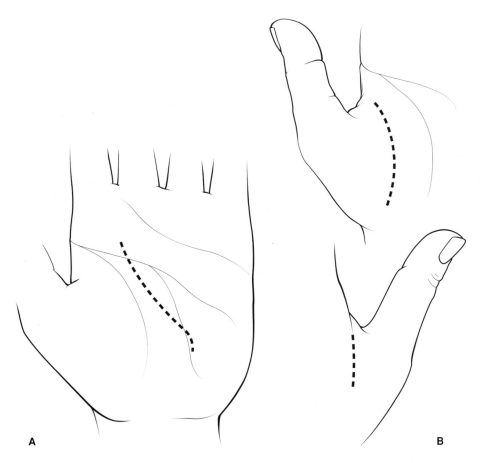

A

B

FIGURE 84.6. Drainage incisions. **A:** Gently curved longitudinal approach to the midpalmar space. **B:** Combined volar and dorsal approach for a thenar space abscess. Volar incision parallels the thenar crease. Care is taken to protect the motor branch of the median nerve.

irrigation catheter and drain, and irrigated for 48 to 72 hours. Intravenous antibiotics are indicated, as well as splinting and elevation. Hand therapy is started after the catheter and drain are removed.

Necrotizing Fasciitis

Necrotizing fasciitis is a life-threatening, rapidly progressive infection of the subcutaneous tissue and fascia. It occurs most commonly in diabetic patients, intravenous drug abusers, and other immunocompromised populations (11). Patients may present initially with a low-grade cellulitis, but cyanotic or bullous changes in the skin soon follow in a typically toxic-appearing patient. An area of cutaneous anesthesia often follows the spread of underlying subcutaneous infection. Fat necrosis is followed by vascular thrombosis, then myonecrosis of associated muscle. Cutaneous vessels are often the last structures affected, thus the appearance of the overlying skin may be misleadingly benign.

Classically, these infections were thought to be caused by *Streptococcus* sp. The majority of these cases are now known to be due to mixed infections of aerobes and anaerobes. The process also can be caused by *Clostridium* sp., with characteristic gas formation in the tissues, demonstrated by crepitus on physical examination and air in the tissues on radiographs.

Necrotizing fasciitis requires aggressive, radical debridement of all nonviable tissue back to bleeding wound margins. Secondary reconstruction of defects is commonly required after the infection is controlled. Patients will often need daily return to the operating room for repeated debridement until the process is under control, and amputation above the area of involvement may be necessary to save a patient's life. The

wounds must be left open between debridements. Silvadene creme is excellent for local antibiotic effect and to keep exposed tendons from desiccating.

High doses of systemic intravenous antibiotics are clearly indicated for necrotizing fasciitis, but it cannot be overemphasized that surgical treatment is the key to saving function in the affected limb and, ultimately, the patient's life. Hyperbaric oxygen therapy should be considered as an adjunct if available.

CHRONIC INFECTIONS

Chronic Paronychia

A paronychia may present as a chronic process, with an indurated, erythematous eponychium and occasional drainage from the nail fold. This occurs more frequently in diabetic patients and in those with frequent occupational exposure to a moist environment, such as food service handlers with frequent immersion of the hands in water. *Candida albicans* is the most common pathogen responsible (12).

These infections can be difficult to treat. Medical management begins with application of topical antifungal and steroid preparations. Removal of a thickened, deformed nail plate may improve results. Should these efforts fail, eponychial marsupialization can be performed. A crescent-shaped portion of skin overlying the proximal nail bed is excised beginning 1 mm proximal to the distal edge of the nail fold and extending proximally for 5 mm. All granulation tissue is removed down to the germinal matrix, which is left undisturbed. Daily dressing changes are performed until the wound closes by secondary intention.

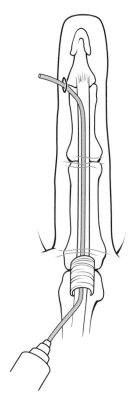

ceptible. *Staphylococcus* is the most common pathogen, but many isolates have been reported, including *Haemophilus* sp. in young children.

Patients may present with a chronically draining wound, and a prior history of trauma is usually elicited. Most will display erythema, pain, and swelling along the course of a bone in the hand. Radiographs may be difficult to differentiate from demineralization that can occur in wound infections without bone invasion. Bone scan, computed tomography (CT), or magnetic resonance imaging (MRI) can support the diagnosis when in question, but bone biopsy and culture are the gold standard for confirming the diagnosis. Superficial swabbing is an inadequate culture technique.

Treatment of osteomyelitis often requires long-term antibiotic therapy. Most authors recommend continuing antibiotics for as long as symptoms persist, with 4 to 6 weeks of therapy as a minimum. Some cases may require treatment for as long as 6 months. Antibiotic coverage should be broad at first, then narrowed, based on bone culture sensitivities. Necrotic bone should be curetted back to bleeding, viable bone stock when performing the biopsy. Even with aggressive surgical treatment and appropriate antibiotic therapy, amputation rates as high as 39% have been reported. Amputation may be the preferred treatment in severe cases so as to avoid subsequent stiffness and disuse in the adjacent digits of the involved hand.

FIGURE 84.7. Catheter irrigation of flexor tenosynnitis. The catheter is inserted proximally and a small Penrose drain inserted distally.

Osteomyelitis

Osteomyelitis is a destructive infection of bone. It develops as the result of direct extension of an adjacent wound infection, septic arthritis, flexor tenosynovitis, or after open fracture, although hematogenous seeding can occur. Bone that has been rendered avascular as a consequence of trauma is most sus-

Onychomycosis

Although typically seen by dermatologists or primary care physicians, patients with onychomycosis, also known as tinea unguium, may occasionally present to a hand surgeon. Infected nails will appear thickened and discolored, and may eventually separate from the nail bed. The nail may appear flaky, or crumble into a powdery substance.

Trichophyton rubrum is the most common cause of onychomycosis in the United States. The infection either invades the distal edge of the nail plate and extends proximally under the nail plate, or begins at the eponychial fold and extends distally. *Candida albicans* may infect the nails as well, particularly in diabetics. Onychomycosis caused by *Candida* involves the entire thickness of the nail plate.

It is important to obtain fungal cultures prior to initiating antifungal therapy. The onychomycosis caused by *T. rubrum* and *C. albicans* may be impossible to differentiate clinically, and the antifungal agents used for each organism are different. *T. rubrum* responds best to oral terbinafine, whereas *C. albicans* can be treated with topical nystatin, miconazole, or econazole, or oral ketoconazole, itraconazole, or griseofulvin.

Removal of the nail plate may improve response for extensively involved nails. The nail plate can be separated from the nail bed by inserting a fine hemostat under the nail plate and gently spreading, then pulling firmly to detach the nail. Alternatively, a Freer elevator can be used to elevate the nail plate, paying particular care to angle away from the nail bed. This is easily tolerated with digital block anesthesia. Oral or topical antifungal therapy is then initiated, and a new nail should grow within 3 to 6 months. Limited resection of the involved portion of a nail reduces the duration of oral antifungal therapy by 50%.

Viral Infections

Warts are infections of the epidermis caused by the human papillomaviruses (HPVs). Two types of warts are commonly seen in the hand. Common warts (verruca vulgaris) represent 95% of hand warts and have the characteristic raised appearance.

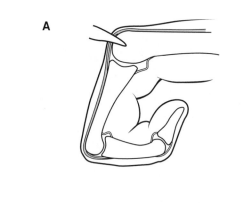

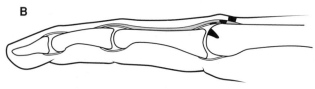

FIGURE 84.8. Human bite injury. **A:** When a tooth pierces the clenched fist of an attacker, it penetrates the skin, tendon, joint capsule, and the metacarpal head. **B:** When the finger is extended by swelling and at surgery, the four puncture wounds do not correspond.

The surface of the wart is rough, with a cauliflowerlike appearance. Flat warts, also known as plane warts (verruca plana), appear as minimally elevated lesions with smooth surfaces. Flat warts account for the remaining 5% of warts, but are much more common on the sole of the foot.

Although the diagnosis of warts is often straightforward, the treatment may be challenging. Half of warts occurring in children will resolve spontaneously within 1 year, and 90% will resolve within 5 years. Thus relatively conservative management is recommended in children. Adults are more likely to require more aggressive treatment. In immunocompromised adults, warts are more difficult to treat than in normal adults, and carry a small risk of transformation into squamous cell carcinoma, particularly flat warts.

The most common treatment options for warts include keratolytic therapy, cryotherapy, and surgical excision. Laser ablation, electrocautery, and intralesional injection with bleomycin or 5-fluorouracil have also been described.

Keratolytic therapy is well tolerated by patients and success rates of 70% have been reported. However, patients must be willing to continue treatment for several days to several weeks. The wart is painted with a salicylic acid preparation daily and allowed to slough off. Alternatively, the wart is covered with a small piece of 40% salicylic acid tape (Mediplast), which can be wrapped in waterproof tape such as Coban. This is repeated every 24 to 48 hours.

Cryotherapy can be used for warts refractory to more conservative management, or when the patient is unwilling to comply with a protracted course of treatment. Liquid nitrogen is typically used without local anesthesia. The burning pain produced is usually well tolerated by adults, but not children.

Warts may be treated surgically when other options have failed or been refused by the patient. The lesion can be curetted and a salicylic acid agent applied to the margins. Warts can also be excised, but care must be taken to ensure an adequate margin to prevent recurrences. A minimum of a 1-mm margin is suggested.

Mycobacterial Infections

Although relatively uncommon, mycobacterial infections are in the differential diagnosis of chronic nodular skin lesions, draining sinus tracts, tenosynovitis, or septic arthritis refractory to treatment. Mycobacteria are notoriously difficult to culture, and infectious disease consultation is recommended when treating patients with suspected tuberculous infections. Although at least 10 different mycobacteria have been implicated in hand infections, the majority of cases are caused by *Mycobacterium tuberculosis*, *M. marinum*, *M. kansasii*, and *M. terrae*. *M. leprae*, the causative agent in Hansen disease, is considered separately. When the diagnosis is in doubt, a tissue biopsy is obtained in addition to a representative culture from the lesion.

Typical (Tuberculous) Mycobacterial Infections

Typical mycobacterial infections include those caused by *M. tuberculosis* and *M. bovis*, the former being the most common. These infections have decreased in frequency, paralleling the decline in pulmonary tuberculosis. While tuberculosis has a predilection for synovium, it can produce skin lesions, osteomyelitis, or arthritis. Coexisting pulmonary and extrapulmonary tuberculosis is uncommon, thus chest radiographs will usually be normal. A purified protein derivative (PPD) skin test will usually be positive. The mainstay of treatment is multidrug therapy with antituberculous agents, just as in pulmonary tuberculosis.

Atypical Mycobacterial Infections

Although the number of typical mycobacterial infections of the hand continue to decline, the number of infections caused by atypical mycobacteria increase yearly. The majority of cases are caused by *M. marinum*, *M. kansasii*, and *M. terrae*. Skin tests are usually negative.

M. marinum is found in warm water, both salt and fresh, and has been found in cultures from fish tanks, swimming pools, boats, piers and stagnant water. It is endogenous to fresh and saltwater marine life. *M. marinum* grows best at 87.8°F (31°C), thus it thrives in human extremities. Infection can result from a break in the skin, which can be very superficial, and contact with fish, contaminated water, or other source of the organism. Treatment includes minocycline and trimethoprim-sulfamethoxazole, with drug-resistant strains requiring multidrug therapy similar to pulmonary disease. Surgical debridement may be indicated when sinus tracts leading to bone or joint fail to close.

MIMICS OF INFECTION

Many conditions are known to mimic infections in the hand and upper extremity, and the clinician should be aware of these to avoid misdiagnosis with potentially disastrous results. Thorough discussion of these conditions is beyond the scope of this text, but a general familiarity is important when evaluating an acute lesion of the hand.

Neoplasms may resemble large abscesses at presentation, and can represent metastatic disease such as renal cell carcinoma or melanoma, or primary tumors such as sarcoma. Obviously, a well-planned biopsy is preferable to an incision and drainage in the middle of the night for these cases. Inflammatory processes, including gout, pseudogout, rheumatic and psoriatic arthritis, and erosive osteoarthritis can all mimic septic arthritis or tenosynovitis. Dactylitis associated with sickle cell disease can resemble osteomyelitis. Spider bites, foreign-body reactions, and injection injuries can mimic cellulitis and closed-space infections. **The lesion most commonly misdiagnosed as an infection is pyoderma gangrenosum, an inflammatory process of unknown etiology that can be associated with systemic diseases such as Crohn disease and ulcerative colitis.**

Consideration of these conditions when assessing an acute inflammatory complaint in the upper extremity may help avoid misdiagnosis. When in doubt, keep in mind the adage to "biopsy what you culture, and culture what you biopsy."

References

1. Neviaser RJ. Acute infections. In: Green D, ed. *Operative Hand Surgery*. Philadelphia: Churchill Livingstone; 1999: 1034.
2. Brook I. Paronychia: A mixed infection. Microbiology and management. *J Hand Surg [Br]*. 1993;18:358.
3. Zook EG. Discussion of "fungal infections of the perionychium." *Hand Clin*. 2002;18:643–646.
4. Perry AW, et al. Fingerstick felons. *Ann Plast Surg*. 1988;20:249.
5. Louis DS, Silva J Jr. Herpetic whitlow: Herpetic infections of the digits. *J Hand Surg*. 1979;4:90–94.
6. Hurst LC, et al. Herpetic whitlow with bacterial abscess. *J Hand Surg*. 1991;16A:311–313.
7. Neviaser RJ. Tenosynovitis. *Hand Clin*. 1989;5:525.
8. Kanavel AB. *Infections of the Hand*. 7th ed. Philadelphia: Lea & Febiger; 1939.
9. Basadre JO, Parry SW. Indications for surgical debridement in 125 human bites to the hand. *Arch Surg*. 1991;126:65.
10. Snyder CC. Animal bite wounds. *Hand Clin*. 1989;5:571.
11. Gonzalez MH. Necrotizing fasciitis and gangrene of the upper extremity. *Hand Clin*. 1998;14:635–645.
12. Canales FL, et al. The treatment of felons and paronychias. *Hand Clin*. 1989;5:515–523.

CHAPTER 85 ■ TENOSYNOVITIS

HOOMAN SOLTANIAN

Tendonitis is an inflammatory process involving a tendon and can happen to any tendon. *Tenosynovitis* is the inflammation of a tendon and its synovial lining. This chapter discusses the tendons commonly involved in the hand and forearm.

The requirement for both stability and precise movements in the hand demands the exact positioning of the force vectors exerted by the tendons with minimal friction during excursion. Fibrous structures, tendon sheaths, and fibro-osseous channels, such as annular and cruciform pulleys, maintain the proper direction of tendon pull. The synovial lining of tendons and their guiding structures minimize the friction. Injury, scarring, or inflammation will increase friction, impair movement, and cause pain. The symptoms of tenosynovitis worsen with swelling, quite often upon awakening from sleep, since a long period of muscle inactivity increases edema. The size discrepancy between the tendon and its sheath causes increased friction, which, in turn, leads to more inflammation and clinical symptoms. Untreated, the pathophysiologic changes can enter a *vicious cycle* (Fig. 85.1).

A subgroup of patients has the tendency to suffer from multiple areas of inflammation and tenosynovitis (mesenchymal syndrome) (1). Recently, many of these patients are erroneously brand marked as "suffering from cumulative trauma disorder." There is no sound scientific proof indicating that repetitive motion alone causes tissue damage or inflammation.

GENERAL PRINCIPLES OF TREATMENT

The treatment for the first occurrence of tenosynovitis is commonly conservative. The most effective treatment is local steroid injection into the involved sheath (triamcinolone 3 to 4 mg). This has the advantage of almost no systemic and minimal local side effects. If severe mechanical locking is present, steroid injection has minimal benefit. Generally, it is recommended not to administer more than two injections into the same area. If the first injection fails to resolve the symptoms, there is no indication for a second injection shortly thereafter. This patient should be considered for surgical release. One should avoid high doses of steroids because of the possibility of soft-tissue atrophy and skin pigment disturbance.

Nonsteroidal anti-inflammatory agents are indicated for temporary treatment of the pain and cases of systemic disorders, such as rheumatoid arthritis, underlying the occurrence of tenosynovitis.

Splinting is usually unnecessary unless it is needed for short-term pain management. Heavy loading of the affected tendon(s) should be avoided until the signs and symptoms of inflammation have subsided.

TENDON SHEATH INJECTION TECHNIQUE

The area of inflammation is identified by careful examination. Using a small amount of local anesthetic intradermally allows for more accurate and less painful placement of the needle. The needle is inserted without the syringe attached through the tendon sheath. Needle placement is confirmed by gentle movement of the tendon in question. At this point, the syringe containing the steroid and a small amount of local anesthetic is attached. If during the injection high resistance is encountered, the needle is advanced slowly toward the floor of the sheath until the resistance decreases.

Immediate improvement of the pain because of the local anesthetic effect confirms both the diagnosis and correct location of the injection. The patient should be advised that there may be a temporary worsening of the pain secondary to the increased volume within the sheath and that the patient's symptoms will not start to improve until the third or fourth day after injection.

DIGITAL FLEXOR TENOSYNOVITIS ("TRIGGER FINGER")

Two flexor tendons enter the corresponding fibro-osseous tunnel at the level of the distal palmar crease (Fig. 85.2). That is the area of tenderness in stenosing flexor tenosynovitis. Often a painful nodule is palpable over the tendon and moves with the tendon excursion. This is the thickened and inflamed region of the tendon, which can be large enough to cause locking of the finger. While the finger is completely extended, the thickened area is within the flexor sheath. With flexion the tendon moves proximally and the nodule exits the fibro-osseous tunnel. The digit can be locked in this position if the nodule is large enough to stop the distal movement of the tendon. During the early phase, increasing tension of the extensors may be able to overcome the blockage at the level of the first annular pulley, and the nodule enters the sheath with an abrupt motion, which causes the "triggering." This process is usually painful.

In mild cases with no significant mechanical blockage, conservative treatment is indicated. Refractory cases require surgical intervention with release of the A-1 pulley (Fig. 85.2), which is best done through a longitudinal incision under local anesthesia and pneumatic cuff. The incision is made directly over the affected tendon. Minimal dissection is required to expose the tendon sheath. The neurovascular bundles on either side of the tendon are protected with gentle retraction. The A-1 pulley is incised from proximal to distal to create a funnel-shaped entry to the flexor sheath. Attention should be paid to the A-2 pulley, which has to be preserved at all costs if one wants to avoid postoperative bowstringing of the tendon and an intrinsic plus

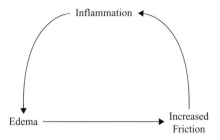

FIGURE 85.1. Vicious cycle of edema and inflammation.

digit. The complete release is confirmed by asking the patient to flex the digit and monitoring the excursion of the tendon. Multiple digits are addressed through separate incisions at the base of each finger. A transverse incision has a higher potential for complications (bleeding, nerve injury, etc.).

In the case of flexor tenosynovitis of the index finger the incision in the A-1 pulley should be made on the radial side of the structure to avoid medial displacement of the tendon with undue ulnar pull on the finger. The patient should keep the hand elevated for the first 24 hours after the operation. After that, gentle range of motion of the finger is encouraged.

Flexor pollicis longus (FPL) presents a special anatomic challenge with the radial digital nerve crossing the tendon on its way to the carpal tunnel proximal to the A-1 pulley. The procedure is performed through a transverse incision at the volar metacarpophalangeal flexion crease. The neurovascular bundle can be very superficial and special attention should be given to its protection. The A-1 pulley should be transected under direct visualization. The surgeon should refrain from blind advancement of the scissors in a proximal direction to avoid injuring the radial digital nerve.

CONGENITAL TRIGGER THUMB

The congenital trigger thumb involves the FPL tendon at birth. The diagnosis is usually missed at birth because of the normal clenched fist posture of the newborn. It is usually diagnosed by the age of 6 months. Differential diagnosis includes congenital clasped thumb, abnormal extensor tendons, and spasticity. There is a pathologic thickening of the tendon at the metacarpophalangeal (MCP) flexion crease (Notta's node). The deformity can be monitored untreated up to age 6 months because (a) some cases spontaneously resolve, (b) the risk of anesthesia is much higher before 1 year of age than after, and (c) the risk of a permanent deformity during this period is minimal. There is significant incidence of bilateral involvement (25% to 33%) (2,3).

The tendon is released through a transverse incision at the MCP crease. Both neurovascular bundles are identified and protected. The pulley is then released and the tendon is retracted to assure unrestricted excursion. No attempt is made to decrease the size of the tendon. The skin is closed with absorbable intradermal sutures. In bilateral cases, both FPL tendons are released at the same time.

FIRST EXTENSOR COMPARTMENT TENOSYNOVITIS (DE QUERVAIN TENOSYNOVITIS)

The first extensor compartment contains the abductor pollicis longus (APL) and extensor pollicis brevis (EPB) tendons (Fig.

85.3). There is high degree of anatomic variation in the position and number of APL tendons. It is not uncommon to find separation of the EPB and APL tendons by a septum, which may explain the lack of improvement with steroid injection into one of the subcompartments. For the same reason, during the surgical treatment the surgeon has to confirm complete release of the involved tendons.

Patients with de Quervain tenosynovitis present with pain on the radial side of the wrist just proximal to the radial styloid. Complete adduction of the thumb, ulnar deviation of the wrist, and MCP flexion of the thumb increase the tension on the tendons of the first extensor compartment and evoke a sharp pain in that area (Finkelstein test). If this maneuver is performed in steps (ulnar deviation of the wrist and passive adduction of the carpometacarpal [CMC] joint followed by passive flexion of the MCP joint), it is possible to determine whether the APL or the EPB tendon is involved. If the adduction causes pain, it is likely that the APL is the source of the symptoms; if the flexion of the MCP joint provokes the pain, it is likely that the EPB is the culprit.

The first treatment step is steroid injection. Surgical release of the first compartment is reserved for refractory cases. During the surgery one has to be cognizant of the branches of the radial sensory nerve. Damage to these branches can cause painful neuromas and dysesthesia of the dorsum of the hand. A transverse incision is made over the first dorsal compartment. The subcutaneous tissue is dissected in blunt fashion parallel to the radial nerve branches. The fibrous retinaculum is incised on its dorsal extent to preserve a volar edge. This decreases the likelihood of painful volar subluxation of the APL tendon postoperatively. The APL tendon is inspected in its entirety and retracted to expose the EPB tendon, which is released as well.

INTERSECTION SYNDROME

Tenosynovitis of the extensor carpi radialis brevis (ECRB) and extensor carpi radialis longus (ECRL) within the second extensor compartment causes pain and swelling on the dorsal forearm proximal to the wrist. This is the area where the APL and EPB muscles cross over the ECRB and ECRL tendons. Strenuous activities requiring wrist extension, such as weight lifting and rowing, can aggravate the symptoms. Conservative therapy includes steroid injection into the point of maximum tenderness (second compartment) and modification of activities with occasional short-term splinting of the wrist in mild extension.

Decompression of the second dorsal compartment is the surgical treatment. Postoperative splinting of the wrist in moderate extension for up to 2 weeks decreases the potential for extensor bowstringing.

EXTENSOR POLLICIS LONGUS TENDONITIS

The EPL tendon crosses through the third extensor compartment. Its muscle belly is parallel to the common digital extensors of the fourth compartment, but the tendon curves in the radial direction around the Lister tubercle to run parallel to the first metacarpal bone. This is an area of increased friction and a common location for EPL tendonitis.

The exact placement of small amount of local anesthetic will help with establishing the diagnosis. If the process fails to respond to steroid injection into the third dorsal compartment, the EPL tendon is transposed subcutaneously radial to the Lister tubercle. The third compartment is closed to avoid relocation of the tendon. Small branches of superficial radial nerve should be protected during the operation.

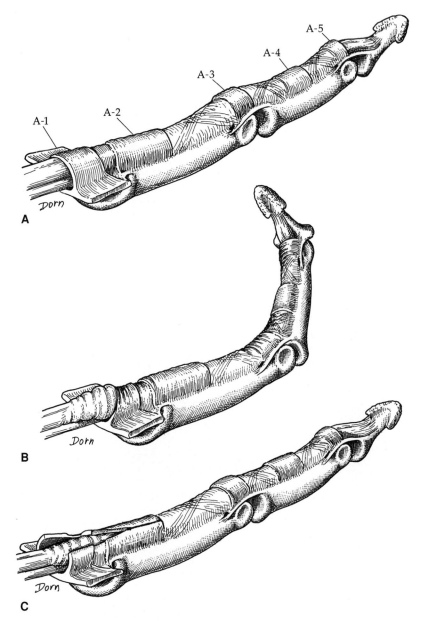

A-1 A-2 A-3 A-4 A-5

Dorn

A

Dorn

B

Dorn

C

FIGURE 85.2. The anatomic relationship between the flexor tendons and the pulley system in the digits. **A:** During extension the affected portion of the tendon is within the sheath. **B:** With flexion, the thickened area of the flexor tendon moves proximally out the sheath. **C:** After longitudinal split of the A-1 pulley, the entrance into the sheath is converted into a funnel configuration. The enlarged tendon can easily move distally. From Beasley RW. *Beasley's Surgery of the Hand.* New York: Thieme; 2003, with permission.

EXTENSOR CARPI ULNARIS TENOSYNOVITIS

Extensor carpi ulnaris (ECU) tendonitis is not uncommon. It should be considered in cases of ulnar sided wrist pain. Because triangular fibrocartilage complex (TFCC) is closely related to the floor of the ECU tendon sheath, it is sometimes very difficult to differentiate between ECU tendonitis and TFCC injury. Complete relief of the pain by injecting a small amount of local anesthetic into the sixth dorsal compartment confirms the diagnosis. Most cases improve with local steroid injections.

The surgical treatment should preserve the volar support of the tendon so it would not subluxate around the ulnar head with wrist extension and supination. Because this instability can be very difficult to correct, the first attempt should be a size reduction of the ECU tendon. In persistent cases, the tendon can be rerouted through the fourth extensor compartment (4).

FLEXOR CARPI RADIALIS TENOSYNOVITIS

The flexor carpi radialis (FCR) tendon enters a fibro-osseous canal at the wrist crease, which includes a rather sharp curve over the ridge of the trapezium. Pain in this area can have multiple causes and other diagnoses, such as a ganglion cyst, undetected scaphoid fracture, and basilar joint arthritis, should be entertained. In addition to meticulous examination, injecting a small amount of local anesthetic into the FCR sheath at this level establishes the diagnosis.

If the conservative therapy, including splinting and steroid injection, is ineffective, surgical release of the FCR sheath is indicated. During the release one should be aware of the palmar branch of the median nerve, which runs along the FCR tendon. The area of contact between the tendon and the trapezium should be inspected for signs of degenerative arthritis and bone spur formation, which should be removed.

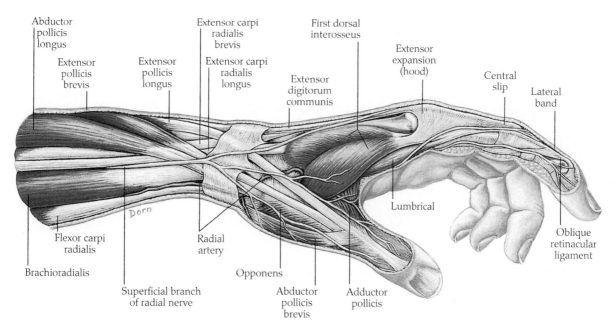

FIGURE 85.3. Lateral extensor compartments. Note the close relationship between the radial nerve branches and the first extensor compartment. From Beasley RW. **Beasley's Surgery of the Hand**. New York: Thieme; 2003, with permission.

LATERAL EPICONDYLITIS ("TENNIS ELBOW")

Lateral epicondylitis is an inflammation of the origin of the ECRB from the humerus. In addition to local tenderness over the lateral epicondyle, the grip strength is usually decreased because of synergistic action of the wrist extensors. The course of the disease can be insidious. Symptoms can be exacerbated by activities requiring power grip and wrist extension. Lateral epicondylitis is not limited to tennis players. Occasional radial nerve compression may coexist, which should be differentiated and treated separately.

Lateral epicondylitis should be treated conservatively at first, including modification of activities, local steroid injection, splinting, and the use of an elastic band at the border of the proximal and middle third of the muscle. The latter would transfer the load to a more distal location of the muscle rather than its origin. Quite often this condition resolves with time (burned out tendonitis). If steroid injections provide significant relief for an extended period of time, they can be repeated without the concern for the ECRB tear. Weakening and tearing of the origin of the ECRB are the goals of the surgical treatment (see below). The likelihood for other side effects of localized steroid injection should be minimal if the medication is injected properly.

Repeated courses of lateral epicondylitis and failed conservative therapy call for surgical intervention. Through a longitudinal incision over the lateral epicondyle the extensor mass is exposed. The ECRL is the superficial muscle that is incised and spread apart to expose the ECRB origin, which can be replaced by granulation tissue as a product of chronic or recurrent inflammation. However, this is not always present. The origin of the ECRB and the periosteum are excised. Any extension of the muscle over to the joint capsule is released as well. The incision in the ECRL is repaired and the skin is closed. The wrist should be splinted in extension for comfort for 2 weeks. After this period, strengthening exercises start.

MEDIAL EPICONDYLITIS ("GOLFER'S ELBOW")

Medial epicondylitis is much less common than lateral epicondylitis. It involves the origin of the pronator-flexor mass from the medial epicondyle. Careful examination will confirm the diagnosis and differentiate it from cubital tunnel syndrome, which occasionally coexists with medial epicondylitis.

The treatment parallels that of lateral epicondylitis. Surgical intervention includes the detachment of the origin of the pronator-flexor mass and excision of the periosteum. The ulnar nerve and its branches should be protected. Submuscular transposition of the nerve is only indicated if signs and symptoms of ulnar nerve compression within the cubital tunnel exist.

References

1. Nirschl RP. Mesenchymal syndrome. *Va Med Mon.* 1969;96:659–662.
2. Fahey JJ, Bollinger JA. Trigger-finger in adults and children. *J Bone Joint Surg Am.* 1954;36-A:1200–1218.
3. Wood VE, Sicilia M. Congenital trigger digit. *Clin Orthop.* 1992;285:205–209.
4. Beasley RW. *Beasley's Surgery of the Hand.* New York: Thieme; 2003.

CHAPTER 86 ■ COMPRESSION NEUROPATHIES IN THE UPPER LIMB AND ELECTROPHYSIOLOGIC STUDIES

CHARLES R. EFFRON AND ROBERT W. BEASLEY

OVERVIEW

A notable increase in the diagnosis of upper limb compression neuropathies has occurred in the past two decades, reflecting (a) more jobs requiring highly repetitive hand tasks, (b) increased awareness of the symptoms in the general population, and (c) financial incentives afforded by governmental and private-sponsored disability plans and by tort (product liability) and workers' compensation litigation.

All the clinician's skills are required to distinguish symptomatic nerve entrapment from other neurologic entities, such as radiculopathy, brachial plexopathy, myelopathy, and other central nervous system disorders, that can mimic peripheral nerve entrapment. Painful rheumatologic and orthopedic disorders may also incorrectly suggest peripheral nerve entrapment. Psychological entities, such as somatoform and factitious disorders, as well as malingering, may be considered as well.

Nontraumatic compression neuropathies in the upper limbs occur at specific locations based on anatomic factors. The most common site of ulnar nerve compression is at the elbow, typically within the ulnar groove or at the cubital tunnel at the free edge of the flexor carpi ulnaris. Much less commonly, the ulnar nerve is entrapped at one of several locations at the wrist. The median nerve is most commonly compressed in the carpal canal of the wrist. Much less frequently, the median nerve may be compressed at the proximal forearm by fibromuscular bands of the flexor digitorum superficialis or pronator teres. An acute compression neuropathy of the radial nerve against the humerus is well recognized. Less often appreciated is subacute or chronic entrapment of the radial nerve in the region of the supinator muscle. The sensory branch of the radial nerve can be compressed by scar tissue secondary to operative procedures at the wrist and distal forearm, and less often by compression at the midforearm by the brachioradialis. There obviously is no focal preponderance for mononeuropathies caused by direct trauma such as a fracture, penetrating wound, or compartment syndrome.

When large, myelinated nerve fibers undergo compression, the response depends on the duration. Acute, brief compression results in a focal conduction block as a result of local ischemia, clinically experienced first as paresthesia and then weakness (e.g., tourniquet injury). This type of injury is reversible if the duration of compression is transient. More prolonged focal compression results in a change in the myelin sheath surrounding the nerve axon. Known as focal demyelination, this process is caused by mechanical compression rather than by ischemia, and typically results in a greater involvement of motor than sensory nerve fibers. Clinical and electrophysiologic signs of focal demyelination usually resolve within a period of weeks to months.

Injury to the axons themselves appears as the duration of compression increases beyond several hours. **The nerve axon begins to degenerate distal to the site of compression or injury, a process termed *wallerian* degeneration.** Recovery requires regrowth of the axon, beginning proximally, which is a slow process. Chronic nerve entrapment causes mixed demyelinating and axonal injury resulting from a combination of mechanical distortion of the nerve, ischemic injury, and impaired axonal flow.

Electrophysiologic testing best exemplifies an extension of, and never a substitute for, a thorough history and physical examination.

Electrophysiologic testing typically comprises two different types of tests, needle electromyelography and nerve conduction. Nerve conduction testing aids in the differentiation of axonal injury and demyelinating injury. The term *electromyelography* is typically, though incorrectly, used in physicians' reports as a synonym for multiple parts of the electrophysiologic assessment. It is more accurate and appropriate to refer to electromyelography and nerve conduction separately as the two tests have different sensitivities and specificities for diagnosing nerve injury.

Electrophysiologic tests are valuable in both localization and characterization of nerve injury. Testing permits differentiating between a focal mononeuropathy, a radiculopathy, and a plexopathy, or the discovery of a more diffuse process, such as a systemic peripheral neuropathy or motor neuron disorder.

Nerve conduction assesses both sensory and motor nerves. A voltage simulator is applied to the skin over different points of the nerve to be tested. The evoked response is recorded from a surface electrode overlying the muscle belly (motor response) or nerve (sensory response). Rarely, a needle is used as the recording electrode. Parameters measured include latency and amplitude, and may also include the duration and area of the sensory or motor action potential. Conduction velocity is calculated across a specific segment.

With a demyelinating lesion, stimulation distal to the focal site of demyelination results in a normal amplitude, distal latency, and duration of the compound muscle action potential (CMAP). Stimulation proximal to the site of demyelination results in a conduction velocity decreased by more than 10 meters per second and an amplitude reduced by more than 20%.

In cases of complete conduction block, a normal response is obtained to distal stimulation but no response is obtained to stimulation proximal to the site of entrapment. Axonal degeneration results in diminished amplitude of the response with relative preservation of the conduction velocity and distal latency until the number of surviving axons has been severely reduced. The amplitude is reduced regardless of whether the nerve is stimulated proximal or distal to the site of nerve entrapment.

The electromyelogram (EMG) assesses only the motor component of the nerve. This test consists of inserting a needle into a muscle and assessing resting electrical activity while acquiring data in real time. The parameters measured include the resting electrical activity (i.e., the presence of abnormal spontaneous activity such as fibrillations and positive sharp waves) and voluntary motor unit analysis to assess duration, amplitude, configuration, and recruitment after the injury.

Demyelination affects recruitment but does not result in abnormal spontaneous activity. Axonal injury results in both abnormal spontaneous activity and diminished recruitment. With reinnervation, there will be a change in the appearance of the voluntary motor units. A caveat is that abnormal spontaneous activity is not seen on needle electromyelography during the first week after an insult and is not reliably seen until 2 weeks after the insult.

SPECIFIC UPPER LIMB COMPRESSION NEUROPATHIES

Median Nerve Compression

Low Median Nerve Compressions

By far the most frequently encountered compression neuropathy in the upper limb is median nerve compression in the carpal tunnel (CT). Carpal tunnel syndrome (CTS) basically is not a neurologic disorder; instead, it is a mechanical compression caused by an idiopathic synovitis of the digital flexor tendons accompanying the nerve through the fixed space of the rigid CT. Compressions can occur in this region as a result of other causes, the most frequent being herniation of a ganglion cyst of the carpus into the tunnel, but those compressions are not CTS.

CTS occurs more frequently among women and typically is first manifested by numbness of the middle finger and the adjacent side of the ring finger upon awakening from sleep, during which there has been no muscular activity to prevent accumulation of fluids in the tissues. At this early stage, it is easily relieved by a few grasping exercises and shaking of the hand. As the duration of CTS increases, one is awakened from sleep by discomfort, numbness extending into the thumb and index finger, and difficulty getting relief from exercises. Eventually the patient develops constant numbness and pain. Pain and tenderness may develop on the anterior wrist at the CT entrance (the Durkin sign) and symptoms often are aggravated by elevation of the hand, as in blow-drying the hair or holding the steering wheel of a car. **Significantly, skin sensibility is not disturbed in the distribution of the palmar cutaneous branch of the median nerve to the base of the palm as this branch of the nerve is subcutaneous and does not pass through the CT.** The Phalen test is not an absolute test but is highly reliable for diagnosis of CTS. The wrist is passively flexed and the time before provoking or aggravating sensory symptoms (particularly the pad of the middle finger) is noted. The shorter that time, the more advanced the disorder. Atrophy of the thenar opponens muscle group is associated only with axonal damage, but even then it is rarely a complaint.

Electrodiagnostic studies (EDSs) are very reliable for evaluation of suspected CTS, but atypical cases exist and thus there are no absolute electrophysiologic norms. In questionable cases, careful clinical evaluations supersede EDSs. Occasionally symptomatic relief from cortisone injected into the CT may help to clarify the situation, but cortisone injection is acceptable treatment only for acute and circumstantial CTS, such as in the terminal weeks of a pregnancy.

The only definitive treatment for CTS is surgical expansion of the CT by transection of the transverse carpal ligament. It is an outpatient procedure performed with a low median nerve block anesthetic. The surgery has minimal risk and is associated with highly predictable recovery, even for advanced cases. However, the time for recovery is not predictable and varies from immediate to several months. The best approach for decompression is a short incision at the base of the palm, parallel to the skin crease of the thenar eminence but ulnar to the course of the palmar branch of the median nerve. This provides direct visualization of the median nerve even if an anomaly is present. Endoscopic decompressions are advocated by some, but are less safe and have no advantage over the described incision. One author (RWB) has seen patients with complications of endoscopic release, including incomplete decompressions, injury, and even complete transaction of the median and ulnar nerves. The two short incisions are collectively as long as the safer longitudinal incision used for direct nerve exposure.

If neurologic recovery does not occur after CT release, incomplete decompression is the most probable cause, although a proximal median nerve compression should be considered. Approximately 68% of patients following CT decompressions have an ill-defined deep aching in the base of the palm. This has been called "pillar pain," but does not explain the pathology. In our experience this is caused by a synovitis of a radiographically normal scaphotrapezial joint and the direct injection of a steroid into that joint consistently gives lasting relief.

Proximal Forearm Median Compression Neuropathies

Proximal forearm median nerve compressions are not as rare as generally believed. **The onset is insidious and is suggested when the early sensory disturbances are greater on the thumb and index finger (in contrast with the middle finger in typical CTS), and include symptoms in the distribution of the palmar cutaneous branch of the median nerve to the base of the palm.** Increased pain in the proximal forearm and greater hand numbness with sustained power gripping, rather than nocturnal distress, is usually the greatest complaint. Gripping tightens the fibrous origin of the finger superficial flexor muscles (flexor digitorum superficialis [FDS]) beneath which the median nerve passes. Pronator teres stress against resistance does not exacerbate symptoms. Tenderness of the median nerve, lying next to the brachial artery and crossed by the FDS origin 4 to 5 cm distal to the elbow skin crease, is typical and is accompanied by a Tinel sign referred into the thumb or index finger. **A positive Phalen test may be found, without other evidence suggesting CTS, because of the "double-crush phenomenon."** Although the anterior interosseous (AI) nerve is part of the median nerve at this level, it is rarely involved. Because of this lack of motor involvement and the great depth of the nerve in the forearm, EDSs are in general of little help with diagnosis except by excluding the diagnosis.

These neuropathies, although inflammatory disorders, rarely resolve with corticosteroid administration. Surgical decompression is the definitive treatment. The incision should be just distal to the elbow, oblique and parallel to the proximal margin of the pronator teres (PT) muscle, which is readily palpated. With retraction, an external neurolysis of the nerve is performed proximally to a point about 2 cm above the elbow. Dissection is extended along the anterior surface of the nerve through the few thin fibers of the PT deep margin crossing the nerve. The nerve is exposed as it passes beneath the fibrous sling of the FDS origin, which is the location of the pathology. If a deep head of the PT is present, it is detached to preclude possible AI nerve symptoms from postoperative inflammation in the area. In more than 90 proximal median nerve compressions with pain and hand sensory disturbances on whom one author (RWB) has operated with consistent relief of symptoms, only two had even a suggestion of pathologic contribution from the PT. Both of these had absent deep heads of the PT, but did have a strong fibrous band along the muscle's deep margin, which may have contributed to nerve compression. **Thus the term "pronator syndrome" appears to be a misnomer and better supplanted with "proximal forearm median nerve compressions."** Immediate and dramatic relief of systems can be expected following decompression.

Anterior Interosseous Neuropathies

Immediately distal to the elbow the AI nerve separates from the deep surface of the median nerve. It passes the two heads of the PT, if both are present, and can have its conducting capacity impaired by kinking if the deep head of the PT is large. The impairment is not by compression as usually expressed. **Unlike the posterior interosseous division of the radial nerve, almost every case of AI neuropathy follows forearm injury, such as a muscle tear from unaccustomed strenuous work or lifting.** As such, there is a rapid onset of symptoms and soreness in the forearm. Because the AI is the motor nerve to the flexor pollicis longus (FPL) and index digitorum profundus muscles, weakness of either or both may be found and documented by EDS. Supportive care and corticosteroid injections with observation for 4 to 6 weeks is usually accepted management, **but the degree of recovery is unpredictable, whether or not definitive surgical treatment (detachment or resection of the deep head of the PT muscle) is performed.** Subsequent tendon transfers to restore function are often required.

Ulnar Nerve Compressions Neuropathies

The ulnar nerve is a continuation of the medial cord of the brachial plexus (C8–T1) and, like the median nerve, is susceptible to compression neuropathies at proximal and distal levels.

Low Ulnar Nerve Compression or Guyon Tunnel Syndrome

At the wrist the ulnar nerve passes with the ulnar artery from the forearm, alongside the pisiform bone, into the hand. This passage is referred to as the Guyon tunnel, and unlike the CT, contains no tendons. **Compression neuropathies in this location are almost unknown unless there has been direct trauma to the area.** Pseudoaneurysms of the ulnar artery may cause ulnar nerve compression in the Guyon tunnel and are characterized by sudden onset of severe pain. Within the tunnel, the motor division of the ulnar nerve begins its separation from the palmar sensory portion, innervates the hypothenar muscles, and passes laterally around the hook of the hamate across the palm for distribution to intrinsic muscles. Measurement of lateral pinch between thumb and side of index finger accurately reflects the strength of the ulnar innervated muscles. **With compression of the ulnar nerve in the Guyon tunnel, sensory disturbances will be to the palmar surfaces of the small and adjacent side of the ring finger, but not to their dorsal surfaces.** Dorsal skin innervation of these fingers is carried by a branch of the ulnar nerve, which separates from the main nerve, 4 to 5 cm proximal to the Guyon tunnel and passes dorsally in the subcutaneous tissues just distal to the styloid process of the ulna. With the large motor component of the ulnar nerve and relatively superficial location, EDSs provide precise measurement signals and are usually diagnostic of this disorder.

Treatment of Guyon tunnel syndrome is surgical decompression with special care to avoid injury to the dorsal division which does not pass through the tunnel. **The safest way to pre-** serve the dorsal division is to identify initially the ulnar artery branches to the ring and small fingers in the proximal palm and to dissect from distal to proximal along them, progressively unroofing and decompressing the Guyon tunnel. Dramatic relief usually follows unless an injury has caused direct nerve damage.

Cubital Tunnel Syndrome

The cubital tunnel is the strong fibrous conduit through which the ulnar nerve (called the cubital nerve in many countries) passes posterior to the elbow. Although true nerve compressions do occur here, nerve adhesions more often are encountered that prevent the nerve's gliding with elbow flexion and thus produces stretch ischemia that impairs nerve conduction. The vast majority of cases occur spontaneously with no documented history of trauma. **Sensory disturbances involve both palmar and dorsal surfaces of the ring and small fingers.** Acute flexion of the elbow for 30 seconds or so usually accentuates the sensory symptoms. As with low ulnar lesions, ulnar innervated intrinsic muscle weakness can readily be measured, and gross atrophy of these muscles is associated with advanced cases. A strong Tinel sign is consistently elicited at the posterior elbow and referred to the small finger. **If there are sensory disturbances of the forearm skin, investigation of the neck or brachial plexus is indicated.** Reliable electrophysiologic indications of ulnar neuropathy at the elbow include demonstration of a more than a 10-smsec drop in cranial nerve V across the elbow segment and/or a >20% reduction in CMAP amplitude.

Treatment in the early stages may involve changing the patient's sleeping posture. An acutely flexed elbow can cause symptoms. A simple static elbow extension splint usually breaks such a habit. Direct trauma activities such as resting the arm on the elbow while taking telephone calls may also produce symptoms. However, chronic cases and those with documented axonal damage and muscle atrophy are helped only by appropriate surgery, which includes transposition of the nerve anterior to the axis of rotation of the elbow so that elbow flexion relaxes rather than stretches the nerve. Simple unroofing of the cubital tunnel does not deal with the problem of nerve adhesions. Subcutaneous transpositions leave the nerve superficial and subject to trauma and painful subluxation across the medial epicondyle. Efforts to prevent the latter by suturing a strip of fascia from the PT muscles across the transposed ulnar nerve should be avoided because of an unacceptably high rate of complications. **By far, the best operation for cubital tunnel syndrome is a submuscular anterior transposition, carefully dissecting along physiologic planes and avoiding injury to the medial antebrachial cutaneous nerve to the forearm.** The most common failure of this operation is a result of kinking of the ulnar nerve as it enters the forearm distal to the medial epicondyle because of inadequate distal mobilization. Although it is undesirable to inject nerves already in trouble, the procedure can be performed with local infiltration anesthetics, if general anesthesia is medically contraindicated. **For all cases, the rate and the degree of recovery of liberated ulnar nerves are substantially less predictable than for the median or radial nerves.**

Radial Compression Neuropathies

The radial nerve, unlike both median and ulnar nerves, has no anatomic arrangement at the wrist level that predisposes to its entrapment. It has three areas where it is vulnerable to inflammatory or compression pathology: (a) the entire radial nerve in the proximal forearm, (b) the posterior interosseous division at the proximal margin of the supinator muscle, and

(c) the superficial sensory branch as it emerges from beneath the brachioradialis muscle to become subcutaneous in the midforearm.

Proximal Radial Nerve Compressions

Radial nerve compressions at the elbow have been reported, purportedly caused by a fibrous band from the shaft of the humerus that crosses the nerve to the lateral epicondyle. If this entity exists, it is exceedingly rare. **Radial neuropathies at the elbow or distally will have no disturbance of the radial wrist extensor muscles (extensor carpi radialis brevis [ECRB] and extensor carpi radialis longus [ECRL]) as their motor nerves separate from the radial nerve proximal to the elbow.** However, thickening of the radial nerve epineurium as a result of inflammation will be encountered and will disturb function of the superficial sensory branch of the nerve, the posterior interosseous (PI) motor division to the digital extensor muscles, or both. Radial nerve pathology in this area has been referred to as "radial tunnel syndrome," but this is a misnomer as there are no structures resembling walls of a tunnel, only soft muscle tissues adjacent to the nerves. Just distal to the elbow the radial nerve is regularly crossed by several large veins, the "leash of Henry," but these do not appear to compress the nerve.

Symptoms typically have an insidious onset with soreness of proximal–lateral forearm muscles. If only the superficial sensory division of the nerve is involved, symptoms are mild with some paresthesia or numbness on the dorsal–lateral aspects of the hand. If pain radiating to the neck and shoulder is severe and there is a profound sense of "heaviness" of the arm, the PI division of the nerve is involved, as is discussed subsequently. With only moderate symptoms limited to the superficial (sensory) division of the nerve, a trial of systemic steroids and rest of the arm usually is considered. Spontaneous remission has been reported. Only rarely will symptoms, limited to the sensory branch of the radial nerve alone, be progressive, severe, or recalcitrant enough to indicate surgical decompression.

Posterior Interosseous Nerve Compressions

Two varieties of pathology of the PI nerve are encountered. The rare one is a spontaneous onset of weakness of the digital extensor muscles innervated by the nerve. Unlike the anterior interosseous nerve, rarely is there a documented history of trauma to the proximal forearm. **Resisted passive flexion of the middle finger usually aggravates discomfort and, because the nerve is primarily motor, an EDS usually documents the diagnosis.**

Because spontaneous recovery for mild cases of PI neuritis are not infrequent, a few weeks of observation is warranted, but severely symptomatic or protracted cases need surgical decompression. Unfortunately the rate or degree of recovery is relatively unpredictable and subsequent tendon transfers often are needed.

The more common variety of PI compression also occurs spontaneously but is characterized by persistent and severe pain from the forearm radiating into the neck and shoulder, despite our being taught that this is a "motor" nerve. Profound heaviness of the arm is so frequent a complaint that one author (RWB) once wrote about it under the title "The Heavy Arm Syndrome." If the patient turns in sleep to the involved side, the patient will awaken. Maximum tenderness is in the proximal forearm, about 5 to 6 cm distal to the elbow skin crease where the PI nerve passes beneath the fibrous proximal margin of the supinator muscle. Digital pressure intensifies the radiating pain dramatically. The same is true for active supination of the forearm while it is being passively held in pronation. The majority of cases have no sensory disturbance in the distribution of the superficial branch of the radial nerve, but occasion-

ally inflammation will "spill over" causing mild disturbance. The diagnosis is basically from careful, and often serial, evaluations. EDS are of little help although occasionally increased polyphasic patterns are found in the extensor indicis proprius (EIP) muscle to which terminal branches of the PI nerve distribute.

Spontaneous remission may occur when symptoms are minor but usually only after many months of misery. In the majority of cases, there has been an extended failure of diagnosis. These cases need surgical decompression, which has little risk, very low morbidity, and is typically followed by prompt relief from the pain.

The incision is made directly over the radial nerve starting 2 cm distal to the elbow crease. It is carried through the subcutaneous tissues with as little damage to cutaneous nerves as possible. After opening the fascia of the "extensor mobile wad" muscles (ECRB, ECRL, and brachioradialis [BR]), passive extension and flexion of the wrist will enable one to identify the physiologic plane between the BR and the radial wrist extensor muscles. In this plane, the tissues can be atraumatically separated and the superficial branch of the radial nerve readily visualized. A careful external neurolysis is performed. Proximally a careful microneurolysis is done along the branches of the PI nerve, which pass deep to the proximal margin of the supinator muscle. No gross pathology will be seen, although the tissues being separated have a "tacky" resistance. Because the pathology is under the fibrous proximal margin of the supinator muscle, it is not seen until that sling is severed longitudinally. Even then the pathology is usually only a subtle reduction in nerve size, but generally the operation is followed by immediate and dramatic relief of even chronic pain.

Wartenberg Syndrome

The superficial (sensory) branch of the radial nerve passes distally in the forearm beneath the BR muscle to the midforearm where it turns laterally into the subcutaneous tissues along the distal radius. At the point of exit from beneath the muscle, a compression of the nerve can develop, causing local pain and sensory disturbance to the dorsal–lateral skin of the hand. This condition is referred to as Wartenberg syndrome and does not develop spontaneously, but is an infrequent complication of trauma to the midforearm. The diagnosis is made by history, the finding of a strong Tinel sign at the point of exit of the nerve from beneath the BR muscle, and sensory disturbance in the nerve's distribution. As the BR is a supinator muscle, pain is accentuated by attempting this motion while the forearm is passively pronated. Treatment is through a short incision at the site of entrapment indicated by the Tinel sign. The nerve is carefully protected and the fibrous margin of the BR muscle is transected several times at 1-cm intervals to relieve all tension. The prognosis is excellent.

Thoracic Outlet Syndrome

Thoracic outlet syndrome (TOS) refers to neurologic or vascular disorders that occur where divisions of the brachial plexus and the subclavian artery pass from the neck into the arms through the interscalene triangle. The sides of the triangle are anterior and medial scalene muscles and the first rib. **Many respected authorities question even the existence of this syndrome, and if it is a reality, it is so extremely rare as to dictate extreme caution in entertaining the diagnosis.**

The typical suspect for the condition is an obese, lethargic woman with heavy pendulous breasts, poor posture, and emotional or psychiatric issues. The neurologic symptoms are ill-defined and inconsistent, except they tend to be of the lower roots (ulnar nerve) of the brachial plexus. Patients will complain of having the greatest distress with activities in which the arms are overhead. **Some will have a cervical rib, but this is**

not pathognomonic of the alleged syndrome. Nor is an abnormal arteriogram pathognomonic. EDS data from most cases fall within the average ranges.

The diagnosis of TOS so precarious that a conservative attitude about treatment should be maintained. Efforts should be directed toward weight reduction, general fitness, and posture correction. Reduction mammoplasty should also be considered. In the rare case for which surgical treatment is warranted, transaxillary first rib resection is the method of choice. Unfortunately, far too many patients are seen who have undergone multiple procedures for a diagnosis of TOS only to be progressively more symptomatic after each procedure.

CHAPTER 87 ■ THUMB RECONSTRUCTION

CHARLES J. EATON

Efforts to restore the structure, function, and appearance of the thumb span the history of hand surgery (1). Staged, pedicled toe-to-thumb transfer without microvascular anastomosis, now only of historical interest, was performed by Nicoladoni in 1898. Forms of phalangization, osteoplastic reconstruction, pollicization, and pedicled digital transfers date back 100 years. Digital neurovascular island flaps and free toe transfers, developed 50 and 40 years ago, respectively, are established techniques now in common use.

INDICATIONS

Loss of thumb function impairs the entire upper limb, and carries a high priority for reconstruction. Despite this, some patients accommodate well to thumb amputation, and therefore reconstruction is indicated for selected cases. Even a replanted thumb, which would appear to be the best possible reconstruction, is not always more functional than an amputation properly revised at the same level (2). Thumb reconstruction is technically demanding, and patient motivation and accommodation are critical factors for good outcome. Strong contraindications to elective thumb reconstruction include significant vascular disease, short life expectancy, chronic pain with disuse of the limb, unreconstructable sensory loss, unrealistic patient expectations, and other contraindications dictated by the common sense of the surgeon.

EVALUATION

Because the key functions of the thumb are always in relation to the rest of the hand, thumb reconstruction is considered in the context of the entire hand. As with any digital injury, initial evaluation includes an assessment of soft tissue deficits, bone loss, condition of joints, the nail bed, zone of tendon injuries, and neurologic status. In addition, the following points relevant to thumb reconstruction are considered:

1. *What is the status of the basal joint?* The thumb carpometacarpal joint is evaluated clinically and radiographically. An injured, stiff, or painful basal joint is a poor foundation for a new thumb, but salvage by arthroplasty may be a possibility (Fig. 87.1).
2. *Is there a first web space contracture or skin deficit?* Web space contracture may be a result of unappreciated skin loss, scar contractures, abductor muscle destruction or paralysis, basal joint pathology, adductor/flexor muscle contracture, or a combination of the above. **Preliminary correction of such contractures should be considered (Fig. 87.2), recognizing that first web space contractures often cannot be fully corrected, even with determined surgical efforts.**

3. *Are there problems with the remaining digits?* Optimum length, mobility, and position of the thumb are all judged in relation to the remaining fingers. A stiff reconstructed thumb may not make useful contact with stiff, short, or insensate fingers. On the other hand, a damaged and otherwise useless finger may be suitable for transfer either as a free transfer (Fig. 87.3), pollicization (Fig. 87.4), or an on-top plasty thumb lengthening (Fig. 87.5).
4. *Has the patient developed maladaptive patterns of use?* Heroic efforts at thumb reconstruction will be unrewarding if the patient has developed a fixed pattern of not using remaining parts of the mutilated hand. This tendency to become functionally "one-handed" is particularly frequent if the situation is long standing or has been complicated by chronic pain.
5. *Do the patient's complaints match the apparent deficit?* Patients with thumb amputation may have less obvious impairments contributing to the restricted use of the hand. Crush/avulsion injuries may result in a wide zone of deep scarring, with prolonged stiffness, swelling, intrinsic tightness and swelling, and compression neuropathies.
6. *What are the patient's expectations?* Although thumb function is the primary reconstructive goal, concerns about social presentation and aesthetics may be equally important. A technical triumph to the surgeon may be seen as a grotesque deformity by the patient. Photographs of other reconstructed thumbs may help some patients understand what is being recommended, but even this must be done carefully to avoid creating false expectations.

If it appears that a patient is likely to be disappointed with the result and especially the appearance of a reconstructed thumb, a lifelike prosthesis, which involves no irreversible procedures, may be the best recommendation if technically feasible (see Chapter 93).

TYPES OF DEFICIENCIES

Thumb deficiencies are considered as either *amputation* or *component loss* (Fig. 87.6). Component loss includes soft tissue coverage or segmental loss of neurovascular, tendon, or skeletal components. Reconstruction may be either *emergency* (possible replantation), *urgent* (fresh open wound), *subacute* (unhealed wounds), or *elective* (healed wounds). Timing of reconstruction is important. The likelihood of septic or flap-threatening complications are greatest when surgery is performed in the subacute healing period (3). **As with any extremity injury, reconstructive priorities are first *healing* (blood supply, stable skeleton, mobile soft-tissue cover) and then *function* (nerve function, passive range of motion, active range of motion).**

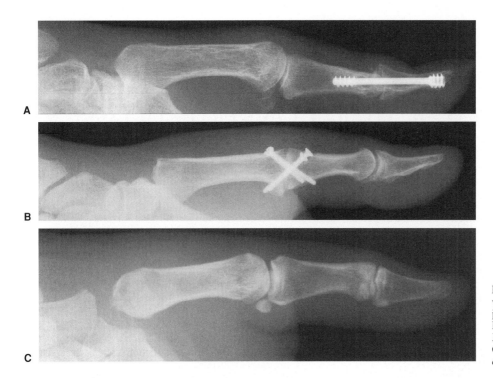

FIGURE 87.1. The most common salvage procedures for unreconstructable joint injuries are arthrodeses. **A:** Interphalangeal arthrodesis. **B:** Metacarpophalangeal arthrodesis. **C:** Soft-tissue arthroplasty of the carpometacarpal joint.

Component Losses

Skeletal injuries are managed by anatomic reduction and fixation. Nonreconstructible injuries of the interphalangeal or metacarpophalangeal joints are treated with arthrodesis, but carpometacarpal injuries are best salvaged with soft-tissue arthroplasty (Fig. 87.1). *Soft-tissue loss* of the thumb is managed as for other digits, with skin grafts or flaps as indicated by the particular defect. *Composite loss* of soft tissue and skeletal elements requires urgent soft-tissue cover with skeletal stabilization and possible bone grafting. **As with any mangling limb injury, the best time to proceed with completion of amputation is at the first operation.**

Reconstructing component loss requires an appropriate flap. Because sensory perception is key to effective use of the thumb, innervated flaps are much preferred for contact area resurfacing, but their availability is limited. *Innervated flaps* appropriate for the thumb include the Moberg palmar advancement flap, the Holevich first dorsal metacarpal flap from the index finger, heterodigital neurovascular sensory "island" flaps, and free finger or toe pulp flaps (Figs. 87.3, 87.7, and 87.8). Standard local digital flaps may be used as well, including V-Y advancements, dorsal transposition, and dorsal or volar cross-finger flaps. *Noninnervated regional flaps*, such as posterior interosseous (Fig. 87.2), radial forearm (Fig. 87.9), and intrinsic muscle flaps (Fig. 87.10), are appropriate for complex proximal and web space defects. Choice of the specific flap depends on the size, location, and orientation of the defect, condition of donor sites, and the surgeon's experience. Table 87.1 lists my preferences for flap coverage of thumb defects.

Unique pitfalls in the management of *degloving* or circumferential soft-tissue loss deserve special mention. If circumferential soft-tissue loss extends *proximal* to the base of the proximal phalanx, the distal phalanx will eventually be lost to avascular necrosis despite flap cover, and primary interphalangeal disarticulation should be considered. Denuded skeleton should be covered in a tubed or closed flap (Fig. 87.9), not buried in a pocket. Planning the flap with a thin template may be misleading: The flap must be designed wide enough to allow for the thickness of the flap itself, and also to allow for flap swelling.

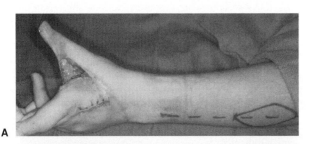

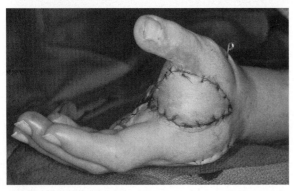

FIGURE 87.2. First web space contracture release with reverse pedicled posterior interosseous artery island flap. **A:** Defect and flap design. **B:** After flap insert.

Amputation

Whenever possible, replantation should be considered for thumb amputation.

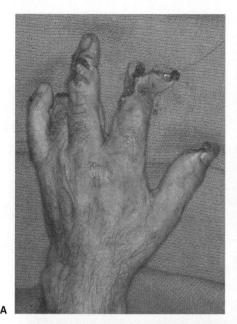
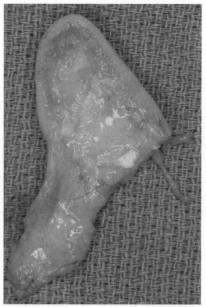
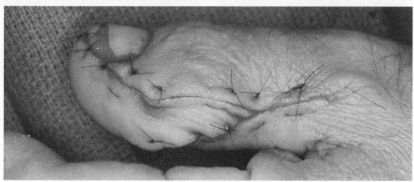

FIGURE 87.3. Emergency thumb pulp resurfacing with free pulp flap harvested from a ring finger amputated in the same accident. **A:** Initial injury with amputated ring finger and loss of thumb soft tissue. **B:** Tissue harvested from amputated part. **C:** Thumb after flap transfer.

Amputation Distal to the Metacarpophalangeal Joint

If there is a functional remnant of the proximal phalanx (Fig. 87.6), primary reconstructive goals are length, stability, and adequate web space (Fig. 87.11). Choices include bone graft with a local flap, osteoplastic reconstruction, phalangization, distraction lengthening, pedicled transfer of a damaged finger remnant to the thumb, or toe-to-thumb transfer (Figs. 87.4 and 87.12 to 87.15).

Amputation Proximal to the Metacarpophalangeal Joint

When the level of amputation is at or proximal to the metacarpophalangeal joint, the thumb ray does not project beyond the web space skin. Functionally, this is a complete thumb amputation, but there is the potential for functional reconstruction pivoting (literally) on having a good basal joint with sufficient metacarpal length and thenar muscle to control it (Fig. 87.6). Options when loss is through the distal metacarpal include osteoplastic reconstruction, pedicled finger remnant transfer, pollicization, and free toe transfer. A proximal metacarpal amputation retains the basal joint but has no intrinsic muscles. With this or an amputation including the basal joint, there are two options: (a) if the fingers are functioning well, provide a stable, static post to oppose the fingers, or (b) full-finger pollicization.

ESTABLISHED THUMB RECONSTRUCTION PROCEDURES

Many procedures for thumb reconstruction have been described. Table 87.2 summarizes the preferred procedure in various circumstances.

Osteoplastic Thumb Reconstruction

Best Indication/Unique Advantages

Partial or distal subtotal amputation may necessitate this procedure. No digit is sacrificed.

Disadvantages and Special Requirements

Multiple staged procedures may be required. Results may be unaesthetic: can be bulky, floppy, and without a thumb nail. Additional neurovascular flap is required for sensibility.

Technique

Osteoplastic reconstruction involves the combination of a bone graft and flap to lengthen the thumb remnant (Fig. 87.14). It typically involves three procedures: lengthening the skeleton with an iliac crest bone graft covered in a tubed distant flap; flap

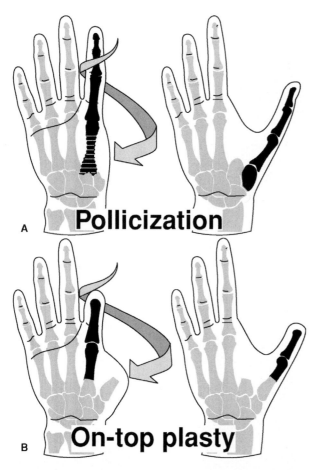

A: **Pollicization**

B: **On-top plasty**

FIGURE 87.4. Pedicled digital transfer to the thumb position. **A:** Total reconstruction of the thumb may be achieved with pollicization of the index finger, which provides the thenar muscle replacements in addition to the entire thumb skeletal ray. **B:** Pedicled transfer of a previously damaged or amputated digit (on-top plasty) may be used to lengthen a partial or distal subtotal thumb amputation.

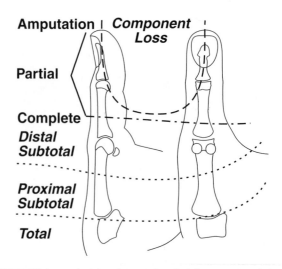

FIGURE 87.6. Level of thumb loss. Thumb defects are classified as either component loss or amputation. Amputations are grouped as partial or complete, and complete amputations can be identified as distal subtotal (retaining the entire metacarpal), proximal subtotal (retaining basal joint but not thenar muscles), and total, with loss of the basal joint.

pedicle division; and transfer of a neurovascular sensory island flap from the ulnar side of the middle finger to the thumb's pinch contact surface. Additional debulking flap revisions are usually required. There are many donor-site variations, including reversed pedicled forearm flaps (radial or posterior interosseous), primary neurovascular island transfer, and combinations with dorsal hand flaps. A variety of free tissue transfers may be used, including the excellent "wraparound" toe transfer, which is discussed below (see Wraparound Toe Transfer) (4).

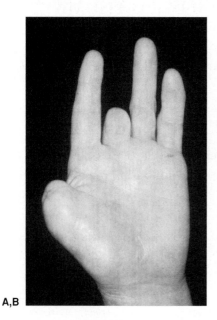
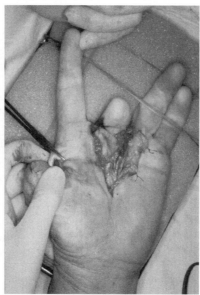
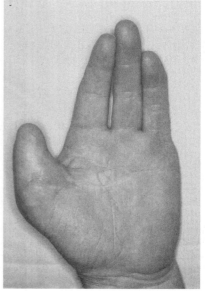

FIGURE 87.5. On-top plasty damaged middle finger remnant is transferred to the thumb, combined with a ray resection. **A:** Initial appearance of the hand. **B:** Mobilization of remaining middle finger. **C:** Final result with long thenal thumb and middle finger ray resection.

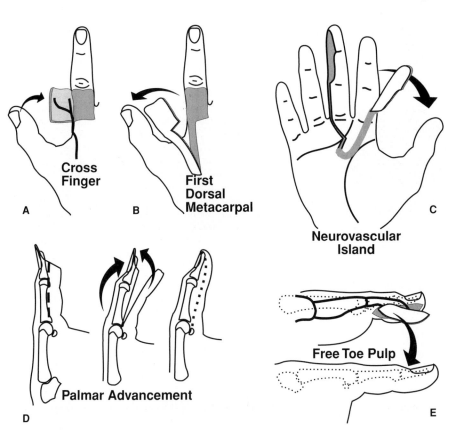

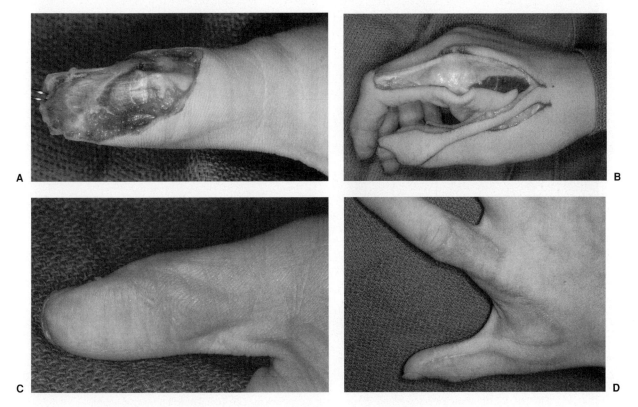

FIGURE 87.7. Sensory flaps for thumb reconstruction. Innervated flaps applicable to the thumb include (**A** and **B**) dorsal flaps from the index finger, including branches of the superficial radial nerve, (**C**) digital neurovascular island transfer, (**D**) Moberg palmar advancement, and (**E**) free neurovascular toe pulp flaps.

FIGURE 87.8. Holevich flap. The dorsal index finger skin may be mobilized on a narrow skin or subcutaneous pedicle for transfer to the thumb. This flap has been used to resurface the distal half of the palmar skin, including the entire pulp surface. **A:** Defect of thumb pulp. **B:** Transfer of flap from index finger. **C:** Palmar view of result. **D:** Dorsal lateral view of result.

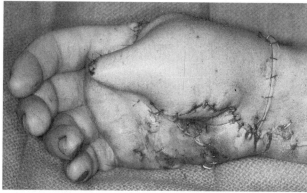

FIGURE 87.9. Circumferential thumb resurfacing with contralateral free radial forearm flap.

ticularly if the web is converted to a cleft by an aggressive Z-plasty.

Technique

This is a web-deepening procedure, results of which are so often disappointing that it is rarely a good recommendation in view of today's alternatives (Fig. 87.12). To allow creation of the cleft, the adductor muscle insertion is detached and repositioned proximally, and the first web space is deepened with a Z-plasty. Correction of an associated first web space contracture may require stripping of the entire ulnar border of the first metacarpal and capsulotomy of the basal joint. The mechanical advantage of the adductor is progressively lessened with more proximal reattachment. If the index finger has been partially amputated or is too damaged to transfer for thumb lengthening, it should be resected to increase the web space.

Phalangization

Best Indication/Unique Advantages

Thumb lengthening by finger transfer is a possible consideration (rare) if the thumb is *nearly* long enough, such as base of proximal phalanx. Usually this is a single-stage operation.

Disadvantages and Special Requirements

Phalangization may not provide much functional improvement, and may result in a very unnatural appearance, par-

Metacarpal Distraction Lengthening

Best Indication/Unique Advantages

Distal subtotal amputation (region of metacarpophalangeal [MCP] joint) is an indication for this procedure and there is little or no donor defect except scar.

Disadvantages and Special Requirements

Only limited lengthening is possible, and absolute cooperation is required.

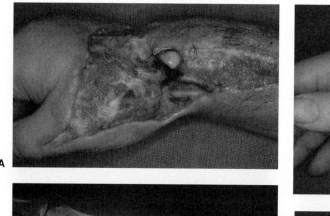

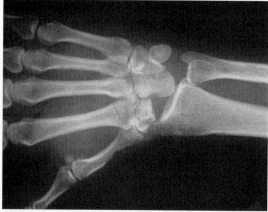

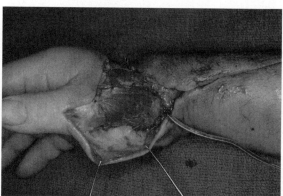

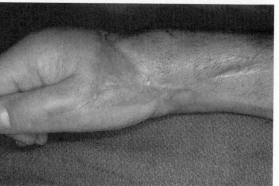

FIGURE 87.10. Thumb metacarpal resurfacing with a muscle flap. This complex wound was a complication of dialysis access surgery. After debridement and proximal row carpectomy, the abductor pollicis brevis muscle was disinserted and transposed dorsally to cover the exposed metacarpal and remaining carpus. **A:** Defect. **B:** Abductor pollicis brevis coverage of exposed bone. **C:** Radiograph showing proximal row carpectomy. **D:** Final result.

TABLE 87.1

FLAP SELECTION FOR SOFT-TISSUE DEFECTS OF THE THUMB

Location	Site of defect requiring flap cover		
	Distal phalanx	Proximal phalanx	Both phalanges
Dorsal or radial	Cross-finger from index or middle	Local thumb, cross-finger	First dorsal metacarpal
Palmar	Moberg palmar advancement, volar cross-finger from middle	Local thumb, first dorsal metacarpal	Distant
Ulnar	Cross-finger from ring or small	Local thumb	Distant
Circumferential	Regional or distant: radial forearm, pedicled groin, posterior interosseous, toe flap		

Technique

After osteotomy, the thumb's metacarpal is slowly lengthened using progressive adjustments of an external fixator in the manner introduced by Ilizarov for the lower limbs (Fig. 87.15). The metacarpal is exposed through a longitudinal incision, and the fixator placed, a *corticotomy* made circumferentially and subperiosteally through the metacarpal shaft. Efforts are made to minimize medullary bone disruption. After 1 week, distraction is begun at a rate of 1 mm per day. If any proximal phalanx exists, the MCP joint will be progressively flexed unless stabilized with a strong Kirschner pin. In small children, new bone growth from the periosteum and medullary bone may adequately fill in the distraction gap, but interposition bone grafting is usually required for adults once maximum lengthening is achieved. Generally, this should incorporate MCP joint arthrodesis and removal of sesamoid bones. Once healed, more bone and soft-

tissue removal can result in a much more pleasing part, which also lends itself to prosthetic fitting if desired.

On-Top Plasty

Best Indication/Unique Advantages

Amputation in the area of the MCP joint is an indication for this procedure, which will enhance the value of a damaged finger.

Disadvantages and Special Requirements

The appropriate finger is infrequently available, and this procedure narrows the palm. Transferred injured parts carry a higher risk of a complication.

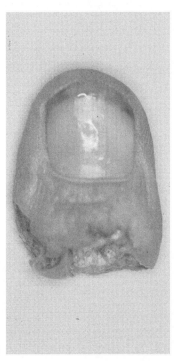
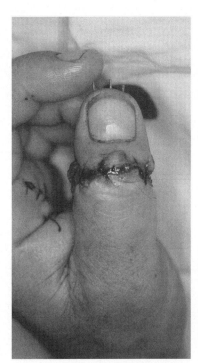
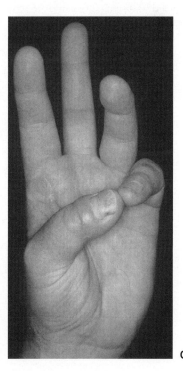

A,B   **C**

FIGURE 87.11. Thumb amputation through the interphalangeal joint treated with replantation and interphalangeal joint fusion. **A:** Amputated part. **B:** Replanted part. **C:** Functional result.

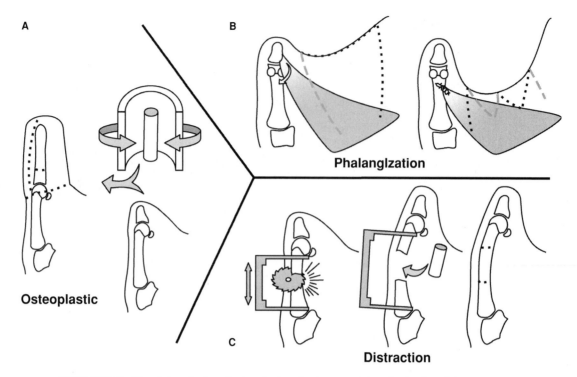

A

B

Phalangization

Osteoplastic

C

Distraction

FIGURE 87.12. Thumb lengthening. Options for lengthening a partial or distal subtotal thumb amputation with the least donor-site morbidity include (**A**) osteoplastic reconstruction, (**B**) phalangization, and (**C**) metacarpal distraction lengthening.

Technique

On-top plasty refers to the neurovascular pedicle transfer of the distal segment of a damaged or partially amputated finger to lengthen the thumb (Figs. 87.4 and 87.5). If the metacarpal of the transformed finger is not needed, usually it is removed by ray resection. Preoperative arteriography may be helpful in planning for some patients.

Pollicization

Best Indication/Unique Advantages

The best indication is proximal subtotal or total amputation. **This procedure is the only satisfactory means of basal joint reconstruction and results in extensive physiologic sensory restoration.**

TABLE 87.2

CHOICES OF TECHNIQUE FOR THUMB RECONSTRUCTION

	Partial	Distal subtotal	Proximal subtotal or complete
Isolated, acquired	Distraction Wraparound osteoplastic	Osteoplastic Distraction wraparound Great toe (adult) Second toe (child)	Pollicization Skin flap, then second toe + metacarpal
Single mutilated finger	On-top plasty	On-top plasty	Pollicization
Multiple mutilated fingers	Distraction Osteoplastic Toe transfer	Osteoplastic Toe transfer	Pollicization Skin flap, then second toe + metacarpal
Cosmetic concerns	Prosthesis	Prosthesis	Prosthesis
Manual labor	Osteoplastic Distraction	Toe transfer	Pollicization
Congenital—child	Distraction	Distraction Second toe transfer	Pollicization Second toe transfer
Congenital—adult	Prosthesis	Prosthesis	Prosthesis
No transferrable digit	Osteoplastic	Osteoplastic	Osteoplastic

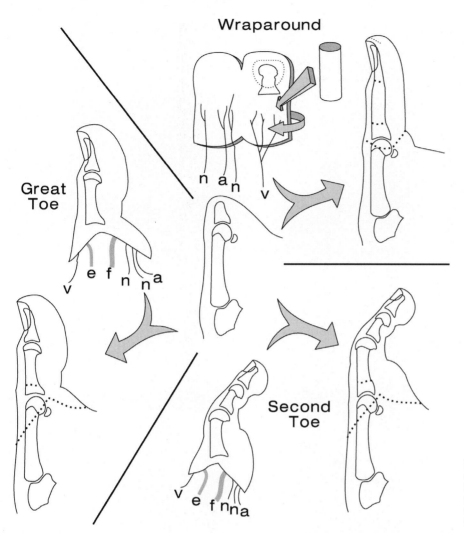

Wraparound

Great Toe

Second Toe

FIGURE 87.13. Toe transfer for thumb reconstruction. Many variations of toe transfer exist, but the most commonly used are the great toe, second toe, and wraparound toe transfers. a, Artery; e, extensor tendon; f, flexor tendon; n, nerve; v, vein.

Disadvantages and Special Requirements

This procedure narrows the palm.

Technique

Pollicization refers to the neurovascular pedicle movement of a finger, often with its metacarpal, for thumb reconstruction (Fig. 87.6). For congenital absence of the thumb, a simplified modification is recommended (4). The index finger is basically recessed by resection of a segment of the second metacarpal base, then pronated about 130 degrees and projected in palmar abduction at its fixed base. Incisions are planned to convert dorsal or palmar skin into a web between middle finger and the new thumb. The extensor tendons must always be shortened as part of the primary procedure. Flexor tendons, in contrast, follow a circuitous route, and length adjustments are performed secondarily if necessary. Structures receive new identities: The extensor digitorum communis becomes the abductor pollicis longus; the extensor indicis becomes the extensor pollicis longus; the first dorsal interosseous becomes the abductor pollicis brevis; the first palmar interosseous becomes the adductor pollicis; the metacarpal head and the proximal and middle phalanges become the trapezium and the metacarpal and proximal phalanges, respectively.

For a proximal thumb amputation, with an intact basal joint, the proximal phalanx of a transferred index finger may be fused to the base of the remaining first metacarpal (5). Obviously, there are an infinite number of variations required for

individual circumstances, but common to all is preservation of intact nerves for critical sensibility, although in adults it has cortical mislocation. **Secondary surgery will be needed for approximately 50% of patients undergoing pollicization, yet in the right circumstances and for the right indication, results will be superior to that of all other available alternatives.**

Toe-to-Thumb Transfers

Best Indication/Unique Advantages

A toe-to-thumb transfer is performed when most of a well-controlled first metacarpal is present but length is needed. Advantages include (a) a good level of sensory recovery, (b) bone growth continues, and (c) that it is a single-stage operation.

Disadvantages and Special Requirements

Foot disability may occur, and the thumb always looks like a toe.

Technique

With the majority of toe-to-thumb transfers, a skin deficit on the hand is encountered. If the recipient site has skin grafts or tight scars, plans should be made for adequate soft tissue prior to the transfer operation (Figs. 87.13 and 87.16).

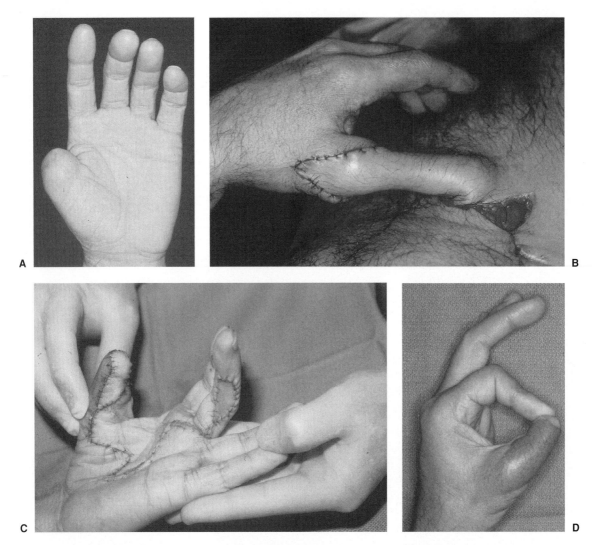

FIGURE 87.14. Osteoplastic thumb reconstruction. Partial amputation, lengthened with an iliac crest bone graft wrapped in a tubed pedicled inferior epigastric flap. After flap division, innervation is provided with a neurovascular sensory island flap transferred from the ring finger. **A:** Initial appearance. **B:** Tubed inferior epigastric flap. **C:** Sensory island flap **D:** Final result. (Case of R. W. Beasley.)

Preoperative arteriography of the hand and foot are generally recommended. Skeletal reconstruction for correct length is tailored to match the defect. Second toe transfers generally are favored for children, and great toe transfers are favored for adults (6), although there is no universal agreement about this, and there are individual considerations for each case.

Toe-to-thumb operations can be performed by one or two teams. The level of toe osteotomy is a convenient reference point from which lengths of skin, tendons, nerves, and vessels may be measured. Recipient vessels in the hand are exposed first to verify their adequacy and to define the necessary donor pedicle length. The radial artery is preferred. Once satisfactory recipient vessels are isolated, foot dissection commences. A racquet-shaped incision is made, which gives more dorsal than plantar skin. Veins are dissected first, elevating thin skin flaps proximally and carefully freeing the venous pedicle up to the skin margin of the toe. Branches of the deep venous system are followed to the deep and variable arterial system. The dorsalis pedis and first dorsal metatarsal artery are dissected to the flap. The plantar digital nerves are small and short compared to those of the thumb, and intraneural dissection of the common digital nerve may be needed. Tendons are severed proximally to allow tendon repairs at a distance from vascular and skele-

tal work. Normal metatrarsophalangeal joint range of motion is hyperextended relative to the thumb metacarpophalangeal joint. If the metatarsophalangeal joint is included in the reconstruction, an oblique metatarsal osteotomy should be used to increase flexion for more natural thumb function. Although the reconstructed thumb is usually pronated, the degree is determined for each case to function best with remaining fingers. If opponensplasty is needed, it can be performed as a primary or secondary procedure. If the vascular pedicle crosses the wrist, a midlateral path is preferred to avoid tension from wrist motion, and end-to-side arterial anastomoses are preferred. Second toe donor sites can usually be closed primarily, and this is facilitated by resection of the second metatarsal. Great toe donor-site closure often requires a skin graft. Donor-site morbidity is small, but cannot be dismissed entirely (7).

Wraparound Toe Transfer

Best Indication/Unique Advantages

For amputation near the MCP joint or distal to it, this is the procedure of choice. It results in the most normal-appearing reconstruction from the foot.

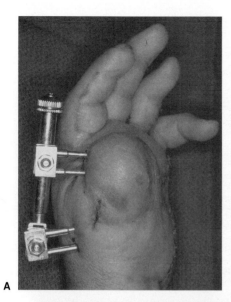
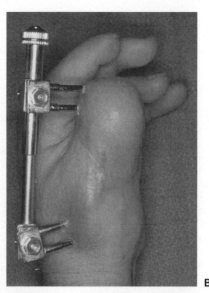

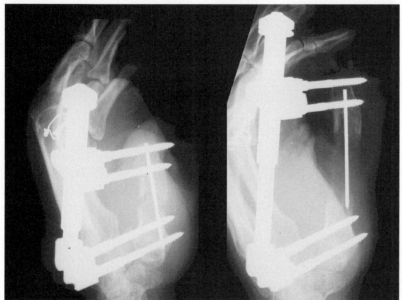

FIGURE 87.15. Distraction lengthening. This patient had undergone a traumatic metacarpophalangeal level thumb amputation, covered in a groin flap, in addition to multilevel injuries of the wrist and all fingers. After metacarpal corticotomy, a distraction fixator was used to lengthen the metacarpal, followed by interpositional bone grafting. A: Distractor applied. B: After lengthening. C: Bone graft placement.

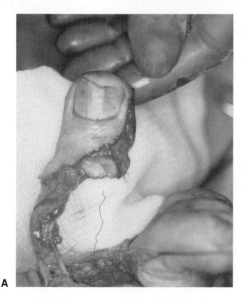
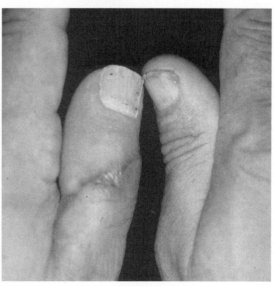

FIGURE 87.16. Toe-to-thumb transfer. Modified wraparound great toe transfer for a degloving injury. A: Toe flap isolated. B: Final result.

Disadvantages and Special Requirements

This technically complex and demanding procedure results in limited functional improvement when used without an MCP joint. It requires an iliac bone graft.

Technique

Wraparound toe transfer is a hybrid of great toe transfer and osteoplastic reconstruction (8) (Fig. 87.13). During harvest, the great toe is filleted, leaving on the foot the medial toe skin out to the tip and its skeleton to the base of the toenail. The isolated free flap for transfer to the hand includes the distal half of the distal phalanx with the plantar, lateral, and dorsal tissues, including the toenail. This complex is wrapped around a bone graft, which spans the gap between the remaining thumb skeleton and the distal phalanx of the transferred toe. The donor-site defect is closed with the medial toe flap, a cross-toe flap from the second toe, and a dorsal skin graft. The ultimate fingernail is narrowed by resection of the germinal matrix from each side. There are no tendon repairs. The typical end result is a more narrow and thumblike reconstruction than is achieved with a great toe transfer, and the great toe length is almost fully preserved.

References

1. Littler JW. On making a thumb: one hundred years of surgical effort. *J Hand Surg.* 1976;1:35.
2. Goldner RD, Howson MP, Nunley JA, et al. One hundred eleven thumb amputations: replantation vs. revision. *Microsurgery.* 1990;11:243.
3. Godina M. Early microsurgical reconstruction of complex trauma of the extremities. *Plast Reconstr Surg.* 1986;78:285.
4. Morrison WA, O'Brien BM, MacLeod AM. Thumb reconstruction with a free neurovascular wrap-around flap from the big toe. *J Hand Surg.* 1980;5:575.
5. Buck-Gramcko D. Thumb reconstruction by digital transposition. *Orthop Clin North Am.* 1977;8:329.
6. Stern PJ, Lister GD. Pollicization after traumatic amputation of the thumb. *Clin Orthop.* 1981;155:85.
7. May JW, Bartlett SP. Great toe-to-hand free tissue transfer for thumb reconstruction. *Hand Clin.* 1985;1:271.
8. Lipton HA, May JW, Simon SR. Preoperative and postoperative gait analyses of patients undergoing great toe-to-thumb transfer. *J Hand Surg.* 1987;12:66.

CHAPTER 88 ■ TENDON TRANSFERS

ROBERT W. BEASLEY

Tendon or muscle transfers follow a basic concept of reconstructive surgery: Nothing new is created but functional parts, or those that can be made functional, are rearranged into the best possible working combination. **Tendon transfers involve detachment of the tendon distally, mobilization without damage to the neurovascular pedicle, and rerouting it to a new distal attachment.** In no area is a thorough knowledge of functional anatomy more essential. The procedures are among the most interesting, diversified, challenging, and rewarding of upper limb surgery.

Littler (1) has given a brief but historic summary of the development of tendon transfer surgery and pointed out that the partially paralyzed limb offers a unique opportunity to gain a working knowledge of hand dynamics. In 1867, Duchenne used faradic current to study the physiology of motion, but it was only with World War I that real progress in clinical application was made. Classic contributions were made by Jones in England (1912), Meyer in Berlin (1916), and Steindler (1918) in America (5). Bunnell and others made refinements with the surge of interest attending World War II (1939–1945), but the landmark publication that set the standard was in 1949 by Littler (5), and it is still applicable today.

Occasionally, a muscle proper rather than just the tendon may be transferred. An example is transfer of the abductor digiti minimi on an intact neurovascular pedicle for thumb opponensplasty (7). More recently this has been performed as free composite tissue transfers by microvascular technique.

BASIC TENETS

The basic principles for all successful tendon transfers can be summarized as follows:

1. Tendon transfers involve the redistribution, not the creation, of new power units. Muscle power is transferred from less important to more important functions so as to improve the system overall.
2. Simplicity in mechanical design predisposes to good results, whereas complexity mitigates against them. More than one change of direction cannot be introduced into the system.
3. Even simple-appearing actions are the results of complex interaction of prime movers, antagonists, and numerous stabilizers (prime movers and antagonists in balanced opposition). Every joint between the muscle's origin and new insertion must be stabilized, or with contraction, the system will buckle. When inadequate muscle is available for stabilization, joints of lesser importance require arthrodesis.
4. If any one of the three major nerves to the hand and forearm are lost, the potential for good reconstruction exists, but if two of the three nerves are lost, a major functional impairment is inevitable. Any worthwhile reconstruction will entail a major simplification of mechanical design.

5. Normal skin sensibility is always desirable, so long as it is above a protective level, but decreased sensibility does not preclude the usefulness of tendon transfers.
6. With interruption of motor nerves, muscle imbalance is immediate, but not deformity. Deformity develops from persistent imbalance and can usually be prevented by appropriate splinting, etc.

INDICATIONS FOR TENDON TRANSFERS

Neurologic Deficits

Poliomyelitis is no longer the most frequent indication for tendon transfers. Rather, paralysis of healthy muscle, usually from nerve injury, is the most frequent indication. Prompt consideration of tendon transfers is indicated if (a) the prognosis for neurologic recovery is poor even with nerve repair, (b) muscles have been destroyed, or (c) nerve grafts have been required to restore nerve continuity. Tendon transfers do not prevent recovered function of a paralyzed muscle if an unanticipated degree of neurologic recovery occurs.

Loss of Muscle–Tendon Unit or as an Alternative to Tendon Repair

Muscles can be directly destroyed or their tendons hopelessly damaged, as with rheumatoid arthritis. For these cases, restoration of an important function may best be accomplished by tendon transfer (Fig. 88.1).

Other Indications

Treating spastic disorders may rarely incorporate tendon transfers. Results are unpredictable because the transferred unit does not have normal neurologic control. It is difficult to treat peripherally an essentially central nervous system problem. Arthrodesis is far more frequently used to improve balance of spastic patients.

EVALUATION AND ESTABLISHMENT OF GOALS

As with most areas of medicine, evaluation and accurate diagnosis begins with taking a detailed and accurate history. Not only does this provide information about the mechanism of injury, but much is learned about the patient, such as intellectual capacity, expectations, and motivation. The patient generally will interpret these efforts as expression of concern, so it goes far toward establishing good rapport.

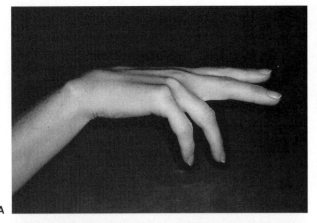

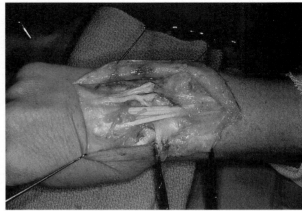

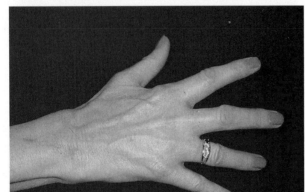

FIGURE 88.1. Tendon transfer for rheumatoid arthritis. **A:** Rupture of extensor digiti minimi and extensor digitorum communis to ring and small fingers as a result of rheumatoid synovitis/arthritis. **B:** Surgical exposure of the rheumatoid-ravaged wrist with ruptured tendons seen toward top of picture. **C:** Restoration of ring- and small-finger extensor by transfer of the distal segments of their ruptured tendon into the side of the intact extensor tendons to middle and index fingers.

Task Analysis and Establishment of Goals

Obviously every patient wants the affected hand to return to its normal status, but most often this is outside the realm of reality. Consequently, it is important that the basis for judgment of care be the crippled hand as presented rather than the normal hand. For elective cases, it is important to sort out the complaints and arrange them in order of priority. With subsequent reference to this list, progress will be appreciated that otherwise would be unrecognized.

Motivation

Motivation is no less a factor for obtaining good results from tendon transfers than it is in any other surgical hand procedure. The patient who shows little interest and/or unrealistic expectations is a poor candidate for surgical repairs. **In general, never do an elective operation that you "had to sell."**

PREREQUISITES TO SURGERY

Open Wounds

In general, a patient is not a candidate for tendon transfers if there are open wounds that could predispose to infection.

Soft-Tissue Coverage

Transferred tendons will glide only if transplanted through mobile, unscarred, healthy tissues. The transfer usually entails subcutaneous rerouting or flap-tissue replacement to provide such coverage. Wounds should be thoroughly healed before consideration is given to tendon transfer.

Precede Transfers with Maximum Joint Mobilization

One rarely gains more active range of motion from tendon transfers than the preoperative passive range of motion.

Skeletal Stabilization

Usually skeletal stabilization requiring arthrodesis should be performed prior to tendon transfers. The exception is a wrist fusion, because observations of the tenodesis effects from wrist flexion–extension is essential to judging tension of the tendon transfer.

Restore Sensibility

When possible restoration of at least protective sensibility should precede tendon transfers. Skin sensibility is not absolutely necessary for tendon transfers to be useful, but it is desirable.

SELECTION OF MUSCLES FOR TRANSFER

Availability

Having established the functional needs and goals and that the patient is emotionally a suitable candidate, the next step is to develop the plan that will best meet those needs (1). A detailed inventory of the existing assets is generated by grading the power of each muscle in the limb on a 0 to 5 scale, 0 being no active movement, 1 being ability to move against gravity, 2 being movement but too weak for any basic tasks, 3 being weak but useful power, 4 being near-normal power, and 5 being fully normal power. Essentially, only muscles of 4 and 5 power ratings are suitable for tendon transfers.

Control

A muscle for transfer should be nonspastic, have good volitional control, and be an independently functional unit, such as the finger superficial flexor muscles or the extensor indicis proprius.

Amplitude of Excursion

The muscle to be transferred must have an adequate amplitude of excursion for its new job or be situated so that it can be enhanced by tenodesis as it crosses an actively controlled joint. Most often this joint will be the wrist.

Anatomic Location

To be considered for tendon transfer a muscle must be so located that its transfer is anatomically and mechanically feasible. The rerouting should be as direct as possible between the muscle's origin and its new insertion. Otherwise, as it begins to function, it will work into a straight line of pull and become too slack. Never is more than one change of direction workable, and simplicity of mechanical design predisposes good results.

Synergism

Muscles that automatically contract simultaneously are referred to as synergistic. One of the many examples of this is wrist extension with finger flexion to grasp. Because of the way our muscle control system works, synergism does not have the importance once ascribed to it. From a control point of view, any muscle can function well at a new task and the ease with which it adapts to it is determined basically by how useful is the new function, not the muscle original function.

Expendability

If a muscle is given a new duty, we must be certain that it will be of more benefit to the patient than keeping the muscle in its normal situation.

RELATION OF MUSCLE LENGTH TO POWER OUTPUT

A muscle's power output is greatest at its resting length and diminishes with either stretching or redundancy as illustrated by the Blix curve. A muscle can shorten approximately 40% by contraction and at that point, power output ceases. It can be stretched approximately 40% before it ruptures, and measurements are deceptive as the energy required for stretching can be substantially recovered, making muscle output appear to be artificially increased (5). For example, when grasping, the wrist positions itself for tenodesis of the finger flexor muscles to maintain a range of optimal muscle power output depending on the size of the object being grasped or pinched.

TENDON TRANSFERS FOR DESTROYED MUSCLE–TENDON UNITS

In many circumstances, a tendon transfer to restore function may be more feasible than trying to restore the normal system (Fig. 88.2). An example illustrating a frequent application of this fact is tendon transfer of an extensor pollicis longus tendon following a fracture of the distal radius (Fig. 88.3).

TENDON TRANSFERS FOR SPECIFIC PALSIES

Radial Nerve Palsies

Radial nerve losses are divided into high and low nerve disruptions. Low lesions are essentially posterior interosseous palsies, without loss of wrist extension. They demonstrate loss of thumb extension–abduction and finger extension at their metacarpophalangeal (MCP) joints, the intrinsic muscles providing interphalangeal extension. **The favored scheme of transfers for low radial nerve lesions is the flexor carpi ulnaris (FCU) to extensor digitorum communis (EDC), the extensor indicis longus (EIP), and the extensor pollicis longus (EPL) as a common unit.** With normal median- and ulnar-controlled antagonist muscles, independent action of each of these muscles' function is observed. The extensor digiti minimi is not included, unless there is no EDC slip to the small finger, as it results in excessive small finger abduction. Tension for each of the transfers is adjusted according to observation with wrist passive extension and flexion. An option is to repower the abductor pollicis longus (APL) with the palmaris, but I have yet to have a patient complain about APL loss. **Remember that simplicity generates good results.** If the FCU is unavailable for transfer, two finger superficial flexor muscles, not their tendons, can be brought through the interosseous membrane, using one for the thumb and the other for the combined fingers.

Extensors

High radial nerve palsies demonstrate the losses of low nerve lesions with the addition of total loss of active wrist extension as a result of paralysis of the extensor carpi radialis longus (ECRL) and brevis (ECRB). The ECRB is both the most central and the prime wrist extensor, so the transferred tendon is sutured into the ECRB. **Transfer of the median innervated pronator teres (PT) into the ECRB works so reliably that it is essentially a classic transfer for restoring active wrist extension** (Fig. 88.4). With the PT's insertion into the ECRB over the

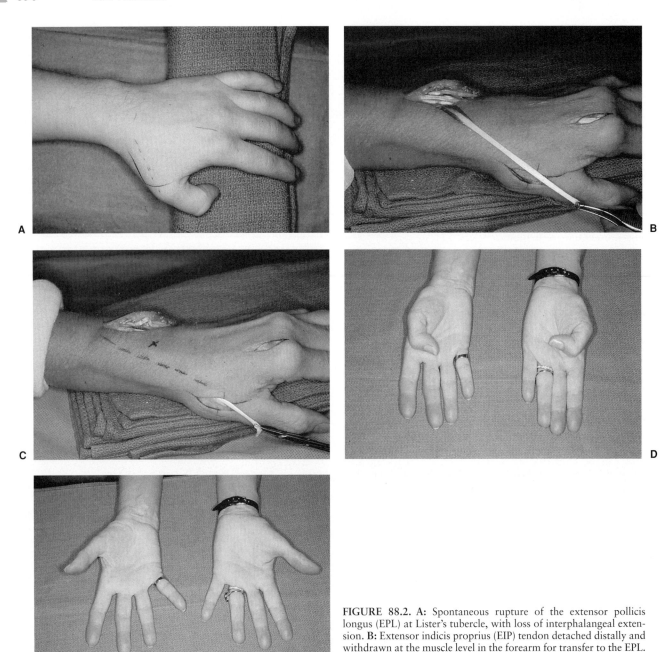

FIGURE 88.2. A: Spontaneous rupture of the extensor pollicis longus (EPL) at Lister's tubercle, with loss of interphalangeal extension. **B:** Extensor indicis proprius (EIP) tendon detached distally and withdrawn at the muscle level in the forearm for transfer to the EPL. **C:** EIP rerouted subcutaneously, avoiding friction against the Lister's tubercle. The tendons are joined in the soft subcutaneous tissue over the first metacarpal. **D, E:** Functional recovery of thumb extension.

radius superficial to its normal insertion, there is no loss of active forearm pronation as a result of this transfer.

Ulnar Nerve Palsies

Ulnar nerve lesions may be high or low, with the low lesions being of tremendous importance as there is interruption of innervation of all interosseous muscles and of the lumbricals of the ring and small fingers, as well as all intrinsic muscles of thumb adduction. Approximately 35% of patients have sufficient overlap in the thenar eminence from the median nerve so as not to be significantly troubled by weakened thumb adduction power. A "claw deformity" of hyperextension of MCP joints with flexion of the proximal interphalangeal (PIP) joints does not occur with the middle and index fingers, as their lumbrical muscles are median innervated. With weakened thumb

adduction, MCP hyperextension with a compensatory hyperflexion of the thumb's interphalangeal (IP) joint may be observed; that is, the Froment sign.

The difference between a high and a low ulnar palsy is that the high lesion has weakness of flexion of the distal joint of the small finger from denervation of its flexor digitorum profundus muscle. With median and radial innervated muscles functioning, loss of the FCU is not missed. The vast majority of ulnar nerve palsies occur at the elbow (cubital tunnel). Low lesions at the Guyon tunnel adjacent to the pisiform bone are not only rare, but almost unknown unless there has been direct trauma to that area.

With ulnar palsies there is paralysis of all interosseous muscles, lumbricals of the ring and small fingers, and muscles of thumb adduction. The clinical manifestation of thumb weakness of adduction varies greatly, depending on the amount of median nerve overlap into adductor muscle group.

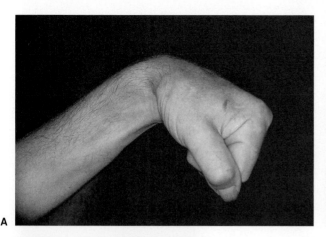
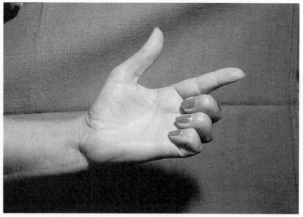

A

B

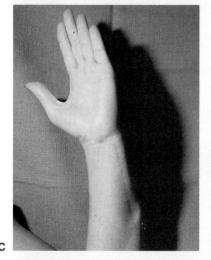
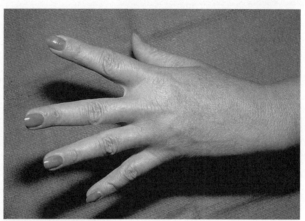

C

D

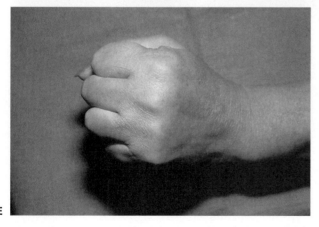

E

FIGURE 88.3. Tendon transfers for radial nerve palsy. **A:** High radial nerve palsy with paralysis of both wrist and digital extensor muscles. The pronator teres was transferred to the extensor carpi radialis brevis to restore wrist extension, and the flexor carpi ulnaris (FCU) was transferred to the combined extensor digitorum communis, extensor indicis proprius, and EPL. **B:** Motion is a result of the prime mover, the antagonist, and the stabilizers. After transfer of the FCU to the combined digital extensor, the index finger can point alone, as the antagonist (intact flexors) of the middle, ring, and small fingers prevent their extension. **C:** Restored wrist and digital extension. Note the long incision required to mobilize the FCU for dorsal transfer. **D, E:** Postoperative full, active extension and unimpaired digital flexion.

Approximately 35% of patients with complete ulnar palsy have sufficient median innervation to the superficial head of the flexor pollicis brevis for clinically satisfactory thumb adduction. **Tendon transfer for ulnar palsy to the fingers can be only incomplete, with restoration of MCP flexion and correction of "clawing," whereas the normal independent function of each interosseous muscle cannot be restored.** The best transfer to restore active MCP finger flexion is with the two slips of a superficial flexor being divided to provide four slips, one for each finger, passed anterior to the intercapsular (intermetacarpal) ligaments and inserted into the flexor tendon sheath's A-2 pulley. Inserting them into the interosseous tendons (lateral bands) alongside the proximal phalangeals risks excessive PIP exten-

sion and "swan neck" deformities, and putting them into bone is excessively traumatic (Fig. 88.5).

If thumb adduction power requires augmentation, this generally is done with transfer of a finger superficial flexor tendon. Ideally, the line of pull should be across the palm tangential to the thumb. The problem is that no functioning muscle lies sufficiently distal for this line of pull, so a tendon transfer has to be taken around a "pulley" for a 90-degree change of direction. **The best of the available compromises is to leave a finger superficial flexor in the carpal tunnel, using the distal edge of the transverse carpal ligament as a pulley.** This is not distal enough to be mechanically correct, but the power of those muscles is so great that a functional level of thumb adduction is restored.

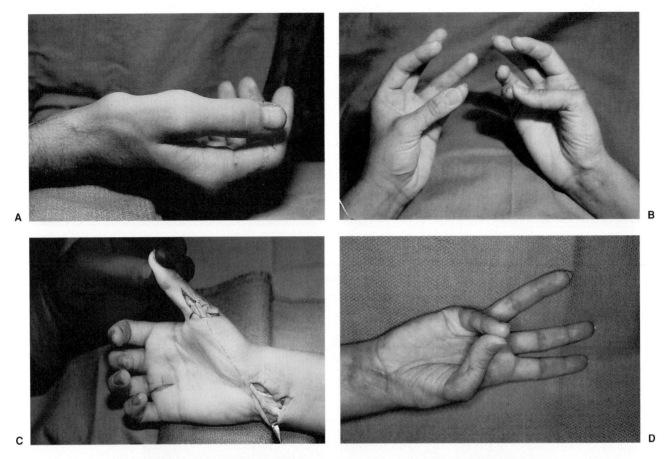

FIGURE 88.4. A: Thenar muscle opponens group atrophy from median nerve injury, without ulnar nerve thenar overlapping innervation. **B:** Opponens palsy seen on right prevents flat pulp-to-pulp opposition to finger pulp. **C:** Classic opponens transfer rerouting the superficial flexor tendon from the ring finger around the FCU (but not around the ulnar artery and nerve) to change its direction of pull to that of the paralyzed abductor pollicis brevis muscle. **D:** Postoperation illustration of restored thumb opposition and good pulp-to-pulp pinch.

Among other schemes advocated for thumb adduction is to carry a tendon graft dorsally, down between the metacarpals, into the palm, and across to the thumb. This is too complex, subject to tendon adhesion fixation, and rarely satisfactory.

Median Nerve Palsies

As with radial and ulnar nerve lesions, two types of lesions will be encountered, that of high and low levels.

Low Median Nerve Palsies

Functional impairment from a low median nerve lesion is predominantly loss of skin sensibility on the working surfaces of the thumb, index, middle, and adjacent side of the ring fingers. These are the areas needed for refined manipulations. The muscle loss of the thumb is that of positioning or opposition and there is a 35% probability of this not being a problem because of ulnar nerve overlap into the superficial head of the flexor pollicis brevis.

If augmentation of thumb opposition is needed, there are several satisfactory options available. The vector force for the three paralyzed muscles is along the abductor pollicis brevis (4). **The method most often used to restore thumb opposition is transfer of a ring or middle finger superficial flexor, rerouting it around the FCU at the pisiform for its change of direction, and**

carrying it subcutaneously over the paralyzed abductor pollicis brevis (APB) for a line of pull directly toward the pisiform (Fig. 88.4). The tendon must be passed around the FCU superficial to the ulnar artery and nerve to avoid compression. An alternative is to bring a finger superficial flexor from the carpal tunnel through a window cut in the transverse carpal ligament and then to the thumb. This procedure has a substantially greater risk of restrictive adhesions.

The major problem common to all schemes for restoration of thumb opposition is adequate pronation and rotation needed for a flat pulp-to-pulp pinch between the thumb and finger pads. Thumb pronation requires great power because the powerful ulnar innervated adductor pollicis is a thumb supinator. In an effort to resolve this problem many distal transfer insertions have been proposed, such as carrying the tendon transfer dorsally across thumb's proximal phalangeal base and inserting into the collateral ligament on the medial side of the MCP joint. Most often a flexor digitorum superficialis (FDS) tendon is used for these transfers, but others have been reported. The functionally independent EIP is excellent. Usually it is routed around the ulnar side of the wrist, but it can be brought through a large opening cut in the interosseous membrane. The abductor digiti quinti (ADQ) muscle can be mobilized on its intact neurovascular pellicle and transferred into the thenar eminence over the paralyzed APB, but the downside of this complex procedure is an unattractive mass across the base of the palm.

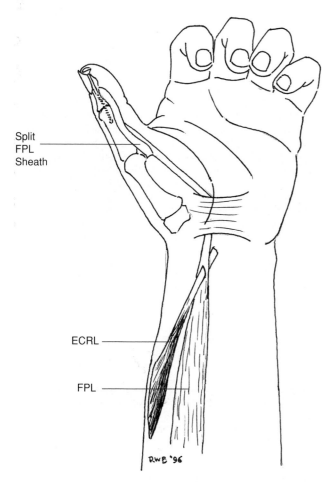

Split FPL Sheath

ECRL

FPL

RWB '96

FIGURE 88.5. Scheme for maximum use of the four muscles functioning distal to the elbow with C5–C6 tetraplegia. Less important joints are stabilized by arthrodesis. Available muscle power is transferred through normal routes. The scheme provides MCP flexion to initiate the finger flexion arc for small-object pinch, as well as independent PIP flexion to accommodate larger objects. Full active finger extension is independent of wrist motion—not an inefficient tenodesis system.

Perhaps the best solution to this problem of restoring good thumb pronation is to transfer the insertion of the deep head of the flexor pollicis brevis from the medial to the lateral side of the first MCP joint. Technically this is difficult, as it is conducted in a small and deep space and great care must be exercised not to injure one of the neurovascular bundles beneath which it is carried.

High Median Nerve Palsies

In addition to the losses of a low nerve lesion, high median nerve palsies involve paralysis of both superficial and deep interphalangeal flexors of the index and middle fingers and the IP joint of the thumb. **Interphalangeal flexion of the index and middle fingers can be restored by suturing their profundus tendons into that of the ring and small fingers, which are ulnar innervated.** If much greater power is needed, it can be provided by transfer of the ECRL to the group. **Excellent restoration of thumb IP flexion can be provided by transfer of the functionally independent EIP into the flexor pollicis longus (FPL).** The tendon junction should be in the forearm amid soft, mobile tissues.

High median nerve palsy also results in very weak forearm pronation. If this needs augmentation, the extensor carpi ulnaris (ECU) can be withdrawn from its sheath and rerouted anteriorly across the forearm and attached into the radius dor-

sally. Another option is to transfer the biceps insertion from the medial to the lateral side of the radius.

Tendon Transfers for Combined Nerve Palsies

Remember this basic principle: If function of any two of the hand's major nerves is lost, reconstruction approaching normal is absolutely precluded and any useful reconstruction requires a great simplification of mechanical design (8). Loss of critical skin sensibility with median nerve losses precludes ability for fine manipulations even if functional muscle rebalancing can be achieved. Although only combined median ulnar palsies are discussed here, the principles are applicable to other combinations.

Low Combined Median Ulnar Palsies

Restoring thumb opposition should be considered only if a good flexion–extension arc can be restored to the fingers. Such restoration requires active finger MCP flexion as a minimum, otherwise finger flexion will start at the distal interphalangeal (DIP) joints, with the fingers rolling up and their pads never facing that of the thumb in opposition. If these requirements cannot be met, it is far better to accept the simple scheme of the thumb adducting against the side of the fully flexed index finger, the "key pinch." However, with low lesions the valuable finger superficial flexors usually are available for tendon transfers. Having them available is a strong indication for their repair if severed in a classic anterior wrist laceration. Usually the FDS of the middle finger is large enough to be split into four slips, one restoring active MCP flexion to a finger for initiation on its flexion there. With combined median ulnar palsies the thumb has lost function of the median innervated muscle for its positioning and the ulnar innervated group for adduction power. In theory, a single tendon transfer along the vector line between these two groups should be useful, but in practice, it provides grossly inadequate power for usefulness. It is trying to do too much with too little. Many schemes to cope with this situation are possible but, generally, arthrodesis of the first MCP joint with carefully considered thumb projection is best and certainly the most reliable.

High Combined Median Ulnar Palsies

In addition to the losses of low lesions, those at a high level have loss of all finger and thumb flexion and sensibility to the critical working surfaced of the palmar skin. Tendon transfers results are very poor functionally, assisting at best. Having only radially innervated muscles with which to work, it is best to fuse the base of the thumb in a carefully selected projection from the palm and to concentrate available functioning muscles to restore finger motion. Several possibilities exist according to the exact situation, but MCP finger flexion usually can be restored by tendon grafts powered by the brachioradialis and interphalangeal finger flexion by transfer of the ECRL to the four-finger flexor digitorum profundus (FDP) tendons as a single unit. The thumb can be provided with independent IP flexion by the EIP. If forearm pronation needs augmentation, it can be provided by ECU transfer or by change of the biceps insertion from the medial to the lateral side of the radius.

HAND RECONSTRUCTION FOR PARALYSIS CAUSED BY SPINAL CORD INJURIES

C5–C6 is the highest level of spinal cord injury for which impressive reconstructions are possible (3). The important thing is the level of cord injury, which may vary considerably from the level of vertebral fractures. Patients with C5–C6 cord injuries have good shoulder control and strong elbow flexion by the biceps but no active elbow extension. Distal to the elbow they typically have only four functioning muscles. If only one muscle is functioning, it is the brachioradialis, followed by the pronator teres, then by the ECRL, and, finally, by the ECRB. If wrist extension is weak, the important ECRB will be weak, and to take the ECRL for a tendon transfer would be disastrous. Skin sensibility in both radial and median nerve distributions is usually not disturbed, but that of the ulnar nerve area is almost anesthetic. If only the brachioradialis is functioning, it can be useful if transferred to the ECRB to provide active wrist extension. Wrist arthrodesis is the last thing to consider for these patients.

When the cord lesion is lower than C5–C6, the digital extensors will be functioning and the situation is essentially that of combined median ulnar paralysis. There are two basic types of reconstruction for C5–C6 cord-injured patients: simple lateral pinch with the thumb and the more complex tripod-type reconstructions.

Key Pinch Reconstructions

Simple adduction of the thumb against the side of the fully flexed, and thus stable, index finger was championed by Moberg (9). It has the advantages of simplicity and predictability, and requires only a single operation. Yet pinch is weak; thumb extension–abduction is not active, but is by wrist tenodesis and it does not use the available functioning units to near their potential. The thumb IP joint is stabilized, either by arthrodesis or by putting a screw across it, and thumb adduction is provided by transfer of the ECRL into the paralyzed FPL. The proximal FPL sheath is opened so that the FPL "bowstrings" to increase its moment arm or force for thumb MCP joint flexion (Fig. 88.6).

Tripod-Type Reconstruction

The other basic type of reconstruction restores some precision-type pinch with thumb-finger pad approximations and generally some type of active finger grasping capability. Obviously there must be good median nerve skin sensibility for this type of reconstruction even to be considered. With four muscles functioning, it is possible to restore active finger extension without relying on wrist tenodesis.

Several designs are feasible, but space restraints here are such that I shall present the one I developed, which optimally uses the few available functioning units (3). It provides finger extension and flexion at both the MCP and PIP joint levels, independent of each other and without a requirement of wrist tenodesis. In addition, it creates the capability for small-object manipulations between the pads of the thumb and index-middle fingers. The downsides of the design are that it is complex, with little margin for error, and that it usually is done in three surgical stages: skeletal stabilization, restoration of flexor systems, and, finally, the extensor mechanisms (3). However, it should be feasible to combine the skeletal stabilization and extensor restoration stages together. In this design, the thumb is fixed by arthrodesis in a carefully planned projection from the palm so that its pad can be met by the pads of the remobilized index and middle fingers. The scheme is unique in that power is transferred through the tendons of paralyzed muscles free of adhesions as they are in their normal beds, and the MCP and PIP joint can be flexed independently to accommodate various-size objects. Full finger extension is independent of wrist movement. A composite illustration of the whole system is shown in Figure 89.5.

RESTORATION OF ACTIVE ELBOW EXTENSION

With paralysis of the triceps, the elbow is unstable and incapable of active extension. Restoration of these capabilities is helpful and generally feasible by extending the posterior deltoid muscle, using strong tendon grafts as substitutes for the triceps. The chief objection to this operation is that the elbow must be immobilized in full extension for 6 weeks, after which permissible flexion can be increased by only about 5 degrees per week.

POSTOPERATIVE MANAGEMENT FOR TENDON TRANSFERS

Transferred tendons must be protected carefully from disruption by rigid cast or splinting for at least 4 to 6 weeks, with the length of time being determined by the amount of stress to which they will be subject. This requires special efforts with children, as they promptly become uninhibited as soon as pain ceases. Flexor tendons require protective immobilization for

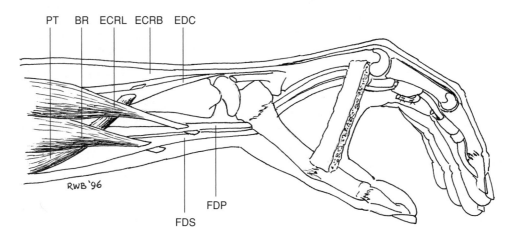

PT   BR   ECRL   ECRB   EDC

FDS

FDP

RWB '96

FIGURE 88.6. Scheme of the simple lateral "key pinch" (Moberg) for C5–C6 tetraplegia. Restored thumb adduction is against the side of the immobile index finger, which has sufficient lateral stability to serve as an anvil. Opening is by wristdrop tenodesis of the EPL attached to the radius proximal to the wrist joint.

3 to 4 weeks, after which active but unresisted movement is encouraged. In general, extensor systems require longer protection not because they heal differently, but because their antagonists are the powerful flexors. No transfer should be submitted to full stress for at least 8 weeks after the transfer.

RE-EDUCATION OF TRANSFERRED MUSCLES

The difficulty of "re-educating" into use of a tendon transfer is inversely related to the usefulness of the new arrangement. Most tendon transfers that have been well-considered and skillfully done almost immediately and automatically function at their new task with no "re-education." This is readily understandable if one considers that the normal control system is basically an extremely rapid "trial-and-error" operation that is guided by constant monitoring of progress toward desired goals. If progress is unsatisfactory, the cortex will recruit other muscle combinations until the desired results occur. A patient with loss of sensory feedback who is blindfolded to block visual input will have illegible handwriting because of their loss of a critical link in the muscle control system.

References

1. Beasley RW. Principles of tendon transfers. *Orthop Clin North Am.* 1970; 1:433.
2. Beasley RW. Tendon transfers for radial nerve palsy. *Orthop Clin North Am.* 1970;1–439.
3. Beasley RW. Surgical treatment of hands for C5-6 tetraplegia. *Orthop Clin North Am.* 1983;14893.
4. Brand P. Tendon transfers for median and ulnar paralysis. *Orthop Clin North Am.* 1970;1–447.
5. Brand P. Tendon transfer reconstruction for radial, ulnar, median and combined paralysis. Principles and techniques. In: McCarthy J, ed. *Plastic Surgery.* Philadelphia: WB Saunders; 1990 .
6. Litter JW. Tendon transfers and arthrodesis is combined median and ulnar nerve paralysis. *J Bone Joint Surg.* 1949;31A:225.
7. Littler JW, Cooley S. Opposition of the thumb and its restoration by abductor digiti quinti transfer. *J Bone Joint Surg.* 1963;45A:1389.
8. Littler JW. Restoration of power and stability to the partially paralyzed hand. In: Converse JM, ed. *Reconstructive Plastic Surgery.* Philadelphia: WB Saunders; 1979.
9. Moberg E. The current state of surgical rehabilitation of the upper limb in tetraplegia. *Paraplegia.* 1987;25:351.

CHAPTER 89 ■ CONGENITAL HAND ABNORMALITIES

MIHYE CHOI, SHEEL SHARMA, AND OTWAY LOUIE

Congenital hand anomalies vary over a spectrum from scarcely noticeable to an absent upper extremity. It is incumbent on the surgeon to decide if further work-up is required for associated anomalies, if surgical intervention is necessary, and what the timing of surgery should be. This chapter presents an overview of the relevant embryology, classification, and treatment of the most common congenital hand abnormalities.

EMBRYOLOGY

The upper limb buds form on the lateral wall of the embryo 4 weeks after fertilization. These buds consist of mesodermal cells covered by ectoderm, and develop into a complete limb under the guidance of three signaling centers: (a) the apical ectodermal ridge (AER); (b) the zone of polarizing activity (ZPA); and (c) the nonridge ectoderm. Each controls growth and patterning along a specific orthogonal axis.

The apical ectodermal ridge is located at the distal aspect of the developing limb and is required for growth in a proximal-to-distal direction. Removal of the AER results in growth arrest and a truncated limb. Moreover, the earlier the AER is removed, the more proximal the defect.

The zone of polarizing activity is a group of mesodermal cells at the posterior limb bud, which functions in anterior-to-posterior limb development. Transplantation of posterior cells to the anterior border of the normal limb results in a mirror duplication of the limb. The ZPA cells act through the Sonic hedgehog (*Shh*) gene (1).

The nonridge ectoderm, also known as the Wingless-type (Wnt) signaling center, controls patterning in the dorsal–ventral axis. It is required for alignment of the limb in a dorsal orientation (dorsalization).

CLASSIFICATION

Although multiple classification schemes of upper limb abnormalities exist, the most widely accepted is that of Swanson (Table 89.1), which categorizes congenital hand abnormalities based on their embryologic origin as well as their clinical manifestation. It has been accepted by the American Society for Surgery of the Hand, as well as the International Federation of Societies for Surgery of the Hand.

Failure of Formation of Parts (Developmental Arrest)

Failure of formation can be transverse or longitudinal. Transverse arrests result in truncated limbs at various levels, most commonly at the midforearm. Generally, there is no role for surgical intervention and, with unilateral involvement, these children seldom require prostheses. Rarely, distraction lengthening and phalangeal transfer may be indicated. More recently, toe-to-hand transfers have been performed.

There are four kinds of longitudinal arrest: preaxial, postaxial, central, and intercalary. Preaxial and postaxial arrest leads to the radial and ulnar club hand, respectively. Central arrest leads to a cleft hand. Intercalary arrest leads to phocomelia, where an intervening segment of limb is absent.

Preaxial Deficiency: Radial Club Hand

Radial dysplasias occur in 1 in 55,000 births. They are typically sporadic and unilateral, more common in males, and more common on the right side. Radial dysplasias are commonly associated with syndromes including Fanconi anemia, thrombocytopenia absent radius (TAR) syndrome, Holt-Oram syndrome (associated with cardiac septal defects), and VATER (vertebral abnormality, anal imperforation, tracheoesophageal fistula, radial, ray, or renal anomalies vertebral, anus, tracheoesophageal, radial, and renal abnormalities) syndrome (2,3). **The presence of these syndromes *must* be evaluated prior to any surgical reconstruction.**

The clinical manifestation of radial club hand is a shortened forearm with radial deviation at the wrist. The pathology affects all structures on the preaxial side of the limb: skeleton, musculotendinous units, joints, neurovascular structures, and soft tissues.

Based on the severity of the deformity, Bayne and Klug classified radial dysplasia into four categories (4) (Table 89.2).

Functional Considerations. In radial aplasia, the carpus lacks support from the distal radius, and the ulna is inadequate to provide stability. This causes the wrist to deviate radially. The forearm flexors worsen the radial deviation and the unopposed action of the wrist and finger flexors cause palmar displacement. The flexor muscles are short, stiff, and often fibrotic. The radial nerve and vessels are deficient and the median nerve is often subluxed toward the concave side. The ulna is also always deficient. Prehension is abnormal, caused by the deficiency of the thumb.

Management. Early manipulation emphasizing elbow flexion and ulnar deviation of the wrist is taught to the parents. Mild type I dysplasia may only require splinting. After evaluation for associated anomalies, surgical options are considered. In types I and II dysplasia with an unstable wrist, distraction lengthening of the radius is recommended. Centralization or radialization are the treatments of choice in severe type II, and in types III and IV; repair should be performed at 6 to 12 months of age. Preoperative splinting to achieve passive flexion of the elbow should be performed. In centralization, the angulation in the forearm is corrected by freeing the distal ulna, cutting a corresponding slot in the carpus, and stabilizing the wrist by passing a pin from the third metacarpal

TABLE 89.1

SWANSON CLASSIFICATION OF CONGENITAL UPPER LIMB ABNORMALITIES

I. Failure of Formation of Parts
Transverse
Longitudinal
   Radial club hand
   Cleft hand
   Ulnar club hand
   Phocomelia
II. Failure of Differentiation or Separation of Parts
Synostosis
Radial head dislocation
Symphalangism
Syndactyly
Contracture
   Arthrogryposis
   Trigger finger
   Clasped thumb
   Camptodactyly
   Clinodactyly
   Windblown hand
   Kirner deformity
III. Duplication
Polydactyly
IV. Overgrowth
Macrodactyly
V. Undergrowth
Thumb hypoplasia
Madelung deformity
VI. Congenital Constriction Ring Syndrome
VII. Generalized Skeletal Abnormalities and Syndromes

to the ulna. A complementary tendon transfer of the radial flexor-extensor mass to the extensor carpi ulnaris is performed (Fig. 89.1). In radialization, the distal ulna is aligned with the second metacarpal and a dynamic transfer of the flexor–extensor mass from its insertion to the radial side of the carpus is performed (5). The key to the success of the operation lies in the rebalancing of forces by tendon transfers. For associated severe thumb hypoplasia or aplasia, pollicization is considered, usually 6 months after centralization or radialization.

TABLE 89.2

CLASSIFICATION OF RADIAL DYSPLASIA

	Type	Characteristics
I	Short radius	Radius has a normal appearance but is shorter than the ulna
II	Hypoplastic radius	Distal and proximal epiphyses present but defective hypoplastic radius
III	Partial absence of radius	The proximal, middle, or distal portion of the radius is absent
IV	Total absence of radius	The most severe and common type

Postaxial Deficiency: Ulnar Club Hand

Compared to radial deficiency, the incidence of ulnar ray deficiency is quite rare, with the incidence varying between 1 per 100,000 and 7.4 per 100,000 live births (6). Typically, the defect is more common in males, unilateral, and left-sided. Unlike radial club hand, it is rarely associated with defects in other organs. Although the cause of ulnar ray deficiency is unknown, it is hypothesized by Cole and Manske to be a defect in the zone of polarizing activity.

The anatomic findings in ulnar ray deficiency include a short, bowed radius with a hypoplastic or absent ulna. The Bayne classification is the most commonly used (Table 89.3).

Because of the small number of patients with ulnar ray deficiency, a consensus on the ideal treatment has not been reached. Hand deformities should be treated, as improvement in function may result. Excision of the ulna anlage, which theoretically could remove an ulnar deviating force, has been promoted by some, and discouraged by others. Creation of a one-bone forearm for types I and II can stabilize and improve function in those with a hypoplastic ulna. Humeral osteotomy remains an option for those with radiohumeral synostosis (7).

Central Deficiency: Cleft Hand

A longitudinal deficiency of the central rays results in cleft hand. Cleft hands are classified as typical or atypical.

The typical cleft hand contains a deep V-shaped central defect secondary to hypoplasia of the long ray. The defect is typically bilateral and inherited. Association with foot clefts is common. In contrast, atypical clefts present as a U-shaped defect secondary to absence of the index, long, and ring fingers. They are unilateral and inheritance sporadic. Association with foot clefts are relatively rare; however, atypical clefts have been documented in Poland syndrome. Atypical clefts are now known to be a form of symbrachydactyly.

Snow and Littler described the original technique for correcting typical clefts. The index ray is transposed into the central defect, deepening the first web space. A palmar-based skin flap is then used to recreate the first web space. More recently, Upton modified this technique to avoid problems with necrosis of the narrow-based palmar flap. He described a circumferential incision around the base of the index finger, with extensions radially and ulnarly at the level of the new digitopalmar flexion crease. After wide exposure, the first dorsal interosseus muscle is released, the index finger transposed, and the transverse intermetacarpal ligament recreated.

Intercalary Deficiency: Phocomelia

Intercalary arrest results in phocomelia, where an intervening segment of the limb is absent. The arm or forearm may be missing, with a normal hand. The use of thalidomide in the first trimester of pregnancy resulted in a marked increase in this deformity. Surgery is usually not indicated.

Failure of Separation or Differentiation of Parts

Syndactyly

Syndactyly is one of the most common congenital hand deficiencies, with an incidence of 1 per 2,000 to 2,500 live births. There is a strong familial tendency: 10% to 40% cases are inherited as a result of a dominant gene with variable penetrance. Males are affected twice as frequently as females. The third web is the most commonly involved, followed by the fourth and second webs. Association with Poland or Apert syndrome is common. The embryologic etiology of syndactyly is thought

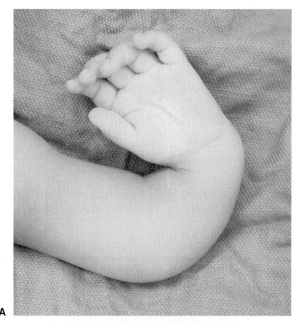

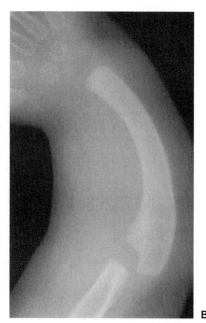

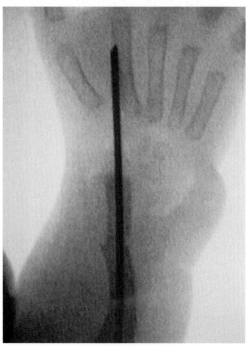

FIGURE 89.1. Radial Club Hand. **A:** Preoperative photograph. **B:** Preoperative radiograph. **C:** Radialization. The second metacarpal was placed in alignment with the ulna, with a retrograde Kirschner wire holding fixation. A corrective osteotomy of the ulna shaft was performed.

to be related to (a) failure of digital patterning, (b) failure of apoptosis, or (c) failure of AER regression.

Fusion can be limited to skin and soft tissue (simple), or include bone (complex). It may involve either the entire digit (complete), or a portion of the finger (incomplete). Complicated syndactyly refers to complex cases that involve some degree of synostosis. Finally, acrosyndactyly refers to fusion of the distal tips of the digits.

Timing of Surgery. Separation as early as 6 months is indicated when syndactyly involves digits of unequal length (i.e., the ring and little fingers). Early separation is also required in complex syndactyly and cases of acrosyndactyly. The timing of all other cases of syndactyly remains somewhat controversial; most advocate surgical correction before age 18 months, whereas others prefer to wait until after this age.

The principles of correction include (a) separation of the digits, (b) creation of a web space, (c) skin coverage, and (d) immobilization.

Separation is carried out via dorsal and volar zigzag incisions creating interdigitating flaps (Fig. 89.2). The nail fusion can be corrected by opposing Z-flaps as described by Buck-Gramcko. After making the incisions, the neurovascular bundles are identified prior to completing the separation. The web can be created using either a large dorsal flap or double opposing triangular flaps from dorsal and volar aspects. The flaps are then interdigitated. There will always be residual raw areas both proximally and on the sides of digits; these should be grafted with skin obtained from the groin crease. To avoid vascular compromise to a single digit, it is critical that separation should not be performed simultaneously on adjacent webs. The authors recommend immobilizing the child's arm in an above-elbow cast until the grafts heal.

Complex syndactyly is a feature of Apert syndrome (see Chapter 25). The Apert hand can be classified into three categories as shown in Table 89.4.

TABLE 89.3

CLASSIFICATION OF ULNAR DEFICIENCY

Type	Characteristics
I Hypoplasia of the ulna	Presence of distal and proximal ulnar epiphysis
II Partial aplasia of the ulna	Absence of the distal or middle one third of the ulna
III Total aplasia of the ulna	Complete absence of the ulna
IV Radiohumeral synostosis	Synostosis of radius to humerus

Types I and II Apert hands should be corrected in two stages: in the first stage, the position of the thumb is corrected with an osteotomy and a three-finger hand is created by separating the second and fourth webs. The second stage involves separation of the remaining digits. The timing of correction of the synostosis between the fourth and fifth metacarpal is disputable. Type 3 deformities may be accompanied with recurrent nail infections, and thus may require separation of the nail prior to formal syndactyly correction.

Symphalangism

Symphalangism is failure of differentiation of the interphalangeal joint. Although the distal interphalangeal joint can be involved, symphalangism of the proximal interphalangeal joint is more common. Inheritance is autosomal dominant. Anatomically, there is no joint capsule. On radiographs, a clear joint space is seen, although ankylosis can appear after adolescence.

The most commonly affected digit is the little finger, followed by the ring, long, and index fingers, respectively. Treatment is usually not required as the hand with isolated symphalangism functions quite well; surgical options include arthrodesis to obtain a more functional position. Arthroplasty and free vascularized joint transfers have also been performed.

Congenital Trigger Thumb

In trigger thumb, there is an inability to extend the interphalangeal joint. A nodule is palpable over the flexor aspect of the metacarpophalangeal joint (Notta node). This differs from a *clasped thumb* in which the metacarpophalangeal joint is also affected.

Spontaneous resolution of the triggering can occur in a third of the affected children by 1 year of age. However, surgical correction is recommended before the age of 3 years so as to avoid any deformity. Treatment involves division of the A-1 pulley, confirming full mobility of the interphalangeal joint at the operation. The digital nerves should be carefully identified.

Clinodactyly

Clinodactyly is defined as curvature of a digit in a radioulnar plane. The most common form is radial deviation of the little finger at the distal interphalangeal (DIP) joint. It occurs as a result of the presence of a *delta phalanx*, a trapezoid-shaped middle phalanx resulting from an abnormal epiphysis. Clinodactyly rarely interferes with function, and treatment is not indicated for aesthetic reasons. In cases of severe angulation with functional problems, a wedge osteotomy can be performed to correct the deformity, but not before 5 to 6 years of age, when the bones are reasonable in size.

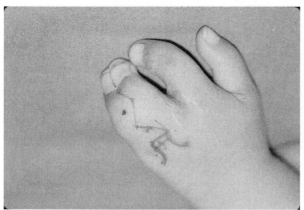

A

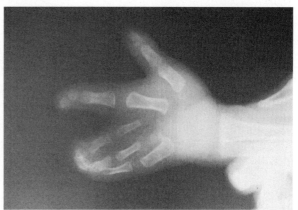

B

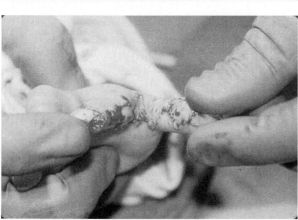

C

FIGURE 89.2. Syndactyly. **A:** Preoperative markings for Brunner incisions in a case of syndactyly. **B:** Radiograph showing complex complete syndactyly. **C:** Postoperative result after release.

Camptodactyly

Camptodactyly is congenital flexion deformity of the proximal interphalangeal joint. The little finger is most commonly involved. There are two types: one that appears in infancy with an equal sex incidence and a second that presents in adolescent girls. Function is rarely impaired, and patients mostly seek consultation regarding its appearance. Skin shortening, tight retinaculum cutis, short sublimis, abnormal lumbricals, lateral band adhesions, central slip anomalies, and bony defects can all be present in these cases. The *extensor deficit* should be measured with the metacarpophalangeal joint in extension and flexion to rule out intrinsic tightness. Splinting may be attempted to correct the deformity. Surgical correction is only indicated in a rapidly progressing deformity. Skin shortage is treated with Z-plasties. The abnormal retinaculum and lateral bands are freed from the phalanx. A short sublimis is lengthened and any abnormal lumbrical insertion is released. An extensor tendon transfer has also been suggested for extensor deficits.

Duplications

Polydactyly can occur either as an isolated malformation or as part of a syndrome. There are at least 119 disorders that contain polydactyly: 97 are syndromic, and 22 are nonsyndromic.

TABLE 89.4

APERT HAND ABNORMALITIES

Type	Characteristics
I	Thumb and little fingers are free; other digits form a central mass
II	Only the thumb is free; there is a central digital mass with a common nail and fourth web syndactyly, the so-called spade deformity
III	The rosebud hand, in which the thumb and the digital mass are fused together and share a common nail

For simplification, these subgroups of congenital hand anomalies can be divided into (a) radial (preaxial), (b) central, and (c) ulnar (postaxial). Mixed polydactyly refers to simultaneous radial and ulnar polydactyly, whereas crossed polydactyly occurs with involvement of both hands and feet.

Radial Polydactyly

The incidence of radial polydactyly is approximately 0.08 per 1,000 live births, and is exemplified by thumb duplication. The Wassel classification scheme is the most commonly used (Fig. 89.3).

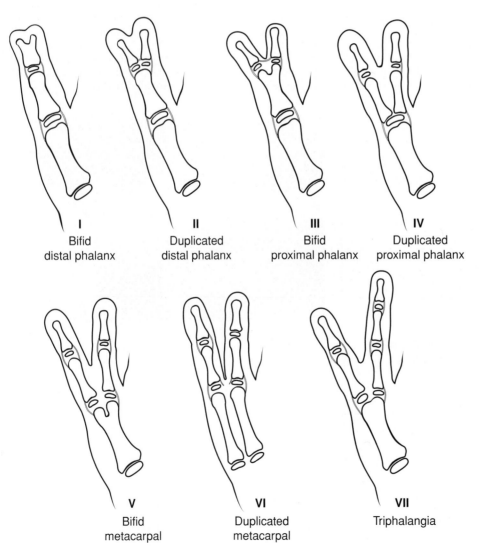

I
Bifid distal phalanx

II
Duplicated distal phalanx

III
Bifid proximal phalanx

IV
Duplicated proximal phalanx

V
Bifid metacarpal

VI
Duplicated metacarpal

VII
Triphalangia

FIGURE 89.3. Thumb duplication: Wassel classification.

Types I and II Wassel thumbs can be treated by removal of one of the duplicate thumbs or the Bilhaut-Cloquet procedure, which consists of excision of the central wedge of the duplicated thumb segment and bringing the remaining segments together (8). Type IV is the most common (43%). Treatment involves ablation of the radial thumb, followed by reconstruction of the radial collateral ligament and intrinsic thenar tendons (Fig. 89.4). Type VII triphalangeal thumbs are treated with the goal of retaining the most functional thumb, regardless of whether it is tri- or biphalangeal.

Central Polydactyly

Included within the term *central polydactyly* are duplications of the index, long, and ring fingers. Inheritance is autosomal dominant. The supernumerary digit is often fused to its adjacent digit. Odd transverse phalanges bridging two adjacent digits have been described. Surgical treatment of central polydactyly can be difficult and the results often suboptimal. The goal is to ablate the duplicated digit with augmentation of the retained digit. Given the complex nature of these deformities, multiple operations are often required.

Ulnar Polydactyly

Temtamy and McKusick divided ulnar polydactyly into well-developed (type A) and rudimentary (type B). Type A is a well-formed supernumerary digit, whereas type B is typically a small and pedunculated skin tag. There is a male predominance and a higher prevalence in African Americans (9). True type A digits require operative amputation, with reconstruction of key structures (i.e., ulnar collateral ligament and ab-

ductor digiti minimi). Type B skin tags can be ligated in the nursery.

Overgrowth or Gigantism

Macrodactyly, or digital gigantism, refers to the enlargement of all elements of an involved digit. Lipofibromatous hamartomas, with excessive fat in all tissues, are characteristic. Single or multiple digits can be involved; the index finger is most frequently affected. The defect is more common in males and the majority of cases are unilateral. Two forms exist: (a) static, where there is enlargement at birth with subsequent proportionate growth, and (b) progressive, where there is increasingly disproportionate enlargement with age.

Children presenting early with mild enlargement are candidates for debulking and epiphysiodesis to arrest skeletal growth. Untreated patients who present later in childhood are more difficult to manage, often requiring shortening and debulking. Distal amputation may be required for severe cases.

Undergrowth or Hypoplasia (Hypoplastic thumb)

The hypoplastic thumb fails to extend to the midaspect of the proximal phalanx of the index finger. It can occur as an isolated deformity, or as part of a broader radial deficiency. Functional limitations in pinch and grasp can result, depending on the severity of the defect. The classification system of Blauth is most commonly used (Table 89.5).

The critical determinant in choosing between reconstruction and ablation is the presence of a carpometacarpal joint. A

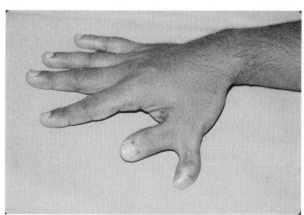

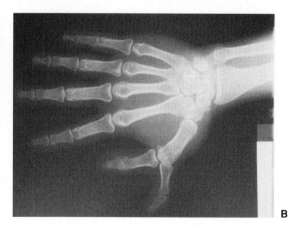

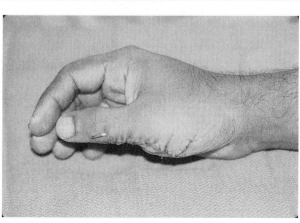

FIGURE 89.4. Thumb duplication. **A:** Duplicated thumb. **B:** Type IV duplicated proximal phalanx. **C:** Postoperative result after excision of the more hypoplastic digit and reconstruction of the remaining digit.

TABLE 89.5

BLAUTH CLASSIFICATION OF HYPOPLASTIC THUMB

Type	Characteristics
I	Mild hypoplasia, all structures present
II	Absence of thenar muscles
III	Absence of thenar muscles, abnormal extrinsic tendons, and skeletal hypoplasia: subdivided into presence of (a) stable carpometacarpal joint and (b) unstable carpometacarpal joint
IV	Pouce flottant; the floating thumb
V	Total aplasia of the thumb

stable basal joint allows reconstruction, whereas an unstable or absent carpometacarpal joint requires ablation. Type I defects rarely require operative intervention. Type II defects can be treated with opponensplasty, release of the first web space, and ulnar collateral ligament reconstruction. Type IIIA defects can be managed similarly, with the addition of extensor tendon transfers. Types IIIB, IV, and V defects are treated with pollicization (10).

Pollicization repositions the index finger to act as a thumb. The ulnar neurovascular bundle to the index finger is freed by ligating the radial artery to the long finger. The A-1 and A-2 pulleys are divided, releasing the flexor tendons, and the extensor tendons are mobilized by dividing any junctura. The metacarpal is divided, and the index finger rotated 150 degrees into pronation and 40 degrees into abduction. The metacarpal head is rotated 70 degrees, and fixed to its base using ab-

sorbable sutures. The interosseous muscles are attached to the lateral bands of the extensor mechanism.

Congenital Constriction Band Syndrome

The incidence of congenital constriction band syndrome is 1 per 15,000. Inheritance is sporadic, although association with other anomalies, such as club feet or cleft lip and palate, has been described. The etiology remains unknown; both extrinsic (i.e., constricting amniotic band) and intrinsic causes have been proposed.

The clinical presentation varies greatly. Anything from shallow grooves in the skin to complete amputations can be found. Patterson classified constriction bands into four types: (a) simple constrictions only; (b) constrictions with distal deformity; (c) constrictions with fusion of distal parts (acrosyndactyly); and (d) intrauterine amputation (11).

Treatment varies depending on the extent of the deformity. Mild simple constrictions may not require any treatment. More severe simple constrictions, as well as those with distal deformity, can be treated with Z-plasty (Fig. 89.5). The procedure is staged, with only half the circumference corrected at the first operation to prevent vascular compromise. The remaining constriction is corrected at a second operation. Those with acrosyndactyly are treated early; separation of the fused digits allows unimpeded growth. Management of intrauterine amputations is tailored to the deformity. A functional amputation may not require surgical intervention. Distraction lengthening with bone grafts and toe-to-hand transfers have been performed for severe defects. Fetoscopic lysis of amniotic bands has been performed in utero (12).

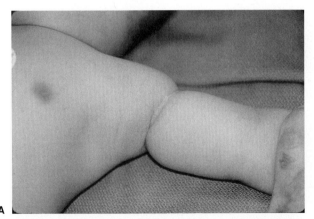

A

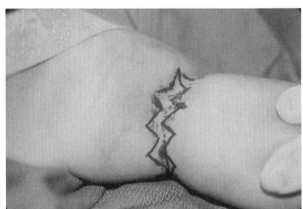

B

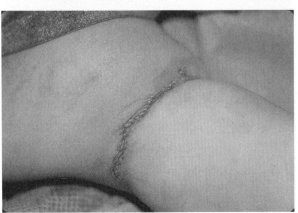

C

FIGURE 89.5. Constriction band syndrome. **A:** Simple constriction ring. **B:** Preoperative markings for release. **C:** Postoperative result after release.

References

1. Riddle RD, Johnson RL, Laufer E, et al. Sonic hedgehog mediates the polarizing activity of the ZPA. Cell. 1993;75:1401–1416.
2. Smith PJ.In: *Lister's The Hand: Diagnosis and Indications*. 4th ed. Churchill Livingstone; 2002: 457.
3. Flatt AE.In: *The Care of Congenital Hand Anomalies*. 2nd ed. St. Louis: Quality Medical Publishing: 1994.
4. Bayne LG, Klug MS. Long-term review of the surgical treatment of radial deficiencies. *J Hand Surg.* 1987;12A(2):169–179.
5. Buck-Gramcko D. Radialization as a new treatment for radial club hand. *J Hand Surg* [Am]. 1985;10:964–968.
6. Froster UG, Baird PA. Upper limb deficiencies and associated malformations: a population based study. *Am J Med Genet.* 1985;1:499–510.
7. Miller JK, Wenner SM, Kruger LM. Ulnar deficiency. *J Hand Surg* [Am]. 1986;11:822–829.
8. Bilhaut M. Guerison d'un pounce bifide par un nouveau procede operatoire. *Congres Francais de Chir.* 1890;4:576.
9. Rayan GM, Frey B. Ulnar polydactyly. *Plast Reconstr Surg.* 2001;107:1449.
10. Kozin SH. Upper-extremity congenital anomalies. *J Bone Joint Surg Am.* 2003;85:1564–1576.
11. Patterson TS. Congenital ring constrictions. *Br J Plast Surg.* 1961;14: 1.
12. Quintero RA, Morales WJ, Philips J, et al. In utero lysis of amniotic bands. *Ultrasound Obstet Gynecol.* 1997;10:316–320.

CHAPTER 90 ■ DUPUYTREN'S DISEASE

M. FELIX FRESHWATER

Unlike the patient seeking cosmetic surgery, a patient rarely arrives in a plastic surgeon's office stating, "I have Dupuytren's disease and want surgery as soon as possible." More commonly, the patient is concerned about the malignant potential of a palmar thickening or mass, or about the inexorable contracture of one or more digits that is interfering with function. The initial consultation provides the plastic surgeon with the opportunity to educate the patient about his disease and treatment choices.

This chapter discusses Dupuytren's disease and includes current theories about the etiology, pathologic anatomy, available surgical treatment, expected results, and attendant complications.

NORMAL ANATOMY

In the past three decades, we have learned much about the normal anatomy of the palmar fascia. This is primarily a result of the anatomic work of Stack and McGrouther. Stack studied cross-sectional anatomy in fetuses. McGrouther dissected a series of fresh and preserved cadavers with Dupuytren's disease using an operating microscope with magnification up to 10× power. He discovered that the palmar fascia was composed of a three-dimensional matrix of transverse, longitudinal, and vertical skin ligaments. McGrouther hypothesized that this matrix enables the skin on the working surface of the hand to better withstand compressive and shear forces while still allowing the digits to move (Fig. 90.1).

PATHOLOGIC ANATOMY

McGrouther was able to correlate the nodules, pits, cords, and joint contractures that extended from the palm into the phalanges.

Dupuytren's Disease versus Dupuytren's Contracture

Dupuytren's disease is the development of scar tissue in the palm and digits. This scar tissue is different from ordinary scar tissue because it contains proportionally more immature type 3 collagen than normally occurring type 1 collagen, which is found in the palmar fascia. Initially, pits or nodules of scar tissue develop in the palm, but most progress to form cords of scar tissue that involve digits as well as the first web space. The cords result in contraction of the metacarpophalangeal joint. As they progress, the proximal interphalangeal joints contract with hyperextension of the distal interphalangeal joints, resulting in a pseudoboutonnière deformity. McFarlane described three types of pathologic cords: the pretendinous cord that develops from the pretendinous band; the lateral cord that develops from the lateral sheet; and the spiral cord that is caused by the confluence of the pretendinous band with the spiral band and lateral

digital sheet. The spinal cord wraps around the neurovascular bundle, placing it at greater risk during surgery.

The first web space cord can cause an adduction contracture of the thumb. When the cords of scar tissue result in joint stiffness, the process is called Dupuytren's contracture.

We know that pits or nodules form in the palm and can rest peacefully for years or, over the course of time, they can progress to the formation of cords that extend into the digits.

Myofibroblasts are found in all stages of Dupuytren's disease. Chiu and McFarlane believe that contractile elements in the myofibroblasts that contain α smooth muscle actin adhere to each other via desmosomal attachments on each cell wall. However, myofibroblasts alone cannot explain the degree of contracture that develops in Dupuytren's disease let alone in Dupuytren's contracture. The effect of mechanical compression of scar tissue has been hypothesized to result in its hypertrophy. This theory has been supported by recent tissue culture research suggesting that Dupuytren's disease fibroblasts have a delayed response to achieving tensional homeostasis. Regression of Dupuytren's contracture via the release of tension in the cords has been described and is part of the rationale for various treatment modalities.

WHO IS AT RISK FOR DEVELOPING DUPUYTREN'S DISEASE?

Dupuytren's disease has a genetic predisposition. The population at greatest risk for Dupuytren's disease is of northern European descent. It is extremely rare in black patients. A landmark epidemiologic study was performed by Mikkelsen in 1969, in a small, isolated, Norwegian coastal town. Almost 16,000 of the town's 27,000 inhabitants older than age 16 years were examined. The prevalence of Dupuytren's disease was 10.5% for men and 3.1% for women. However, the ratio of men to women uniformly decreased from 8:1 in the 40- to 44-year-old age group to 1:1 in the 85- to 89-year-old age group. The International Federation of Societies for Surgery of the Hand (IFSSH) undertook an epidemiologic study of 1,150 patients who consulted hand surgeons worldwide. Among the conclusions of this study were the following:

■ The typical patient was a 57-year-old male with a 10-year history of Dupuytren's disease.
■ The disease was bilateral with one hand being more severe, and severity being unrelated to hand dominance.
■ The patient is unlikely to admit any diathesis factors.
■ In females, the disease had a later onset and was less severe.
■ Japanese had later onset, fewer diathesis factors, and less-severe disease.
■ Unilateral disease was less severe.
■ Alcoholism and epilepsy were associated with more severe disease, trauma was associated with less severe disease.

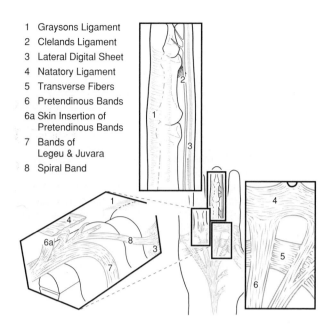

1 Graysons Ligament
2 Clelands Ligament
3 Lateral Digital Sheet
4 Natatory Ligament
5 Transverse Fibers
6 Pretendinous Bands
6a Skin Insertion of
   Pretendinous Bands
7 Bands of
   Legeu & Juvara
8 Spiral Band

FIGURE 90.1. Anatomy of the palmar and digital fascia. A thorough knowledge of the anatomy of the palmar and digital fascia in the normal palm and finger is essential for an understanding of the patterns of anatomic distortion in the hand with Dupuytren's contracture.

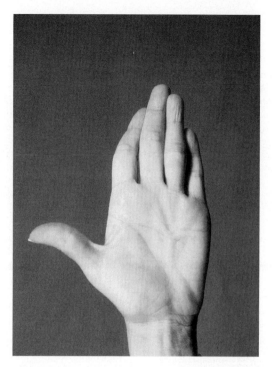

FIGURE 90.2. Case report of traumatic palmar fasciitis. This now 54-year-old female court reporter fell while jogging 17 years prior to this photograph. She developed a hematoma at the intersection of her fourth ray with the proximal palmar crease. The hematoma was replaced by a painful palmar mass that was diagnosed by an orthopedic surgeon as a "ganglion." Eventually the pain resolved; however, 10 years later the patient developed the bands that are visible in the photograph. They are asymptomatic and do not interfere with her ability to consistently report verbatim more than 250 words per minute.

Other factors have been implicated in the development of Dupuytren's disease, including alcoholism, drug therapy for epilepsy, diabetes, and smoking. It is thought that these factors are related to their respective metabolic effects. Repetitive trauma, however, has not been implicated as a cause. A single traumatic event can cause traumatic palmar fascitis (TPF) in some patients with a genetic predisposition (Fig. 90.2). TPF is histologically indistinguishable from Dupuytren's disease. Factors that distinguish traumatic palmar fascitis from Dupuytren's disease include the following:

- TPF can result from a relatively trivial palmar wound or blunt trauma.
- TPF occurs in young patients.
- TPF progresses unpredictably, but can occur within days of the event.
- The lesion from TPF is often painful, sometimes burning, and fails to respond to either systemic or locally injected steroids.
- TPF has a high incidence of postsurgical recurrence.

Recently research has focused on the exact genetic mechanism for the development of the disease with involvement of the Zf9 transcription factor gene that increases transforming growth factor-beta 1 (TGF-β_1), a cytokine that stimulates fibroblast proliferation and extracellular matrix deposition.

THE INITIAL CONSULTATION

A pertinent history is mandatory. As previously noted, the patient usually presents with one of two chief complaints caused by Dupuytren's disease. Either the patient has a nodule or cord and is concerned about its malignant potential, or has a contracture and is concerned about loss of hand function. The history should include a determination of family history of Dupuytren's disease. Merely asking about Dupuytren's disease is insufficient because the disease is frequently misdiagnosed. An older relative with "arthritis" may have had Dupuytren's contracture. It is important to ascertain the duration of the patient's nodules or cords. If the patient has developed a contracture, the examiner should assess the rate the contracture is progressing.

A thorough hand examination should be performed with particular attention to palpating the hand and digits for any asymptomatic nodules or cords. Frequently, the patient is unaware of pathology in the first web space, which may not be apparent until the examiner palpates it and compares radial abduction in both hands. One must accurately measure the sensory status of the digits because a patient with Dupuytren's disease may have underlying median neuropathy that can present postoperatively as an unrecognized cause of complex regional pain syndrome. Furthermore, if a patient develops a postoperative neuropathy, it is important to know the baseline preoperative sensibility. This enables the surgeon to advise the patient of the potential for recovery from a postoperative neurapraxia that can develop if there has been a longstanding joint contracture. Accurate measurement of joint range of motion is mandatory. These measurements allow the surgeon to follow the patient's condition should surgery be deferred. Postoperatively, joint measurements are useful for measuring the rate of recovery.

If the surgeon notes contracture of a proximal interphalangeal joint, the surgeon should test that joint for attenuation of its extensor mechanism. This is accomplished by having the patient fully flex his or her wrist. The examiner uses his or her digit on the dorsum of the proximal phalanx to flex the metacarpophalangeal joint of the digit being examined. This creates a tenodesis effect on the central slip and, if it is not intact, an extensor lag will develop. If the patient cannot extend the joint in this manner, postoperative splinting of the joint will be necessary.

WHAT DO YOU COUNSEL THE PATIENT?

Patients are informed that the rate of progression cannot be predicted. For example, decades may pass before a nodule progresses to a cord and then to a contracture. A useful means of empowering the patient and allowing the patient to be involved in the patient's own treatment planning is the "tabletop test," which was developed by Hueston. In this form of self-examination, the patient is advised to return for treatment when the patient can no longer place his or her hand flat on a table.

A discussion of surgical risks and complications should include the following points:

1. Surgery for Dupuytren's contracture is akin to an antibiotic rather than a vaccine. In other words, just as an antibiotic may cure a bacterial infection, surgery may cure the immediate problem of joint contracture. However, unlike a vaccine that prevents the contraction of a disease, surgery does not prevent either its recurrence in the operative site or the extension of Dupuytren's disease to elsewhere in the hand.
2. Surgery has inherent risks beyond the anesthetic risks, including the following:
   a. Wound infection;
   b. Bleeding or hematoma formation;
   c. Numbness from either direct injury to or stretching of digital nerves;
   d. Tissue necrosis, including flap necrosis;
   e. Vascular problems ranging from cold intolerance to gangrene from either direct injury to or stretching of digital arteries;
   f. Stiffness from either regression of released joints or stiffness of uninvolved joints;
   g. Pain ranging from postoperative incisional pain to the dreaded complication of complex regional pain syndrome.

The surgeon should discuss these risks with the patient, be sure that all of the patient's questions are answered, and not rely on the patient's completing a consent form as being the sole basis for these risks having been understood by the patient.

WHAT DO YOU DO IN THE OPERATING ROOM?

A complete description of the types of surgery available to treat Dupuytren's contracture is beyond the scope of this chapter and there are excellent descriptions of worthwhile techniques by other authors. There are five types of surgical treatment for the diseased fascia.

1. Fasciotomy, which was the procedure performed by Dupuytren's in the early 19th century without anesthesia or aseptic technique. This is typically reserved for the frail, elderly patient who is not a candidate for major surgery and postoperative rehabilitation. It is the simple division of any cords in the palm and can even be performed percutaneously. Typically, fasciotomy is performed in these patients to improve skin hygiene and make custodial care more facile. The rationale for performing fasciotomy is that it relieves longitudinal traction, albeit temporarily.
2. Radical fasciectomy, which was popularized in England after World War II. It was based on the premise that Dupuytren's disease was like a tumor and complete excision of the palmar fascia would improve function while lessening recurrence or extension. Sadly, this procedure produced many surgical cripples. **Fortunately, it has been abandoned.**
3. **Limited fasciectomy, which is the most common form of treating Dupuytren's contracture today.** Only the diseased tissue in the palm and digits is excised and local flaps are fashioned as needed in order to minimize unfavorable scar formation. The technique is predicated on the fact that there is no skin deficiency in Dupuytren's contracture so that rearrangement of the skin by Z-plasties, Y–V plasties, and combinations thereof, is sufficient to relieve the tension that incites the progression of the Dupuytren's disease. The open palm technique of McCash is a modification of the limited fasciectomy technique in which the palm is allowed to heal by secondary intention. It was developed to lessen the dreaded consequences of hematoma formation and flap necrosis.
4. Dermofasciectomy with skin grafting, which is the removal of the diseased fascia and its overlying skin. It is reserved for three specific circumstances—when treating patients with recurrent disease; when replacing flaps of uncertain viability; and when treating younger patients with a very strong diathesis.
5. Segmental aponeurectomy, which is the removal of approximately 1-cm segments of the diseased cords and nodules without skin undermining.

TREATING THE CONTRACTURES

Metacarpophalangeal Joints

Because these joints are cam shaped, their collateral ligaments are stretched in flexion. Thus when the pretendinous cords are released, the metacarpophalangeal joints readily return to extension.

Proximal Interphalangeal Joints

These joints are less forgiving than the metacarpophalangeal joints. Despite careful release of the cords that are causing the contracture, the proximal interphalangeal joints may have intrinsic structural tightness that limits their satisfactory release. Furthermore, if these joints have been severely flexed for years, attempts to completely correct the contracture may result in stretching of the neurovascular structures, resulting in further damage to or even loss of the digit.

WHAT ARE THE EXPECTED RESULTS?

Although there are many retrospective studies by different authors describing their clinical experiences, there is a dearth of useful studies discussing the results of surgical treatment.

A recent prospective trial supports the theory that longitudinal tension incites the development of Dupuytren's disease. Half the patients were treated by fasciotomy through a transverse incision and the other half had a Z-plasty performed after the fasciotomy. The patients were followed for 2 years, but the trial had to be stopped because the recurrence rate was statistically significantly greater in the first group.

The most comprehensive epidemiologic study was described by McFarlane using the IFSSH data. **He concluded that no** matter which procedure was performed, the results of metacarpophalangeal joint release were satisfactory, but the degree of proximal interphalangeal joint correction was less if the open palm technique had been performed. He also found that no matter which technique had been employed, the recurrence rate was between 50% and 60%. The variables that contributed to the worse results were alcoholism, extensive involvement, and the open palm technique.

Many authors have dealt with the problem of proximal interphalangeal joint correction. Techniques ranging from gentle manipulation to arthroplasty have been advocated. A prospective study of patients with proximal interphalangeal joints with contractures of 60 degrees or more divided them into two groups. The first group had fasciectomy performed and the second group had additional surgery to release the joints. Both groups had identical postoperative therapy. At 6-month follow-up examination there was no statistical difference in the results.

WHAT DOES THE FUTURE HOLD FOR ALTERNATIVE TREATMENT?

Various forms of nonsurgical treatment of Dupuytren's disease have been tried. The most promising modality is an enzymatic fasciotomy via the injection of clostridial collagenase. Clinical trials have been conducted suggesting that improvement will occur within 1 month of a single injection, that metacarpophalangeal joints respond better than interphalangeal joints, and that there were fewer recurrences during a 4-year follow-up period.

Suggested Readings

Badalamente MA, Hurst LC, Hentz VR: Collagen as a clinical target: nonoperative treatment of Dupuytren's's disease. *J Hand Surg.* 2002;27A:788–798.

Bayat A, Watson JS, Stanley JK, et al. Genetic susceptibility to Dupuytren's disease: association of Zf9 transcription factor gene. *Plast Reconstr Surg.* 2003;111:2133–2139.

Beasley RW. Dupuytren's's disease. In: Beasley RW, ed. *Beasley's Surgery of the Hand.* New York: Thieme; 2003:468–487.

Beyermann K, Prommersberger KJ, Jacobs C, et al. Severe contracture of the proximal interphalangeal joint in Dupuytren's's disease: does capsuloligamentous release improve outcome? *J Hand Surg.* 2004;29(B):240–243.

Bisson MA, Mudera V, McGrouther DA, et al. The contractile properties and responses to tensional-loading of Dupuytren's's disease-derived fibroblasts are altered: a cause of contracture? *Plast Reconstr Surg.* 2004;113:611–621.

Brickley-Parsons D, Glimcher MJ, Smith RJ, et al. Biochemical changes in the collagen of the palmar fascia in patients with Dupuytren's's disease. *J Bone Joint Surg Am.* 1981;63:787–797.

Brody GS, Peng STJ, Landel RF. The Etiology of Hypertrophic Scar Contracture: Another View. *Plast Reconstr Surg* 1981;67:673–684.

Burge P, Hoy G, Regan P, et al. Smoking, alcohol and the risk of Dupuytren's's contracture. *J Bone Joint Surg Br.* 1997;79:206–210.

Chiu HF, MacFarlane RM. Pathogenesis of Dupuytren's contracture: a correlative clinical-pathological study. *J Hand Surg.* 1978;3A:1–10.

Citron N, Hearnden A. Skin tension in the aetiology of Dupuytren's disease: a prospective trial. *J Hand Surg.* 2003;28B:528–530.

Furnas DW. Dupuytren's contracture in a black patient in East Africa. *Plast Reconstr Surg.* 1979;64:250–251.

Gabbiani G, Majno G. Dupuytren's's contracture: fibroblast contraction? An ultrastructural study. *Am J Pathol.* 1972;66:131–146.

Hueston JT. Regression of Dupuytren's contracture. *J Hand Surg.* 1992;17B:453–457.

Hueston JT. The table top test. *Med J Aust.* 1976;2:189–190.

Hurst LC and Badalamente MA. Associated Diseases in McFarlane RM, McGrouther DH, and Flint MH eds. *Dupuytren's Disease: Biology and Teatment.* Edinburgh: Churchill Livingstone, 1990:253–260.

McFarlane RM. Patterns of diseased fascia in the fingers in Dupuytren's contracture. Displacement of the neurovascular bundle. *Plast Reconstr Surg.* 1974;54:31–44.

McFarlane RM. The results of treatment. In: McFarlane RM, McGrouther DH, Flint MH, eds. *Dupuytren's Disease: Biology and Treatment.* Edinburgh: Churchill Livingstone; 1990:387–412.

McFarlane RM, Botz JS, Cheung H. Epidemiology of surgical patients. In: McFarlane RM, McGrouther DH, Flint MH, eds. *Dupuytren's Disease: Biology and Treatment.* Edinburgh: Churchill Livingstone; 1990:201–238.

McGrouther DA. Dupuytren's contracture. In: Green DP, Hotchkiss RN, Pederson WC, eds. *Green's Operative Hand Surgery.* 5th ed. New York: Churchill Livingstone; 2005:159–186.

McGrouther DA. *The Hand.* 1984;14:215–236.

Moermans JP. Long-term results after segmental aponeurectomy for Dupuytren's disease. *J Hand Surg.* 1996;21B:797–800.

Stack HG. *The Palmar Fascia.* London: Churchill Livingstone; 1973.

Smith P, Breed C. Central slip attenuation in Dupuytren's contracture: a cause of persistent flexion of the proximal interphalangeal joint. *J Hand Surg.* 1994;19(A):840–843 .

CHAPTER 91 ■ REPLANTATION IN THE UPPER EXTREMITY

NEIL F. JONES

Replantation describes the re-attachment of a *completely amputated* part by restoration of arterial inflow and venous outflow, whereas revascularization describes restoration of arterial inflow or venous outflow, or both, to an *incompletely amputated* part, no matter how small the point of attachment.

Following the first successful replantation of an upper arm amputation by Malt and McKhann in 1962, the first successful replantation of an amputated thumb was performed in 1968 by Komatsu and Tamai. Since then replantation teams have been organized in most major hospitals, and microsurgical techniques have become an integral part of the training of plastic surgeons and hand surgeons, leading directly to the evolution of elective microsurgical free tissue transfer.

INDICATIONS

In general, any patient with an amputation involving the upper extremity is a candidate for replantation, but ideal candidates have sharp, guillotine-type amputations of the thumb, multiple digits, hand, wrist, and forearm that are minimally contaminated (Table 91.1). The decision to proceed with replantation of an amputated part can only be made by an experienced microsurgeon or hand surgeon. Because the patient and family naturally expect a miraculous result, it is important that the referring physician explain that the patient is being transferred for evaluation by an experienced microsurgeon to determine whether replantation is possible, rather than raising their hopes unrealistically. When faced with a difficult decision regarding replantation, the surgeon should consider whether the function of the hand can be improved by replantation when compared to closing the amputation stump and future fitting of a prosthesis.

CONTRAINDICATIONS

Contraindications to replantation may be either absolute or relative (Tables 91.2 and 91.3).

ABSOLUTE CONTRAINDICATIONS

Significant Associated Injuries

Digital amputations are rarely associated with other major injuries, but major amputations of the arm are frequently associated with head, chest, and abdominal injuries. These may be life-threatening and may preclude replantation of the upper extremity amputation.

Multiple Injuries within the Amputated Part

If there are segmental amputations at multiple levels in the amputated extremity (Fig. 91.1A), or if there is extensive crushing or degloving of the amputated part (Fig. 91.1B), replantation is contraindicated. Clinical inspection of the amputated part is correlated with radiographs that may reveal fractures at multiple levels. In the digits, a red line along the lateral aspect of the finger—the "Chinese red streak sign"—is indicative of an avulsion of the digital artery and usually precludes successful replantation. Similarly, coiling or tortuosity of the digital arteries when the digit is inspected under loupe magnification is also evidence of an avulsion mechanism and indicates extensive damage along the digital artery.

Systemic Illness

Finally, elderly patients with previous history of a myocardial infarct, heart failure, chronic obstructive pulmonary disease, or insulin-dependent diabetes may not be candidates for prolonged surgery and anesthesia.

RELATIVE CONTRAINDICATIONS

Age

Elderly patients may have significant systemic disease, but more importantly, the recovery of tendon and nerve function in the replanted digit is poorer than in a younger patient and there is the added risk of producing stiffness in the interphalangeal joints of adjacent uninjured fingers. Arteriosclerosis is relatively rare in the arteries of the upper extremity but can occasionally complicate the anastomoses of the radial and ulnar arteries during replantation at the wrist level in an elderly patient.

Replantation in young children may be more technically demanding because of the small caliber of the vessels and the propensity for vasospasm, but every effort should be made to replant a digit in a child, as the digit will continue to grow and the results of the tendon and nerve repairs are so much better than in an adult (1,2).

Avulsion Injuries

With avulsion injuries, there is usually extensive damage to the digital arteries and digital nerves both proximal and distal to the level of amputation (Fig. 91.2). Experimentally, actual injury to the digital artery has been shown to extend as far as 4 cm from the site of transection when examined by

TABLE 91.1

AMPUTATIONS SUITABLE FOR REPLANTATION

Thumb
Multiple digits
Transmetacarpal
Wrist
Forearm
Single digit in children

TABLE 91.3

RELATIVE CONTRAINDICATIONS TO REPLANTATION

Patient's advanced age
Avulsion injuries
Prolonged warm ischemia time
Massive contamination
Patient's psychological problems
Single-digit amputation

electron microscopy compared with 0.8 cm under the operating microscope. Injuries resulting from rodeo or waterskiing demonstrate obvious avulsions of nerves and tendons, with long segments of these structures hanging from the amputated digit (Fig. 91.2C). In contrast, the digital arteries are usually avulsed distally from within the digit, sometimes all the way to the trifurcation of the digital artery at the level of the distal interphalangeal joint. Replantation will only be successful if a normal lumen of digital artery can be found before the artery trifurcates. In addition, replantation requires the use of interposition vein grafts or transposition of a neurovascular bundle from an adjacent digit (3).

The most extreme example of an avulsion injury is the so-called ring avulsion injury. These injuries range from circumferential lacerations at the level of the proximal phalanx with thrombosis or transection of the dorsal veins and both digital arteries (Fig. 91.3) to complete degloving of the soft-tissue envelope of the digit or amputation of the digit through the distal interphalangeal joint (Fig. 91.4). The Urbaniak classification of ring avulsion injuries has been expanded by Kay et al. (4) into four categories (Table 91.4).

Arterial revascularization usually requiring interposition vein grafts is necessary for class IIa and class IIIa injuries whereas class IIv and class IIIv injuries require venous anastomoses. Class IV complete degloving or complete amputations require a full replantation procedure. Approximately 75% of classes II, III, and IV ring avulsion injuries can be successfully salvaged by revascularization or replantation.

Prolonged Warm Ischemia Time

Muscle is the tissue most susceptible to ischemia and undergoes irreversible changes after 6 hours at room temperature. Because a proximal forearm or upper arm amputation contains significant muscle mass, it is vitally important that such amputations be cooled as quickly as possible, and if necessary, reperfused through arterial shunts to reduce the warm and cold ischemia times. **Because digits do not contain muscle, they have a much longer ischemic tolerance.** With multiple digital amputations, cases have been reported of successful replantation after 33 hours of warm ischemia, and after 94 hours of cold ischemia. A hand amputation has been successfully replanted after 54 hours of cold ischemia.

TABLE 91.2

ABSOLUTE CONTRAINDICATIONS TO REPLANTATION

Significant associated injuries
Multiple injuries within the amputated part
Systemic illness

Massive Contamination

Surgical debridement precedes any major upper extremity replantation, but occasionally, massive contamination in farm injuries or tissue impregnation by oil or grease in machine injuries preclude replantation because of the risk of infection and overwhelming sepsis. In rare situations in which the distal part is devascularized and the zone of injury is extensive, massively contaminated, or ill defined, temporary ectopic implantation of the distal part with anastomoses to the thoracodorsal artery and vein is a reasonable option. The proximal stump can then be treated with conservative debridement and after healing has been achieved, the distal part can be electively replanted onto the healed stump several months later.

Psychological Problems

Self-inflicted amputations, usually of the hand or wrist, may foreshadow a later successful suicide attempt. These patients require an emergency psychiatric evaluation prior to any decision regarding replantation.

Single-Digit Amputations

Although a single-digit amputation should always be replanted in children (Fig. 91.5), replantation of a single digit in an adult remains controversial. **Even though viability can be restored after amputation proximal to the proximal interphalangeal (PIP) joint, digital motion is compromised because of the adhesions associated with flexor tendon repairs in zone II, resulting in less than satisfactory flexion at the PIP and distal interphalangeal (DIP) joints. Replantation of an index finger amputation proximal to the PIP joint in an adult is almost universally unrewarding, because the brain excludes the index finger and substitutes the middle finger for thumb–middle finger pinch.** Similarly, replantation of a single middle, ring, or small finger may interfere with the motion of the other two fingers because of the common origin of the flexor digitorum profundus tendons. However, replantation of a single-digit amputation through the middle phalanx distal to the insertion of the flexor digitorum sublimis tendon, or through the distal phalanx, may provide excellent sensory return, with maintenance of full flexion at the PIP joint.

TRANSFER TO A REPLANTATION SERVICE

Once the surgeon has decided, usually by telephone, that the patient and the amputated part are suitable for potential replantation, the referring physician should ensure that hemorrhage from the amputation stump has been stopped by

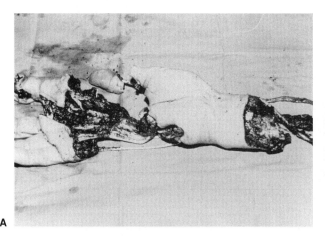

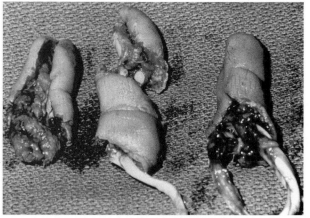

FIGURE 91.1. Contraindication to replantation. **A:** A multisegmental amputation through the distal forearm, palm, and within the thumb and index finger sustained in an agricultural injury is an absolute contraindication to replantation. **B:** Extensive lacerations and crushing of these three digits precludes replantation.

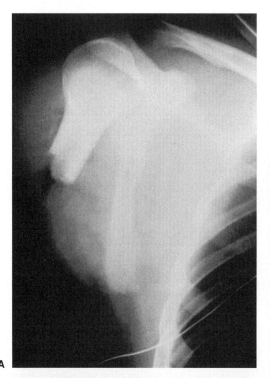

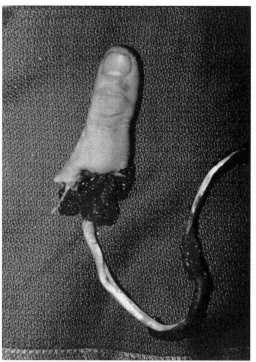

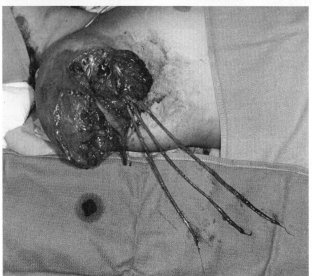

FIGURE 91.2. Avulsion injuries. **A** and **B:** Avulsion of the right upper extremity through the proximal third of the humerus in a snowmobile accident resulted in avulsion of the median, ulnar, and radial nerves. Replantation is contraindicated. **C:** Typical avulsion amputation of the thumb at the level of the metacarpophalangeal (MCP) joint with avulsion of the flexor pollicis longus from the musculotendinous junction in the forearm. Contrary to other avulsion amputations, every attempt should be made to replant a thumb avulsion.

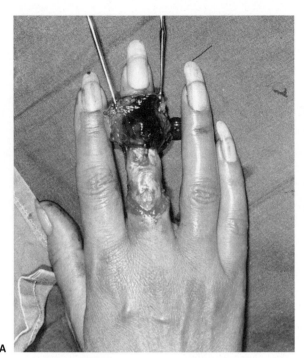
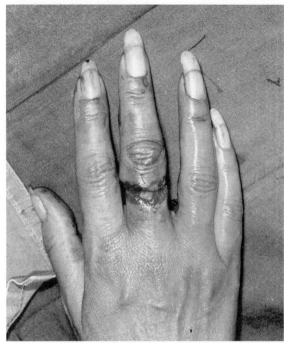

A

B

FIGURE 91.3. Class II ring avulsion injury of the right long finger with partial degloving of the soft-tissue envelope and transection of all dorsal veins and both digital arteries, but without an associated phalangeal fracture.

application of a pressure dressing and elevation, and that fluid resuscitation has been instituted if necessary. Tetanus prophylaxis may be required and broad-spectrum intravenous antibiotics are begun. The amputated part is wrapped in sterile gauze moistened with lactated Ringer solution, sealed in a plastic bag, and placed in a container of water and ice at a temperature of 39.2°F (4°C). The surgeon should also advise the referring physician of the urgency of transfer of the patient and amputated part either by ambulance or, occasionally for major replantations, by helicopter.

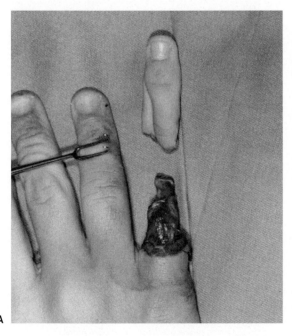
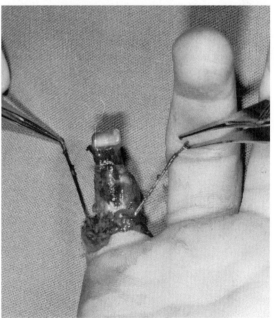

A

B

FIGURE 91.4. Class III ring avulsion injury of the dominant right small finger in an 11-year-old girl. The digital nerves and arteries were avulsed at the level of the distal interphalangeal joint and replantation could not be completed.

TABLE 91.4

CLASSIFICATION OF RING AVULSION INJURIES (4)

Class I	Circulation adequate, with or without skeletal injury
Class IIa	Arterial circulation inadequate, no skeletal injury
Class IIv	Venous circulation inadequate, no skeletal injury
Class IIIa	Arterial circulation inadequate with fracture or joint injury
Class IIIv	Venous circulation inadequate with fracture or joint injury
Class IV	Complete amputation

EVALUATION FOR REPLANTATION SURGERY

A member of the replantation team should obtain a history from the patient, including the patient's age, hand dominance, occupation, and pre-existing systemic illness. A description of the mechanism of injury usually allows the surgeon to determine whether the amputation was caused by a sharp transection or a crushing or avulsion mechanism. Physical examination is performed to exclude other injuries. Radiographs of the amputated part and the proximal extremity should be obtained if they have not already been sent with the patient. It is important to exclude any associated fractures in the limb proximal to the level of amputation. Routine investigations include a chest radiograph, electrocardiogram, complete blood count, and electrolytes. Blood typing and cross-matching are necessary for all major replantation procedures.

PREPARATION OF THE AMPUTATED PART

If the surgeon decides that the patient and the amputated part fulfill the criteria for replantation, the amputated part and radiographs are taken to the operating room so that the amputated part can be prepared while the patient is being made ready for anesthesia and surgery. The amputated part is cleaned with routine bacteriocidal solution and placed on a small operating table. If there is gross contamination, the part can be irrigated with pulsatile jet lavage. All of the structures in the amputated part are then identified and tagged, initially under loupe magnification and later under the operating microscope.

Skin Incisions

In an amputated digit, two midlateral incisions are made so that anterior and posterior skin flaps can be mobilized to provide access to the radial and ulnar neurovascular bundles. For ring avulsion injuries, a single dorsal midline incision may be used. For arm and forearm amputations, the incisions are not placed directly over the nerves and arteries, because it is likely that primary closure will not be possible and it is better not to place skin grafts directly over the repaired arteries and nerves. The incisions in the amputated part and in the amputation stump can be staggered so that the flaps can be transposed in a Z-plasty fashion during final closure. Contused skin margins and contaminated subcutaneous tissue are sharply debrided.

Debridement

In major forearm and upper arm amputations, it is difficult to determine how much of the muscle will eventually remain

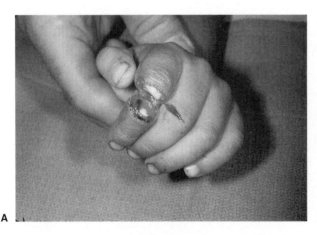

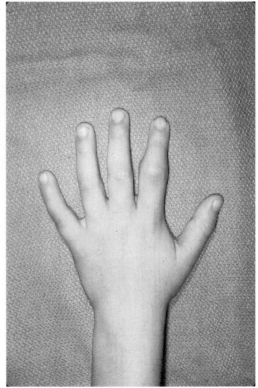

FIGURE 91.5. Replantation of a single-digit amputation in a child should always be attempted and is usually associated with very satisfactory flexor tendon function, sensory return, and relatively normal growth. In this 2-year-old child, a steel door severed all structures from the dorsum of the left index finger through the proximal interphalangeal (PIP) joint, leaving only a small pedicle of palmar skin.

viable. Contused, lacerated, or contaminated muscle is sharply debrided. Irrigation with heparinized lactated Ringer solution through a catheter inserted into one of the inflow arteries can be used to determine which portions of the muscles will remain viable once arterial inflow is restored. Any muscle that does not "weep" the lactated Ringer solution should be aggressively excised as it will not be perfused after the arterial and venous anastomoses are completed. **Fasciotomies are usually required in upper arm and forearm amputations, and are designed over the anterior and posterior forearm muscle compartments and over the second and fourth metacarpals to decompress the intrinsic muscle compartments.**

Tagging of Neurovascular Structures

Under loupe magnification or the operating microscope, the two digital arteries and the radial and ulnar digital nerves are identified through the midlateral incisions and traced in a distal-to-proximal direction to identify the digital nerves and arteries at the level of the amputation. With avulsion amputations, there may be tortuosity of the digital arteries, which should be traced, until the arterial lumen appears normal under the operating microscope. In some avulsion injuries, the digital artery is not present at the level of the amputation and has been avulsed from within the digit. The surgeon must find the distal end of the digital artery, and replantation will require interposition vein grafts. The two digital arteries and two digital nerves are identified with an 8-0 nylon marking suture or small metallic clips to allow easier identification later in the surgery. To distinguish between the digital artery and the digital nerve, either both ends of the suture or a single end of the suture can be left long. The digital nerves are cut 1 to 2 mm distal to the level of the amputation until a normal-appearing fascicular pattern is seen. Similarly the digital arteries are cut with the microdissecting scissors and the vessel lumen dilated with a vessel dilator. Serial sectioning is continued distally until a normal-appearing lumen of the digital artery is seen under the operating microscope.

The dorsal skin flap is elevated distally in the plane between the subcutaneous tissues and the underlying extensor tendons to visualize the dorsal veins within the subcutaneous tissues. The dorsal skin is then elevated 1 to 2 mm from the level of the amputation to identify two or three veins, which are again tagged with 8-0 nylon sutures as small clips.

In upper arm and forearm amputations, the brachial, radial, and ulnar arteries, together with the median, ulnar, and radial nerves and several large subcutaneous veins, are identified and tagged.

Preparation of Flexor and Extensor Tendons

The extensor tendon in the amputated digit does not usually retract and can be gently elevated from the underlying periosteum for a distance of 5 mm. The flexor digitorum profundus and flexor digitorum sublimis tendons may be apparent at the level of the amputation or may be found more distally in the digit, depending on the position of the hand at the time of amputation. The flexor tendon sheath is incised to identify the two flexor tendons, but care should be taken to preserve at least 50% of the A-2 and A-4 pulleys. The ends of the two flexor tendons are cut sharply with a scalpel to debride any ragged or contaminated tendon. A core suture of 4-0 braided nylon may be placed into the flexor digitorum profundus tendon prior to bony fixation of the amputated part, as it may become more difficult to place this core suture later in the replantation sequence.

Bony Shortening and Fixation

Bony shortening is an integral component of replantation surgery in all upper extremity amputations, as it potentially allows primary nerve repair and end-to-end vessel anastomoses. Depending on the level of amputation, the surgeon decides whether bony shortening should be performed on the amputated part only, on the amputation stump only, or in both places. However, it is important to maintain the mobility of the metacarpophalangeal (MCP), PIP, and DIP joints, and the insertion of the flexor and extensor tendons.

The periosteum on the amputated bone is elevated. A small hole is made in a piece of Esmarch bandage or surgical glove, and the bone end is placed through this hole to protect the soft tissues during bony resection. The bone is then cut transversely, using a power saw. In forearm amputations, the radius and ulna may require 2.5 to 5 cm of shortening, and in upper arm amputations, the humerus may require 4 to 8 cm of shortening to allow primary nerve and muscle repair.

Rigid internal fixation is the technique of choice in replantation surgery, primarily to allow early protected motion of the adjacent joints. Type A intraosseous wiring or 90-90 intraosseous wiring is used for replantations through the phalanges. Longitudinal K-wires or minicompression plates are best for transmetacarpal amputations. Rigid fixation of the radius and ulna requires 3.5-mm dynamic compression plates, and fixation of the humerus requires 4.5-mm plates (5). These plates or intraosseous wires may be applied to the bone within the amputated part prior to fixation of the part to the amputation stump.

If the amputation passes through a joint, primary arthrodesis accomplishes both bony shortening and bony fixation. This is especially indicated in amputations of the thumb at the level of the MCP joint (Fig. 91.6) and amputations of the hand at the level of the radio-carpal joint. However, for amputations of the digit through the metacarpophalangeal joints, an alternative option is immediate placement of a silastic implant arthroplasty to preserve motion at this joint.

Hemostasis

Finally, hemostasis is achieved in the amputated part by bipolar coagulation as this can be difficult once revascularization is performed. Hemostasis is particularly important in transmetacarpal amputations where branches of the deep metacarpal arteries may bleed profusely, as well as in forearm amputations. The amputated part is now ready for replantation and is wrapped in gauze moistened with ice-cold lactated Ringer solution.

PREPARATION OF THE AMPUTATION STUMP

The patient is usually placed under continuous axillary block anesthesia using 0.5% bupivacaine (Marcaine) or under general anesthesia. A urinary catheter is inserted because of the length of the procedure. A padded tourniquet is applied around the upper arm for all amputations other than those through the humerus itself. Debridement, identification, and tagging of all structures is performed exactly as described for the amputated part. The flexor tendons may have retracted proximally and after retrieval can be held out to a suitable length by transfixion with a 23-gauge needle. A similar core suture of 4-0 braided nylon can be placed into the proximal stump of the

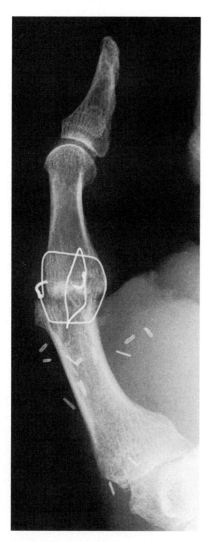

FIGURE 91.6. Postoperative radiograph following thumb replantation showing primary arthrodesis of the MCP joint using 90-90 intraosseous wiring.

flexor digitorum profundus tendon prior to replantation. After identification of the digital arteries, they can be mobilized more proximally into the palm. The ends of the digital arteries are then sharply cut with microdissecting scissors and the vessel lumen is dilated with vessel dilators. The arteries are serially sectioned until a normal-appearing intima is seen under the operating microscope.

After debridement, identification, and tagging of all structures, the tourniquet is deflated to assess the force of arterial inflow. Distal traction is applied to each proper or common digital artery using jeweller's forceps, and if there is a good "spurt" test, each digital artery is occluded with a single vessel clamp. If there is poor inflow through the proximal arteries, this may be a result of vasospasm or because of more proximal compression of the ulnar artery in Guyon's canal. The digital arteries can be bathed with 2% lidocaine (Xylocaine) or papaverine to relieve vasospasm. In transmetacarpal amputations, it is better to release the ulnar artery through the Guyon's canal and expose the entire superficial palmar arch.

Finally, hemostasis is achieved in the proximal stump, especially in transmetacarpal, forearm, and upper arm amputations.

TECHNIQUE OF REPLANTATION

Once the surgeon has established that there is good proximal arterial inflow and sufficient time (20 minutes) has elapsed since the previous tourniquet deflation, the tourniquet is re-inflated as this will facilitate bony fixation and repair of the flexor and extensor tendons and digital nerves.

Although the following sequence of repair during digital replantation has been advocated:

1. Bony fixation
2. Repair of periosteum
3. Extensor tendon repair
4. Flexor tendon repairs
5. Arterial anastomoses
6. Nerve repairs
7. Venous anastomoses
8. Skin closure

the sequence can vary, depending on the surgeon's preference. **It is probably more logical to perform the bony fixation, flexor and extensor tendon repairs, and the digital nerve repairs under the tourniquet, and then complete the replantation with the venous anastomoses and digital artery anastomoses.**

Bone Fixation

The distal amputated part is aligned with the proximal stump and fixation completed using compression plates for the humerus, radius, and ulna; longitudinal K-wires or minicompression plates for the metacarpals; and Lister type A intraosseous wiring or 90-90 intraosseous wiring for the phalanges. For amputations through the metacarpophalangeal joint of the thumb or through the radiocarpal joint at the wrist, primary arthrodesis is performed using similar techniques (Fig. 91.6).

Periosteum

If possible, the dorsal periosteum is repaired using 5-0 absorbable suture. This probably enhances bony union, but more importantly may prevent extensor tendon adhesions at the site of bony fixation.

Extensor Tendon

The extensor tendon is then repaired using 4-0 nonabsorbable, interrupted mattress or figure-of-eight sutures.

Flexor Tendons

The hand is then turned over and the palmar periosteum repaired with 5-0 absorbable sutures. **If possible, both flexor digitorum profundus and flexor digitorum sublimis tendons are repaired.** The flat flexor digitorum sublimis tendon is repaired with interrupted mattress or modified Kessler sutures of 4-0 braided nylon. The two core sutures previously placed into the proximal and distal stumps of the flexor digitorum profundus tendon are then tied and the tendon repair completed with a circumferential epitendinous running suture using 6-0 nylon. The same meticulous technique should be used for repair of the flexor tendons for a replant as in an isolated zone II flexor tendon repair so as to provide the best possible circumstances for independent gliding of the flexor tendons following replantation.

Nerve Repair

Under the microscope, the proximal and distal digital nerves are coapted by an epineurial repair using 9-0 or 10-0 nylon sutures. In more proximal amputations at the wrist, forearm, or upper arm level, group fascicular repair of the median, ulnar, and radial nerves is performed using 9-0 nylon sutures. Obviously, the median, ulnar, and radial nerve repairs are performed without tension, and this is usually possible because of the previous bony shortening.

Venous Anastomoses

If the usual tourniquet time of 120 minutes has not been exceeded during bony fixation, extensor and flexor tendon repairs, and the nerve repairs, the venous anastomoses can be started under the tourniquet. Otherwise the tourniquet is deflated and the venous and arterial anastomoses performed with the tourniquet down. Two or three dorsal veins in each digit are anastomosed end-to-end using standard microsurgical techniques, usually using 10-0 nylon sutures. If there is any tension whatsoever on the venous anastomoses when the proximal and distal stumps of the vein are introduced into the approximator clamp, interposition vein grafts should be considered. For transmetacarpal amputations and amputations at the level of the wrist, at least three or four dorsal veins should be anastomosed, approximately two veins for each artery. **Performing the venous anastomoses before the arterial anastomoses reduces blood loss and avoids performing the venous anastomoses in a pool of blood once arterial inflow has been restored.**

However, the arterial anastomoses must be performed before the venous anastomoses

1. if there has been a long ischemic interval;
2. in distal amputations in which restoration of arterial inflow allows easier identification of the distal veins;
3. in upper arm and proximal forearm replantations where there is a significant mass of devascularized muscle, in which event, the arterial anastomoses must *always* be performed first and the patient allowed to bleed from the open veins in the distal part before completing the venous anastomoses. Otherwise, if the venous anastomoses were completed first, the acidotic, hyperkalemic venous blood returning to the systemic circulation from the reperfused ischemic muscle could (occasionally) result in cardiac arrest.

Arterial Anastomoses

The adventitia is removed from the ends of the digital arteries and the lumen dilated with vessel dilators. If the digital arteries can be approximated under minimal tension using a double approximator clamp, direct end-to-end anastomoses are performed using interrupted 9-0 or 10-0 nylon sutures. If there is excessive tension, or if there is a definite segmental gap between the proximal and distal ends of the artery, then interposition vein grafts are necessary. Most digits can be successfully replanted by anastomosis of only one digital artery, but it is preferable to repair both arteries. In the forearm, both the radial and ulnar arteries should be repaired. Instead of conventional end-to-end sutured anastomoses, the Precise Anastomotic Coupler (3M Company, Minneapolis-Saint Paul, MN) may be used for anastomosis of the radial and ulnar arteries at the wrist, the common digital arteries in the hand, and the veins over the dorsum of the hand. Couplers may save time compared with conventional sutured anastomoses, especially when multiple anastomoses have to be performed.

Interposition Grafts

Interposition vein grafts may be required in the following three circumstances (6):

1. To preserve a functional joint when bony shortening cannot be performed.
2. In avulsion or crush injuries where there is an extensive zone of injury along the artery.
3. To facilitate positioning of the hand in order to perform the microsurgical anastomoses.

In thumb amputations where the ulnar digital artery is usually the dominant arterial blood supply to the thumb, it is necessary to hypersupinate the hand in order to perform an end-to-end anastomosis of the ulnar digital artery. It is much easier to anastomose an interposition vein graft to the ulnar digital artery while the amputated thumb is on the back table. The interposition vein graft then can be anastomosed to the princeps pollicis artery on the dorsum of the first web space, which is a much more convenient position both for the surgeons and the operating microscope.

Harvesting of Vein Grafts

Vein grafts can be harvested from the anterior aspect of the distal forearm for digital replantations, or from the dorsum of the foot and lower leg for forearm vessels. Vein grafts should be harvested under tourniquet control with bipolar coagulation or fine suture ligation of small branches. A suture is placed on the distal end of the vein graft to orientate the direction of flow and further sutures may be placed along the length of the vein graft to prevent torsion. Y-shaped vein grafts may be harvested to facilitate the anastomosis of a single common digital artery to the digital arteries of two adjacent digits (Fig. 91.7).

Arterial Grafts

An inherent disadvantage of vein grafts is that the proximal (outflow) end of a vein graft is usually of larger caliber than the distal (inflow) end; consequently, there may be a discrepancy between the proximal (outflow) end of a vein graft and the distal digital artery. For this reason, Godina advocated the use of interposition arterial grafts harvested from the subscapular-thoracodorsal-circumflex scapular and serratus arterial system. This branching system also provides a mechanism to graft a single inflow common digital artery to two distal digital arteries. Lister also recommended using the posterior interosseous artery as an interposition arterial graft.

Composite Venous Grafts

Finally, a composite venous flap, consisting of a small skin flap and a subcutaneous vein, can be harvested from an adjacent finger or from the dorsum of the foot to provide an interposition vein graft for a segmental defect in the venous outflow of a digital replant, especially if there is also an associated skin defect.

Vein Graft Anastomoses

Many interposition vein grafts or arterial grafts can be anastomosed to the distal digital artery in the amputated part on a back table prior to bony fixation. Alternatively, the interposition graft is anastomosed end-to-end to the proximal digital artery, or end-to-side to the superficial palmar arch or to the radial or ulnar artery at the wrist. After completion of this proximal anastomosis, the microsurgical clamps are released

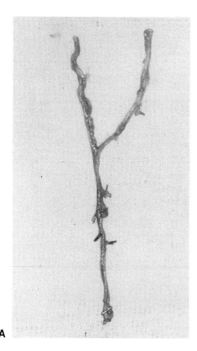

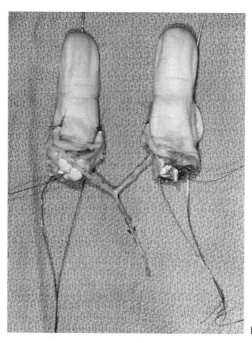

A

B

FIGURE 91.7. A Y-shaped vein graft harvested from the dorsum of the foot can be anastomosed on a back table to the digital arteries of two adjacent digits to facilitate multiple digit replantation.

to allow flow into the interposition vein graft or arterial graft. This sequence has the advantage of confirming the patency of the proximal anastomosis and in addition avoids torsion of the graft and allows accurate estimation of the length of graft required to reach the distal vessel. The distal anastomosis can then be performed end-to-end with arterial blood remaining within the graft, or, alternatively, a single microvascular clamp can be applied proximal to the proximal anastomosis and the blood irrigated out of the graft with heparinized saline. Finally, if the vein graft is too long, it may kink, which could result in eventual occlusion of the vein graft and an unsuccessful replant, especially in the fingers. Consequently, if there is any kinking, either the proximal or distal anastomosis should be revised with a shorter length of graft.

Reperfusion of the Amputated Part

Once the arterial anastomoses or interposition vein grafts are complete, the microsurgical clamps are released. All anastomoses are bathed with a solution of 2% lidocaine (Xylocaine) and papaverine, and the extremity is irrigated with warm saline. Successful restoration of perfusion to the amputated digit or extremity is then assessed by return of turgor and color to the distal pulp and capillary refill in the distal phalanx. In addition, bright red bleeding should be seen at the edges of the amputated part. The patency of each arterial and venous anastomosis is tested using the Acland test, stripping a segment of vessel with two vessel dilators distal to the anastomosis followed by release of the proximal vessel dilator.

If the digit or hand does not "pink-up," there are three possibilities:

1. Vasospasm
2. Technical problems at the arterial anastomoses
3. Inadequate proximal arterial inflow.

Vasospasm can be relieved by lidocaine (Xylocaine) or papaverine and by warming the extremity. If the Acland patency test reveals poor flow distal to an anastomosis, then the anastomosis is explored and redone, or a vein graft interposed. If there is poor inflow proximal to the anastomosis, this either

may indicate vasospasm that can be relieved pharmacologically or may mandate placement of a vein graft from a larger, more proximal, inflow artery such as the superficial palmar arch or the radial or ulnar arteries at the wrist.

Alternatively, if the digit becomes swollen and cyanotic with rapid capillary refill, the surgeon should examine the venous anastomoses under the operating microscope. Although vasospasm is a potential cause, it is much more likely that venous outflow is occluded because of a technical problem at one of the anastomoses, and this requires either revision of the anastomosis or insertion of a small vein graft to relieve any tension at the anastomosis.

Closure

Once the surgeon is satisfied with perfusion of the extremity, the skin is closed. Tight closure is avoided because this will compress the venous outflow and lead to secondary venous thrombosis. Skin flaps can be transposed as Z-plasties, or small, split-thickness skin grafts can be applied, even directly over arterial or venous anastomoses or vein grafts. If at any time during skin closure the fingertip loses its pinkish color or becomes dusky, then excessive tension is compromising either arterial inflow or venous outflow. Sutures must be removed and a split-thickness skin graft applied or the wound allowed to granulate. It is vitally important that dressings remain loose and not be applied circumferentially. Finally, the extremity is immobilized in a plaster-of-Paris splint and elevated.

POSTOPERATIVE CARE AND MONITORING

Smoking

The patient should not be allowed to smoke because of the potentially detrimental effect of the vasoconstrictive mechanism of nicotine (7).

Antithrombotic Medications

On release of the microsurgical clamps a bolus of 40 mL of dextran 40 is given intravenously followed by a continuous infusion of dextran 40 at 25 mL per hour for 5 days (based on a 70-kg adult). Aspirin 80 mg is given daily and antibiotics are continued for several days at the discretion of the surgeon. **Heparin anticoagulation is not used in most replantations except in special circumstances where there has been an extensive crushing injury or where there have been prolonged difficulties restoring arterial inflow or venous outflow.** The dose of continuous intravenous heparin is adjusted based on the activated partial thromboplastin time. However, heparin may cause hemorrhage within the replant itself, producing edema and swelling that inevitably results in compression of the arterial or venous anastomoses and eventually secondary thrombosis.

Clinical Observation

Experienced nursing staff should monitor the perfusion of the replant hourly for 48 hours by inspection of the color of the fingertip and capillary refill. If the fingertip becomes pale with slow capillary refill, arterial thrombosis or vasospasm of the arterial inflow is suspected. A swollen and blue fingertip with increased capillary return indicates venous congestion caused by constrictive dressings or thrombosis of the venous anastomoses.

Monitoring Techniques

More objective techniques of postoperative monitoring of perfusion following replantation include temperature monitoring, laser Doppler flowmetry, transcutaneous partial pressure of oxygen (Po_2), and pulse oximetry. Differential temperature monitoring by comparison of the temperature of the replanted digit with an adjacent normal digit or the contralateral hand is the most popular method. **A temperature drop of 3.6°F (2°C) or an absolute temperature of less than 86°F (30°C) mandates immediate re-exploration of the arterial and venous anastomoses.** A pulse oximeter probe secured to the distal phalanx is the simplest technique for postoperative monitoring and provides continuous recordings of the pulse rate and the oxygen saturation within the digit. Loss of the pulse rate indicates arterial occlusion whereas a fall in the oxygen saturation below 90% usually indicates venous occlusion.

RE-EXPLORATION

If clinical examination or a more objective monitoring technique suggests that perfusion is compromised, the surgeon should initially check that congealed blood within the dressings has not become constricting. All dressings are removed and if any sutures appear tight, they are cut immediately. If there is no improvement in color and capillary refill of the fingertip, the patient should be returned immediately to the operating room for re-exploration of the arterial and venous anastomoses. Thrombosis of one or more of the anastomoses may be obvious, but otherwise a patency test should be performed distal to each anastomosis. **If there is either thrombosis or lack of flow, the anastomosis is taken down and revised, which almost always necessitates the use of an interposition vein graft.** Providing that compromised perfusion is detected in a timely manner, revision of the anastomoses is often successful. In cases of venous congestion where no further venous anastomoses can be performed, the nail plate is removed, the nail bed roughened, and heparin-soaked pledgets applied to promote venous bleeding. Alternatively, serial application of leeches can occasionally salvage replants compromised by venous congestion.

REPLANTATION FOR SPECIFIC LEVELS OF AMPUTATION

Distal Phalanx

With sharp amputations through the distal phalanx, replantation may be a superior option to other forms of fingertip coverage (8). Although it can be technically demanding because of the small size of the distal arteries, successful replantation restores a virtually normal appearance and satisfactory sensibility if the digital nerves can be approximated (Fig. 91.8). A 0.028 or 0.035 K-wire is passed retrograde through the distal fragment of the distal phalanx and the amputated distal phalanx is partially sutured with one or two sutures along its palmar surface to temporarily stabilize the distal fragment. One digital artery and the two digital nerves are repaired under the operating microscope. The distal phalanx is then reduced and the K-wire drilled antegrade to just beneath the articular surface of the distal phalanx, or, if necessary, across the distal interphalangeal joint into the middle phalanx.

Finding a suitable vein in the replanted distal phalanx may be a problem. Occasionally after release of the tourniquet, a small vein can be identified dorsally just proximal to the nail fold and a single venous anastomosis performed. Alternative solutions to prevent venous congestion include removal of the

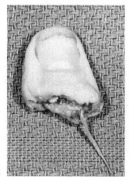
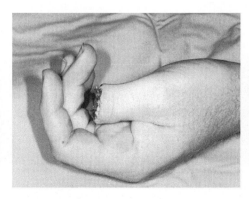
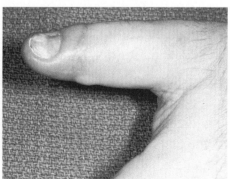

A,B   C

FIGURE 91.8. Successful replantation of an amputation through the distal phalanx of the left thumb.

nail plate and application of heparin-soaked pledgets, temporary application of leeches, or the creation of an arteriovenous anastomosis between the other distal digital artery and a proximal vein. Finally, the dorsal skin and nail bed are loosely repaired.

Middle Phalanx

Good functional results can be achieved after replantation of digital amputations through the middle phalanges distal to the insertion of the flexor digitorum sublimis tendon, because PIP joint flexion can be maintained and the return of sensation is relatively good after repair of the digital nerves (9).

Proximal Phalanx

The results of replantation of amputations through the proximal phalanges are compromised by tendon adhesions in zone II. Consequently, it is vitally important to use the same

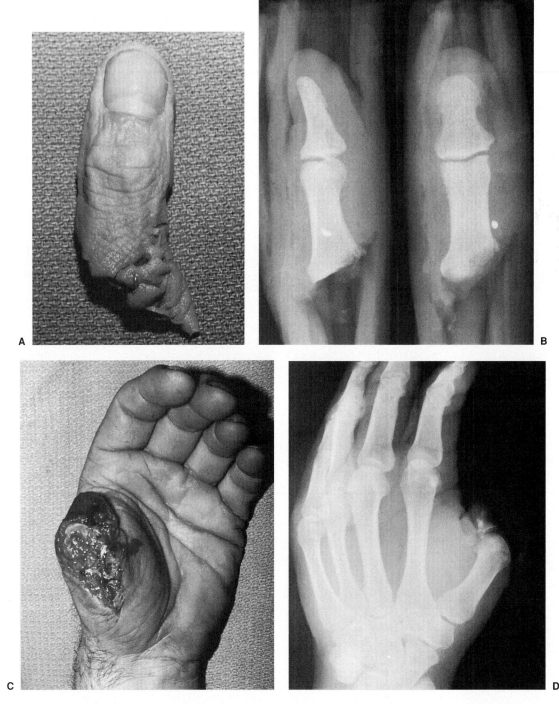

FIGURE 91.9. Amputation of the thumb, which is usually in the region of the MCP joint, is an absolute indication for replantation and is associated with excellent functional results. **A:** Amputated part. **B:** Radiograph of amputated part. **C:** Amputation stump. **D:** Radiograph of amputation stump.

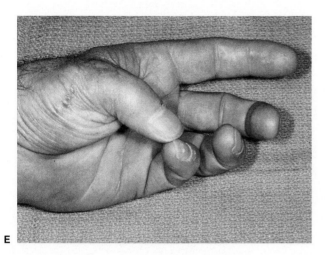

FIGURE 91.9. (*Continued*) E: Postoperative result.

meticulous technique to repair the flexor digitorum profundus and flexor digitorum sublimis tendons in a replanted finger as in an isolated zone II flexor tendon repair. If K-wires are used for bony fixation, they should not transfix the MCP or PIP joints so that early gentle passive and active range-of-motion exercises can be instituted.

Destruction of the articular cartilage at the PIP joint mandates arthrodesis of the PIP joint in a functional position. PIP joint arthrodesis can be accomplished by the same techniques of bony fixation—either 90-90 intraosseous wiring or Lister type A intraosseous wiring. The PIP joint of the index finger is usually arthrodesed in a position of 20 degrees of flexion, and the PIP joints of the middle, ring, and small fingers at angles of 30, 40, and 50 degrees, respectively.

Multiple Digits

With multidigit amputations through the proximal or middle phalanges, the surgeon can either perform the replantation in a digit-by-digit sequence or in a structure-by-structure sequence. In the first technique, all the structures in a single finger are repaired before proceeding to replant the subsequent digits. In the structure-by-structure technique, the same structure is repaired in all the replanted digits sequentially. For example, bony fixation of all the digits is performed followed by repair of all the flexor tendons and so on. Which technique is used depends on the surgeon's preference, but a structure-by-structure sequence may be faster and associated with a slightly improved survival rate (10). If a structure-by-structure approach is selected, the digital arteries in each digit are repaired last so that repair of other structures is not obscured by bleeding and there is less swelling.

Replantation should always be attempted when more than two digits are amputated, even though the circumstances may be less than ideal. Such "salvage" replantations may involve transposition of an amputated digit to replace a more important digit that cannot be replanted. For example, if in a multiple-digit amputation the thumb is so badly damaged that it cannot be replanted, one of the other digits (occasionally) can be replanted in the thumb position to provide a better functional reconstruction of the hand. Similarly, transposition of a longer amputated digit from the ulnar side of the hand may preserve a more appropriate length of a digit on the more important radial side of the hand, or may allow PIP joint motion to be maintained in the transposed replanted digit. Most importantly, vein grafts, nerve grafts, skin grafts, and even small

free skin flaps or free joint transfers can be salvaged from a nonreplantable digit to reconstruct an adjacent digit.

Thumb

Because the thumb contributes 40% to the overall function of the hand, all thumb amputations should be considered candidates for replantation (Fig. 91.9) (11). The majority of thumb amputations occur at or distal to the MCP joint and because the thumb is relatively unprotected by the other digits, avulsion amputations are relatively common, such as in waterskiing and rodeo injuries (Fig. 91.2C).

Specific considerations for replantation of the thumb include the following:

1. Bony fixation of amputations through the MCP and IP joints;
2. Use of interposition vein grafts to facilitate positioning of the thumb for completion of the arterial anastomoses; and
3. Use of immediate tendon transfers for avulsion injuries.

If the thumb amputation involves disarticulation through the MCP or interphalangeal (IP) joint, bony shortening is performed on either side of the joint and primary arthrodesis of the joint is performed using either crossed K-wires, tension band wiring, or intraosseous wiring in a position of slight flexion (Fig. 91.6).

The ulnar digital artery of the thumb is usually the dominant arterial blood supply to the thumb and it is usually much easier to anastomose an interposition vein graft end-to-end to the ulnar digital artery during preparation of the thumb on the back table. The vein graft can then be anastomosed to the radial artery on the dorsal aspect of the thumb–index finger web space in a much more convenient position for completing the arterial anastomosis than having to hypersupinate the hand. If the radial digital artery to the thumb is of satisfactory caliber, it can also be repaired end-to-side to the same vein graft "upstream" to the anastomosis of the vein graft to the ulnar digital artery.

In avulsion injuries of the thumb, if the extensor pollicis longus and flexor pollicis longus tendons have been avulsed from their musculotendinous junction, immediate tendon transfers can be performed using the extensor indicis proprius to the extensor pollicis longus and the flexor digitorum sublimis from the ring finger to the flexor pollicis longus. Obviously, these tendon transfers are only performed if the avulsion amputation does not involve the interphalangeal joint.

Transmetacarpal

Excellent functional results can be achieved following replantation of transmetacarpal amputations. Care must be taken during bony fixation to prevent malrotation of an individual digit because rotation at the metacarpal level translates into a greater functional deficit than a similar degree of malrotation further distally in the digit. Bony fixation can be achieved very simply by longitudinal K-wires in children (Fig. 91.10) or with rigid internal fixation using plates and screws in adults. At least 1 cm of bony shortening should be performed to prevent secondary intrinsic tightness in the fingers. In addition, because the distal portions of the interosseous muscles have lost both their nerve and blood supply, they should be completely debrided, which may lead to some degree of clawing of the fingers. **The carpal tunnel and Guyon's canal should be released prophylactically during the initial preparation of the**

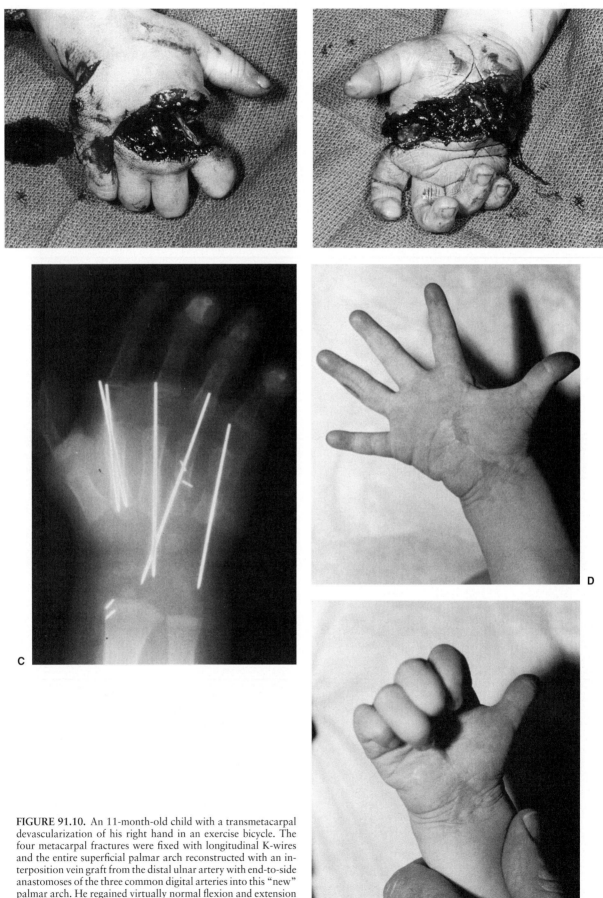

FIGURE 91.10. An 11-month-old child with a transmetacarpal devascularization of his right hand in an exercise bicycle. The four metacarpal fractures were fixed with longitudinal K-wires and the entire superficial palmar arch reconstructed with an interposition vein graft from the distal ulnar artery with end-to-side anastomoses of the three common digital arteries into this "new" palmar arch. He regained virtually normal flexion and extension of the fingers. Five years after the operation, despite good sensation, he still had cold intolerance.

amputation stump so that postoperative swelling does not result in compression of the median nerve or, more importantly, the ulnar artery. Finally, branches of the deep metacarpal arteries should be identified both in the distal amputated part and in the amputation stump, and ligated to prevent postoperative hemorrhage causing a hematoma after revascularization is completed.

Wrist

Obviously, replantation at the transcarpal level is technically much easier than replantation of amputations across the palm or out in the digits because the radial and ulnar arteries and dorsal veins are much larger than the common digital and proper digital arteries and veins. Specific considerations for amputations at the level of the wrist include the technique of bony shortening, the need for fasciotomies of the intrinsic muscles, and whether primary nerve repair or delayed secondary nerve grafting is required.

There are three choices for bony shortening of amputations around the level of the wrist:

1. Partial or total carpectomy and primary arthrodesis of the wrist. This is especially indicated if the radiocarpal joint is destroyed or in a young, working man.
2. Proximal row carpectomy if the distal articular surface of the radius is preserved.
3. Shortening osteotomy of the radius and Darrach resection of the distal ulna if the level of amputation is just proximal to the distal articular surface of the radius.

Regardless of the time required to revascularize the hand, fasciotomies of the thenar, hypothenar, and interosseous muscle compartments must be performed.

Primary epineurial or group fascicular repair of the median, ulnar, and superficial radial nerves is optimal if bony shortening allows this option. Otherwise, the nerve ends should be tagged and group fascicular nerve grafting performed as a secondary procedure a few weeks later.

Forearm and Upper Arm

Because more proximal amputations through the forearm and upper arm are rarely caused by a sharp guillotine-type mechanism, there is usually extensive damage to the adjacent muscles. Radical debridement of the muscles in the amputated part and in the stump is essential to prevent secondary infection and overwhelming sepsis. Debridement of forearm and elbow amputations should be performed under a sterile tourniquet, but a tourniquet cannot really be used for amputations above the elbow. Fasciotomies of the anterior and posterior forearm compartments are an absolute necessity, and release of the transverse carpal ligament and fasciotomies of the intrinsic muscles in the hand may also be necessary, if there is excessive swelling of the hand, or if increased compartmental pressures are measured after reperfusion of the hand.

It is vital to re-establish arterial inflow as quickly as possible in amputations of the upper arm and forearm. If the ischemia time has been prolonged, it is probably beneficial to re-establish arterial inflow using a temporary vascular shunt from the proximal brachial artery into the distal brachial artery or radial artery. This temporary arterial shunt will allow reperfusion of the extremity while debridement, identification of tendons and nerves, and bony fixation are completed. Alternatively, if the ischemic time is relatively short, rigid bony fixation can be performed after radical debridement followed immediately by arterial repair.

The amount of bony shortening should be sufficient to allow primary repair of the median, ulnar, and radial nerves, but may also facilitate skin closure over the vital structures. Rigid internal fixation is achieved with 4.5-mm dynamic compression plates for the humerus and 3.5-mm dynamic compression plates for the radius and ulna.

The arterial anastomosis is performed immediately after bony fixation and before the venous anastomoses are performed. After arterial inflow has been re-established, the veins in the distal part are allowed to bleed to prevent this venous blood, which contains high concentrations of potassium and lactic acid, from reaching the systemic circulation and potentially triggering a cardiac arrest. Three to four venous anastomoses are then performed, but prior to release of the microsurgical clamps on the venous anastomoses, the patient is given intravenous sodium bicarbonate, again to neutralize the potential acidosis. The obvious disadvantage of re-establishing arterial inflow before venous outflow is that blood loss may be considerable and is usually underestimated.

The flexor and extensor muscles or tendons are then repaired, followed by epineurial or group fascicular repair of the median, ulnar, and radial nerves. If bony shortening was insufficient to allow primary nerve repair, the nerve ends should be tagged and sural nerve grafts performed as a secondary procedure (Fig. 91.11).

The skin should be loosely approximated to cover the anastomoses and nerve repairs. If necessary, meshed split-thickness skin grafts can be harvested to provide complete coverage. Occasionally, an emergency free skin or muscle flap may be required to provide coverage of vital structures in those amputations in which there has been extensive skin loss.

Unlike replantations in the hand, successful replantations through the forearm and upper arm usually require a "second-look" operation 48 to 72 hours later to check for infection and to ensure that no further debridement of the wound is necessary.

The best functional results are achieved with replantations through the distal forearm and wrist, because the extrinsic flexor and extensor muscles remain innervated and satisfactory sensory return can be expected in young individuals.

COMPLICATIONS

Replantation in the upper extremity may be associated with a relatively high rate of complications (Table 91.5).

Malunion and Nonunion

Whitney et al. (12) reported an overall 50% incidence of bony problems and a 16% rate of nonunion in digital replantations fixed with tetrahedral wiring or K-wires, but this high complication rate might be reduced by improved techniques of rigid internal fixation using 90-90 intraosseous wiring or miniplate fixation.

Joint Stiffness

Stiffness of the MCP, PIP, and DIP joints remains a problem because of edema and swelling in the replanted digit. The surgeon should avoid using longitudinal K-wires to transfix joints, and the hand therapist should begin gentle passive range-of-motion exercises when the dressings are changed 5 to 7 days postoperatively. It is important to encourage active and passive range-of-motion exercises of the joints of adjacent noninjured digits, otherwise these, too, can become stiff.

Tendon Adhesions

Replantations, especially at the level of the proximal phalanges and at the wrist, are associated with restricted range of motion as a result of adhesions around the flexor tendon repairs. Meticulous repair of the flexor tendons and early protected active flexion protocols for tendon rehabilitation may reduce the restriction. Secondary tenolyses or two-stage flexor tendon grafting may significantly increase the total active range of motion of a replanted digit.

Muscle Contractures

Intrinsic muscle contracture may develop after replantation proximal to the wrist, and ischemic contracture of either the forearm flexor or extensor muscles may compromise successful replantation at the forearm or elbow level. Intrinsic muscle contractures can be treated by release of a portion of the intrinsic tendon or by an intrinsic muscle slide. Loss of intrinsic muscle function might be restored by conventional tendon transfers.

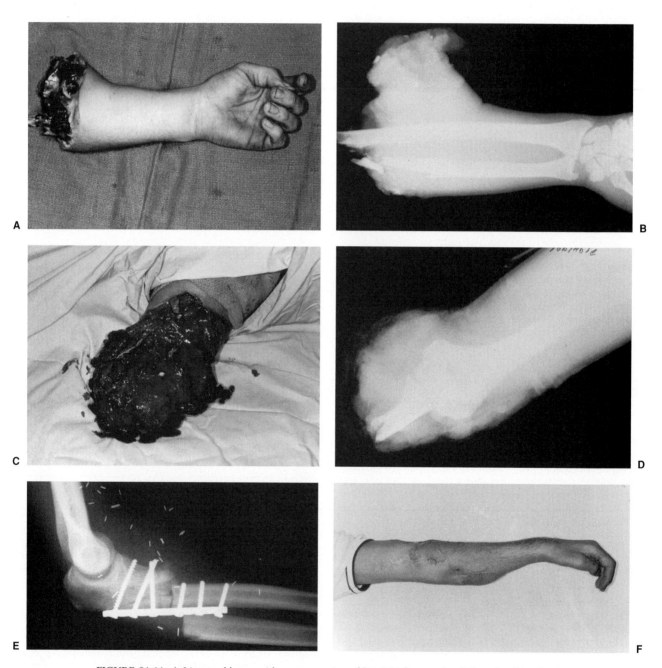

FIGURE 91.11. A 21-year-old man with an amputation of his right forearm just below the elbow by a triple-bladed saw in a lumber mill. He underwent creation of a one-bone forearm with osteosynthesis of the distal radius to the proximal ulna. Excellent wrist flexion and extension and finger flexion and extension were regained. After secondary sural nerve grafting of the median nerve and a tendon transfer for abduction of the thumb he recovered protective sensibility and returned to work driving heavy plant machinery.

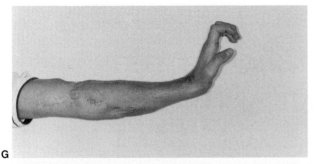

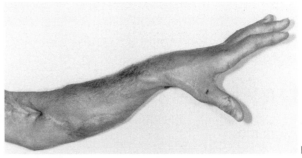

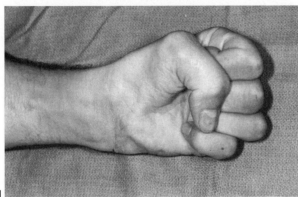

FIGURE 91.11. (*Continued*)

Sensory Return and Cold Intolerance

Sensory return (13) after upper extremity replantation is dependent on the level of amputation and whether bony shortening has allowed primary nerve repair. Replantation at the level of the middle phalanx is obviously associated with a better return of sensation than is replantation at the level of the upper arm. Gelberman et al. showed that return of digital sensibility is related primarily to the level of blood flow in the replanted finger and then to the level of amputation, the mechanism of injury, and the patient's age. In their study, 46% of digital replantations regained two-point discrimination better than 10 mm, but this was not as good as the two-point discrimination achieved after digital nerve repair alone. A pulse pressure below 70% of the contralateral digit was associated with poor two-point discrimination of 15 mm or greater and severe cold intolerance. Pain on exposure to cold (cold intolerance) after replantation is a significant problem, but does not appear to be any more disabling than after simple closure of the amputation stump. Functional outcome, especially after major upper extremity amputations, is crucially dependent on bony shortening to allow primary nerve repair and, hopefully, return of sensation in the hand and digits (14,15). Chen stated that "a viable upper extremity replantation without return of sensation is not a functional success."

TABLE 91.5

COMPLICATIONS OF REPLANTATION

Malunion and nonunion
Joint stiffness
Tendon adhesions
Muscle contractures
Poor sensation
Cold intolerance

References

1. Cheng GL, Pan DD, Yang ZX, et al. Digital replantation in children. *Ann Plast Surg*. 1985;15:325.
2. Daigle JP, Kleinert JM. Major limb replantation in children. *Microsurgery*. 1991;12:221.
3. Alpert BS, Buncke HJ, Brownstein M. Replacement of damaged arteries and veins with vein grafts when replanting crushed, amputated fingers. *Plast Reconstr Surg*. 1978;61:17.
4. Kay S, Werntz J, Wolff TW. Ring avulsion injuries: Classification and prognosis. *J Hand Surg*. 1989;14A:204.
5. Meuli H, Meyer V, Segmuller G. Stabilization of bone in replantation surgery of the upper limb. *Clin Orthop*. 1978;133:179.
6. Greenberg BM, Cuadros CL, Jupiter JB. Interpositional vein grafts to restore the superficial palmar arch in severe devascularizing injuries of the hand. *J Hand Surg*. 1988;13A:753.
7. Wilson GR, Jones BM. The damaging effect of smoking on digital revascularisation. Two further case reports. *Br J Plast Surg*. 1984;37:613.
8. Foucher G, Norris RW. Distal and very distal digital replantations. *Br J Plast Surg*. 1992;45:199.
9. May JW, Toth BA, Gardner M. Digital replantation distal to the proximal interphalangeal joint. *J Hand Surg*. 1982;7:161.
10. Camacho FJ, Wood MB. Polydigit replantation. *Hand Clin*. 1992;8:3, 409.
11. Schlenker JD, Kleinert HE, Tsai T. Methods and results of replantation following traumatic amputation of the thumb in sixty-four patients. *J Hand Surg*. 1980;5:63.
12. Whitney TM, Lineaweaver WC, Buncke HJ, et al. Clinical results of bony fixation methods in digital replantation. *J Hand Surg*. 1990;15A:328.
13. Yamauchi S, Nomura S, Yoshimura M, et al. A clinical study of the order and speed of sensory recovery after distal replantation. *J Hand Surg*. 1983;8:545.
14. Kleinert HE, Jablon M, Tsai T. An overview of replantation and results of 347 replants in 245 patients. *J Trauma*. 1980;20:390.
15. Tamai S. Twenty years' experience of limb replantation-review of 293 upper extremity replants. *J Hand Surg*. 1982;7:549.

CHAPTER 92 ■ UPPER LIMB ARTHRITIS

ALAMGIR ISANI

Arthritis falls into two general categories. By far the most common is the degenerative group, (e.g., osteoarthritis) characterized by primary articular destruction. The second major group has inflammation as the primary feature, with bone/cartilage destruction being secondary. Rheumatoid arthritis is a typical example of the latter.

DEGENERATIVE JOINT DISEASE

Degenerative arthritis is a general term incorporating common idiopathic osteoarthritis (Fig. 92.1), aggressive erosive osteoarthritis (Fig. 92.2), and traumatic arthritis, development of which is attributed to injury. All are chronic, progressive arthropathies characterized by degeneration of cartilaginous joint surfaces and by hypertrophy of bone at the articular margins. A strong family history of similar problems, especially among females is typical. Inflammation may be surprisingly minimal, in contrast to rheumatoid arthritis, which is characterized primarily by painful inflammation of the synovial membranes of joints and tendon sheaths, with joint destruction being secondary. Furthermore, osteoarthritis occurs in an older age group than does rheumatoid disease. Degenerative arthritis is by far the most frequently encountered arthropathy in the hands, and most commonly begins in the basal joint of the thumb or distal interphalangeal joints.

An uncommon but dramatic variant of primary osteoarthritis is erosive osteoarthritis. Exhibiting clinical and pathologic manifestations similar to those of rheumatoid disease, with violent inflammatory episodes, this variant mysteriously causes total destruction of individual joints without any pathology in adjacent joints (Fig. 92.2).

Traumatic Arthritis

Traumatic arthritis is considered a separate entity, even though the clinical, radiographic, and histologic characteristics are indistinguishable from spontaneously occurring osteoarthritis. By definition, there must be a clear history of specific injury to the joint. Degenerative osteoarthritis, in contrast, is spontaneous and is attributable to the "wear and tear" associated with daily use and for which genetic factors are apparent. The distinction is not clear-cut, and the term *traumatic arthritis* is applied in some cases in the sense that trauma may have accelerated a normally occurring degenerative process. Often, the issue of delineation between traumatic and degenerative arthritis is of more legal than clinical concern.

Incidence and Clinical Presentation of Degenerative Arthritis

All types of degenerative arthritis are characterized by joint deformity, both clinically and radiographically, localized tenderness, variable pain, and eventual restriction of joint motion. Pathologically, there is destruction of cartilage on opposing surfaces of normal joints. Anti-inflammatory medications may give transient improvement in symptoms, but once the articular surfaces are destroyed, there is no possibility of spontaneous recovery or permanent relief of symptoms by conservative or nonsurgical treatment. The basic indication for treatment is pain, and the individual tolerance to pain is highly variable. The symptoms are evaluated on an individual basis in the context of age, health, and occupation. **Although radiographs are diagnostic, there is essentially no correlation between the degree of disease they illustrate and the pain each individual experiences.**

Osteoarthritis is common. Approximately 10% of adults older than age 50 years have significant symptomatic osteoarthritis. An even greater percentage of them have radiographically demonstrable but asymptomatic disease. The prevalence increases with age and in postmenopausal women, and there is clearly a familial predisposition. Occupational influences are controversial, but in the legal arena have been linked to repetitive mechanical use, at least to the extent that such activity aggravates a naturally developing disorder.

The initial manifestation of primary osteoarthritis occurs in weight-bearing joints of the legs or back, or in joints of the hands, where it characteristically involves the carpometacarpal joint at the base of the thumb and the distal interphalangeal joints of the fingers.

Pathogenesis

Although the pathogenesis remains unresolved, primary osteoarthritis is considered a wear-and-tear phenomenon with the progressive loss of cartilage and exposure and later destruction of underlying bone. The synovial tissue is minimally affected. The progressive destruction of articular cartilage is the sine qua non of osteoarthritis.

Degenerative Arthritis of Basal Joints of the Thumb

The term *basal joint of the thumb* is used imprecisely to refer to either the metacarpal–trapezial, the scaphotrapezial, or both of these joints (pantrapezial). The first metacarpal–trapezial joint has opposing, reciprocally concave articular surfaces. The double-saddle configuration of this special joint allows a tremendous range of motion in flexion–extension and abduction–adduction planes, and also permits some axial rotation. The joint is stabilized by capsular structures and the strong volar carpometacarpal ligament, which securely tethers the base of the metacarpal to the carpus. Additionally, dynamic stability is provided by muscle and tendon units disposed circumferentially around the first metacarpal.

884

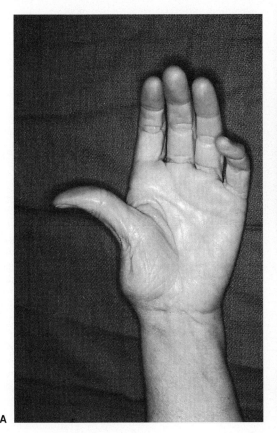
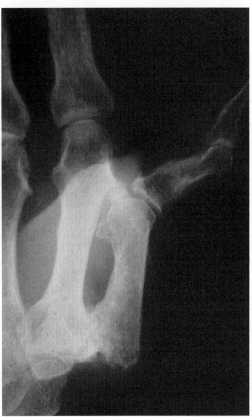

FIGURE 92.1. A: Typical metacarpal-trapezial deformity of advanced thumb basal joint idiopathic osteoarthritis with subluxed and flexed first metacarpal-trapezial joint and reciprocal metacarpophalangeal (MCP) hyperextension. **B:** Radiographs demonstrating the advanced pathology of this case.

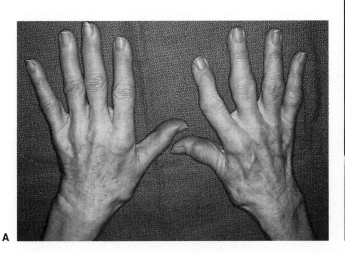
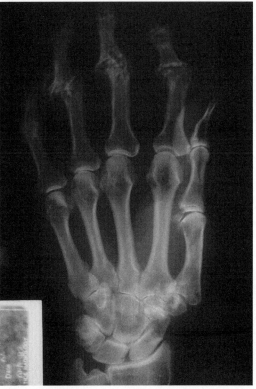

FIGURE 92.2. A and B: Clinical and radiographic findings of erosive osteoarthritis showing marked destruction of the proximal interphalangeal joints.

Pathogenesis

The thumb is the key unit for opposition, pinch, and precision manipulation. These functions impose special demands at each joint. Motion at the interphalangeal and the metacarpophalangeal (MCP) joints occurs primarily in the flexion–extension axis. In contrast, the metacarpocarpal joint has to be widely adaptive in order to position the thumb effectively for its range of activity. With thumb motion, the distribution of force vectors is uneven, being concentrated disproportionately along the dorsal facet of the trapezium, where capsular support is weakest. The abductor pollicis longus tendon, which inserts at the base of the first metacarpal, reinforces this weak capsule, but it also is a powerful force for subluxation of the base of the metacarpal. Although these anatomic and mechanical alterations contribute to basal joint arthrosis, poorly understood biologic and genetic factors also influence the predisposition of certain individuals to the disease process. The preponderance of postmenopausal women with this disease is a paradox as most older women impose relatively low stress demands on their hands.

Clinical Presentation

The chief symptoms of degenerative arthritis of either joint at the base of the thumb are pain and swelling, aggravated by use and relieved by rest. Pain is typically of a piercing type, provoked especially by twisting motions and lasting only moments until the late stages of the disease when deep and constant aches are typical. A frequent early complaint is the "loss of strength" and inability to perform simple tasks such as turning a key or opening a jar top. The natural history is generally one of gradual, but progressive, deterioration, with variable periods of pain remission. In general, this common disorder is not an indication of generalized, disabling arthritis, although there is often asymptomatic evidence of osteoarthritic damage to other joints, especially in distal finger joints.

Physical examination reveals swelling, tenderness, and variable crepitation directly over the first metacarpal (MC) and/or scaphotrapezial joints. Subluxation is common, and passive reduction reproduces the typical piercing pain. With advanced destruction, the joints may become fixed in adduction/flexion with reciprocal MCP joint hyperextension (Fig. 92.1). With loss of motion, pain frequently diminishes. Axial compression and rotation of the thumb metacarpal may elicit a painful grinding.

Radiographic Findings

Radiographic evidence of degenerative arthritis may precede clinical manifestations by several years, often with an episode of trauma apparently initiating symptoms. In other cases, radiographic changes are not detected in patients with early symptoms. **As noted earlier, radiographically demonstrated joint destruction correlates poorly with the severity of clinical symptoms, and it is the latter that determines treatment.**

Classic radiographic findings include narrowing of the joint space as cartilage deteriorates, marginal bone erosions, subchondral sclerosis or condensation of bone, reactive cystic changes, and marginal bone hypertrophy with osteophyte or spur formation (Fig. 92.1B).

Collapse Deformity

A multiarticulate system, such as the thumb, is prone to a mathematically predictable pattern of collapse, according to the principle elaborated by Landsmeer (1). **In short, each joint in a multiarticulate system (such as a finger), when subjected to longitudinal compression, will buckle in a sequentially opposite direction, forming a zigzag collapse pattern.** With pro-gressive thumb basal joint flexion/adduction and subluxation, a compensatory hyperextension of the MCP joint develops (Fig. 92.1B).

Stages of Thumb Basal Joint Degenerative Disease

Clinical staging, as suggested by Burton et al. (2), is a helpful guide to management and is briefly reviewed.

Stage I is associated with a lax joint and is characterized by pain. Stress radiography often documents pathologic joint subluxation whereas standard radiographs often reveal minimal, if any, pathology. Intolerable pain associated with long periods of writing is the most typical chief complaint, and the patients often are young. Tenderness over the joint and pain as its subluxation is passively reduced may be the only abnormal physical finding.

Stage II is characterized by more intense and more constant symptoms, chronic joint subluxation, and radiographic changes of joint space narrowing, subchondral bone sclerosis, and/or cystic changes with minor osteophyte formation.

Stage III of pantrapezial arthrosis is characterized by pain and weakness at a level that impedes many activities and frequent extension of the process into neighboring joints. Often pain is felt deep in the thenar eminence and radiates up the forearm. Although there is little correlation between radiographic findings and of symptoms, films at this stage will demonstrate joint destruction.

Stage IV is characterized by pantrapezial arthritic destruction, joint subluxation, and a zigzag deformity of MC joint flexion and MCP hyperextension (Fig. 92.1B). Functional impairment is severe with impaired range of motion, but the loss of motion may be accompanied by a reduction in pain.

Treatment of Thumb Basal Joint Arthritis

Treatment is determined by the severity of symptoms and disability for each individual patient.

Conservative Treatment. A trial of nonsurgical therapy helps to establish rapport and confidence, but pain reduction is only transient. Such measures include immobilization with a splint, direct steroid injections into the involved joints, and altered work activity to reduce forceful and strenuous use of the thumb. Oral nonsteroidal anti-inflammatory medications during periods of acute exacerbations are occasionally helpful.

Surgical Treatment. Once the cartilaginous articular surfaces are destroyed, relief can only be provided by surgical separation of the denuded bones. Persistent intractable pain and progressive handicap that is not responsive to conservative measures constitute the primary indications for surgical treatment. The basic types of operation for this are briefly described in the following material.

Ligament reconstruction. When symptoms warrant repair for stage I disease, extra-articular ligament reconstruction, using a portion of the flexor carpi radialis tendon, is the preferred treatment. Ligamentous stabilization of the subluxating joint halts the otherwise inexorable progression of the degenerative process.

Arthrodesis. Arthrodesis of an arthritic first MC joint is a reasonable option only if one can be certain that the pathology is confined to that specific joint, such as a late complication of a Bennett fracture. Currently, arthrodesis (fusion) (Fig. 92.3A) is infrequently employed, being recommended occasionally for traumatic arthritis of the trapezial–metacarpal joint of young patients engaged in heavy labor. If the diagnosis of localized disease is correct, relief of pain is predictable, but the arthrodesis significantly restricts motion, requires a prolonged period of immobilization, and the nonunion rate is substantial.

Treatment of Stages II to IV Arthritis. Resection of the trapezium relieves pain but does not prevent thumb shortening, instability at its base, and weakness. **Consequently, some**

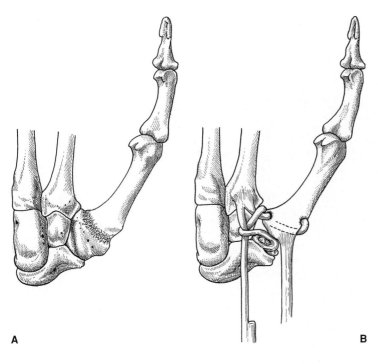

A

B

FIGURE 92.3. A: Schematic of fusion of the trapeziometacarpal joint. **B.** Schematic of trapezial excisional arthroplasty with ligament suspension using a split portion of the flexor carpi radialis tendon.

type of trapezial resection arthroplasty with ligament reconstruction (Fig. 92.3B) is the most frequently employed surgical treatment of thumb basal joint arthritis today. It predictably relieves pain and preserves most mobility; in addition, recovery is relatively rapid.

Implant arthroplasty is the term used when some kind of material is placed in the space created by trapezial resection in an effort to prevent shortening. Such materials have included fascia, tendon, silicone, and Vitallium. Until recently, silicone rubber spacers were most often used (3). Clinical results were generally good, but development of synovitis and local cystic bone degeneration from silicone particles, along with concern about the long-term effects of silicone implants, resulted in abandonment of their use. Despite this, if an old implant has to be removed after thorough encapsulation and healing, its removal has not proved to compromise significantly the good functional recovery. The most accepted operation today is trapezial resection with a tendon suspension of the thumb's metacarpal to the base of the index metacarpal, which gives stability and prevents excessive shortening (2,4). Stuffing tendon or fascia into the space created by trapezial removal alone will not prevent thumb shortening. After about 4 weeks of immobilization, progressive remobilization and muscle rehabilitation exercises are started. These are among the most rewarding and satisfying of reconstructive operations.

Interphalangeal Joint Arthritis

Osteoarthritis tends to develop insidiously and affects multiple distal interphalangeal (DIP) finger joints. In contrast, erosive osteoarthritis tends to single out and rapidly destroy one of the proximal interphalangeal joints in a violent manner (Fig. 92.2). Because of the common occurrence of osteoarthritis of DIP joints, even patients with severe deformity may have surprisingly little pain or impairment of use. The chief concern is frequently the disturbing appearance, a fact that patients may not readily acknowledge. The knobby appearance of the distal joints is caused by osteophytes and hard connective-tissue nodules called Heberden nodes. Infrequently, similar subcutaneous

nodules develop at the proximal interphalangeal (PIP) joints, where they are called Bouchard nodes.

Treatment of typical distal interphalangeal joint osteoarthritis is dictated by the degree of symptoms. Rest provided by restriction of activities and splinting is the mainstay of initial treatment. Oral anti-inflammatory medications should be tried, but response is unpredictable and often poor. Intra-articular steroid injections are transiently helpful for the majority of cases. With supportive measures for symptomatic relief, acute episodes often go into spontaneous remission. **Surgery is indicated for intractable pain or deformation of alignment severe enough to interfere with effective function.** The presence of Heberden or Bouchard nodes, although aesthetically displeasing, are infrequently, in themselves, an indication for excision. Because implant arthroplasties for distal joints have limited success, arthrodesis in a functional position is the treatment of choice. This provides relief of pain, improved alignment, and better appearance.

The treatment of mild degenerative arthritis of PIP joints is intra-articular injection of steroids and splinting for rest. **Surgery is the only option for advanced or recalcitrant cases, but a truly good solution does not exist.** Joint fusion offers the most reliable means of relieving pain but results in total loss of motion at the joint. PIP joint fusion is least disturbing for the index finger. The index works against the thumb in order to pinch, for which PIP mobility is not required. The lack of pain and good stability are more important than flexion for the index and middle fingers. For the ring and small fingers, which are principally involved in power grasp, loss of PIP mobility from arthrodesis is much more debilitating and has to be considered carefully and individually.

The success of implant arthroplasty at the PIP joints is determined chiefly by the condition of the adjacent tendons, ligaments, and supporting soft-tissue structures. When these are in good condition, an implant arthroplasty is clearly more desirable than arthrodesis for a destroyed PIP joint of the middle, ring, or small finger. Because these joints have little axial loading, silicone spacers in the shape of a hinge continue to be used. When supporting soft-tissue structures are in good condition, a stable joint with an extension/flexion arc of 60 to 80 degrees frequently is achieved.

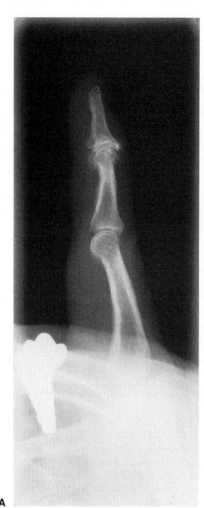
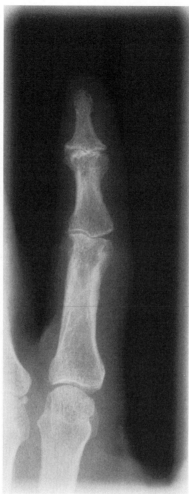

A

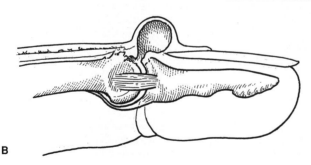

B

FIGURE 92.4. A: Radiographic demonstration of osteoarthritic changes in the DIP joint giving rise to synovitis, the cyst, and its pressure damages to the skin and fingernail germinal matrix. **B:** Typical synovial (mucous) cyst with fingernail deformity, which developed in response to irritation of osteoarthritic osteophyte at the interphalangeal joint.

Associated Disorders

A common complication of osteoarthritis at the DIP is a dorsal synovial cyst, commonly referred to as a "mucous cyst," with or without fingernail deformity (Fig. 92.4). These cysts develop in response to irritation of arthritic osteophytes at the margins of the arthritic joint. The pressure of the expanding cyst thins the overlying skin and damages the germinal matrix of the fingernail, resulting in its progressive deformity. Recurrent inflammation is common. The risk, aside from fingernail deformity, is infection communicating directly into the arthritic joint and troublesome chondritis. Surgical correction requires synovectomy with excision of the cyst, debridement of osteophyte from the arthritic joint margins, and repair of the skin defect, usually with local flaps and occasionally supplemented with a skin graft. The technical challenge is removal of the osteophytes from the dorsal margin of the base of the distal phalanx without detaching the insertion of the attenuated extensor tendon.

Metacarpal Boss

A metacarpal boss results from degenerative arthritis of the second and/or third metacarpocarpal joints, and is often mistaken for a dorsal ganglion cyst. Symptoms include deep aching and variable tenderness, accentuated by compression or torsion with activities such as golf. Localized tenderness, with pressure aggravating the symptoms, is the key to diagnosis. Usually, a boss can be illustrated with lateral-oblique wrist radiographs showing subtle dorsal joint lipping and/or narrowing of space in the tender joint.

In the majority of cases, no treatment is required. Direct steroid injections into the joint and rest are employed. When symptoms persist but are not severe, surgical excision of only the dorsal lipping of joint margins down to healthy articular cartilages will generally give relief, provided these joints are stable. When there is joint instability or if symptoms are severe, arthrodesis is required for predictable pain relief.

RHEUMATOID ARTHRITIS

Rheumatoid arthritis (RA) is a systemic autoimmune disease of uncertain etiology, which is characterized primarily by synovial inflammation with secondary skeletal destruction (Fig. 92.5). Polyarticular involvement is the rule, with an age prevalence between 20 and 40 years and a female preponderance. Although synovial and articular tissues are focal target structures, the immunologic disorder frequently affects disparate visceral organs such as the heart, pericardium, and lungs. Juvenile rheumatoid arthritis is a particularly aggressive variant that affects teenage children.

The clinical course of rheumatoid arthritis (also known as polyarthritis) is extremely varied in terms of distribution, severity, rapidity of progression, and ultimate damage. In most cases, the diagnosis will have been established and medical treatment initiated before the surgeon is consulted. However, RA must be considered in any patient with ill-defined and persistent joint inflammation and pain. Variation in early symptoms is the rule rather than the exception, with onset occasionally being heralded by unexplained, painful swelling of a single joint. At this stage, minimal if any derangement of laboratory tests, except perhaps an elevated erythrocyte sedimentation rate, is common. The course of rheumatoid arthritis is as unpredictable as its onset, but when progressive, the diseased synovium causes both enzymatic and mechanical destruction of tendons, laxity and attenuation of ligamentous support systems of joints, and eventual enzymatic degradation of articular cartilage and subchondral bone. The ultimate deformities are as varied as the presentation of the disease.

Rheumatoid Synovitis

Rheumatoid synovitis damages extensor and flexor tendons. Joint destruction and shifts in alignment result in abnormal frictions and vector forces on the tendons traversing them. The extensor tendons are usually most involved over the dorsal aspect of the wrist, where a boggy swelling of diseased synovium

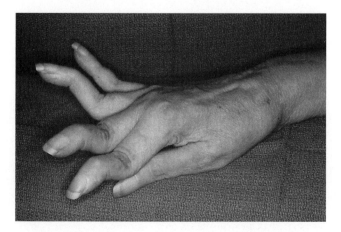

FIGURE 92.5. Hand ravaged by severe rheumatoid arthritis.

may be visible with an hourglass configuration, proximal and distal to the extensor retinaculum. As the tendons are attenuated, even a simple act, such as snapping fingers together or lifting a cup, may result in tendon ruptures and loss of extension of one or more fingers, most often those on the ulnar aspect of the hand. **The risk of tendon rupture is so high that prophylactic tenosynovectomy to minimize probability of tendon ruptures should be considered if the tenosynovitis has not responded to medical treatment over a period of 4 to 6 months.** While not absolute, synovectomy reduces substantially the chance of tendon rupture, especially at the wrist level (5). Synovectomy is usually performed in conjunction with other needed repairs, such as realignment of a subluxed wrist.

A painless, and thus deceptive, variant of rheumatoid synovitis that occurs along extensor tendons at the wrist and dorsal hand is termed *villonodular synovitis*. It presents insidiously as a soft, ill-defined, but prominent mass about the digital extensor tendons at the wrist level. Typically painless, without the usual inflammatory signs of soreness, redness, or increased temperature, this entity causes spontaneous tendon rupture in some cases but is unpredictable, and spontaneous remissions can occur. Synovectomy is considered if the mass persists for more than 6 months.

Flexor tenosynovitis usually presents with pain, swelling, decreased wrist motion, and impaired finger flexion. Classic carpal tunnel syndrome very rarely indicates rheumatoid involvement. Synovectomy is not indicated for the classic carpal tunnel syndrome, which demonstrates a dry, tenacious type of flexor synovitis. Occasionally with symptoms of carpal tunnel syndrome, a wet, proliferative, and invasive synovitis (rheumatoid type) is unexpectedly encountered. For such cases a thorough flexor synovectomy is indicated to minimize risk of tendon ruptures. The proliferative synovitis may extend distally into the fibro-osseous flexor tendon sheaths of the fingers, causing a "trigger finger" (see Chapter 82) to be the presenting symptoms of the disease.

Wrist Synovitis

Dorsal tenosynovitis is usually visible, but radiocarpal and intracarpal rheumatoid synovitis leading to progressive and serious cartilage and bone destruction is less readily apparent. Pain with diffuse swelling and diminishing range of motion are typical, and progressive destruction with loss of ligament integrity leads to anterior wrist subluxation, loss of carpal height, and collapse. The malalignment of the wrist greatly increases the chance tendons rupture.

Prominent ulnar side wrist pain is frequently encountered owing to synovitis and destruction of the distal radioulnar joint (DRUJ). Typically, the loss of soft-tissue support results in painful dorsal DRUJ instability and subluxation.

Attritional ruptures of the extensor tendons to the ulnar digits from the sharp end of the distal ulna are common. Prophylactic synovectomy with distal ulna resection offers the best probability of prevention, while also relieving pain at the DRUJ. Flexor tendon ruptures at the proximal wrist are relatively infrequent. **Although synovectomy does not always prevent tendon ruptures, in conjunction with DRUJ resection, it is consistently effective in alleviating wrist pain.**

Wrist arthrodesis may be required for advanced wrist destruction and collapse. However, the alternative of thorough synovectomy followed by 4 to 6 weeks of wrist immobilization often results in a fibrous union that has some resiliency, remains aligned, and is stable, as the forces on it are of such low magnitude. Wrist collapse and deviation profoundly affect function at the metacarpophalangeal finger joints, shifting forces of both extensor and flexor tendons ulnarward, to become a factor in the typical ulnar finger drift of advanced rheumatoid arthritis.

Rheumatoid Disease of Fingers

Metacarpophalangeal joint problems frequently herald the onset of rheumatoid arthritis and may begin as an unexplained and single painful and swollen joint without radiographic changes. Less often it may be "triggering" a finger or early ulnar finger deviation. With progressive disease, the hypertrophic synovitis attenuates and weakens the joint-supporting structures. With weakened joint capsule and ligaments accompanied by intrinsic muscle tightness, a volar subluxation of the proximal phalanges occurs. Deforming forces, including an ulnar shift of the flexor tendons traversing the MCP joints, cause progressive ulnar finger drift. As deformity increases, the extensor tendons sublux from their central and dorsal position over the MCP joints and migrate eventually to the respective ulnar intermetacarpal gullies. This results in further ulnar drift, loss of MCP joint extension, and eventually volar dislocation of the proximal phalanges.

Synovectomy of diseased MCP joints usually relieves pain, but is often of short-term benefit, as it does not address the imbalance of intrinsic muscle tightness. Treatment is by MCP joint resection, which shortens the skeleton and provides relative lengthening of the intrinsic muscle system. MCP joint resection is combined with a thorough synovectomy and dorsal repositioning of the extensor tendons over the joints to restore active extension. Like the PIP joints, the MCP joints have low axial loading, and so silicone spacers are used as interposition arthroplasties. These combined procedures offer the best possibility for lasting improvement.

Proximal interphalangeal joint complications of the rheumatoid process are common and disabling. Complications include central slip disruption, leading to boutonnière deformity or intrinsic muscle tightness, and progressive disruption of joint support tissues, causing swan-neck deformities. Treatment is difficult because direct repairs cannot satisfactorily be accomplished with the diseased, disrupted tissues. Interposition arthroplasty for the PIP joints is rarely feasible in rheumatoid arthritis because success depends on good connective tissue support. As a result, arthrodesis of a badly diseased PIP joint in a more functional position is the only realistic option. In practice, simple pinning of the joint in the selected position for 4 to 6 weeks is usually sufficient without a formal arthrodesis.

Rheumatoid Disease of the Thumb

The thumb is a separate functional unit. Although RA destruction at the basal joint can be severe, unlike osteoarthritis, RA rarely causes pain in that site. Fixed flexion deformity from intrinsic muscle contractures or gross instability of the thumb MCP and/or interphalangeal (IP) joints generally is the greatest problem. In most cases, arthrodesis is the only option, but provides impressive functional improvement. As the MCP joint develops a flexion contracture, a reciprocal hyperextension of the thumb IP joint follows. If symptomatic, arthrodesis offers the only worthwhile treatment.

PSORIATIC ARTHRITIS

Psoriatic arthritis (6) is a seronegative arthropathy associated with psoriatic skin changes, although initially the latter may be difficult to locate. Rheumatoid factor and antinuclear antibodies are usually absent. Joint involvement may be monoarticular but more commonly is polyarticular. Fortunately, the vast majority of patients with characteristic dermal psoriasis never develop associated arthropathies. Any joint in the body may be affected, but hand involvement is common and often is associated with onychodystrophy. The clinical presentation is characterized by moderately painful joint stiffness, weakness, and insidious but progressive flexion contractures.

Pain is usually not as severe as with rheumatoid arthritis. Radiographic articular destruction is evident with chronic joint involvement although bone stock and density remain normal. **Treatment of psoriatic arthritis is essentially medical and supportive, with splinting and functional adaptions of prime importance in the early stages to retard the progression of joint contractures and destruction,** for which occasional arthrodesis in a better position is worthwhile. Most patients with psoriatic arthritis requiring surgical treatment are managed in a manner similar to that required for rheumatoid disease.

ARTHRITIS OF SYSTEMIC LUPUS ERYTHEMATOSUS

As the name implies, disseminated lupus erythematosus (systemic LE) is a seropositive systemic autoimmune disorder with multiorgan involvement and a characteristic photosensitive cutaneous facial rash. Musculoskeletal involvement is common and frequently severe and progressive. The periarticular soft tissues are primarily involved, with resulting generalized ligamentous laxity and joint incompetence leading to progressive deformity. Unlike rheumatoid disease, articular and skeletal structures are basically spared, with little radiographic change, even when deformity is severe. Raynaud phenomenon, with pain and cold intolerance, is a common accompaniment, and may be among a patient's early symptoms.

As the disease progresses with development of deformities, appearance of the hands has much in common with that of rheumatoid arthritis, except that generally there is much less gross synovitis even as deformities become severe. The biomechanical needs for treatment are also similar to those for rheumatoid disease, but the response to surgical repair is different. Appropriate repair of rheumatoid-deformed hands always incorporates soft-tissue reconstructions, which generally are predictable and followed by imperfect, but at least rewarding, long-term improvement. In contrast, soft-tissue repair of the hand affected with lupus deformities does not provide long-term improvement, and results are consistently disappointing. **Thus, one must be extremely conservative with regard to surgical indications, undertaking only an absolute minimum of soft-tissue repairs.** This makes selective arthrodesis the mainstay of treatment.

GOUTY ARTHRITIS

Gout is a metabolic disorder characterized by hyperuricemia and clinically manifests as an acute monoarticular inflammatory condition. Approximately 90% of patients with gout are men, and the metatarsophalangeal joint of the big toe is involved in approximately 50% of cases. Diagnosis is usually based on clinical grounds, aided by elevated uric acid blood levels and identification of the urate crystals in joint fluid or tophi. The therapeutic response to colchicine is dramatic.

The characteristic histologic lesion is the tophus, which is a nodular deposit of monosodium urate crystals with an associated foreign body reaction. The clinical signs of an acute attack are a painful, swollen, exquisitely tender and hot joint. **Surgical intervention is restricted to removing larger tophi that are unsightly or a mechanical hindrance to joint motion.** Occasionally, joint destruction of the interphalangeal joints is so great that an arthrodesis in a functional position is warranted.

Pseudogout affects older people and is characterized by acute recurrent arthritis involving larger joints. It is always accompanied by chondrocalcinosis of the affected joint. Identification of calcium pyrophosphate crystals in the joint aspirate is diagnostic of pseudogout.

References

1. Landsmeer JM. Anatomical and functional investigation of the articulations of the fingers. *Acta Anat*. 1955;24(Suppl):1.
2. Burton RI, Pellegrini VD. Surgical management of basal joint arthritis of the thumb: II. Ligament reconstruction with tendon interposition arthroplasty. *J Hand Surg*. 1986;11:324.
3. Swanson A. Disabling arthritis at the base of the thumb: treatment by resection of the trapezium and flexible (silicone) implant arthroplasty. *J Bone Joint Surg*. 1972;54A:456.
4. Eaton RO, Glickel SZ, Littler IW. Tendon interposition arthroplasty for degenerative arthritis of the trapezius in metacarpal joint of the thumb. *J Hand Surg*. 1985;IOA:645.
5. Millender LH, Nalebuff B. A. Preventive surgery—Tenosynovectomy and synovectomy. *Orthop Clin North Am*. 1969;6:765.
6. Belsky MR, Feldon PF, Millender LH, et al. Hand involvement in psoriatic arthritis. *J Hand Surg*. 1982;7:203.

CHAPTER 93 ■ UPPER LIMB AMPUTATIONS AND PROSTHESES

ROBERT W. BEASLEY AND GENEVIEVE DE BESE

Despite the impressive advances in reparative surgery, management of amputations remains an important part of upper limb surgery. The negative aura that surrounds amputations favors rapid disposition of the problem, but it should be looked upon as a rehabilitative operation, leaving the parts in the best possible condition for prosthetic development, if that is contemplated. Initial treatment substantially determines long-term outcome, so the surgeon assuming responsibility for initial care should be knowledgeable about prosthetic requirements. The goal for the remaining limb is that it heal pain-free and be left in as useful a condition as possible (Fig. 93.1). The treating surgeon should not "go as far as he can" and then refer the patient for prosthetic development. Thoughtful consideration of the total impact of amputations is as important as the physical impairment on which attention tends to be centered. Survival of the part is not always in the patient's best interest, even if technically possible. Although each case needs individual consideration, some basic guidelines are useful.

The greater the number of injured parts, the less likely one is to amputate damaged parts to which vascularity can possibly be restored. **In general if any four of the six basic parts (skin, vessels, skeleton, nerves, and extensor and flexor tendons) are irreparably damaged, amputation is considered.** The concept of elective levels of amputation has given way to saving all length feasible, at least initially. If amputation is just distal to a normal or minimally damaged joint, a flap for wound closure to preserve length may be indicated. This is especially true for the elbow, through the base of the proximal phalanx of the thumb or base of the middle phalanx of fingers.

Severed nerves are cut short while under tension so the ends retract into healthy tissues. It is not a question of preventing neuromas, as they are inevitable, but of preventing neuroma symptoms. Chronic pain problems are rare among patients who enjoyed primary wound healing and early active motion. Sharp spicules of severed bone are smoothed and, if joint condyles are present, they are tapered to avoid a bulbous end of the finger, which is unsightly and may prevent top-quality prosthetic development (Fig. 93.1).

AESTHETIC CONSIDERATIONS

The hands, like the face, are constantly exposed to scrutiny, portray personality, and are major communicators. Amputation is not a cosmetic issue, but one of disfigurement. To ignore or deny that disfigurement is of real socioeconomic importance is unrealistic, as confirmed by the United States Supreme Court.

PATIENT RESPONSE TO AMPUTATIONS

Function is considered in the global sense of how well the individual achieves an independent, adjusted, and productive life, not simply the ability for pinch or grasping. The tendency is to overestimate physical impairment while neglecting the total impact on an individual. Regardless of whether persistent disability is a result of physical or emotional factors, the economic consequences are the same. Also note that the patient's total response to loss bears almost no relation to the actual amount of physical loss. It cannot be assumed that a patient with only a finger tip amputation will make a rapid recovery and adjustment.

Response to amputations can be considered in three basic phases. The first phase is one of denial and disbelief. This is a short phase during which the patient gets lots of attention, and most patients handle it well. The second phase is recognition of reality and is usually characterized by anxiety about the future and sometimes anger with a sense of being "victimized." It is a period of many consultations, with emotional turmoil and seeking "miracle" solutions. It also is the phase in which enlightened guidance can be most helpful. The third phase of emotional responses goes in one of two directions. The majority of patients make appropriate accommodation to their losses and fully use their remaining assets, whereas a few find "a new friend" on whom they can blame failures or who can act as a vehicle for secondary gains. Successful help in the latter case is generally very discouraging.

CLASSIFICATION OF HAND AMPUTATIONS

The variety of hand amputations is infinite, but organizing them into four major categories is useful for discussion of the subject. There is overlapping of the groups, but the majority of amputations fall primarily into one of the categories.

Lateral (Radial) Amputations

Radial amputations involve primarily the thumb and/or index finger, the "fine manipulations" unit of the hand. If there is a functional thumb, but substantial loss of the index finger, the patient will subconsciously shift to a thumb-middle finger small-object-handling unit. There was a time when "ray" index resection (through the base of the second metacarpal) was strongly advocated for index finger amputations proximal to the neck of the proximal phalanx, but it is infrequently performed now. If about 12 mm or more of proximal phalanx

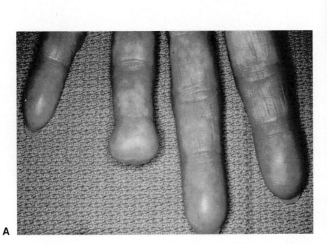
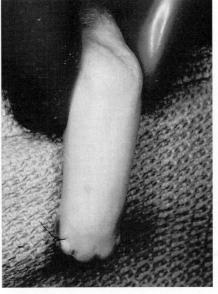

FIGURE 93.1. **A:** Bulbous finger amputation is unsightly and precludes prosthetic fitting. **B:** Amputation closure with taper and good soft-tissue coverage, which is socially presentable.

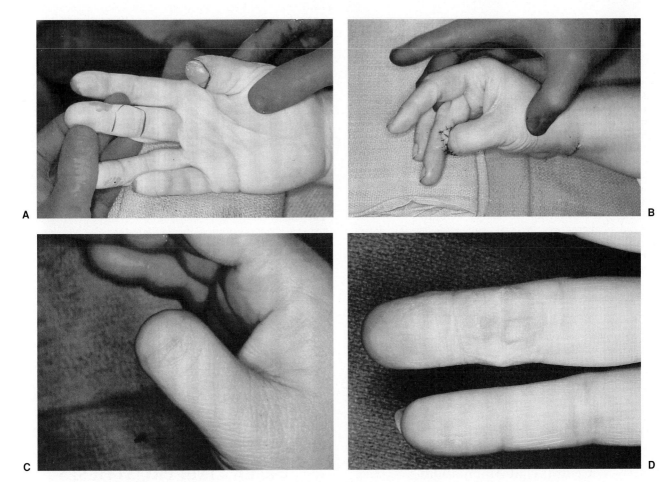

FIGURE 93.2. **A:** Distal thumb amputation healed with unstable and painful scar. **B:** Volar cross-finger flap from middle finger attached. **C:** Repair with tissue of perfect match, good pulp, and good recovery of sensibility. **D:** Middle finger flap donor-site repair with skin grafts from wrist.

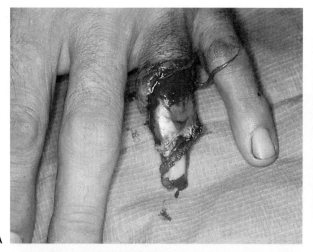

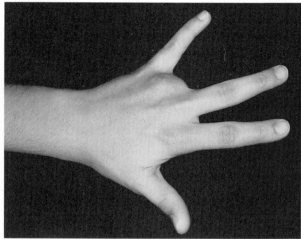

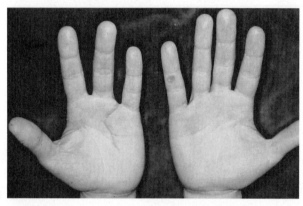

FIGURE 93.3. A: Ring avulsion injury. B: Essential amputation too short to be useful. C: Fourth ray resection. Balance restored and gap in palm eliminated by transposition of small finger onto the base of the metacarpal.

distal to the interdigital web is present, a finger prosthesis with passively changeable contour can be developed for most patients. **With this development, ray index resection as part of primary treatment is rarely, if ever, indicated.** The proximal interphalangeal (PIP) joint of the fingers is most important and in general should be saved, even if a flap for wound closure is required.

Preservation of length for thumb amputations is almost always indicated and very often requires a flap to accomplish. Traditionally this was by a dorsal flap from the adjacent index finger, but the donor-site mutilation. Beasley (1981) developed an alternative, the volar cross-finger flap (Fig. 93.2). Thumb amputations proximal to the metacarpophalangeal (MCP) joint are usually best treated by one of the numerous reconstructive procedures (see Chapter 88).

Medial (Ulnar) Amputations

The ring and small fingers, with some contribution from the middle finger, constitute the power grasping unit of our hands. To be effective they need length and a good flexion–extension arc. This functional unit is of much more value than that generally accorded to it. If the ring finger is lost, balance is improved by transposition of the small finger on to the fourth metacarpal with advancement to reduce gross shortness compared to the adjacent middle finger (Fig. 93.3).

Central Unit Amputations

Machines such as punch presses can cause central amputations, limited to the ring and/or middle fingers and their metacarpals.

While both pinch and grasping capability is preserved, these losses are troublesome because of small objects rolling from the palm and, of course, they are aesthetically disturbing. Surgical help is limited to the provision of soft-tissue coverage and displacement of sensitive neuromas. Some may be candidates for prosthetic development, especially for the deformity, but for technical reasons this is usually short of satisfactory. If any finger has a length of 12 to 15 mm distal to the interdigital web, preservation of length is important and often requires flap closure. With middle finger ray resection (through its metacarpal), index finger transposition onto the base of the third metacarpal gives excellent restoration of balance to the hand (Fig. 93.4).

Transverse Amputations

Physical impairment increases geometrically as the level of amputation becomes more proximal. Commonly encountered is transverse amputation of all fingers through their metacarpals, but with an uninjured thumb. There should be a conservative attitude about constructing a unit to oppose the thumb by flap-bone-grafts or by toe transfers. These procedures for the unilateral amputee badly accentuate the disfigurement, rarely improve needed capability significantly, and often preclude prosthetic development, which most patient's will choose if aware of what is available today.

UPPER LIMB PROSTHESES

The most basic axiom concerning prostheses is that more of them replace missing parts. The purpose is to minimize the

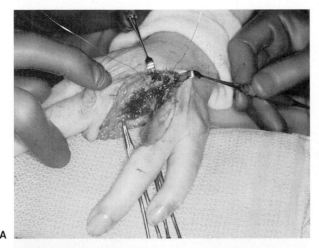

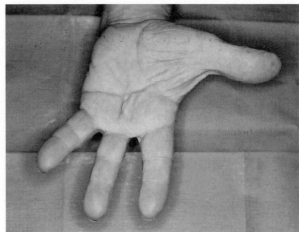

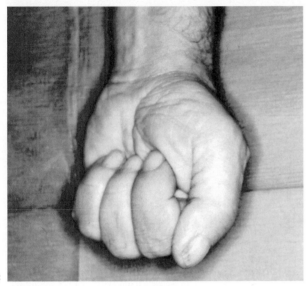

FIGURE 93.4. A: Middle finger ray resection leaves central gap in hand. **B** and **C:** Index finger transposition to base of third metacarpal restores balance and good function to hand.

physical, emotional, social, and economic consequences of the loss.

Despite impressive surgical advances, there are situations for which a prosthesis, alone or in combination with surgical repair, offers the best option. A realistic master plan should be agreed upon, surgery done with the same care and skill used in any reconstructive procedure, and a prosthesis fabricated to the highest standards (Fig. 93.5).

Except in wartime, major bilateral upper limb amputations are rare. Even unilateral total hand amputations are infrequent. The big numbers are in digital and partial hand amputations and there is increasing awareness that to be acceptable in most circumstances today, each must have a socially acceptable presentation. With the constant shifting of the workers into service industries, deformity is recognized as a real socioeconomic handicap, not a cosmetic issue (Fig. 93.6). This has been confirmed by the United States Supreme Court (*Arlene vs. Nassau County*, 1987).

Unilateral versus Bilateral

Fortunately, bilateral total hand amputations are rare. Although bilateral amputees suffer socioeconomically as do unilateral amputees, for the bilateral cases the physical impairment is so extreme as to overshadow other considerations. Their management is beyond the scope of this overview, but in general there is still a tendency to overestimate physical impairment to the neglect of emotional and total impact of losses.

Specificity of Prostheses

It is essential to recognize that any prosthesis can meet only specific and limited needs. The term "artificial hand" should be discarded as it implies unrealistic expectations. Also, the same patient may need different types of prostheses for different occasions. For example, one might need a rugged and ugly clamping device for the factory, but a mechanically simpler, passively adjustable prosthesis of near-normal appearance for business and social occasions. The prime needs of each patient should be determined accurately and prostheses targeted to these needs. This minimizes unrealistic expectations, disappointments, and failures.

Congenital versus Acquired Losses

A child born without a hand (agenesis) does not experience the sense of physical impairment of one with an acquired amputation that disrupts learned functional patterns. With agenesis, techniques may be different, but to that individual they seem normal. The basic problem of almost all those with congenital defects is not physical, but development of a strong

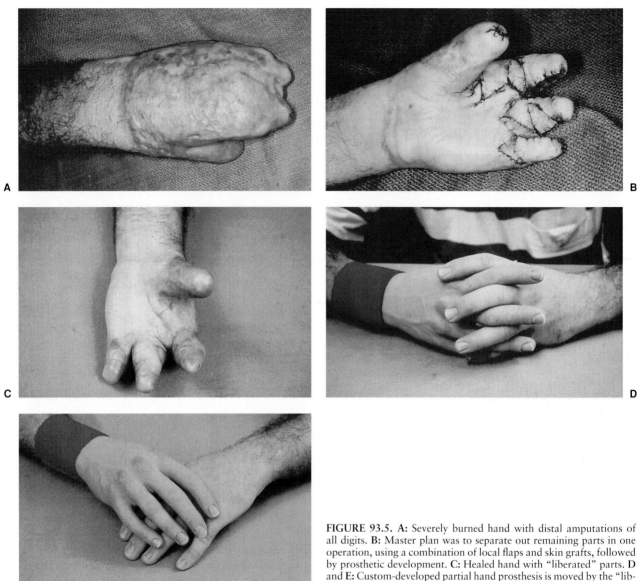

FIGURE 93.5. A: Severely burned hand with distal amputations of all digits. **B:** Master plan was to separate out remaining parts in one operation, using a combination of local flaps and skin grafts, followed by prosthetic development. **C:** Healed hand with "liberated" parts. **D** and **E:** Custom-developed partial hand prosthesis is moved by the "liberated" short digits and also restores near-normal social presentation. (Courtesy of American Hand Prostheses, Inc., New York, NY.)

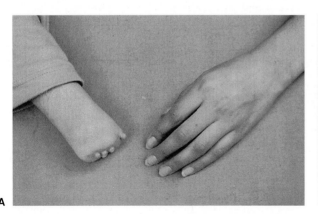

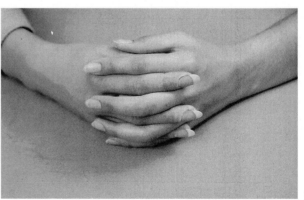

FIGURE 93.6. A: Unilateral hand agenesis. Having grown up this way, the patient has no sense of physical impairment, so the essential problems are emotional and social adjustment. **B:** A first-class, precisely adjustable prosthesis is the only means of giving a normal social presentation. (Courtesy of American Hand Prostheses, Inc., New York, NY.)

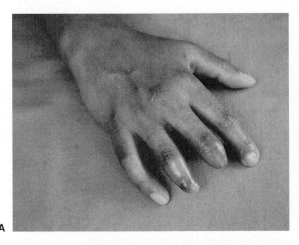

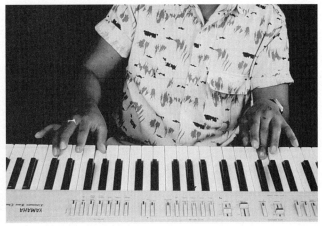

FIGURE 93.7. **A:** Distal finger amputations of professional musician. **B:** Precise-fitting digital prostheses restores their tips to where the brain, through learned patterns, expects them to be, resulting in unconscious or automatic control. (Courtesy of American Hand Prostheses, Inc., New York, NY.)

and secure personality in face of being "different." The family is the prime influencing factor on early personality development and if their manner reflects the child's being inferior, the child will firmly adopt this attitude. Appropriate prostheses may eventually be helpful in dealing with a sense of inferiority (Fig. 93.6), but is not applicable in the early formative years when it is the family and not the child who need guidance. Prostheses should be considered when the child, not the parents, demands it. With infrequent exceptions, this is rarely before age 10 to 12 years, when social awareness is heightened.

Levels of Amputation

Generally the more distal the level of amputation, the more useful will be prosthetic fitting. This is because the more distal the amputation, the more sensory feedback systems will be functioning to give automatic control. Traditional teaching is that finger prostheses are "cosmetic" and only impair capability. In fact, a digital prosthesis of high quality, as available today, fits so perfectly that both position and pressure feedback is provided. Combined with the prosthetic finger tip being where the brain expects it to be, this results in a remarkable degree of subconscious control and can be among the most helpful of prostheses (Fig. 93.7).

Aesthetic Considerations

The issue is whether the disfigurement is so great as to disturb the purpose of encounters, break the line of thought, or is genuinely grotesque. It is unrealistic to deny that disfigurement is of real socioeconomic importance. It has nothing to do with "cosmesis," which is changing something normal to have better appearance in one's opinion.

There are two areas of consideration. One is the area of artistic factors (size, shape, color, etc.), which the artist can duplicate remarkably. The other area, and of equal or greater importance, is the ability to do ordinary tasks in the expected manner. Improving physical capability should be an important design concern for all hand prostheses to reduce the conspicuousness of the disfigurement.

Types of Prostheses

There are only two basic types of hand prostheses, active (mechanical) or passive (purposely without internal mechanical

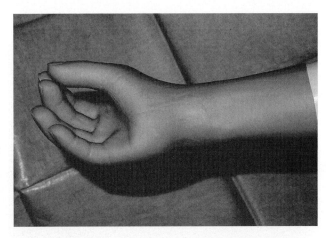

FIGURE 93.9. The most commonly used externally powered active prosthesis is a myoelectrically controlled, opening and closing electric clamp, but it has none of the manipulating capabilities of our hands. No currently available externally powered active prosthesis has a good, socially acceptable appearance.

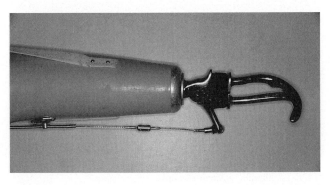

FIGURE 93.8. Split-hook active prosthetic terminal device is rugged and easily positioned, but for many is not socially acceptable.

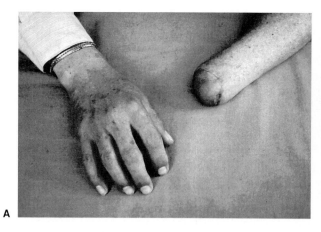
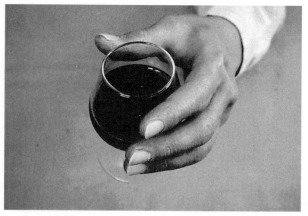

FIGURE 93.10. A: Wrist disarticulation. **B:** The light, stain-resistant silicone prosthesis with passively adjustable digital armatures can be pressed around light objects while simultaneously restoring social presentation. (Courtesy of American Hand Prostheses, Inc., New York, NY.)

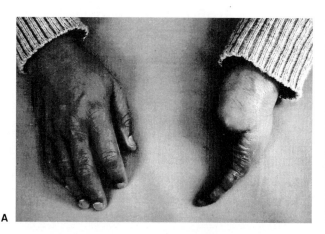
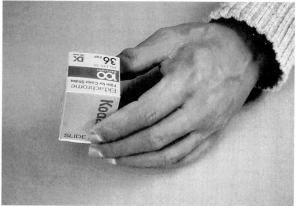

FIGURE 93.11. A: Blast injury leaving only the small finger. **B:** The single remaining finger placed in the middle finger position of a fine partial prosthesis has its usefulness vastly enhanced. (Courtesy of American Hand Prostheses, Inc., New York, NY.)

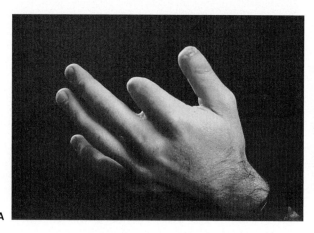
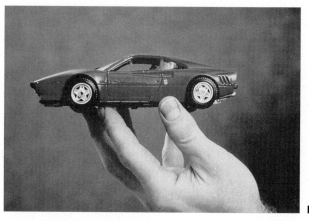

FIGURE 93.12. A: Thumb and index finger amputations. **B:** Manipulating capability and social presentation improved by precise-fitting digital prostheses. (Courtesy of American Hand Prostheses, Inc., New York, NY.)

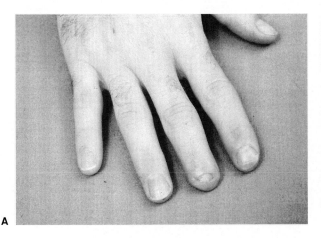

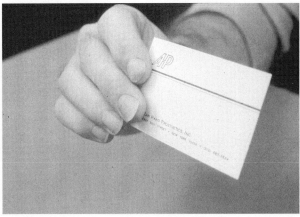

A   B

FIGURE 93.13. **A:** A mutilated distal phalanx and fingernail. **B:** The unique sub-mini digital prosthesis covers only the distal phalanx, is thin like a surgeon's glove to transmit sensibility, and provides for the first time a practical and secure methods of attaching a prosthetic fingernail to an intact distal phalanx. (Courtesy of American Hand Prostheses, Inc., New York, NY.)

units, although changing of their configuration with the other hand is often desirable). Active prostheses are no more than simple clamping devices that have none of the manipulating capability characteristic of our hands. They may be body powered (Fig. 93.8) or externally powered. Of the latter, only electric motors have proven to be practical because of ready availability of recharging facilities, but they deliver energy slowly, make noise, and have no subconscious control because there is no sensory feedback The control system that is almost exclusively used is the myoelectric system, which is velocity based rather than position and force directed, so activities are essentially visually guided. Their greatest virtue for unilateral hand amputees is that great clamping forces can be generated and suspension straps for below-elbow amputees are eliminated. Aesthetically, myoelectric hands are poor because of their shape, the thumb moving straight away from the index and middle finger pads rather than in an arc laterally, and their slow, abnormal, and noisy motion of parts (Fig. 93.9). Considerable improvement in the artistic aspects can result from covering with a high-quality, custom-made silicone glove.

During the phase of emotional turmoil, looking for miracle devices, most unilateral above-elbow amputees try myoelectric hand prostheses, but the majority eventually opt for the lightweight, lifelike passive prosthesis constructed with a passively positionable elbow joint, which makes the prosthetic forearm useful for many activities.

Passive prostheses purposefully have no internal mechanical units, but best meet the needs of the vast majority of hand amputees today as the big numbers are in partial hand and digital amputations. While not containing motors, the digits of passive prostheses can be constructed with armatures that permit change in their configuration by the normal hand. The introduction of microhinged rather than wire armatures was a major advance, as the problem of breakage from metal

fatigue and the necessity for firm anchorage of their proximal ends was eliminated (Fig. 93.10).

Partial hand prostheses provide prosthetic parts against which remaining normal one can work (Fig. 93.11). The variety of losses encountered is innumerable, but the principles are the same.

Digital prostheses are among the most rewarding, not only for restoring excellent social presentation, but for enhancing capability as a result of their substantial subconscious control. With the loss of both interphalangeal joints, the digital prosthesis can be fabricated with a passively adjustable, multihinged armature (Fig. 93.12).

Until recently all finger prostheses were made to cover the whole finger, even if a good proximal interphalangeal joint were present. The technological breakthrough of the Bio-Chromatic (American Hand Prosthetics, New York, NY) coloring system led to development of the superb "mini" prosthesis for fingers with intact PIP joints (Fig. 93.7). In turn, this led to the sub-minidigital prosthesis for loss of part of the distal phalanx or even damaged or lost fingernails (Fig. 93.13).

Suggested Readings

Baumgartner R. Active and carrier-tool prostheses for upper limb amputations. *Orthop Clin North Am.* 1981;12:955.

Beasley R. *Hand Injuries.* Philadelphia: WB Saunders; 1981.

Beasley R. Reconstructive surgery in the management of congenital anomalies of the upper extremities. In: Swinyard C, ed. *Limb Development and Deformity.* St. Louis: Charles Thomas; 1969.

Beasley R, de Bese G. Upper limb amputations and prostheses. *Orthop Clin North Am.* 1986;17:395.

Brown P. The rational selection of treatment for upper extremity amputations. *Orthop Clin North Am.* 1981;12:893.

Simpson D. Extended physiologic proprioception. In: *Symposium on Upper Extremity Prostheses and Orthoses.* Goteborg, Sweden: 1971.

Page numbers followed by *f* indicate figures; *t* indicate tabular material.